Conditioning *for* Strength *and* Human Performance

SECOND EDITION

Conditioning *for* Strength *and* Human Performance

T. JEFF CHANDLER, EdD, CSCS*D, NSCA-CPT, FNSCA, FACSM
Editor in Chief, Strength and Conditioning Journal
Professor and Department Head, HPER
Jacksonville State University
Jacksonville, AL

LEE E. BROWN, EdD, CSCS*D, FNSCA, FACSM
Professor, Strength and Conditioning
Department of Kinesiology
Director, Center for Sport Performance
California State University, Fullerton
Fullerton, CA

Wolters Kluwer | Lippincott Williams & Wilkins
Health
Philadelphia • Baltimore • New York • London
Buenos Aires • Hong Kong • Sydney • Tokyo

Acquisitions Editor: Emily Lupash
Product Manager: Linda G. Francis
Editorial Assistant: Zachary Shapiro
Design Coordinator: Teresa Mallon
Illustration Coordinator: Susan Caldwell
Manufacturing Coordinator: Margie Orzech
Prepress Vendor: SPi Global

Printed in China

Library of Congress Cataloging-in-Publication Data

Conditioning for strength and human performance / [edited by] T. Jeff Chandler, Lee E. Brown.—2nd ed.
p. ; cm.
Includes bibliographical references and index.
ISBN 978-1-4511-0084-6
I. Chandler, T. Jeff. II. Brown, Lee E., 1956-
[DNLM: 1. Physical Fitness—Problems and Exercises. 2. Exercise—Problems and Exercises. 3. Exercise Therapy—Problems and Exercises. QT 18.2]
613.7'1—dc23

2011040482

LWW.com

9 8 7 6 5 4 3 2

RRS1206

DEDICATION

Lee E. Brown: For Theresa, thank you for carrying me all these years, without you I am nothing.

T. Jeff Chandler: To my wife, Pam, and my family. Thank you all for your continued love and support.

FOREWORD

The ultimate goal of strength and conditioning coaches and personal trainers is to enhance human performance, both in athletes and in fitness enthusiasts. *Conditioning for Strength and Human Performance* provides the necessary knowledge base these professionals require. This text is appropriate for strength and conditioning professionals working with the general population in which a major goal of a conditioning program is to enhance general health and physical fitness, as well as for professionals working in high school and collegiate athletic settings where the major goal of a conditioning program is to enhance physical performance in athletic events.

Some texts for the strength and conditioning profession claim to be based in research and science. Hearsay and popular ideas, however, often make up a significant portion of the topics covered. The contributors to *Conditioning for Strength and Human Performance* have all based the material covered in their respective chapters in research and science, which is an important aspect of the development not only of strength and conditioning professionals but also of the profession itself.

Included in the first part of the text is information related to physiology, anatomy, and biomechanics, all presented in a clear, understandable manner. This information is necessary for the sound development of strength and conditioning programs. The remainder of the text presents chapters addressing virtually all aspects of administration of strength and conditioning programs, chapters on the various types of strength and conditioning (weight training, aerobic training), and chapters dedicated to unique aspects of strength and conditioning programs. These special topics give the reader of *Conditioning for Strength and Human Performance* sound information related to unique aspects of developing strength and conditioning programs. For example, readers will find chapters concerning spotting of resistance training exercises, plyometrics, speed and agility, the role of strength and conditioning in injury prevention and rehabilitation, ergogenic aids, and the use of implements other than traditional machines, barbells, and dumbbells in strength and conditioning programs. These unique chapters are written by individuals well-known for their knowledge in these specialized areas of the strength and conditioning field.

It is important to note that the authors of the chapters in this text are a mix of sport scientists, strength and conditioning coaches, and practitioners, giving the work a balance between sound sport science information and its application in the development of strength and conditioning programs. I recommend this text to all individuals working in the strength and conditioning profession.

Steven J. Fleck, Ph.D.

PREFACE

PURPOSE AND AUDIENCE

Conditioning for Strength and Human Performance is an entry-level textbook for courses covering strength training, conditioning, and personal training. This course is usually offered in the junior or senior year and has several recommended prerequisites, including anatomy and physiology, exercise physiology, and biomechanics. The textbook begins with a review of the basic science applied to training and conditioning and then moves to practical application of these basic science principles. An important option for the course instructor is a laboratory component with many activities that can be taught in the "lab" (weight room/exercise facility). The primary audience for this book consists of students in kinesiology, exercise science, athletic training programs, and preprofessional tracks such as premedicine, prephysical therapy, and prephysician assistant. Exercise science and related majors often include areas of study related to careers as a personal trainer and strength and conditioning coach.

The body of knowledge in the field of strength training and conditioning is growing rapidly. One reason we decided to produce this text was to provide students in the field with up-to-date information from this growing body of research. The field of strength training is dynamic and will continue to grow and change. Previously held beliefs will be challenged; some will stand and some will fall.

The second edition of this text contains several updated chapters and four new chapters with information that is very important to our field: Evidence-Based Practice (Chapter 12); Periodization (Chapter 14); Sport Psychology (Chapter 18); and Gender Issues in Strength (Chapter 19). We feel the current edition of the text is comprehensive yet understandable and applicable to the practicing strength and conditioning coach.

Another reason we prepared this text was to disseminate knowledge, perhaps in a somewhat different way than has been done previously. Learners have different learning styles, and we hope that we have provided learning opportunities for all types of learners.

The knowledge we have gained as professionals should not be proprietary. We do not "own" the information that we have learned, and we should freely share it with others. In fact, if the discipline of strength training and conditioning is to grow and flourish as it should, we must all take responsibility for passing on the most current body of knowledge in our field.

CHAPTER FEATURES

The pedagogical elements of the text were designed to present the basic material in a clear and concise manner as well as to challenge students to go beyond the textbook and seek information to answer more complex questions. Some students will learn best from reading and studying the figures and key terms. Some students will learn best by listening to instructors' lectures, and some will learn best from the application questions and activities recommended in the text. We encourage all students to participate in all of the activities provided, realizing that each student will learn best when information is presented in a style that suits him or her best. Since there is no universal best learning style, instructors are encouraged to use a variety of activities to disseminate the information in this text.

The text includes several pedagogical features to aid in the comprehension and retention of material. They provide numerous opportunities for students to apply the material in the context of their careers.

KEY POINTS

Key points are succinct statements of important information. They briefly summarize the main concepts of a specific section of the text. Each key point is set apart in the body of the text along with the expanded text containing specific information.

REAL-WORLD APPLICATION

These boxes contain analogies or metaphors that link theoretical concepts to practical application, or practical tips. They relate the chapter content to the real world.

Q & A FROM THE FIELD

This is a simulated "ask-the-expert" column. The questions come from the point of view of a professional in a field appropriate to each chapter.

MAXING OUT

These questions or activities designed to stimulate critical thinking appear at the ends of the chapters. They are based on real-life scenarios and may contain challenging content that students may not be able to answer based on the preceding chapter. They will take students above and beyond what they have just read.

CASE EXAMPLE

Case examples walk students through the design and implementation of a program. They are based on the following template:

1. Background
2. Recommendations/Consideration
3. Implementation
4. Results

LEARNING RESOURCES

Conditioning for Strength and Human Performance, Second Edition, provides numerous opportunities for students to reinforce their learning. Using the scratch-off code on the inside front cover of the book, students can access thePoint website for the book. There they will find a set of nearly 200 quiz questions that will help them to test their retention of the material. A practical exam uses video clips to demonstrate various exercises, and multiple-choice questions allow students to practice identifying exercises and ensuring proper form. Students can further apply their knowledge of the text through additional case examples and lab assignments, which put the book's content into context and provide a link to their future careers.

Instructors' resources are available on the website (http://thepoint.lww.com/ Chandler). Included in the instructors' resources are the following valuable assets:

- PowerPoint lecture outlines by chapter
- Test generator
- Image bank
- Answers to "Maxing Out" activities from the chapters

We have included many improvements to the second edition of Conditioning for Strength and Human Performance based to a large extent on your recommendations. The editors therefore encourage you, both instructors and students, to continue to send us feedback on the usefulness of each component of the text. Together, we can continue to make a significant contribution to the field of strength training and conditioning.

T. Jeff Chandler and Lee E. Brown

USER'S GUIDE

This User's Guide introduces you to the many features of ***Conditioning for Strength and Human Performance.*** Taking full advantage of these features, you not only read about strength and conditioning, you become involved in activities that help you learn and put your knowledge into practice.

This second edition of *Conditioning for Strength and Human Performance* was created and developed to explain how one can train for maximum performance, the knowledge of which builds off of an understanding of the basic science that serves as a foundation for strength and conditioning. The book also aims to help students put this science into practice with information about testing, assessment, exercise techniques, and program development. Please take a few moments to look through this User's Guide, which will introduce you to the tools and features that will enhance your learning experience. Each chapter is loaded with features that help you focus on the key points, deepen your knowledge, and apply your new skills.

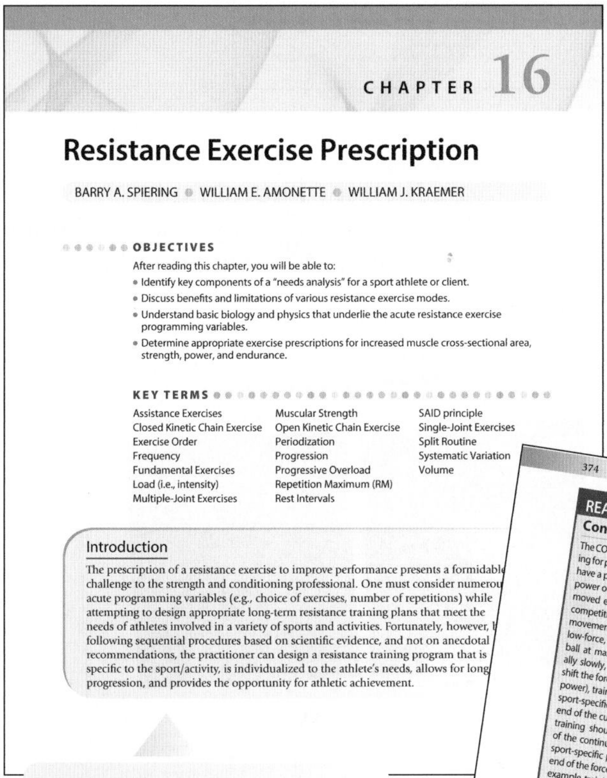

CHAPTER 16

Resistance Exercise Prescription

BARRY A. SPIERING • WILLIAM E. AMONETTE • WILLIAM J. KRAEMER

OBJECTIVES

After reading this chapter, you will be able to:

- Identify key components of a "needs analysis" for a sport athlete or client.
- Discuss benefits and limitations of various resistance exercise modes.
- Understand basic biology and physics that underlie the acute resistance exercise programming variables.
- Determine appropriate exercise prescriptions for increased muscle cross-sectional area, strength, power, and endurance.

KEY TERMS

Assistance Exercises	Muscular Strength	SAID principle
Closed Kinetic Chain Exercise	Open Kinetic Chain Exercise	Single-Joint Exercises
Exercise Order	Periodization	Split Routine
Frequency	Progression	Systematic Variation
Fundamental Exercises	Progressive Overload	Volume
Load (i.e., intensity)	Repetition Maximum (RM)	
Multiple-Joint Exercises	Rest Intervals	

Introduction

The prescription of a resistance exercise to improve performance presents a formidabl[e] challenge to the strength and conditioning professional. One must consider numerou[s] acute programming variables (e.g., choice of exercises, number of repetitions) while attempting to design appropriate long-term resistance training plans that meet the needs of athletes involved in a variety of sports and activities. Fortunately, however, b[y] following sequential procedures based on scientific evidence, and not on anecdotal recommendations, the practitioner can design a resistance training program that is specific to the sport/activity, is individualized to the athlete's needs, allows for long[-term] progression, and provides the opportunity for athletic achievement.

Introductions beginning each chapter explain why the material is important to you and give you a preview of what you'll find in the chapter.

Real-World Application Boxes demonstrate how to apply what you learn to real-world training situations.

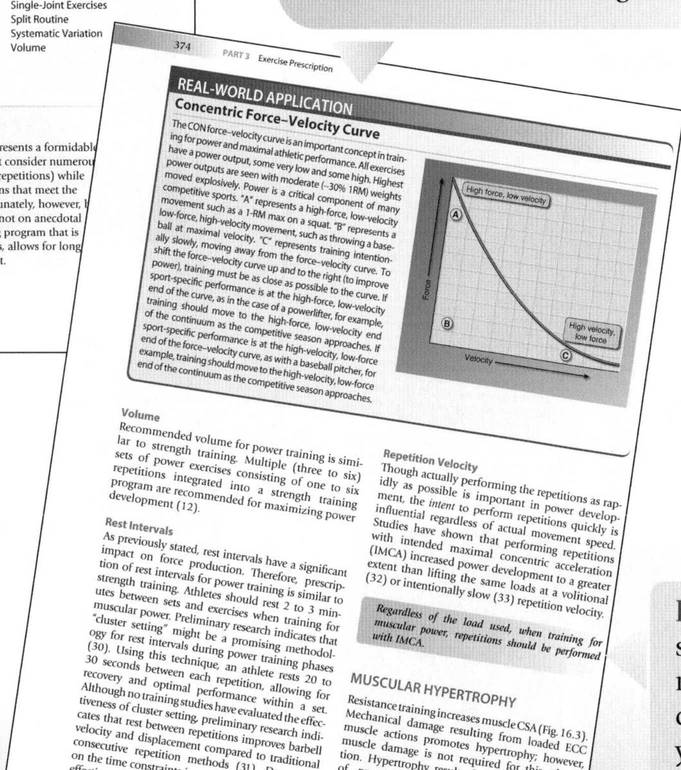

374 PART 3 Exercise Prescription

REAL-WORLD APPLICATION

Concentric Force–Velocity Curve

The CON force–velocity curve is an important concept in training for power and maximal athletic performance. All exercises have a power output, some very low and some high. Highest power outputs are seen with moderate (~30% 1RM) weights moved explosively. Power is a critical component of many competitive sports. "A" represents a high-force, low-velocity movement such as a 1-RM max on a squat. "B" represents a low-force, high-velocity movement, such as throwing a baseball at maximal velocity. "C" represents training intentionally slowly, moving away from the force–velocity curve. To shift the force–velocity curve up and to the right (to improve power), training must be as close as possible to the curve. If sport-specific performance is at the high-force, low-velocity end of the curve, as in the case of a powerlifter, for example, training should move to the high-force, low-velocity end of the continuum as the competitive season approaches. If sport-specific performance is at the high-velocity, low-force end of the force–velocity curve, as with a baseball pitcher, for example, training should move to the high-velocity, low-force end of the continuum as the competitive season approaches.

Volume

Recommended volume for power training is similar to strength training. Multiple (three to six) sets of power exercises consisting of one to six repetitions integrated into a strength training program are recommended for maximizing power development (12).

Rest Intervals

As previously stated, rest intervals have a significant impact on force production. Therefore, prescription of rest intervals for power training is similar to strength training. Athletes should rest 2 to 3 minutes between sets and exercises when training for muscular power. Preliminary research indicates that "cluster setting" might be a promising methodology for rest intervals during power training phases (30). Using this technique, an athlete rests 20 to 30 seconds between each repetition, allowing for recovery and optimal performance within a set. Although no training studies have evaluated the effectiveness of cluster setting, preliminary research indicates that rest between repetitions improves barbell velocity and displacement compared to traditional consecutive repetition methods (31). Depending on the time constraints in training, this could be an effective technique, especially for the Olympic lifts.

Repetition Velocity

Though actually performing the repetitions as rapidly as possible is important in power development, the *intent* to perform repetitions quickly is influential regardless of actual movement speed. Studies have shown that performing repetitions with intended maximal concentric acceleration (IMCA) increased power development to a greater extent than lifting the same loads at a volitional (32) or intentionally slow (33) repetition velocity.

Regardless of the load used, when training for muscular power, repetitions should be performed with IMCA.

MUSCULAR HYPERTROPHY

Resistance training increases muscle CSA (Fig. 16.3). Mechanical damage resulting from loaded ECC muscle actions promotes hypertrophy; however, muscle damage is not required for this adaptation. Hypertrophy results from an accumulation of proteins via increased rate of synthesis, decreased degradation, or both (34). Following a bout of resistance exercise, protein synthesis elevates at 2 to 3 hours, peaks at approximately

Key Points summarize and reinforce key concepts that you need to know.

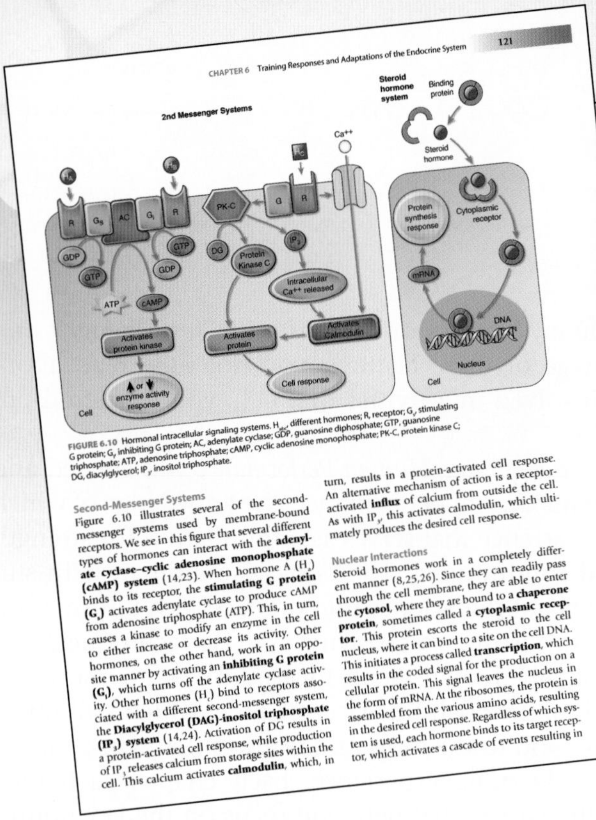

CHAPTER 6 Training Responses and Adaptations of the Endocrine System 121

FIGURE 6.10 Hormonal intracellular signaling systems. H, different hormones; R, receptor; G_s, stimulating G protein; G_i, inhibiting G protein; AC, adenylate cyclase; GDP, guanosine diphosphate; GTP, guanosine triphosphate; ATP, adenosine triphosphate; cAMP, cyclic adenosine monophosphate; PK-C, protein kinase C; DG, diacylglycerol; IP_3, inositol triphosphate.

Second-Messenger Systems

Figure 6.10 illustrates several of the second-messenger systems used by membrane-bound receptors. We see in this figure that several different types of hormones can interact with the **adenylate cyclase–cyclic adenosine monophosphate (cAMP) system** (14,23). When hormone A (H_a) binds to its receptor, the **stimulating G protein** (G_s) activates adenylate cyclase to produce cAMP from adenosine triphosphate (ATP). This, in turn, causes a kinase to modify an enzyme in the cell to either increase or decrease its activity. Other hormones, on the other hand, work in an opposite manner by activating an **inhibiting G protein** (G_i), which turns off the adenylate cyclase activity. Other hormones (H_c) bind to receptors associated with a different second-messenger system, the **Diacylglycerol (DAG)-inositol triphosphate (IP_3) system** (14,24). Activation of DG results in a protein-activated cell response, while production of IP_3 releases calcium from storage sites within the cell. This calcium activates **calmodulin**, which, in turn, results in a protein-activated cell response. An alternative mechanism of action is a receptor-activated **influx** of calcium from outside the cell. As with IP_3, this activates calmodulin, which ultimately produces the desired cell response.

Nuclear Interactions

Steroid hormones work in a completely different manner (8,25,26). Since they can readily pass through the cell membrane, they are able to enter the **cytosol**, where they are bound to a **chaperone protein**, sometimes called a **cytoplasmic receptor**. This protein escorts the steroid to the cell nucleus, where it can bind to a site on the cell DNA. This initiates a process called **transcription**, which results in the coded signal for the production on a cellular protein. This signal leaves the nucleus in the form of mRNA. At the ribosomes, the protein is assembled from the various amino acids, resulting in the desired cell response. Regardless of which system is used, each hormone binds to its target receptor, which activates a cascade of events resulting in

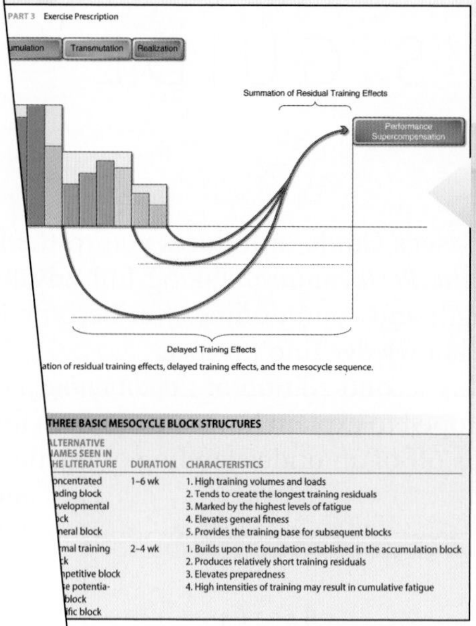

PART 3 Exercise Prescription

...ation of residual training effects, delayed training effects, and the mesocycle sequence.

THREE BASIC MESOCYCLE BLOCK STRUCTURES

...LTERNATIVE ...AMES SEEN IN ...HE LITERATURE	DURATION	CHARACTERISTICS
...oncentrated ...ading block ...evelopmental ...ck ...neral block	1–6 wk	1. High training volumes and loads 2. Tends to create the longest training residuals 3. Marked by the highest levels of fatigue 4. Elevates general fitness 5. Provides the training base for subsequent blocks
...mal training ...k ...petitive block ...e potentia- ...block ...fic block	2–4 wk	1. Builds upon the foundation established in the accumulation block 2. Produces relatively short training residuals 3. Elevates preparedness 4. High intensities of training may result in cumulative fatigue

Figures and **Charts** are a fast and easy way to get a quick overview of key relationships and key information.

Full Color Photographs help you learn exactly how you should perform specific training techniques.

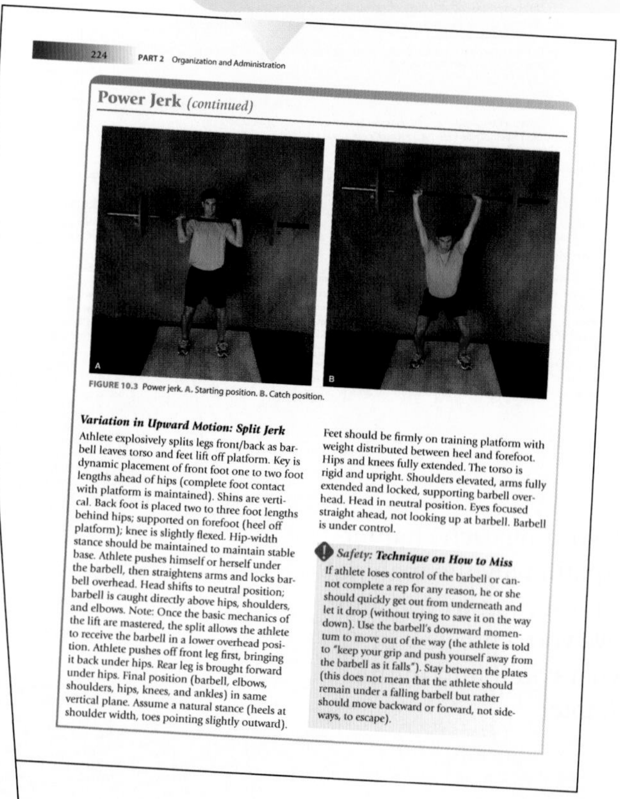

224 PART 2 Organization and Administration

Power Jerk *(continued)*

FIGURE 10.3 Power jerk. A. Starting position. B. Catch position.

Variation in Upward Motion: Split Jerk

Athlete explosively splits legs front/back as barbell leaves torso and feet lift off platform. Key is dynamic placement of front foot one to two foot lengths ahead of hips (complete foot contact with platform is maintained). Shins are vertical. Back foot is placed two to three foot lengths behind hips; supported on forefoot (heel off platform); knee is slightly flexed. Hip-width stance should be maintained to maintain stable base. Athlete pushes himself or herself under the barbell, then straightens arms and locks barbell overhead. Head shifts to neutral position; barbell is caught directly above hips, shoulders, and elbows. Note: Once the basic mechanics of the lift are mastered, the split allows the athlete to receive the barbell in a lower overhead position. Athlete pushes off front leg first, bringing it back under hips. Rear leg is brought forward under hips. Final position (barbell, elbows, shoulders, hips, knees, and ankles) in same vertical plane. Assume a natural stance (heels at shoulder width, toes pointing slightly outward).

Feet should be firmly on training platform with weight distributed between heel and forefoot. Hips and knees fully extended. The torso is rigid and upright. Shoulders elevated, arms fully extended and locked, supporting barbell overhead. Head in neutral position. Eyes focused straight ahead, not looking up at barbell. Barbell is under control.

Safety: Technique on How to Miss

If athlete loses control of the barbell or cannot complete a rep for any reason, he or she should quickly get out from underneath and let it drop (without trying to save it on the way down). Use the barbell's downward momentum to move out of the way (the athlete is told to "keep your grip and push yourself away from the barbell as it falls"). Stay between the plates (this does not mean that the athlete should remain under a falling barbell but rather should move backward or forward, not sideways, to escape).

Sequence Boxes present step-by-step instruction and illustration of exercises and movements you will use with the athletes you train.

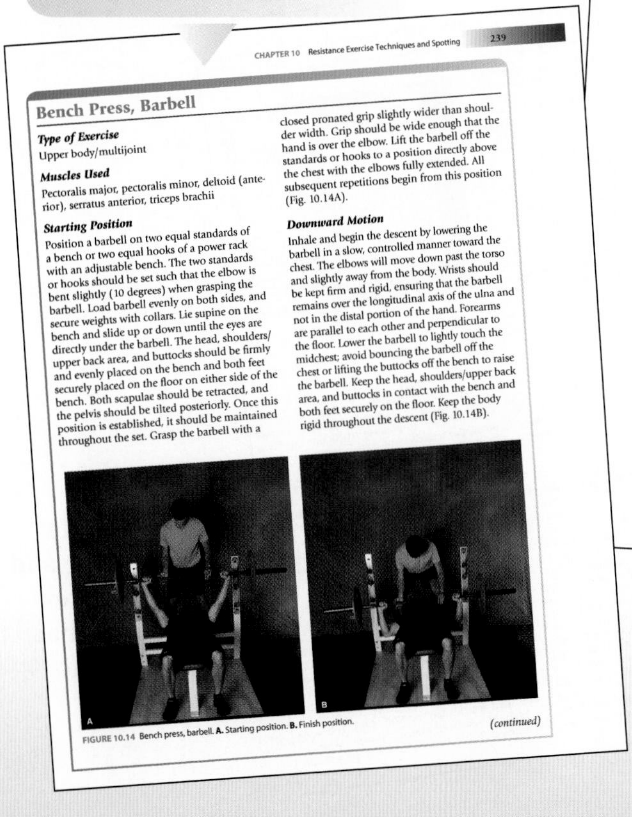

CHAPTER 10 Resistance Exercise Techniques and Spotting 239

Bench Press, Barbell

Type of Exercise

Upper body/multijoint

Muscles Used

Pectoralis major, pectoralis minor, deltoid (anterior), serratus anterior, triceps brachii

Starting Position

Position a barbell on two equal standards of a bench or two equal hooks of a power rack with an adjustable bench. The two standards or hooks should be set such that the elbow is bent slightly (10 degrees) when grasping the barbell. Load barbell evenly on both sides, and secure weights with collars. Lie supine on the bench and slide up or down until the eyes are directly under the barbell. The head, shoulders/upper back area, and buttocks should be firmly and evenly placed on the bench and both feet securely placed on the floor on either side of the bench. Both scapulae should be retracted, and the pelvis should be tilted posteriorly. Once this position is established, it should be maintained throughout the set. Grasp the barbell with a closed pronated grip slightly wider than shoulder width. Grip should be wide enough that the hand is over the elbow. Lift the barbell off the standards or hooks to a position directly above the chest with the elbows fully extended. All subsequent repetitions begin from this position (Fig. 10.14A).

Downward Motion

Inhale and begin the descent by lowering the barbell in a slow, controlled manner toward the chest. The elbows will move down past the torso and slightly away from the body. Wrists should be kept firm and rigid, ensuring that the barbell remains over the longitudinal axis of the ulna and not in the distal portion of the hand. Forearms are parallel to each other and perpendicular to the floor. Lower the barbell to lightly touch the midchest; avoid bouncing the barbell off the chest or lifting the buttocks off the bench to raise the barbell. Keep the head, shoulders/upper back area, and buttocks in contact with the bench and both feet securely on the floor. Keep the body rigid throughout the descent (Fig. 10.14B).

FIGURE 10.14 Bench press, barbell. **A.** Starting position. **B.** Finish position.

(continued)

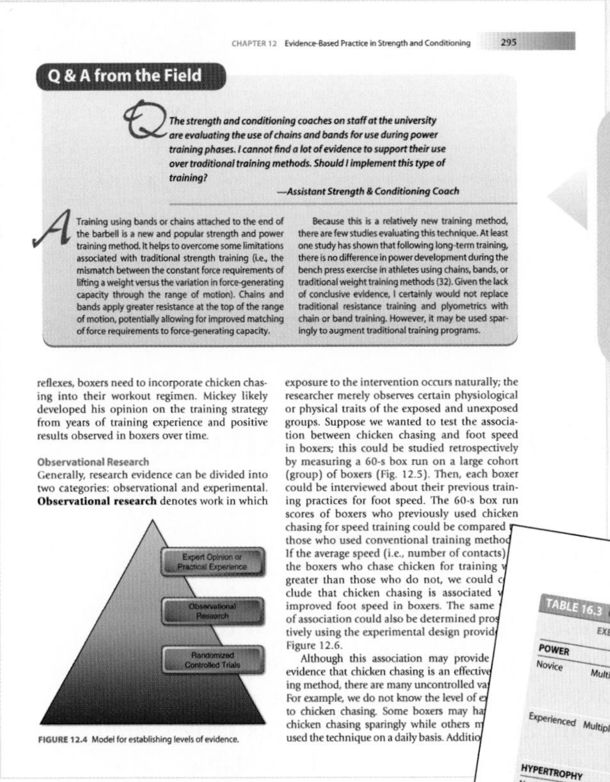
CHAPTER 12 Evidence-Based Practice in Strength and Conditioning 295

Q & A from the Field

Q The strength and conditioning coaches on staff at the university are evaluating the use of chains and bands for use during power training phases. I cannot find a lot of evidence to support their use over traditional training methods. Should I implement this type of training?

—Assistant Strength & Conditioning Coach

A Training using bands or chains attached to the end of the barbell is a new and popular strength and power training method. It helps to overcome some limitations associated with traditional strength training (i.e., the mismatch between the constant force requirements of lifting a weight versus the variation in force-generating capacity through the range of motion). Chains and bands apply greater resistance at the top of the range of motion, potentially allowing for improved matching of force requirements to force-generating capacity.

Because this is a relatively new training method, there are few studies evaluating this technique. At least one study has shown that following long-term training, there is no difference in power development during the bench press exercise in athletes using chains, bands, or traditional weight training methods (32). Given the lack of conclusive evidence, I certainly would not replace traditional resistance training and plyometrics with chain or band training. However, it may be used sparingly to augment traditional training programs.

reflexes, boxers need to incorporate chicken chasing into their workout regimen. Mickey likely developed his opinion on the training strategy from years of training experience and positive results observed in boxers over time.

Observational Research

Generally, research evidence can be divided into two categories: observational and experimental. **Observational research** denotes work in which exposure to the intervention occurs naturally; the researcher merely observes certain physiological or physical traits of the exposed and unexposed groups. Suppose we wanted to test the association between chicken chasing and foot speed in boxers; this could be studied retrospectively by measuring a 60-s box run on a large cohort (group) of boxers (Fig. 12.5). Then, each boxer could be interviewed about their previous training practices for foot speed. The 60-s box run scores of boxers who previously used chicken chasing for speed training could be compared to those who used conventional training methods. If the average speed (i.e., number of contacts) of the boxers who chase chicken for training is greater than those who do not, we could conclude that chicken chasing is associated with improved foot speed in boxers. The same type of association could also be determined prospectively using the experimental design provided in Figure 12.6.

Although this association may provide evidence that chicken chasing is an effective training method, there are many uncontrolled variables. For example, we do not know the level of exposure to chicken chasing. Some boxers may have used chicken chasing sparingly while others may have used the technique on a daily basis. Additio

FIGURE 12.4 Model for establishing levels of evidence.

Q & A from the Field is a simulated ask-the-expert column that offers you fresh insight and perspective by answering questions posed by students and professionals.

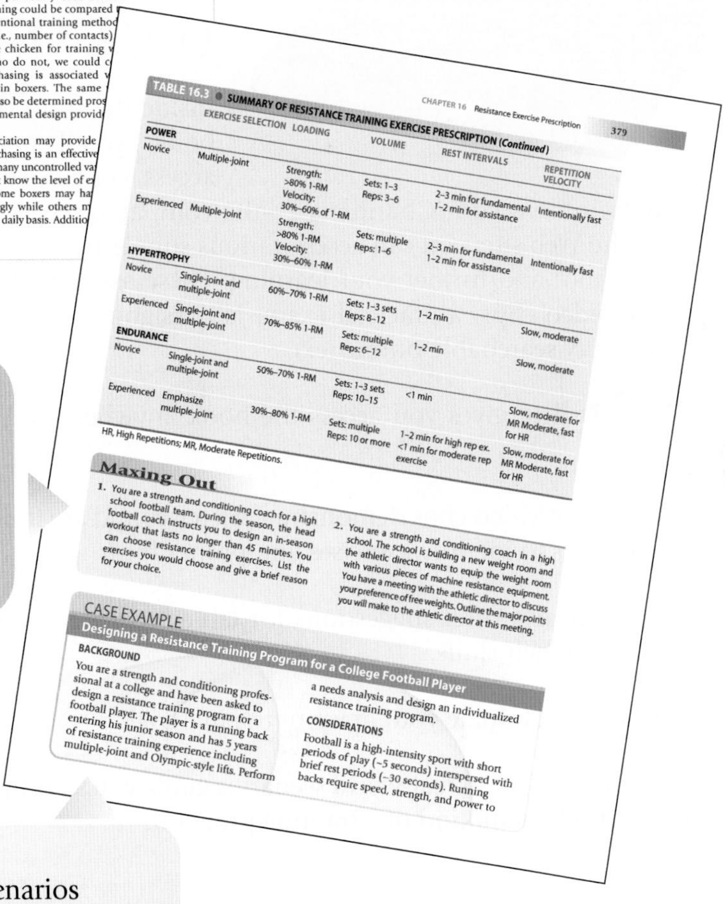
CHAPTER 16 Resistance Exercise Prescription 379

TABLE 16.3 ● SUMMARY OF RESISTANCE TRAINING EXERCISE PRESCRIPTION (Continued)

	EXERCISE SELECTION	LOADING	VOLUME	REST INTERVALS	REPETITION VELOCITY
POWER					
Novice	Multiple-joint	Strength: >80% 1-RM Velocity: 30%–60% of 1-RM	Sets: 1–3 Reps: 3–6	2–3 min for fundamental 1–2 min for assistance	Intentionally fast
Experienced	Multiple-joint	Strength: >80% 1-RM Velocity: 30%–60% 1-RM	Sets: multiple Reps: 1–6	2–3 min for fundamental 1–2 min for assistance	Intentionally fast
HYPERTROPHY					
Novice	Single-joint and multiple-joint	60%–70% 1-RM	Sets: 1–3 sets Reps: 8–12	1–2 min	Slow, moderate
Experienced	Single-joint and multiple-joint	70%–85% 1-RM	Sets: multiple Reps: 6–12	1–2 min	Slow, moderate
ENDURANCE					
Novice	Single-joint and multiple-joint	50%–70% 1-RM	Sets: 1–3 sets Reps: 10–15	<1 min	Slow, moderate for MR Moderate, fast for HR
Experienced	Emphasize multiple-joint	30%–80% 1-RM	Sets: multiple Reps: 10 or more	1–2 min for high rep ex. <1 min for moderate rep exercise	Slow, moderate for MR Moderate, fast for HR

HR, High Repetitions; MR, Moderate Repetitions.

Maxing Out

1. You are a strength and conditioning coach for a high school football team. During the season, the head football coach instructs you to design an in-season workout that lasts no longer than 45 minutes. You can choose resistance training exercises. List the exercises you would choose and give a brief reason for your choice.
2. You are a strength and conditioning coach in a high school. The school is building a new weight room and the athletic director wants to equip the weight room with various pieces of machine resistance equipment. You have a meeting with the athletic director to discuss your preference of free weights. Outline the major points you will make to the athletic director at this meeting.

CASE EXAMPLE

Designing a Resistance Training Program for a College Football Player

BACKGROUND

You are a strength and conditioning professional at a college and have been asked to design a resistance training program for a football player. The player is a running back entering his junior season and has 5 years of resistance training experience including multiple-joint and Olympic-style lifts. Perform a needs analysis and design an individualized resistance training program.

CONSIDERATIONS

Football is a high-intensity sport with short periods of play (~5 seconds) interspersed with brief rest periods (~30 seconds). Running backs require speed, strength, and power to

Maxing Out Boxes help you use your new skills and knowledge to solve problems based on real-life scenarios.

Case Examples set forth a range of scenarios and then guide you step-by-step through the design and implementation of a training program.

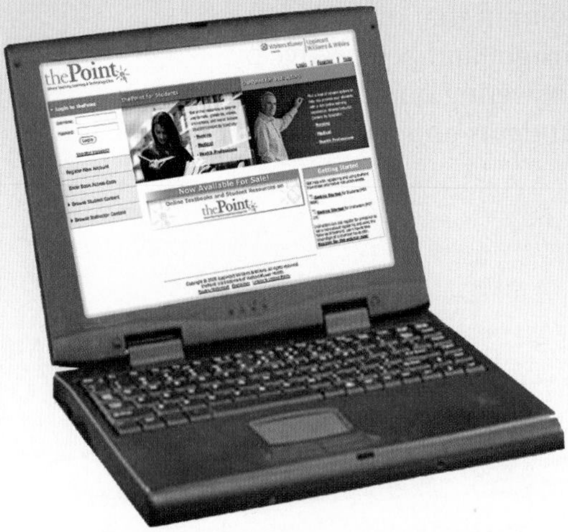

Student Resources

thePoint

Inside the front cover of your textbook, you'll find your personal access code. Use it to log on to **http://thePoint.lww.com/Chandler2e**—the companion Web site for this textbook. On the Web site, you can access various supplemental materials available to help enhance and further your learning. These assets include an interactive quiz bank, video clips, a practical exam, lab assignments, and case studies, as well as the fully searchable online text.

Full Text Online gives you access the book anywhere you have an internet connection.

Practical Exam video clips demonstrate exercises and are followed by multiple choice questions to identify exercises and proper form.

Lab Assignments offer suggestions for lab activities for you to practice and further develop their skills.

Quizzes let you evaluate your grasp of the material.

Case Studies based on real-world scenarios guide you step-by-step through the design and implementation of a training program.

REVIEWERS

CAROL COLE, MS
Associate Professor
Exercise, Nutrition & Sport Sciences
Sinclair Community College
Dayton, OH

FRANCES FLINT, PhD, CAT(C), ATC
Coordinator-Athletic Therapy
Kinesiology and Health Science
York University
Toronto, ON Canada

SOPHIE MABRY, MA
Human Performance Program Director
Human Performance
Arapahoe Community College
Littleton, CO

DOUG SMITH, PhD
Associate Professor
Health and Human Performance
Oklahoma State University
Stillwater, OK

THOMAS STORER, PhD
Professor
Kinesiology
El Camino College
Torrance, CA

TIMOTHY TAFT, MD
Professor
Orthopaedics
The University of North Carolina at Chapel Hill
Chapel Hill, NC

MALCOLM T. WHITEHEAD, PhD
Assistant Professor
Health and Human Performance
Northwestern State University
Natchitoches, LA

JASON WINCHESTER, PhD
Assistant Professor
Health, Rec., and Tourism
George Mason University
Manassas, VA

CONTRIBUTORS

CLINT ALLEY, MS
Huntington, WV

WILLIAM E. AMONETTE, PhD, CSCS
Fitness & Human Performance Program
University of Houston-Clear Lake
Houston, TX

JOSE ANTONIO, PhD, FNSCA, FACSM, FISSN
CEO—International Society of Sports Nutrition
Assistant Professor—Nova Southeastern University
Davie, FL

C. ERIC ARNOLD, PhD
Associate Professor
Department of Physical Therapy
College of Health Professions
Marshall University
Huntington, WV

TRAVIS W. BECK, PhD
Assistant Professor
Department of Health and Exercise Science
University of Oklahoma
Norman, OK

JAKE BLEACHER, MS, PT, OCS, MTC, CSCS
Board Certified Specialist in Orthopaedic Physical Therapy
The Ohio State University Sports Medicine Center
Columbus, OH

W. BRITT CHANDLER, MS, CSCS*D
Managing Editor
Strength and Conditioning Journal
Lexington, KY

JARED W. COBURN, PhD, CSCS*D, FNSCA, FACSM
Professor
Department of Kinesiology
California State University, Fullerton
Fullerton, CA

HERBERT A. DEVRIES, PhD, FACSM
Professor Emeritus
University of Southern California
Los Angeles, CA

TODD S. ELLENBECKER, DPT, MS, SCS, OCS, CSCS
Clinic Director, Physiotherapy Associates Scottsdale Sports Clinic
Scottsdale, Arizona
National Director of Clinical Research, Physiotherapy Associates
Memphis, TN
Director of Sports Medicine, ATP World Tour

KIRK L. ENGLISH, MA
Division of Rehabilitation Sciences
University of Texas Medical Branch
Galveston, TX

TAMMY K. EVETOVICH, PhD
Professor
Department of Health, Human Performance, and Sport
Wayne State College
Wayne, NE

ANDREW C. FRY, PhD, CSCS, FNSCA
Professor & Chair
Department of Health, Sport & Exercise Sciences
Director of Research
Research & Coaching Performance Team
University of Kansas
Lawrence, KS

JOHN F. GRAHAM, MS, FNSCA
Director
Department of Community and Corporate Fitness
Lehigh Valley Health Network
Allentown and Bethlehem, PA

G. GREGORY HAFF, PhD, CSCS*D, ASCC, FNSCA
Senior Lecturer Strength and Conditioning
School of Exercise, Biomedical and Health Sciences
Edith Cowan University, Joondalup, Western Australia

DISA L. HATFIELD, PhD, CSCS
Assistant Professor
The University of Rhode Island
Kingston, RI

ALLEN HEDRICK, MA, CSCS*D, RC, FNSCA
Head Strength and Conditioning Coach
Athletic Department
Colorado State University-Pueblo
Pueblo, CO

KRISTI R. HINNERICHS, PhD, ATC
Assistant Professor
Department of Health, Human Performance, and Sport
Wayne State College
Wayne, NE

JAY R. HOFFMAN, PhD, CSCS, FACSM, FNSCA
Professor
Sport and Exercise Science
University of Central Florida
Orlando, FL

TERRY J. HOUSH, PhD, FNSCA, FACSM
Professor
Department of Nutrition and Health Sciences
Director, Human Performance Laboratory
University of Nebraska-Lincoln
Lincoln, NE

EDWARD JO, MS, CSCS
Graduate Research Assistant
Department of Nutrition, Food, and Exercise Sciences
The Florida State University
Tallahassee, FL

ANDY V. KHAMOUI, MS, CSCS
Graduate Research Assistant
Department of Nutrition, Food, and Exercise Sciences
The Florida State University
Tallahassee, FL

DUANE V. KNUDSON, PhD
Professor and Chair
Department of Health and Human Performance
Texas State University
San Marcos, Texas

MARK KOVACS, PhD, CSCS
Department of Health, Physical Education, and Sport Science
WellStar College of Health and Human Services
Kennesaw State University
Kennesaw, Georgia
Coaching Education & Sport Science
USTA Player Development, Inc.
Boca Raton, Florida

WILLIAM J. KRAEMER, PhD, CSCS, FACSM, FNSCA
Professor
Departments of Kinesiology, Physiology and Neurobiology, and Medicine
School of Medicine
Human Performance Laboratory
University of Connecticut
Storrs, CT

MELISA LEMUS, MPT, MS, CSCS
Core Academy of Tennis
St. Louis, Missouri

SCOTT K. LYNN, PhD
Assistant Professor
Department of Kinesiology
California State University, Fullerton
Fullerton, CA

MOH H. MALEK, PhD, CSCS*D, FACSM, FNSCA
Associate Professor
Director: Integrative Physiology of Exercise Laboratory
Eugene Applebaum College of Pharmacy & Health Sciences
Wayne State University
Detroit, MI

SUSAN MERRIMAN, MS, PT, OCS
Physiotherapy Associates Scottsdale Sports Clinic
Scottsdale Arizona

GUILLERMO J. NOFFAL, PhD, CSCS
Associate Professor
Department of Kinesiology
California State University, Fullerton
Fullerton, CA

JOE ROGOWSKI, MS, ATC, CSCS
Sport and Exercise Science
University of Central Florida
Orlando, FL

ABBIE E. SMITH, PhD, CSCS*D, CISSN
Assistant Professor, Applied Physiology Laboratory
Department of Exercise and Sports Science
University of North Carolina Chapel Hill
Chapel Hill, NC

BARRY A. SPIERING, PhD, CSCS
Assistant Professor
Department of Kinesiology
California State University, Fullerton
Fullerton, CA

TRACI A. STATLER, PhD, CC AASP
Assistant Professor
Department of Kinesiology
California State University, Fullerton
Fullerton, CA

MARGARET E. STONE, MS, FNSCA, ASCC
Director, Center of Excellence for
Sport Science and Coach Education
East Tennessee State University
Johnson City, TN

MICHAEL H. STONE, PhD, FNSCA, FEL.UKSCA, ASCC
Graduate Program Director/KLSS
Exercise and Sport Science Laboratory Director
Center of Excellence for
Sport Science and Coach Education
East Tennessee State University
Johnson City, TN

LEM TAYLOR, PhD, CISSN
Assistant Professor
Department of Exercise & Sport Science
Director, Exercise Biochemistry Lab
University of Mary Hardin-Baylor
Belton, TX

N. TRAVIS TRIPLETT, PhD, CSCS*D, FNSCA
Professor
Director, Graduate Program
Department of Health, Leisure, and Exercise Science
Appalachian State University
Boone, NC

COLIN WILBORN, PhD
Assistant Professor
Department of Exercise & Sport Science
University of Mary Hardin-Baylor
Belton, TX

FEATURE CONTRIBUTORS

VANESSA L. CAZAS, MS, CSCS
Center for Sport Performance
California State University
Fullerton, CA

BRITT CHANDLER, MS, CSCS, NSCA-CPT
Managing Editor,
Strength and Conditioning Journal
Lexington, KY

JAMES J. TUFANO, MS, CSCS
Center for Sport Performance
California State University
Fullerton, CA

ACKNOWLEDGMENTS

In an extensive work such as this book, many individuals play critical roles. We would like to specifically thank editorial product managers Andrea Klingler and Linda Francis. We would like to acknowledge the efforts of Britt Chandler for his work in developing the ancillaries for this text.

Lee Brown would like to acknowledge the support of his graduate students and the faculty of the Department of Kinesiology at California State University, Fullerton. Jeff Chandler would like to acknowledge the support of students and faculty of the Department of Health, Physical Education, and Recreation at Jacksonville State University, Jacksonville, Alabama.

We are fortunate to be involved with an outstanding group of colleagues in the field of strength training and conditioning. We acknowledge their many contributions to the field and their continued hard work to move our discipline forward.

TJC & LEB 2012

CONTENTS

PART four Special Topics 421

PART

one two three four

Basic Science

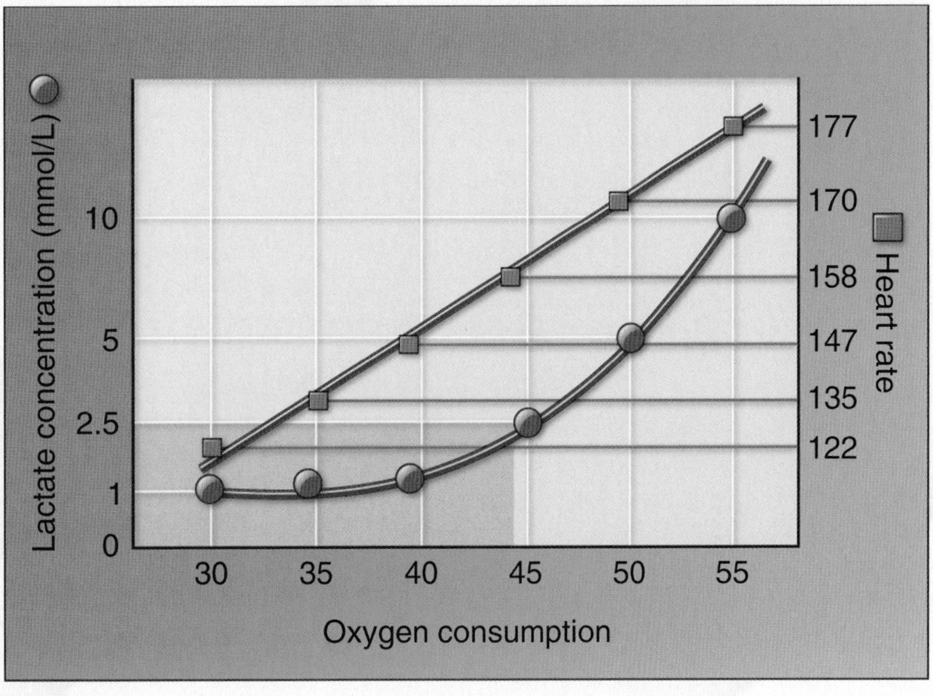

CHAPTER 1

Bioenergetics

C. ERIC ARNOLD ● T. JEFF CHANDLER

OBJECTIVES

After completing this chapter, you will be able to:

- Understand the basic concepts related to energy production for human movement and athletic performance.
- Understand the role of enzymes in catalyzing chemical reactions.
- Recognize and identify the energy systems and their role in human athletic performance.
- Understand the role of lactic acid and lactate in human athletic performance.
- Identify anabolic and catabolic reactions in the production of energy.
- Demonstrate an understanding of the limiting factors in human athletic performance.
- Understand the concept of oxygen consumption related to the production of energy.
- Understand the concept of metabolic specificity as related to human athletic performance.

KEY TERMS

Activation Energy
ADP + Pi
Anabolic
ATP
Blood Lactate
Bioenergetics
Carbohydrate
Cardiorespiratory Endurance
Catabolic
Chemical Energy
Cytoplasm
Deaminated
Electron Transport System (ETS)
Endergonic
Energy
Energy Charge of the Cell
Enzyme
Excess Postexercise Oxygen Consumption (EPOC)
Exergonic
Gluconeogenesis
Krebs Cycle
Lactate Shuttle
Mechanical Energy
Mitochondria
Nitrogen
Oxygen Consumption
Oxygen Deficit
Phosphate
Phosphofructokinase (PFK)
Q10 Effect
Radiant Energy
Rate-Limiting Enzyme
Reactant
Steady State
Specificity of Training
Substrate
Thermodynamics

Introduction

Human movement requires **energy**, and energy is vital for athletic performance. **Bioenergetics** is the flow of energy in biological systems and is a key consideration during exercise. For any physical activity, energy must be generated and used by the body to accomplish the task. The source of energy influences the ability of the sprinter to complete the 100-m dash or the marathoner to complete a run. Understanding metabolism, specifically the energy systems that are used during various types of exercise, is vital in developing effective activity-specific conditioning programs. With a basic knowledge of bioenergetics, the student can understand specific chemical reactions that take place in skeletal muscles and how energy from the chemical reactions fuel muscles during exercise.

Bioenergetics is the study of sources of energy in living organisms and how that energy is ultimately utilized.

The food we eat contains energy in the form of **chemical energy**. We store this chemical energy in our body in the forms of glycogen, fat, and protein. Ultimately, the chemical energy stored can be released to provide energy to produce adenosine triphosphate (ATP). ATP is the most important source of energy to support muscle contraction during exercise.

The structure of ATP is composed of an adenine group, a ribose group, and three phosphate groups joined together (Fig. 1.1). The formation of the ATP occurs by combining adenosine diphosphate (ADP) and inorganic phosphate (Pi). This process requires a substantial amount of energy, which must be captured from the food we eat.

ATP is the high-energy molecule responsible for muscular contraction and other life-sustaining metabolic reactions in the human body.

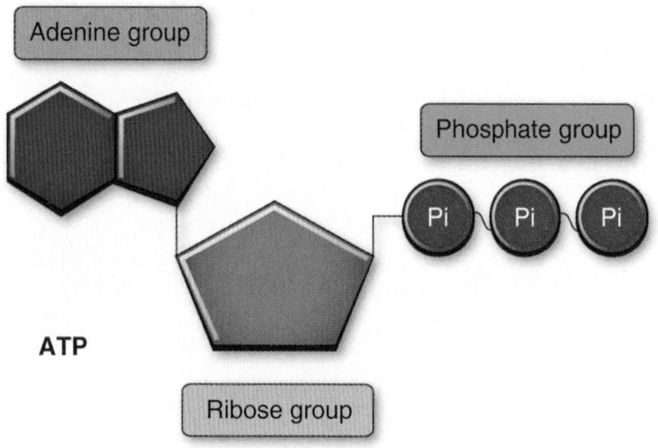

FIGURE 1.1 The basic structure of ATP. Energy is stored in the three phosphate bonds.

ATP is a high-energy molecule that stores energy in the form of chemical bonds. Energy is released when the chemical bonds that join ADP and Pi together to form ATP are broken (Fig. 1.2). The chemical energy derived from the breaking of the chemical bonds provides energy for performing various types of physical activity.

Metabolism is the sum total of **anabolic** and **catabolic** processes. A catabolic process breaks larger compounds into smaller compounds. In metabolism, this involves the breakdown of substances such as carbohydrate for the purpose of providing fuel for

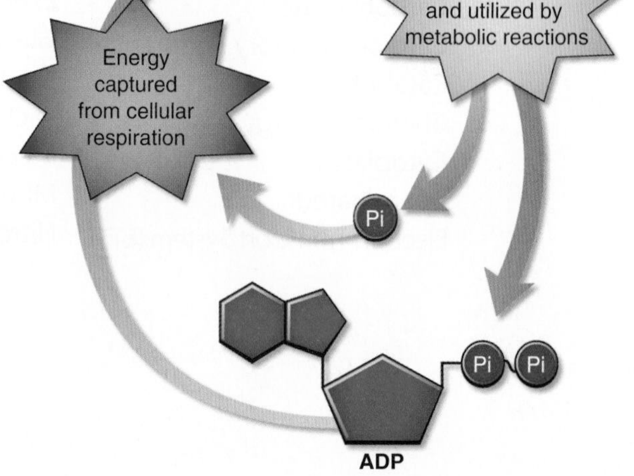

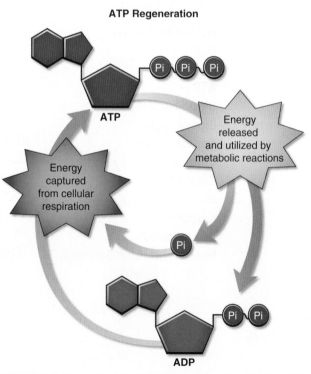

FIGURE 1.2 Regeneration of ATP. Energy is released when ATP is broken down into ADP and Pi. ATP is regenerated from ADP and energy captured from food.

the muscles during exercise. An anabolic reaction builds larger compounds from smaller compounds.

Metabolism = Catabolism + Anabolism.

ENZYMES

Enzymes are protein-structured molecules that speed or facilitate certain chemical reactions by lowering the **activation energy** of a chemical reaction (1). Activation energy is considered an energy barrier that must be overcome for a chemical reaction to occur (Fig. 1.3). The enzyme does not become a part of the product but remains intact as an enzyme.

A chemical reaction is classified as either an **exergonic** or an **endergonic** reaction. An exergonic reaction gives off energy and an endergonic reaction absorbs energy from its surroundings. During a 100-m sprint, ATP is being broken down in the muscle and energy is being released (exergonic reaction) and utilized by the muscles (endergonic reaction) that are being actively recruited during the activity. An exergonic reaction is illustrated in Figure 1.4 where A → B is a spontaneous downhill reaction. In this example, the energy level of the **reactant**(s) (**ATP**) is greater than that of the **product**(s) (**ADP + Pi**) (1).

An endergonic reaction is illustrated in Figure 1.5 where C → D is a nonspontaneous uphill reaction (1). In this example, the energy level of the product(s) is greater than the reactant(s) (1). The C → D transition will not occur unless an enzyme is present to lower the energy of activation (1). The energy of activation serves as an energy barrier to the chemical reaction (1).

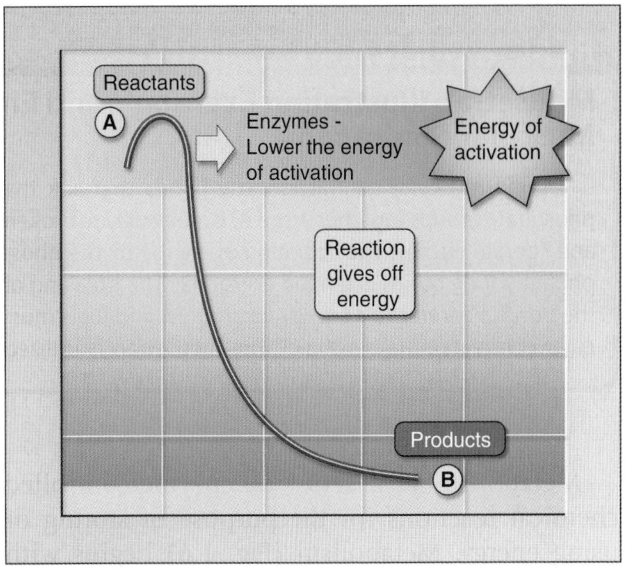

FIGURE 1.4 Exergonic chemical reaction. In this reaction, the energy level of the reactant(s) is greater than that of the product(s).

The following biochemical reaction is instrumental in muscular contraction:

ATP → ADP + Pi + Energy

ATPase is the enzyme that catalyzes this reaction.

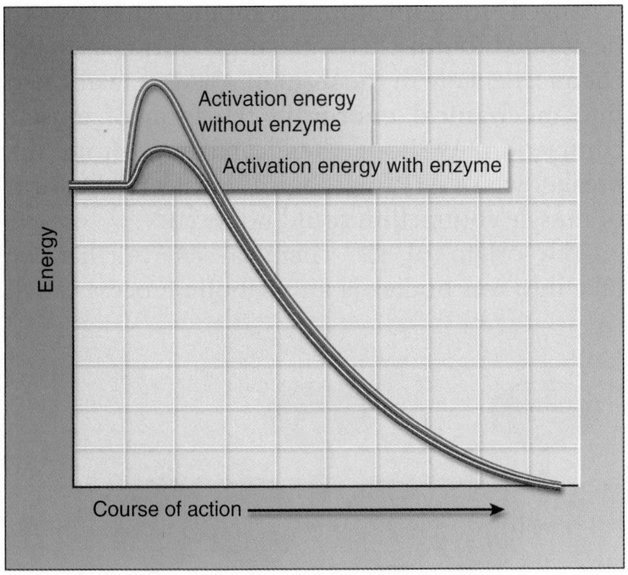

FIGURE 1.3 Energy of activation. An enzyme lowers the amount of energy that must be overcome for a chemical reaction to occur.

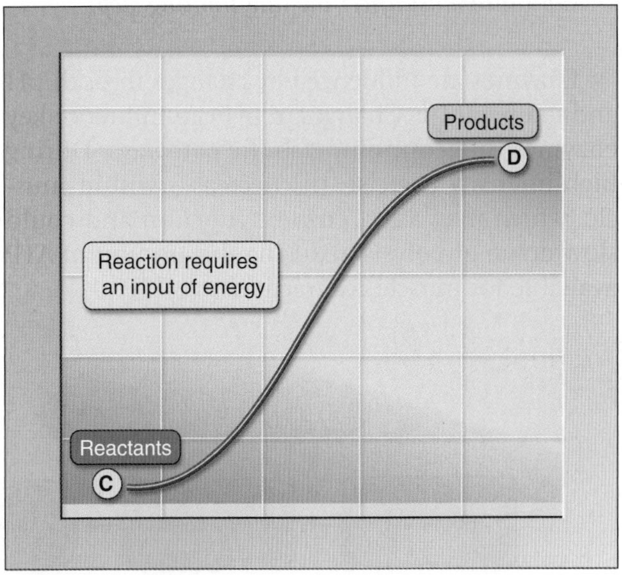

FIGURE 1.5 Endergonic chemical reaction. In an endergonic chemical reaction, the energy level of the product(s) is greater than that of the reactant(s).

REAL-WORLD APPLICATION

Mousetrap Illustrating Exergonic and Endergonic Biochemical Reactions during Muscular Contraction

During muscular contraction, the bonds that link the phosphate groups together in the ATP molecule are broken and liberate energy. The liberation of energy by the phosphoanhydride bonds is termed exergonic. The breaking of the bonds liberates this energy (exergonic) and fuels muscular contraction (endergonic). The mousetrap is utilized to illustrate both exergonic and endergonic biochemical reactions. Pulling the mousetrap spring back creates stored energy in the spring, and when the spring is released, an exergonic reaction occurs. The endergonic reaction is illustrated by the snapping of the mousetrap (trap consuming the energy).

Metabolism is a series of enzyme-controlled chemical reactions for the purpose of storing or using energy. Metabolism (Fig. 1.6) begins with a **substrate**, which is the beginning material in the reaction. In each step, the substrate undergoes a chemical change catalyzed by enzymes. At each step, the substrate is modified, and the modified compounds are referred to as intermediates. In the final step, the resulting compound is referred to as the product.

In a series of metabolic reactions, one enzyme is generally referred to as the "rate-limiting" enzyme. A **rate-limiting enzyme** is defined as an enzyme that catalyzes the slowest step in a series of chemical reactions (Fig. 1.7). Generally, the rate-limiting enzyme catalyzes the first step in the series of chemical reactions.

To stimulate or inhibit a series of reactions, a substance must affect the rate-limiting step.

Enzymes are influenced by changes in both pH and temperature. Changes in pH can influence key enzymes that control metabolic pathways. During high-intensity exercise, pH decreases within muscle, which may affect enzyme function and could slow down glycolysis, reducing the amount of ATP available for muscle contraction.

Temperature can have an important effect on enzymatic reactions. This effect is studied by changing the temperature in multiples of 10 °C and is referred to as the **Q10 effect**. Increasing the temperature by 10 °C doubles the speed of the enzymatic reaction. From a practical perspective, warming up the muscles prior to engaging in physical activity allows the athlete to take advantage of the Q10 effect.

THE "CREATION" OF CHEMICAL ENERGY

Where does energy come from? Energy is neither created nor destroyed but can be changed from one form to another. This concept reinforces the first law of **thermodynamics**, the physical science dealing with energy exchange, where energy is "changed" from one form to another. This law can be applied to muscle contraction. During exercise, chemical energy in the form of ATP is transformed into **mechanical energy** in the form of muscle contraction. Without chemical energy from the breakdown of ATP, mechanical energy in the form of muscle contraction could not occur.

The origin of the chemical energy that we take into our bodies is an anabolic process called

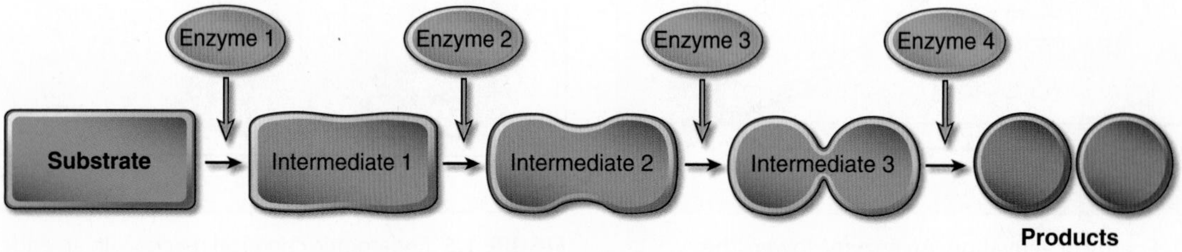

FIGURE 1.6 Metabolism. In this metabolic pathway, enzymes facilitate chemical reactions that change a substrate to intermediates and, finally, to a product.

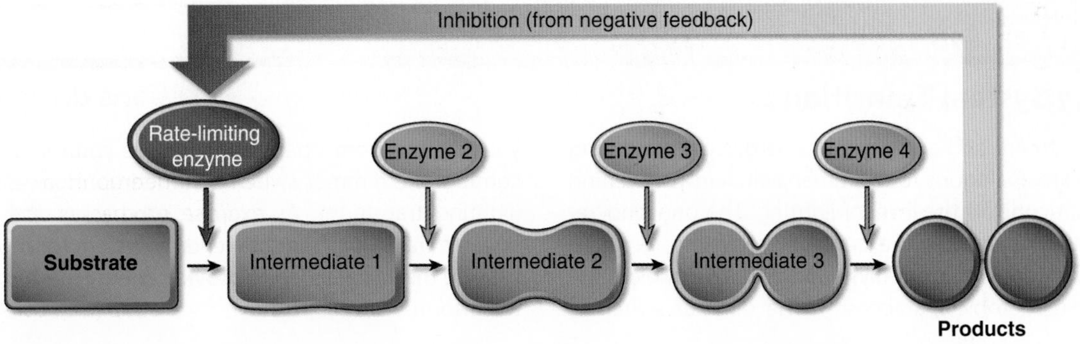

FIGURE 1.7 Inhibition of a chemical reaction. A rate-limiting enzyme is inhibited by the final product of the reaction through the negative feedback mechanism.

photosynthesis. In photosynthesis, green plants, in the presence of sunlight and chlorophyll, take carbon dioxide and water and change them into **carbohydrate** (a carbon/hydrogen/oxygen compound) with oxygen given off into the atmosphere. It is this reaction that converts the sun's energy to chemical energy that we need to live and also replenishes the oxygen supply in our atmosphere. This carbohydrate compound formed in green plants is the basic form of energy needed by man. This carbon structure can be modified through anabolic reactions to form fats, which also contain carbon, hydrogen, and oxygen, and proteins, which contain carbon, hydrogen, oxygen, and **nitrogen**.

ENERGY SYSTEMS

There are three distinct yet closely integrated energy systems that operate together in a coordinated fashion to provide energy for muscle contraction. The three energy systems are the phosphocreatine system, the anaerobic glycolytic system, and the oxidative system. The phosphocreatine and anaerobic glycolytic systems provide ATP at a high rate to support muscle contraction during short bursts of high-intensity exercise such as a 200-m sprint. However, the supply of ATP by the phosphocreatine and anaerobic glycolytic energy systems is limited (Table 1.1).

Three energy systems provide ATP for muscular work: the phosphocreatine system, the anaerobic glycolytic system, and the oxidative system.

The oxidative system predominates during low to moderate exercise intensity when oxygen is available to the muscle. At lower exercise intensities such as during walking, ATP demand is low, and energy can be supplied at a high enough rate through the oxidative energy systems (2). At higher exercise intensities, ATP demand is high, and energy cannot be supplied solely by oxidative metabolism (2). The anaerobic glycolytic system, therefore, must fill this gap between the phosphocreatine system and the oxidative system. During high-intensity exercise, the supply of ATP must be derived from the phosphocreatine and anaerobic glycolytic energy systems.

TABLE 1.1 ● THE ENERGY SYSTEMS AND THEIR APPROXIMATE CONTRIBUTIONS TO VARIOUS DURATIONS OF EXERCISE AT MAXIMAL INTENSITY (1)

ENERGY SYSTEM	DURATION
Phosphocreatine system	0–10 s
Phosphocreatine system and glycolytic system (slow)	10–30 s
Glycolytic system (fast)	30 s to 2 min
Glycolytic system (fast) and oxidative system	2–3 min
Oxidative system	<3 min and rest

REAL-WORLD APPLICATION

Energy System Transition

The recruitment and activation of energy systems during exercise are analogous to a dimmer switch in your dining room that controls the level of lighting. The phosphocreatine energy system is the first energy system recruited followed by anaerobic glycolysis and oxidative phosphorylation (e.g., aerobic metabolism). The dimmer switch in your dining room operates in that as you request more lighting, the dimmer switch is turned up more and more (lighting transition). As exercise progresses, the energy systems transition from one energy system to the next to provide the ATP needed to provide energy for the muscles to perform.

It is important to note that all three energy systems are active at a given point in time, but one system will predominate based on the conditions at that time (Fig. 1.8). Each energy system operates like a dimmer switch in that they are not completely turned off but transition from one energy system to the next based on energy requirements of the muscle during exercise. Exercise intensity, duration, and the mode of exercise play an instrumental role in determining which energy system will predominate during exercise. However, exercise intensity plays the most important role in dictating which energy system is activated.

Exercise intensity is the most important variable related to which energy system is activated to produce ATP for muscular work.

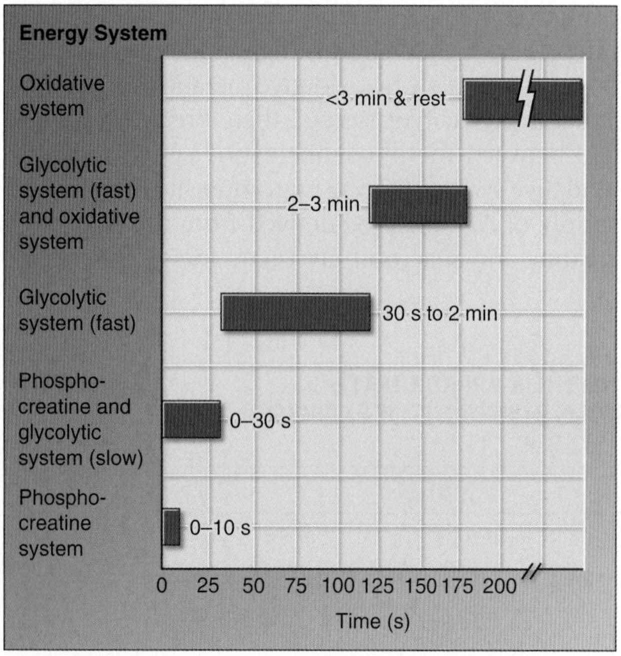

FIGURE 1.8 The energy systems and their approximate contributions to various durations of exercise at maximal intensity. Note the overlapping and timing of the various energy systems.

Exercise intensity is prescribed using a percentage of maximal oxygen consumption (% $\dot{V}O_{2max}$). Maximal oxygen consumption is defined as the greatest amount of oxygen utilization that occurs during dynamic exercise and is measured in either $mL \cdot kg^{-1} \cdot min^{-1}$ or $L \cdot min^{-1}$. For example, an individual may be prescribed exercise that requires 70% of his or her $\dot{V}O_{2max}$. Understanding when a specific energy system is turned on during various activities and or sporting events can assist the strength coach in developing programs that are metabolically specific.

THE PHOSPHOCREATINE SYSTEM

ATP is broken down to release energy (a catabolic process) and can be regenerated from its component parts, an adenosine group and three **phosphate** groups. Conversely, energy is required to add a phosphate group to an adenosine group, which is an anabolic process.

When muscular energy is needed for a short period of time, the phosphocreatine system is capable of supplying most of the needed ATP. The phosphocreatine system will also supply energy in the beginning stages of all types of exercise. ATP is produced in the phosphocreatine system

BOX 1.1

Characteristics of the Phosphocreatine System

1. Involves only one chemical step
2. Catalyzed by the enzyme creatine kinase (CK)
3. Very fast chemical reaction
4. One ATP generated per creatine phosphate molecule
5. Lasts for 5 to 10 seconds at maximal intensity
6. Anaerobic
7. Fatigue associated with creatine phosphate depletion
8. The dominant energy system in speed and explosive power events

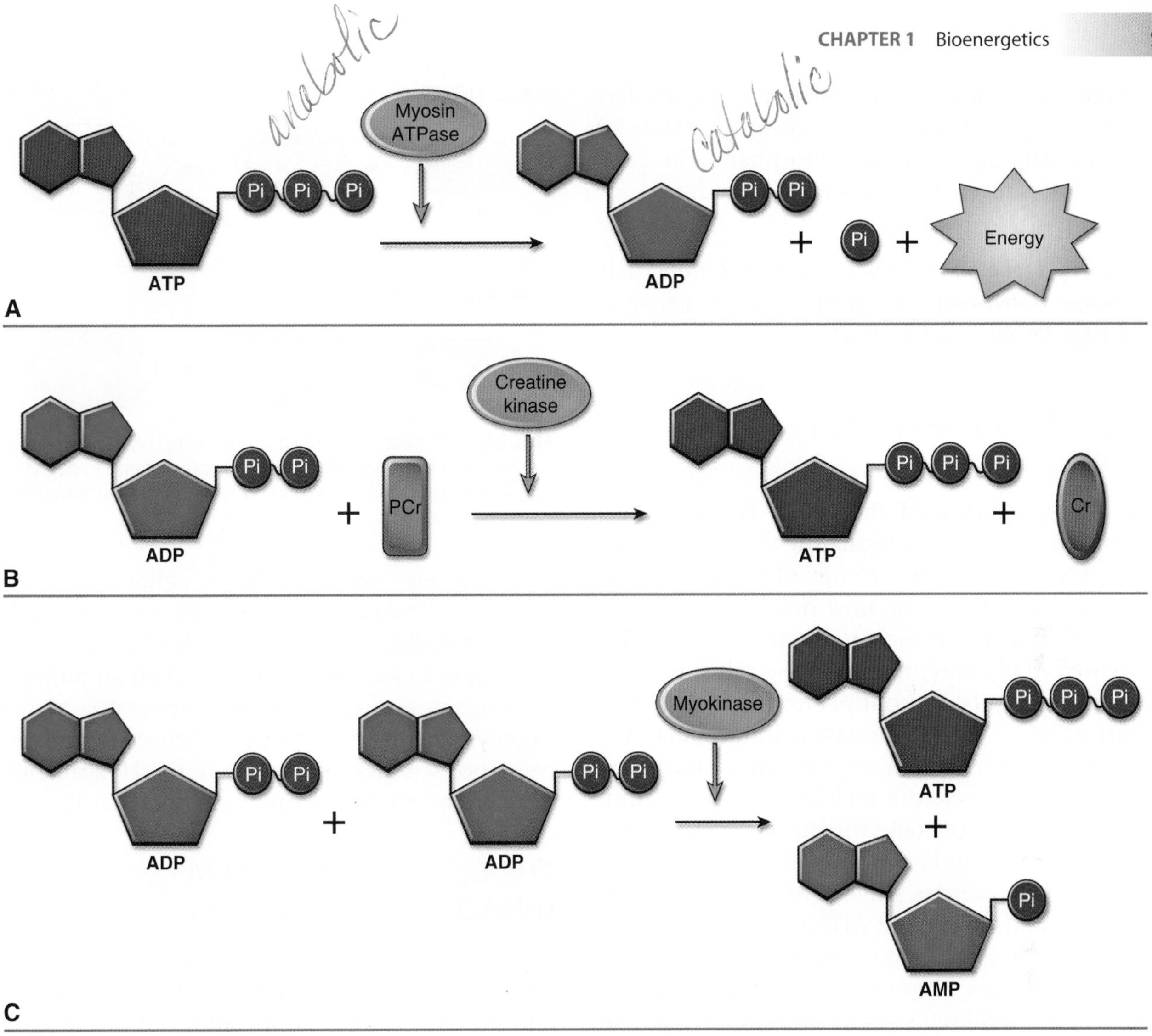

FIGURE 1.9 Reactions of the phosphagen system. **A.** Myosin ATPase reaction. **B.** CK reaction. **C.** Myokinase reaction.

anaerobically (without oxygen present). There are three basic reactions in the phosphocreatine system (Fig. 1.9). When physical activity is initiated, ATP stored in the muscles is utilized. All activities are initiated anaerobically, as it takes time to begin to produce ATP aerobically. The phosphocreatine system can regenerate ATP anaerobically, allowing anaerobic activity to proceed at a maximal or near-maximal level, but only for a short period of time.

$$(\mathbf{PCr + ADP \leftrightarrow ATP + Cr})$$

The first step in the phosphocreatine system is the breakdown of ATP to ADP + Pi in the presence of the enzyme myosin ATPase. This reaction produces energy for muscle contraction anaerobically. Some ATP is stored in the muscles to perform this task. As mentioned, the initiation of all activity depends on this stored ATP. Following the initial breakdown of ATP, there are two reactions that regenerate ATP anaerobically. These reactions are often named by the enzymes that catalyze the reactions: the CK reaction and the myokinase reaction.

$$\mathbf{PCr + ADP \leftrightarrow ATP + Cr}$$

In the CK reaction, phosphocreatine is combined with ADP in the presence of the enzyme CK to form new ATP.

$$\mathbf{ADP + AMP \xrightarrow{\text{Creatine kinase}} ATP}$$

A second reaction that can regenerate ATP anaerobically over the short term is the myokinase reaction, which regenerates ATP from two ADP. This reaction results in the production of one ATP and one adenosine monophosphate (AMP). The production of AMP is important to the control of metabolism, as AMP is a potent stimulator of glycolysis.

$$\mathbf{ADP + ADP \xrightarrow{\text{Myokinase}} ATP + AMP}$$

In summary, energy from carbohydrates (or fats or proteins) is stored in the chemical bonds of ATP between adenosine and phosphate (Fig. 1.9). When ATP is regenerated, energy is stored.

When a phosphate group is removed from ATP, energy is released. ATP is the ultimate source of energy for muscular contraction.

REGULATION OF ENERGY PRODUCTION

The **energy charge of the cell** (ATP/ADP ratio) plays an integral role in regulating the phosphocreatine system. The energy charge of the muscle cell provides information on how much energy (ATP) is available in the muscle to support the activity. Increased ADP concentration in the cell stimulates CK, the key regulatory control enzyme of the phosphocreatine system. An increase in intracellular ATP inhibits CK, thus decreasing the rate of the enzymatic reaction. Therefore, high levels of ADP stimulate CK, which accelerates the breakdown of PCr + ADP → ATP + Cr and provides energy for short-term high-intensity exercise. High levels of ADP in the muscle would reflect that ATP is being extensively used by the muscle for providing energy for generating force as in a 200-m run. Low levels of ADP in the muscle would reflect that ATP is not being used at a high level as in walking at a slow pace.

Postexercise phosphocreatine resynthesis occurs between 2 and 3 minutes of recovery (2) using the phosphocreatine energy shuttle. This process involves shuttling Cr and PCr between sites of utilization (e.g., myofibrils) and sites of regeneration (e.g., **mitochondria**). When specifically training recovery of the phosphocreatine system, it may be advantageous for the athlete performing 40-yd sprints to allow for a 2- to 3-minute recovery to optimize phosphocreatine resynthesis (3). This would also apply to resistance training when an athlete is training for recovery of the phosphocreatine system. Allowing adequate recovery time between sprints and resistance sets would provide more ATP availability through the phosphocreatine chemical reaction.

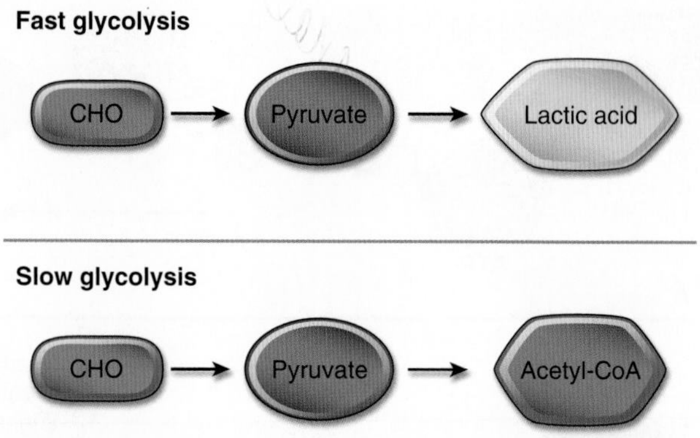

FIGURE 1.10 Reactions of fast and slow glycolysis. Pyruvate is converted to lactic acid if no oxygen is present and to acetyl-CoA in the Krebs cycle if oxygen is present. CHO, carbohydrate.

THE GLYCOLYTIC SYSTEM (ANAEROBIC GLYCOLYSIS)

The glycolytic system involves the breakdown of carbohydrate anaerobically to produce energy. Fats and proteins cannot be metabolized in the glycolytic system. The carbohydrate (the substrate) comes from either blood glucose or glycogen stored in the liver or muscles. There are two types of glycolysis, fast glycolysis and slow glycolysis (Fig. 1.10). Slow glycolysis is sometimes referred to as "aerobic glycolysis" (1). Adaptations in the ability of muscle tissue to utilize specific substrates depend to a large extent on the muscle fiber type (Table 1.2).

TABLE 1.2 ● SKELETAL MUSCLE FIBER TYPES RELATED TO SUBSTRATE AND ENERGY SYSTEMS

	TYPE I	TYPE IIA	TYPE IIX
Phosphocreatine stores	Low	High	High
Glycogen stores	Low	High	High
Triglyceride stores	Low	Intermediate	Low
Myosin ATPase activity	Low	High	High
Glycolytic enzyme activity	Low	High	High
Oxidative enzyme activity	High	Low	Low

TABLE 1.3 ● KEY ENZYMES IN ANAEROBIC GLYCOLYSIS

GLYCOGEN PHOSPHORYLASE	DEGRADES GLYCOGEN INTO GLUCOSE
Hexokinase	First committed step in glycolysis, converts glucose to glucose 6-phosphate
PFK	Rate-limiting enzyme in anaerobic glycolysis
Lactate dehydrogenase	Conversion step from pyruvate to lactate

BOX 1.2

Characteristics of Glycolytic System

1. Eighteen chemical reactions, six are repeated
2. Twelve chemical compounds, eleven enzymes
3. PFK is the rate-limiting enzyme
4. Fast, but not as fast as creatine phosphate system
5. Two ATPs if glucose is the substrate, three ATPs if glycogen is the substrate
6. Anaerobic
7. One- to two-minute duration at high (not maximal) intensity
8. Fatigue associated with decreased pH reflecting an increase in hydrogen ions
9. Predominant energy system in high-intensity non-maximal exercise, for example, 800-m run.

Fast glycolysis breaks down glucose to pyruvate and eventually to lactic acid anaerobically with the net production of two ATPs. If glycogen is the substrate, one ATP is saved, and there is a net production of three ATPs. Key enzymes in anaerobic glycolysis are provided in Table 1.3.

Slow glycolysis is the path the pyruvate takes if sufficient oxygen is present for aerobic metabolism. When oxygen is present, pyruvate is changed through a series of biochemical reactions to acetyl-CoA, the first compound in the Krebs cycle. Slow glycolysis prepares the carbon compound (pyruvate) to enter the aerobic pathway. Glycolytic reactions take place, for the most part, in the **cytoplasm** of the cell, the watery medium between the cell membrane and the nucleus. The final step in slow glycolysis, pyruvate to acetyl-coA, takes place in the mitochondria.

Anaerobic glycolysis produces a net gain of two ATPs, but it has the ability to proceed when there is no O_2 present.

The control enzyme of the glycolytic system is **phosphofructokinase (PFK)**. PFK is the rate-limiting enzyme that controls the rate of glycolysis. PFK is inhibited by high levels of ATP, phosphocreatine, citrate, free fatty acids, and a markedly decreased pH. PFK is stimulated by high concentrations of inorganic phosphate (Pi), ADP, phosphate, and ammonia, and is strongly stimulated by AMP.

THE OXIDATIVE SYSTEM

The oxidative system aerobically oxidizes or "burns" carbohydrates (or other carbon-containing structures obtained from fat or protein). The preferred fuels for aerobic metabolism are carbohydrates and fats, but protein can be **deaminated** (removing the amino group, the nitrogenous component of the carbon/hydrogen/oxygen/nitrogen compound) and oxidized aerobically. The oxidative system is a complex process that involves two parts: the **Krebs cycle** (citric acid cycle) (Fig. 1.11) and the **electron transport system (ETS)** (Fig. 1.12). The Krebs cycle is a complex series of enzyme-controlled metabolic

REAL-WORLD APPLICATION

ATP Investment and Generation Phases in Glycolysis

In the initial phases of anaerobic glycolysis, two ATPs must be invested into the system, and four ATPs are eventually produced, for a net gain of two ATPs. This investment of ATPs is like an investment in a particular stock (e.g., IBM stock), and ATP generation is like a profit gained from that particular stock. So a net total of two ATPs are generated from the metabolism of one glucose molecule in glycolysis. Glycolysis is similar to investing in a stock where you invest $200 and get back $400 at the end of the quarter. Therefore, you have a net gain of $200, or double what you had when you initially invested in the stock.

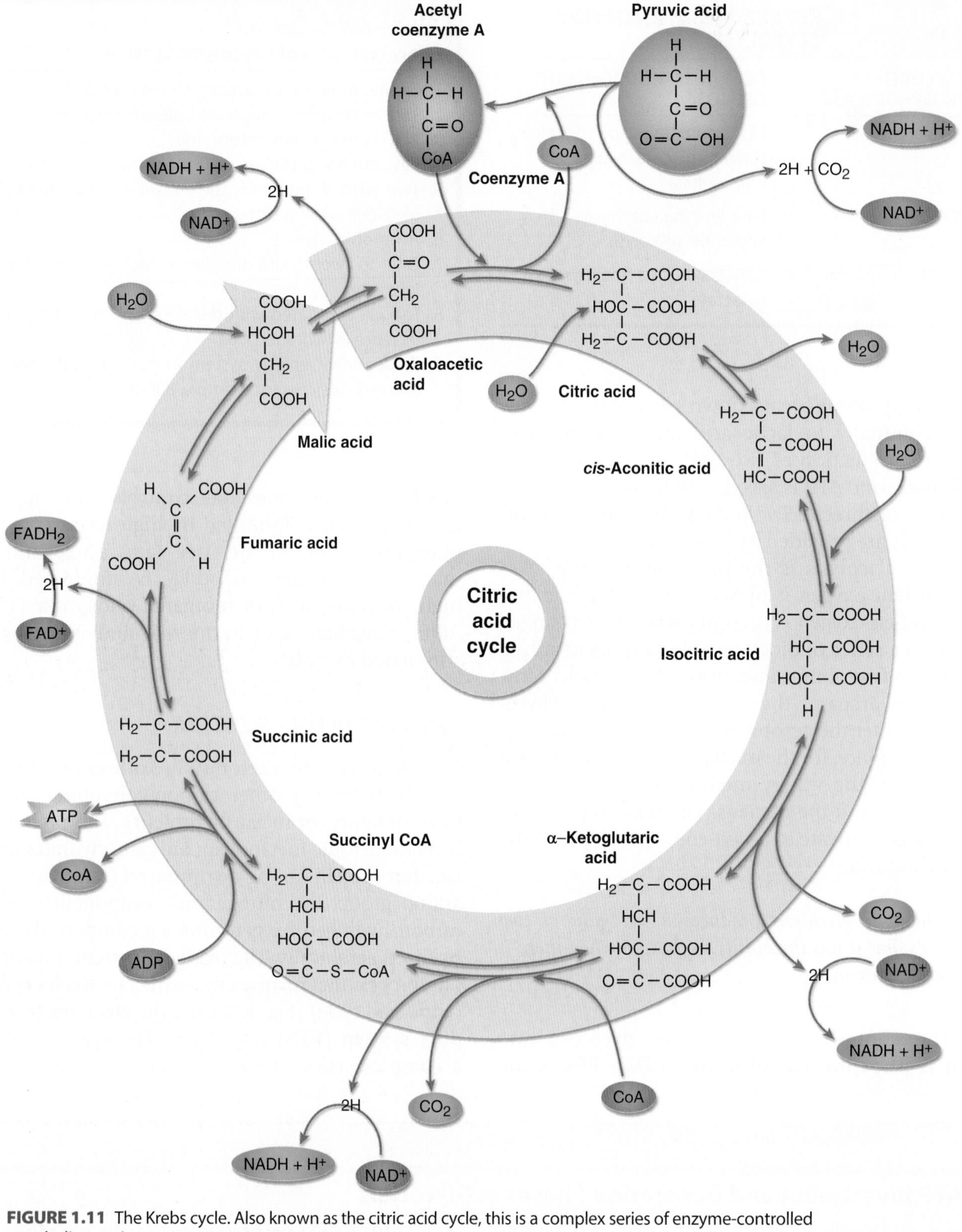

FIGURE 1.11 The Krebs cycle. Also known as the citric acid cycle, this is a complex series of enzyme-controlled metabolic reactions.

reactions. The Krebs cycle is located in the mitochondria, which is the site of aerobic ATP production.

The Krebs cycle plays an integral role in oxidizing carbohydrates, fats, and proteins. The electron transport chain is located in the inner membrane of the mitochondria and is responsible for the aerobic production of ATP. The Krebs cycle generates electrons in the form of hydrogen

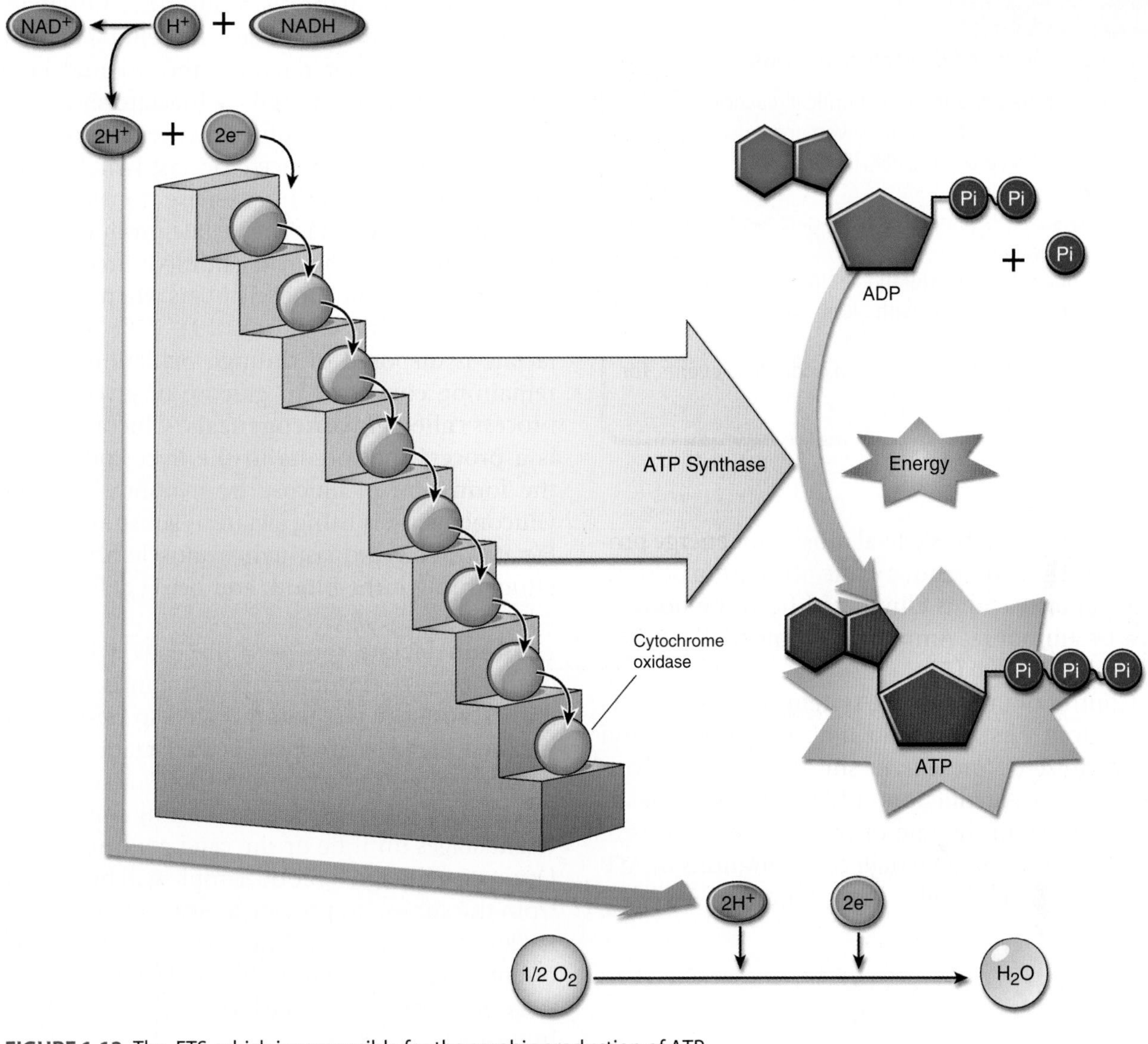

FIGURE 1.12 The ETS, which is responsible for the aerobic production of ATP.

ions shuttled through the ETS by electron carriers (flavin adenine dinucleotide [FAD^+] or nicotinamide adenine dinucleotide [NAD^+]). It is in the ETS that many ATP molecules are generated. Aerobic metabolic reactions take place in the mitochondria, an organelle inside the cell membrane in the cytoplasm. One molecule of glucose oxidized aerobically produces approximately 38 ATPs (1).

***The aerobic system can produce many more ATPs per molecule than the anaerobic system, but it cannot produce ATP rapidly; the intensity must remain at or below* steady state.**

Fats can also be oxidized aerobically to form ATP. First, fats are broken down into glycerol and free fatty acids. The free fatty acids enter the mitochondria, and through a process called beta-oxidation, they are degraded to acetyl-CoA and hydrogen atoms, with the acetyl-CoA entering the Krebs cycle directly.

Although it is not a preferred source of energy, protein can be broken down and oxidized aerobically. First proteins are catabolized into their smaller components, amino acids. Amino acids can then be deaminated. The carbon/hydrogen/oxygen portion of the compound can be converted to glucose through gluconeogenesis, pyruvate, and other Krebs cycle intermediates. The contribution of amino acids to energy production is minimal for anaerobic activities, but may contribute up to 18% of the energy requirements for aerobic exercise (4). Branched-chain amino acids are the major

BOX 1.3

Characteristics of Oxidative System

1. One hundred twenty-four chemical reactions
2. Thirty compounds, twenty-seven enzymes
3. Rate-limiting enzymes, PFK, ID, CO
4. Slow
5. Thirty-six ATPs generated from glucose, thirty-seven via glycogen
6. Potentially limitless duration at lower intensity
7. Fatigue associated with fuel depletion (muscle glycogen)
8. Predominant energy system in endurance events, for example, marathon

amino acids used by skeletal muscle for energy production. The nitrogenous waste, the amino portion of the amino acid, is eliminated from the body as urea or ammonia. Ammonia is potentially a contributor to fatigue (5).

Control of the oxidative system is related to several factors. First, adequate amounts of FAD^+ and NAD^+ must be present to shuttle hydrogen ions into the ETS. A reduction in FAD^+ and NAD^+ leads to a decrease in the rate of oxidative metabolism. The ETS is inhibited by high concentrations of ATP and stimulated by high concentrations of ADP (1).

LACTATE

The lactic acid formed as a result of fast glycolysis is immediately buffered and changed into a salt, lactate. While lactic acid is certainly associated with fatigue, lactate becomes a substrate that can be converted back into pyruvate and used in the Krebs cycle, particularly in the heart and in slow-twitch muscle fibers (4,6).

The lactic acid produced during heavy exercise is rapidly converted to lactate. Lactate is a useful metabolic compound that can be transported to the liver and changed to glucose in a process called gluconeogenesis. It can then be used by the body as fuel during exercise.

Lactate was once perceived as a metabolic waste product; however, lactate is now considered an important fuel source. The **lactate shuttle** hypothesis proposed by Brooks (7) explained that lactate played a key role in the distribution of carbohydrate energy among various tissues and cellular compartments. Brooks later renamed the original lactate shuttle hypothesis the cell–cell lactate shuttle (8). The cell–cell lactate shuttle involves the transportation of lactate produced by fast-twitch muscle fibers (type IIx) during exercise to slow-twitch muscle fibers (type 1). The lactate produced by the fast-twitch muscle fibers is shuttled directly to the adjacent slow-twitch muscle fibers where oxidation occurs. According to Brooks (9), 75% to 80% of lactate is disposed of through oxidation with the remaining converted to glucose or glycogen in a process called **gluconeogenesis**. Gluconeogenesis is a process that occurs in the liver and involves the formation of glucose from noncarbohydrate. Gluconeogenesis using lactate as substrate involves lactate leaving the fast-twitch muscle fibers, circulating through the blood, and being delivered and taken up by the liver.

Blood lactate can be utilized as a laboratory test to predict endurance performance. The common laboratory test incorporated to estimate this maximal steady-state speed is the lactate threshold. To determine the lactate threshold, a subject will run on a treadmill at various running speeds at different stages until he or she can't continue further. During each stage, a blood sample will be obtained from the subject to provide a measure of the blood lactate concentration. The lactate threshold represents the point where blood lactate begins to increase in a nonlinear fashion at a specific exercise intensity (Fig. 1.13).

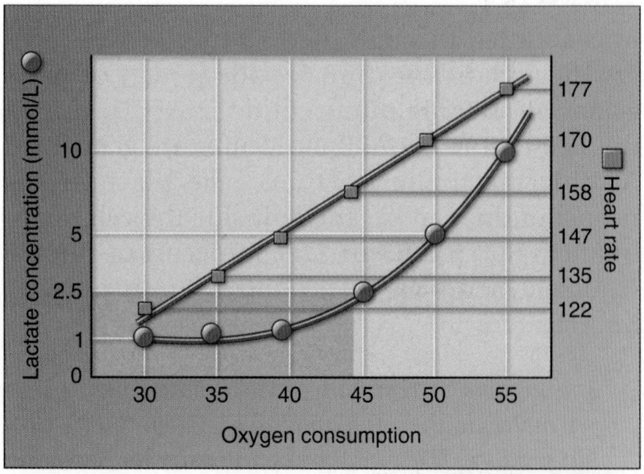

FIGURE 1.13 The lactate threshold, which represents the point where blood lactate begins to increase in a nonlinear fashion at a specific exercise intensity (18). As the exercise intensity increases, blood levels of lactic acid begin to accumulate in an exponential fashion.

Q & A from the Field

Q ***I have always heard that lactic acid makes you fatigued. Is that true?***

A Lactic acid is a by-product of anaerobic metabolism. Anaerobic exercise is by definition of high intensity, and the end product will be lactic acid. Also by definition, high-intensity anaerobic exercise will lead to fatigue rather rapidly. In one sense, the production of lactic acid parallels fatigue. It may also be that molecules of lactic acid interfere with efficient muscle contraction. Lactic acid is also responsible for the immediate burning in muscle that is exercising at a high intensity. This burning is not to be confused with the delayed onset of muscle soreness that occurs over the next 24 to 48 hours, which is not due to lactic acid. The lactic acid that is produced is quickly buffered to lactate. Lactate can be transported to the liver and converted to glucose. Lactate is a useful energy source for recovery from intense anaerobic exercise.

The lactate threshold is an important factor in performance. If two athletes participating in an aerobic event have the same Vo_{2max}, the athlete with the highest lactate threshold will be likely to win the race.

The running speed at which the lactate threshold occurs is used as a predictor of performance (10). The measure of the maximal steady-state running speed is beneficial in predicting success in distance running events from 2 miles to the marathon (6,11–15).

SUMMARY OF CATABOLIC PROCESSES IN THE PRODUCTION OF CELLULAR ENERGY

Figure 1.14 summarizes the breakdown of food (catabolic process) for the production of energy. The food we eat is composed of fats, carbohydrates, or proteins. Carbohydrates are broken down into blood glucose. The blood glucose can either be used for energy or stored as glycogen. When glycogen stores in the liver and muscles are full, the glucose is stored as fat. The glucose, through glycolysis, is converted to pyruvic acid and then either lactic acid if no oxygen is present (fast glycolysis) or acetyl-CoA if oxygen is present in the cell. The acetyl-CoA then goes into the Krebs cycle and the ETS to produce ATP with the eventual end products of CO_2 and H_2O.

Fats and proteins can both be used for energy. Fats are catabolized into glycerol and fatty acids. The glycerol can be converted to pyruvate and enter into glycolysis. Fatty acids undergo beta oxidation and are converted to acetyl-CoA and enter the Krebs cycle.

Proteins are catabolized into amino acids. The amino acids are deaminated with the amino group being secreted as urea. The resulting carbon compound can be converted to pyruvate, acetyl-CoA, or other Krebs cycle intermediates.

Q & A from the Field

Q ***What energy system will be most efficient in cross country skiing?***

A Efficiency is relative to the task. Because cross-country skiing is a long distance event the aerobic energy system will be the most efficient. The aerobic energy system is the most efficient at producing ATP over a continuous period of time, since it can produce approximately 38 ATPs per molecule of glucose. The anaerobic pathways will be much less efficient as they lack the capacity to sustain ATP production over a long period of time.

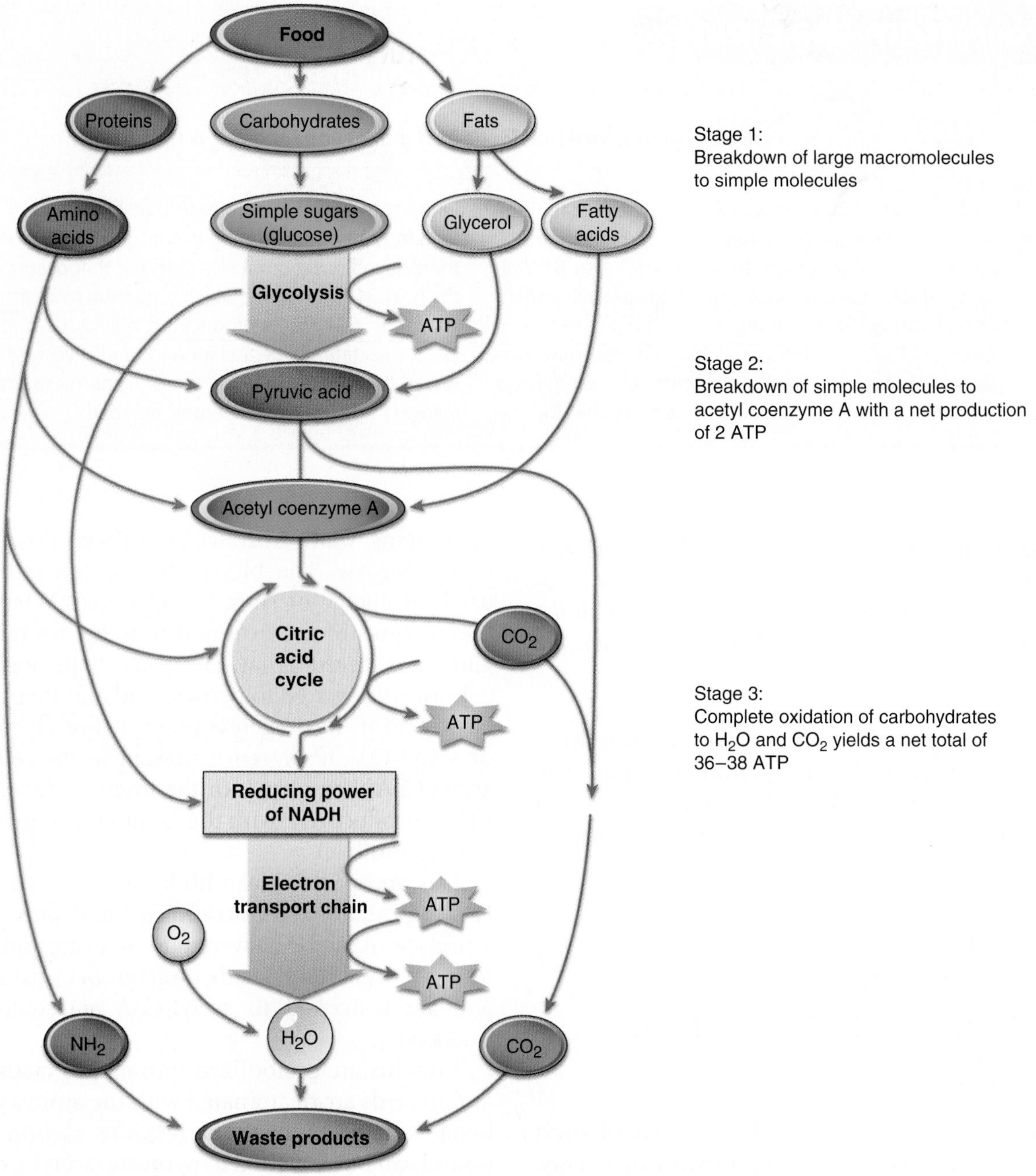

FIGURE 1.14 Summary of catabolic processes involved in the breakdown of food to energy.

EFFICIENCY OF THE ENERGY-PRODUCING PATHWAYS

Efficiency of the energy-producing pathways depends on the demands of the activity. At first glance, it may appear that the aerobic pathway is the most efficient as it produces many more ATP molecules than the anaerobic pathways. There are, however, different ways to calculate efficiency. The simplest method of looking at the efficiency of each metabolic system is relative to the task at hand. If the task is a 100-m sprint, the oxidative system is very inefficient as it does not have the time needed to produce ATP. Likewise, if the task is a marathon, the anaerobic pathways will be much less efficient as they lack the capacity to produce ATP over a long period of time. Using this logic, the anaerobic energy systems are the most efficient at producing ATP immediately. The aerobic energy system is the most efficient for producing ATP over a continuous period of time.

REAL-WORLD APPLICATION

Efficiency of Energy Systems: Is the Aerobic System or the Anaerobic System More Efficient?

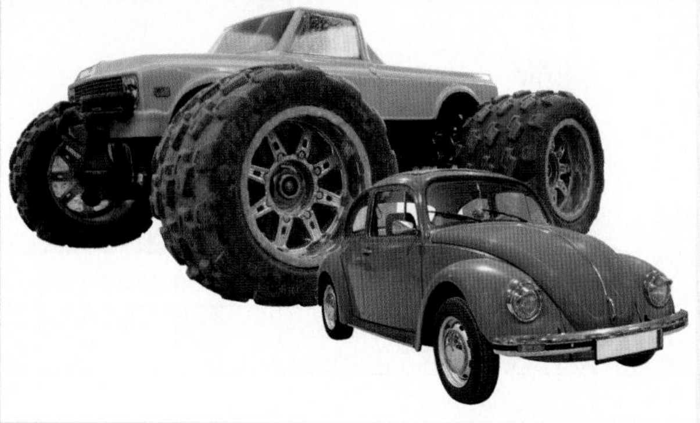

Efficiency must be related to a specific task. For example, an economy car is more economical or efficient in terms of miles per gallon than a 4 × 4 "monster truck" for traveling cross country, but the truck is more efficient at carrying or pulling a heavy load or climbing a steep hill. Efficiency must be viewed as task specific. The anaerobic energy systems are most efficient at producing ATP rapidly. The aerobic system is very inefficient at producing ATP if the demand is immediate. The aerobic energy system is more efficient at producing ATP over a longer duration and a lower workload. The anaerobic system, like the truck, is inefficient at performing low-intensity work over a long period of time. The aerobic system, like the economy car, is inefficient at performing at a high intensity such as pulling heavy loads or climbing a steep hill.

LIMITING FACTORS OF PERFORMANCE

Factors that limit performance from the metabolic standpoint will relate to the buildup of metabolic byproducts (lactic acid and possibly ammonia), the depletion of PCr, or the depletion of substrate (fats, carbohydrates, or proteins). Obviously, the limiting metabolic factor in a given activity will depend on the energy system involved in the activity, which is determined basically by the intensity and duration of the activity (Table 1.4). A low-intensity activity such as a long-distance run will result primarily in the depletion of muscle and liver glycogen.

High-intensity activities that are not repeated without a great deal of rest have essentially no metabolic limiting factors. In repeated high-intensity activities, muscle glycogen, ATP/PC, and a decrease in pH are all possible limiting factors. The hydrogen ions given off from the buildup of lactic acid has been shown to decrease force production in skeletal muscle (16), possibly by competing with the binding sites on troponin.

TABLE 1.4 ● METABOLIC FACTORS THAT LIMIT PERFORMANCE

ACTIVITY	PRIMARY LIMITING FACTORS
Marathon	Muscle glycogen, liver glycogen
High-intensity repeated (10 × 40 yd)	ATP, muscle glycogen, decreased pH
High intensity (400 m)	Decreased pH

OXYGEN CONSUMPTION

Oxygen consumption is the ability of the body to take in and use oxygen to produce energy. Oxygen consumption can be estimated using a metabolic cart that can measure the oxygen content of the inspired and expired air. Maximal oxygen consumption is considered a measure of **cardiorespiratory endurance**. Maximal oxygen consumption is also called Vo_{2max}, which can be measured in milliliters/kilogram/body weight ($mL \cdot kg^{-1}$) or in liters/minute ($L \cdot min^{-1}$). Measuring Vo_{2max} in $mL \cdot kg^{-1} \cdot min^{-1}$ is used when comparing two individuals because body weight influences maximal oxygen consumption. Liters per minute is used when just comparing an individual from one test to the second test. From a practical perspective, a coach develops a training program for his or her cross-country athletes and desires to see what impact it has had on their Vo_{2max}. Prior to the training program, the coach obtains a baseline measure of Vo_{2max} and then the training program begins. Therefore, the coach would have his or her athletes perform a second Vo_{2max} test to determine if any significant changes occurred in their respective values.

An important addition to the $\dot{V}O_{2max}$ test would be the ability to obtain blood lactate levels during the test. The coach would have his or her athletes run on a treadmill at various speeds where a blood lactate sample would be obtained at each stage of the protocol. Information obtained from the $\dot{V}O_{2max}$ would include: (a) at what $\dot{V}O_2$ did the lactate threshold occur? (b) at what percentage of the $\dot{V}O_{2max}$ did the lactate threshold occur? (c) at what running speed did the lactate threshold occur? and (d) what heart rate (subjects would need a heart rate monitor) was achieved at the lactate threshold? The information provided could assist both the coach and the athlete in tailoring a specific program based upon their $\dot{V}O_{2max}$, indicating at what point and or percentage of the $\dot{V}O_2$ the lactate threshold (LT) occurred and what maximal heart rate was achieved at the LT.

In the recovery from anaerobic work, energy (ATP) is supplied aerobically.

Because it takes time for the oxidative system to begin to produce adequate ATP to support an aerobic activity, all exercise is supported initially by anaerobic metabolism. The initial portion of energy supplied anaerobically is termed the **oxygen deficit**. After exercise, this "shortfall" must be replenished aerobically. This replenishment of the anaerobic system is termed the oxygen debt, or **excess postexercise oxygen consumption (EPOC)**(17). The term EPOC is more accurate than oxygen debt. The term debt implies a direct replacement of the deficit or initial shortfall. EPOC supports a number of metabolic processes that are in effect postexercises. EPOC must support (a) the elevated HR during recovery, (b) elevated respiration rate during recovery, (c) elevated metabolism for heat dissipation, (d) elevated metabolism for the breakdown of hormones released during exercise, (e) the resynthesis of ATP and CP stores, (f) resynthesis of glycogen from lactate, and (g) the resaturation of body tissues (blood and muscle tissue) with oxygen (18,19).

Oxygen consumption, oxygen deficit, and EPOC are depicted for aerobic work in Figure 1.15. Exercise where the oxygen supply is equal to the oxygen demand is termed steady-state exercise. In aerobic exercise, anaerobic metabolism supplies energy for the first few minutes, creating an oxygen deficit. Although part of this deficit can be paid back during the activity, the deficit must be repaid after exercise. Again, the energy for this postexercise metabolic activity comes from aerobic sources. With anaerobic activity, note that the oxygen deficit is much larger because the demand for energy is greater than in the initial stage of aerobic activity.

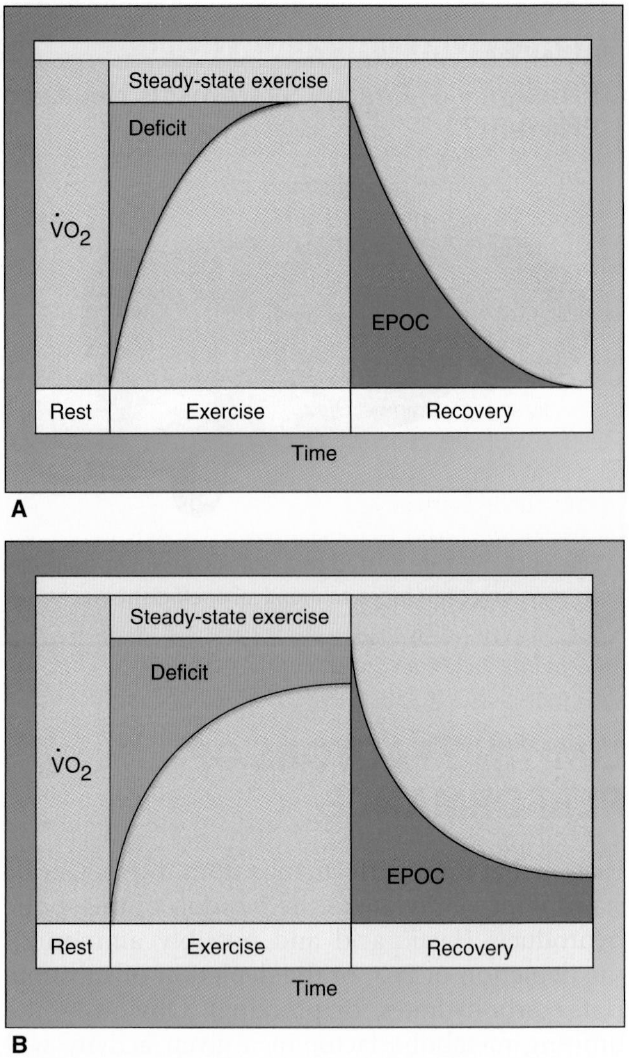

FIGURE 1.15 Oxygen deficit and EPOC for **(A)** aerobic exercise and **(B)** anaerobic exercise.

METABOLIC SPECIFICITY

Specificity of training is a key concept in the field of training and conditioning. If training is to be specific to an actual sport or activity, then the training must focus on the same metabolic energy pathways used in the sport or activity. It is important to note that all energy systems are active to some degree all

BOX 1.4

Examples of Specificity of Training

1. If the average tennis point is 6 seconds, and the average intensity is 60% of maximum, it does not mean that all training should be done for 6 seconds at 60% of maximum intensity. Some points are shorter, and some are longer. Some points are more intense, and some points are less intense. Duration and intensity, then, should be used to determine a reasonable range within which a majority of the training should fall. Progression, from general training to metabolically specific training, is also a factor.
2. Football players predominately perform short bursts of high intensity. The short burst of activity requires the phosphocreatine and anaerobic glycolytic energy systems. Devising a conditioning program that includes sprint/agility activities at 5 to 10 seconds of sustained high-intensity exercise would activate the phosphocreatine system. The anaerobic glycolytic energy system would be activated during the longer sprints (30 seconds to 2 minutes).

of the time. Also, the intensity of the activity is also a key determining factor in the energy system utilized.

Training energy systems involves manipulating both the intensity and the duration of the activity. Metabolic specificity does not mean that *all* training is exactly the same intensity and duration as the activity. Most activities are difficult to classify exactly in terms of intensity and duration. A basic understanding of metabolism and bioenergetics is a key to understanding the field of conditioning and applying that knowledge to improve human performance.

Summary

The concepts of bioenergetics are keys to understanding human performance as well as the exercise prescriptions that will enhance performance. The source of energy for a specific sport or activity depends on the intensity and the duration of the activity, among other factors. Bioenergetics is a complex process breaking down food and changing it to the energy we need to move. Since human adaptations to training are specific to the type of training, we must learn to train athletes in such a way that the appropriate energy systems are stressed specific to the demands of the sport or activity.

Maxing Out

1. Energy system training is sport specific and may be specific to positions within a sport. Consider a soccer player. What are some things you need to consider when planning a metabolically specific training program for a soccer player? How would the program of a goalie differ from that of a midfielder?
2. What happens to the excess carbohydrate we consume in our diet when muscle glycogen stores are full?
3. What is the fate of lactic acid produced during exercise?

REFERENCES

1. Brooks GA, Fahey TD, Baldwin K. *Exercise Physiology: Human Bioenergetics and Its Applications*. Boston, MA: McGraw Hill; 2005.
2. Spriet LL, Howlett RA, Heigenhauser GJF. An enzymatic approach to lactate production in human skeletal muscle during exercise. *Med Sci Sports Exerc*. 2000;32(4):756–763.
3. Harris RC, Edwards RHT, Hultman E, et al. The time course of phosphocreatine resynthesis during recovery of the quadriceps muscle in man. *Pfluegers Arch*. 1976;97:392–397.
4. Brooks GA. Amino acid and protein metabolism during exercise and recovery. *Med Sci Sports Exerc*. 1987;19:S150–S156.
5. Smith SA, Montain SJ, Matott RP, et al. Creatine supplementation and age influence muscle metabolism during exercise. *J Appl Physiol*. 1998;85:1349–1356.
6. Costill D, Thompson H, Roberts E. Fractional utilization of the aerobic capacity during distance running. *Med Sci Sports*. 1973;5:248–252.
7. Brooks GA. The lactate shuttle during exercise and recovery. *Med Sci Sports Exerc*. 1986;18:360–368.
8. Brooks G. Intra- and extra cellular lactate shuttles. *Med Sci Sports Exerc*. 2000;32(4):790–799.
9. Brooks GA. Lactate shuttles in nature. *Biochem Soc Trans*. 2002;30(2):258–264.
10. Bassett DR Jr, Howley ET. Limiting factors for maximum oxygen upatke and determinants of endurance performance. *Med Sci Sports Exerc*. 2000;32(1):70–84.
11. Farrell P, Wilmore J, Coyle EF, et al. Plasma lactate accumulation and distance running performance. *Med Sci Sports*. 1979;11:338–344.
12. Foster C. Blood lactate and respiratory measurement of the capacity for sustained exercise. In: Maud P, Foster C, eds. *Physiological Assessment of Human Fitness*. Champaign, IL: Human Kinetics; 1995.
13. Lafontaine T, Londeree B, Spath W. The maximal steady state versus selected running events. *Med Sci Sports Exerc*. 1981;13:190–192.
14. Lawler J, Powers S, Dodd S. A time saving incremental cycle ergometer protocol to determine peak oxygen consumption. *Br J Sports Med*. 1987;21:171–173.
15. Lehmann M, Burg A, Kapp R, et al. Correlations between laboratory testing and distance running performance

in marathoners of similar ability. *Int J Sports Med.* 1983;4:226–230.
16. Hermansen L. Effect of metabolic changes on force generation in skeletal muscle during maximal exercise. In: Porter R, Whelan J, eds. *Human Muscle Fatigue*. London, UK: Pitman Medical; 1981.
17. Gaesser GA, Brooks GA. Metabolic bases of excess post oxygen consumption. *Med Sci Sports Exerc.* 1984;10(1):29–43.
18. Borsheim E, Bahr R. The effect of exercise intensity, duration, and mode on excess post oxygen consumption. *Sports Med.* 2003;33(14):1037–1060.
19. Mole PA. Exercise metabolism. In: Bove AA, Lowenthal DT, eds. *Exercise Medicine: Physiological Principles and Clinical Application*. New York: Academic Press; 1983:43–88.

CHAPTER 2

The Cardiorespiratory System

JAY R. HOFFMAN ● JOE ROGOWSKI

OBJECTIVES

After completing this chapter, you will be able to:

- Assess and analyze blood pressure readings.
- Understand the P-QRS-T Complex.
- Explain the changes in cardiac output during exercise.
- Discuss the redirection of blood flow in response to exercise.
- Explain the effects of the environment on the cardiorespiratory system.

KEY TERMS

Assist
Bohr Effect
Bradycardia
Cardiac Cycle
Cardiac Output
Cardiovascular Drift
Chronotropy
Concentric Hypertrophy
Depolarization
Diastasis
Diastole
Diastolic Blood Pressures
Eccentric Hypertrophy
Ejection Fraction
Ejection Phase
End-Diastolic Volume
End-Systolic Volume
Erythropoietin
Expiration
Ficks Equation
Frank-Starling Mechanism
Hypertrophic Cardiomyopathy
Hyperventilation
Hypervolemia
Hypohydration
Hypoxia
Inspiration
Intercalated Discs
Interventricular Septum
Intropy
Myocardium
Partial Pressure
P-QRS-T Complex
Repolarization
Stroke Volume
Systole
Systolic Blood Pressure
Trachycardia
Valsalva Maneuver
Ventilation
Ventilatory Equivalent

Introduction

The primary role of the cardiorespiratory system is to meet the energy demands of the body. As energy demands increase, as might be expected during exercise, the cardiorespiratory system is able to compensate by increasing the amount of oxygen that is consumed and the volume of blood that can be pumped into the circulation. During prolonged exercise training, physiological systems are able to adapt to the increased demands that are placed upon it. These adaptations are specific to the type of exercise stimulus that is presented. This chapter reviews the cardiovascular and respiratory system, as well as the changes that are seen during acute exercise and adaptations that are seen during prolonged training. In addition, environmental factors that affect cardiorespiratory function are also discussed.

CARDIOVASCULAR SYSTEM

The cardiovascular system consists of an elaborate network of vessels that comprise the circulatory system and a powerful pump (the heart) that is responsible for providing for the delivery of oxygen and nutrients to active organs and muscles and in removing waste products of metabolism. The heart is a four-chambered muscular organ that is located in the midcenter of the chest cavity. Its anterior border is the sternum, while posteriorly it borders the vertebral column. The lungs are situated on the heart's lateral borders, and inferior to the heart is the diaphragm.

MORPHOLOGY OF THE HEART

The heart muscle, referred to as the **myocardium**, is similar in appearance to striated skeletal muscle. However, the fibers of the myocardium are multinucleated and interconnected end to end by **intercalated discs**. These discs contain desmosomes that maintain the integrity of the cardiac fibers during contraction and gap junctions that allow for a rapid transmission of the electrical impulse that signals for contraction. The structure of the myocardium can be thought of as three separate areas: atrial, ventricular, and conductive. The atrial and ventricular myocardium function quite similarly as skeletal muscle, in that they will contract in response to electrical stimuli. However, in contrast to skeletal muscle fibers, an electrical stimulus of only a single cell in either chamber will result in an action potential being rapidly spread to the other cells of the atrial and ventricular myocardium resulting in a coordinated contractile mechanism. In addition, the cardiac fibers in each of these areas can function separately. The conductive tissue that is found between these chambers provides a network for the rapid transmission of conductive impulses allowing for coordinated action of both the atrial and the ventricular chambers.

The structural detail of the heart can be seen in Figure 2.1. There is a striking difference in the anatomy and physiology of the right and left sides of the heart that relate to their specific functions. The right side of the heart receives blood from all parts of the body (right atria), while the right ventricle pumps deoxygenated blood to the lungs through the pulmonary circulation. The left side of the heart receives oxygenated blood from the lungs (left atria) and pumps this blood from the left ventricle into the aorta and through the entire systemic circulation. The left ventricle is an ellipsoidal chamber surrounded by thick musculature that provides the power to eject the blood through the entire body. The right ventricle, however, is crescent shaped with thin musculature reflecting the reduced ejection pressures seen in this ventricle (25 mm Hg) compared to approximately 125 mm Hg in the left ventricle at rest. A thick solid muscular wall or **interventricular septum** separates the left and right ventricles.

Blood flow from the right atria to right ventricle goes through the tricuspid valve (consisting of three cusps or leaflets that allow only a one-directional flow of blood). The bicuspid or mitral valve allows blood flow between the left atria and the left ventricle. The semilunar valves located on the arterial walls on the outside of the ventricles prevent

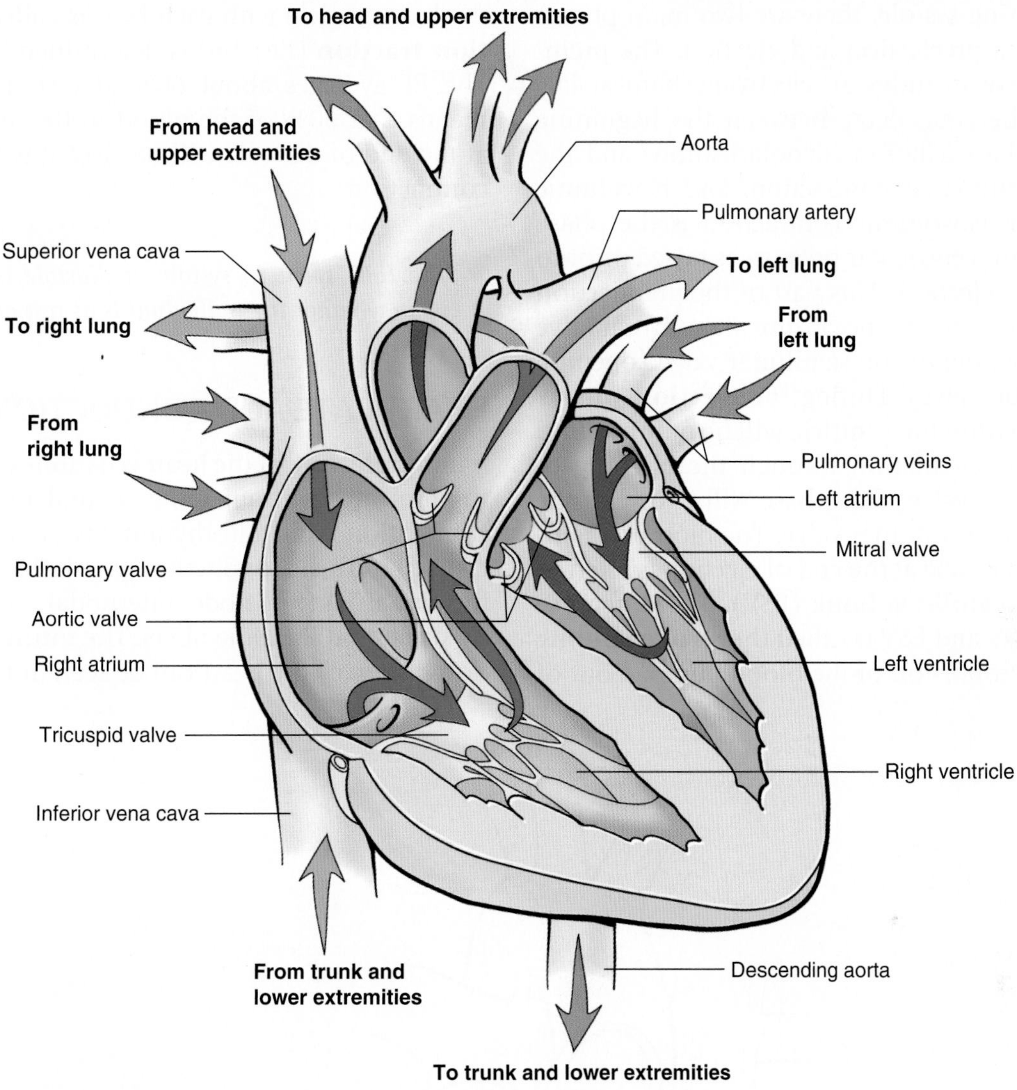

FIGURE 2.1 Anatomy of the heart.

blood from flowing back into the heart between contractions. During systole, the cusps lie against their arterial wall attachments; however, during diastole or retrograde flow, the cusps fall passively inward, sealing the lumen.

CARDIAC CYCLE

The contraction phase in which the atria or ventricles expel the blood in their chambers is called **systole**. The relaxation phase in which these chambers refill with blood is referred to as **diastole**. One complete revolution of systole and diastole is referred to as a **cardiac cycle**. At rest, the heart spends most of its time (~60%) filling with blood (diastole) and less time (~40%) expelling the blood (systole). However, during exercise, this situation is reversed, with most of the cardiac cycle spent in systole. During systole, the tricuspid and mitral valves are closed. However, blood flow from pulmonic and systemic circulation continues into the atria. As systole ends, the atrioventricular (AV) valves rapidly open and the blood that has accumulated in the atria flows quickly into the ventricles accounting for 70% to 80% of the ventricular filling. There are three specific periods occurring diastole. The initial third is one of rapid filling; the middle third is characterized by very little blood flow into the ventricle and is referred to as **diastasis**; and during the final third, ventricle filling is completed with an additional 20% to 30% of blood pumped into the ventricle as the result of atrial systole.

The volume of blood in the ventricle at the end of diastole is called the **end-diastolic volume**

(EDV). During systole, there are two main phases that occur: a preejection and ejection. The preinjection phase includes an electromechanical lag, which is the time delay between the beginning of ventricular excitation (depolarization) and the onset of ventricular contraction, and isovolumic contraction. Isovolumic contraction is the phase in which intraventricular pressure is raised prior to the onset of ejection. This part of the preinjection phase occurs between the closure of the mitral valve and the opening of the semilunar valve (opening of the aortic valve). During the **ejection phase**, the blood within the ventricle will be pumped into the systemic circulation through the opening of the semilunar valve. This phase will end with the closing of the semilunar valve. The blood remaining in the ventricle at the end of ejection is referred to as **end-systolic volume** (ESV). The difference between EDV and ESV is called the **stroke volume** (SV). The proportion of the blood pumped out of the left ventricle with each beat is called the **ejection fraction** (EF) and is determined by SV/EDV. The EF averages about 60% at rest. This simply means that 60% of the blood in the left ventricle at the end of diastole will be ejected with the next contraction.

The time spent in systole or diastole is dependent upon whether the individual is at rest or exercising.

HEART RATE AND CONDUCTION

A unique feature of the heart is its ability to contract rhythmically without either neural or hormonal stimulation. This autorhythmicity is due to a specialized intrinsic conduction system that consists of the sinoatrial (SA) node, internodal pathways, the AV node, and Purkinje fibers. The intrinsic conduction system of the heart can be seen in Figure 2.2.

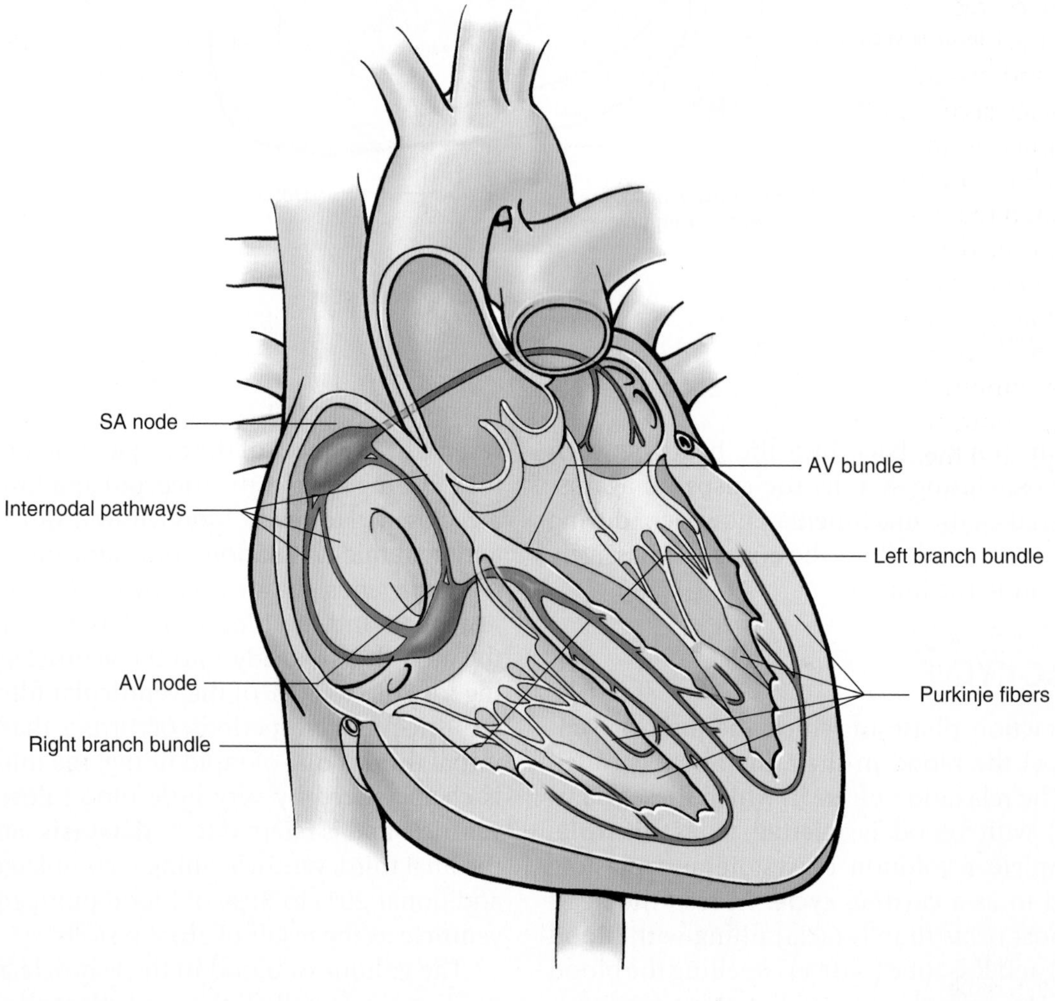

FIGURE 2.2 Intrinsic conduction system of the heart.

The SA node is located in the right atrium and is a collection of specialized cells that are capable of generating an electrical impulse. Because of this distinctive ability, it is appropriately nicknamed the pacemaker of the heart. Once an impulse leaves the SA node, it propagates leftward and downward spreading through the atria syncytium of first the right and then the left atria through internodal pathways merging onto the AV node located toward the center of the heart on the lower right atrial wall.

The AV node, or the AV junction (composed of the AV node and the Bundle of His), delays transmission of the impulse for a 10th of a second. This slight delay of ventricular excitation and contraction will allow for the atria to contract and also permit a limitation in the number of signals that are transmitted by the AV node. This appears to serve as a protective mechanism for the ventricles from atrial tachyarrhythmias. The Bundle of His is found distally in the AV junction and divides into a right and left segments (bundle branches), which transmit the electrical impulses to the right and left ventricles, respectively. The Purkinje fibers are found on the distal tips of the right and left bundle branches and extend their fibers into the walls of the ventricles accelerating the conduction velocity of the impulse to the rest of the ventricle. The conduction velocity of the Purkinje fibers may increase fourfold than that seen at the Bundle of His.

As mentioned earlier, the SA node, AV node, and Purkinje fibers have the inherent ability for spontaneous initiation of the electrical impulse. However, the autonomic nervous system can also influence the rate of impulse formation (referred to as **chronotropy**), contractile state of the myocardium (**inotropy**), and the rate of spread of the excitation impulse. The sympathetic and parasympathetic nervous systems, as well as certain hormones, can influence cardiac contractility. The atria are well supplied with both sympathetic and parasympathetic neurons, while the ventricles are primarily innervated by sympathetic neurons. Sympathetic stimulation releases the catecholamines epinephrine and norepinephrine from sympathetic neural fibers. These neural hormones accelerate heart rate by increasing SA node activity and increase both atrial and ventricular contractile force. Increases in heart rate are termed **tachycardia**.

Parasympathetic stimulation through the vagus nerves releases the neurohormone acetylcholine, which has a depressant effect on SA node activity and decreasing atrial contractile force. Decreases in heart rate are termed **bradycardia**. Sympathetic stimulation may increase heart rate by over 120 bpm and strength of contraction by 100%, while maximal vagal stimulation may decrease heart rate by 20 to 30 bpm and lower strength of contraction by approximately 30% (1).

THE ELECTROCARDIOGRAM

The **P-QRS-T complex** is the typical pattern that is associated with electrocardiogram (ECG) interpretation (Fig. 2.3). Einthoven, a Dutch physician and scientist who was credited with the invention of the ECG in the early part of the 20th century, wanted to be mathematically correct with his description of ECG wave patterns. It is said that he admired the work of Descartes, the inventor of analytical geometry. Descartes labeled successive points on a curve starting with the letter "P". Therefore, Einthoven thought the letter "P" would be an appropriate means of labeling the first wave on an ECG (2).

It is through the ECG that we are able to detect abnormalities of the electrical activity of the heart. The basic principles of this pattern are addressed

Q & A from the Field

Q *My resting heart rate is about 45 beats per minute (bpm). I am a distance runner. Is that too low?*

A A low resting heart rate can be an indication of cardiac problems. In the case of a healthy athlete, the answer is probably not. Regular participation in aerobic exercise often results in a decreased resting heart rate, approximately 5 to 25 bpm. This is due to both the increased efficiency of the heart and the adaptations to the nervous system that affect heart rate. There appears to be a smaller reduction in heart rate from resistance training. The effects of resistance training on heart rate appear to be related to the volume and intensity of training.

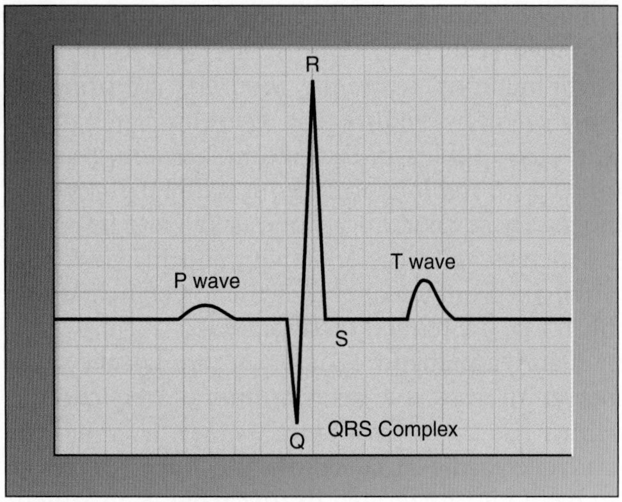

FIGURE 2.3 Normal ECG.

in this section. In addition, the differential diagnosis of the athletic heart is briefly examined. Since a normal ECG is based on a nonathletic population, there is much confusion in regard to the athletic heart because of the similarities it has to an abnormal ECG. Unfortunately, this is an area that is often misunderstood due to the lack of research currently available to the medical community.

The ECG is composed of 12 electrode leads that are placed on specific sites of the body (Fig. 2.4). The sites of these leads are typically the arms, legs, and chest. The stimulation of the heart is recorded by these electrodes and the electrical signal that is recorded is presented by wave patterns (P-QRS-T complex). We have all seen a heart rate belt that picks up one's training pulse. This is just one chest lead that gives one number (bpm). With the 12-lead ECG, you have many more leads that provide more data regarding the electrical activity of the heart. It transfers the information into this P-QRS-T wave complex, which provides an indication of the normal or abnormal functioning of the heart.

Stimulation of cardiac tissue is a continuous sequence of a process referred to as **depolarization** and **repolarization**. The contraction of the atria and ventricles occurs when the cardiac cells are depolarized. As it was previously mentioned, this corresponds with the atria and ventricles pumping blood. The relaxation phase, allowing the cardiac cells to return back to normal resting state, is the repolarization. In the ECG, this is represented with the depolarization of the atria (P wave) followed by the depolarization of the ventricles (QRS complex) and then a return to resting state or repolarization (ST, T, and U waves).

The P Wave

The P wave is the depolarization of the atria beginning with the SA node and spreading from the right atria to the left atria. Some abnormal P wave ECG readings include

- Prolonged P wave
  - Enlarged atria
- Absent or retrograde P wave
- Retrograde meaning the pacemaker of the heart is starting at the AV junction and the initiation of the heart beat is flowing backward (retrograde)
- Increased or decreased amplitude of P wave
  - Indicative of hypokalemia or hyperkalemia

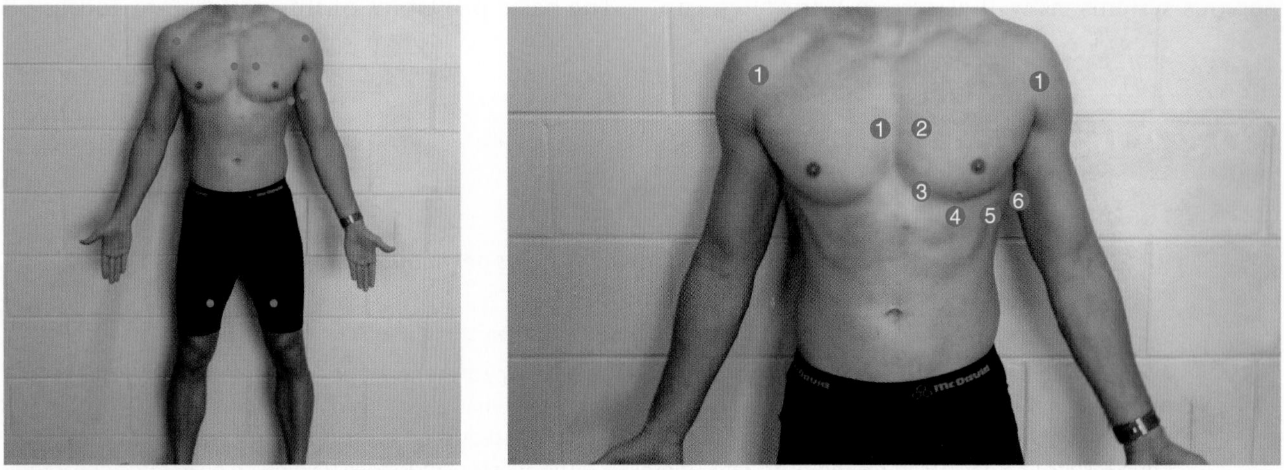

FIGURE 2.4 ECG electrode placement.

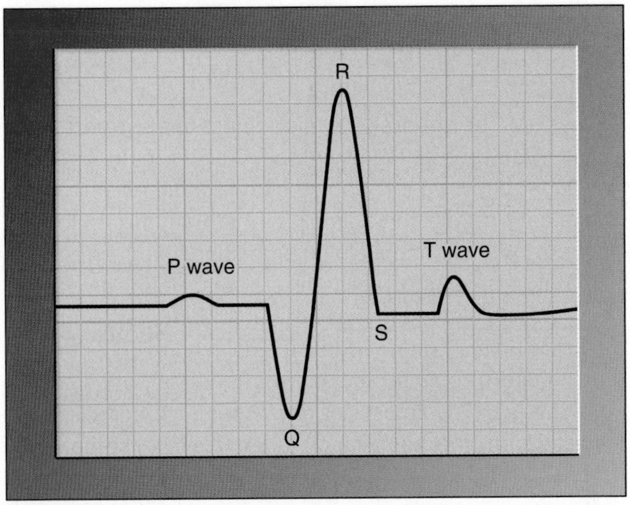

FIGURE 2.5 Wide QRS complex. Because of the fast depolarization/stimulation of the ventricles, the QRS complex is typically narrow. When there is an abnormality like a ventricular bundle branch block, the QRS complex is wide, representing a delayed ventricular response.

Hypokalemia can be an issue in athletics as a result of poor potassium intake, excessive perspiration, or gastrointestinal issues resulting in diarrhea. Some of the other signs and symptoms of this condition are muscle cramping and extreme fatigue.

QRS Complex

The QRS complex represents the depolarization of the ventricles, where the blood is being ejected from the heart. Even though it appears to be complex, the QRS represents this single event. The direction of the electrical impulse will indicate whether the deflection will be positive or negative. The first negative deflection is the Q wave. The first positive deflection is the R wave and the following negative deflection is the S wave. Some abnormal QRS wave readings:

- Conduction delay resulting in wide QRS complex (Fig. 2.5)
  - Bundle branch block
  - Electrolyte disturbance
  - Ischemia
- Decreased amplitude of complex
  - Chronic lung disease
  - Obesity
- Increased amplitude of R waves (Fig. 2.6)
  - Ventricular hypertrophy (athletic heart) or hypertrophic cardiomyopathy (HCM)
- Abnormal Q waves
  - Myocardial infarction

Because of the fast response of the Purkinje fibers in the ventricles, the QRS complex depolarizes quickly. For this reason, we see (delays) in the QRS complex conduction (delays) resulting in an abnormal ECG. In the case of left and right ventricular hypertrophy, it is important to be aware that thin, young, and athletic individuals will demonstrate tall voltage in the R waves of the chest leads. It is difficult sometimes to differentiate between someone who is a well-conditioned athlete versus someone who has ventricular hypertrophy. It is usually recommended that the individual in question receives further testing in the form of an echocardiogram to make the differential diagnosis. Even then, it may still be difficult to diagnose.

T Wave

After the depolarization of ventricles and the resulting QRS complex, the T wave represents the

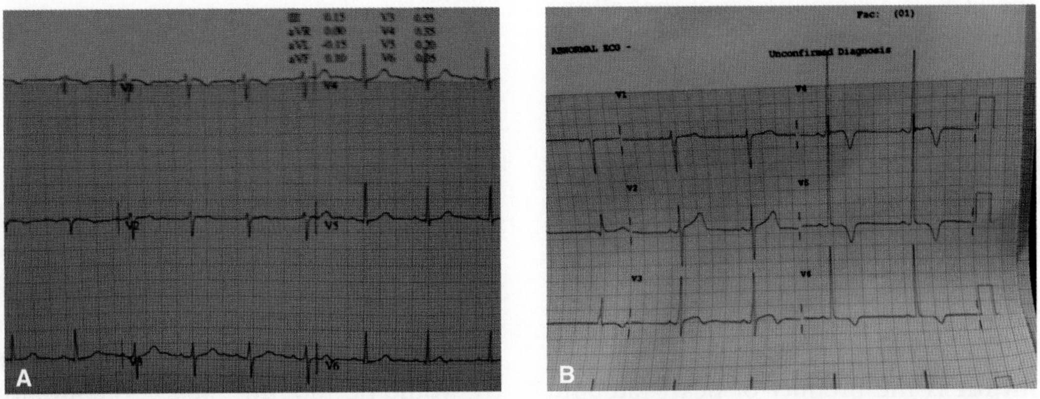

FIGURE 2.6 Increased amplitude of R wave. **A.** This shows the normal ECG of a professional basketball player. **B.** This shows an abnormal ECG strip of a professional basketball player. Note the very tall R waves in V4, V5, and V6. Also, a significantly inverted T wave can be seen, which can be indicative of hypertrophic obstructive cardiomyopathy.

beginning of ventricular repolarization. T waves are normally asymmetrical in shape with the asymmetry occurring toward the end of the wave in the form of a peak (Fig. 2.7A). A symmetrical T wave may be indicative of a myocardial infarction. Many times, the S wave and T wave are looked at collectively. This is referred to as the ST segment. In addition, the Q wave and T wave are also sometimes grouped to provide the QT interval. Some T wave abnormal ECG findings include

- T wave inversion
  - Myocardial ischemia
  - Myocarditis
  - Young patient
  - Arrhythmogenic right ventricular dysplasia (ARVD)
- Tall T wave
  - Acute myocardial ischemia "tombstones"
- ST-segment depression
  - Right and left ventricular hypertrophy
  - Non–Q wave MI
  - Subendocardial ischemia
- ST-segment elevation
  - Pericarditis
- Conduction delay of the QT interval (Fig. 2.7B)
  - Long QT syndrome

It is noteworthy to realize that many abnormalities are not limited to one lead or one ECG wave. More often than not, several leads and ECG waves are affected. For example, someone with HCM might present a tall R wave in the QRS complex and an inverted T wave, which are present in all lateral chest leads. Additionally, someone who is unhealthy may be suffering from several different cardiac issues making diagnosis more complicated. However, the ECG is a simplified tool that allows the practitioner a quick glimpse into the function of the heart as seen in the P-QRS-T complex.

The ability to interpret the P-QRS-T complex may assist in the detection of abnormalities in cardiac cycle.

CARDIAC OUTPUT

Cardiac output is the product of heart rate and SV. It refers to the amount of blood pumped by the heart in 1 minute. Cardiac output responds to the energy demands of the body. In the average adult male (regardless of training status), the total volume of blood pumped out of the left ventricle per minute at rest is approximately 5 L. If an individual's resting heart rate is 70 bpm, SV would need to be approximately 71 mL · beat^{-1}. In the endurance athlete, heart rate is generally much lower at rest due to a greater vagal tone and reduced sympathetic drive. If the heart rate of this athlete was 50 bpm, SV would be 100 mL · beat^{-1}. A comparison of the cardiac output in trained and sedentary males can be seen in Table 2.1. The mechanism that drives

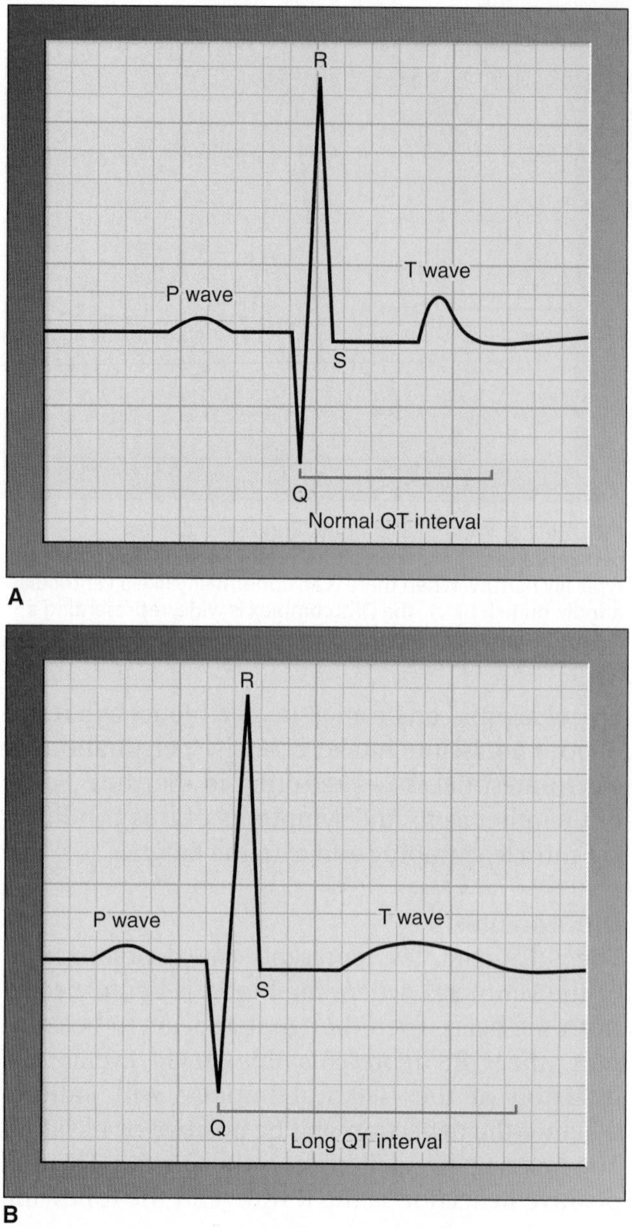

FIGURE 2.7 A. Normal T wave. **B.** Conduction delay of QT interval.

TABLE 2.1 ● CARDIAC OUTPUT AT REST IN SEDENTARY AND ENDURANCE-TRAINED MEN

	CARDIAC OUTPUT = (L)	HEART RATE × (BEATS · min^{-1})	STROKE VOLUME (mL)
Sedentary	5	70	71
Trained	5	50	100

this particular adaptation is not entirely clear but is likely related to the increased vagal tone seen consequent to endurance training and to morphological adaptations of the heart.

VASCULATURE

The vascular system is composed of a series of vessels that carry oxygenated blood away from the heart (arterial system) to the tissues and return deoxygenated blood from the tissues back to the heart (venous system). The heart has its own coronary vascular system that is responsible for supplying the myocardium with oxygen and nutrients. The arterial system receives the blood from the left ventricle of the heart and distributes it throughout the body. Blood is first ejected from the left ventricle into a thick, elastic vessel called the aorta. From the aorta, the blood is then circulated throughout the body via a network of arteries, arterioles (small arterial branches), metarterioles (smaller branches), and capillaries. The walls of the arteries are both strong and thick to withstand the rapid transport of blood under high pressure to the tissues. The thickness of these vesicles prevents any gaseous exchange from occurring between them and the surrounding tissues. In addition, the arterial vasculature system is innervated by the sympathetic nervous system, allowing it to be effectively stimulated for regulating blood flow. As blood reaches the tissues, it becomes diverted to smaller branches of the arterial system. At the end of the metarterioles (the smallest arterial vessel) are the microscopic capillaries. The capillaries are approximately 0.01 mm in diameter and consist of a single layer of endothelial cells. Because of this small diameter, the rate of blood flow decreases as the blood circulates toward and into the capillaries. In addition, there is an extensive branching of the capillary microcirculation creating a large surface area between the capillary vasculature–surrounding tissues. The combination of a large surface area, slow rate of blood flow, and a thin layer of endothelial cells make the capillaries an ideal place for gas exchange between the blood and the tissues.

As the blood leaves the capillaries, it enters the venous circulation. Similarly to the arterial system, the venous system is composed of vessels of various sizes that get larger as they get closer to the heart. Deoxygenated blood leaving the capillaries enters venules (small veins) that increase the rate of blood flow (due to the smaller cross-sectional area of the venous system in comparison to the capillary system). The blood is transported back to the heart via the superior vena cava (venous blood returning from areas above the heart) and the inferior vena cava (venous blood returning from areas below the heart). The deoxygenated blood then enters the right atrium, goes through to the right ventricle, and is pumped to the lung to be reoxygenated and subsequently transported back into the left side of the heart to be circulated through the arterial circulation.

During rest, blood flow is controlled by the autonomic nervous system and is primarily distributed to the liver, kidneys, and brain. However, during exercise, there is a redistribution of blood flow to the exercising muscles. The muscles may receive 75% or more of the available blood at the expense of the other organs. In combination with a greater cardiac output, the exercising muscles may receive up to a 25-fold increase in blood flow. The flow of blood to the muscles and organs at rest and during exercise can be seen in Figure 2.8.

During exercise, blood flow will be diverted from organs to exercising muscles.

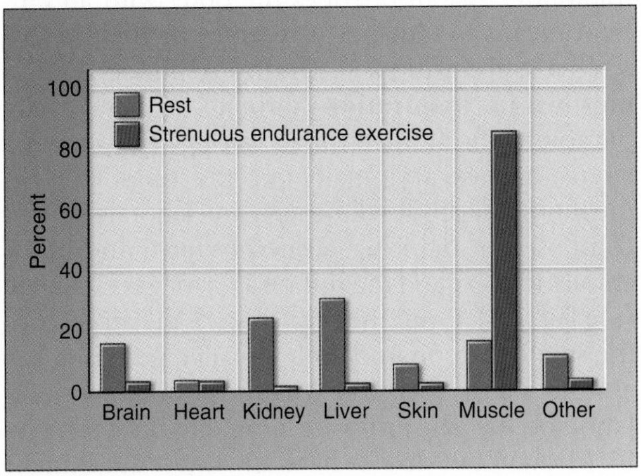

FIGURE 2.8 Distribution of cardiac output.

BLOOD PRESSURE

During each contraction, blood is pumped into the aorta from the left ventricle (systole). The pressure within the aorta under normal resting conditions reaches approximately 120 mm Hg. This measurement is referred to as the **systolic blood pressure** and represents the strain against the arterial walls during ventricular contraction. Since the pumping action or contraction of the left ventricle of the heart is pulsatile in nature, the arterial pressure will fluctuate from an elevated level during systole to a lower level during the heart's relaxation phase known as diastole. **Diastolic blood pressures** are approximately 80 mm Hg at rest and provide an indication of the peripheral resistance, or ease at which blood flows into the capillaries. As blood flows through the systemic circulation, pressure will continue to fall and reach approximately 0 mm Hg as it reaches the right atrium. The decrease in arterial pressure during each segment of the systemic circulation is directly proportional to the vascular resistance in that segment. Changes in the resistance of the systemic circulation are quite important in the regulation of blood flow.

Blood pressure may reach unsafe levels during exercise. It is important to understand both normal and abnormal changes in blood pressure as related to various types of exercises.

RESPIRATORY SYSTEM

The coordination between the cardiovascular and respiratory system provides the body with an efficient means to transport oxygen to the tissues and remove carbon dioxide. During respiration, air is breathed in (**inspiration**) through the nasal cavity or mouth. The air then travels through the pharynx, larynx, trachea, and finally into the lungs. Once in the lungs, the air flows through an elaborate system composed of branches termed bronchi and bronchioles that expand the surface area for gas exchange (see Fig. 2.9). From the bronchioles, the air reaches the smallest respiratory unit, the alveoli. It is at the alveoli that gas exchange with the pulmonary circulation occurs. The lungs are located in the chest cavity (thorax) but do not have any direct attachment to the ribs or any other bony structure. Instead, they are suspended by pleural sacs that connect to both the lungs and the thoracic cavity. Between the pleural sacs and the lungs, a fluid is present to prevent friction from occurring during respiration.

During inspiration, the muscles of the thoracic cavity (diaphragm and external intercostal muscles) contract causing the thorax to expand. As a result, the lungs stretch and initiate a reduction in air pressure within the lungs. As pressure within lungs is reduced to levels below that seen on the outside, the pressure gradient will cause air to rush inside the lungs. During exercise, additional muscles (i.e., pectoralis, sternocleidomastoid) can be recruited causing a greater movement of the thorax creating an even larger lung expansion.

When air is breathed out (**expiration**), the inspiratory muscles relax, or during forced expiration, contraction of the internal intercostal and abdominal muscles will cause the thorax to return to its normal position. As a result, the pressure within the lungs expands to levels above that seen outside, causing expiration to occur.

Change in pressure is the primary mechanism in which air and gases flow into and out of the lungs and through the entire respiratory and circulatory systems. For **ventilation** to occur (process of inspiration and expiration), only slight changes in pressure between the lungs and the outside environment need to occur. For instance, standard atmospheric pressure is 760 mm Hg, and only slight changes in intrapulmonary pressure (pressure within the lungs) are needed to cause air to be inhaled. During ascent to altitude, this process is not as simple and will be explained in much greater detail later.

PRESSURE DIFFERENTIALS IN GASES

In addition to changes in pressure that causes inspiration and expiration, pressure differentials in the gases that comprise the air we breathe will be the primary impetus causing oxygen and carbon dioxide exchange. The air we breathe is composed of a mixture of gases. Each gas will exert a pressure in proportion to its concentration in the gas mixture, known as its **partial pressure**. The air that we breathe is composed of 79.04% nitrogen, 20.93% oxygen, and 0.03% carbon dioxide. At sea level, in which atmospheric pressure is 760 mm Hg, the partial pressure of oxygen is 159.1 mm Hg (20.93% and 760 mm Hg) and carbon dioxide is 0.2 mm Hg (0.03% × 760 mm Hg).

As the air reaches the alveoli, the partial pressures of the gases in the alveoli and the partial

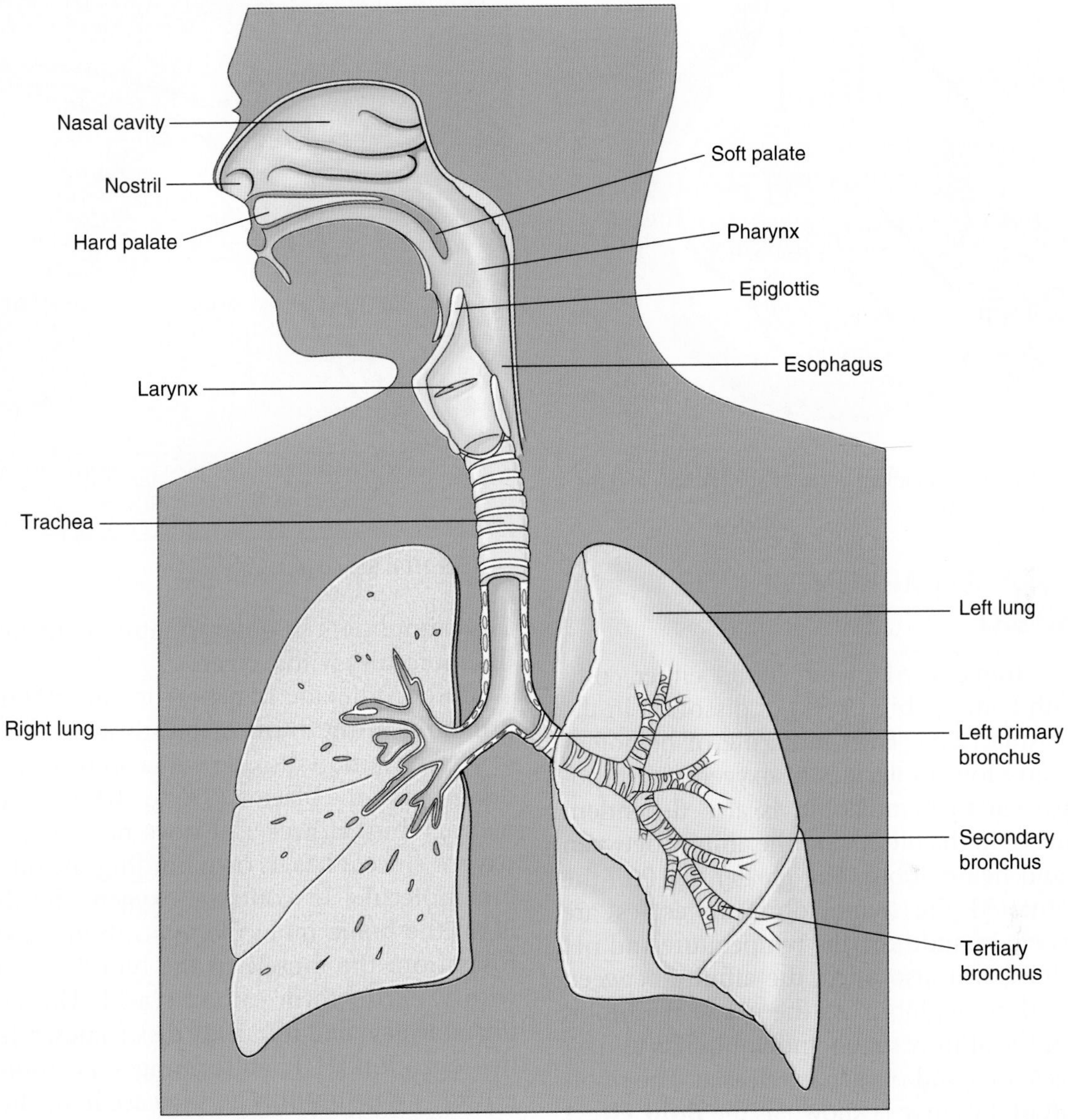

FIGURE 2.9 Anatomy of the respiratory system.

pressures of the gases in the blood create a pressure gradient (see Fig. 2.10). This is the basis of gas exchange. If the partial pressures of the gases on either side of the membrane were equal, no gas exchange would occur. The greater the pressure gradient, the faster the gases will diffuse across the membrane. As inspired air moves into the alveoli, the partial pressure of oxygen (Po_2) is between 100 and 105 mm Hg (this is due to mixing of air within the alveoli). At the pulmonary capillary, blood has been stripped of most of its oxygen by the tissues. Typically, the Po_2 at the pulmonary capillary level is between 40 and 45 mm Hg. As a result, the pressure gradient favors oxygen going from the alveoli to the capillary. In addition, the pressure gradient of carbon dioxide favors exchange from the capillary to the alveoli where it can be exhaled from the body during expiration. The pressure gradient for carbon dioxide is not as great at the capillary–alveoli membrane as it is for oxygen. Nevertheless, carbon dioxide diffuses quite easily across the membrane, despite the low pressure gradient, due to greater membrane solubility than oxygen.

Gas exchange occurring at the capillary and alveoli and between the capillary and the tissue is the result of pressure differentials that cause oxygen or carbon dioxide to diffuse from an area of high concentration to one of low concentration.

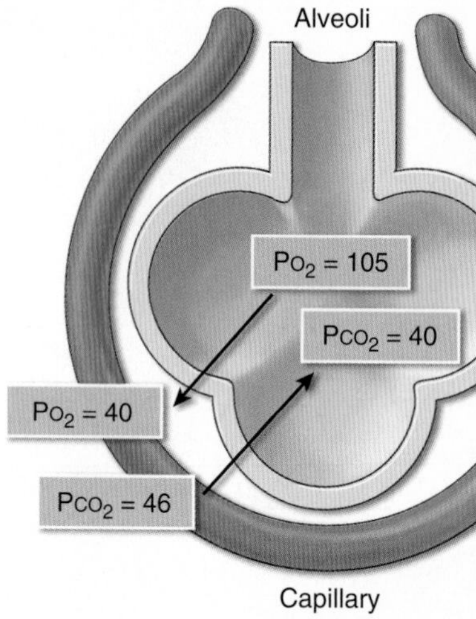

FIGURE 2.10 Pressure gradient between the capillary and the alveoli within the lungs.

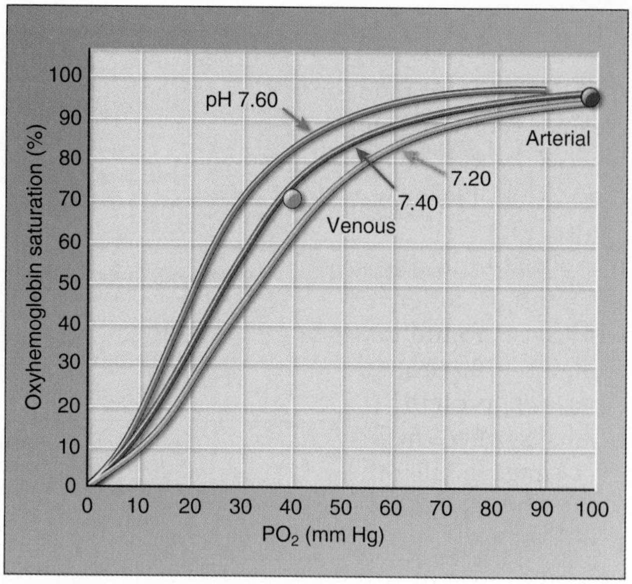

FIGURE 2.11 Bohr effect.

OXYGEN AND CARBON DIOXIDE TRANSPORT

Oxygen is transported in the blood either combined with hemoglobin (98%) or dissolved in the blood plasma (2%). Each molecule of hemoglobin can carry four molecules of oxygen. The binding of oxygen to hemoglobin is also dependent upon the Po_2 in the blood and the affinity between oxygen and hemoglobin. The greater the Po_2, the more saturated the hemoglobin molecules are with oxygen. In addition, the temperature and pH of the blood will also affect the affinity between oxygen and hemoglobin. As the pH of the blood decreases, the affinity that hemoglobin has to oxygen is decreased and oxygen is released. The rightward shift of the curve is known as the **Bohr effect** (see Fig. 2.11) and is important during exercise when a greater amount of oxygen is needed in the active musculature. On the other hand, when the pH is high, as it would be in the lungs, there is a greater affinity between oxygen and hemoglobin; this is important in order to saturate the hemoglobin molecules with oxygen.

Carbon dioxide transport in the blood occurs primarily in the form of bicarbonate ion (~60% to 70%). Carbon dioxide will also be transported, dissolved in the plasma (7% to 10%), or bound to hemoglobin. However, it does not compete with oxygen since it has its own binding site on the globin molecule. In contrast, oxygen's binding site is on the heme molecule. As carbon dioxide diffuses from the muscle to the blood, it combines with water to form carbonic acid. This is a very unstable acid and it quickly dissociates, releasing a hydrogen ion (H^+) and forming a bicarbonate ion (HCO_3^-). The result is an increase in acidity, causing hemoglobin to lose its affinity for oxygen and increases oxygen's rate of diffusion into the tissues.

Gas exchange is affected by changes in pH and temperature.

REAL-WORLD APPLICATION

Increasing Maximal Oxygen Consumption

Athletes of many sports aim to increase their level of maximal oxygen consumption. In the past, coaches have instructed their athletes to perform long slow distance (LSD) training with the goal of increasing Vo_{2max}. However, in recent years, it has been observed that interval training results in Vo_2 increases similar to, or even greater than, traditional LSD training. Therefore, it may be beneficial to incorporate interval training into a conditioning program for athletes whose sports rely on the adenosine triphosphate/creatine phosphate and glycolytic systems, yet participate in competition for prolonged periods of time.

BLOOD

Blood is a viscous fluid that is composed of cells and plasma. More than 99% of the cells in the blood are red blood cells, the remainder being white blood cells. Plasma is part of the extracellular fluid of the body. It is quite similar in composition to interstitial fluid that is found between tissue cells. The primary difference being the amount of protein that is found between the two fluids (plasma contains ~7% protein, while interstitial fluid contains ~2% protein). The percent of the blood that is cells is called the hematocrit. The hematocrit for the average man is approximately 42, while that for the average woman is approximately 38. In other words, 42% of the blood is composed of cells in men and 38% in women. The remaining component is plasma.

CARDIOVASCULAR RESPONSE TO ACUTE EXERCISE

Oxygen consumption ($\dot{V}O_2$) is elevated during acute exercise to meet the higher energy needs of the exercising muscle. As exercise intensity increases, a greater demand for energy is met by an increase in the cardiac output and/or by a greater oxygen extraction from the vasculature (a greater a-$\bar{v}O_2$ difference). During the early stages of exercise, increases in both heart rate and SV occur quite rapidly to bring about elevations in cardiac output. Figure 2.12 demonstrates the effects of varying intensities of exercise on heart rate, SV, and cardiac output.

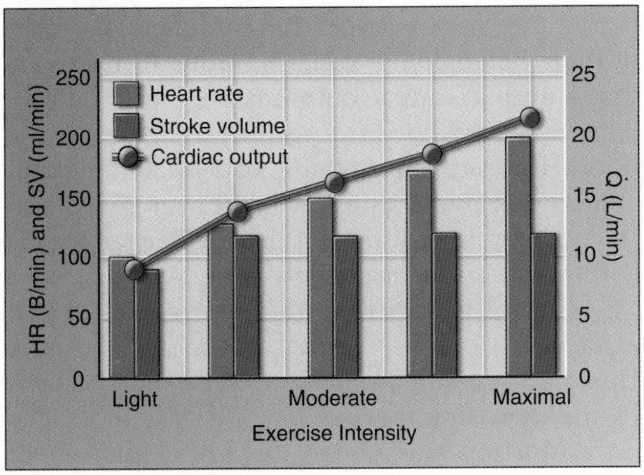

FIGURE 2.12 Effect of exercise intensity on heart rate, SV and cardiac output. HR, heart rate; SV, stroke volume; Q, cardiac output.

CARDIAC OUTPUT

Cardiac output at rest is approximately 5 L. However, during maximal endurance exercise, cardiac output may increase upward to 20 L in young, sedentary men, whereas in young, endurance-trained male athletes, cardiac output may reach 40 L. In examining this considerable difference in cardiac output, we can see that the maximal heart rate for both of these individuals (assuming that both men are 20 years old) will be approximately 200 bpm (maximal heart rate = 220 − age). Thus, a difference in SV must account for the large differences seen in cardiac output. In our example, the SV of the sedentary male would be approximately 100 mL · beat^{-1}, while the SV in the endurance-trained athlete may reach 200 mL · beat^{-1}.

The importance of a large cardiac output for the endurance athlete is reflected by the linear relationship seen between cardiac output and oxygen consumption (3). This relationship is seen not only in adults but also reported in children and adolescents (4) and between trained and untrained individuals (5).

Increases in cardiac output during exercise is the result of changes in SV and heart rate. SV and heart rate respond differently to various types of training.

HEART RATE

Heart rate elevation during exercise is primarily controlled by sympathetic stimulation from the brain's higher somatomotor centers. The heart rate response is directly proportional and linear to the intensity of exercise. As intensity of exercise increases, heart rate will continue to increase until it reaches a plateau. It is at this point that the individual has apparently reached his or her maximal level.

Initial increases in heart rate are also related to a withdrawal of parasympathetic input. This occurs during low-intensity exercise. As exercise continues in duration, or increases in intensity, a greater sympathetic stimulation is seen and becomes the driving force in elevating heart rate. Sympathetic activation occurs from feedback mechanisms in peripheral, mechanical, and chemical receptors that monitor changes in pH, hypoxia, temperature, and other metabolic variables that can alter sympathetic drive.

As heart rate increases, the volume of blood that is pumped into the circulation will increase. However, there is a limitation to this effect. As heart rate rises above a certain level, the strength of each contraction may decrease due to a metabolic overload. More importantly, the greater rate of contraction results in less time spent in diastole. The time between contractions becomes so reduced that there is not a sufficient time for the blood to flow from the atria to the ventricles. Thus, the total volume of blood made available to the circulation is reduced. This is why, during artificial electrical stimulation, the heart rate will only be elevated to between 100 and 150 bpm. However, elevations in heart rate from sympathetic stimulation will result in a heart rate between 170 and 250 bpm. The difference being that sympathetic stimulation will also result in a stronger systolic contraction, decrease the time during systole, and thereby allow a greater time for filling during diastole.

Decreases in resting heart rate likely reflect changes in sympathetic and parasympathetic stimulation.

STROKE VOLUME

Increases in SV are accomplished early during exercise primarily through an increase in left ventricular EDV. This rapid augmentation of SV is due to the **Frank-Starling mechanism**, which is related to the increased volume of blood that returns to the heart during exercise. With a greater volume of blood returning to the heart, the ventricles will become stretched to a greater extent than normal and will respond with a more forceful contraction. This stronger contraction will result in a greater volume of blood entering the systemic circulation with each heart beat. This mechanism appears to occur early on during exercise and at a relatively low level of exercise intensity. The Frank-Starling mechanism may cause an approximate 30% to 50% increase in SV (6). As exercise continues, increases in EDV will reach a plateau while exercise intensity is still at a submaximal intensity. Further increases in SV are attributed to the enhanced left ventricular contractile function (controlled by enhanced sympathetic stimulation), resulting in a greater decrease in end-systolic ventricular volume.

There are two mechanisms that appear to be responsible for the increase in EDV during exercise. The initial mechanism involves the use of the exercising muscles as a pump to increase the rate of return of the blood to the heart. Interestingly, this would be expected to increase the pressures within the ventricular cavity during filling, thereby raising diastolic pressure. However, this does not occur in the healthy heart, and in contrast, the relaxation seen in the left ventricle reduces the ventricular pressure below that of the left atrium. This will cause the mitral valve to open and the onset of ventricular filling. As mentioned earlier, the enhanced sympathetic response during exercise will increase the relaxation time during diastole. During this time, the increase in size of the left ventricle causes a further reduction in pressure creating a suctioning effect drawing additional blood into the chamber. This facilitation of the suctioning mechanism by sympathetic drive is the secondary mechanism that contributes to the increased SV and is crucial in the recruitment of Frank-Starling mechanisms (6).

CARDIAC DRIFT

As exercise duration is prolonged, or when exercise is performed in a hot environment, a gradual increase in heart rate and a decrease in SV may occur even when exercise intensity is maintained. This is referred to as **cardiovascular drift** and is thought to occur from a greater percentage of circulating blood being diverted to the skin in an attempt to dissipate body heat as a result of an increased core temperature. The greater concentration of blood in the periphery and a loss of some plasma volume to the sweat will result in a reduced blood return to the heart. This decrease in EDV will result in a reduced SV. Heart rate will be elevated to compensate for the change in SV and to maintain cardiac output.

a-vo_2 DIFFERENCE

During rest, each liter of blood contains approximately 200 mL of oxygen in an individual with a normal hemoglobin concentration. Considering that a normal cardiac output is 5 $L \cdot min^{-1}$ at rest, approximately 1 L of oxygen is available to the body. However, only 250 mL, or 25%, of the available oxygen is actually extracted from arterial blood (a-vo_2 difference) during rest leaving the remaining 750 mL of oxygen available as a reserve.

As might be expected, during exercise, oxygen extraction from the arterial blood is increased. Up to 75% of the available oxygen may be used by the exercising muscles. The increase in oxygen extraction appears to be related to the intensity of exercise and may be further enhanced following endurance training programs. The ability to extract oxygen from the blood and the total blood volume available to the muscles is critical in determining the aerobic capacity of the individual. This is reflected by the **Fick equation**:

$$\dot{V}o_{2max} = \text{Maximal cardiac output} \times \text{Maximal a-}\bar{V}o_2 \text{ difference}$$

Interestingly, there may be very little difference between moderately trained individuals and endurance athletes in the ability to extract oxygen, despite large differences in $\dot{V}o_{2max}$. Therefore, the primary factor determining aerobic capacity is likely cardiac output.

DISTRIBUTION OF CARDIAC OUTPUT

During exercise, most of the circulating blood is diverted to the active muscles (see Fig. 2.2). The extent of this shunting will be dependent upon the environmental condition and possibly other factors including the type of exercise and fatigue. The shunting of blood is generally accomplished by diverting blood flow from organs or areas of the body that can tolerate a reduction in blood flow to the exercising muscles. However, certain organs such as the heart cannot function without a normal blood flow and will not compromise its blood supply during exercise.

BLOOD PRESSURE

Blood pressure typically increases in a linear fashion during dynamic exercise such as walking, jogging, or running. In the healthy individual, this increase is seen only in the systolic response. The systolic blood pressure response appears to be buffered to a large extent by the decrease in peripheral resistance caused by the vasodilation in the vasculature of the exercising muscles (7). The decrease seen in peripheral resistance also appears to account for the minimal to no change observed in diastolic pressures. Diastolic pressure may also decrease during higher intensity bouts of exercise.

During exercise that involves the upper body only, both systolic and diastolic blood pressures are higher than when exercise is performed with only the legs (8). This is thought to occur because of the relatively smaller muscle mass and vasculature of the arms. Even when these vessels are maximally dilated, it does not appear to have the same effect on peripheral resistance compared with lower body exercise. The higher pressor response seen with upper body exercise has important implications in determining the exercise prescription for individuals exercising with coronary heart disease.

During resistance exercise, large increases in both systolic and diastolic blood pressures can be seen (9–11). During maximal efforts that involve a large muscle mass, intra-arterial blood pressures exceeding 350/250 mm Hg in healthy young men have been reported (10). The large pressor response seen during resistance training is a combination of vascular compression within contracting muscles and a Valsalva maneuver. The magnitude of the pressor response is also related to the relative size of the muscle mass involved and the intensity of the effort. Blood pressure will increase with each repetition in a set to failure and then drop rapidly to below resting levels after the last repetition (10,11). This is a transient decrease and is likely

Q & A from the Field

Q *Can resistance training be harmful to the heart? I heard it can cause an enlarged heart.*

A The heart is a muscle, and exercise, including resistance training, increases the workload on the heart. The heart can hypertrophy just like any other muscle. Body builders and weightlifters can get an enlarged heart, which by itself does not cause any heart problems. Resistance training will cause your heart muscle to thicken without enlargement of its cavity. This enables the heart to work better under the increased intrathoracic pressure that occurs with anaerobic exercise. Other causes of an enlarged heart (certain diseases) are associated with specific heart problems. Endurance exercise may decrease the size of an "enlarged heart" and has other benefits as well.

related to the large vasodilation of the vasculature that was occluded during muscle contraction and may contribute to the dizziness that may be experienced after an intense exercise session.

A major portion of the large pressor response seen during resistance training is attributed to a **Valsalva maneuver** (7). During a Valsalva maneuver, there is a rapid increase in intrathoracic pressure, which results in an increase in both systolic and diastolic blood pressures (9). However, if the Valsalva maneuver is maintained, within several seconds, the systolic and diastolic pressures will begin to drop because of the reduced diastolic filling caused by impaired venous return. Although often contraindicated during resistance exercise, the Valsalva maneuver may in fact be quite beneficial and have a protective effect in healthy resistance-trained individuals (7,12). The increase in intrathoracic pressure seen during the Valsalva maneuver will provide stabilization to the spinal column and reduce left ventricular transmural pressure (afterload) (13). This contrasts to the high afterload that is normally expected when systolic pressures are elevated. In addition, the increase in intrathoracic pressure is also transmitted to the cerebral spinal fluid, which will reduce the transmural pressures of the cerebral vessels preventing vascular damage at the time of peak peripheral resistance (12).

During exercise, systolic blood pressure is expected to increase relative to changes in exercise intensity; however, diastolic blood pressure will remain the same or decrease slightly.

PULMONARY VENTILATION DURING EXERCISE

During submaximal exercise, ventilation will increase linearly with oxygen uptake. The increase in oxygen consumption is primarily the result of an increase in tidal volume (amount of air inspired or expired during a normal breathing cycle). As exercise intensity is elevated, the increase in oxygen consumption may rely more on increasing the breathing rate. During steady-state exercise, minute ventilation (liters of air breathed per minute) will plateau when the demand for oxygen is met by supply. The ratio of minute ventilation to oxygen consumption is termed the ventilatory equivalent and is symbolized by V_E/V_{O_2}. During submaximal exercise, the ventilatory equivalent in healthy individuals is approximately 25:1 (14). That is, 25 L of air is breathed in for every liter of oxygen. This ratio may be slightly higher in children (15) and also be affected by the mode of exercise (swimming vs. running) (16). However, during maximal exercise, minute ventilation increases disproportionately in relation to oxygen uptake, and the ventilatory equivalent may reach as high as 35 to 40 L of air per liter of oxygen consumed in the healthy adult.

CARDIOVASCULAR ADAPTATIONS TO TRAINING

Prolonged participation in exercise programs results in a number of cardiovascular adaptations that are specific to the type of exercise program used. Endurance training and resistance training are modes of training that represent two distinctly different physiological demands that are placed on the cardiovascular system. Although many of the cardiovascular adaptations observed in these training programs are similar, others are quite different. A summary of these adaptations can be seen in Table 2.2 and are discussed in this section.

CARDIAC OUTPUT AND STROKE VOLUME

Increases in $\dot{V}\mathbf{O}_{2max}$ are characteristic of endurance training programs. These increases are generally accompanied by increases in cardiac output and an improved extraction capability within skeletal muscle (increase in a-vo_2). Improvement in oxygen extraction is related to the greater perfusion capabilities of exercising muscle. Since maximal heart rates are unaffected by training and will not differ between elite endurance athletes and age-matched sedentary individuals, increases in cardiac output are primarily the result of improved SV.

Endurance training is a potent stimulus for increasing SV both at rest and during maximal exercise. Increases in SV are related to an enlarged ventricular chamber (referred to as **eccentric hypertrophy**) caused by a chronic increased ventricular filling seen during endurance exercise. This increased preload is thought to relate to the expanded plasma volume associated with such training (17,18).

Resistance training results in little to no change in cardiac output. Although significantly greater

TABLE 2.2 ● CARDIOVASCULAR ADAPTATIONS TO PROLONGED ENDURANCE AND RESISTANCE TRAINING

	Endurance Training		Resistance Training	
	REST	**EXERCISE**	**REST**	**EXERCISE**
Heart Rate	D	NC	D or NC	NC
Stroke Volume	I	I	I or NC	I or NC
Cardiac Output	NC	I	NC	I or NC
Blood Pressure				
Systolic	D or NC	D or NC	D or NC	D or NC
Diastolic	D or NC	D or NC	NC	D or NC
Morphological Adaptations				
Left Ventricular Mass	I	I		
Left Ventricular Diameter	I	I or NC		
Wall Thickness				
Left ventricle	I	I		
Septum	I	I		

I, decrease; D, decrease; NC, no change.

SVs have been reported in elite-level weightlifters when compared to recreational lifters (19), the increase in SV seen in these athletes appeared to be more of a factor of a larger body size than a training adaptation (20).

Increases in cardiac output following prolonged endurance training are the result of an increased SV.

HEART RATE

A decrease in resting heart rate and a relative decrease in heart rate at any given submaximal $\dot{V}O_{2max}$ are commonly found adaptations in endurance training programs (21,22). The decrease in heart rate during submaximal exercise is likely subsequent to improved SV and also is reflective of an improved exercise economy. The mechanism regulating training-induced bradycardia is not thoroughly understood but is likely related to a change in the balance between sympathetic and parasympathetic activity. In addition, a decrease in the intrinsic rate of firing of the SA node following long-term training has also been suggested to be a factor in the bradycardic response to long-term training (23).

BLOOD PRESSURE

In normotensive individuals, resting systolic or diastolic pressures are generally unresponsive to endurance training programs. However, based on a number of epidemiological studies and other investigations examining exercise and hypertension, it appears that exercise is a potential stimulus for reducing both systolic and diastolic blood pressure in hypertensive individuals (24). The reduction in resting blood pressure appears to occur during endurance exercise programs that occur at frequencies between three and five sessions per week and that are of at least 30 minutes in duration and between 50% and 70% of $\dot{V}O_{2max}$ (24,25).

During endurance exercise, the blood pressure response has been shown to decrease for a given level of exercise intensity (7). However, this is likely related to the initial conditioning level of the individual. Well-conditioned endurance athletes likely need to train at a high intensity of exercise for a prolonged duration and to see such adaptations.

Resistance training appears to result in no change or a slight decrease in resting blood pressure (26), but a significant decrease in the blood pressure response during resistance exercise at the same absolute load (27,28). Any decrease in resting blood pressure subsequent to resistance training is likely the result of a decrease in body fat and possible reduction in the sympathetic drive to the heart (similar to what may drive the reduction in blood pressure during endurance exercise) (29).

Changes in resting blood pressure is dependent upon the individual's initial conditioning level.

CARDIAC MORPHOLOGY

An athlete's heart is quite large in comparison to a recreationally trained or sedentary individual. For many years, a debate was waged whether this enlarged heart in athletes was a consequence of pathological disease or physiological adaptation. However, the technological advances during the past 30 years have allowed for a much closer examination of the physiological adaptations of the heart in conjunction with prolonged training.

During prolonged training, the heart will adapt to match the workload placed on the left ventricle in order to maintain a constant relationship between systolic cavity pressure and the ratio of wall thickness to ventricular radius (30). Adaptations to the morphology of the heart are governed by the law of Laplace that states that wall tension is proportional to pressure and the radius of curvature (31). During a pressure overload, common to resistance exercise programs, the septum and posterior wall of the left ventricle increase in size to normalize myocardial wall stress. During a volume overload, common to endurance training programs, the increase is predominantly in the internal diameter of the left ventricle (increasing the size of the cavity), with a proportional increase in both the septum and the posterior wall of the ventricle. Both endurance training and resistance training are at either ends of the spectrum concerning the volume and pressure stresses placed upon the heart. However, most sports have a parallel impact on both cavity dimension and wall thickness (32). In these sports, athletes are performing a combination of aerobic and anaerobic training resulting in cardiovascular adaptations associated with both an enlarged diastolic cavity dimension and a larger wall thickness. In the sports that primarily emphasize a single form of training, the morphological changes of the heart may be more extreme.

Endurance-trained athletes have been shown to have a greater than normal left ventricular internal diameter, with normal to slightly thicker walls (32–35). This type of left ventricular hypertrophy is termed eccentric hypertrophy and is considered to be a normal physiological response to a volume overload (greater EDVs) consistent with prolonged endurance training.

Resistance-trained athletes on the other hand have normal internal diameters, but significantly thicker ventricular walls (19,34,36,37). This type of hypertrophy is referred to as **concentric hypertrophy** and at times may approach levels that are seen in **hypertrophic cardiomyopathy** (a disease of the myocardium that is associated with large thickening of the septum and posterior wall at the expense of cavity size, greatly impairing left ventricular function). Importantly, the concentric hypertrophy seen in the resistance-trained athlete does not impede on the internal diameter of the ventricle. In addition, the type of hypertrophy seen in cardiomyopathy is usually asymmetric, whereas in resistance-trained or power athletes, the change in wall size is generally symmetrical. Figure 2.13 compares morphological changes in the left ventricle between endurance- and resistance-trained individuals.

Left ventricular mass in highly trained athletes are on an average 45% greater than in age-matched control subjects (33). This increase in mass is related to the increases in left ventricular internal diameter and ventricular wall thickness. When examined relative to changes in body mass or body surface area, the significantly greater ventricular mass is still present. Some studies have suggested that differences are more prevalent in elite athletes than in athletes of lesser caliber (20).

Morphological changes of the heart are dependent upon the type of training program performed.

RESPIRATORY ADAPTATIONS TO TRAINING

For the most part, the respiratory system is not a limiting factor in providing a sufficient amount of oxygen to the exercising muscles. However, similar to most other physiological systems in the body, the respiratory system can also adapt to physical exercise in order to maximize its efficiency. In general, lung volume and capacity change very little as the result of physical exercise. It does appear that during maximal exercise vital capacity may increase slightly, but this may be related to the

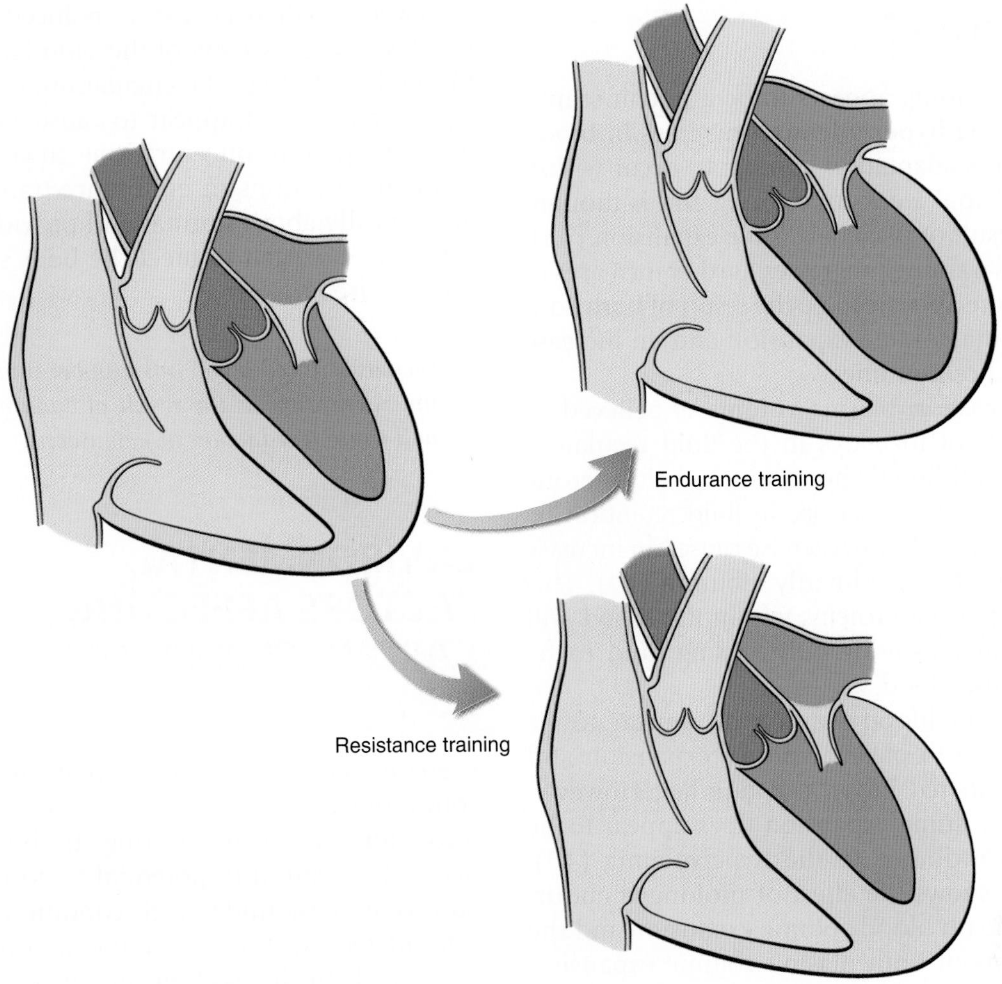

FIGURE 2.13 Caricature of morphological adaptations of the left ventricle subsequent to endurance and resistance training.

slight decrease seen in residual volume (amount of air remaining in the lungs following a maximal expiration) (38).

Respiratory capacity does not appear significantly affected by physical exercise.

VENTILATORY EQUIVALENT AND MINUTE VENTILATION

Endurance training appears to reduce the **ventilatory equivalent** (i.e., amount of air is inspired at a particular rate of oxygen consumption) during submaximal exercise (39,40). As a result, the oxygen cost of exercise attributable to ventilation is reduced. This benefit may be realized by a reduction in fatigue of the ventilatory musculature and greater oxygen availability to the exercising muscles (41).

Minute ventilation also appears to decrease during submaximal exercise following prolonged endurance training, reflecting on the improved exercise efficiency resulting from such training. However, during maximal exercise, endurance training appears to cause minute ventilation to increase. During maximal exercise, minute ventilation is thought to increase in relation to increases in $\dot{V}O_{2max}$ (42). In untrained subjects, minute ventilation can increase from 120 L · min^{-1} to about 150 L · min^{-1} after training (38). In addition, minute ventilation in highly trained endurance athletes may increase to 180 L · min^{-1} and has been reported to be as high as 240 L · min^{-1} in elite rowers (38).

BLOOD VOLUME ADAPTATIONS TO TRAINING

Endurance training appears to be a potent stimulus for causing **hypervolemia** (increases in blood volume). This adaptation appears to occur within the initial 2 to 4 weeks of training and is thought to be the result of plasma volume expansion (43). However, as training progresses, further increases in blood volume appears to be the result of both continued plasma volume expansion and an increase in red blood cell number.

The increase in plasma volume is believed to be the result of increases in the fluid regulatory hormones, antidiuretic hormone, and aldosterone that bring about an increase in fluid retention by the kidneys. In addition, exercise causes an increase in plasma proteins, primarily albumin (44). This increase in plasma proteins within the blood will cause a greater osmotic pull causing fluid to be retained in the blood.

Increases in blood volume do appear to be the result of both plasma volume expansion and an increase in red blood cell number. However, the plasma volume expansion does appear to be a greater contributor to the hypervolemia (45). Figure 2.14 shows the effect of prolonged endurance training on blood volume expansion and the contributions of both plasma volume expansion and increases in red blood cell number. Although both plasma volume and red blood cell volume increase, they do not increase proportionally. Thus, hematocrit will decrease. A reduced hematocrit will lower the viscosity of the blood and facilitate blood flow through the circulation. Reductions in hematocrit do not appear to cause a concern for low hemoglobin concentrations. In fact, hemoglobin concentrations in endurance-trained athletes are typically above normal and provide an ample capacity of oxygen to meet the body's needs during exercise.

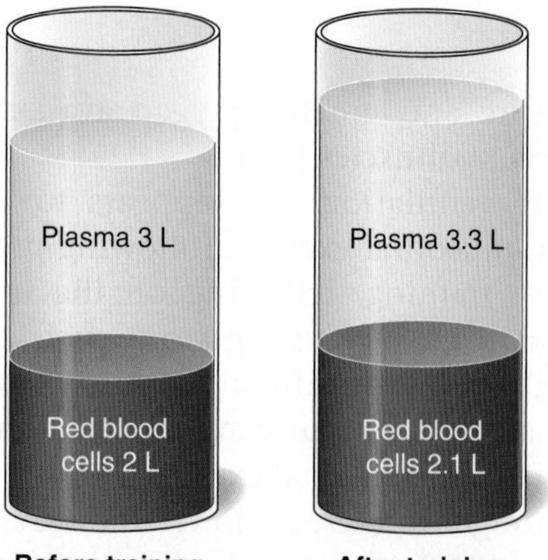

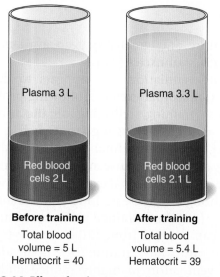

FIGURE 2.14 Effect of endurance training on blood volume, plasma volume, and hematocrit. (Reprinted with permission from Hoffman JR. *Physiological Aspects of Sport Training and Performance*. Champaign, IL: Human Kinetics; 2005:55.)

Increases in red blood cell number and plasma volume expansion as the result of endurance training will cause a reduction in hematocrit.

ENVIRONMENTAL FACTORS AFFECTING CARDIORESPIRATORY FUNCTION

Exercise performed under severe environmental conditions can cause a large strain on the cardiorespiratory system in meeting the body's oxygen needs. In addition to potential performance limitations, exercise under such conditions poses significant risks to the health and well-being of the individual. In this section, discussion focuses on the effects of exercising in the heat and altitude has on cardiorespiratory function.

CARDIORESPIRATORY RESPONSE TO EXERCISE IN THE HEAT

During exercise in the heat, a large volume of circulating blood (up to 7 L · min^{-1}) is diverted to the skin to help dissipate the increase in body heat (46). As blood flow to the skin is increased, the peripheral vasculature becomes compliant and engorged with blood creating blood pools (47). Blood pooling in the periphery causes a reduction in venous return and subsequently a decrease in cardiac filling. The resulting cardiovascular strain is reflected by a decrease in SV. To compensate, the heart rate must increase in order to maintain cardiac output. In addition, blood flow from splanchnic and renal areas is further reduced to compensate for the greater blood flow that is diverted to the exercising muscle and periphery for heat dissipation (46).

To combat elevations in body temperature resulting from exercising in the heat, sweat rate will increase to enhance evaporative cooling. This adds to the cardiovascular strain by causing a greater reduction in blood volume (48). However, as blood volume becomes reduced, it will result in less blood being made available to the periphery, and as a result, sweat output will decline and the body's ability to dissipate heat will be reduced. Consequently, core temperature will rise, and in combination with a reduced blood volume, cardiovascular strain becomes elevated and the risk for heat illness is increased. When exercise in the heat is further complicated with a body water deficit, the resulting dehydration will exacerbate the physiological strain.

During intense exercise in the heat, blood flow must be redistributed to accommodate the competing interests of thermoregulation and skeletal muscle function.

A body water deficit has significant implications for cardiovascular function. **Hypohydration** (an existing body water deficit) results in a reduction in plasma volume. As a consequence, less blood is available to both exercising muscle and the skin. In addition, decreases in plasma volume are also associated with a reduction in SV (49). To compensate, the heart rate will increase in order to maintain normal blood flow. However, depending upon the magnitude of the body water deficit, the increase in heart rate may be insufficient to fully compensate for the lower SV. As a result, cardiac output will also be reduced (49,50). However, it does appear that cardiac output can be maintained at higher degrees of hypohydration if it occurs in the absence of a thermal strain (51).

Cardiovascular function can be compromised during exercise in the heat by the reduction SV.

EFFECT OF ALTITUDE ON THE CARDIORESPIRATORY RESPONSE

As one ascends above sea level, the partial pressure of oxygen (PO_2) becomes reduced. Remember that the pressure gradient between arterial PO_2 and tissue PO_2 is approximately 64 mm Hg at sea level (the difference between an arterial PO_2 of 104 mm Hg and a tissue PO_2 of 40 mm Hg). This creates a pressure gradient causing oxygen to diffuse easily into the tissues. However, at altitude, a reduction in arterial PO_2 will cause a decrease in the pressure gradient reducing the diffusion capability of oxygen from the vasculature into the tissue. For instance, at an elevation of 2,500 m, the arterial PO_2 drops to about 60 mm Hg, with the tissue PO_2 remaining at 40 mm Hg, creating a pressure gradient of only 20 mm Hg. This 70% reduction in the pressure gradient will cause a significant reduction in the speed at which oxygen moves between the capillaries and tissues. The reduction in the pressure gradient between the vasculature and the tissues has important implications in maintaining exercise performance during exercise at altitude. To compensate for the reduced PO_2 at altitude, breathing rate is increased. However, as breathing rate increases (**hyperventilation**), the partial pressure of carbon dioxide (PCO_2) in the alveoli also becomes reduced. As a result, the stimulus to maintain a high rate of ventilation may be removed since PCO_2 is an integral part of the driving force behind hyperventilation.

To compensate for the reduced oxygen availability at altitude, elevations in cardiac output occurs at rest and during exercise. The primary mechanism resulting in the increased cardiac output appears to be an increase in heart rate. Heart rate has been shown to increase between 40% and 50% at rest without any change in SV (52). Even during exercise, the increase in cardiac output appears to be primarily the result of an increase in heart rate. In contrast to what is normally seen during exercise at sea level, during exercise at altitude, SV will decrease (52). The decrease in SV is apparently from a reduction in plasma volume that is observed within a short time following arrival at altitude (53,54).

During initial exposure at altitude (observed at elevations above 3,000 m), decreases in plasma volume appear to be the result of both diuresis and natriuresis (increased sodium excretion) (55). The diuresis may be explained by the large evaporative heat loss caused by ventilation of dry inspired air at altitude. The natriuresis appears to be the result of a neural stimulation of the kidney to decrease the reabsorption of sodium due to the **hypoxic** (low oxygen) stimulus (55). Even during prolonged exposure to altitude, plasma volume will still remain below normal levels, and studies examining individuals who reside at altitude have reported lower plasma volumes in comparison to residents of sea level communities (56). Thus, acclimatization does not seem to have any significant effect on a return of blood volume to preexposure levels.

Changes in the partial pressure of oxygen as the result of ascending to altitude will impair gas exchange in the lungs and tissues.

Cardiorespiratory Changes from Prolonged Exposure at Altitude

During the first few days at altitude, changes in the respiratory response can be seen. Initially, breathing rate is increased while arterial Po_2 decreases. However, after a few days at altitude, arterial Po_2 begins to rise as Pco_2 values fall. The ventilatory rate though will continue to rise as a result of changes in the ventilatory response to CO_2 levels and in the sensitivity of the carotid body. The carotid body is situated above the bifurcation of the carotid artery. It serves as a sensor of oxygen saturation in the blood, and its location is ideal for this role since it receives a large blood supply allowing it to respond to oxygen saturation and not to oxygen content (57). The increased sensitivity of the carotid body appears to have a biphasic response. The initial response may be a decrease in the hypoxic ventilatory response during the first 3 to 5 days of altitude exposure, but following these initial days of exposure, an increase in the ventilatory response is seen (57).

In addition to changes in the ventilatory response, another component of respiratory adaptation to altitude may be in the diffusion capacity of oxygen. After 7 to 10 weeks of altitude exposure, diffusion capacities are reported to increase between 15% and 20% (56). Although much of this improved diffusion capacity may be accounted for by increases in hemoglobin concentrations, other studies comparing individuals permanently residing at altitude to individuals residing at sea level have also reported significant differences in oxygen diffusion capacities between these population groups (58). These differences may be related to the larger lung volumes developed through exposure to chronic hypoxia and the subsequent development of greater surface area for oxygen diffusion (59).

Altitude and temperature each elicit various physiological responses specific to the environment.

After several weeks of altitude exposure, cardiac output remains similar to those values observed at sea level. However, similar to what occurs during an acute exposure to altitude, increases in cardiac output following extended stays at elevation also appear to be primarily attributed to increases in heart rate. SV though continues to remain reduced (60). One of the best known adaptations to prolonged exposure to altitude is the increase in the number of red blood cells per unit volume of blood. Exposure to hypoxic conditions results in the release of the hormone erythropoietin. **Erythropoietin** is responsible for stimulating red blood cell (erythrocytes) production and is seen to increase within 2 hours of exposure to altitude and reaches a maximum rate of increase at about 24 to 48 hours (61). After 3 weeks of exposure to altitude, erythropoietin concentrations appear to return to baseline levels, but not until they have contributed to an approximate 20% to 25% increase in packed cell volume (62). Increases in red cell mass continue to increase even after erythropoietin returns to normal levels (62). However, the mechanism that underlies this continued increase is not known. This physiological adaptation to altitude is one of the reasons why many endurance athletes live at altitude and train at sea level.

As red cell volume increases, so does the blood's hemoglobin concentration. This increase allows for a greater amount of oxygen to be carried per unit volume of blood. However, as red cell volume and hemoglobin concentration increase, the viscosity of the blood will also increase presenting an inherent danger associated with these physiological adaptations associated with altitude.

Summary

In this chapter, we saw the effect of acute exercise on cardiac function and how the heart will compensate for the increased energy demands of exercising muscles. This compensation is manifested by changes in cardiac output, regulated in part by enhanced sympathetic drive and increased venous return. In addition, blood flow is diverted from nonexercising muscles and nonessential organs to exercising muscles to provide for greater oxygen delivery. Differences in the acute cardiac response between endurance and resistance training programs were also discussed. Discussion also focused on the coordinated relationship between the cardiovascular and the respiratory systems and the effect both acute and prolonged training has on their function. In addition, the effects of prolonged training on both cardiovascular and respiratory adaptations were discussed and focus was directed on how these adaptations are dependent upon the type of training program employed. Finally, the effects of environmental stresses were also reviewed. Specific discussion was directed at acute exercise in the heat and at altitude, and adaptation to prolonged exposure to altitude was also briefly reviewed.

Maxing Out

1. You are responsible for training a university's club ski team in Colorado, but most of the members are traveling to Florida during winter break. The first competition of the ski season is in the second week of January. When do you advise your athletes to return to the mountains and what physiological changes may happen when they are on vacation?
2. After an unusually hot and humid summer, one of the players on the team complains to you about having a higher heart rate than normal. You investigate the issue and discover that many of the players have resting heart rates approximately 10 beats higher than they did 3 months ago. What may have caused the problem and how might you go about fixing it?
3. One of your athletes mysteriously loses consciousness during an intense lifting session that consists of sets of two to three repetitions. His teammates report that his face turned very red during his final repetition during a set of dead lifts. What may have caused this to happen?

REFERENCES

1. Adamovich DR. *The Heart. Fundamentals of Electrocardiography, Exercise Physiology and Exercise Stress Testing*. Freeport, NY: Sports Medicine Books; 1984
2. Hurst, JW. Naming of the waves in the ECG, with a brief account of their genesis. *J Am Heart Assoc.* 1998;98:1937–1942.
3. Lewis SF, Taylor WF, Graham RM, et al. Cardiovascular responses to exercise as functions of absolute and relative work load. *J Appl Physiol.* 1983;54:1314–1323.
4. Cunningham DA, Paterson DH, Blimkie CJ, et al. Development of cardiorespiratory function in circumpubertal boys: a longitudinal study. *J Appl Physiol.* 1984;56:302–307.
5. Saltin B, Astrand PO. Maximal oxygen uptake in athletes. *J Appl Physiol.* 1967;23:353–358.
6. Bonow RO. Left ventricular response to exercise. In: Fletcher GF, ed. *Cardiovascular Response to Exercise*. Mount Kisco, NY: Futura Publishing Co, Inc; 1994:31–48.
7. MacDougall JD. Blood pressure responses to resistive, static, and dynamic exercise. In: Fletcher GF, ed. *Cardiovascular Response to Exercise*. Mount Kisco, NY: Futura Publishing Co, Inc.; 1994:155–174.
8. Toner MM, Glickman EL, McArdle WD. Cardiovascular adjustments to exercise distributed between the upper and lower body. *Med Sci Sports Exerc.* 1990;22:773–778.
9. MacDougall JD, McKelvie RS, Moroz DE, et al. Factors affecting blood pressure response during heavy weightlifting and static contractions. *J Appl Physiol.* 1992;73:1590–1597.
10. MacDougall JD, Tuxen D, Sale DG, et al. Arterial blood pressure response to heavy resistance exercise. *J Appl Physiol.* 1985;58:785–790.
11. Sale DG, Moroz DE, McKelvie RS, et al. Comparison of blood pressure response to isokinetic and weight-lifting exercise. *Eur J Appl Physiol.* 1993;67:115–120.
12. McCartney N. Acute responses to resistance training and safety. *Med SciSports Exerc.* 1999;31:31–37.
13. Lentini AC, McKelvie RS, McCartney N, et al. Assessment of left ventricular response of strength trained athletes during weightlifting exercise. *J Appl Physiol.* 1993;75:2703–2710.
14. Wasserman K, Whipp BJ, Davis JA. Respiratory physiology of exercise: metabolism, gas exchange, and ventilatory control. *Int Rev Physiol.* 1981;23:149–211.
15. Rowland TW, Green GM. Physiological responses to treadmill exercise in females: adult-child differences. *Med Sci Sports Exerc.* 1988;20:474–478.
16. McArdle WD, Glaser RM, Magel JR. Metabolic and cardiorespiratory response during free swimming and treadmill walking. *J Appl Physiol.* 1971;30:733–738.
17. Carroll JF, Convertino VA, Wood CE, et al. Effect of training on blood volume and plasma hormone concentrations in the elderly. *Med Sci Sports Exerc.* 1995;27:79–84.
18. Convertino VA, Keil LC, Bernauer EM, et al. Plasma volume, osmolality, vasopressin, and renin activity during graded exercise in man. *J Appl Physiol.* 1981;50:123–128.
19. Pearson AC, Schiff M, Mrosek D, et al. Left ventricular diastolic function in weight lifters. *Am J Cardiol.* 1986;58:1254–1259.
20. Fleck SJ. Cardiovascular adaptations to resistance training. *Med Sci Sports Exerc.* 1988;20:S146–S151.
21. Blomqvist CG, Saltin B. Cardiovascular adaptations to physical training. *Annu Rev Physiol.* 1983;45:169–189.
22. Charlton GA, Crawford MH. Physiological consequences of training. *Cardiol Clin.* 1997;15:345–254.
23. Schaefer ME, Allert JA, Adams HR, et al. Adrenergic responsiveness and intrinsic sinoatrial automaticity of exercise-trained rats. *Med Sci Sports Exerc.* 1992;24:887–894.
24. Seals DR, Hagberg JM. The effect of exercise training on human hypertension: a review. *Med Sci Sports Exerc.* 1984;16:207–215.
25. Fagard RH. Exercise characteristics and the blood pressure response to dynamic physical training. *Med Sci Sports Exerc.* 2001;33:S484–S492.
26. Goldberg L, Elliot DL, Kuehl KS. A comparison of the cardiovascular effects of running and weight training. *J Strength Cond Res.* 1994;8:219–224.
27. McCartney N, McKelvie RS, Martin J, et al. Weight-training-induced attenuation of the circulatory response of older males to weight lifting. *J Appl Physiol.* 1993;74:1056–1060.

28. Sale DG, Moroz DE, McKelvie RS, et al. Effect of training on the blood pressure response to weight lifting. *Can J Appl Physiol.* 1994;19:60–74.
29. Fleck SJ, Kraemer WJ. *Designing Resistance Training Programs.* Champaign, IL: Human Kinetics; 1997.
30. Shapiro L. The morphological consequences of systemic training. *Cardiol Clin.* 1997;15:373–379.
31. Ford LE. Heart size. *Circ Res.* 1976;39:299–303.
32. Spirito P, Pelliccia A, Proschan M, et al. Morphology of the "athlete's heart" assessed by echocardiography in 947 elite athletes representing 27 sports. *Am J Cardiol.* 1994;74:802–806.
33. Maron BJ. Structural features of the athletic heart as defined by echocardiography. *J Am Coll Cardiol.* 1986;7:190–203.
34. Morganroth J, Maron BJ, Henry WL, et al. Comparative left ventricular dimensions in trained athletes. *Ann Intern Med.* 1975;82:521–524.
35. Pelliccia A, Maron BJ, Spataro A, et al. The upper limit of physiologic cardiac hypertrophy in highly trained elite athletes. *N Engl J Med.* 1991;324:295–301.
36. Fleck SJ, Henke C, Wilson W. Cardiac MRI of elite junior Olympic weight lifters. *Int J Sports Med.* 1989;10:329–333.
37. Menapace FJ, Hammer, WJ, Ritzer TF, et al. Left ventricular size in competitive weight lifters: an echocardiographic study. *Med Sci Sports Exerc.* 1982;14:72–75.
38. Wilmore JH, Costill DL. *Physiology of Sport and Exercise.* Champaign, IL: Human Kinetics; 1999.
39. Girandola RN, Katch FL. Effects of physical training on ventilatory equivalent and respiratory exchange ratio during weight supported, steady-state exercise. *Eur J Appl Physiol.* 1976; 21:119–125.
40. Yerg JE II, Seals DR, Hagberg JM, et al. Effect of endurance exercise training on ventilatory function in older individuals. *J Appl Physiol.* 1985;58:791–794.
41. Martin B, Heintzelman M, Chen HI. Exercise performance after ventilatory work. *J Appl Physiol.* 1982;52:1581–1585.
42. McArdle WD, Katch FI, Katch VL. *Exercise Physiology. Energy, Nutrition, and Human Performance.* 4th ed. Baltimore, MD: Williams & Wilkins; 1996:417–456.
43. Convertion VA. Blood volume: its adaptation to endurance training. *Med Sci Sports Exerc.* 1991;23:1338–1348.
44. Yang RC, Mack GW, Wolfe RR, et al. Albumin synthesis after intense intermittent exercise in human subjects. *J Appl Physiol.* 1998;84:584–592.
45. Green HJ, Sutton J, Coates G, et al. Response of red cells and plasma volume to prolonged training in humans. *J Appl Physiol.* 1991;70:1810–1815.
46. Rowell LB. *Human Circulation Regulation during Physical Stress.* New York: Oxford University Press; 1986.
47. Sawka MN, Wenger CB, Young AJ, et al. Physiological responses to exercise in the heat. In: Marriott BM, ed. *Nutritional Needs in Hot Environments.* Washington, DC: National Academy Press; 1993:55–74.
48. Sawka MN, Pandolf KB. Effects of body water loss on physiological function and exercise performance. In: Gisolfi CV, Lamb DR, eds. *Fluid Homeostasis during Exercise. Perspectives in Exercise Science and Sports Medicine.* Vol. 3. Indianapolis, IN: Benchmark Press; 1990:1–38.
49. Nadel ER, Fortney SM, Wenger CB. Effect of hydration on circulatory and thermal regulation. *J Appl Physiol.* 1980;49:715–721.
50. Sawka MN, Knowlton RG, Critz JB. Thermal and circulatory responses to repeated bouts of prolonged running. *Med Sci Sports Exerc.* 1979;11:177–180.
51. Sproles CB, Smith DP, Byrd RJ, et al. Circulatory responses to submaximal exercise after dehydration and rehydration. *J Sports Med Phys Fitness.* 1976;16:98–105.
52. Vogel JA, Harris CW. Cardiopulmonary responses of resting man during early exposure to high altitude. *J App Physiol.* 1967;22:1124–1128.
53. Singh MV, Rawal SB, Tyagi AK. Body fluid status on induction, reinduction and prolonged stay at high altitude on human volunteers. *Int J Biometeorol.* 1990;34: 93–97.
54. Wolfel EE, Groves BM, Brooks GA, et al. Oxygen transport during steady-state submaximal exercise in chronic hypoxia. *J Appl Physiol.* 1991;70:1129–1136.
55. Honig A. Role of arterial chemoreceptors in the reflex control of renal function and body fluid volumes in acute arterial hypoxia. In: Acher H. O'Regan RG, eds. *Physiology of the Peripheral Arterial Chemoreceptors.* 1983; 395–429.
56. West JB. Diffusing capacity of the lung for carbon monoxide at high altitude. *J Appl Physiol.* 1962;17:421–426.
57. Ward MP, Milledge JS, West JB. *High Altitude Medicine and Physiology.* London, England: Chapman and Hall Medical; 1995.
58. Dempsey JA, Reddan WG, Birnbaum ML, et al. Effects of acute through life-long hypoxic exposure on exercise pulmonary gas exchange. *Respir Physiol.* 1971;13:62–89.
59. Bartlett D, Remmers JE. Effects of high altitude exposure on the lungs of young rats. *Respir Physiol.* 1971;13: 116–125.
60. Reeves JT, Groves BM, Sutton JR, et al. Operation Everest II: preservation of cardiac function at extreme altitude. *J Appl Physiol.* 1987;63:31–539.
61. Eckardt K, Boutellier U, Kurtz A, et al. Rate of erythropoietin formation in humans in response to acute hypobaric hypoxia. *J Appl Physiol.* 1989;66:1785–1788.
62. Milledge JS, Coates PM. Serum erythropoietin in humans at high altitude and its relation to plasma renin. *J Appl Physiol.* 1985;59:360–364.

CHAPTER 3

The Neuromuscular System: Anatomical and Physiological Bases and Adaptations to Training

JARED W. COBURN • TRAVIS W. BECK • HERBERT A. DEVRIES • TERRY J. HOUSH

OBJECTIVES

After completing this chapter, you will be able to:

- Identify the structures of a neuron.
- Grasp the feedback mechanisms of proprioception.
- Differentiate types of muscle fibers.
- Chronologize the sliding filament theory of muscle contraction.
- Explain the neural and muscular adaptations to resistance training.

KEY TERMS

A Band
Acetylcholine (ACh)
Actin
Action Potential
Adenosine Diphosphate (ADP)
Adenosine Triphosphate (ATP)
Antagonist Coactivation
Axon
Bilateral Deficit
Concentric Muscle Action
Corpus Striatum
Crossbridge Recycling (Crossbridge Recharging)
Cross-Education (Cross-Training)
Dendrites
Dynamic Constant External Resistance (DCER)
Eccentric Muscle Action
Electromyography (EMG)
End Bulb
Endolymph
Endomysium
Epimysium
Extrapyramidal System
Growth Hormone
H Zone
Hyperplasia
Hypertrophy
I Band
Intrafusal (IF) Muscle Fibers
Inverse Myotatic Reflex
Isokinetic Muscle Action
Isometric Muscle Actions
Kinesthesis
Lower Motor Neurons
Motor Unit
Motor Nuclei
Motor (Efferent)
Motor Endplate
Motor Neuron
Monosynaptic Reflex
Myelin
Myosin ATPase
Myosin Crossbridge
Myofilaments
Myoneural Junction (Neuromuscular Junction)
Myosin
Myotatic
Neural Adaptations
Neuron
Nodes of Ranvier
Peak Torque
Proprioception
Proprioceptive–Cerebellar System
Pyramidal Tracts

Pyramidal System
Rate Coding
Rate of Force Development (RFD)
Recruitment
Red Nucleus
Reflex
Repetition Maximum (RM)
Saltatory Conduction
Sarcolemma
Sarcomere
Sarcoplasm
Sarcoplasmic Reticulum (SR)
Schwann Cells
Sensory (Afferent)
Size Principle
Sliding-Filament Theory
Substantia Nigra
Synapse
Synapses
Testosterone
Transverse Tubules (T Tubules)
Troponin
Tropomyosin
Utricle
Upper Motor Neurons
Vestibular Receptors
Z Line

Introduction

The nervous system can be divided anatomically into the central (brain and spinal cord) and peripheral (outside of the spinal cord) systems or functionally into the somatic (voluntary) and autonomic (involuntary) systems. The autonomic nervous system is composed of the sympathetic and parasympathetic systems, which control the involuntary functioning of various internal organs, the circulatory system (including vasoconstriction and vasodilation), and the endocrine glands. Voluntary human movement, however, is controlled by the somatic nervous system. When we decide to perform a muscle action, the electrical activity that eventually leads to muscle contraction originates in the motor cortex of the brain and travels through the central and peripheral systems to the muscle.

The nervous system controls both voluntary and involuntary functions. Voluntary human movement is controlled by the somatic nervous system, while the involuntary functioning of internal organs, circulatory system, and endocrine glands is controlled by the autonomic nervous system.

THE NEURON

A nerve cell, or **neuron**, is the basic structural unit of the nervous system. Billions of neurons are in the nervous system; usually, several neurons are interconnected by **synapses** (junctions between neurons) to form pathways for conducting nervous impulses. The neurons that conduct sensory impulses from the periphery to the central nervous system are called **sensory, or afferent**, neurons. The neurons that conduct impulses from the central nervous system to the muscles are called **motor, or efferent**, neurons. Although neurons are microscopic in diameter, one cell can be up to approximately 3 ft in length, such as a neuron that extends from the spinal cord to a muscle of the foot.

Familiarizing yourself with the structure of a neuron will aid in understanding the function of the neuron and the pathways of neural impulses.

The typical motor neuron (Fig. 3.1) includes a cell body, **dendrites** (which receive impulses and conduct them to the cell body), and an **axon** (which conducts the impulses away from the cell). The cell body of the motor neuron, which innervates skeletal muscle, lies in the gray matter in the ventral horn of the spinal cord; its axon joins many axons from other motor neurons (and many sensory axons) to form a spinal nerve. Such a nerve is thick enough to be seen in gross dissection. The motor neuron branches and rebranches into many twigs, each of which innervates one muscle fiber.

One characteristic of many neurons is the presence of **myelin**, which surrounds the axon as a

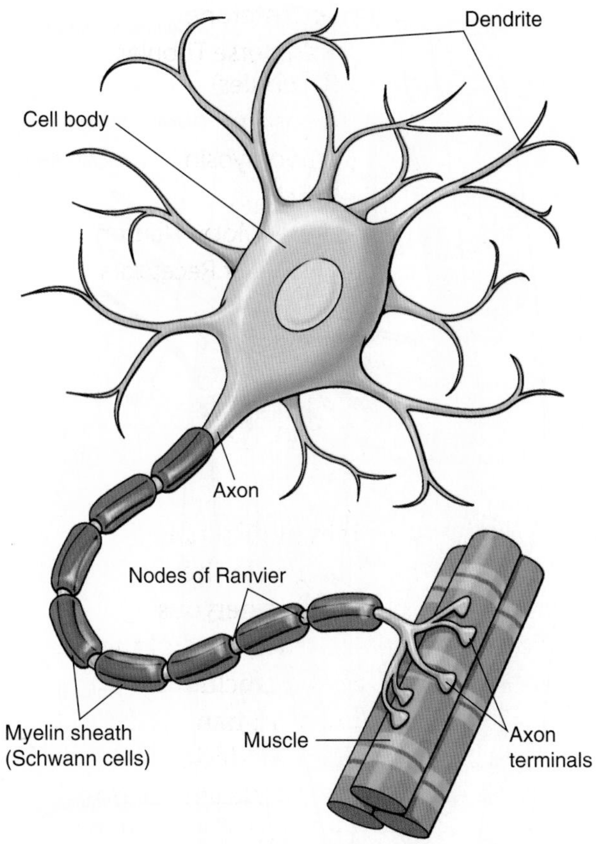

FIGURE 3.1 The neuron and its components. Each neuron consists of dendrites, a cell body, and an axon.

sheath. It is a fatty white substance produced by **Schwann cells** in the peripheral nervous system. The myelin sheath is laid down in segments along the length of the axon, resulting in gaps called **nodes of Ranvier**. In myelinated axons, the velocity whereby the action potential is conducted is increased because it jumps from one node of Ranvier to the next. This is called **saltatory conduction**. Generally speaking, the thicker the myelin sheaths around an axon, the greater the conduction velocity of an action potential.

Neurons conduct electrical impulses to and from the central nervous system.

REFLEXES AND INVOLUNTARY MOVEMENTS

A **reflex** is most simply defined as an involuntary motor response to a given stimulus. An illustration is the automatic, unthinking leg extension response when a physician taps the patellar tendon with a rubber mallet. In this simplest form, a reflex consists of a discharge from a sensory (afferent) nerve ending, with the impulses traveling over the sensory nerve fiber to a synapse in the spinal cord with a motor (efferent) neuron. When the motor neuron is stimulated to discharge, impulses travel over its axon to the muscle, causing it to move. This simple reflex arc is called the **myotatic** or stretch reflex; because it involves only one synapse in the spinal cord, it is called a **monosynaptic reflex**. Other more complex reflexes (such as removing the hand from a hot surface) can involve multiple neurons and synapses.

A reflex is an involuntary response to a given stimulus.

PROPRIOCEPTION AND KINESTHESIS

Optimal coordination of motor activity by the central nervous system depends on a constant supply of sensory feedback during the movement. This feedback of sensory information about movement and body position is called **proprioception**. The receptors for proprioception are of two types: vestibular and kinesthetic.

The **vestibular receptors** are found in the inner ear and respond to the movement of a fluid called **endolymph**. Indirectly, the inertia of the endolymph provides data to the brain regarding rotational acceleration or deceleration of movement, as in twisting or tumbling. Movement itself, however, is not recognized. For example, moving at almost the speed of sound in an airliner produces no sensation unless a change of direction or velocity occurs.

The vestibular system also includes an inner ear structure called the **utricle**, which provides data regarding positional sense. Specialized structures in the utricle respond to linear acceleration and tilting and thus are the source of data that inform us of our posture and orientation in space. For example, sensory information from the utricle is responsible for our ability to tell whether we are standing up or lying down, even with our eyes closed.

The kinesthetic or muscle sense is crucial to our ability to properly execute movement; it provides information about what our limbs or body segments are doing without our having to look. For example, most individuals have no difficulty touching their noses with their index fingers, even when blindfolded. Furthermore, one can usually make reasonably accurate guesses about the weight of an object by lifting it.

The two primary receptor structures that serve **kinesthesis** (sense of movement and body part location in space) are muscle spindles and Golgi tendon organs. Muscle spindles are large enough to be visible to the naked eye and are widely distributed throughout muscle tissue. Their distribution, however, varies from muscle to muscle. In general, muscles used for intricate movements (such as finger muscles) have many muscle spindles, while muscles involved primarily in gross movements have few.

Proprioceptors provide sensory feedback to the nervous system regarding the stretch and tension of skeletal muscle.

In humans, each spindle includes from five to nine **intrafusal (IF) muscle fibers**. These IF fibers should not be confused with skeletal (extrafusal [EF]) muscle fibers, which cause muscle contraction. The IF fibers of the muscle spindles are innervated by gamma motor neurons, while EF (skeletal) fibers are innervated by alpha motor neurons. Alpha motor neurons make up about 70% of the total efferent fibers; gamma motor neurons make up the remaining 30%. The structure of a muscle spindle is shown in Figure 3.2. It is important to note that the muscle spindles are oriented parallel to the EF fibers.

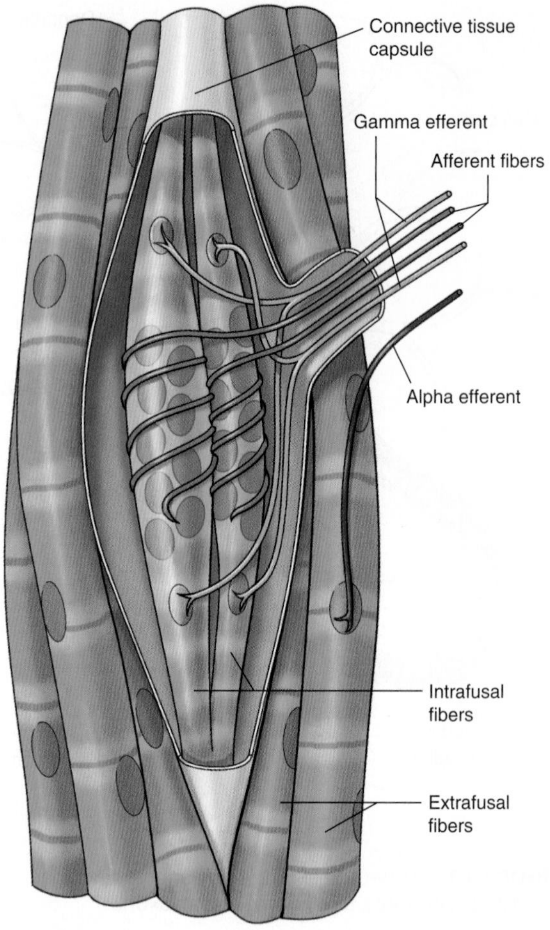

FIGURE 3.2 Muscle spindle. This sensory receptor is sensitive to stretch and helps to monitor muscle length.

Because IF fibers lie lengthwise, parallel with the skeletal (EF) fibers, an externally applied stretch results in stretching the IF as well as the EF fibers. Thus, stretching results in a sensory afferent discharge from the muscle spindles leading to contraction of the muscle that was stretched. This response underlies the stretch or myotatic reflex when a physician strikes the patellar tendon.

The Golgi tendon organ (Fig. 3.3) is found in the musculotendinous junction and lies in series with the EF (skeletal) muscle fibers. Therefore, active shortening of the muscle (contraction) causes the Golgi tendon organ to discharge, while the muscle spindle discharges only when the muscle is stretched. The muscle spindle ceases to fire when contraction begins because it is in parallel with the EF muscle fibers and is thus unloaded as soon as the EF fibers shorten in contraction.

The primary functional difference between the muscle spindle and the Golgi tendon organ is that the muscle spindle facilitates contraction, whereas the Golgi tendon organ inhibits contraction, not only in the muscle of origin but also in the entire functional muscle group. Thus, the Golgi tendon organ may provide a protective mechanism that prevents damage to muscle tissue or a joint during extreme contractions. The activity of the Golgi tendon organ that prevents overstressing the tissues is called the **inverse myotatic reflex**.

Proprioception involves sensory feedback about movement and body position. Kinesthesis is sometimes called muscle sense and involves the functions of muscle spindles and Golgi tendon organ.

HIGHER NERVE CENTERS AND VOLUNTARY MUSCULAR CONTROL

Voluntary muscular activity is controlled by three primary systems: the pyramidal system, the extrapyramidal system, and the proprioceptive–cerebellar system.

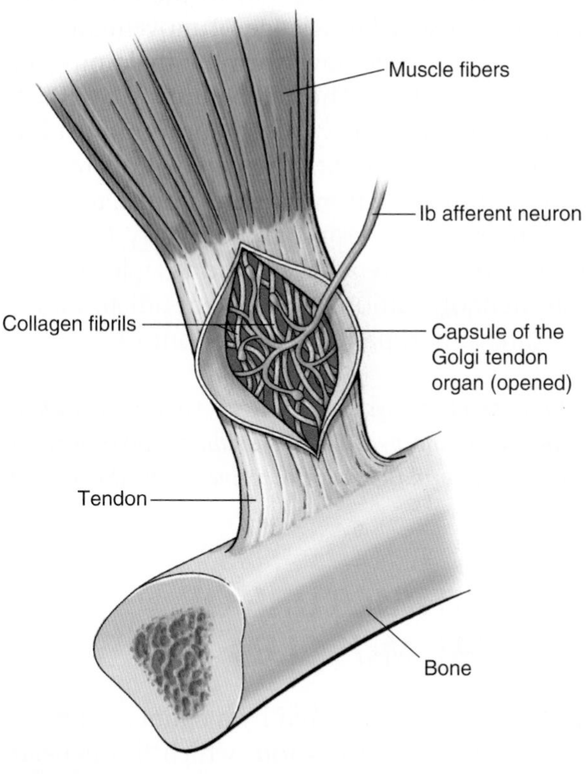

FIGURE 3.3 Golgi tendon organ. Located at the musculotendinous junction, this sensory receptor monitors tension.

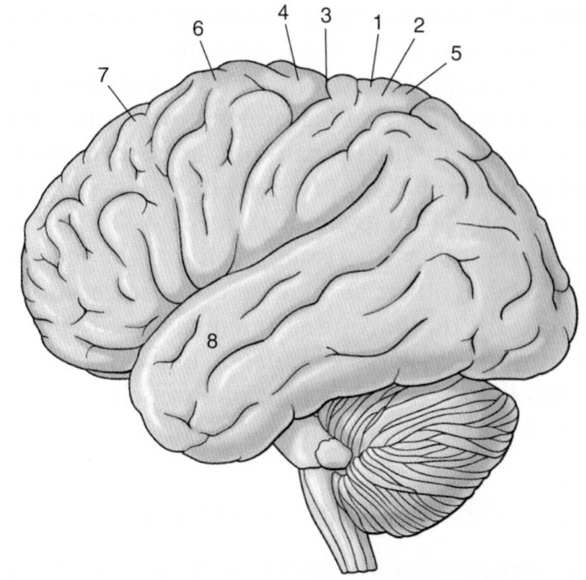

FIGURE 3.4 The areas of the human cerebral cortex involved in the pyramidal and extrapyramidal systems. The pyramidal system originates mainly in area *4* (motor cortex) of the brain and controls specific, voluntary movements. The extrapyramidal system (mainly area *6*, but also areas *1* to *3*, *5*, *7*, and *8*) is concerned with large, general movement patterns and posture control.

THE PYRAMIDAL SYSTEM

Electrical stimulation and clinical observations have been used to identify the functions of the various parts of the cerebral cortex. The most commonly used architectural map of the human cortex that relates location to function is that of Brodmann (Fig. 3.4).

The **pyramidal system** originates in large pyramid-shaped neurons found mainly in area 4, often called the motor cortex, of the Brodmann map. The axons of the motor neurons with cell bodies in area 4 form large descending motor pathways, called

REAL-WORLD APPLICATION

The Physiology of Stretching

It has been theorized that stretching can improve performance and prevent injury. It is also important, however, to consider how to stretch. Specifically, we must consider the effect of the muscle spindle on flexibility and stretching.

A muscle that is stretched rapidly with a jerky motion will respond by contracting. The magnitude and rate of this contraction vary directly with the magnitude and rate of the movement that causes the rapid stretch. This contraction is a result of the myotatic or stretch reflex. The rapidly applied stretch causes activation of the muscle spindles located between the skeletal (EF) muscle fibers. This rapid stretch causes an afferent impulse to be carried by a sensory neuron to the spinal cord, where the neuron synapses with a motor neuron. The motor neuron then carries an impulse back to the skeletal muscle, causing it to contract. The important point is that if, in an attempt to stretch the muscle, the stretch is applied with a bouncing, jerky motion, the result is activation of the myotatic reflex. This causes a contraction of the very muscle that is the object of the attempted stretch. This can lead to less than optimal stretching at best and injury at worst.

Static stretching, on the other hand, in which the stretch is applied slowly, does not invoke the myotatic reflex. By moving slowly into the stretched position, activation of the muscle spindles is avoided. This allows the muscle to relax while being elongated, leading to a more effective stretch.

pyramidal tracts, that go directly (in most cases) to synapses with the motor neurons in the ventral horn of the spinal cord. The neurons with cell bodies in the brain are called **upper motor neurons**, while those in the spinal cord are called **lower motor neurons**. Approximately 85% or more of the neurons of the pyramidal tract cross from one side to the other (decussate), some at the level of the medulla, others at the level of the lower motor neuron. The motor cortex is oriented by movement, not by muscle. That is, stimulation of the motor cortex results not in a twitch of one muscle but in a smooth synergistic movement of a group of muscles.

THE EXTRAPYRAMIDAL SYSTEM

The **extrapyramidal system**, or the premotor cortex, originates primarily in area 6 of Brodmann's area. Some of the fibers descending in the extrapyramidal tracts, however, originate in other areas of the cortex, such as areas 1, 2, 3, 5, and 8.

The descending tracts from the premotor cortex are more complex than those from the motor cortex. These neurons do not synapse directly with the lower motor neurons but travel through relay stations called **motor nuclei**. The most important motor nuclei are the **corpus striatum**, **substantia nigra**, and **red nucleus**. Some neurons, however, also go by way of the pons to the cerebellum.

Important functional differences exist between the pyramidal and extrapyramidal systems. For example, electrical stimulation of area 4 produces specific movements, while stimulation of area 6 produces only gross movement patterns. Thus, it is likely that learning a new skill in which conscious attention must be devoted to the movements (as in learning a new gymnastic move, where every aspect of the movement is contemplated) involves area 4. As an individual becomes more skilled, the origin of the movement is thought to shift to area 6 (often, gymnasts do not have to concentrate on their feet but rather on very general patterns of movement). Area 4, however, still participates as a relay station, with fibers connecting area 6 to area 4.

THE PROPRIOCEPTIVE–CEREBELLAR SYSTEM

Kinesthesis and the vestibular system involve the sensory functions of the **proprioceptive–cerebellar system**. Typically, the pathway associated with vestibular proprioception leads directly or indirectly (via the medulla) to the cerebellum. Conscious sensory knowledge of movement from kinesthesis, however, travels via the thalamus, cortex, and cerebellum. The cerebellum is central to the gathering of sensory information on position, balance, and movement. The cerebellum receives sensory information from muscles, joints, tendons, and skin as well as visual and auditory feedback. Thus, the loss of cerebellar function can lead to the impairment of volitional movements, disturbances of posture, and impaired balance control.

Three primary systems control voluntary human movement: the pyramidal system, the extrapyramidal system, and the proprioceptive–cerebellar system.

GROSS STRUCTURE OF SKELETAL MUSCLE

A skeletal muscle is covered by a connective tissue sheath called the **epimysium**, which lies beneath the skin, subcutaneous adipose tissue, and superficial fascia. The epimysium merges with the connective tissue of the tendon, which allows the force produced by muscular contraction to be transmitted through the connective tissues to the tendon and bone, resulting in movement.

Skeletal muscle cells or muscle fibers are oriented in bundles called fasciculi. Each fasciculus, which contains from a few muscle fibers to several hundred, is surrounded by a connective tissue sheath called the perimysium. Figure 3.5 illustrates these and other gross and microscopic structures of skeletal muscle.

The gross structures of skeletal muscle are important for transducing the force of muscular contraction to the tendon and bone, resulting in movement.

MICROSCOPIC STRUCTURE OF SKELETAL MUSCLE

Surrounding each muscle fiber is a delicate connective tissue sheath known as the **endomysium**. Thus, the endomysium surrounds a single fiber, the perimysium surrounds a fasciculus, and the epimysium surrounds the whole muscle. The force produced within a muscle fiber is transferred in series

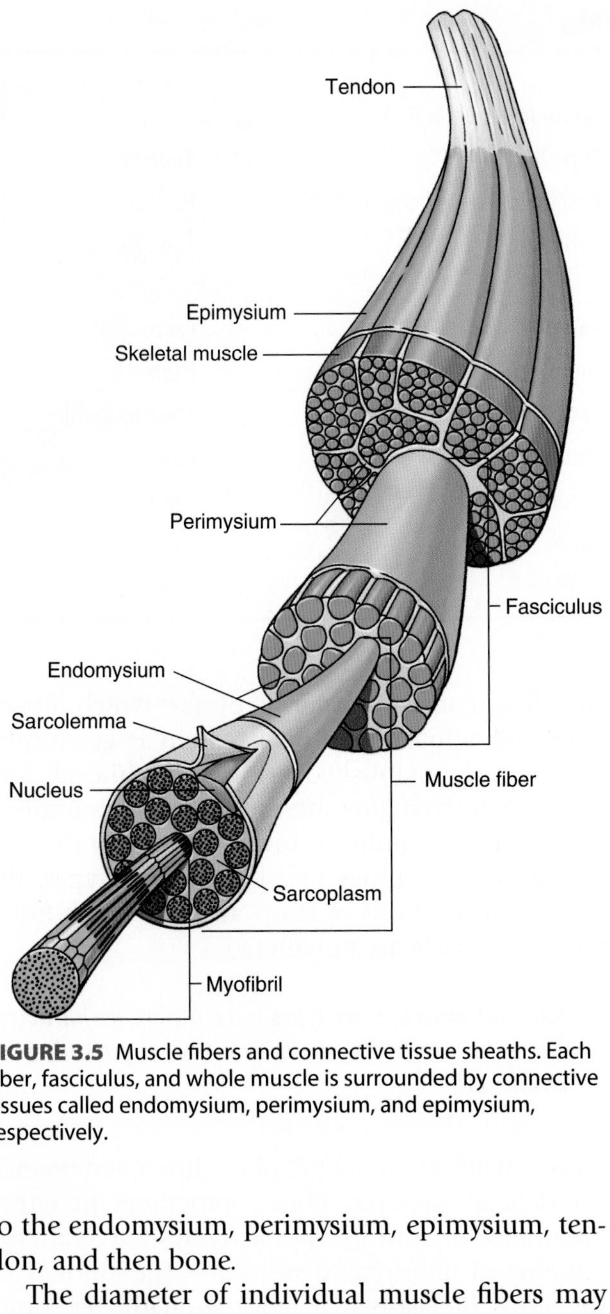

FIGURE 3.5 Muscle fibers and connective tissue sheaths. Each fiber, fasciculus, and whole muscle is surrounded by connective tissues called endomysium, perimysium, and epimysium, respectively.

to the endomysium, perimysium, epimysium, tendon, and then bone.

The diameter of individual muscle fibers may vary from approximately 10 to 100 µm (1,000 µm = 1 mm), while the length may range from 1 mm to the length of the whole muscle. The thickness of the fiber is related to the amount of force that the fiber can produce, and each muscle has fibers of characteristic size. For example, the eye muscles have fibers with a small diameter, while the fibers of the quadriceps femoris muscles are large.

STRUCTURE OF THE MUSCLE FIBER

Each skeletal muscle fiber is surrounded by a cell membrane known as the **sarcolemma**. Situated just inside the sarcolemma are many nuclei, which direct protein synthesis within the cell. The fluid part, or cytoplasm, of the muscle cell is known as the **sarcoplasm**. Much of the sarcoplasm is occupied by column-like structures known as myofibrils. Alternating light and dark bands run the length of the myofibrils. The strict alignment of these bands from one myofibril to another is what gives the muscle fiber its characteristic striated appearance under the light microscope.

Muscle fibers may vary greatly in size and length yet have the same structures (i.e., cell membrane, cytoplasm) as other cells in the body.

MUSCLE FIBER TYPES

In the past, muscle fibers were classified based simply on their appearance. Red fibers were considered to be well suited for endurance activities, such as those involving long-term contractions.. White fibers, however, were considered to be specialized for speed of contraction yet susceptible to fatigue. Recently, the identification of types of skeletal muscle fiber through the use of histochemical techniques has made it possible to examine the chemical constituents of these fibers, thereby providing the means for correlating their structure and function.

Two to as many as eight different muscle fiber types have been identified. The nomenclature for describing the various fiber types has been based on their appearance, function, biochemical properties, and histochemical properties. The older fast-twitch (white) versus slow-twitch (red) fiber-type classification system has become inadequate, since there are two subtypes of fast-twitch fibers that are physiologically and histochemically different. Thus, the new nomenclature (proposed by Peter et al.) (1) for three different muscle fiber types is based on the function and biochemical properties of the fiber.

The three primary fiber types in human skeletal muscle are slow oxidative (SO), fast oxidative glycolytic (FOG), and fast glycolytic (FG) (1). These fiber types are also identified as type I, type IIA, and type IIB, respectively, by Dubowitz and Brooke (2). The former nomenclature, however, is more descriptive, since it provides information about the characteristics and functioning of the various fiber types. For example, SO fibers have a slow twitch speed and favor oxidative (aerobic) energy production, while FG fibers have a fast twitch speed and favor

TABLE 3.1 ● CHARACTERISTICS OF MUSCLE FIBER TYPES

NOMENCLATURE			
Older systems	Red slow-twitch (ST)	White fast-twitch (FT)	
Dubowitz and Brooke (2)	Type I	Type IIA	Type IIB
Peter et al. (1)	Slow, oxidative (SO)	Fast, oxidative glycolytic (FOG)	Fast, glycolytic (FG)
MHC content	Type I	Type IIA	Type IIX
CHARACTERISTICS			
Speed of contraction	Slow	Fast	Fast
Strength of contraction	Low	High	High
Fatigability	Fatigue resistant	Fatigable	Most fatigable
Aerobic capacity	High	Medium	Low
Anaerobic capacity	Low	Medium	High
Size	Small	Large	Large
Capillary density	High	High	Low

glycolytic (anaerobic) energy production. Table 3.1 compares the naming systems and lists the characteristics of muscle fiber types.

Developments in gel electrophoresis techniques have now allowed researchers to classify muscle fibers based on their myosin heavy chain (MHC) isoform content. The results from this fiber type classification system have been shown to be similar to those from traditional histochemistry techniques (3). However, the MHC isoform content of a muscle fiber has been shown to be important for determining its performance in strength/power activities (4). These techniques have led to the discovery that in humans, fibers typed as IIB based on histochemistry are typed as IIX based on MHC content. Thus, a more contemporary fiber classification scheme in humans is type I, IIA, and IIX.

The basic functional unit of the neuromuscular system is the **motor unit**, which consists of a motor neuron (nerve) and all the muscle fibers that it innervates. All of the fibers within a particular motor unit are of the same type, although the fibers from different motor units are intermingled. In small muscles, a single motor unit may consist of only a few fibers; in large muscles, each motor unit may comprise several hundred fibers.

The patterns of fiber-type distribution in the various muscles are related to the function(s) of the muscle. For example, postural muscles must be fatigue resistant and therefore are usually composed mainly of SO fibers. The ocular muscles, however, do not contract for extended periods and therefore consist primarily of fast-twitch fibers. Each individual's fiber-type pattern is genetically determined, established prior to adulthood, and probably unchanging thereafter. Although training may result in significant improvements in the performance capabilities of all three fiber types, the relative proportions of slow- and fast-twitch fibers within a muscle are not altered.

Skeletal muscle fiber types have different characteristics that are utilized under different physiological situations.

Different athletic activities place different demands on skeletal muscles. Elite competitors in either endurance or sprint/power activities have extreme patterns of fiber-type distribution (i.e., mostly of the slow- or fast-twitch type). Nonathletes, however, usually have a fairly even pattern of fiber-type distribution.

STRUCTURE OF THE MYOFIBRIL AND THE CONTRACTILE MECHANISM

The **sarcomere** is the functional unit of the myofibril (Fig. 3.6). It extends from one **Z line** to an adjacent Z line. The sarcomere comprises two **myofilaments** (contractile proteins), **myosin**, and **actin**, which lie parallel to one another. The myosin filament is approximately twice as thick as the actin

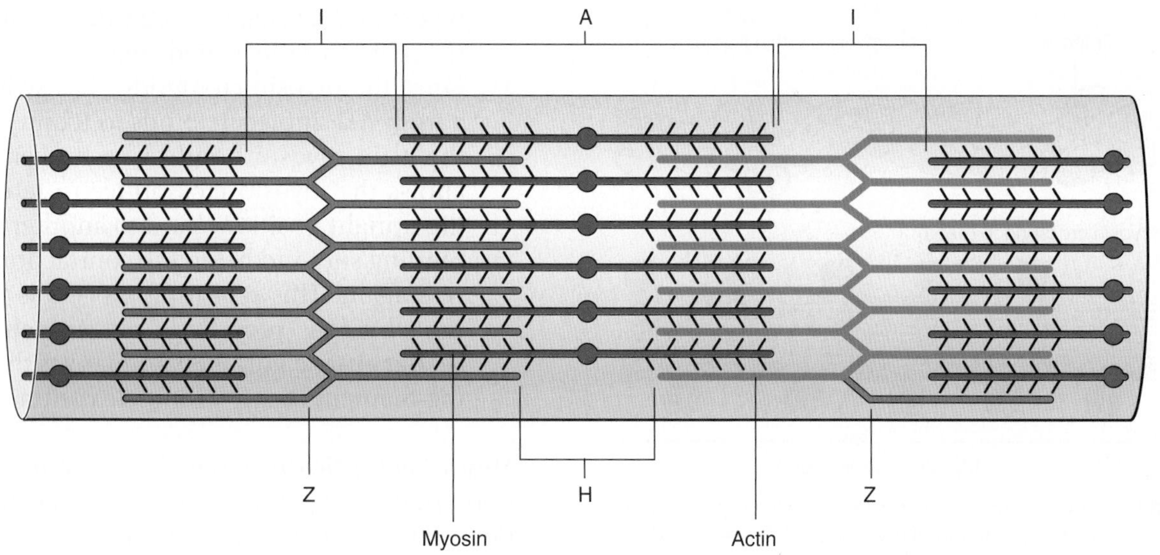

FIGURE 3.6 A sarcomere extends from Z line to Z line. The sarcomere is the functional unit of the myofibril.

filament and defines the length of the **A band**. It is the A band that forms the dark part of the striation effect. The actin filaments are longer than the myosin filaments and extend inward from the Z lines toward the center of the sarcomere. Within the A band is a lighter region known as the **H zone**, the area of the A band that does not contain actin filaments. The **I band** is the area between the ends of the myosin filaments. Because it is less dense than the A band, the I band is also lighter in color. These alternating areas of greater and lesser optical density are what give skeletal muscle its characteristic "striped" or "striated" appearance.

Understanding the sliding filament theory can help you understand the synchronization between the neural and muscular systems in both muscle action and muscle relaxation.

THE SLIDING-FILAMENT THEORY OF MUSCLE CONTRACTION

The **sliding-filament theory** has been used to describe the mechanics of muscle contraction. It states the following

1. Voluntary muscle contraction is initiated in the cortex of the brain.
2. Typically, the electrical current, or **action potential**, travels via an upper **motor neuron** and synapses with a lower motor neuron in the ventral horn of the spinal cord.
3. The action potential passes along to the end of a lower motor neuron (**end bulb**) and causes the release of the stimulatory neurotransmitter **acetylcholine (ACh)**. The intersection between a lower motor neuron and a muscle fiber is called the **myoneural junction or neuromuscular junction**.
4. The ACh is released into a small gap between the motor neuron and the muscle fiber called the **synapse**. The ACh then binds to receptor sites on the muscle fiber membrane at a location called the **motor endplate**.
5. The binding of ACh with the receptors at the motor endplate causes an action potential to spread along the muscle fiber's sarcolemma.
6. The action potential travels along the sarcolemma and down channels that lead into the muscle fiber, called **transverse tubules or t tubules**.
7. The action potential travels down the t tubules and intersects an intracellular structure called the **sarcoplasmic reticulum (SR)** . One function of the SR is to store calcium. When stimulated by the action potential, the SR releases calcium into the fiber's sarcoplasm.
8. The calcium binds to a protein called **troponin**, which is bound to another protein

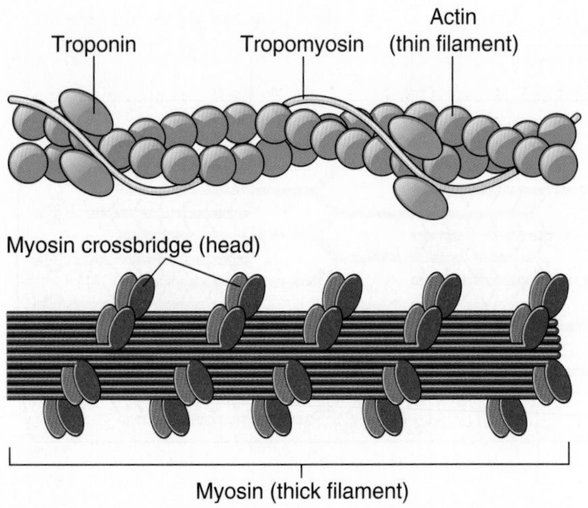

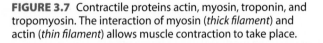

FIGURE 3.7 Contractile proteins actin, myosin, troponin, and tropomyosin. The interaction of myosin (*thick filament*) and actin (*thin filament*) allows muscle contraction to take place.

called **tropomyosin**. Under resting conditions, the contractile proteins actin and myosin are separated by the presence of tropomyosin. The binding of calcium to troponin changes the shape of the tropomyosin molecule and uncovers the binding sites on the actin molecule. Figure 3.7 illustrates these contractile proteins.

9. The **myosin crossbridge**, or myosin head, then binds with the binding site on the actin molecule.
10. The breakdown of **adenosine triphosphate (ATP)** to **adenosine diphosphate (ADP)** is required for muscular contraction. Multiple theories have been put forward regarding the way in which the energy liberated from the breakdown of ATP contributes to muscular contraction (5). The traditional sliding-filament theory indicates that the binding of the actin and myosin filaments activates an enzyme called **myosin ATPase**, which breaks down an ATP molecule bound to the myosin crossbridge. The breakdown of ATP liberates energy that causes the myosin crossbridge to swivel toward the center of the sarcomere. As the myosin molecule swivels, it pulls the actin molecules and Z lines of the sarcomere together. This causes a shortening of the sarcomere, or muscular contraction. More recent evidence suggests that even when the muscle is in a rested state, the myosin head stores the energy from ATP breakdown. This suggests that it is the binding of the myosin crossbridge to actin that allows for the release of this stored energy.
11. Once the myosin crossbridge has swiveled, a fresh ATP molecule binds to it and causes the actin/myosin bond to be broken. This allows the myosin crossbridge to return to the upright position, bind to another actin-binding site, and begin the contraction process again. This repeating process is called **crossbridge recycling or crossbridge recharging**. Figure 3.8 summarizes the sliding-filament theory of muscle contraction.

Muscle contraction is initiated by the central nervous system and generated at the molecular level through interaction of the contractile proteins actin and myosin.

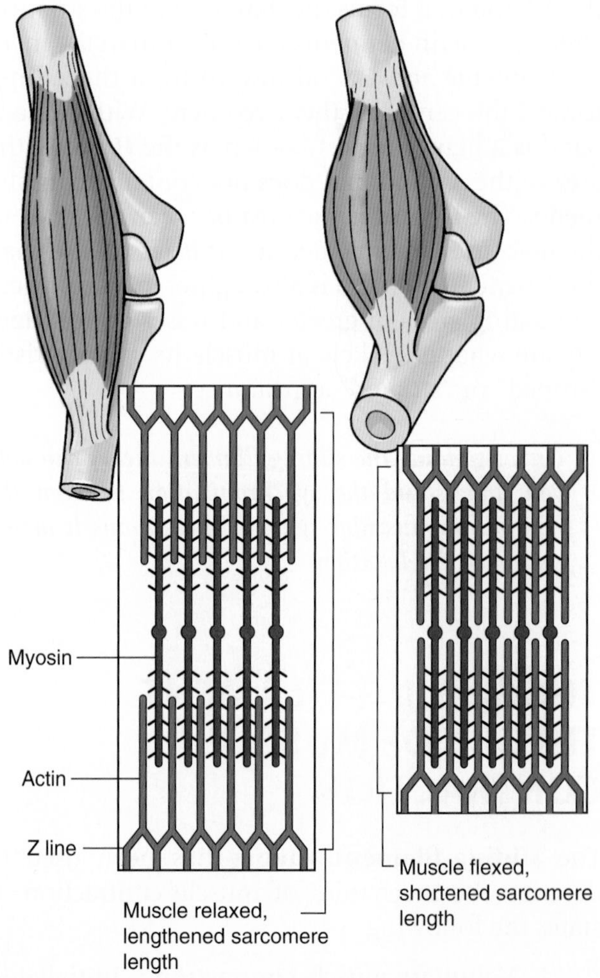

FIGURE 3.8 The sliding-filament theory of muscle contraction. This theory proposes that the filaments slide past each other during muscle contraction without themselves changing in length.

GRADATION OF FORCE

The central nervous system controls the gradation of muscular force by varying the number of motor units activated, or motor unit **recruitment**, and by increasing or decreasing the firing frequency of the active motor units, or **rate coding** (Fig. 3.9). The recruitment of motor units generally follows what is called the **size principle**, according to which increasingly forceful contractions are achieved by the recruitment of progressively larger motor units. Smaller motor units are typically composed of SO fibers and have the lowest stimulus thresholds for contraction. Thus, smaller motor units are active during low-intensity contractions. Increasingly forceful contractions, however, require the recruitment of larger motor units containing fast-twitch fibers. In addition, active motor units can produce greater force by firing at higher frequencies (rate coding). The relative contributions of recruitment or rate coding to increasing force production vary from muscle to muscle. In general, large muscles with mixed fiber types, such as the quadriceps, tend to rely on recruitment to a greater degree than do small muscles, such as those in the finger, which rely more on rate coding.

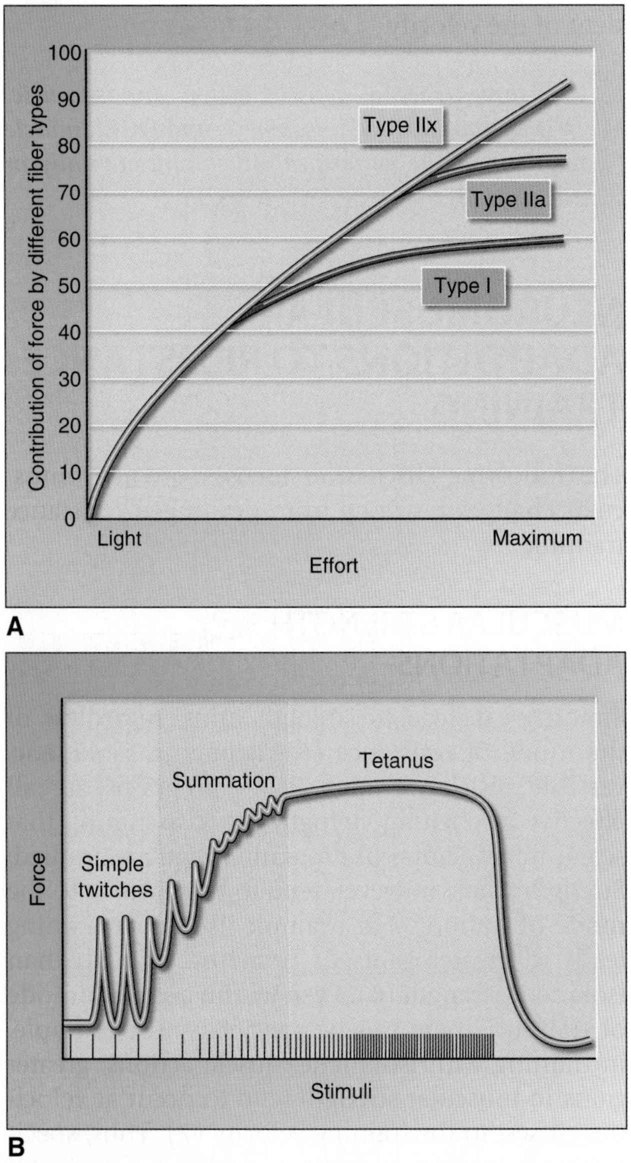

FIGURE 3.9 Contributions of **(A)** motor unit recruitment and **(B)** firing rate to force production. The nervous system uses these two methods to vary the force production of whole muscles.

Muscle force is modulated through two mechanisms: motor unit recruitment and rate coding. The relative contributions of these two mechanisms to force production vary in different muscles.

TYPES OF MUSCLE ACTIONS

The term *muscle contraction* implies muscle shortening. Muscles, however, can produce force while shortening, lengthening, or maintaining a given length. The term *muscle action* is therefore more accurate and descriptive. Muscle action types include isometric, dynamic constant external resistance (DCER), isokinetic, concentric, and eccentric muscle actions.

ISOMETRIC MUSCLE ACTIONS

Isometric muscle actions involve production of force without movement at the joint or shortening of the muscle fibers. Very few athletic activities involve isometric muscle actions; thus, isometric strength does not predict success in sporting activities very well. Isometric strength is also joint angle–specific owing to varying degrees of overlap of the actin and myosin filaments as well as biomechanical factors. In comparing isometric strength between individuals, the joint angle at which the isometric muscle action is performed is an important consideration.

DYNAMIC CONSTANT EXTERNAL RESISTANCE MUSCLE ACTIONS

The muscle actions that occur during the lifting of free weights have traditionally been referred to as isotonic muscle actions. During such an action, a muscle generates a constant amount of force throughout a range of motion. Force production by a muscle, however, rarely remains constant as the joint angle changes. Thus, the term **dynamic constant external resistance (DCER)** muscle actions more accurately describes the muscle actions occurring during this type of movement. Although the weight being lifted remains constant (constant external resistance) with changes in the joint angle, the force produced by the muscle is changing, or dynamic.

DCER strength is usually expressed in terms of a **repetition maximum (RM)** load. An RM load is the maximum amount of weight that can be lifted for a specified number of repetitions. For example, a 1-RM load is the maximum amount of weight that can be lifted through the full range of motion for only one repetition, whereas a 6-RM load is the maximum amount of weight that can be lifted for six repetitions but not seven. Typically, DCER strength testing involves a trial-and-error procedure where progressively heavier weights are attempted until the 1-RM is determined. Because strength is joint angle–specific, DCER strength is limited by the weakest point in the range of motion; therefore, the 1-RM load is the maximum weight that can be lifted at the weakest point in the range of motion.

ISOKINETIC MUSCLE ACTIONS

An **isokinetic muscle action** is a dynamic movement that occurs at a constant velocity. Typically, isokinetic muscle actions are performed on a dynamometer, a device that accommodates the counterresistance based on the amount of torque being produced. This allows movement to occur at a constant velocity regardless of torque production. Isokinetic strength testing has advantages over both isometric and DCER testing because, during a maximal isokinetic muscle action, maximum torque (**peak torque**) is produced throughout the entire range of motion.

CONCENTRIC AND ECCENTRIC MUSCLE ACTIONS

A **concentric muscle action** occurs when a muscle produces torque (technically, the muscle produces force, resulting in torque around the joint) and shortens. When a muscle lengthens while producing torque, it is performing an **eccentric muscle action**. Both DCER and isokinetic muscle actions can be performed concentrically and eccentrically (Fig. 3.10). The force produced concentrically decreases as velocity increases. When the velocity of a concentric muscle action is low, both slow- and fast-twitch fibers contribute to force production; at higher velocities, the rate of muscle shortening is too great for the slow-twitch fibers to contribute to torque production. Because the slow-twitch fibers are "unloaded" at high velocities, fewer muscle fibers contribute to torque production; therefore, torque is decreased. On the other hand, eccentric strength changes little with increased velocity. During eccentric muscle actions, the myosin cross-bridges are pulled apart from the actin molecules. In theory, the amount of force necessary to pull the myosin heads from the actin molecules is independent of the velocity.

The three types of muscle action are isometric, DCER, and isokinetic. Isokinetic and DCER muscle actions may be performed either concentrically or eccentrically.

NEUROMUSCULAR ADAPTATIONS TO RESISTANCE TRAINING

The following discussion focuses on neuromuscular changes resulting from prolonged resistance training.

MUSCULAR STRENGTH ADAPTATIONS

Training can lead to strength gains, regardless of the mode of resistance (6). Isometric, isokinetic, variable resistance, and DCER programs are all effective at eliciting strength gains, assuming that scientific principles of program design are applied. Strength gains, however, tend to be sensitive to the mode of training. For example, isometric training leads to greater gains in isometric strength than isokinetic strength (6). Even within a specific mode of training, there can be specificity. For example, in training with isokinetic muscle actions, greater gains in muscular strength tend to occur at velocities closest to the training velocity (7). Thus, specificity of training must be considered if the goal of a resistance-training program is to transfer the newly developed strength to other activities, such as sport, recreational, or occupational pursuits.

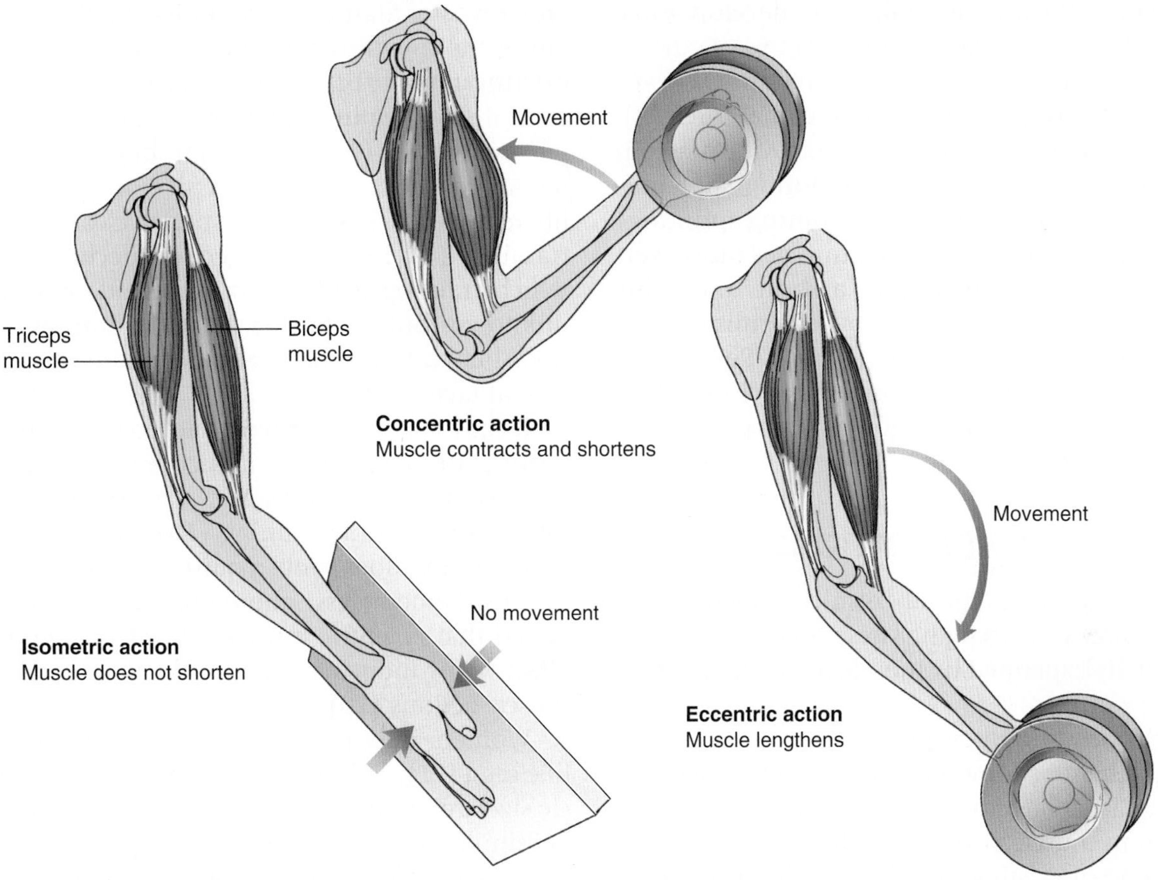

FIGURE 3.10 Types of muscle actions. Muscle may produce force while shortening, lengthening, or maintaining a constant length.

Strength gains resulting from resistance training tend to be specific to the type of training performed.

In terms of the absolute weight lifted, men tend to be stronger than women. This is because men are usually bigger and have more muscle mass. Women tend to be about 40% to 50% as strong as men in upper body movements and 50% to 80% as strong in lower body movements (6). When strength is expressed relative to muscle cross-sectional area, however, there are no sex-related differences in muscular strength (8) (Fig. 3.11). Thus, for a given amount of muscle, men and women produce the same amount of force.

The quality of muscle is the same for men and women. In addition, men and women respond to resistance training in a similar manner.

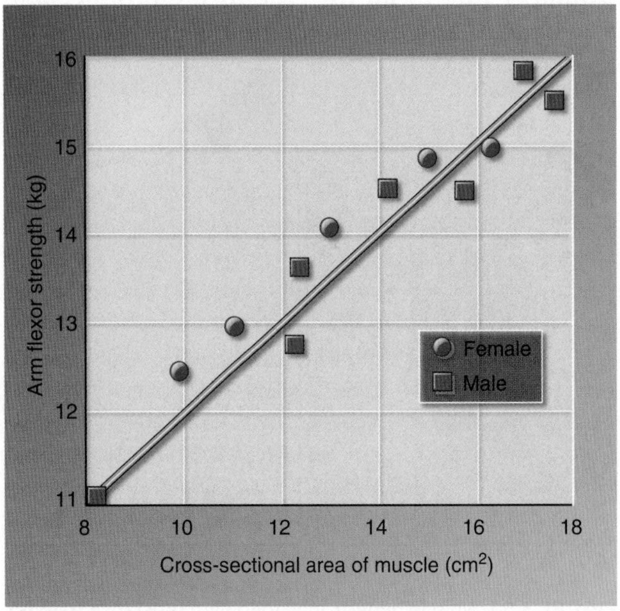

FIGURE 3.11 Muscle strength per unit of cross-sectional area of human muscle. There is no qualitative difference in strength per unit of muscle size between the genders.

For many athletes, the ability to develop force rapidly is as important, if not more so, as developing maximal force. It usually takes in excess of 0.3 to 0.4 seconds to generate maximal force (9). Because time is limited during many sport activities (i.e., 0.22 to 0.27 seconds during shot putting and 0.101 to 0.108 seconds during sprinting) (10,11), however, the activated muscles must exert as much force as possible in a short time. This capability can be measured by determining the **rate of force development (RFD)** . Performing "power" or "explosive" training exercises (plyometrics, cleans, pulls, weighted jumps, etc.) can increase the RFD (12).

MUSCLE FIBER ADAPTATIONS

Resistance training typically results in increases in muscle size and strength. These adaptations may be partially explained by muscle fiber adaptations.

Hypertrophy and Hyperplasia

Perhaps the most obvious adaptation to resistance training is enlargement of the trained muscles. Growth in muscle size can result from an increase in the size of existing muscle fiber (**hypertrophy**) or an increase in the number of muscle fibers (**hyperplasia**).

Substantial evidence supports muscle fiber hypertrophy as the primary mechanism of increasing muscle size (13) (Fig. 3.12). This increase is primarily due to an increase in the number and size of actin and myosin filaments (14). The actin and myosin filaments are added to the periphery of the myofibrils, resulting in enlargement of existing myofibrils. Once the myofibril reaches a critical size, it splits, yielding two or more daughter myofibrils (14). Although both slow- and fast-twitch fibers increase in size, the fast-twitch fibers appear to be more responsive to resistance training (14,15). The precise mechanism by which training leads to muscular adaptations is unknown, but it appears to be a complex interplay between mechanical, metabolic, and hormonal factors (16–18).

It has been suggested that eccentric muscle actions are necessary to induce muscle hypertrophy. Hypertrophy, however, can occur following concentric-only training (19), suggesting that hypertrophy does not require eccentric muscle actions. Nonetheless, numerous studies have suggested that eccentric muscle actions may be more effective for inducing hypertrophy than concentric muscle actions (20).

Women respond to resistance training much like men (21). Although the absolute gains in muscle size are greater in men, the percentage increases are similar for the two sexes (22,23).

Evidence from studies of laboratory animals suggests that hyperplasia may contribute to resistance training–induced increases in muscle size (24,25). Although there is some conflicting information (26), the general consensus in humans is that hypertrophy accounts for the training-induced increase in muscle size and that hyperplasia is probably of little or no significance (6).

Hypertrophy is the primary mechanism by which muscles increase in size.

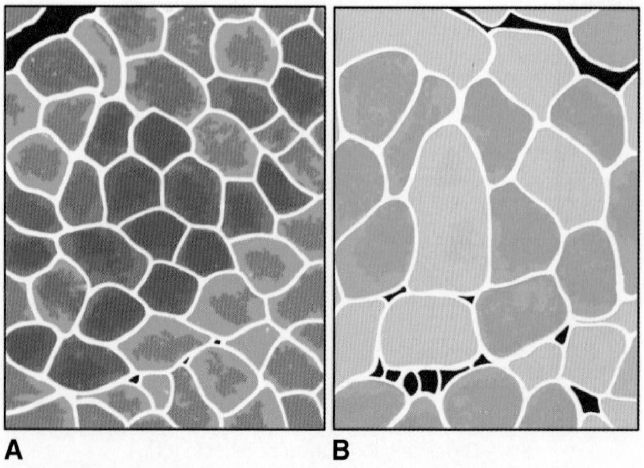

FIGURE 3.12 Muscle hypertrophy following resistance training. **A.** Before training. **B.** After training. Hypertrophy results from an increased content of contractile protein (actin and myosin) in muscle.

Muscle Fiber Transformation

The possibility that training can alter muscle fiber types has intrigued exercise scientists and resistance-training practitioners for years. The transformation of a type I (SO) fiber to a type II (FOG or FG) fiber, or vice versa, has obvious implications for strength and power performance. To date, the evidence suggests that heavy resistance training can transform only muscle fibers within a given muscle fiber type, that is, from type IIX to IIA (15,27). Transformation of type IIX to type IIA fibers occurs rapidly with heavy resistance training (28). The functional implication of this transformation, however, is unclear.

Q & A from the Field

Q ***The head coach of our women's volleyball team is hesitant to implement a resistance-training program for our team. He doesn't believe that female athletes can gain strength and muscle size, like male athletes can. My previous experience is with conditioning male athletes. Is it true that females are less trainable than males when it comes to resistance training?***

—Undergraduate student intern

A There is every reason to believe that female athletes will adapt to resistance training in a manner similar to male athletes. The typical female athlete will be smaller, weaker, and have less muscle mass than her male counterpart. Her gains in size and strength will also be less than those of the male if expressed on an absolute basis, that is, weight lifted in pounds. When size and strength gains are expressed as a percentage increase relative to initial values, however, the female will experience gains that are comparable to those of her male counterpart. Female muscle is of the same quality as that of male muscle and is just as trainable.

NERVOUS SYSTEM ADAPTATIONS

Although muscles produce force, it is the nervous system that provides for the activation of muscle tissue. It is not surprising, therefore, that resistance-training programs lead to adaptations in both the nervous and muscular systems.

Evidence of Neural Adaptations

Several pieces of evidence point to the role of **neural adaptations** in resistance training. For example, increases in muscular strength may occur without accompanying increases in muscular size (29). If there is no increase in the size of the muscle fibers producing force, the logical conclusion is that adaptations within the nervous system are responsible for the observed strength gains.

It has been shown that the early gains in strength following initiation of a resistance-training program often occur in the absence of muscle hypertrophy (30). Previously untrained subjects may have difficulty in fully activating their motor units, and strength gains resulting from the first several weeks of resistance training have been attributed to learning to recruit those units (30). Although neural adaptations are often associated with the early phase of resistance training (30), one study found that 2 years of training led to significant increases in strength and power despite minimal changes in muscle fiber size in competitive Olympic weight lifters (29). Weight lifters compete within body-weight categories and often want to develop increased strength without changes in muscle mass that might lead to changes in body weight (6). Thus, neural adaptations are an essential mechanism of strength increase among these athletes.

Early gains in strength are due to neural factors, while long-term gains in strength are primarily due to hypertrophy.

Performing resistance training with one limb can lead to strength increases in the untrained limb on the opposite (contralateral) side of the body (31–33). This phenomenon is known as the **cross-education or cross-training** effect. The strength gain in the untrained limb is typically equal to or <60% of that in the trained limb (33). The cross-education effect demonstrates specificity of training. For example, unilateral resistance training for one leg will increase the strength of the contralateral leg but not the contralateral arm. There is also specificity with regard to muscle action type. Training with concentric muscle actions leads to greater gains in the untrained limb when tested concentrically than eccentrically (33). Theories to explain this cross-education effect include (a) neural activation of the corresponding muscles on both sides of the body, (b) activation of muscle of the contralateral limb to maintain stability during unilateral muscle actions, or (c) some unidentified spinal mechanism (33).

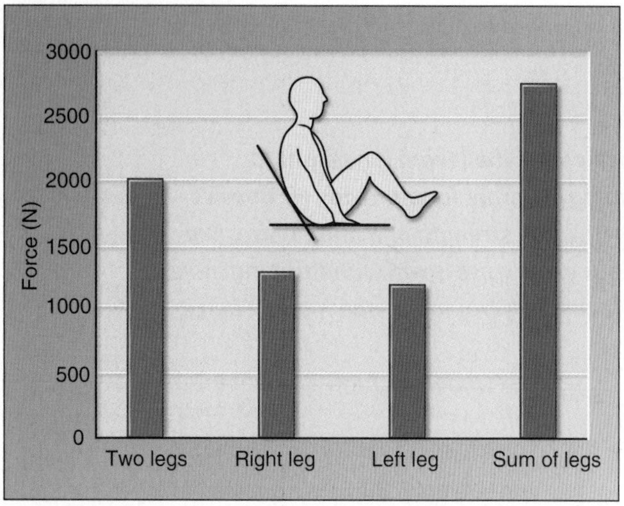

FIGURE 3.13 The bilateral deficit, showing that the bilateral force (two legs) is less than the sum of the left and right legs acting separately (sum of legs).

Force measured with both limbs concurrently (bilaterally) is typically less than the sum of the force developed by each limb independently (unilaterally) (34) (Fig. 3.13). This **bilateral deficit** may be the result of less activation to each muscle group during bilateral activation than to either muscle group activated maximally alone (35). This suggests that there is an inhibitory mechanism that limits maximal activation during bilateral muscle actions. Training with bilateral muscle actions reduces the bilateral deficit, bringing bilateral force production close to the sum of unilateral force production (36).

Cross education and the reduction of the bilateral deficit provide evidence of neural adaptations to resistance training.

Electromyographic Evidence of Neural Adaptations

Electromyography (EMG) records and quantifies the electrical activity in the muscle fibers of activated motor units (37) (Fig. 3.14). It reflects the number of motor units activated and their firing rates (37). Typically, isometric muscle actions are characterized by linear or curvilinear increases

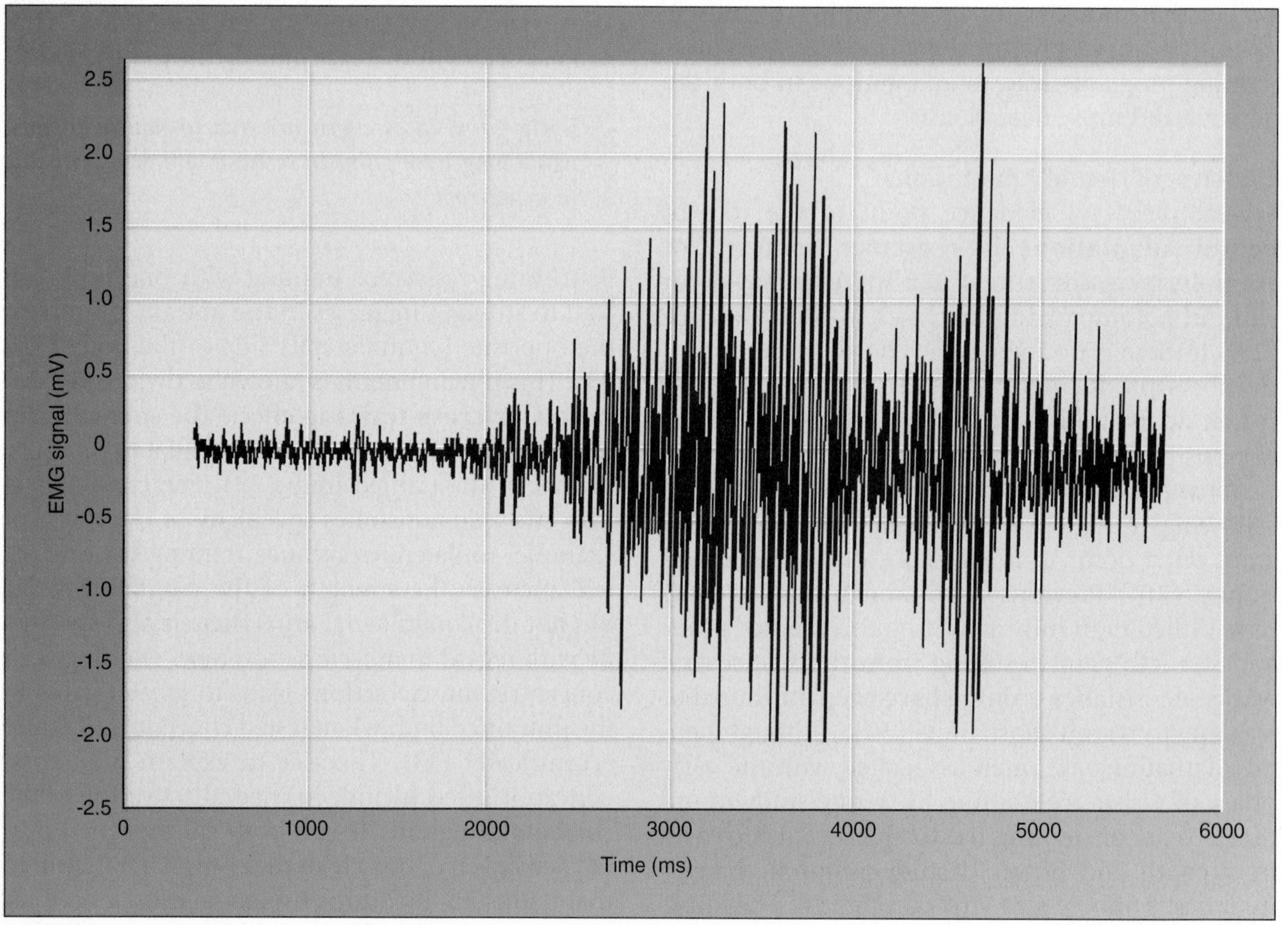

FIGURE 3.14 Raw EMG signal. EMG is the recording of muscle action potentials.

in EMG amplitude with torque (or force) (38). Therefore, an increase in maximal EMG activity would reflect an increase in motor unit activation (a neural adaptation). The increase in EMG activity may result from increased numbers of active motor units (i.e., high-threshold motor units), increased motor unit firing rates, or motor unit synchronization.

Numerous investigations have shown increases in EMG activity as a result of resistance training (39–41). Untrained individuals (those unfamiliar with a resistance training exercise) may not be able to recruit the highest-threshold motor units (types IIA and IIB) (39). This is indicative of an inability to fully activate the agonist muscle(s). An increase in the ability to recruit these high-threshold motor units can increase the expression of muscular strength. For example, type IIB motor units make up only about 5% of the total number of motor units of the triceps brachii, but these units contain approximately 20% of the total number of muscle fibers (37).

Increasing the firing rate of motor units can also affect the force produced by activated motor units. Motor units can increase their force 10-fold by altering their firing rates (42). Not surprisingly then, resistance training has been shown to increase motor unit firing rates after training (43).

Increased synchronization of motor units has been observed after strength training (44). The more synchronous the firing of motor units, the more motor units will be firing at any given time. Theoretically, this might lead to an increase in maximal force production, although some evidence suggests that asynchronous firing of motor units may be more effective than synchronous firing in producing force during submaximal muscle actions (45). Thus, the role of synchronization of motor unit firing in force production remains unclear (6).

> *Increased neural drive results from increased motor unit recruitment, increased motor unit firing rate, or synchronization of motor unit firing.*

A maximal muscle action of an agonist muscle or muscle group is typically accompanied by simultaneous activation of the antagonist muscle or muscle group (37). This is known as **antagonist coactivation** (or cocontraction). For example, a maximal voluntary contraction of the elbow flexors (agonists) may also involve activation of the elbow extensors (antagonists). This coactivation reduces the net torque in the intended direction, reducing performance on the strength test. Coactivation may be a strategy used to help stabilize a joint, particularly if the individual is inexperienced or uncertain about lifting a load (46). Strength training reduces coactivation of antagonist muscle groups, leading to an increase in the expression of muscular strength (47).

METABOLIC ADAPTATIONS

Some evidence points to increased fuel availability following resistance training. One study showed increases in ATP (18%), PC (25%), and glycogen (66%) levels following 5 months of heavy resistance training (48). Another study showed increased activity levels of several key enzymes involved in anaerobic energy metabolism (creatine kinase, myokinase, and phosphofructokinase) (49). Others, however, concluded that strength training does not increase ATP or PC levels (50) or lead to increased activities of enzymes associated with the phosphagen, glycolytic, or oxidative energy systems (51). Differences between studies may be due to the pretraining status of subjects, muscles examined, and variations in the design of the training programs (6).

ENDOCRINE ADAPTATIONS

The two hormones most important for resistance-training adaptations are **testosterone** and **growth hormone**. It has been shown that an acute bout of resistance exercise can increase circulating levels of these anabolic hormones (52), which are sensitive to program design variables such as load and rest period. Testosterone, for example, was elevated following the use of both 5-RM loads with 3-minute rest periods and 10-RM loads with 1-minute rest periods. Growth hormone, however, was highest following a 10-RM load with 1-minute rest periods between multiple sets.

Reports conflict regarding chronic changes in circulating levels of testosterone following resistance training. Some studies have reported increased resting levels of testosterone (28,29), while others have not (53). Discrepancies may be attributed to differences in the volume and intensity of the training programs employed (54) and training status (55). Circulating levels of growth hormone do not appear to change with resistance training (56). The cumulative effect of acute increases in growth hormone following resistance-training sessions may be the most important mechanism leading to adaptations. It should be noted that changes in the number of receptors for a given hormone may alter the effects of that hormone on protein synthesis. For example, resistance training has led to an increase in the number of androgen receptors in rats (57). This type of adaptation can lead to an increased hormonal effect on the cell in the absence of changes in circulating concentrations.

> ***Both acute and chronic changes in the levels of circulating testosterone and growth hormone may occur following resistance training. These changes appear to be sensitive to the design of the training program, such as load and rest period between sets.***

Summary

The nervous system is complex; it may be divided into central (brain and spinal cord) and peripheral (motor and sensory neurons) components. Motor neurons conduct nervous impulses from the central nervous system (brain and spinal cord) to peripheral structures, such as skeletal muscles, while sensory neurons conduct nervous impulses from peripheral structures to the central nervous system. A reflex is an involuntary motor response to a given stimulus. Of the many types of reflexes, the myotatic (stretch) and inverse myotatic reflexes are especially important for those cultivating strength and conditioning.

The individual fibers comprising skeletal muscle are arranged into bundles called fasciculi. Each fiber, fasciculus, and whole muscle is surrounded by connective tissues called endomysium, perimysium, and epimysium, respectively. These connective tissues transmit the force of muscle contraction to the tendons, which are attached to bones and cause movement. The sliding-filament theory of muscle contraction describes how actin and myosin interact to cause contraction and thus force production.

The three muscle fiber types found in humans are slow oxidative (SO), fast oxidative glycolytic (FOG), and fast glycolytic (FG). These fiber types differ from one another based on their contractile and metabolic characteristics. The relative proportions of each fiber type differ among people and are largely determined by genetics.

Resistance training increases muscle size and strength. *Hypertrophy* refers to an increase in cell size and is thought to be the primary mechanism by which muscles are enlarged with training. The nervous system also adapts to chronic heavy resistance training. Evidence of neural adaptations include the cross-education (cross-training) effect, reduction of the bilateral deficit, increased electromyographic activity, and reduced antagonist coactivation.

Maxing Out

1. You are working with a group of track athletes who want to estimate the percentage of fast-twitch muscle fibers in their quadriceps muscles, but you do not have access to the technology required for a muscle biopsy. You know that Thorstensson and Karlsson (58) developed a fatiguing isokinetic leg-extension test to estimate the percentage of fast-twitch fibers in the quadriceps muscles. In this test, the subject performs 50 consecutive maximal isokinetic leg extensions at 180 degrees · s^{-1} and the percent decline in peak torque is used to estimate the percentage of fast-twitch muscle fibers through the following equation:

   Percent fast-twitch fibers
   = (percent decline – 5.2)/0.9

   Percent decline
   = ([initial peak torque – final peak torque]/ initial peak torque) × 100

   Estimate the percentage of fast-twitch muscle fibers for subjects with declines of 25%, 40%, 67%, and 83%.
2. A previously inexperienced weight trainer has completed the first 2 weeks of a resistance-training program designed to increase muscle size and strength. The athlete approaches you and expresses frustration that she does not see any sign of an increase in muscle size or fat-free body mass. Considering the time course of contributions from neural adaptations versus hypertrophy, explain to the athlete why this is normal following just 2 weeks of resistance exercise.
3. An athlete is intrigued that he is not able to exert as much force during higher- versus lower-speed concentric muscle actions despite making a maximal effort under each condition. Explain why there is a negative relationship between force and velocity for concentric muscle actions.

REFERENCES

1. Peter JB, Barnard RJ, Edgerton VR, et al. Metabolic profiles of three fiber types of skeletal muscle in guinea pigs and rabbits. *Biochemistry* 1972;11(14):2627–2633.
2. Dubowitz V, Brooke MH. *Muscle Biopsy: A Modern Approach.* Philadelphia, PA: W.B. Saunders Company; 1973.
3. Fry AC, Allemeier CA, Staron RS. Correlation between percentage fiber type area and myosin heavy chain content in human skeletal muscle. *Eur J Appl Physiol Occup Physiol.* 1994;68(3):246–251.
4. Schilling BK, Fry AC, Chiu LZ, et al. Myosin heavy chain isoform expression and in vivo isometric performance: a regression model. *J Strength Cond Res.* 2005;19(2):270–275.
5. Pollack GH. *Muscles and Molecules: Uncovering the Principles of Biological Motion.* Seattle, WA: Ebner and Sons Publishers; 1990.
6. Fleck SJ, Kraemer WJ. *Designing Resistance Training Programs.* Champaign, IL: Human Kinetics; 2004:xiii, 377.
7. Coyle EF, Feiring DC, Rotkis TC, et al. Specificity of power improvements through slow and fast isokinetic training. *J Appl Physiol.* 1981;51(6):1437–1442.
8. Ikai M, Fukunaga T. Calculation of muscle strength per unit cross-sectional area of human muscle by means of ultrasonic measurement. *Int Z Angew Physiol.* 1968;26(1):26–32.
9. Zatsiorsky VM. Biomechanics of strength and strength testing. In: Komi PV, ed. *Strength and Power in Sport.* Oxford, UK: Blackwell Scientific; 2003:439–487.
10. Lanka J. Shot putting. In: Zatsiorsky VM, ed. *Biomechanics in Sport: Performance Enhancement and Injury Prevention.* Oxford, UK; Malden, MA: Blackwell Science; 2000: 435–457.
11. Mero A, Komi PV. Force-, EMG-, and elasticity-velocity relationships at submaximal, maximal and supramaximal running speeds in sprinters. *Eur J Appl Physiol Occup Physiol.* 1986;55(5):553–561.
12. Hakkinen K, Komi PV, Alen M. Effect of explosive type strength training on isometric force- and relaxation-time, electromyographic and muscle fibre characteristics of leg extensor muscles. *Acta Physiol Scand.* 1985;125(4):587–600.
13. Shoepe TC, Stelzer JE, Garner DP, et al. Functional adaptability of muscle fibers to long-term resistance exercise. *Med Sci Sports Exerc.* 2003;35(6):944–951.
14. Goldspink G, Harridge S. Cellular and molecular aspects of adaptation in skeletal muscle. In: Komi PV, ed. *Strength and Power in Sport.* Oxford, UK: Blackwell Scientific; 2003:231–251.
15. Kraemer WJ, Patton JF, Gordon SE, et al. Compatibility of high-intensity strength and endurance training on hormonal and skeletal muscle adaptations. *J Appl Physiol.* 1995;78(3):976–989.
16. Crewther B, Cronin J, Keogh J. Possible stimuli for strength and power adaptation: acute metabolic responses. *Sports Med.* 2006;36(1):65–78.
17. Crewther B, Cronin J, Keogh J. Possible stimuli for strength and power adaptation: acute mechanical responses. *Sports Med.* 2005;35(11):967–989.
18. Crewther B, Keogh J, Cronin J, et al. Possible stimuli for strength and power adaptation: acute hormonal responses. *Sports Med.* 2006;36(3):215–238.
19. Housh DJ, Housh TJ, Johnson GO, et al. Hypertrophic response to unilateral concentric isokinetic resistance training. *J Appl Physiol.* 1992;73(1):65–70.
20. Farthing JP, Chilibeck PD. The effects of eccentric and concentric training at different velocities on muscle hypertrophy. *Eur J Appl Physiol.* 2003;89(6):578–586.
21. Holloway JB, Baechle TR. Strength training for female athletes. A review of selected aspects. *Sports Med.* 1990;9(4):216–228.
22. Brown CH, Wilmore JH. The effects of maximal resistance training on the strength and body composition of women athletes. *Med Sci Sports.* 1974;6(3):174–177.
23. Cureton KJ, Collins MA, Hill DW, et al. Muscle hypertrophy in men and women. *Med Sci Sports Exerc.* 1988;20(4):338–344.
24. Alway SE, Winchester PK, Davis ME, et al. Regionalized adaptations and muscle fiber proliferation in stretch-induced enlargement. *J Appl Physiol.* 1989;66(2):771–781.
25. Gonyea WJ, Sale DG, Gonyea FB, et al. Exercise induced increases in muscle fiber number. *Eur J Appl Physiol Occup Physiol.* 1986;55(2):137–141.
26. Tesch PA, Larsson L. Muscle hypertrophy in bodybuilders. *Eur J Appl Physiol Occup Physiol.* 1982;49(3):301–306.
27. Staron RS, Johnson P. Myosin polymorphism and differential expression in adult human skeletal muscle. *Comp Biochem Physiol B Biochem Mol Biol.* 1993;106(3): 463–475.
28. Staron RS, Karapondo DL, Kraemer WJ, et al. Skeletal muscle adaptations during early phase of heavy-resistance training in men and women. *J Appl Physiol.* 1994;76(3):1247–1255.
29. Hakkinen K, Pakarinen A, Alen M, et al. Neuromuscular and hormonal adaptations in athletes to strength training in two years. *J Appl Physiol.* 1988;65(6):2406–2412.
30. Moritani T, deVries HA. Neural factors versus hypertrophy in the time course of muscle strength gain. *Am J Phys Med.* 1979;58(3):115–130.
31. Farthing JP, Chilibeck PD. The effect of eccentric training at different velocities on cross-education. *Eur J Appl Physiol.* 2003;89(6):570–577.
32. Munn J, Herbert RD, Gandevia SC. Contralateral effects of unilateral resistance training: a meta-analysis. *J Appl Physiol.* 2004;96(5):1861–1866.
33. Zhou S. Chronic neural adaptations to unilateral exercise: mechanisms of cross education. *Exerc Sport Sci Rev.* 2000;28(4):177–184.
34. Cresswell AG, Ovendal AH. Muscle activation and torque development during maximal unilateral and bilateral isokinetic knee extensions. *J Sports Med Phys Fitness.* 2002;42(1):19–25.
35. Howard JD, Enoka RM. Maximum bilateral contractions are modified by neurally mediated interlimb effects. *J Appl Physiol.* 1991;70(1):306–316.
36. Enoka RM. Muscle strength and its development. New perspectives. *Sports Med.* 1988;6(3):146–168.
37. Sale DG. Neural adaptations to strength training. In: Komi PV, ed. *Strength and Power in Sport.* Oxford, UK: Blackwell Scientific; 2003:281–314.
38. Alkner BA, Tesch PA, Berg HE. Quadriceps EMG/force relationship in knee extension and leg press. *Med Sci Sports Exerc.* 2000;32(2):459–463.

39. Aagaard P, Simonsen EB, Andersen JL, et al. Neural inhibition during maximal eccentric and concentric quadriceps contraction: effects of resistance training. *J Appl Physiol.* 2000;89(6):2249–2257.
40. Higbie EJ, Cureton KJ, Warren GL III, et al. Effects of concentric and eccentric training on muscle strength, cross-sectional area, and neural activation. *J Appl Physiol.* 1996;81(5):2173–2181.
41. Narici MV, Roi GS, Landoni L, et al. Changes in force, cross-sectional area and neural activation during strength training and detraining of the human quadriceps. *Eur J Appl Physiol Occup Physiol.* 1989;59(4):310–319.
42. Sale DG, McComas AJ, MacDougall JD, et al. Neuromuscular adaptation in human thenar muscles following strength training and immobilization. *J Appl Physiol.* 1982;53(2):419–424.
43. Kamen G. Resistance training increases vastus lateralis motor unit firing rates in young and old adults. *Med Sci Sports Exerc.* 1998;30(suppl):S337.
44. Felici F, Rosponi A, Sbriccoli P, et al. Linear and non-linear analysis of surface electromyograms in weightlifters. *Eur J Appl Physiol.* 2001;84(4):337–342.
45. Lind AR, Petrofsky JS. Isometric tension from rotary stimulation of fast and slow cat muscles. *Muscle Nerve.* 1978;1(3):213–218.
46. Enoka RM. *Neuromechanics of Human Movement.* Champaign, IL: Human Kinetics; 2002:xix, 556.
47. Hakkinen K, Kallinen M, Izquierdo M, et al. Changes in agonist-antagonist EMG, muscle CSA, and force during strength training in middle-aged and older people. *J Appl Physiol.* 1998;84(4):1341–1349.
48. MacDougall JD, Ward GR, Sale DG, et al. Biochemical adaptation of human skeletal muscle to heavy resistance training and immobilization. *J Appl Physiol.* 1977;43(4): 700–703.
49. Costill DL, Coyle EF, Fink WF, et al. Adaptations in skeletal muscle following strength training. *J Appl Physiol.* 1979; 46(1):96–99.
50. Tesch PA, Thorsson A, Colliander EB. Effects of eccentric and concentric resistance training on skeletal muscle substrates, enzyme activities and capillary supply. *Acta Physiol Scand.* 1990;140(4):575–580.
51. Tesch PA, Komi PV, Hakkinen K. Enzymatic adaptations consequent to long-term strength training. *Int J Sports Med.* 1987;(8 suppl 1):66–69.
52. Kraemer WJ, Fleck SJ, Dziados JE, et al. Changes in hormonal concentrations after different heavy-resistance exercise protocols in women. *J Appl Physiol.* 1993;75(2): 594–604.
53. Hakkinen K, Pakarinen A, Alen M, et al. Serum hormones during prolonged training of neuromuscular performance. *Eur J Appl Physiol Occup Physiol.* 1985;53(4):287–293.
54. Hakkinen K, Pakarinen A, Alen M, et al. Relationships between training volume, physical performance capacity, and serum hormone concentrations during prolonged training in elite weight lifters. *Int J Sports Med.* 1987; (8 suppl 1):61–65.
55. Ahtiainen JP, Pakarinen A, Kraemer WJ, et al. Acute hormonal responses to heavy resistance exercise in strength athletes versus nonathletes. *Can J Appl Physiol.* 2004;29(5):527–543.
56. Kraemer WJ, Staron RS, Hagerman FC, et al. The effects of short-term resistance training on endocrine function in men and women. *Eur J Appl Physiol Occup Physiol.* 1998; 78(1):69–76.
57. Inoue K, Yamasaki S, Fushiki T, et al. Rapid increase in the number of androgen receptors following electrical stimulation of the rat muscle. *Eur J Appl Physiol Occup Physiol.* 1993;66(2):134–140.
58. Thorstensson A, Karlsson J. Fatiguability and fibre composition of human skeletal muscle. *Acta Physiol Scand.* 1976;98(3):318–322.

CHAPTER 4

The Skeletal System

W. BRITT CHANDLER ● CLINT ALLEY ● T. JEFF CHANDLER

OBJECTIVES

After completing this chapter, you will be able to:

- Understand, articulate, and discuss the living nature of bone tissue including the mechanisms for responding to load and stress.
- Recognize and identify the types of tissue found in the human skeletal system.
- Discuss the functions of the skeletal system in general, the functions of specific joint classifications, and the functions of the various anatomical components that comprise the skeletal system.
- Discuss the role of Wolff's law in bone remodeling.
- Recognize the role of Minimal Essential Strain for bone health, growth, and development.
- Discuss the key concepts of training bone in the realm of human performance including the forces applied, the direction of the forces, speed of loading, rest periods, vibration, and other factors.

KEY TERMS

Amphiarthrosis
Appendicular Skeleton
Articular Cartilage
Articulations
Axial Skeleton
Canaliculi
Cartilage
Collagen
Cortical Bone
Diaphysis
Diarthrosis
Distal Insertion
Epiphyseal Discs
Flat Bones
Irregular Bones
Lacunae
Lever
Ligaments
Long Bones
Minimal Essential Strain (MES)
Osteoblasts
Osteoclasts
Osteocytes
Osteonic Canal
Osteons
Osteoporosis
Periosteum
Proximal Insertion
Short Bones
Synarthrosis
Tendons
Trabecular Bone
Wolff's Law

Introduction

The living skeleton is much more than the calcified bones we study in anatomy. It is a dynamic system with living cells that continually remodel bone and respond to the demands placed on it by training and conditioning. Specific protocols of loading and unloading bone tissues cause unique adaptations to bones, ligaments, tendons, and cartilage. **Ligaments** connect one bone to another. **Tendons** connect muscle to bone, and **cartilage** protects the ends of bones. This chapter discusses the anatomy, physiology, and response to training of the skeletal system.

The bones of the skeletal system provide the internal framework of the body; that is, they comprise the levers and articulations that enable us to move. A **lever** is a rigid bar that moves around an axis of rotation. **Articulations**, where one bone meets another bone, allow movement and serve as the axes around which movement occurs. Bones function to protect our vital organs from trauma; they also produce blood cells, including the red blood cells (RBCs) that transport oxygen to our tissues. In addition to all this, bones serve as depositories for the minerals we need to remain healthy.

STRUCTURE OF THE SKELETAL SYSTEM

The human skeleton is divided into two major parts, axial and appendicular (Fig. 4.1). The **axial skeleton** consists of the skull, vertebral column, sacrum, coccyx, ribs, and sternum. The **appendicular skeleton** can be subdivided into the pectoral and the pelvic girdles. The pectoral girdle includes the clavicle and scapula. The pelvic girdle is made up of the coxal bones of the hip. The bones of the appendicular skeletal system form articulations or joints that allow movement when forces are applied by muscles.

The skeletal system is composed of an axial skeleton and an appendicular skeleton.

The body's movement is general in nature (both angular and linear) and can range from locomotion and gross positioning to adept manipulations of the hands and feet.

BONE TISSUE

One way to classify bones is by their appearance (Fig. 4.2). The **long bones** (femur, tibia, humerus, and radius) determine most of the length of the arms and legs, are responsible for most of our mature height, and provide one location for blood cell production. These bones are generally longer than they are wide. **Short bones** (carpals and tarsals) are more cubical in shape. Several adjacent short bones provide the hands and feet with a flexible base for dexterity at the distal articulations. The **flat bones** (ribs, scapula, bones of the skull, and sternum) provide another site for blood cell production and protect the vital organs. Last, **irregular bones** (the vertebrae and maxilla) have different shapes depending on their functions. They may provide multiple facets for articulation and muscular attachment or unique leverage, depending on their location.

To better understand the function and nature of the bone and its relation to physical activity, look first at its structures. Figure 4.3 illustrates these structures.

1. **Osteons**: Predominant structures found in cortical bone that compose the matrix.
2. **Osteocytes**: Bone cells. There are two types of bone cells, osteoclasts and osteoblasts, both located in the lacunae. **Osteoclasts** are responsible for reclaiming calcium for metabolic processes and removing damaged bone. **Osteoblasts** are responsible for depositing new bone matrix to replace the bone removed by osteoclastic activity.
3. **Canaliculi**: Small canals that allow the dissemination of nutrients and metabolites to osteocytes and surrounding tissue.
4. **Lacunae**: Small spaces at the centers of canaliculi, which house the osteocytes.

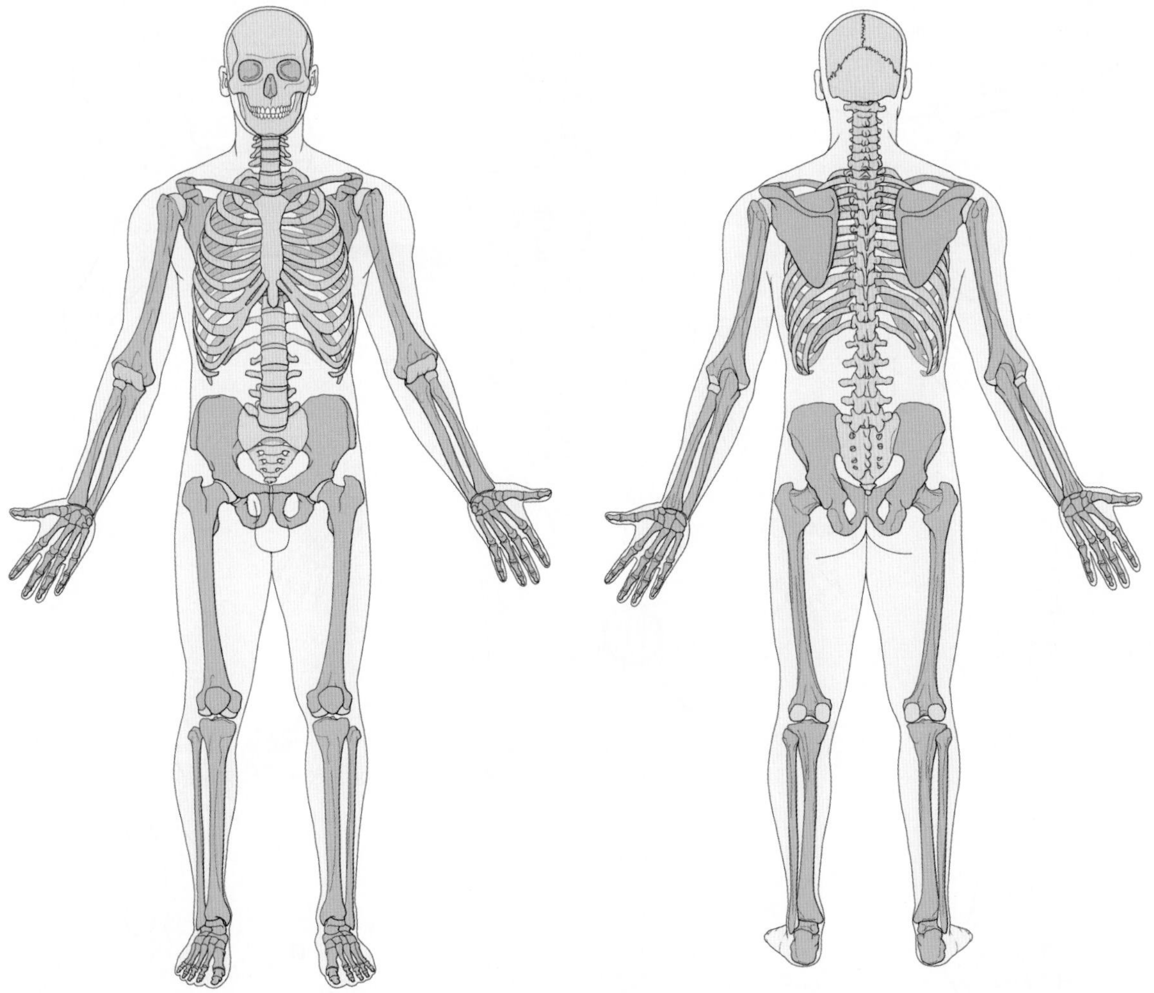

FIGURE 4.1 The axial skeleton and the appendicular skeleton. The axial skeleton consists of the skull, spine, and ribs. The appendicular skeleton consists of the appendages, shoulder girdle, and hip girdle.

5. **Osteonic canal**: A longitudinal canal at the center of the osteon, which provides for the passage of nutrients and metabolic wastes. The osteonic canals house arterioles and venules, which carry blood and nourishment to the bone tissue. Osteonic canals are interconnected by perforating canals running perpendicular to them.

In a magnified cross-sectional view of a mature long bone, the osteonic canals run parallel to the shaft of the long bone and are surrounded by a calcified concentric matrix that fuses them together. Much like the annular concentric rings you see in a crosscut tree, the concentric rings travel outward from the osteonic canal. Canaliculi are strategically placed to disperse fluid to the surrounding tissue. The osteocytes residing in the lacunae are distributed throughout the concentric rings to support the metabolism of specific portions of the bone. All the concentric rings surrounding an osteonic canal form an osteon.

There are two types of bone relative to porosity. **Cortical bone** is highly mineralized and dense, having a low porosity. This type of bone is found in the shafts of long bones and most small, short, irregular bones that are regularly subjected to compressive stresses. **Trabecular bone** is less mineralized, is more porous, and is therefore less dense. It is found at the ends of long bones and is encased in cortical bone, which provides certain advantages in enabling movement. Cortical bone is denser and thus contains more minerals, which add to its weight and rigidity. Because trabecular bone is located at the ends of long bones, the weight at the end of the bone is decreased, thus reducing the force that muscles must generate to move the

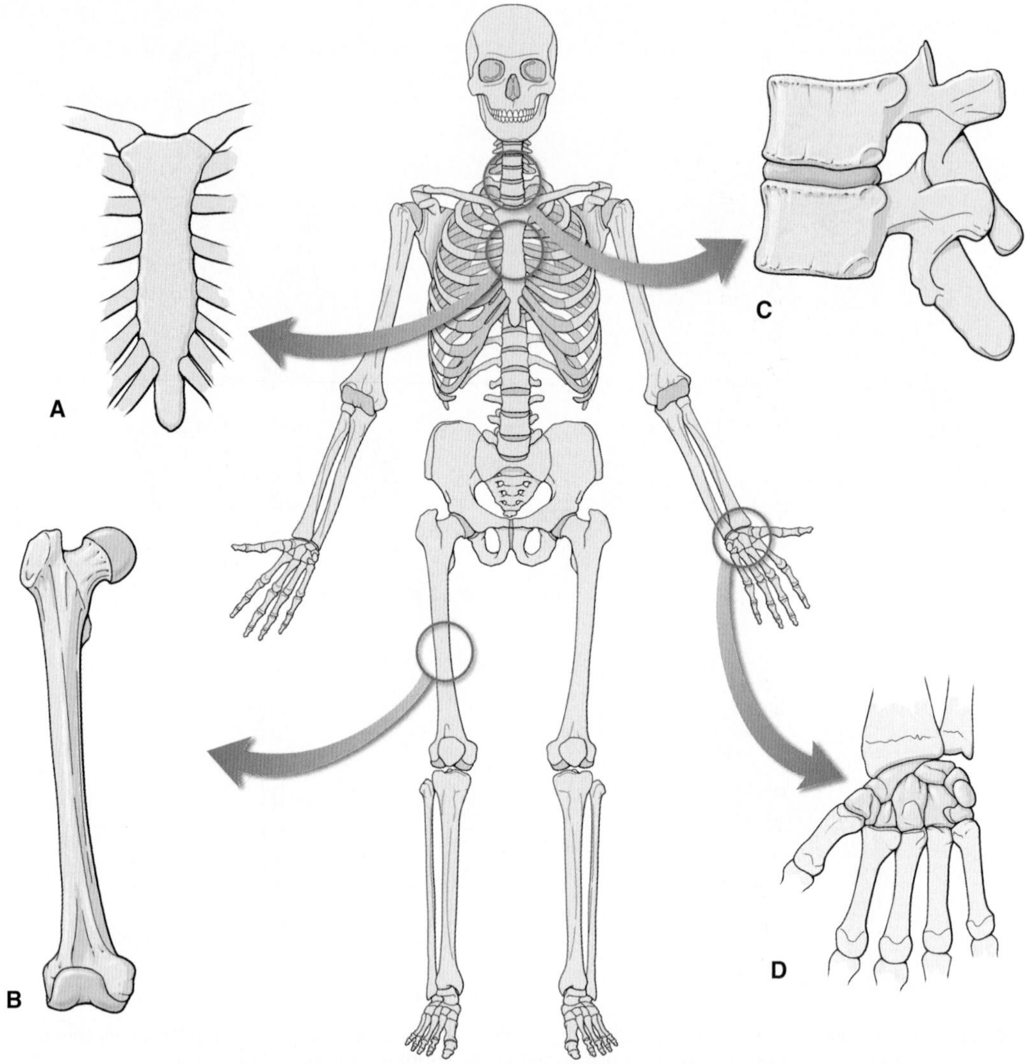

FIGURE 4.2 Classification of bones by their appearance. **A.** The sternum is a flat bone. **B.** The femur is a long bone. **C.** The vertebrae are irregular bones. **D.** The carpals are short bones.

lever. If the entire skeleton were composed of cortical bone, movement would be impaired due to the weight of the bones.

Bone tissue is continually being reabsorbed and reformed, and exercise is a key stimulus for this process. When bone is optimally stressed, osteoblasts deposit minerals, primarily calcium phosphate, on the collagen matrix. **Collagen** is a tough flexible protein found in other connective tissue as well as bone. Particularly in preadolescents and to some extent in adolescents, bone is more flexible because less calcium phosphate has been deposited on the collagen matrix. The **periosteum** is a tough, fibrous outer covering of bone. As we age, our bones continue to grow in circumference because new bone is being developed underneath the periosteum.

Bone tissue is living tissue that is constantly being remodeled. Several factors, including hormonal status, nutritional status, and exercise, determine bone density.

Epiphyseal discs are the site at which bone increases in length. Long bones continue to grow in length up to the time of epiphyseal closure. Prior to epiphyseal closure, bone tissue in this region is more prone to injury from abnormal stresses. Injuries to the epiphysis prior to closure can cause cessation of longitudinal bone growth, which can lead to a limb-length discrepancy. Although resistance training is a concern in this regard, an appropriately designed resistance training program controls the stresses applied to the skeletal system

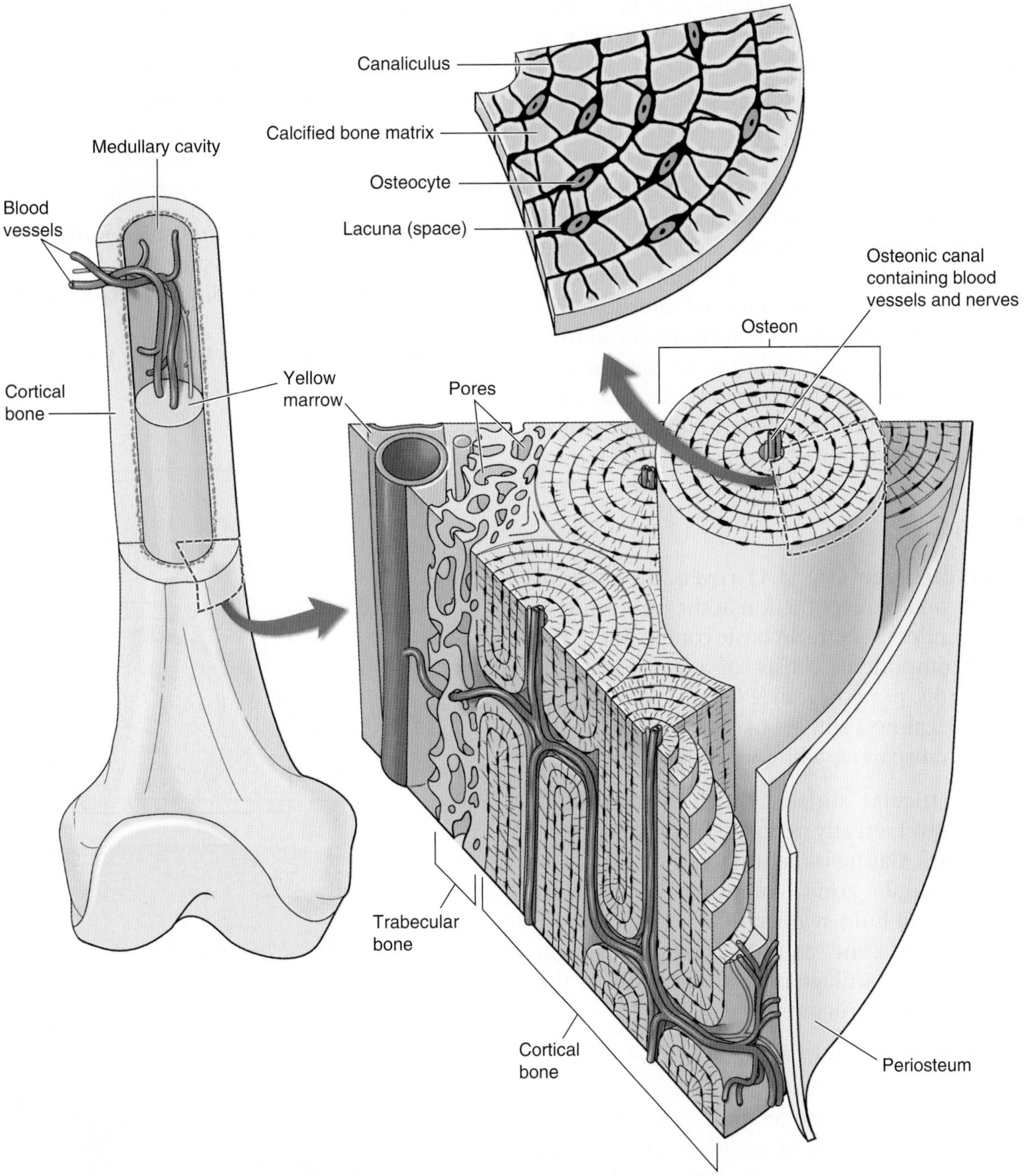

FIGURE 4.3 Longitudinal cross section of a mature long bone. Osteonic canals run longitudinally through long bones. Osteocytes are arranged in concentric circles around the osteonic canal.

more closely than does participation in many sports and activities.

Training exercises performed properly and under proper supervision with spotters should minimize the risk of epiphyseal disc injuries during training.

Appropriately applied forces will strengthen the skeletal system. Building bone density in youth may help to maintain bone density throughout life. Many of the skeletal problems associated with aging are related to decreases in bone density. Some of these problems are related to hormonal or nutritional status. Some problems may be related to our failure to attain maximum bone density as we mature to adulthood.

LIGAMENTOUS TISSUE

Ligaments are composed of tough, fibrous tissue with little elasticity. Ligaments prevent joints from moving in abnormal patterns. By their arrangement, they may allow movement in one plane only or restrict movement in an abnormal direction. In a joint that is inherently lax, as in the shoulder, numerous ligaments function to stabilize the joint in various planes of motion. The ligaments may also serve to fix a bone to another bone where little or no movement is intended, as in the acromioclavicular joint.

CARTILAGE

Articular cartilage (Fig. 4.4) covers the ends of long bones and reduces friction at the joint while it is moving under pressure. In basic composition, the structural components consist of a dense mesh of collagen fibrils, proteoglycan (PG) macromolecules, and water, creating a stiff gel-like substance. The tissue is semitransparent, with four distinct layers:

1. The articular surface, which is superslick. This layer greatly reduces friction between two articulating bone surfaces.
2. The middle zone, composed of collagen fibrils and fluid-swollen PGs
3. The deep zone and the tidemark region where the cartilage matrix meshes with the actual bone structure

By maintaining the fluid content in the tissue at normal levels, the protective and friction-reducing properties of cartilage are retained (1). If the friction-reducing properties of cartilage are lost, this may damage the cartilaginous tissue resulting in eventual deterioration of the joint increasing the potential for injury (2).

ARTICULATIONS

Articulations are where bones join together. At articulations, contact is maintained by cartilage and forces associated with movement of the joint. This arrangement allows bone growth, conversion of angular to linear motion, and dexterity at distal extremities; it also provides for fusion, support summation, and motion as dictated by the location, type, and function of the articulation.

Articulations can be classified by the type of connective tissue used to form the articulation. There are three major classifications of joints: synarthrosis joints, amphiarthrosis joints, and diarthrosis joints. Each type of articulation has specific characteristics in terms of the stability and mobility. A description of the classifications is as follows (Fig. 4.5):

1. **Synarthrosis**: Immovable joints, bound tightly by fibrous tissue
2. **Amphiarthrosis**: Slightly movable joints, cartilaginous
3. **Diarthrosis**: Freely movable joints, synovial

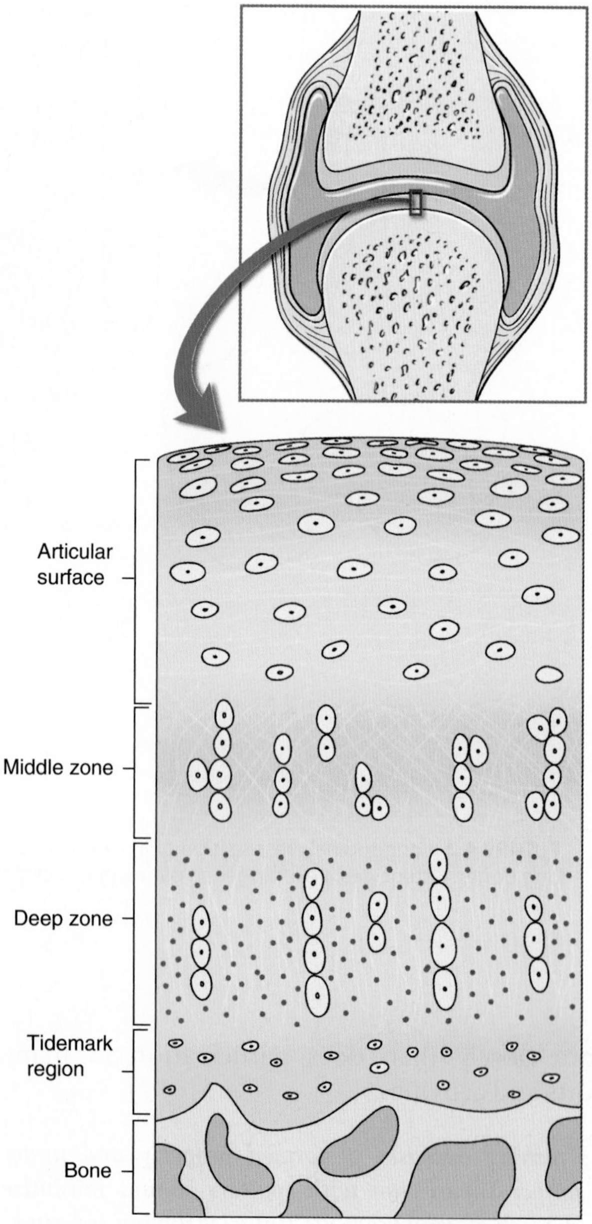

FIGURE 4.4 Layers of articular cartilage. Articular cartilage covers the ends of long bones.

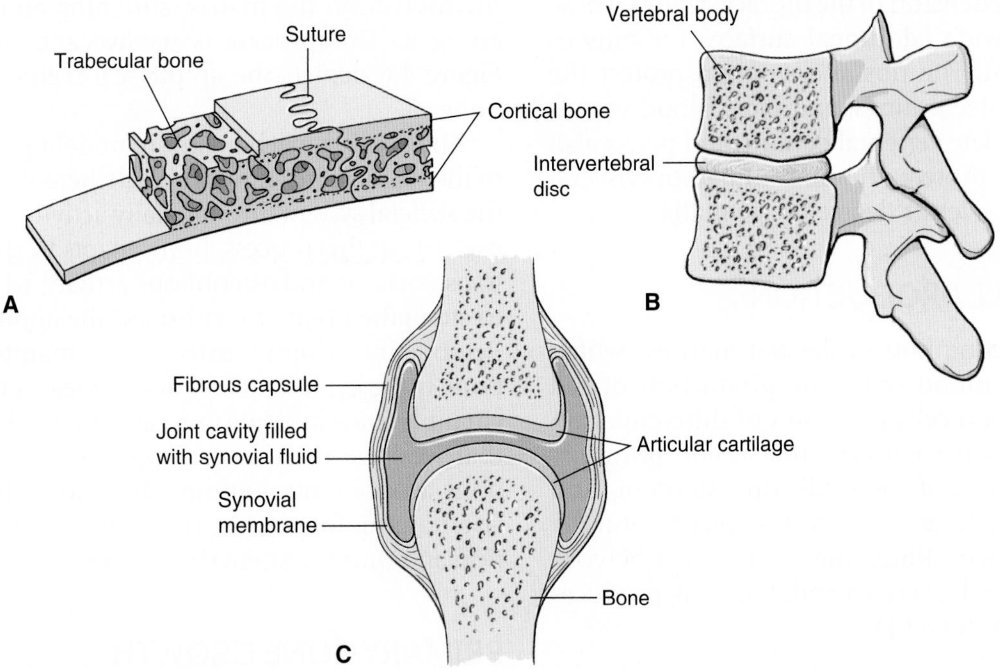

FIGURE 4.5 Types of articulations. **A.** A cranial suture is a synarthrotic joint. **B.** The shoulder is an amphiarthrotic joint. **C.** The knee is a diarthrotic joint.

FUNCTIONS OF THE SKELETAL SYSTEM

The bones of the skeleton provide structure, allow movement, and provide protection for our organs as well as other physiological functions. Let's examine each of these functions in more detail.

STRUCTURE AND PROTECTION

Without bones, we would be incapable of standing, sitting, or moving in general. The length of our long bones determines the length of our body segments. For example, the talus, calcaneus, tibia, and femur make up the length of the leg and allow for ankle and knee flexion, extension, and gross compensation for surface irregularities so that we may stand erect. We can walk on an irregular or uneven surface because the foot can compensate for the slope with this adaptable base of support.

MOVEMENT

Bones provide both a proximal and a distal insertion for muscles, allowing movement when sufficient tension is developed in the muscle that crosses a joint. The **proximal insertion** is closer to the trunk, and the **distal insertion** is farther from the trunk. The bones of the appendicular skeleton and, to a lesser degree, the axial skeleton are arranged as sets of levers with reciprocally shaped surfaces that allow maximal contact to be maintained at the joint during movement. Joints function as axes of rotation around which torque is generated by muscle force.

> ***The structure of the skeletal system allows it to perform one of its essential functions: movement.***

The bones of the skeleton act as a mechanical framework for movement and the attachment of muscles. The irregular bones of the spine (the vertebral bodies) are specifically engineered to bear the summed weight of the body superior to a specific vertebral articulation. Vertebral bodies distribute weight over a large surface area to distribute increasing pressures at each descending vertebral level. The legs, in particular the femur and tibia, are structured such that the cortical portion of the bone resists compressive forces from the weight of the entire body superior to them. The hips can experience as much as six times body weight during normal stair climbing (3). The bones support as much as five times their weight in soft tissue in the normal adult.

One function of the skull and vertebral column is to protect the brain and spinal cord from injury. The thoracic vertebrae have spinous processes that restrict hyperextension in the thoracic region. These processes provide additional surfaces for muscular attachment. The ribs and sternum protect the heart, liver, spleen, lungs, and large blood vessels in the thorax. The vertebral column and pelvis also mechanically protect the abdominal or visceral organs and to a lesser degree the genitalia.

BLOOD CELL PRODUCTION

The spongy bone houses the red marrow, which produces the blood cells. The production of red and white blood cells is a result of differentiation of mature blood stem cells that reside primarily in the flat bones of the skull, ribs, sternum, and the ends of the long bones. As the spleen naturally destroys damaged RBCs, these cells must be continually replaced. Every second, the body produces over 2 million RBCs (4).

GROWTH OF THE SKELETAL SYSTEM

Bone changes in size and functional characteristics via two processes: (a) normal growth and (b) remodeling due to applied loads. Normal growth is largely a function of migration of the epiphysis, resulting in an increase in bone length and diameter prior to skeletal maturity. Chondrocytes secrete a matrix of cartilage and minerals that then deposit themselves on the matrix, stiffening and strengthening it. This process is passive and takes time. Figure 4.6 depicts the epiphyseal region of a long bone.

The second mechanism, remodeling, is a result of the stresses and strains (or lack thereof) applied to the skeletal system through daily activity or planned exercise. In this process, bone adapts to stresses due to osteoclastic and osteoblastic activity, which serves to strengthen bone to withstand the applied forces. Remodeling is more active in the maintenance of bone integrity; it increases and decreases the bone's circumference in relation to activity level. It is here that we have the greatest opportunity to generate bone adaptation to training. By loading in an exercise/training format, we can influence this adaptation and thus the strength of bone.

PRIMARY BONE GROWTH IN THE EPIPHYSIS

At birth, the skeletal system is composed of a cartilaginous framework that has the general form of the skeleton but is not distinguished in proportion, specific structure, or definitive landmarks. In the first stage of growth, calcification of the cartilage framework begins. Development of the periosteum is evidenced by the periosteal bone collar along the center of the shaft and the development of articular cartilage at the ends of the femur. The collar appears as a ring of calcified bone around

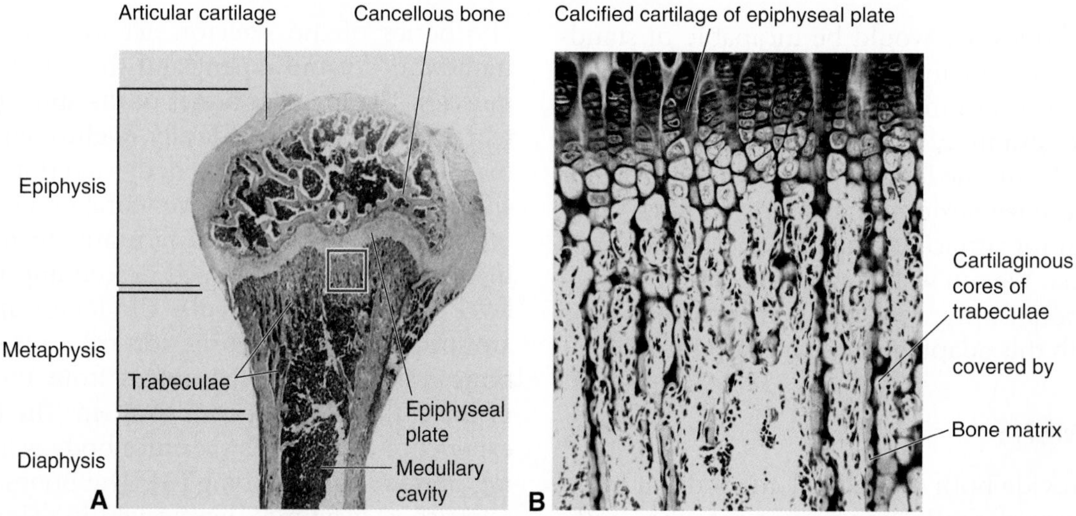

FIGURE 4.6 Epiphyseal growth region **A.** The end of a long bone covered by cancellous bone and articular cartilage. The epiphyseal disc separates the epiphysis from the metaphysis. **B.** A magnified section of the metaphysis undergoing calcification of the cartilaginous matrix. From Cormack DH. *Essential Histology*. 2nd ed. Philadelphia, PA: Lippincott Williams & Wilkins; 2001, with permission.

the shaft at approximately the midline. A short time later, the periosteal bone collar becomes the primary ossification center and epiphyseal capillaries develop in the bone's proximal and distal ends.

Soon the ossification (calcium deposition) of the **diaphysis** or shaft of the bone becomes evident at the center of the shaft, and the epiphyseal plates or growth centers are apparent at the ends of the heavily mineralized centers. As the epiphyseal discs lay down new bone, they migrate toward the distal ends. Still later, additional growth centers originate at both ends, forming the unique structural features of a long bone. The secondary ossification centers lay down spongy bone, which is covered by articular cartilage. As this growth in length is taking place, the layer on the surface just beneath the periosteum is adding to the circumference of the bone in response to the compression, shear, tension, and torsional loading imposed by movement and exercise. Long bones reach their final length in early adulthood, when the epiphyseal discs are completely closed. Figure 4.7 illustrates the transition of bone from cartilaginous to fully ossified.

Chondrocytes are active cells that specialize in the generation of the protein cartilage framework or matrix. In human growth, they synthesize and secrete matrix into the extracellular space (5). Chondrocyte hypertrophy is an active process resulting in increased amounts of intercellular material, including mitochondria and endoplasmic reticulum. Increases in the height of the chondrocyte column are responsible for 44% to 59% of longitudinal bone growth, the remainder being due to matrix synthesis and chondrocyte proliferation. The rate of differentiation of mesenchymal stem cells into chondrocytes is a factor that regulates the synthesis of the matrix and thus the rate of bone growth (5). In addition to the collagen matrix being laid down, osteoclasts and osteoblasts are being differentiated near the epiphysis, where there is a narrow band of cells called the "proliferating region" of the growth plate. Here, chondrocytes multiply and secrete matrix materials, causing migration of the active growth center toward the proximal and distal ends of the long bones. The matrix material is the template for ossification.

ADAPTATIONS OF THE SKELETAL SYSTEM LOADING

Loads applied to the skeletal system cause adaptations to occur that are specific to the type of load.

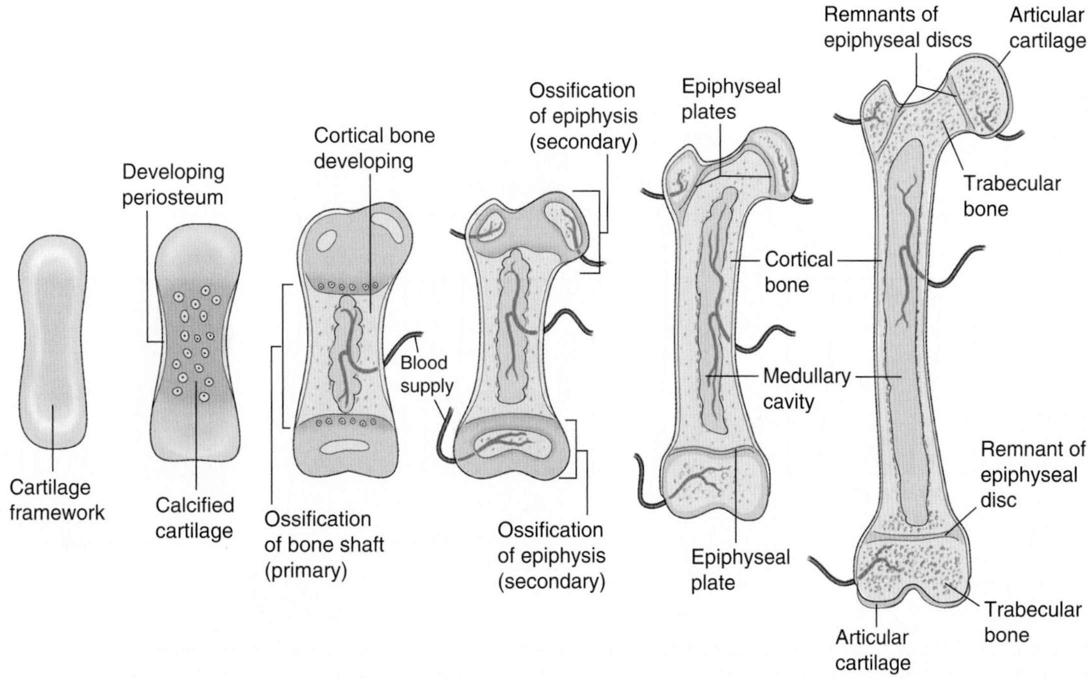

FIGURE 4.7 Prior to ossification, bone begins as a cartilaginous framework.

WOLFF'S LAW

Adaptation to training can be defined according to **Wolff's law**, which states that "the densities, and to a lesser extent, the sizes and shapes of bones are determined by the magnitude and direction of the acting forces applied to bone."

Growth in circumference acts to distribute the compressive forces over an increased cross-sectional area and thus reduces the amount of pressure per square unit of the bone's cross-sectional surface. In animal experiments, growth in regions of higher stresses and strain has been shown to occur (6). These adaptations can actually change the geometry of the bone and thus the response to a repetitive movement or strain. Increased thickness in the direction of force application and bending serves to better accommodate repeated flexion. Bones, like muscles, adapt to progressive overload. If we increase the load, we increase flexion in the bone. Figure 4.8 demonstrates how bone under axial load "bends," stimulating the deposition of bone underneath the periosteum at the specific location where the bending occurred. Weight-bearing exercises are most effective in ensuring the overall health (size and density) of the skeletal system in a healthy individual.

The response of bone tissue to stress is specific to the type of stress applied.

Because the diameter of the bone is enlarged through growth at the outer surface, the space in the center of the bone, required for the marrow, nerves, and blood supply, is not reduced. Since these functions are essential to healthy bone, hypertrophy on the external surfaces does not reduce the functional interior space but does allow increasing load accommodation.

MINIMAL ESSENTIAL STRAIN

Minimal essential strain (MES) is the minimal volume and intensity of loading required to cause an increase in bone density. Approximately 10% of the strain required to fracture the bone is considered the threshold at which new bone formation is triggered (7).The interaction of matrix strain and fluid flow may actually be the interacting source of the remodeling signal in bone tissue (8). Whether the stress comes from exercise or the work environment, bone remodeling will occur if the stress triggers the osteoblasts to migrate to the strained region of bone. The Real-World Application box below provides an analogy to illustrate the concept of bone remodeling.

An exercise program that does not reach the level of MES will be ineffective at promoting bone density.

MES varies by age and individual. An obese individual will have greater loads placed on the skeletal

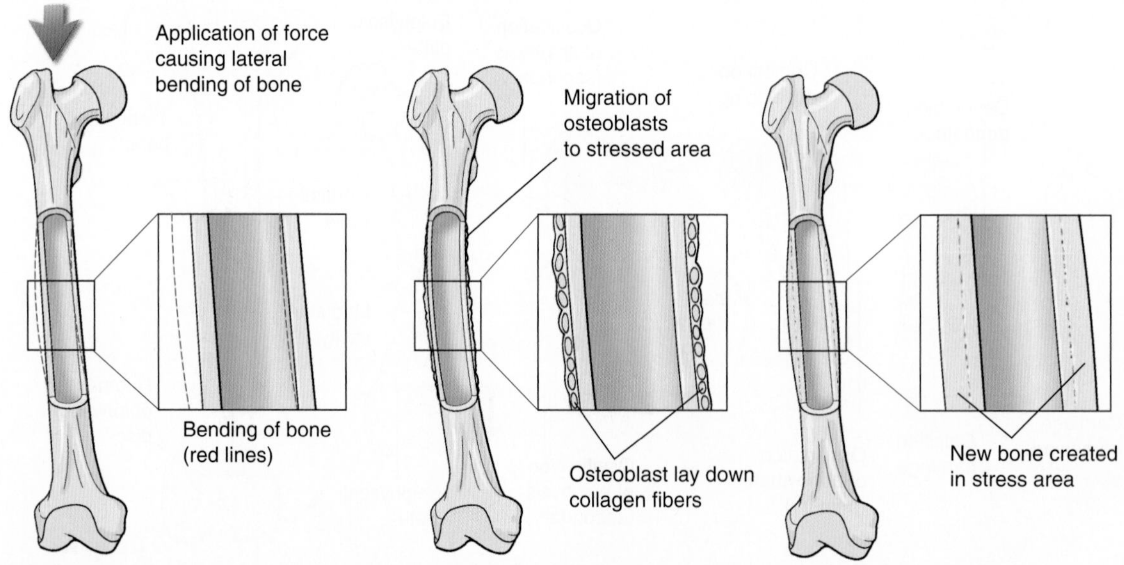

FIGURE 4.8 Wolff's law. If the load and speed of movement are high enough, bone will "bend" under an axial load. This stimulates the deposition of calcium in the specific location of the stress. Therefore, bone responds to "bending" by getting thicker in the direction of the load.

REAL-WORLD APPLICATION

An Illustration for Remodeling Bone: The I Beam

Imagine the strength of an I-beam increased proportionally by increases in thickness of specific portions of the beam. The increases in thickness of the vertical portion of the beam simulate an increase in rigidity from increased bone mineral density (BMD). As you can see, there is an increased difficulty of bending the I-beam on the right versus the left. If bone strength is increased due to increased BMD as a result of remodeling, then the MES would increase as the bone got stronger.

system in normal daily activities than his or her lighter peers. The obese individual, however, will also likely be less active.

Bone density decreases with age, beginning in the third decade. The amount of strain needed to start the remodeling process may occur in the elderly with a decreased load. In a younger, more active population, the requirements of MES should be higher based on higher individual levels of bone density. Therefore, more rigorous exercise may be required to achieve MES in a young, active population. Although stresses applied to bone and subsequent remodeling are ongoing, bone continues to increase in diameter. The total stress required to initiate new bone growth by remodeling is increased if the bone is stronger.

TRAINING ADAPTATIONS TO THE SKELETAL SYSTEM

The response of bone to applied forces is specific to the applied forces. Strain activation changes a small section of exterior bone from the normal state to a state of remodeling. The location of the adaptation is underneath the outer layer of the bone—in the periosteum. The activated area of bone begins resorption or the removal of the damaged bone by osteoclasts. This will take 1 to 3 weeks. Next is a reversal from primarily osteoclastic activity to osteoblastic activity, which takes another 1 to 2 weeks. Osteoblasts start forming new bone by producing matrix in the now cleared resorption area, which takes approximately 3½ months.

Mineralization of bone takes place by the precipitation of calcium phosphate crystals, which bind to and fill in the protein matrix. Calcification increases the diameter of the bone and the thickness of the external cortical bone layer. Calcification of the matrix increases the rigidity of the bone. This adaptation can be stimulated by loading in exercise and can result in an increase in bone density during progress from a less trained to a more trained condition.

Studies in elderly females have shown no significant change in bone density in the femur and forearm after a resistance training period of 5 months or more (9). In animal studies, small changes in bone density result in a significant shift in bone strength (6). In all cases, care should be taken in training the elderly and the untrained so as to reduce the risk of injury. In these populations, acute loading may require less resistance than that perceived to result in the damage or failure of bone.

Q & A from the Field

Q *My mother and grandmother both have osteoporosis. Is there anything I can do to decrease my chances of having osteoporosis when I get older?*

A Heredity is certainly a risk factor. In females, the hormonal changes that accompany menopause are a risk factor. Several lifestyle factors increase the risk of osteoporosis: smoking, nutritional deficiencies, excessive alcohol consumption, and the lack of weight-bearing exercise. Everyone loses some bone density as they age. It is important to maximize bone density when you are younger with a weight-bearing exercise program designed to improve bone density.

THE SKELETAL SYSTEM AND HEALTH

Although balanced growth, proper mineralization, and good training are important indicators of good health, pathologies can occur as a result of specific disorders of or stresses on the skeletal system. This section discusses loss of bone mass, improper alignment, structural damage, and repair of bone.

BONE DENSITY AND HEALTH

Peak bone density is an indicator of long-term skeletal health. It is generally accepted that those who achieve a higher peak bone mass are less at risk for osteoporotic fracture later in life. **Osteoporosis** is a disease characterized by a loss of bone density; it is insidious in that it presents no signs or symptoms until the fracture of a bone that has lost its mineral density occurs. Three distinct populations are at higher risk for osteoporosis: (a) postmenopausal women after about age 50, (b) both men and women after about age 70, and (c) young female athletes who also have eating disorders, in whom it is a component of the female athletic triad (discussed later in this chapter).

We know that the appropriate dose of physical activity can increase BMD throughout our lives (10). Consider the person who achieves higher peak bone density and a larger calcium depot reserve to begin with. As he or she ages, the individual with higher bone density will likely be less prone to developing osteoporosis.

If the bone mineral reserve was small to begin with, reductions in bone mineralization and decreases in strength would reach a critical state more rapidly. Reduced bone mineralization and thus the structural integrity of the bone make the elderly more susceptible to bone breakage. A broken hip in an elderly individual can occur as a break at the neck of the femur under the normal load of locomotion, causing the person to fall. In normal locomotion, the stress on bone can be two to three times that of body weight. These breaks occur because the bone density and strength at a vital load-bearing point are diminished due to increased relative osteoclastic activity.

The higher the bone density achieved in the active years, the better the ability to maintain bone density through the aging process into the regression period. Attention given to diet and exercise in the early years may make the functional difference in the later years (11). Although new bone formation can occur at any time of life, the greatest gains are attained in the preadolescent and adolescent years. Adults who started engaging in load-bearing sports before puberty had 22% greater bone mineral content than did a control group. This is compared with a similar group of adults who first started participating in load-bearing activities in adulthood; although these individuals also had increased bone mineral content, it was only 8.5% greater than that in the control group (11). In the case of the female athletic triad, at the time in life when BMD should be peaking, these athletes are intentionally starving their systems and thus greatly reducing their probability of good bone health in their later years.

SPINAL ALIGNMENT MALADIES

The spinal maladies presented below are related to an improper or exaggerated spinal curve. An exaggerated thoracic curve, the curve of the vertebrae associated with the ribs and cervical area, is called kyphosis. This malady can result in a gross "head forward" posture or "hunchback." Another spinal deformity is the curvature of the lumbar vertebrae called lordosis. Both lordosis and kyphosis occur primarily in the sagittal plane.

A lateral curvature of the spine that can be life threatening in extreme cases is scoliosis, which can occur simultaneously in the frontal and transverse planes (12), resulting in a far more complex diagnosis (Fig. 4.9). This curve is not a mere exaggeration but rather should not exist and serves no function. In an exercising population, we should be aware of these maladies and the restrictions they may impose on the individual. Exercise programs that accommodate or minimize the effects of these disorders should be considered as much as possible.

FEMALE ATHLETIC TRIAD

The female athletic triad is a disease predominantly found in females whose sport, training, or competition is enhanced by a reduced ratio of body fat to lean body mass. Its components are osteoporosis, disordered eating (usually anorexia nervosa), and amenorrhea. Long-distance runners and gymnasts seem particularly susceptible to this malady, although it is also possible that

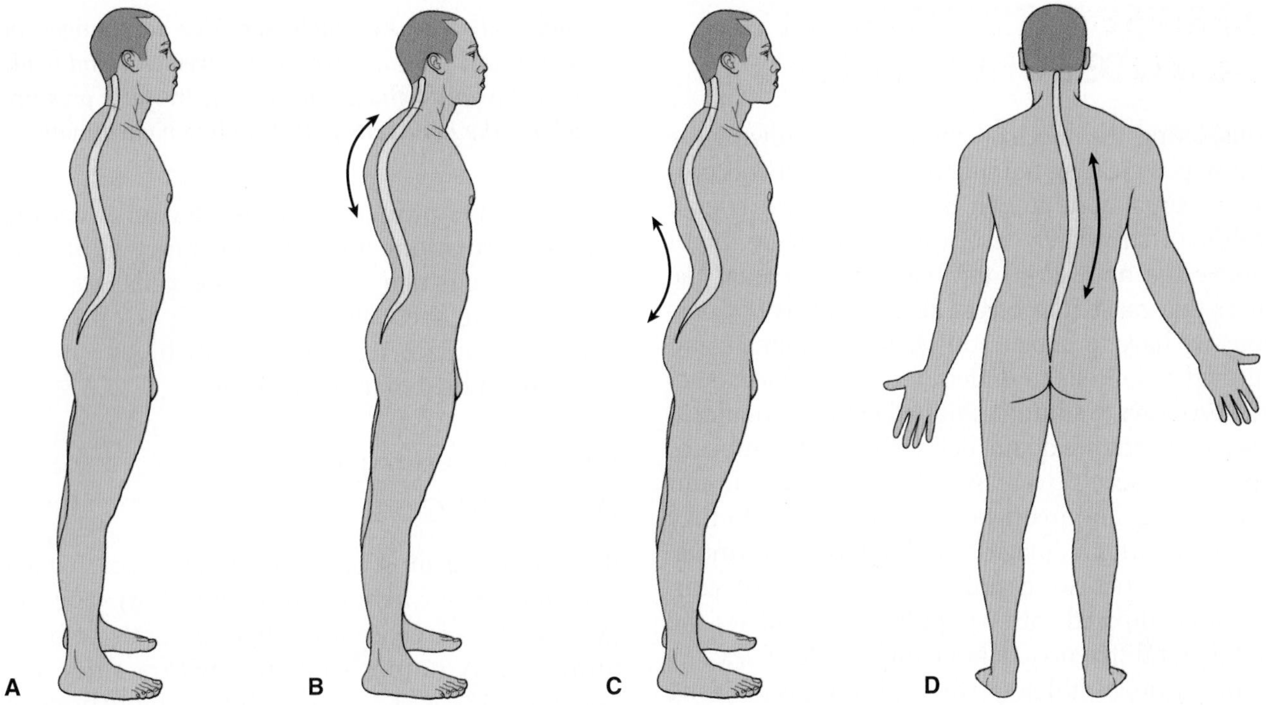

FIGURE 4.9 Skeletal abnormalities of the spine. **A.** Normal spinal alignment. **B.** Kyphosis. **C.** Lordosis. **D.** Scoliosis.

young girls choose these sports to hide their disorder. Addiction to exercise caused by endorphin addiction has also been proposed as a cause of this behavior. Often these athletes attempt to improve their performance by reducing body fat. Reduced body fat improves performance by modifying the strength-to-weight ratio, increasing power, and reducing total workload. When this process is carried to extremes, the female athletic triad can occur.

The three factors that make up this disorder are described as follows:

1. An eating disorder (normally anorexia nervosa) generally accompanied by a distorted body image. An anorexic athlete will see herself as fat even when she has starved herself to a dangerously low level.
2. Osteoporosis is the loss of BMD and destruction of associated matrix materials. Loss of bone tissue can compromise health and make bone brittle. Competitive athletes generate much greater than normal forces in the body, and their bones may not hold up to these forces.
3. Amenorrhea (irregular or complete absence of menses). The athlete reduces nutritional intake to the point where not enough essential fat is left to produce enough female hormones. Estrogen is the major hormone responsible for the balance of osteoclastic and osteoblastic activity. If the athlete cannot produce enough estrogen, osteoclastic activity rises and bone tissue is lost.

A heavy training load (frequently self-imposed) is usually a part of a competitive athlete's training program. The female athlete triad is probably an interaction of overtraining, poor diet, and lack of adequate body fat from which to produce the required hormones to generate the menstrual cycle. It may also be driven by psychological factors, including the desire to be thin (13).

Different types of female athletes were compared in and out of season, looking at factors related to the female athletic triad. Long-term exposure to decreased estrogen levels was nearly associated linearly with decreased BMD. A prolonged exposure to decreased estrogen locally generates compounds that cause an environment favoring the formation of osteoclasts and inhibiting apoptosis in osteoclasts when signaled (14). A lack of tone (normal resting muscle tension) in the muscles, in spite of a high-level training state, can be a key indicator of abnormality. In essence, these athletes starve themselves yet continue to train hard in an effort to improve their performance.

EXERCISE PRESCRIPTION TO PROMOTE BONE DENSITY

Considering the mechanisms of bone growth, the next step is creating training programs that will provide maximal bone growth, bone density, and overall health. To adequately test bone strength, we might remove the bone from the body and measure the forces that cause it to break. Because this is not possible, we have to depend on studies in animals and cultured bone cells to understand the characteristics and responses to stimuli exhibited in these situations. The current studies do not define the exact number of repetitions, sets, percentage of repetition maximum (RM), speed, and frequency of loading, nor do they provide us with a "magic" combination or formula. Generally, when we examine a population of nonathletes compared with a population of athletes, we find major differences in bone mineral densities.

In racquet athletes, we find increased bone density in the dominant arm compared to the nondominant arm (15). Elevated activity levels in the athlete provide musculoskeletal stresses that improve BMD over that of the less active population (10). Currently, we cannot describe the best way to accomplish the desired goal. We can, however, provide some insight into the possible results of specific training programs and their effect on bone density.

LOADING SPEED

Studies have been done to determine the effect of purposely slow training on bone density. Static loading has repeatedly been shown to produce little or no significant effect on new bone growth. Dynamic loading, on the other hand, has been shown to produce significant increases in new bone formation (16).

Bone cells are extremely sensitive to changes in hydrostatic pressure. Training movements and loads that maximize fluctuations in hydrostatic pressure within the bone cells will stimulate bone growth.

This occurs primarily because dynamic loading causes fluctuations in fluid pressure within the lacunar–canalicular system. Bone cells are very responsive to these fluctuations. We can presume that to stimulate new bone growth, our movements must be dynamic in nature.

RATE AND FREQUENCY OF LOADING

Bone responds most effectively to exercises that are dynamic and involve rapid loading (16). The frequency of an exercise also affects the rate of bone formation. A runner who runs with a stride frequency of 90 cycles · min^{-1} will form more bone in the pelvis and lower extremities than will someone who runs with a slower cadence of 60 cycles · min^{-1}.

Dynamic exercise at a high loading rate stimulates bone development. Deliberately slow movements probably will not promote bone adaptation to the same extent as dynamic movements.

DIRECTION OF LOADING AND RESPONSE

In animal experiments using rats, a process of loading the right ulna was applied to the right side of the animal, with the left side unstressed and used as control (6). Data were gathered after a 16-week application of loading. Before and after, dual x-ray

Q & A from the Field

Q ***I have heard that swimming is not a good activity to promote bone density. Is this true? Why? It seems like it would be a very good activity for bone density.***

A Swimming, or any activity in the water, takes place in a semiweightless environment. Astronauts lose bone density through prolonged exposure to a weightless environment. Because swimming is not a weight-bearing activity, it does not provide the minimal stimulus to bone to stimulate growth.

absorptiometry (DEXA) tests were conducted. A modest increase of 5.4% BMD was found. After DEXA, the ulnae were removed and tested for strength in the direction of the loading protocol. It was determined that the increase in maximal amount of force that the bone could support before failing was 64%. So a relatively small increase in BMD can translate into a much greater increase in strength to failure. The majority of bone growth took place consistent with the direction of loading. In keeping with Wolff's law, the stimulus of loading actually changed the geometry of the bone.

> ***Training programs that utilize a variety of movement and loading patterns will probably stimulate bone development to a greater extent.***

INTENSITY OF EXERCISE

Load-bearing activities that place an axial load on the skeleton will induce greater bone formation. Along these lines, exercises such as running or jumping will elicit greater bone formation than walking (17). Dynamic weight-bearing exercises (such as the sport of weightlifting and the Olympic-style lifts) load more of the skeleton per repetition than do, say, arm curls. In animal experiments, the majority of new bone formation (>95%) is stimulated by the first 40 repetitions of an exercise (18). Additional repetitions do not significantly increase the amount of bone that is formed.

> ***Exercises that place an axial load on the skeletal system are probably superior, in terms of improving bone density, to exercises that do not place an axial load on the skeleton.***

Short bouts of exercise followed by rest are better than prolonged workouts (19). The androgen receptors in the body that stimulate new bone growth experience desensitization after a period of time. They need a recovery period before they can be stimulated again to promote bone growth.

Bone takes about 6 to 8 hours to recover its ability to stimulate new bone (19). After the androgen receptors that regulate new bone growth become saturated, they are again available after 6 to 8 hours of rest. Because more receptors are available, full stimulation from the new bout of exercise may result. If a second training session starts before this recovery period, the formation of new bone may be compromised slightly.

FREQUENCY OF TRAINING

It appears it is better to add workouts to the training schedule rather than to extend existing workouts as long as there is enough rest between sessions. Rats that were trained to make 120 jumps five times a week experienced twice as much bone growth in their limbs as did another group that was trained to make 300 jumps twice a week (17). The same number of jumps distributed over a greater number of workouts significantly increased the development of new bone.

VIBRATION

With space travel, it was learned that astronauts lost bone density while in space (20). On the long-duration flights on Mir in the 1990s, cosmonauts lost as much as 20% of their bone density. In a weightless environment, as in space, axial loading of the skeletal system due to gravity does not

Q & A from the Field

Q ***What is the best activity to promote bone density throughout the entire skeletal system?***

A At present, it would appear that moderate- to high-intensity resistance training using a variety of exercises and movement patterns would cause maximum adaptation of the skeletal system. Exercises should load the body axially, such as the bench press for the upper body or the squat for the lower body. Other activities do not stimulate bone density in the entire skeleton. Jogging causes some increase in bone density in the hips but not in the upper body. Tennis may stimulate increases in bone density in the dominant arm but not in the nondominant arm.

occur. One of the contemplated remedies for this problem is vibration. Some information suggests the use of vibration as an alternative or supplemental method of training to maximize or maintain bone density.

When we look at the sensitivity of mature osteocytes to changes in hydrostatic pressure and increased osteoblastic activity, vibration would change the direction and flow of intracellular fluid at a rapid rate. Would the rate be adequate to inspire new bone growth, and if so, what rate would be optimal?

Experimentation to combat the effects of microgravity using vertical vibrational loading to promote bone strength and BMD gains is ongoing (1). Therapeutic applications of vibration to improve or maintain bone density are being investigated in rehabilitation settings (21).

One study used a vibrating platform to manipulate rats with removed ovaries. Hormonal changes after menopause are thought to be at least partly responsible for bone loss in females. Over a 12-week period, the experimenters evaluated the effect of vibration in regard to bone loss and compared the experimental condition to a control condition (22). The results showed less bone loss over a 5-week period in the vibration-trained group compared to the control group.

Vibration as a stimulus for bone growth may promote bone density and prevent its loss under specific conditions.

Some important factors in vibration research include harmonic resonance dynamics, frequency modulation, consistent loading and stimulus application, and study length. Harmonic resonance occurs at certain frequencies of vibration. At some frequencies, tissue damage may occur. Frequency modulation is associated with the construction and application of sonic vibration. The mechanism of applying mechanical vibrational loading must be quantifiable and repeatable.

Summary

Mechanisms within the human body cause adaptation of skeletal tissue in response to imposed stresses (23). The dynamic loading of bone stimulates bone growth. The rate and frequency of loading in animal models has a direct effect on bone growth. Designing conditioning programs to maximize bone growth and development should be specific to the demands of the sport and should include multidirectional loading.

Modest changes in BMD can represent large changes in bone strength. Short bouts with high-intensity loads are probably superior in promoting bone strength. Vibration will promote bone density in certain populations under specific conditions.

Frequent, short, dynamic exercises followed by a minimum of 6 to 8 hours of rest appear to be optimal for the maintenance of bone health in athletes and others. The rest allows the osteoclastic activity to become more prominent than osteoblastic activity. This should be considered in planning training programs or practice sessions where multiple sessions are performed in 1 day.

Maxing Out

1. A nonathletic female expresses concern to you that she may be at risk of bone density disorders as she gets older. Design a conditioning program to promote maximal bone density in this individual.
2. You believe that a female athlete on the track team is at risk for osteoporosis and that she may possibly have an eating disorder complicating the situation. What steps should you take to deal with this situation appropriately?
3. An athlete in a collision sport has a history of bone injuries, primarily stress fractures. He is accustomed to hard training and is experienced in a variety of lifting techniques. He is currently not injured. Plan a resistance training program for this athlete to promote maximal bone density.

REFERENCES

1. Teshima R, Nawata J, et al. Effects of weight bearing on the tidemark and osteochondral junction of articular cartilage. *Acta Orthop Scand.* 1999;70(4):381–386.
2. Olsen S, Oloyede A. A finite element analysis methodology for representing the articular cartilage structure. *Comp Meth Biomech Biomed Eng.* 2002;5(6):377–386.
3. Costigan PA, Deluzio KJ, Wyss UP. Knee and hip kinetics during normal stair climbing. *Gait Posture.* 2002;16(1):31–37.
4. Rothenberg E, Lugo JP. Differentiation and cell division in the mammalian thymus. *Dev Biol.* 1985;112:1–17.
5. Ballock RT, O'Keefe RJ. Current concepts review: the biology of the growth plate. *J Bone Joint Surg.* 2003;85A(4):715–726.

6. Robling AG, Hinant FM, et al. Improved bone structure and strength after long term mechanical loading is greatest is loading is separated into short bouts. *J Bone Min Res*. 2002;17:1545–1554.
7. Frost H. From Wolff's law to the Utah paradigm: insights about bone physiology and its clinical applications. *Anat Rec*. 2001;262:398–419.
8. Nauman E, Wesley C, Chang W, et al. Microscale engineering applications in bone adaptation. *Microscale Thermophys Eng*. 1998;2:139–172.
9. Simpkin A, Ayalon J, Leichter I. Increased trabecular bone density due to bone loading exercises in postmenopausal osteoporotic women. *Calcif Tissue Int*. 1987;40:59–63.
10. Nutter J. Physical activity increases bone density. *NSCA J* 1986;8(3):67–69.
11. Silverwood B. Building healthy bones. *Paediatr Nurs*. 2003;15(5):27–29.
12. Burwell RG. Aetiology of idiopathic scoliosis: current concepts. *Pediatr Rehabil*. 2003;6(3–4):137–170.
13. Bemben DA, Torey D, Buchanan, et al. Influence of type of mechanical loading, menstrual status, and training season on bone density in young women athletes. *J Strength Cond Res*. 2004;8(2):220–226.
14. Chan GK, Duque G. Age-related bone loss: old bone, new facts. *Gerontology*. 2002;48:62–71.
15. McClanahan BS, Harmon-Clayton K, Ward, KD, et al. Side-to-side comparisons of bone mineral density in upper and lower limbs of collegiate athletes. *J Strength Cond Res*. 2002;16(4):586–590.
16. Hert J, Liskova M, Landa J. Reaction of bone to mechanical stimuli. 1. Continuous and intermittent loading of the tibia in rabbits. *Folia Morphol (Praha)*. 1971;19:290–300.
17. Hsieh YF, Turner CH. Effects of load frequency on mechanically induced bone formation. *J Bone Min Res*. 2001;16:918–924.
18. Torvinen S, Kannua P, Sievanen H, et al. Effect of 8-month vertical whole body vibration on bone, muscle performance, and body balance: a randomized controlled study. *J Bone Miner Res*. 2003;18(5):876–884.
19. Rubin C, Lanyon L. Regulation of bone formation by applied dynamic loads. *J Bone Joint Surg*. 1985;66A:397–402.
20. Shackelford LC, Oganov V, LeBlanc A, et al. Bone mineral loss and recovery after shuttle-Mir flights. www.hq.nasa.gov/osf/station/issphase1sci.pdf. Accessed June 24, 2006.
21. Cheung JT, Zhang M, Chow DH. Biomechanical responses of the intervertebral joint to static and vibrational loading: a finite elemental study. *Clin Biomech*. 2003;9:790–799.
22. Flieger J, Karchaolis T, Khaldi L, et al. Mechanical stimulation in the form of vibration prevents post-menopausal bone loss in ovariectomized rats. *Calcif Tissue Int*. 1998;63:510–514.
23. Platen P, Chae E, Antx R, et al. Bone mineral density in top level male athletes of different sports. *Eur J Sport Sci*. 2001;1:5.

CHAPTER 5

Biomechanics of Human Movement

SCOTT K. LYNN ● GUILLERMO J. NOFFAL

OBJECTIVES

After completing this chapter, you will be able to:

- Comprehend units of biomechanical measurements.
- Apply velocity and joint angle specificity to training.
- Understand the length–tension and force–velocity–power relationships.
- Conceptualize Newton's laws of motion and apply them to training.
- Evaluate and compare different modes of resistance.
- Use a fundamental knowledge of biomechanics to be able to progress and regress exercises to appropriate level for any individual.

KEY TERMS

Acceleration
Angular Motion
Biomechanics
Balance
Displacement
Distance
Force
Friction
Gravity
Inertia
Length
Mass
Mechanical Advantage
Momentum
Power
Rotary Inertia
Stability
Stretch-Shortening Cycle
Time
Torque
Velocity
Velocity/Speed Advantage
Weight
Work

Introduction

Biomechanics has been defined as "the study of the structure and function of biological systems using the means and methods of mechanics" (1). This definition divides the word biomechanics into two parts: bio (biological system) and mechanics. In the field of strength and conditioning, the biological system that we are most concerned with is the human body's musculoskeletal system. This involves all tissues directly involved with producing, preventing, or influencing movement (muscles, bones, ligaments, tendons, cartilage, etc.). Also, "mechanics" is defined as the study of the influence of force on bodies. Therefore, this chapter examines how we can manipulate forces in a strength and conditioning setting to produce the desired effect on the structures (tissues) and functions (movements) of the human musculoskeletal system.

Biomechanics is the science of applying mechanical principles to biological systems such as the human body.

For the strength and conditioning specialist, a basic knowledge of biomechanics is essential in order to be able to evaluate human movement and then be able to design and prescribe appropriate movements (exercises) aimed at increasing the overall efficiency of movement. Forces are required to produce any type of human movement and there are various different types of forces and aspects of those forces that must be considered by the strength and conditioning specialist. A sound knowledge of basic mechanical principles will allow for the prescription of appropriate movements at the appropriate intensity to produce the desired movement outcomes without increasing the chance for injury (acute or chronic) of any of the movement structures/tissues.

This chapter will be divided into the following sections:

1. Basic biomechanics: Biomechanical concepts essential to the strength and conditioning specialist will be defined.
2. Human musculoskeletal mechanics: Mechanical characteristics of the human musculoskeletal system that affect movement will be discussed.
3. Biomechanics of resistance: An examination of the biomechanics of various forms of resistance used in a strength and conditioning setting.
4. Progressing/regressing movement: An application of how a basic knowledge of biomechanics can be used to make an exercise easier or harder to suit different individuals.

It should be noted that many terms used in this chapter are not used according to their strict mechanical definition but have been simplified so that their applications in a strength and conditioning setting can be more clearly understood.

BASIC MECHANICS

Biomechanics can be simply defined as the effect of forces on the structure and function of living systems. In the field of strength and conditioning, there are several mechanical concepts that must be understood in order to fully comprehend how to most effectively and safely achieve our training goal. If we think of the simple example of someone lifting a barbell, some of the key mechanical concepts include force, distance, speed, inertia, mass, weight, velocity, acceleration, torque, power, and momentum. Many of these are derived from three basic variables—length, time, and mass (2). The basic unit of **time** is measured in either seconds, minutes, or hours; however, since many sporting or lifting movements are short in duration, they are most often measured in seconds. The basic dimension of **length** (sometimes also referred to as space) is measured in inches, feet, and yards in the United States; but the scientific community has adopted the metric system, which utilizes centimeters, meters, kilometers, and so on. Lastly, the basic dimension of **mass** is commonly measured in kilograms.

To illustrate many of these biomechanical principles, we will examine one of the most basic of exercises, the bench press. First, in the process of lowering the bar to your chest or pushing it back up, the bar moves through space in a slightly curved path. Naturally, if you are a tall individual with long arms, you will be moving it a greater distance than someone with short extremities. Thus, **distance** is defined as the total path traveled by the bar. **Displacement** is defined as a straight line between where the movement started and where the movement ended. Although there is a difference between the two terms (distance vs. displacement) they are most often used interchangeably to describe how far the object has traveled. So, in the bench press example, if a beginner lifter struggles to push the weight up and it does not take a direct line from his or her chest to the finish position, he or she will have pushed the bar a greater distance than a more experienced individual who is able to push it straight up (Fig. 5.1). For the more experienced lifter, the movement was much more efficient as the distance the bar traveled was much smaller.

Similarly, if the beginner lifter took much longer to push the bar up, he or she would also have a lower bar **velocity** (often referred to as speed), which is defined as displacement divided by time. Velocity can be measured in any unit that divides a measure of distance by a measure of time. The most common units used to measure velocity include $m \cdot s^{-1}$, $km \cdot h^{-1}$, $mi \cdot h^{-1}$. Therefore, in order to calculate velocity you must measure the distance the object moved and the time it took to cover that distance. Distance and time can be measured is several different ways, these include the use of a tape measure and timing gates, video equipment, or electronic transducers.

Another illustration of velocity is the example of a sprinter finishing the 100-m race in 10 seconds. This sprinter has achieved an average velocity of 10 $m \cdot s^{-1}$ over the course of the race. This gives the strength and conditioning specialist some information, but in order to tailor appropriate training sessions to improve a sprinter's time, more information, is needed. If we obtained 10 m split times for this race, we could calculate many velocities throughout the race and this would give us much

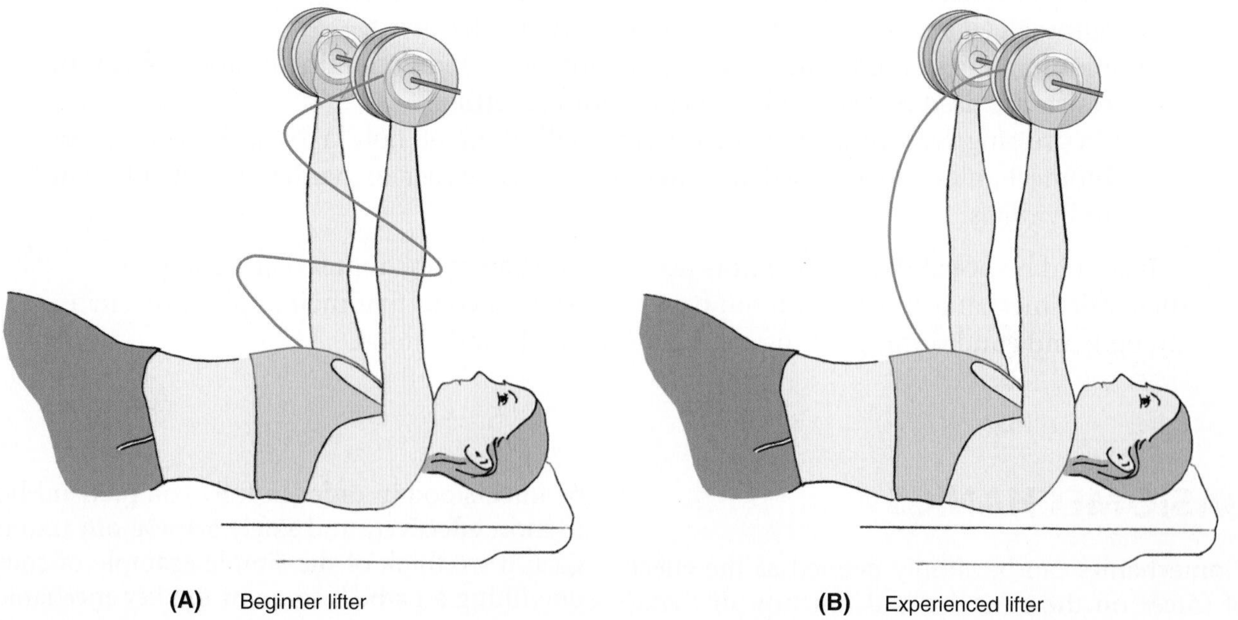

FIGURE 5.1 The path that the barbell travels for (A) a beginner and (B) an experienced lifter. Notice that the distance travelled is much greater for the beginner lifter; however, the displacements are the same.

BOX 5.1

Calculating Average Velocity during Sprint Running

The example is an athlete completing a 30-m sprint. We have electronic timing lights at 10, 20, and 30 m from the starting light gate. The average speed over the last 10 m might be used as an indication of maximum running speed. Let us assume that the times and distances are as follows:

Distance	10	20	30
Time	1.741	2.890	3.995

Velocity is the change in distance over change in time. Therefore, velocity = (30 – 20)/(3.995 – 2.890) = 10/1.105 = 9.05 m · s^{-1}.

BOX 5.2

Calculating Work and Power during Weight Training

Let us use the example of a bench press to demonstrate the calculation of work and power. If the mass of the bar is 80 kg then the weight force that this equates to is 784 N (80 × 9.81). During the repetition, the lifter moves the bar through a distance of 0.70 m and then the work completed is approximately 549 J (80 × 9.81 × 0.7). Now, let us assume that the lift is completed in 1.5 seconds. The average power output during the lift can be calculated as work divided by time, which equals 366 W (549 ÷ 1.5).

more information regarding the portions of the race that need the most work. For example, if there is a large drop in velocity toward the end of the race, the strength and conditioning specialist may need to design a training program to work on the endurance of the athlete to ensure that he or she is better able to maintain the velocity through the finish line. Thus, it becomes increasingly important to examine not just velocity, but how velocity is changing over time.

$$\text{Acceleration} = \text{Velocity} \cdot \text{Time}^{-1}$$

Acceleration is a measure of how velocity changes over time (defined as velocity divided by time). In the bench press example, acceleration or deceleration of the bar is achieved through the application of force. **Force** is defined as a push or pull that moves or tends to move an object. The unit of force in the metric system is the Newton, while in the United States the pound (lb) is more commonly used. The amount of force being applied to an object can be calculated by multiplying mass of the object times its acceleration. **Mass** is a measure of the quantity of matter within the object, and, in the human body, it would be the sum of all the tissues that make up our bodies (bones, muscles, fluids, etc.)

$$\text{Force} = \text{Mass} \cdot \text{Acceleration}$$

Mass can be thought of as a measure of the linear inertia of a body. Inertia is defined as the resistance to changes in motion, and, therefore, an object with a large mass will be more difficult to get moving or to stop once it has begun moving in a straight line than an object with a smaller mass. Mass is often equated to **weight**; however, they differ in that weight is mass multiplied by the acceleration due to gravity (which we assume to be a constant value of 9.81 m · s^{-2} on the earth). Therefore, a person with a mass of 100 kg would weigh 981 N while on earth, while in space in a zero gravity environment this person would be weightless and while standing on the moon this person would weigh 162 N (the acceleration due to gravity on the moon is approximately 1.62 m · s^{-2}). Thus, while the weight

REAL-WORLD APPLICATION

Acceleration Forces in Lifting Weights

One component of acceleration that is constantly acting on the human body and sports implements is acceleration due to gravity. In the example of an arm curl with a dumbbell:

$$F = ma + mg$$

where F, force; m, mass of the dumbbell; a, instantaneous acceleration of the dumbbell; g, acceleration due to gravity (9.81 m · s^{-2}); with a concentric muscle action in the dumbbell curl, gravity is a resistance force that results in negative acceleration. With an eccentric muscle action to lower the dumbbell, the force of gravity results in positive acceleration.

REAL-WORLD APPLICATION

Understanding the Difference between Velocity and Acceleration

An example that most are familiar with involves discussing how you would change velocities while driving your car (i.e., either speed up or slow down). In order to accelerate your car, or increase your car's speed, the accelerator pedal must be pressed. Conversely, in order to decelerate your car, or decrease the speed, you must press on the brakes. Thus, if while traveling at 40 mph you decide to increase your speed to 50 mph, an acceleration is needed. And if you are going at 40 mph and you wish to stop your car (velocity of zero), a deceleration is needed. The rate at which these accelerations/decelerations happen becomes extremely important as well. Assume you are traveling at 40 mph in your car and an animal jumps into the road directly in front of you, you need to decelerate from 40 mph to zero mph in a very short period of time to avoid hitting the animal. This scenario requires an extremely large deceleration as a large change in speed must happen over a short period of time. However, if you are going at the same speed and you see the traffic light change to red 500 yd in front of you, you can apply the brake more lightly and slow down gradually over a longer period of time. Thus, the same change in speed over a longer period of time requires a much smaller magnitude of deceleration. Good athletes generally have to ability to produce large accelerations and decelerations (quick changes in velocities); therefore training the ability to quickly and safely change speeds is important in most athletes.

will change depending on where the individual is standing, the mass will remain constant. It is fitting that the unit of force bears Isaac Newton's name as he has been credited with the discovery of gravity. **Gravity** is a mutually attractive force between two bodies that possess mass. Since the mass of the earth is much greater than that of anything on its surface, it will attract or pull all objects toward its core. Gravity is an important concept for strength and conditioning practitioners, as weight training includes lifting and lowering objects against and with the force of gravity. It should be noted that gravity always pulls objects toward the center of the earth and thus only acts in the vertical direction.

Momentum is the product of mass and velocity and it is an important concept for strength and conditioning specialist, since momentum alone can continue the motion of an object. Unlike previous Aristotelian views that a constant force application was needed to maintain motion, Newton found that an object's inertia (mass) while on the move had a tendency to maintain that motion and only an external force acting on the object will slow it down and eventually stop it. Therefore, the greater the momentum of an object the greater the external forces needed to subsequently stop it.

Momentum = Mass · Velocity

> ***Momentum and inertial patterns of the sport/activity should be mimicked during training.***

There are many ways to increase the intensity of a workout session. Naturally, the most obvious is to increase the amount of weight being lifted. Another simple modification is to increase the number of repetitions to increase the workload. This introduces the concept of **Work**, which is defined as force times displacement and is measured in Joules. As you increase the number of repetitions, you also increase the displacement over which a force has been applied, therefore increasing the amount of work done. If there are two individuals lifting the same amount of weight over the same distance, then these individuals are doing the same amount of work; yet if one of these individuals is capable of producing the lift in a shorter period of time, then it is said that this person is more powerful.

Work = Force · Displacement

Power is calculated in two different ways—as work divided by time or as force multiplied by velocity, and it is measured in Watts. Commonly used "slow-moving" exercises such as the bench press, squat, and dead lift only produce approximately half the power of the faster Olympic lifts (3). As can be seen from the formula, the optimization of both force and velocity is necessary for the greatest power output, and while large loads require large amounts of force to get moving, the movement speed is too low for optimal power. Conversely, lighter loads can be accelerated to high speeds but do not include the necessary force production to achieve greatest power.

Power = Force · Velocity

Power = Work · Time^{-1}

Up to this point we have only been considering movements of objects or the body in a straight line, or what is generally called linear motion; however, many movements take place about an axis or fulcrum and are defined as **angular motion**. In the human body these angular motions occur as our segments (foot, lower leg, thigh, etc.) rotate about axes created at the joints (ankle, knee, hip, etc.). Angular motion is usually measured in degrees, but in some instances can be described in radians (approximately 57 degrees) or revolutions (1 rev = 360 degrees).

Force or power applied is determined by a complex range of neural and mechanical interactions within the muscle, between muscle and tendon, and between muscle and the skeleton.

As discussed above, forces are needed to create linear motion. The angular equivalent of force is a **torque** (T), which is needed to create angular motion, and is expressed in foot-pounds (ft lb) or Newton-meters (N · m).

Torque = Force · Distance (length of the lever arm).

In order to lift a dumbbell, the biceps brachii muscle must produce a torque in the upward direction. How much torque is produced depends on the amount of force being utilized multiplied by the torque arm (which is also referred to as the force arm, lever arm, moment arm, or resistance arm). The torque arm is defined as the perpendicular distance between where the force is being applied (the attachment of the biceps on the bone) and the axis of rotation (the elbow joint). In the example shown in Figure 5.2, lifting the dumbbell through concentric activity of the biceps requires a counterclockwise torque of greater magnitude than the clockwise torque being produced by the dumbbell. That is, force of the biceps multiplied by the torque arm of the biceps has to be greater than the weight of the dumbbell multiplied by the distance this dumbbell is from the axis of rotation in order to produce concentric elbow flexion. If the opposite is true, and the counterclockwise torque created by the dumbbell is greater than the clockwise torque created by the biceps brachii, eccentric elbow extension will be the resulting motion as the muscle will have allowed the dumbbell to "win." Isometric activity would occur when the magnitude of the torque produced by the muscle is equal to the torque produced by the dumbbell.

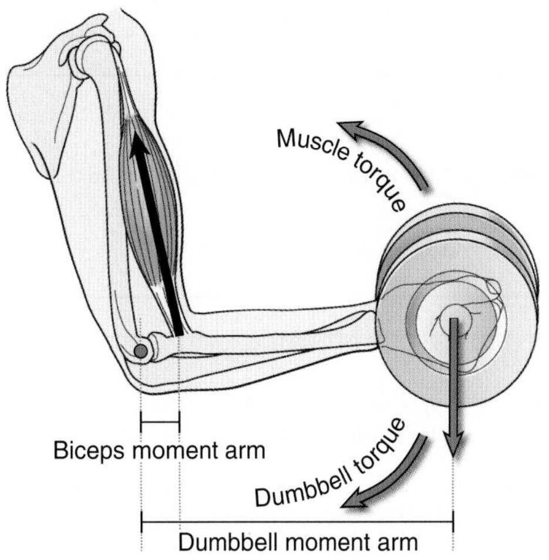

FIGURE 5.2 The biceps muscle torque (counterclockwise) and the torque produced by the dumbbell (clockwise), in an elbow flexion exercise.

This is a very important biomechanical variable for the strength and conditioning specialist as modifying the placement of the weight or resistance from the axis of rotation can be an effective tool in either increasing or decreasing the muscular effort needed to successfully complete a movement. Figure 5.3 demonstrates this concept as Figure 5.3A would require much more muscular torque than Fig. 5.3B to move the same mass. A real-life example of this would be having somebody do leg raises in the supine position with the legs straight and then with the legs bent at the knees. Bending the knees shortens the torque arm distance and decreases the amount of muscular torque needed to perform this exercise.

Whereas **inertia** relates to an object's resistance to being moved or stopped from moving (in a linear sense), **rotary inertia** refers to an object's resistance to being spun (angular motion). Linear inertia can be easily represented by the mass of the object; however, in order to calculate the rotary inertia you need to measure both the mass of the object and how this mass is distributed relative to the axis of rotation. A simple example demonstrating this concept involves asking an individual to run without bending their knees. They will obviously not be able to run nearly as fast as when they are able to flex the knee during the swing phase of the running gait. While the legs themselves are not changing their mass as the hip flexes and extends, the outstretched leg is maintaining the mass of the lower leg and foot relatively far from the hip (axis of rotation) creating a large

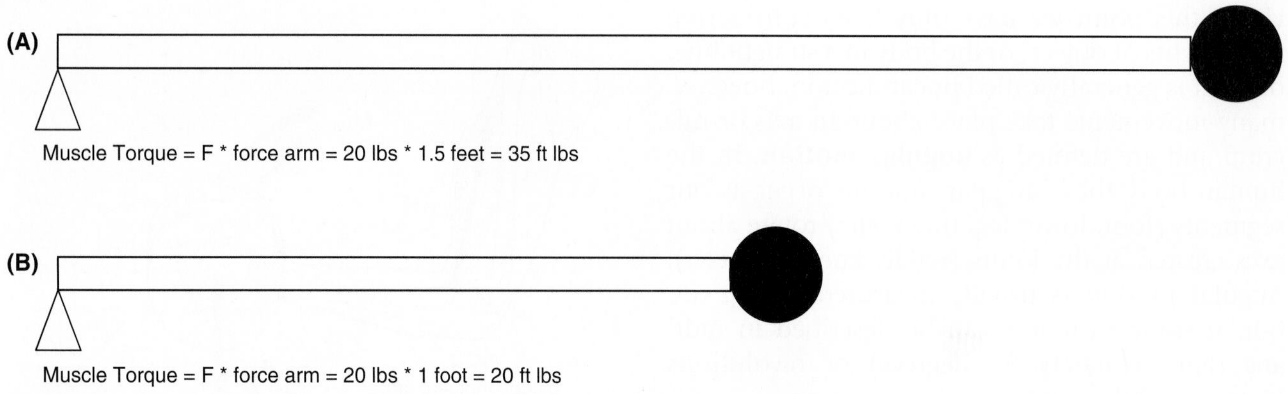

FIGURE 5.3 **A.** A longer force arm with the same mass = more torque required to move the object; **(B)** A shorter force arm with the same mass = less torque required to move the object.

amount of rotary inertia. If instead the runner flexes the knee during the swing phase, this will bring the lower leg and foot closer to the hip (axis of rotation) and in so doing decreasing the rotary inertia and allowing the entire leg to now flex forward at a faster rate. This allows for the person to get through the recovery (swing) phase in a much shorter time and therefore run much faster (Fig. 5.4).

Though this example demonstrates how bringing the mass closer to the axis of rotation promotes faster rotations, there are instances when rotation is not desired and the goal is to increase the rotary inertia. Good examples of this are individuals walking along a tightrope. These daredevils often carry a long pole in their hands that is bent down from weights attached at its ends. The weights serve two purposes: it puts mass far away from the performer and brings the center of gravity of the individual closer to the wire rendering them more stable and less likely to tip over (angular motion) to one side or the other due to the greater rotary inertia (Fig. 5.5).

The term **balance** implies control of equilibrium, whereas **stability** is resistance to loss of equilibrium. One of the ways individuals increase their stability is by increasing their base of support. This base of support is defined as the two-dimensional area formed by the supporting segments of the body (Fig. 5.6). Coaches often ask their players to spread their feet shoulder-width apart rendering them more stable. Increasing the base of support enhances stability because it increases the distance your line of gravity has to move before it is ends up outside this base, causing a loss of balance. Once the line of gravity is outside the base of support, the body will experience a destabilizing torque from the pull of gravity that will tend to topple the body over. Lowering your center of gravity also increases stability by decreasing the magnitude of this destabilizing torque by reducing distance from your center of gravity to your axis of rotation (your feet on the ground). Olympic lifting

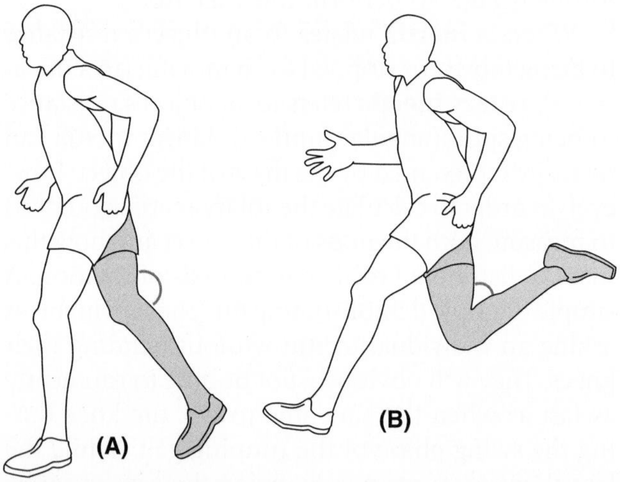

FIGURE 5.4 There is much more knee flexion during the swing phase of running **(B)** than there is when walking **(A)**. This allows the runner to decrease the rotary inertia of the swing leg and move it much faster.

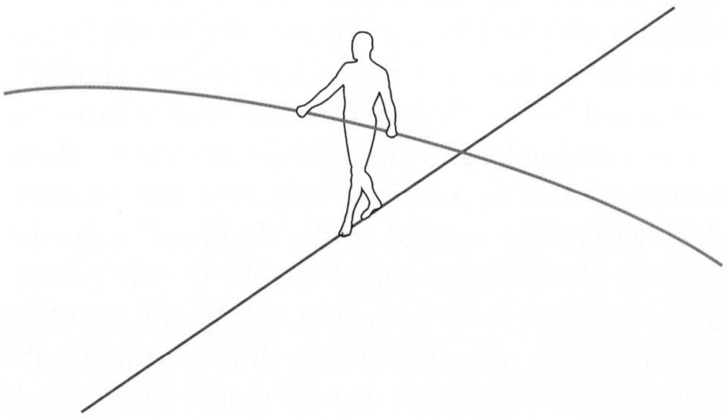

FIGURE 5.5 The pole used by a tightrope walker increases their rotary inertia.

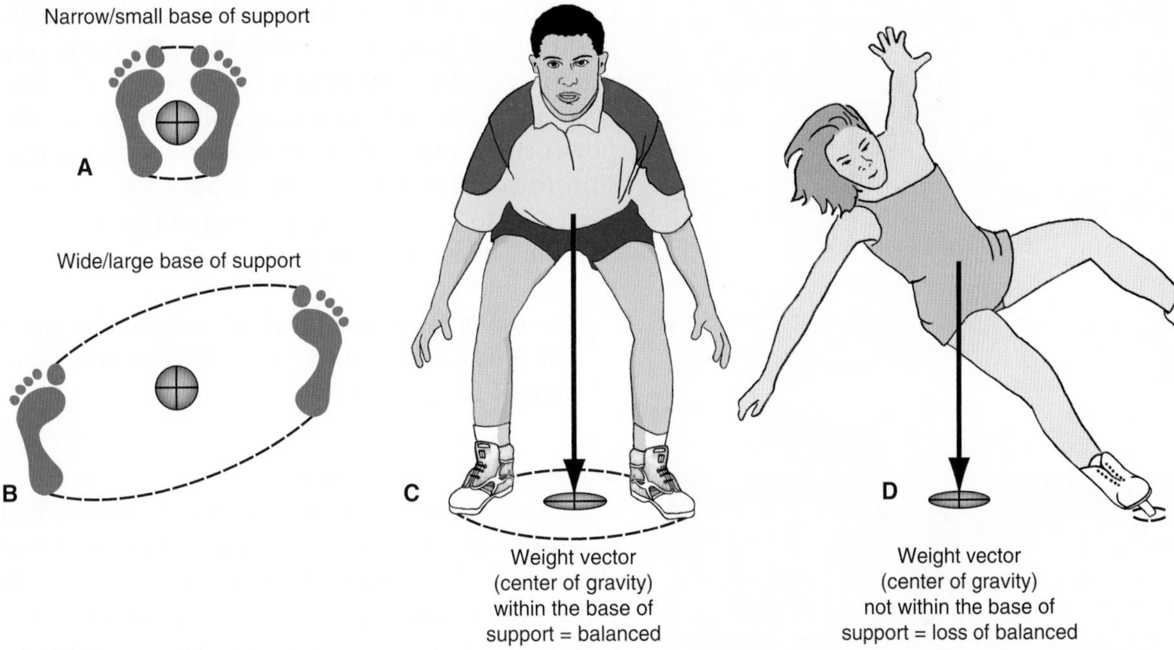

FIGURE 5.6 The position of the center of gravity relative to the base of support determines whole body stability and balance.

competitions require not only for the athlete to lift the weight above their heads but also need to demonstrate control of the weight by balancing it for 3 seconds. This balance is difficult due to the high center of gravity position since it is not uncommon for these athletes to be lifting more than two times their own body weight. Therefore, a shorter lifter would have a stability advantage over a much taller lifter as the same small movement of the load would produce a greater destabilizing torque on the taller lifter. The most unstable foot position possible in a human being is standing on one foot. When standing on one foot our base of support becomes the length or width of the foot, and if the center of gravity falls outside of the dimensions of the foot, there will be a loss of balance. The strength and conditioning specialist can use this foot position during many different exercises to train whole body stability. By training in this very unstable position, one can further develop the body's sensory and muscular recruitment strategies needed to maintain balance. Several pieces of equipment frequently in use in strength and conditioning facilities also have the goal of creating an unstable surface to allow for the training of the ability to maintain balance.

One such recent invention is the BOSU ball (Fig. 5.7). If we stand on the platform side of this ball the base of support becomes the portion of the ball that is in contact with ground. The stability challenge can then be altered by how much air you put in the ball. If the ball is pumped up with a lot of air, it will be very rigid and you will be balancing on a really small area of the ball. This makes maintaining balance more difficult as the base of support is extremely small. To make this challenge easier, you can remove air from the ball so that the ball become softer and more of it then comes in contact with the ground, increasing the base of support.

Friction can sometimes be used to increase the difficulty of a certain task or exercise. The two factors related to friction are the nature of the two surfaces attempting to slide past one another (the coefficient of friction) and the amount of force pressing the two surfaces together (the normal force). Monarch cycle ergometers use increased tension of the belt around the wheel to increase the friction and increase the resistance. Football coaches stand on top of blocking sleds to increase the force pressing the sled to the ground and in so doing making it harder for football players to push the sled across the grass. Application of talcum powder to the hands in order to remove moisture and get a better grip is an example of changing the nature of the surfaces in contact.

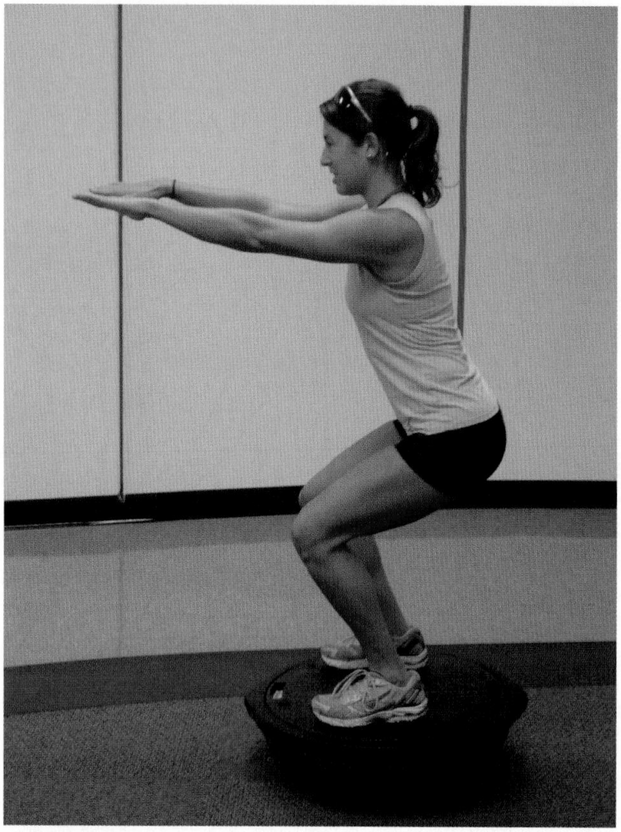

FIGURE 5.7 Using a BOSU ball to alter the size of the base of support during a squatting exercise.

HUMAN MUSCULOSKELETAL MECHANICS

LENGTH–TENSION RELATIONSHIP

There are two types of tissues that can create tension in a muscle: (a) the active component consisting of the acting and myosin muscle proteins and (b) the passive component consisting of the connective tissue within the muscle belly which comes together on either end to form the muscle tendon. The tension/force that can be created by these two different types of tissues changes as the length of the muscle changes throughout a movement (4,5).

The length–tension curve for the active component of muscle is an inverted "U" shape. The peak of this curve (where the maximum active tension/force can be produced) corresponds to the position where the muscle is in an optimal position to allow the most actin/myosin crossbridges. As the muscle is increasingly stretched beyond this length, these crossbridges are torn apart so the amount of tension/force the active component of muscle can produce decreases as the length of the muscle increases. Conversely, as the muscle is shortened from this optimal length, increasing numbers of the actin/myosin crossbridges become overlapped and are no longer able to produce the power strokes that allow for the production of tension/force. Therefore, as the length of a muscle decreases so too does the amount of tension/force that the active component of muscle can produce.

The use of various methods of resistance training can produce force-curve characteristics similar to those of the sport/movement activities.

The passive component of muscle only produces force/tension when the muscle is lengthened. You can think of your muscles as elastic bands. If you shorten an elastic band beyond its resting length it does not create any tension/force. The only way to produce tension/force of an elastic band is to stretch it beyond its resting length so that it then tries to snap back to its original shape. Therefore, when a muscle is shortened the total length–tension curve involves only the inverted U shape of the active component. However, as the muscle is increasingly lengthened, the tendon and connective tissues are stretched beyond their resting length and produce an increasing amount of force with increased lengthening. Therefore, the total tension/force achieved when a muscle is stretched beyond its resting length is the sum of both the active and passive components (Fig. 5.8).

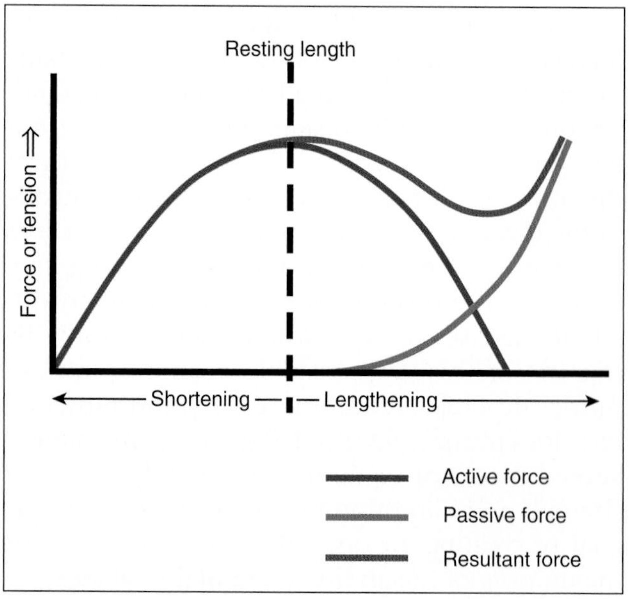

FIGURE 5.8 The active, passive, and resultant forces for the typical muscle length tension curve.

FORCE–VELOCITY–POWER RELATIONSHIP

Although the amount of force a muscle can produce is important, perhaps more important in many human movements is the velocity at which a muscle can develop this force. Often the terms "strength" and "power" are used erroneously interchangeably. Strength refers to a muscles ability to produce force in isometric or slow velocity contractions, whereas power refers to a combination of force production and velocity (6). Training only force development at slow speeds (strength) may have negative implications for a wide range of individuals.

Most sports require the application of maximal power output rather than force.

Obviously, most sporting activities involve high velocity/high power movements and, therefore it may not be effective to train an athlete to only be able to slowly develop extremely large forces. Also, in order to train older adults to avoid falls, we must be concerned with the velocity of muscular contraction as well. If an individual loses his or her balance, he or she must move quickly and adjust the position of his or her center of gravity or take a step to widen the base of support to avoid falling. It has also been shown that as one ages, explosive strength or power decreases more than the maximum isometric strength (7), which makes training these fast muscular contractions essential in older adults. Therefore, an understanding of the relationship between force, velocity, and power presented in Figure 5.9 (5) is essential for the strength and conditioning specialist.

Training at velocities and joint angles specific to the sport/movement activities will result in the greatest carryover to performance.

If a muscle is maximally activated in an attempt to produce movements at different speeds, several important points must be observed:

1. As the speed of concentric contraction increases, the force that can be produced during those contractions decreases. Therefore, the minimum amount of force a muscle can produce is during a fast concentric contraction.
2. Greater tension can be developed during an isometric contraction (velocity = 0) than during any speed of concentric contraction.

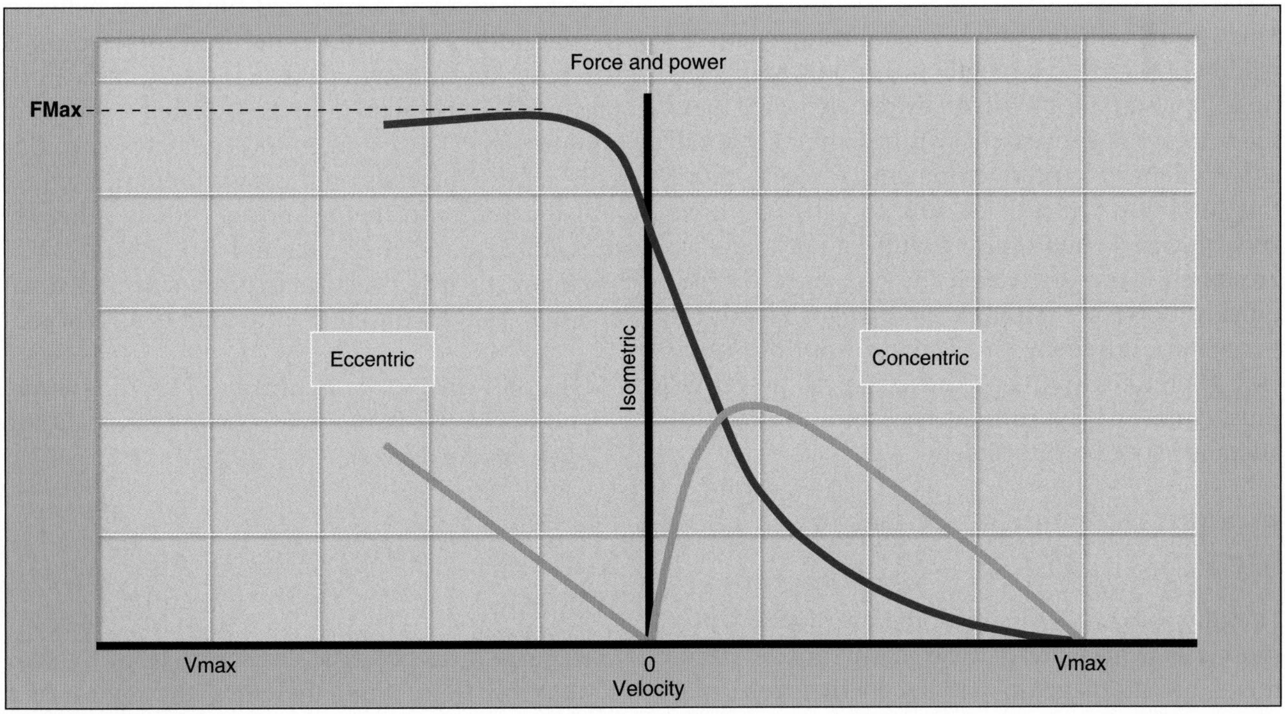

FIGURE 5.9 The force–velocity (*purple*), power–velocity (*orange*) relationship. *Note:* Recent research (Carney et al.) has determined the eccentric force-power relationship.

3. Muscles can generate their greatest forces while resisting motion during eccentric (lengthening) contractions. These eccentric or lengthening velocities are shown as negative velocities (X axis) in Figure 5.9. It should also be noted that forces generated during eccentric contractions also rise slightly and then remain relatively constant as velocity increases.
4. As was mentioned in the Basic Mechanics section, Power = force × velocity. Since force and concentric velocity have an inverse relationship (i.e., as velocity goes up, force goes down), the point of peak concentric power will occur somewhere between an isometric and maximum velocity concentric contraction. The in vitro concentric power curve derived from the force–velocity relationship of skeletal muscle is highly dependent on the movement being tested. Izquierdo et al. (7) demonstrated that the best resistances (forces) for the development of peak power in the upper body were in the range of 30% to 45% of maximum isometric force. However, for explosive lower body movements peak power was observed at 60% to 70% of maximum isometric force.
5. Recent research (Carney et al.) has demonstrated that as eccentric velocity increases, power increases as well in a linear relationship.

This force–velocity–power relationship can be readily observed in strength and conditioning settings. If we attempt to lift an extremely heavy load, the velocity of movement will be extremely small as we will need to produce maximal forces to move this load and will not be able to get it to move very quickly. When training with lighter loads we are much more able to get the resistance moving quickly; however, training with too light a load will necessitate extremely small forces from our muscles. Therefore, in order to achieve peak power we must choose an appropriate resistance to allow for adequate speed of movement.

PHYSIOLOGICAL CROSS-SECTIONAL AREA

The physiological cross-sectional area (PCSA) of a muscle is a measure of how many muscle sarcomeres are arranged in parallel in that particular muscle. This has been shown to determine the maximum force generating capacity of the muscle (8). Therefore a bigger muscle (larger PCSA) can produce more force than a smaller muscle (small PCSA). This is logical as one of the main goals of resistance training is to increase the size and hence the force-producing capacity of our muscles.

One muscle with an extremely large PCSA in the human body is the gluteus maximus muscle (9). With the force-generating capacity of this muscle being so large, many smaller muscles must compensate for it if it is not working efficiently. Therefore, it is important that we train it appropriately as extremely common pathologies such as low back pain have been associated with a loss of neural drive to this muscle—termed "gluteal amnesia" (10).

STRETCH-SHORTENING CYCLE

Most human movements begin with motions in the opposite direction to the intended movement. In a vertical jump, this involves the initial flexion of the knee/hips and dorsiflexion of the ankles used to accelerate the center of gravity downward. This causes an eccentric stretch of the knee/hip extensors and ankle plantarflexors that is quickly turned into a concentric contraction of these same muscles to produce the upward motion of the center of gravity, resulting in the jump. This eccentric stretch followed closely by a concentric shortening has been termed the **stretch-shortening cycle** (SSC) of a muscle. If there is a minimal time delay between the eccentric stretch and concentric contraction, it has been shown that there is an increase in the force produced as compared to an isolated concentric contraction (11). The magnitude of increase in concentric force depends on the movement performed and the resistance being moved, but is generally thought to be in the magnitude of 10% to 20%. Therefore, the SSC is critical in producing high force and high power concentric muscular contractions.

The SSC is inherent in almost all sporting movements and this mechanism is critical for producing high force and power.

JOINT ANGLE AND MUSCULAR TORQUE

Muscles pull on bones at a distance from the axis of rotation (joint) and therefore, they produce a torque that attempts to produce angular motion of the bones to which they are attached. The amount

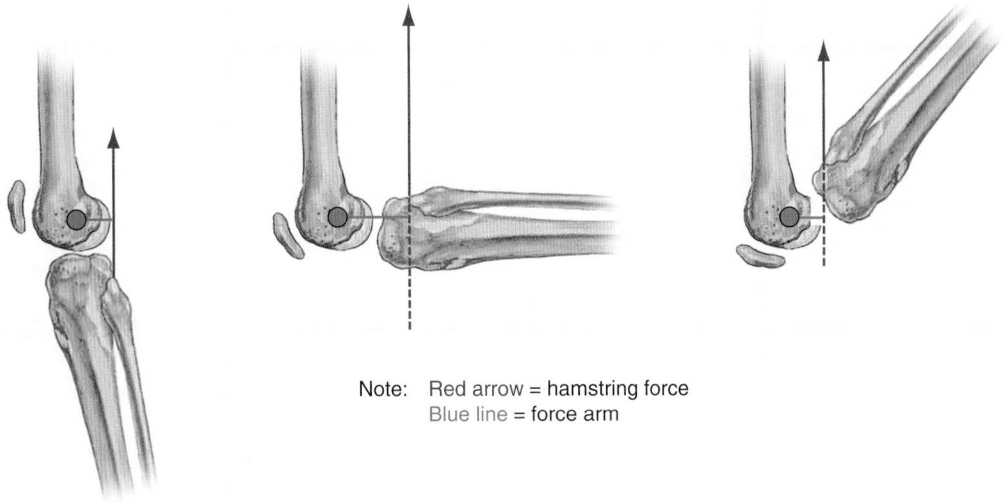

FIGURE 5.10 The change in the torque generating capacity (force arm distance) of the hamstring muscles as the knee joint angle changes.

of torque can be calculated by multiplying the force by the force-arm distance. As a muscle causes movement of the bones, the length of the force arm changes. This means that with the same amount of muscular force, there are changes in the amount of torque generated as the muscle moves the joint through its range of motion. In a simple hinge joint like the elbow/knee, the flexors (biceps brachii/hamstrings) are at a mechanical advantage at a joint angle of 90 degrees as the force arm is the longest in this joint position. As the joint angle increases or decreases, the force arm decreases in length, creating less torque with the same muscular force (Fig. 5.10).

LEVERS

The arrangement of the bones, muscles and joints in the human body create simple machines called lever systems. The anatomical levers of the body cannot be changed, but when the system is well understood, they can be used more efficiently to maximize the muscular efforts of the body (12). The three components of every lever system include the axis (joint), the resistance (weight of the segment being moved and any attached external weight) and the force (muscle force). The location of these three components with respect to one another will determine the type of lever and most importantly, the movement characteristics for which they are best suited. The lever type is determined primarily by which of the three components is located in between the other two. That is, a first class lever has the axis in between the other two, while a second class lever has the resistance in the middle, and finally, a third class lever has the force in between the axis and resistance (Fig. 5.11).

The distances between the axis and the force (force arm [FA]) and the axis and the resistance (resistance arm [RA]) help determine the types of movements that each lever system is best designed to perform. Those levers with a short RA and a long FA are said to have a large **mechanical advantage** (calculated by dividing the FA by the RA). This is because large resistances can be moved short distances with small forces if a lever is used that creates this mechanical advantage. For example, if a 180 lb person wants to move a 900 lb rock, they could do this most effectively by getting a board and wedging it under the rock and then balancing the board on an object really close to the rock (creating the axis of rotation). If the distance between the axis and the rock is 2 ft this creates 1,800 ft-lbs of torque that must be overcome in order to move the rock. Therefore, the person would need to jump on the board 10 ft from the axis to produce the required torque needed to move the large rock, but the resultant displacement and hence the velocity of the rock would not be large.

Human muscle bone levers have the muscles attached really close to the joints creating extremely short FAs. By comparison, our limb segments are relatively long creating much longer RAs. This creates a mechanical disadvantage or a **velocity/speed advantage** (calculated by dividing the RA by the FA) in human muscle bone levers. This is due to the fact that it will take a lot of force to get the resistance moving (mechanical disadvantage), but once we get it moving it will have a much larger displacement

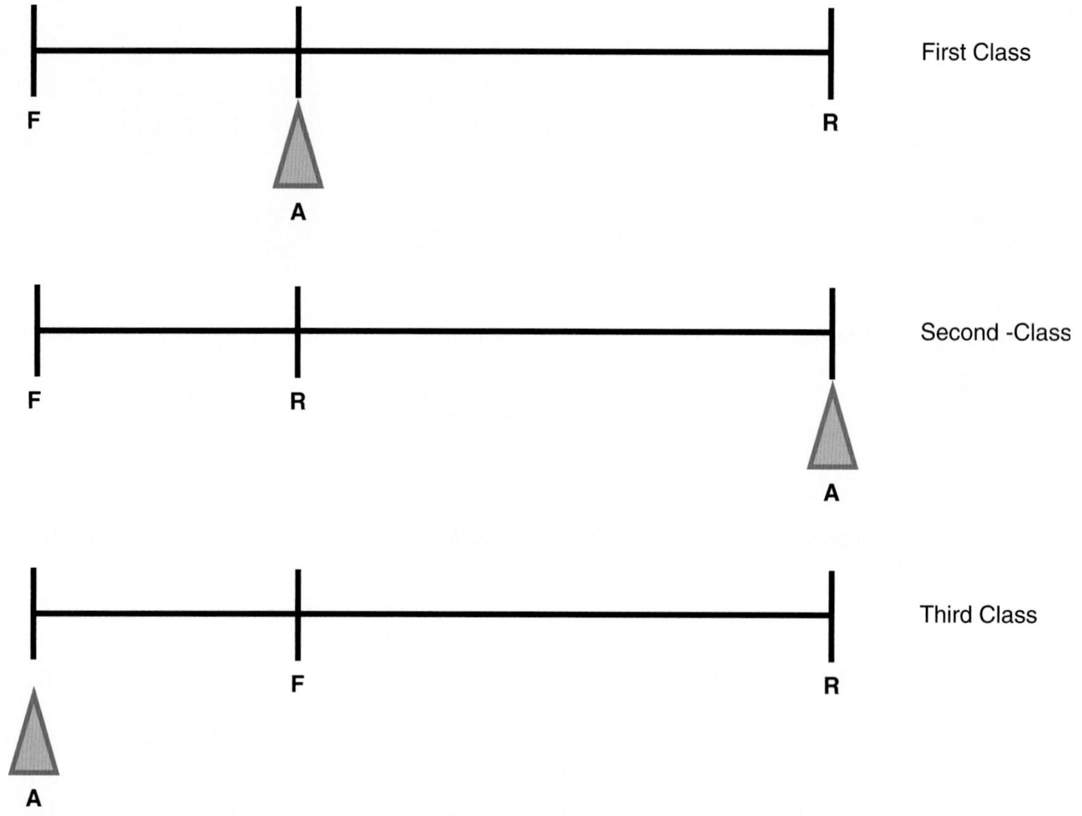

FIGURE 5.11 First class, second class, and third class lever systems.

and hence velocity/speed. This concept is displayed in research that examined the anatomical differences in the ankle/foot between a group of collegiate sprinters and a group of height matched nonathletes (13). It was discovered that the sprinters had longer toes and also had 25% shorter Achilles tendon FAs (Fig. 5.12). Therefore, the sprinters had shorter FA and were also able, with their longer toes, to get the force of the ground pushing back up on their foot further from the axis of rotation at their ankle, creating a longer RA. This creates a greater velocity/speed advantage that may be one mechanical reason why sprinters can run faster than nonsprinters.

The musculoskeletal system is designed for speed and range of motion rather than high force production.

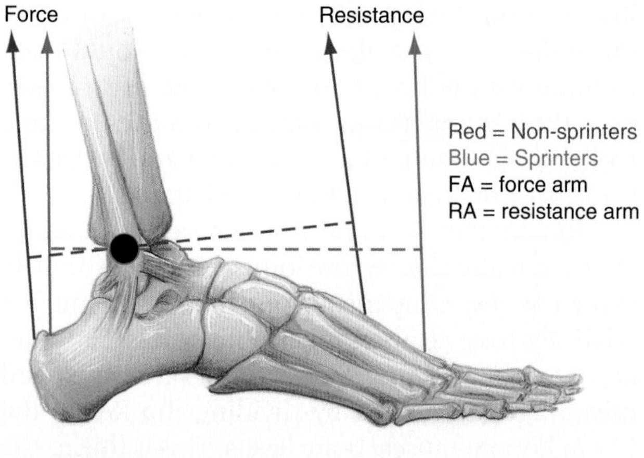

FIGURE 5.12 The differences in anatomy noted by Lee and Piazza (2009) between sprinters and nonsprinters. Sprinters had a shorter force arm and a longer resistance arm, creating a speed advantage.

BIOMECHANICS OF RESISTANCE

In strength and conditioning settings, various forms of resistance have been used to make movements/exercises more challenging. The extra stimulus provided by this resistance can help accomplish the goal of the training session, whether it is simply to make fundamental human movement patterns more efficient or to increase strength, speed, or both (i.e., power). The original and most commonly used form of resistance simply utilizes different forms of mass and the force of gravity. As various technologies have advanced, other forms of resistance have been developed that have certain biomechanical characteristics that are different from mass and provide a different stimulus to the human body during training. The following section will examine several different forms of resistance and discuss how the mechanics of these then produce different training stimuli. This information is important for the strength and conditioning specialist so that the appropriate form of resistance can be used to accomplish the specific functional goal of the training. It is important to tailor the training to the particular goal of the program to ensure success. An appropriate analogy can be drawn to the engines in our automobiles. A formula one car (designed for speed) will require a much different engine than a truck designed to haul and tow large loads. The strength and conditioning specialist needs to choose the appropriate form of resistance to ensure that we are building the correct engines (muscles) to meet the goals of the individual.

The following section will examine the biomechanics of several different forms of resistance, which will be divided into two main categories: (a) those that use mass and the force of gravity as the resistance and (b) those that do not use significant mass and generate the mechanical resistance using other means.

MASS

When using any form of mass as resistance, the most important biomechanical concept that the strength and conditioning specialist must keep in mind is its inherent inertial properties. To be put another way, mass resists changes to its state of motion. So if it is not moving, large forces must be applied to the mass to get it moving, and once it begins moving, less force must be applied to keep it moving. Most overlook the fact that, when performing a lift with a 20-lb dumbbell, the resistance provided to the human body throughout that lift can vary from much greater than 20 lb to overcome the inertia of that mass, to almost zero if the mass is accelerated to a high enough speed during the lift.

The force the person is applying to the mass can best be calculated using the equation $F = \text{ma} + \text{mg}$. The second part of this equation (mg) is constant as the acceleration due to gravity ($g = 9.81\ \text{m} \cdot \text{s}^{-2}$) and the mass remain constant throughout a lift. However, the first half of this equation (ma) is not constant as the mass must be accelerated at the start of the lift and decelerated at the end of the lift. If a mass is moved extremely slowly through the range of motion, the effect of the "ma" term becomes negligible; however, for rapid movements with large changes in speed, this term becomes extremely important and can cause great variation in the resistance felt by the muscles throughout the range of motion. It has been shown that doing high-speed lifts with free-weight resistance requires in excess of 190% of the weight of the load in order to produce these high accelerations (14,15). That means that if doing a bench press with 130 lb, the resistance at the beginning of the concentric phase can actually exceed 250 lb as the momentum of the eccentric phase is quickly absorbed and the bar is accelerated concentrically to a high rate of speed. Then, once the weight is moving at a high rate of speed, the resistance provided to the muscles can decrease to almost zero if the weight is accelerated fast enough that the magnitude of the (m × a) term equals that of the (m × g) term. This gives the lifter the feeling that the bar is temporarily floating and almost thrown into the air, which can be dangerous in a bench press movement. This is demonstrated by studies showing that well-trained athletes can spend up to 52% of the concentric phase of a high speed lift attempting to decelerate and control the trajectory of the load (16), this leads to a decrease in the activity of the muscles producing the movement during this portion of the lift (15).

Two common forms of mass used as resistance in strength and conditioning settings include (a) free weights and (b) gravity-based machines.

Free Weights

Free weights are often thought to include only barbells and dumbbells but can also come in many other forms. Any object that has a mass and allows for 6 degrees of freedom movement of that mass can be considered a "free weight." Other common forms of free weights include: kettlebells, medicine balls, weight vests, weighted ankle/wrist straps, weighted sleds, training ropes, chains, and the simplest form of resistance of all, the individual's own body weight. The biomechanics of these forms of resistance follow the laws of inertia outlined above and always have the resistance acting vertically downward. Therefore, the force needed to move these weights vertically can be determined using the formula $F = \text{ma} + \text{mg}$. The force needed to move these weights horizontally does not need to overcome gravity and therefore can be determined using $F = \text{ma}$. Therefore, adjusting how much a mass is moved horizontally/vertically can be a good method of progressing and regressing many different movements as the amount of gravity that must be overcome during the movement can be altered.

Q & A from the Field

Q ***If the elbow flexors are strongest at 90 degrees of flexion, why is the "sticking point" in the midrange of the movement?***

A The elbow is strongest in flexion at 90 degrees because the length of the force arm, "the perpendicular distance from the muscle insertion to the axis of rotation," is maximal at 90 degrees. However, the RA, the perpendicular distance from the point of force application to the axis of rotation, is also greatest in the midrange of the motion for an isotonic exercise. Although the mechanical advantage of the elbow flexors is greatest at 90 degrees, the increasing length of the RA in a heavy isotonic exercise overcomes this advantage. The sticking point will occur somewhere near 90 degrees of flexion.

Gravity-Based Machines

The resistance of any mass acts vertically down which limits our ability to train certain muscle groups. For example, using mass to train a vertical shoulder press movement is appropriate but in order to train the antagonist movement (i.e., lat pull down exercise), the gravity force needs to be redirected. This is accomplished by machines that use cables and pulleys to allow us to direct the resistance of a mass/gravity upward or horizontally (Fig. 5.13). Older versions of these machines would have the user adjust the resistance by adding/removing weighted plates but newer versions of these machines use pin loaded weight stacks to make the adjusting of the resistance much easier.

Engineers have also attempted to design gravity based machines so that the resistance delivered to the individual better matches our muscles' ability to produce force across the range of motion of the joint. For example, in the free weight bench press we are limited in resistance by the amount we are able to move through our weakest point (sticking point) near the bottom of the lift. Therefore, our

Q & A from the Field

Q ***How can I alter the squat movement pattern to make it more "knee dominant" or more "hip dominant"?***

A Muscle contributions to movement depend on their external loading. During any weight bearing activity, our body weight acts down and pushes our feet into the ground. The ground then pushes back up on us creating a Ground Reaction Force (GRF). In a squat, when the knee and hip are flexed, this GRF falls anterior to the hip and posterior to the knee in the sagittal plane. Therefore, the GRF is trying to push both of these joints into flexion and the extensor muscles must control these torques in the eccentric phase and overcome them in the concentric phase. The distance of this GRF vector from the knee and the hip helps to determine how hard each of these muscle groups will have to work to produce the movement. A more "hip dominant" squat has the GRF acting closer to the knee and further from the hip (increasing the torque on the hip and decreasing the torque on the knee). A more "knee dominant" squat has the GRF acting closer to the hip and further from the knee (increasing the torque on the knee and decreasing the torque on the hip).

There are several ways to alter how much the knee and hip extensors contribute to producing this motion, but all utilize this basic mechanical principle. One simple way to shift the loading onto one joint or the other to change where the mass of the body segments and resistance are located. Doing a counter-balanced squat, where you hold weights in your hands and raise them in front of you as you sit back in the squat, shifts the GRF anteriorly. This makes the exercise more "hip dominant" as it increases the load on the hip extensors and decreases the load on the knee extensors. Conversely, performing a squat where the weights remain on your shoulders keeps the GRF acting more posteriorly, which makes it more "knee dominant" (increases the load on the knee extensors and decreases the load on the hip extensors). (Lynn & Noffal, in press)

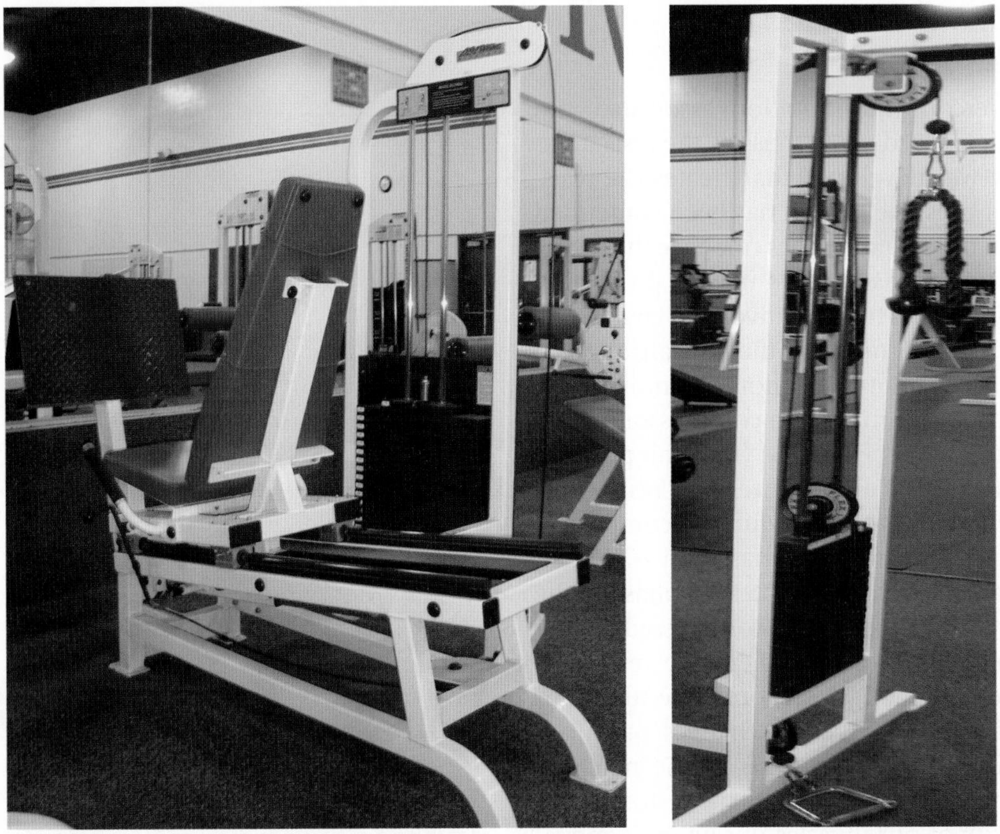

FIGURE 5.13 Two gravity based weight machines that allow the resistance of the mass to be redirected using pulleys.

muscles are not getting challenged appropriately in the upper part of the range of motion.

This was originally overcome by creating machines where the user would start the movement in their weakest position (i.e., the bottom position of the chest press movement), but with the machine lever arm to the weight stack extremely short. As the movement proceeded from bottom to top, the machine's lever arm to the weight stack would increase in length thus also increasing the resistance felt by the user in later stages of the lift. Various other gravity based machines have also attempted to produce a variable amount of resistance throughout a lift using different designs.

One common design uses a cable or chain that wraps over a variable-radius cam and alters the lever arm distance to the resistance (weight stack) as the user moves through the range of motion (Fig. 5.14). Again, this allows for the user to feel more resistance at portions of the lift where the muscles are mechanically strongest and less resistance where the muscles are less optimally positioned. However, all of these machines use mass for the resistance and therefore the speed of movement becomes really important as creating large accelerations of the mass will negate the effects of these variable resistance designs.

Understanding the mechanics underlying a piece of resistance training or conditioning equipment will assist in initial purchase decisions as well as exercise selection.

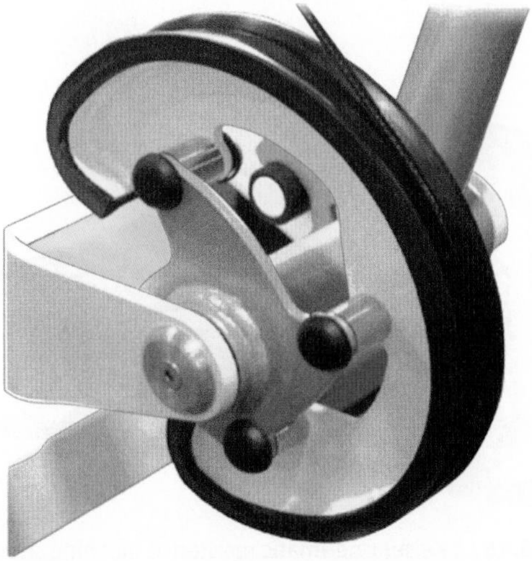

FIGURE 5.14 A variable radius cam.

OTHER FORMS OF RESISTANCE

Pneumatic Resistance

In order to overcome the limitations associated with training at high speed using mass as the resistance, a technology was developed that creates the resistance with air pressure (17). It has been contended that this form of resistance does not have the inherent limitations of mass and its inertial properties. Therefore, high speed training involving large accelerations can be performed and the resistance can be kept relatively constant throughout the movement. The basic technology involves a compressor pumping air into a cylinder (Fig. 5.15) (more air pressure = more resistance, less air pressure = less resistance) equipped with a piston that further compresses the air during the concentric phase and is pushed back out by the air during the eccentric phase of the movement. As the air is further compressed during the concentric phase of movement the resistance increases and this, along with some fine tuning of the force curve using leverage changes produced by engineering the moving parts of the machine appropriately, is thought to match the force producing capacity of our muscles during most movements. The user also has control of the resistance with hand buttons or foot pedals that can increase (pump in more air) or decrease (let air out) the resistance throughout the movement.

There has been a wide range of exercise equipment designed using this pneumatic resistance technology. Some of these include machines designed for high stability that guide the user through the range of motion and train only specific movements (chest press, leg extension, leg press, etc.) (see Fig. 5.16).

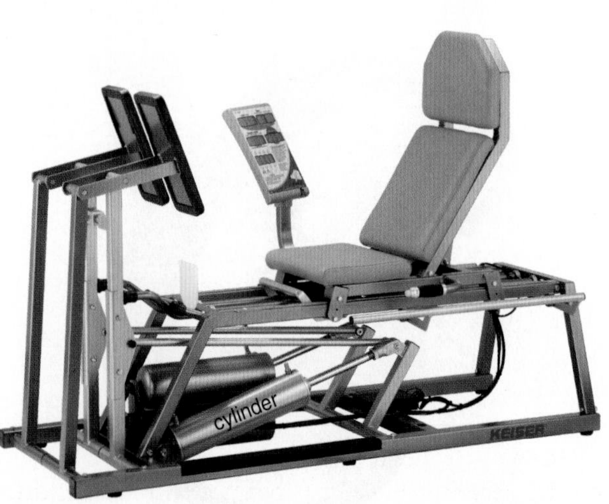

FIGURE 5.15 A Keiser pneumatic resistance machine showing the air cylinder (with the piston inside).

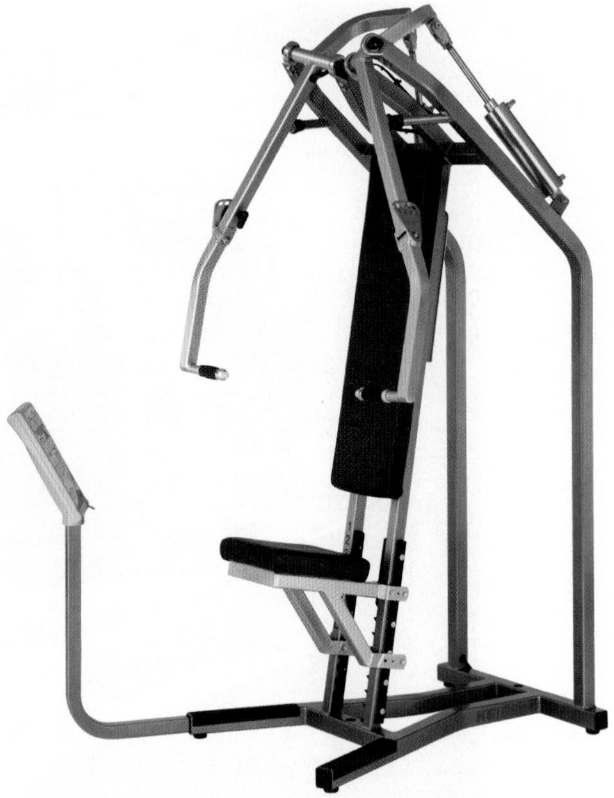

FIGURE 5.16 A pneumatic resistance machine designed for high stability by guiding the user through the range of motion.

There are also cable machines that can be adjusted to provide the resistance in the desired direction for the exercise and allow for a less controlled range of movement (see Fig. 5.17). Finally, there have been power racks designed to be able to incorporate both mass and air resistance in a wide range of total body 6 degrees of freedom movements (bench press, squat, dead lift, power clean, etc.). These can combine different amounts of mass and air resistance (Fig. 5.18) or can be used with negligible mass and only air resistance (Fig. 5.19), depending on the goal of the training session.

Research has shown that pneumatic resistance allows for greater movement velocities and also produces greater muscle activity at the end range of motion as compared to free weights in a bench press movement (18). This is due to the fact that pneumatic resistance contains limited mass and therefore does not develop momentum at high speeds. Athletic movements as well as many movements in everyday life (i.e., regaining equilibrium after a loss in balance) require high speed muscular contractions and velocity specific power production. Therefore, training with pneumatic

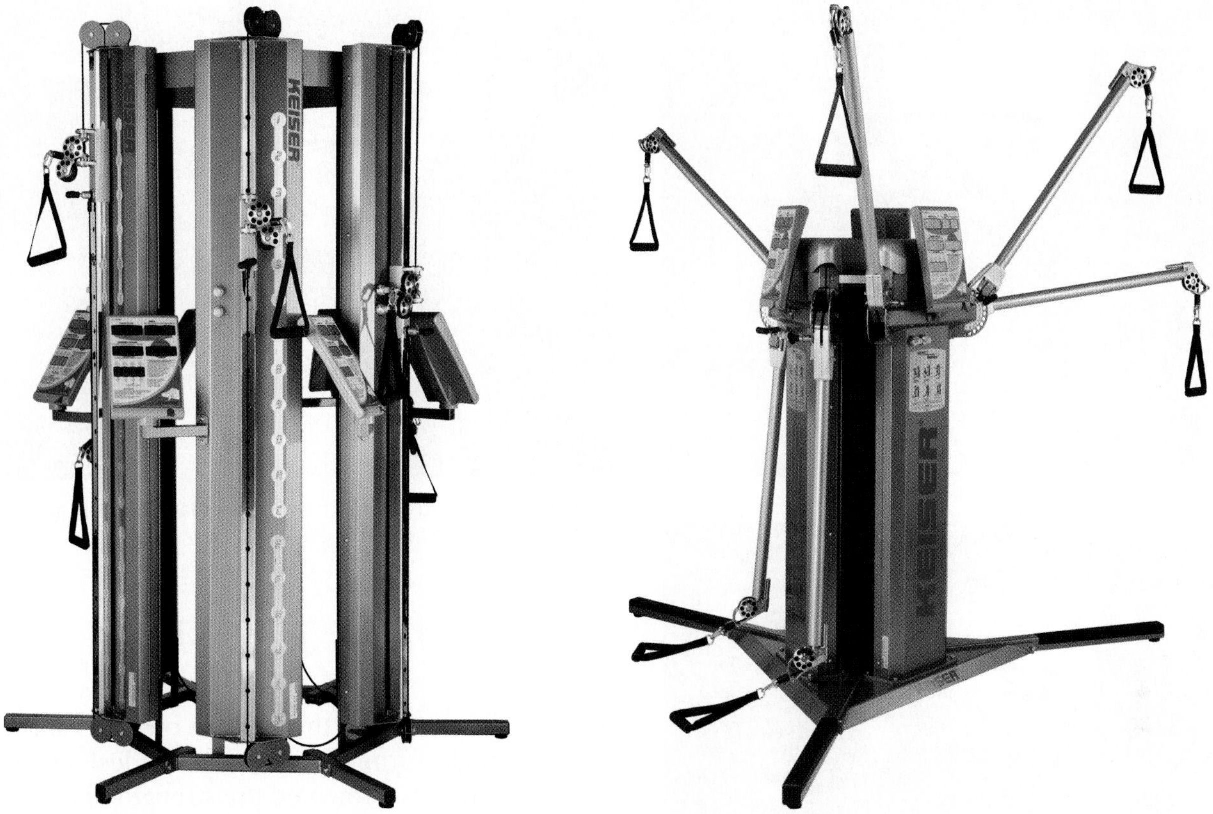

FIGURE 5.17 Adjustable pneumatic resistance machines that allow for the resistance to be directed in any direction and allow for much less control of the range of motion.

resistance could provide some movement specific advantages over free weights. However, this work also suggests that pneumatic resistance reduces the forces required to use the stretch shortening cycle at the end of the eccentric and start of the concentric phase of motion (18). Therefore, further investigation is needed to identify the neuromuscular responses of the human body to this alternate form of resistance.

Hydraulic Resistance

Another form of resistance similar to pneumatics uses fluid (generally oil) to create the resistance. This form of resistance has the movement drive a piston that forces the fluid through a small opening creating the resistance. The difference between pneumatic and hydraulic resistance comes in the compressibility of the fluid being used for the resistance. The air used in pneumatic resistance is compressible and, therefore, the forces put in to compressing it during the concentric phase are returned during the eccentric phase. The oil used in hydraulic resistance is essentially incompressible and, therefore, hydraulic resistance does not provide any eccentric resistance during movement.

It has been shown that greater gains in peak torque can be achieved when movements are trained both concentrically and eccentrically (19). However, an examination of the differences between groups of subjects training with free weights (concentric–eccentric) and hydraulics (concentric only) revealed no differences in velocity, torque, power, or force between groups (20). Therefore, there is some controversy in the literature regarding the usefulness of hydraulic resistance in a training program. It can also be suggested that the elimination of the eccentric phase created with this equipment may have uses for special populations as it may also decrease the muscle soreness experienced by the user.

Elastic Resistance

Various forms of elastic resistance have become extremely common in strength and conditioning settings recently. Elastics provide a variable amount of resistance throughout a movement as the elastic will produce more force the more it is stretched.

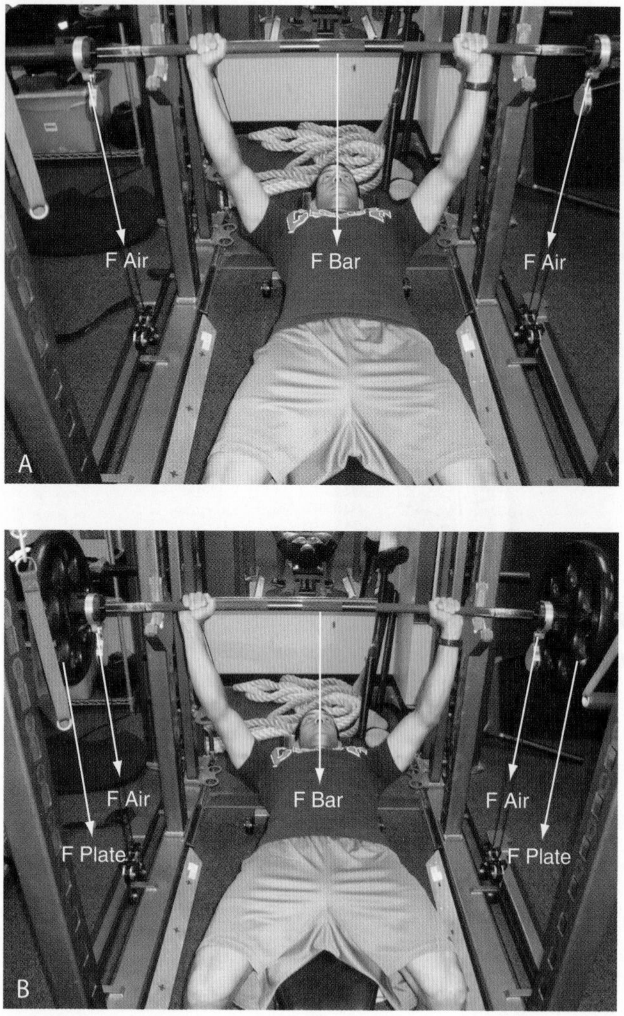

FIGURE 5.18 Combining mass (bar and plates) with pneumatic resistance in a bench press exercise.

It also provides an eccentric resistance as all the force that went into stretching the elastic will be returned as the individual's muscles control the speed at which the elastic is returned to its original length.

Studies comparing the effects of training with elastic resistance to training with mass as a resistance also provide contradictory results. In a sample of sedentary middle aged women, there was found to be no differences in several functional and structural measures between training with elastic resistance versus training with a weight machine (21). Whereas, in a sample of recreationally trained college students, those who trained by simply doing depth jumps (using body weight) increased their vertical jump height, while those who trained with elastic resistance (VertiMax) did not change their jump height after training (22).

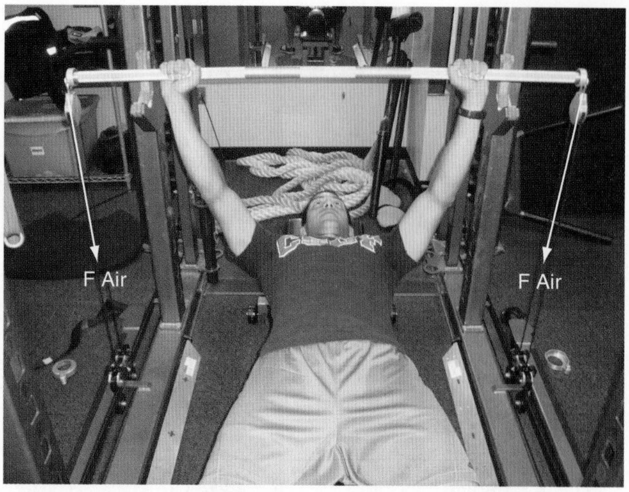

FIGURE 5.19 Using a bar with negligible mass and only air resistance in the bench press exercise.

WHAT FORM OF RESISTANCE IS BEST?

It should be clear from the sections outlined above that no single form of resistance is ideal for all training purposes. However, the strength and conditioning specialist must have a basic knowledge of all forms of resistance and how they can be combined and altered so that an appropriate stimulus can be selected to meet the goal of each individual training program.

PROGRESSING/REGRESSING MOVEMENT

As a strength and conditioning specialist, an important skill is to be able to modify movements/exercises to (a) increase the difficulty of movement to further challenge those who have mastered the basic movement and (b) decrease the difficulty of movement to allow those unable to perform the basic movement a chance to develop the proper strength and/or muscular recruitment strategies.

Progressing and regressing movements/exercises requires a good basic knowledge of many basic biomechanical principles. The simplest progressions and regressions can be performed by simply manipulating the variables of the equation presented in a previous section ($F = ma$). If we assume that progressions would generally involve creating movements that require more force production. This can be accomplished by either increasing the mass or increasing the rate of velocity change during the movement (acceleration or deceleration). Conversely, we could easily regress a movement/exercise by decreasing the mass being moved or by moving more slowly (requiring less accelerations/decelerations). Although this sounds logical, there are other factors that must be kept in mind. For example, moving extremely slowly through a bench press movement may seem like a regression (less accelerations) when it may actually make the exercise more difficult. Newton's First Law (Law of Inertia) tells us that an object in motion wants to remain in motion; therefore, getting the bar moving quickly in certain phases of the lift would require less muscular effort to keep it moving in other phases. This becomes important in overcoming points in the range of motion where the muscle length–tension relationship and angle of pull of muscle are at their least optimal (sticking point). Therefore, simply trying to manipulate the variables of that equation in order to progress/regress movements is not enough. The strength and conditioning specialist needs a much more complete knowledge of biomechanics to be able to tailor movement/exercise difficulty to the level of each individual.

The following section will use the example of the single-leg Romanian dead lift (RDL) in order to illustrate how biomechanical principles can be used to progress or regress a movement/exercise. We will begin with a biomechanical description of the basic movement.

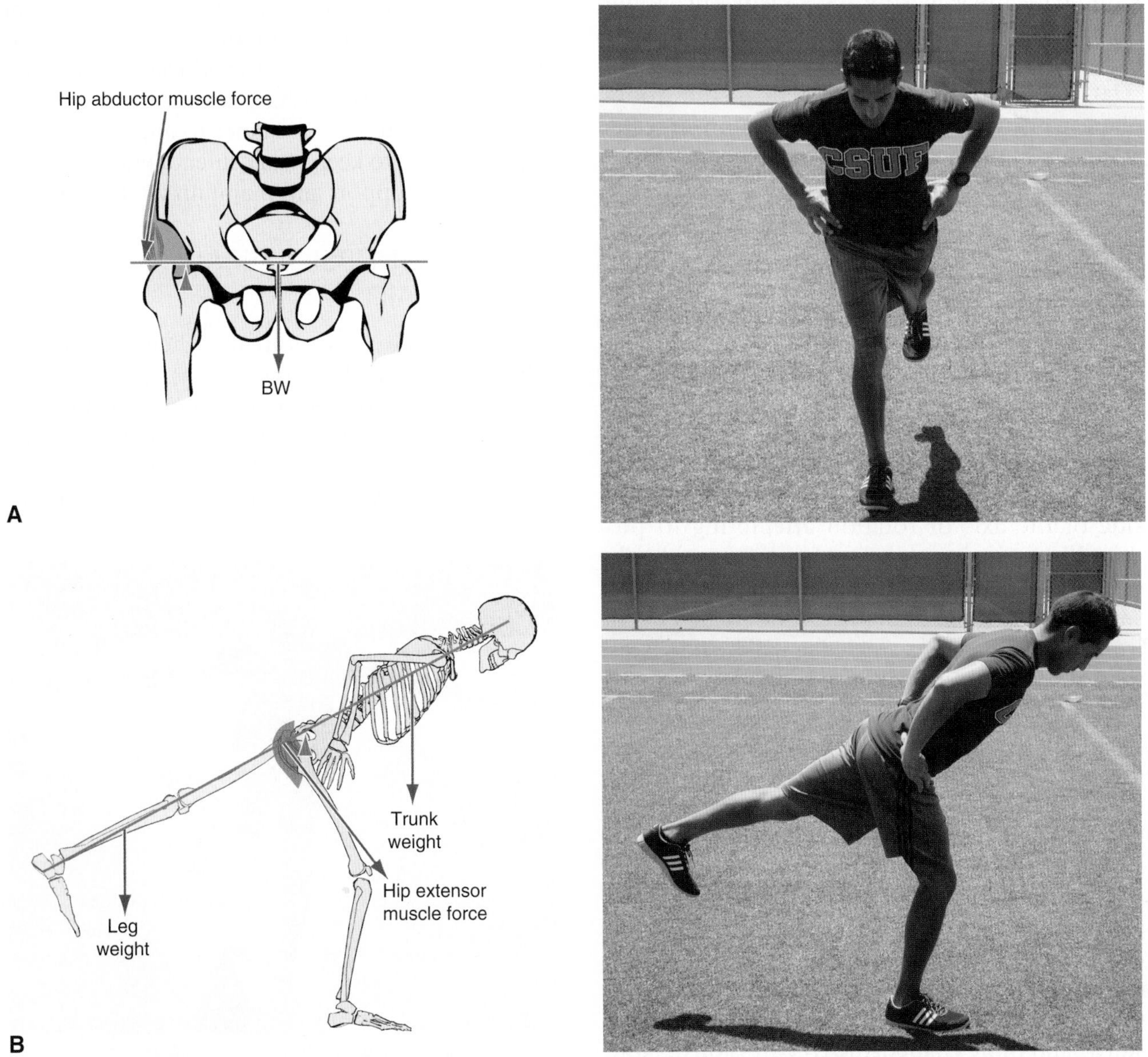

FIGURE 5.20 The basic single-leg Romanian dead-lift exercise.

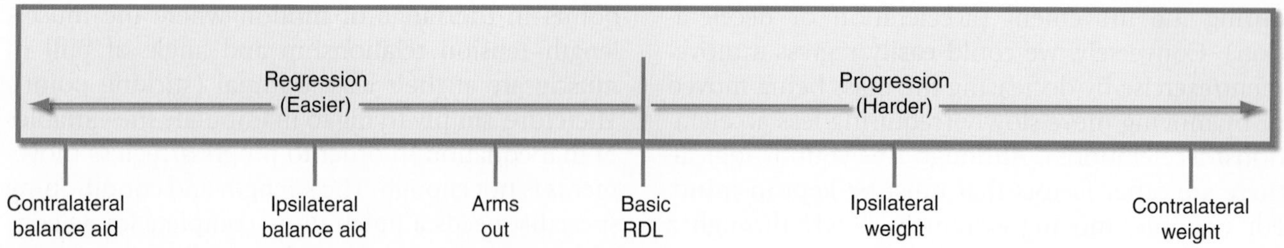

FIGURE 5.21 The single-leg RDL progression/regression continuum.

SINGLE-LEG ROMANIAN DEAD LIFT

This basic exercise (shown in Fig. 5.20) has several main goals when used in a training program. Some of these goals include (a) training the hip abductors to increase frontal plane control of the pelvis, (b) training the hip extensors in the sagittal plane, and (c) to train the balance and proprioceptive systems in single limb stance.

If we examine this movement in the frontal plane, we can see that the axis of rotation is created at the hip of the stance limb. Gravity then pulls on the rest of the body (person's left in Fig. 5.20) and produces a torque that is attempting to spin the pelvis clockwise. The hip abductors then produce a force on the other side of the axis of rotation to counter the body weight (clockwise) torque with the muscular (counterclockwise) torque needed to maintain a steady pelvis.

In the sagittal plane, tilting of the trunk anteriorly creates a clockwise torque attempting to produce flexion at the stance hip. We then have two counterclockwise torques acting on the other side of the axis of rotation attempting to produce hip extension: (a) the torque created by the weight of the contralateral leg (which will be of smaller magnitude than the torque created by the trunk as the mass of a single leg will be much less than the mass of the trunk) and (b) the muscle force created by the hip extensors that is needed to absorb the excess trunk torque in the eccentric phase and overcome it to produce the concentric hip extension needed to return to a standing position.

We will now examine how a good knowledge of biomechanics can be used to create three regressions and two progressions of the basic RDL exercise. The following continuum (Fig. 5.21) shows each of the five exercise modifications that can be used to make the exercise less challenging (regressions) and more challenging (progressions). Note: The further the exercise is to the right, the harder the exercise is; the further the exercise is to the left, the easier the exercise is.

REGRESSION: ARMS OUT

The first basic regression involves doing the exercise with your arms out in a "T" position as shown in Figure 5.22. This simple modification of the exercise spreads your mass out over a larger distance, which increases your rotary inertia in the frontal plane. This increased resistance to angular motion makes it easier to keep your center of gravity within your base of support and maintain your balance.

REGRESSION: IPSILATERAL BALANCE AID

In this middle regression, the client would use a balance aid in the same arm as the stance leg (Fig. 5.23). This regression does not have an effect in the frontal plane as the force produced by the balance aid passes directly through the axis of rotation of the hip and therefore does not increase or

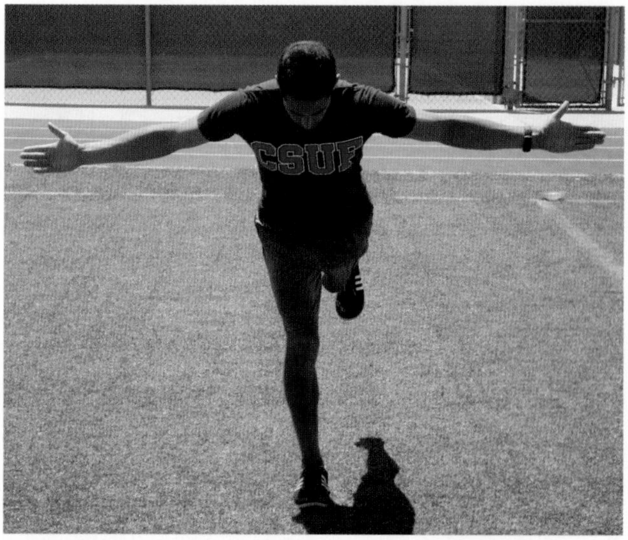

FIGURE 5.22 The single-leg RDL exercise—arms out regression.

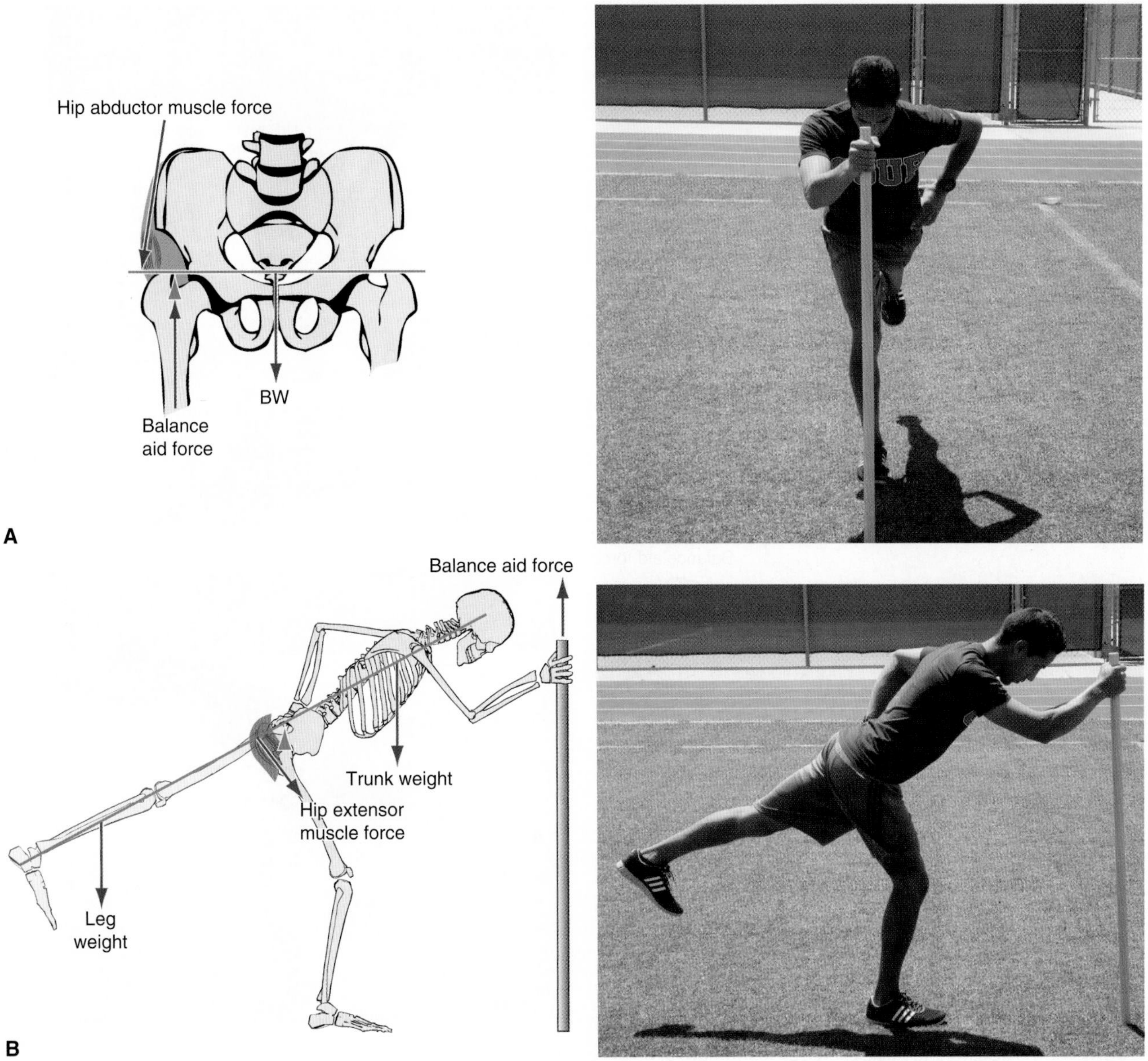

FIGURE 5.23 The single-leg RDL exercise—ipsilateral balance aid regression.

decrease the torque required from the hip abductors. The effect of this regression occurs in the sagittal plane as there is another force to help fight the weight of the trunk that is pulling the stance phase hip into flexion. This decreases the force required from the hip extensors to both slow down the hip flexion in the eccentric phase and to create the hip extension in the concentric phase.

The ipsilateral balance aid would also increase the base of support in the anterior–posterior direction, therefore, making it easier to maintain balance in this direction. However, it does not increase the base of support in the mediolateral direction.

REGRESSION: CONTRALATERAL BALANCE AID

In the third regression, the client would use a balance aid in the opposite arm as the stance leg (Fig. 5.24). This regression makes this exercise easier in both the sagittal and frontal planes. Since the balance aid is still the same distance from the axis of rotation of the hip in the sagittal plane, this regression would have the same effect on the hip extensors as would the ipsilateral balance aid. However, this regression decreases the challenge for the hip abductors in the frontal plane as the balance aid produces an extra counterclockwise torque

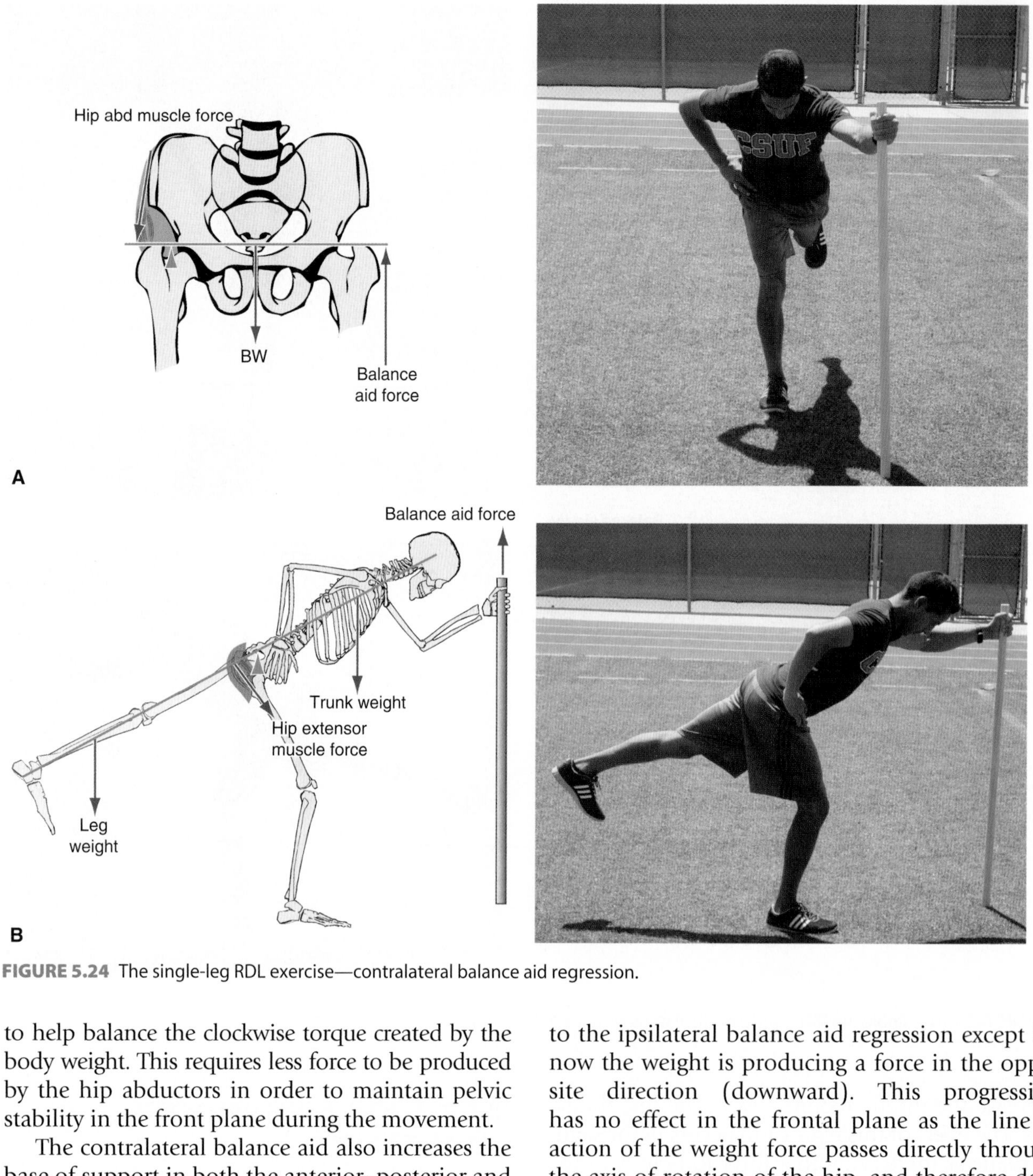

FIGURE 5.24 The single-leg RDL exercise—contralateral balance aid regression.

to help balance the clockwise torque created by the body weight. This requires less force to be produced by the hip abductors in order to maintain pelvic stability in the front plane during the movement.

The contralateral balance aid also increases the base of support in both the anterior–posterior and mediolateral directions. This makes it much easier to maintain the center of gravity within the base of support and maintain balance.

PROGRESSION: IPSILATERAL WEIGHT

The first progression involves adding a weight (generally a dumbbell) to the same hand as the stance leg (Fig. 5.25). This progression is similar to the ipsilateral balance aid regression except for now the weight is producing a force in the opposite direction (downward). This progression has no effect in the frontal plane as the line of action of the weight force passes directly through the axis of rotation of the hip, and therefore does not increase or decrease the torque required from the hip abductors. The effect of this progression occurs in the sagittal plane as the weight produces an extra clockwise torque that must be absorbed by increasing the eccentric and concentric force created by the hip extensors to perform this movement.

The use of various methods of resistance training can produce force-curve characteristics similar to those of the sport.

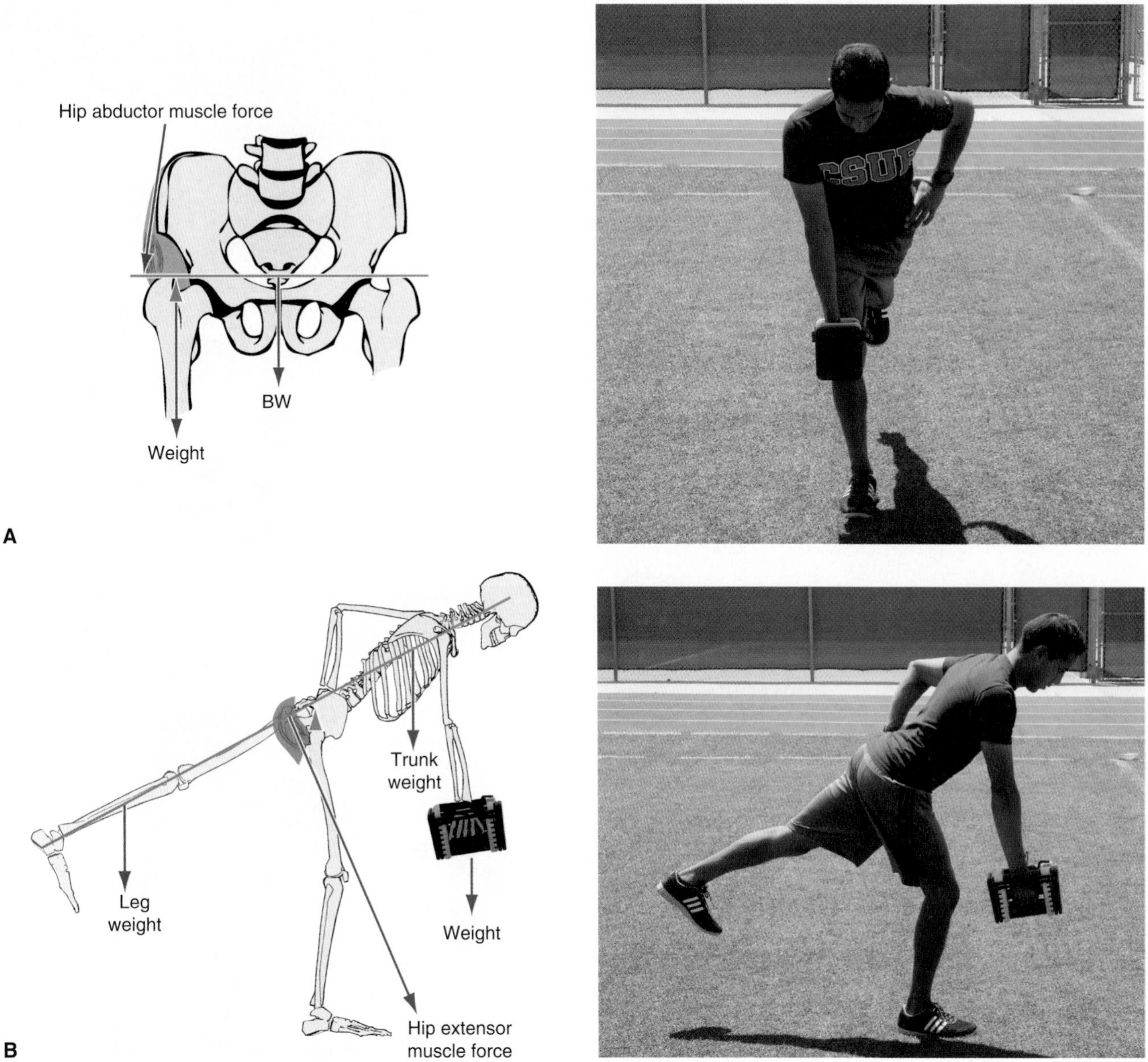

FIGURE 5.25 The single-leg RDL exercise—ipsilateral weight progression.

PROGRESSION: CONTRALATERAL WEIGHT

The second progression involves adding a weight to the opposite hand as the stance leg (Fig. 5.26). This progression makes the exercise more challenging for both the hip extensors and hip abductors. Now, the downward force produced by the weight is also producing a clockwise torque in the frontal plane and therefore the hip abductors must produce a much greater force to keep the pelvis stable. The effect of this contralateral weight in the sagittal plane is the same as with the ipsilateral weight, as the dumbbell is the same distance from the axis of rotation of the hip; therefore, the extra clockwise torque that must be absorbed by increasing the force created by the hip extensors is the same in both progression conditions.

Summary

A good fundamental knowledge of biomechanics is essential for any strength and conditioning professional. This knowledge is imperative in order to ensure the prescribed exercises are tailored to the correct level, using the correct form and amount of resistance, and reinforcing the appropriate movement pattern to achieve the functional goals of the training session as quickly and safely as possible.

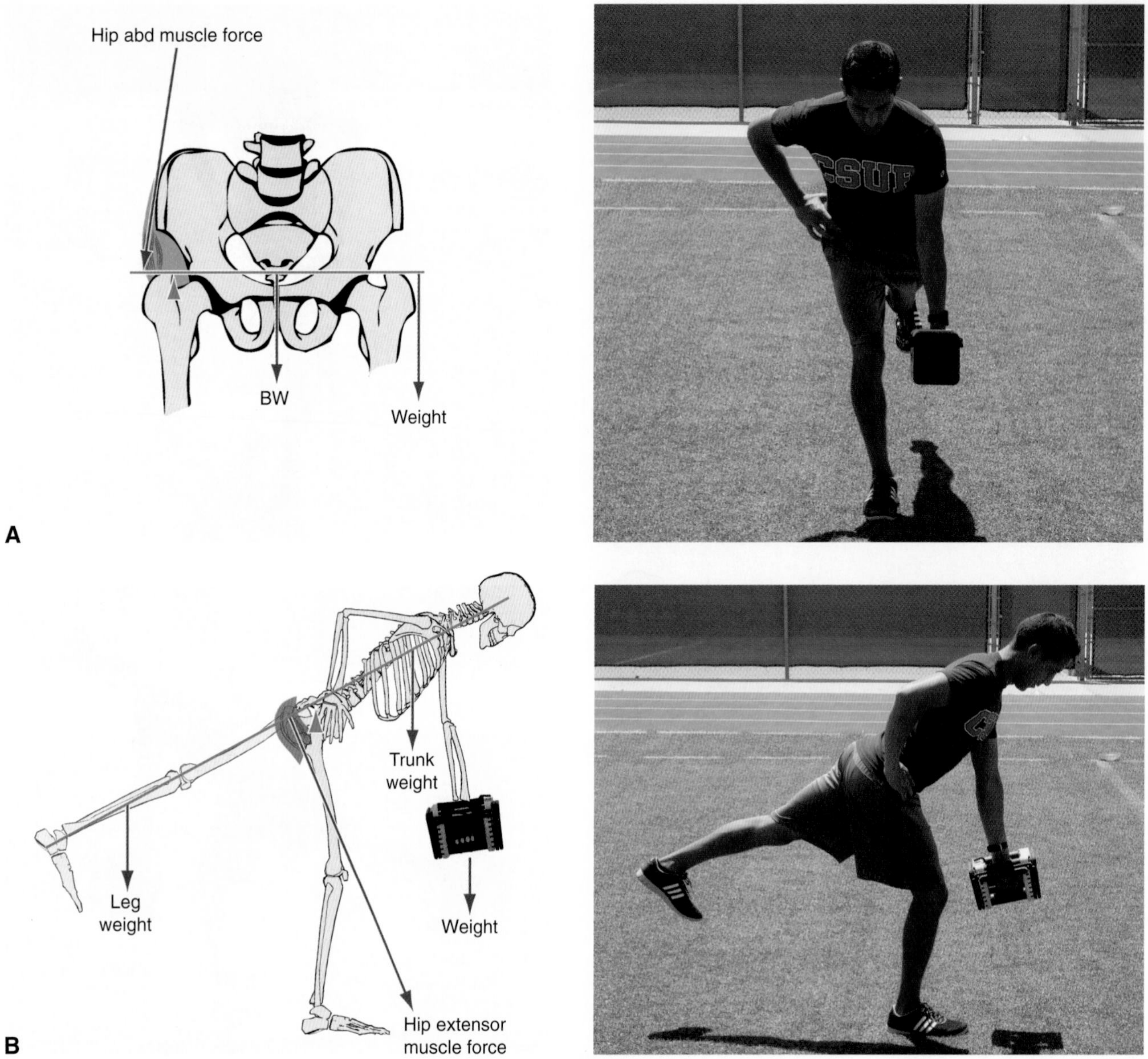

FIGURE 5.26 The single-leg RDL exercise—contralateral weight progression.

Maxing Out

1. You want to incorporate some Olympic lifting into the strength and conditioning program for the volleyball team. Problem is the athletes are having real trouble learning to perform the lifts correctly. How could biomechanics be used to assist you in teaching the athletes?
2. The football coach has told you that he only wants his players completing single joint exercises on pin-loaded resistance machines and at slow speed. His rationale is that he does not want the athletes injured in the weight room. From your biomechanics knowledge you do not believe such a program is optimal but you have to convince the coach. Write a discussion paper outlining the basis for including ground supported, multijoint movements including high speed exercises once the athletes have developed the appropriate patterns of movement and muscle activation strategies.

CASE EXAMPLE

Extending the Application of a Simple Contact Mat Timing System to Derive More Pertinent Mechanical Measurements

BACKGROUND

You have just been employed as a strength and conditioning coach with a small college that has limited performance testing equipment and no current budget to purchase more sophisticated equipment. The program has a simple electronic timing system that can record contact time and flight time during vertical jumping. In the past, only the flight time has been recorded and provided to the athletes and coaches but you would like to provide more extensive information that is more understandable and relevant.

RECOMMENDATIONS/CONSIDERATIONS

One of the problems with just providing flight time is that the athletes cannot really relate to the measure. They want to know how high they have jumped. Also, in terms of quantifying leg power, flight time does not adequately quantify the explosiveness of the athlete or account for athletes of differing body weights. Based on your biomechanics knowledge you recommend to the coaches that the jumps be performed from an approach run, that the athletes jump onto the mat then jump vertically upward for maximum height, landing back on the mat. You also recommend recording body mass. From these additional measures, jump height and power will be calculated.

IMPLEMENTATION

Each sporting squad is tested after a functional movement assessment and prior to a skills session. They are instructed beforehand to avoid strenuous activity for the previous 48 hours.

Measurement of body mass. Body mass is measured in kilograms for each athlete using an electronic scale.

Measurement of Jump Performance. As a group, the athletes are instructed in the correct technique for performing the test.

Stand approximately three strides back from the contact mat. Step into the mat area, landing with both feet on the mat, then jump vertically upwards for maximum height landing back on the mat. The hands are to be held on the hips throughout the test.

At the end of each trial, the contact time and subsequent flight time will be recorded.

CALCULATIONS

Flight to Contact Ratio. A useful and easily calculated measure is simply flight time divided by contact time.

Jump Height. Jump height can be estimated based on the flight time and the assumption of simple projectile motion. The formula is

$$\textbf{Jump height} = (g \times \textbf{flight time}^2)/8$$

where $g = 9.81\ \text{m} \cdot \text{s}^{-2}$

Work Done. Once jump height has been determined, the work done during the concentric phase of the jump can be calculated as

$$\textbf{Work} = F \cdot d = \textbf{mass} \times g \times \textbf{jump height}$$

Absolute Power Output. As we have a measure of contact time prior to the jump, we have an estimate of the time over which the work calculated above was completed. We must assume that the duration of the concentric and eccentric phases are roughly equal as we have no way of measuring this. So the concentric time is equal to the contact time divided by 2. Absolute power is then calculated as the Work done divided by the concentric time.

$$\textbf{absolute power} = \textbf{work} / (\textbf{flight time}/2)$$

Relative Power Output. Relative power output is calculated as absolute power output divided by body mass. This gives an indication of the power to weight ratio for the athlete.

$$\textbf{relative power} = \textbf{absolute power} \cdot \textbf{body mass}^{-1}$$

RESULTS

The following results were obtained on six athletes and the subsequent additional measures calculated. As you can appreciate, the use of biomechanics principles has provided for a much more in depth and relevant analysis of vertical jump performance. This test could then be repeated at various intervals during a training program designed to improve vertical jump performance. This will provide invaluable quantitative feedback regarding whether or not your training is accomplishing its goal with every single athlete.

CASE EXAMPLE (*Continued*)

Extending the Application of a Simple Contact Mat Timing System to Derive More Pertinent Mechanical Measurements

Athlete	A	B	C	D	E	F
Mass (kg)	80	78	82	79	69	74
Contact time (s)	0.561	0.493	0.587	0.534	0.521	0.508
Flight time (s)	0.567	0.587	0.543	0.602	0.511	0.519
Flight:Contact ratio	1.011	1.191	0.925	1.127	0.981	1.022
Jump height (m)	0.394	0.423	0.362	0.444	0.320	0.330
Work done (J)	309	323	291	344	217	240
Absolute power (W)	1,103	1,312	991	1,290	832	944
Relative power ($W \cdot kg^{-1}$)	13.8	16.8	12.1	16.3	12.1	12.8

REFERENCES

1. Hatze H. The meaning of the term: "Biomechanics." *J Biomech.* 1974;7:189–190.
2. McGinnis PM. *Biomechanics of Sport and Exercise.* 2nd ed. Champaign, IL: Human Kinetics; 2005.
3. Garhammer J. A review of power output studies of Olympic and Powerlifting: methodology, performance prediction, and evaluation tests. *J Strength Cond Res.* 1993;7:76–89.
4. Hof AL, Van den Berg JW. EMG to force processing II: Estimation of parameters of the Hill muscle model the human triceps surae by means of a calf ergometer. *J Biomech.* 1981;14:759–770.
5. Hill AV. *The First and Last Experiments in Muscle Mechanics.* Cambridge: Cambridge University Press; 1970.
6. Knudson D. *Fundamentals of Biomechanics.* 2nd ed. New York, NY: Springer; 2007.
7. Izquierdo M, Ibanez J, Gorostiaga E, et al. Maximal strength and power characteristics in isometric and dynamic actions of the upper and lower extremities in middle-aged and older men. *Acta Physiol Scand.* 1999;167:57–68.
8. Gans C. Fiber architecture and muscle function. *Exer Sports Sci Rev.* 1982;10:160–207.
9. Ito J, Moriyama H, Inokuchi S, et al. Human lower limb muscles: an evaluation of weight and fiber size. *Okajimas Folia Anatomica Japonica.* 2003;80(2-3):47–56.
10. McGill S. *Low Back Disorders: Evidence Based Prevention and Rehabilitation.* 2nd ed. Champaign, IL: Human Kinetics; 2007.
11. Wilson GJ, Elliott BC, Wood GA. The effect on performance of imposing a delay during the stretch-shorten cycle movement. *Med Sci Sports Exer.* 1991;23:364–370.
12. Floyd RT. *Manual of Structural Kinesiology.* 17th ed. New York: McGraw Hill; 2009.
13. Carney KR, Brown LE, Coburn JW, Spiering BA, Bottaro M. Eccentric torque-velocity and power-velocity relationships in men and women. European Journal of Sport Science. (in press)
14. Lynn SK, Noffal GJ. Lower Extremity Biomechanics During a Regular and Counter-Balanced Squat. Journal of Strength and Conditioning Research. (In press)
15. Lee SM, Piazza SJ. Built for speed: musculoskeletal structure and sprinting ability. *J Exp Biol.* 2009;212:3700–3707.
16. Cronin JB, McNair PJ, Marshall RN. Force-velocity analysis of strength-training techniques and load: implications for training strategy and research. *J Strength Cond Res.* 2003;17:148–155.
17. Newton RU, Kraemer WJ, Hakkinen K, et al. Kinematics, kinetics, and muscle activation during explosive upper body movements. *J Appl Biomech.* 1996;12:31–43.
18. Elliott BC, Wilson GJ, Kerr GK. A biomechanical analysis of the sticking region in the bench press. *Med Sci Sports Exer.* 1989;21:450–462.
19. Keiser DL. Pneumatic exercising device. US Patent, 4,257,593; 1981.
20. Frost MF, Cronin JB, Newton RU. A comparison of the kinematics, kinetics and muscle activity between pneumatic and free weight resistance. *Eur J Appl Physiol.* 2008; 104:937–956.
21. Lacerte M, deLateur BJ, Alquist AD, et al. Concentric versus combined concentric-eccentric isokinetic training programs—effect on peak torque of human quadriceps muscle. *Arch Phys Med Rehabil.* 1992;73:1059–1062.
22. Hortobagyi T, Katch FI. Role of concentric force in limiting improvement in muscular strength. *J Appl Physiol.* 1990;68:650–658.
23. Colado JC, Triplett NT. Effects of a short-term resistance program using elastic bands versus weight machines for sedentary middle aged women. *J Strength Cond Res.* 2008; 22:1441–1448.
24. McClenton LS, Brown LE, Coburn JW, et al.. The effect of short-term VertiMax vs. depth jump training on vertical jump performance. *J Strength Cond Res.* 2008;22: 321–325.

CHAPTER 6

Training Responses and Adaptations of the Endocrine System

ANDREW C. FRY • DISA L. HATFIELD • JAY R. HOFFMAN

OBJECTIVES

After reading this chapter, you will be able to:

- Familiarize yourself with hormone and neurohormone regulation in the body during rest and exercise.
- Understand how steroid, peptide and amine hormones differ from one another.
- Identify the roles that testosterone, cortisol, growth hormone, and insulin play during and after exercise.
- Describe the acute and chronic adaptations that occur within the endocrine system in response to training.
- Properly predict how hormones can affect various training programs and continue to optimize performance while avoiding overtraining.

KEY TERMS

Acute
Adrenal Cortex
Adrenocorticotropic Hormone (ACTH)
Amine Hormone
Albumin
Alpha Cells
Alpha Receptors
Amino Acids
Analogues
Anabolic Hormone
Adenylate Cyclase–Cyclic Adenosine Monophosphate (cAMP) System
Autocrine
Beta Cells
Beta Receptors
Biocompartments
Biologically Active
Binding Protein
Calmodulin
Catabolic Hormone
Catecholamines Chronic
Chaperone Protein
Chromaffin Cells
Circadian Rhythm
Corticotropin-Releasing Hormone (CRH)
Cross-Reactivity
Cybernetic Regulation
Cytoplasmic Receptor
Cytosol
Degradation
Diurnal Variation
Diacylglycerol (DAG)–Inositol Triphosphate (IP_3) System
Down-Regulation
Endocrine
Endogenous
Enzymes
Exogenous
Fight-or-Flight Response
Free Hormone
Free Testosterone
GH-Inhibiting Hormone
Half-Life ($T_{1/2}$)
Hormone
Hypothalamic–Pituitary Axis
Inhibiting G Protein (G_i)
Influx
Leydig Cells
Lipolysis
Lipophilic
Lipophobic
Messenger Ribonucleic Acid (mRNA)
Metabolism
Neuroendocrine
Neurohormone
Neurotransmitter

- Nocturnal Urine Measures
- Pancreas
- Paracrine
- Peptide Hormone
- Plasma Fluid Shift
- Postreceptor Activity
- Posttranslational Processing
- Precursor Molecule
- Pulsatile
- Quantal Release
- Receptor
- Receptor Density
- Receptor Specificity
- Salivary Concentrations
- Sex Hormone–Binding Globulin
- Signaling Pathway
- Spillover
- Steroid Hormone
- Stimulating G protein (G_s)
- Stress hormone
- Système Internationale (SI)
- Translation
- Transport protein
- Total hormone concentration
- Transcription
- Trophic hormone
- Up-regulation

Introduction

The human body is designed to provide amazing control of its physiological systems during physical exercise and sport performance. Each of these physiological systems is closely regulated and coordinated. The optimal result is an improvement in performance. As with each of the other physiological systems, the hormonal system is closely controlled and responds to exercise and physical activity to assure optimum results. But what exactly is this hormonal, or endocrine, system? How does it work? How can it influence the other systems of the body? Perhaps of most importance to this chapter, how does the endocrine system respond to the short-term requirements of a single bout of exercise, and how does it adapt to the chronic stresses of a long-term training program?

THE ENDOCRINE SYSTEM

The endocrine system helps to maintain homeostasis in the body by regulating hormonal functions. This occurs through the communication between chemicals in the body that regulate different physiological actions. These chemicals are called messengers; they are secreted into the bloodstream and travel to their respective binding sites. Once they have arrived at the designated binding site, they promote changes in cellular functions.

WHAT ARE HORMONES?

Our first challenge is to define the term **hormone**. For the purposes of this chapter, a hormone is a chemical compound that is secreted into the circulation to regulate a biological function at a distant site in the body. A hormone is secreted directly into the bloodstream from a tissue known as an endocrine gland. These glands contain specialized cells designed to create and release their respective hormones. A **neurohormone** is very similar except that it is released from a nerve ending into the circulation. Regardless of the source, the hormones and neurohormones travel to various parts of the body until they reach their target tissues. Once arriving, they can bind, or attach, to specialized receptors on or in the cells of the target tissues. In this manner, hormones are able to influence how the target tissues function.

Hormones are chemical compounds secreted by endocrine tissues and transported via the circulation.

ENDOCRINE TISSUES

Numerous hormones and neurohormones are involved in the proper functioning of a healthy system. Hormones are chemical compounds that are produced by endocrine tissues and typically released into the circulation. Neurohormones are types of hormones that also function as neurotransmitters in the nervous system. Of particular interest for this chapter are those hormones that specifically respond to physical exercise and sport performance. Obviously, numerous endocrine

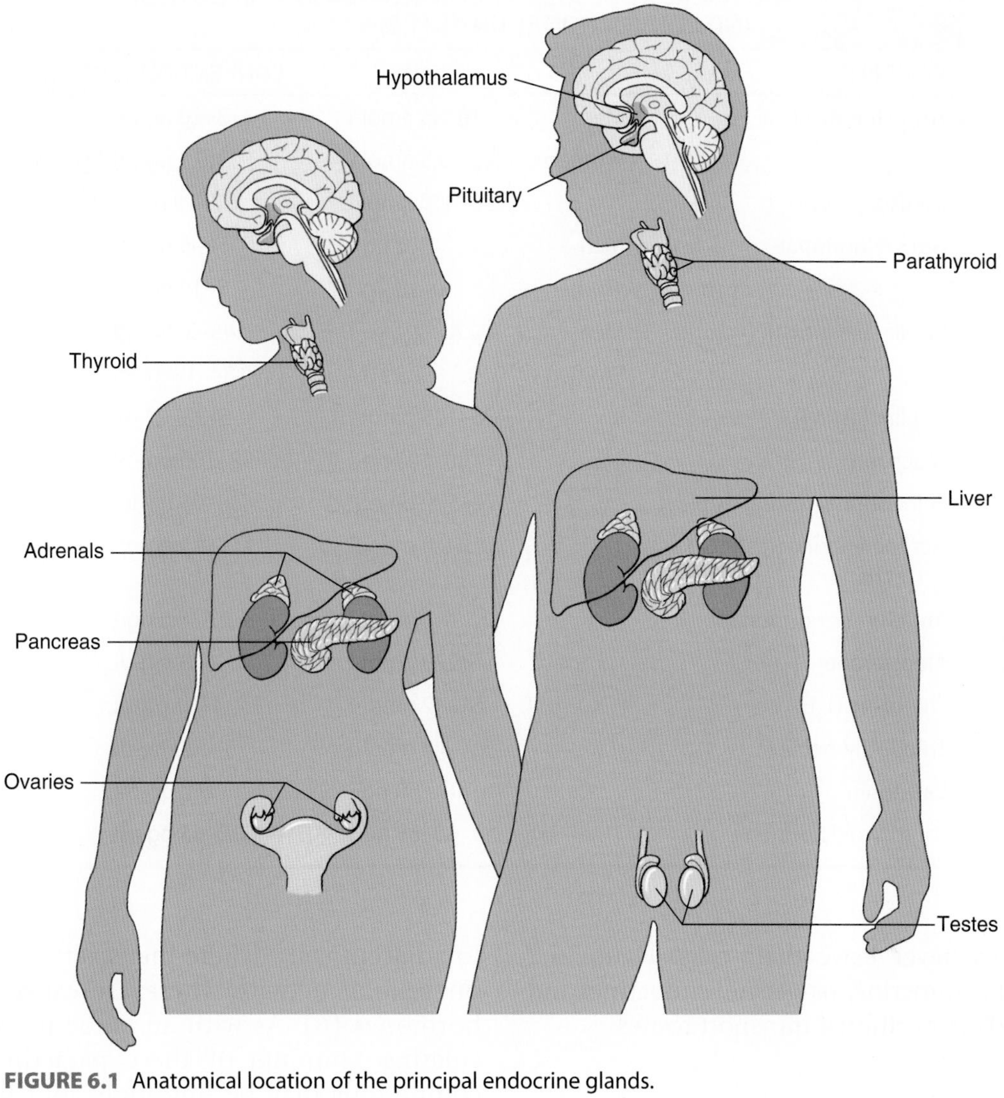

FIGURE 6.1 Anatomical location of the principal endocrine glands.

tissues in the body participate in this process, whether it involves the short-term or sudden **acute** responses to a single bout of exercise or the long-term **chronic** adaptations to regular exercise and training. Figure 6.1 illustrates the endocrine glands and tissues responsible for the hormones and neurohormones discussed in this chapter. These are the tissues that produce the primary hormones examined in this chapter. In general, these tissues release their hormonal products into the circulation, whereby they are transported to their target sites throughout the body. In studying the endocrine and neuroendocrine systems, it is important to be familiar with the various endocrine tissues as well as the normal blood concentrations of the hormones, as listed in Table 6.1 (3,4).

Although those in the medical profession and the related health sciences often use conventional units of measure, scientific reporting requires the use of the measurements defined by the **Système Internationale (SI)**. The SI system is universally recognized by scientists all over the world and provides a logical and systematic method for quantification (4).

HORMONAL TRANSPORTATION ROUTES

Although most of the hormones discussed in this chapter are released into the circulation for transport to their respective targets, other methods of transport exist. Some hormones never leave their

TABLE 6.1 ● TYPICAL ADULT SERUM CONCENTRATIONS IN BOTH SI AND CONVENTIONAL UNITS (1,2)

VARIABLE		SI UNIT	CONVENTIONAL UNIT
Testosterone (4 PM)	Men	10–35 nmol·L^{-1}	3–10 ng·mL^{-1}
	Women	<3.5 nmol·L^{-1}	<0.1 ng·mL^{-1}
Cortisol (4 PM)		50–410 nmol·L^{-1}	2–15 μg·dL^{-1}
Growth hormone	Men	0–5 μg·L^{-1}	0–5 ng·mL^{-1}
	Women	0–10 μg·L^{-1}	0–10 ng·mL^{-1}
Insulin-like growth factor-I	Men	0.45–2.2 kU·L^{-1}	0.45–2.2 U·mL^{-1}
	Women	0.34–1.9 kU·L^{-1}	0.34–1.9 U·mL^{-1}
Insulin (fasting)		35–145 pmol·L^{-1}	5–20 μU·mL^{-1}
Glucagon		50–100 ng·L^{-1}	50–100 pg·mL^{-1}
Epinephrine (resting, supine)		170–520 pmol·L^{-1}	30–95 pg·mL^{-1}
Norepinephrine (resting, supine)		0.3–2.8 nmol·L^{-1}	15–475 pg·mL^{-1}
Antidiuretic hormone		2.3–7.4 pmol·L^{-1}	2.5–8.0 ng·L^{-1}
Aldosterone		<220 pmol·L^{-1}	<8 mg·dL^{-1}
Thyroxine (T_4)		51–42 nmol·L^{-1}	4–11 μg·dL^{-1}
Triiodothyronine (T_3)		1.2–3.4 nmol·L^{-1}	75–220 ng·dL^{-1}
Calcitonin		<50 ng·L^{-1}	<50 pg·mL^{-1}
Parathyroid hormone		10–65 ng·L^{-1}	10–65 pg·mL^{-1}

tissue; others never leave their cells. Figure 6.2 illustrates the autocrine, paracrine, endocrine, and neuroendocrine hormonal transport routes.

Autocrine

When hormones or neurohormones are synthesized in their respective cells, not all are released into the circulation. Certain of these chemical compounds never leave the cell. Instead, they remain within the cell and influence the activity of the cell in some manner. These are called **autocrine** hormones (5). An example of this is insulin-like growth factor-I (IGF-I). IGF-I is produced in many cells of the body and is responsible for many of the actions of growth hormone (GH). IGF-I can be measured from the circulating blood, but some IGF-I never leaves the cell. Although circulating amounts of this hormone are still important, they do not account for the IGF-I that never leaves the cell and functions in an autocrine manner.

Paracrine

Some hormones leave their endocrine cells but never enter the circulation. Instead, they travel to adjacent cells, where they exert their influence on cellular activity. These are called **paracrine** hormones (6). As with an autocrine system, circulating amounts of these paracrine chemical compounds may be important, but they do not account for the portion that never enters the circulation.

Endocrine

This chapter is concerned primarily with endocrine and neuroendocrine mechanisms. The term **endocrine** refers to hormones that are released into the bloodstream or lymph system to control growth, metabolism, mood, and reproduction; **neuroendocrine** refers to hormones that are released into the bloodstream or lymph system following stimulation of the nervous system. Once the chemical compound is released, it travels via the circulation and eventually reaches its target tissue or is broken down to its metabolic by-products. Although many factors influence the concentrations of these hormones in the blood, it is still essential to measure their concentrations in blood to fully understand their roles in physiological function.

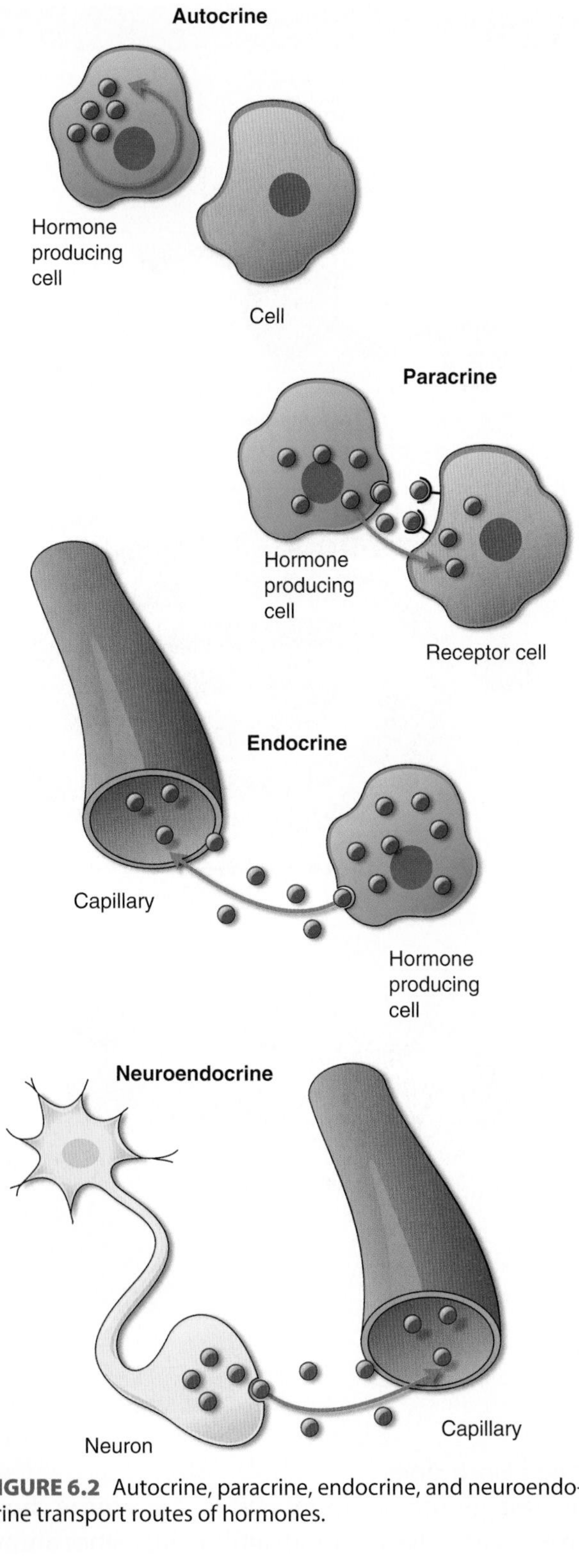

FIGURE 6.2 Autocrine, paracrine, endocrine, and neuroendocrine transport routes of hormones.

> *Once produced, most hormones enter the circulation for transport (endocrine), some travel to adjacent cells (paracrine), and some never leave the cell (autocrine).*

TYPES OF HORMONES

As might be expected, hormones come in different chemical forms (Fig. 6.3). Basically, three chemical structures account for the hormones that most interest us (7).

Steroid Hormones

First are the **steroid hormones**, which all share the same four-carbon ring structure and affect growth and the development of the sex organs. All steroid hormones are made from a cholesterol molecule, which is called a **precursor molecule**. Depending on the endocrine tissue involved, the cholesterol molecule is converted by **enzymes** (proteins serving as catalysts in mediating and speeding a specific chemical reaction) into the final steroid hormone that is to be released. Different endocrine glands have different hormonal enzymes that determine which steroid hormone will be produced. Since the steroid hormones are formed from cholesterol, they are **lipophilic** ("lipid-loving"), which means that they can pass through the lipid membrane of a cell. Pharmaceutical forms of steroids, which are orally ingested or injected (and are called **exogenous** steroids—i.e., coming from outside the body), are typically variations of the hormones naturally produced by the body (which are known as **endogenous** steroids). This chapter deals only with the body's own natural production of these hormones.

Peptide Hormones

A second group of hormones comprises the **peptide hormones**, which consist of chains of **amino acids**, the building blocks of protein. Small chains (of fewer than 20 amino acids) are simply termed *peptides;* larger chains are called *polypeptides*. These hormones can be quite long, as exemplified by GH, which is 191 amino acids long. The shapes of these polypeptides are often determined by their amino acid sequences and by the existence of bonds between certain amino acids. These bonds cause the peptide to configure into the specific shape required for the hormone to function optimally. If any alteration occurs in the chain of amino acids, the hormone's function may be affected. This can occur when one or more of the amino acids in the chain are replaced with a different amino acid or if the peptide chain is cut, resulting in a smaller peptide chain. Sometimes these altered forms of the hormone still have a function,

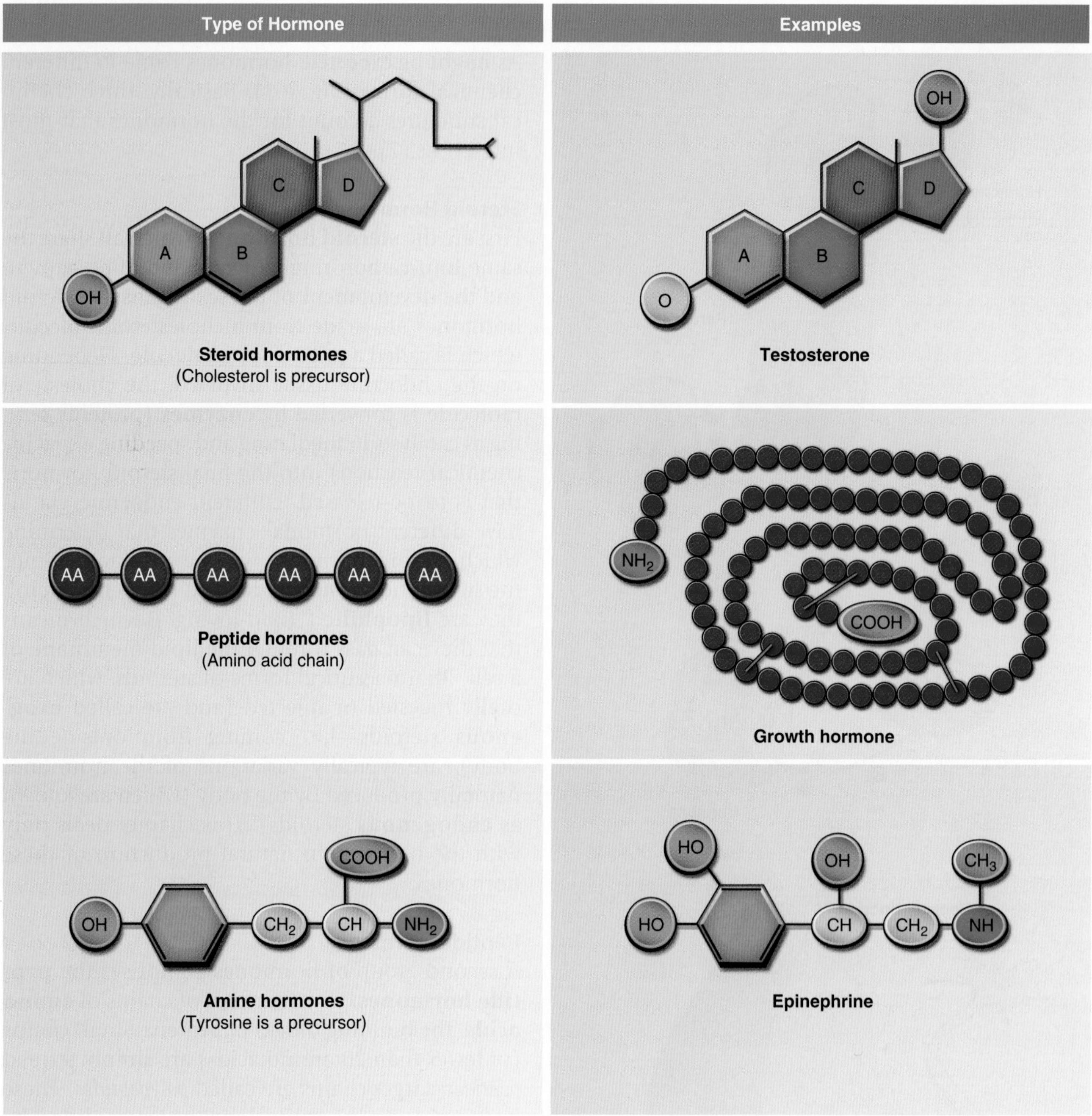

FIGURE 6.3 Different types of hormones include steroid, peptide, and amine.

but it is often different from that of the original hormone. Peptide hormones are more prone to **degradation**, or breakdown of a complex compound into simpler compounds, in the circulation than steroid hormones. Additionally, peptide hormones are **lipophobic** ("lipid-hating"), meaning that they are repelled by lipids and cannot readily pass through the cell membrane. As such, they require a receptor at the membrane permitting them to act.

Amine Hormones

The last group of hormones is the **amine hormones**, characterized by an amine ring. Since amine hormones are derived from amino acids, they are sometimes classified as protein hormones. These hormones are found as either hormones or neurohormones and can be produced and secreted by either endocrine tissues or nerve endings. Some of these compounds also function as neurotransmitters in the nervous system. The typical precursor molecule of amine hormones is the amino acid tyrosine. In the event that tyrosine is not available in adequate quantities, phenylalanine can be converted to tyrosine and then used for the synthesis, or creation, of an amine hormone. Some amine hormones—such as epinephrine (Epi) (also known as adrenaline) and norepinephrine (NE) (noradrenaline)—break down rapidly in the circulation. As such, they must exert their influence on target tissues rapidly. Amine hormones are lipophobic; therefore, like peptide hormones, they require a membrane receptor.

The three types of hormones—steroid, peptide, and amine—are each synthesized differently. Each of the three types has a specific role during exercise.

HORMONE PRODUCTION

As shown in Figure 6.4, each of the three types of hormones is produced in a different manner. A cursory understanding of how one's body makes these hormones can give us a greater appreciation of the complex role they play in human performance.

Production of Steroid Hormones

As mentioned earlier, the synthesis of the different types of steroid hormones is dependent on the various enzymes present in the particular endocrine gland (8,9). The first step is the conversion of cholesterol to pregnenolone in the mitochondria of the cell. This is called the rate-limiting step in the process, since the subsequent steps occur more readily. Once the stimulus for steroid hormone synthesis arrives at the endocrine cell, the process begins with this first step to pregnenolone. Pregnenolone is then transported to the endoplasmic reticulum, where it is converted via several enzymatic steps into the desired steroid. For some of the steroid hormones, additional processing occurs back in the mitochondria. Once the final hormone is completed, it can diffuse through the cell membrane, which consists of two lipid layers. Owing to the hormone's ability

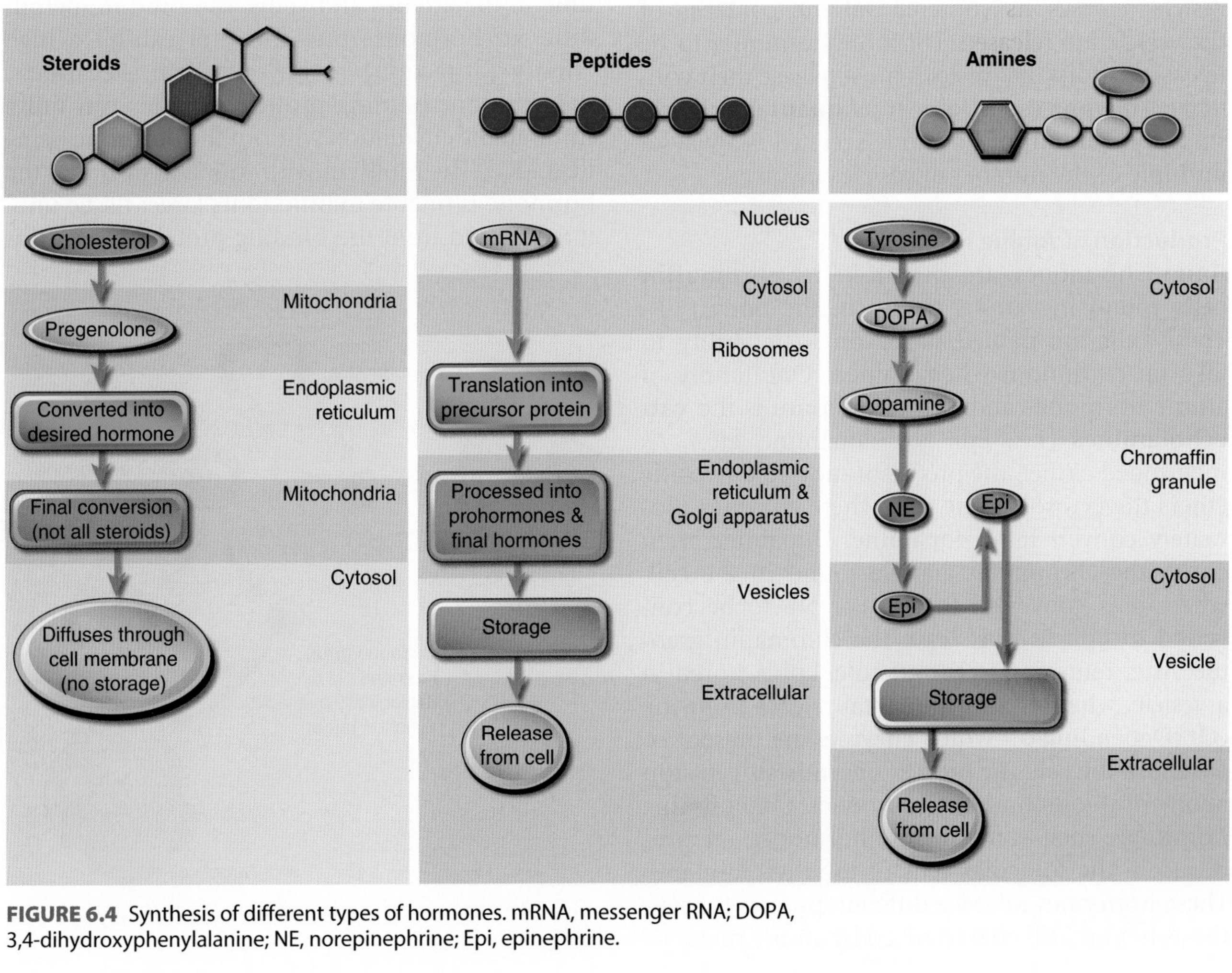

FIGURE 6.4 Synthesis of different types of hormones. mRNA, messenger RNA; DOPA, 3,4-dihydroxyphenylalanine; NE, norepinephrine; Epi, epinephrine.

to exit the cell easily, these hormones are not stored but rather produced as needed.

Production of Peptide Hormones

Peptide hormones are synthesized when the appropriate signal for hormone production results in **messenger ribonucleic acid (mRNA)** being produced in the cell nucleus (9). The mRNA serves as the code indicating which amino acids are needed and in what order. The mRNA is transported to the ribosomes, where the appropriate amino acids are brought and assembled into a precursor molecule in a procedure called **translation**. The precursor molecules are then transported to the endoplasmic reticulum and the Golgi tendon organ for further modification; this process is termed **posttranslational processing**. This often includes splicing the precursor amino acid chain into smaller molecules. Because peptide molecules are lipophobic (repelled by lipids), they cannot pass through the cell membrane. To be released, they must enter storage vesicles in the cell, which can eventually release them to the surrounding environment. When a vesicle releases its contents, all the contents of the vesicle are released. For more hormones to be released, additional vesicles must release their contents. This process is known as **quantal release**, since the amount of hormone secreted is always a multiple of the number of vesicles involved.

Production of Amine Hormones

Amine hormones are produced in **chromaffin cells** found in various tissues in the body (10). These cells are named based on their ability to take up chromium when stained. One family of amine hormones and neurohormones is the **catecholamines** (i.e., Epi, NE, dopamine, etc.). As mentioned earlier, the precursor molecule tyrosine enters the cytosol of the cell, where enzymes ultimately convert it to dopamine. Dopamine then enters the chromaffin granule found in the cell, where it is converted to NE. For NE to be converted to Epi, it must leave the chromaffin granule. After returning to the granule, Epi is stored in a vesicle, where it awaits quantal release from the cell. Depending on which enzymes are present or absent in the cell, the process of synthesis can stop at any of the preliminary hormones. Other amine hormones, such as the thyroid hormones, are produced in the follicular cells of the thyroid gland. These hormones follow a different process for synthesis but are still characterized by amine rings.

HORMONAL TRANSPORT AND BINDING PROTEINS

Once hormones are released into the circulation, they must be transported in a timely fashion to the tissues where they are to act. One problem the hormones encounter is **metabolism** or their degradation. Numerous factors can prevent hormone molecules from ever reaching their targets because of degradation. The time it takes for a hormone to be partially metabolized in the circulation, or for half of it to be degraded, is called its **half-life ($T_{1/2}$)**. Some hormones have a half-life measured in seconds, while the half-lives of others are measured in minutes or hours. To preserve a hormone for longer periods, the hormonal molecule may be protected by becoming attached to a **binding protein**, which preserves the hormone and assists in its transport (Fig. 6.5) (11). Hormones such as steroid and thyroid hormones are bound to these **transport proteins**, while amines and protein hormones are not. **Albumin**, a binding protein made in the liver that helps to maintain blood volume in the arteries and veins, can bind numerous different hormones but does not exhibit a high affinity (attraction) to any of them. Regardless, the hormone-binding protein complex can move through the circulation without the hormone being degraded. The problem with this system is that the hormone is unable to bind to its target tissue until it is released from the binding protein. When this

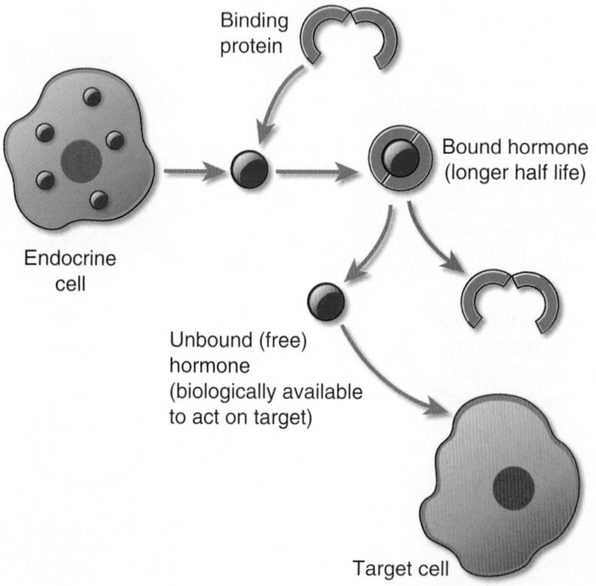

FIGURE 6.5 Binding proteins help protect circulating hormones.

happens, the hormone is considered **biologically active** or available for use during metabolism. The portion of the hormone not bound to a binding protein is called the percent **free hormone**, while the **total hormone concentration** includes both the free and the bound portions. Typically, when binding proteins are used, most of the circulating hormones are bound to a transport protein. For example, only approximately 1% to 2% of the total testosterone in the circulation is free testosterone or not bound to its binding protein.

Binding proteins protect the hormone (bound hormone), but the hormone is biologically active only when it dissociates from the binding protein (free hormone).

FACTORS AFFECTING CIRCULATING CONCENTRATIONS

The concentration of hormones in the blood can be extremely variable, depending on the hormone and on a number of contributing factors (12).

Hormone Production and Release

At first, it would seem that the primary factor would simply be how much hormone is being produced by the endocrine gland. Although this is certainly one factor, the process is much more complicated (Table 6.2). Three sites in the body can contribute to the circulating concentrations. These include the endocrine cell, the circulating blood, and the target tissue. At the endocrine cell, it is not only the rate of hormonal synthesis that matters; additional factors are how much hormone is released and how quickly this occurs.

Hormonal Transport in the Circulation

In the circulation, the binding proteins can affect the availability of a hormone at its target tissue (11). Additionally, hormones are degraded in various tissues, thus affecting how much hormone arrives at the target site. Hepatic clearance is a particularly large factor in this process, but other tissues are involved as well. Concerning exercise, after a vigorous effort, blood may pool in the venous circulation, resulting in less of the hormones circulating to the target tissue. One of the largest factors during exercise is **plasma fluid shifts** (13). Plasma is the fluid portion of blood; during physical exercise, this fluid leaves the blood. This alone can result in a higher hormonal concentration. Contributing factors to this fluid shift include fluid loss via sweating, due to increased arterial pressures and postural changes. Plasma volume shifts of more than 15% have been reported for long-term aerobic exercise as well as resistance exercise (RE). This response is augmented when the exercise occurs in a hot, humid environment.

TABLE 6.2 ● FACTORS AFFECTING HORMONE CONCENTRATIONS

SITE	FACTOR
Endocrine cell	Hormone synthesis Hormone release
Circulation	Method of transport to target tissue Binding proteins Hormonal concentration • Total • Free • Bound Fluid (plasma) shifts Venous pooling Hepatic (kidney) clearance rates Extrahepatic clearance rates Degradation of hormones
Target tissue Receptors	Binding affinity Maximal binding capacity Sensitivity
Intracellular	Second-messenger systems Nuclear receptor adaptations

Source: Reproduced with permission from Kraemer WJ. Endocrine responses and adaptations to strength training. In: Komi PV, ed. *Strength and Power in Sport.* Oxford, UK: Blackwell; 1992:291–304.

Hormonal Activity at the Target Cell

At the target tissue, the properties of the hormone receptors are critical factors (14). **Receptors** are the cellular structures to which the hormones bind, resulting in the appropriate action at the cell. The number of receptors (**receptor density**) available, how readily the hormone attaches to the receptor (affinity), and how sensitive the receptor is to the hormone can vary. Furthermore, **postreceptor activity** can vary. This involves the role of the **signaling pathways** that tell the cell how to respond once the hormone has bound to the receptor. Some of these signals are initiated at the receptors in the cell membrane, while some are initiated in the cell nucleus, depending on the hormone.

Hormones affect their target tissues by binding to hormone-specific receptors. Binding at these receptors initiates the specific cellular responses to the hormone.

TROPHIC HORMONES AND PULSATILITY

For a hormone to be secreted by its endocrine gland, the gland must receive some type of signal. The signal for many hormones is a **trophic hormone** from another endocrine gland or from the nervous system (15). When increased concentrations of a hormone are required, the body detects this need and causes the trophic hormonal signal to be increased. This signal is not based simply on the hormone's concentration. Instead, trophic hormones are released in a **pulsatile** fashion (Fig. 6.6) (16). This means that the hormone is released in periodic bursts. The trophic signal is increased either by increasing the frequency of the pulses or by increasing their magnitude or amplitude. Needless to say, to properly study these signals, many blood samples must be taken to measure pulse frequency and amplitude. For example, the primary trophic hormone for testosterone in males is luteinizing hormone (LH), which is released from the anterior pituitary gland. In turn, LH is regulated by LH-releasing hormone (LH-RH) from the hypothalamus. As such, the control of our hormones is very complex and highly dependent on the signaling pattern of the trophic hormones.

Circulating concentrations are often regulated by trophic hormones that signal the synthesis and release of the hormones. This system is synchronized by a negative-feedback system that can detect the current blood concentrations.

HORMONAL RHYTHMS

Many hormones present different blood concentrations at different times of the day (17). In biological systems, hormonal variations occur over a number of time periods (e.g., hourly, less than every 24 hours, every 24 hours, or at different times of the year [seasonally]). Of particular interest to this chapter are the **circadian rhythms** or daily cycles of physiological processes, also known as the **diurnal variation**. Figure 6.7 illustrates an example of the diurnal variation for cortisol. As shown, baseline concentrations can be quite high late in the typical sleep cycle and early in the morning. Therefore, any interpretation of the hormonal responses to exercise and sport must consider where the baseline values were prior to the physical activity (18,19). Many researchers simply avoid the times of day when hormonal concentrations are elevated (e.g., early morning for cortisol). In addition, when hormonal levels are being studied over a long time, as in a training study, the time of day the blood samples are taken must be kept constant to minimize the effect of diurnal variations.

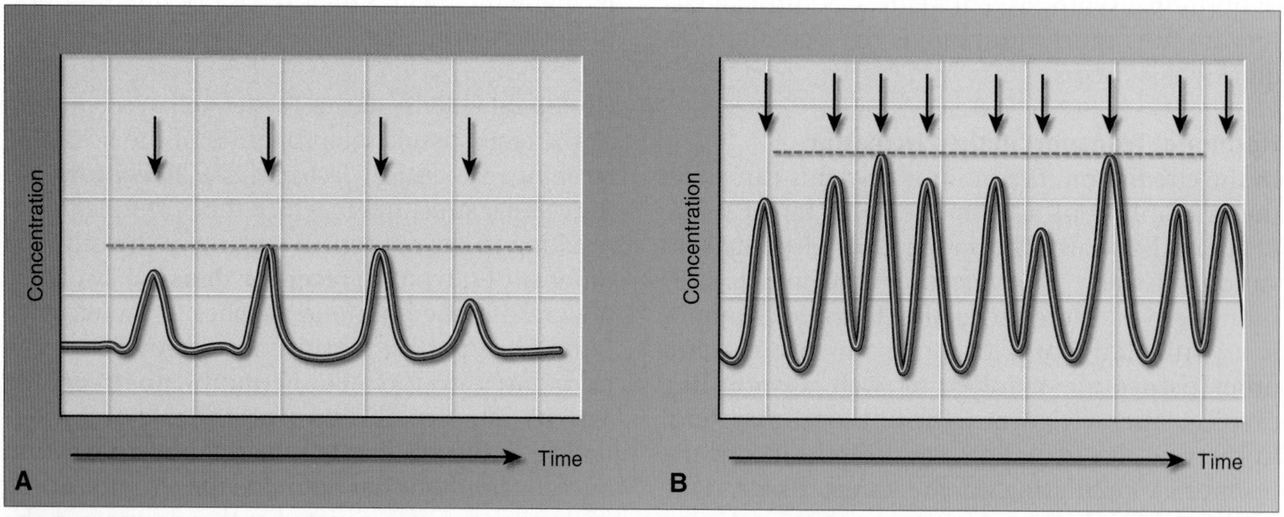

FIGURE 6.6 Pulsatility. Trophic hormones increase their signal by increasing the number and magnitude of pulses. Each *arrow* indicates a trophic hormone pulse. **A.** A basal trophic signal. **B.** An amplified trophic signal. Note that the signal is amplified by increasing both the frequency and the magnitude of pulses.

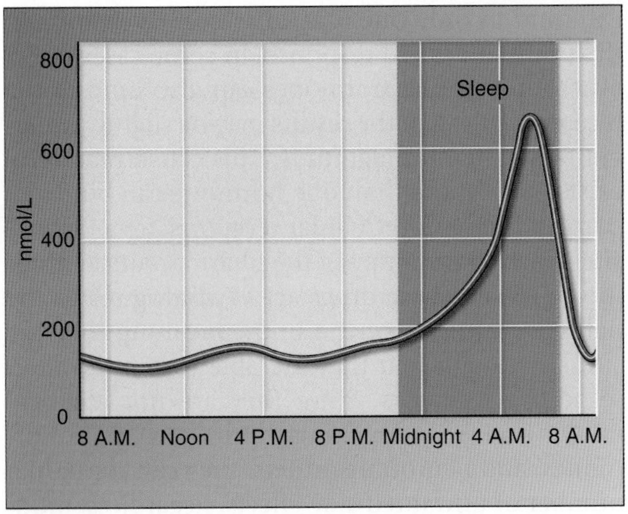

FIGURE 6.7 Examples of the variations of concentrations of cortisol during a typical day. The shaded area indicates a typical sleep cycle. (Modified with permission from Goodman HM. *Basic Medical Endocrinology*. New York: Raven Press; 1998:103.)

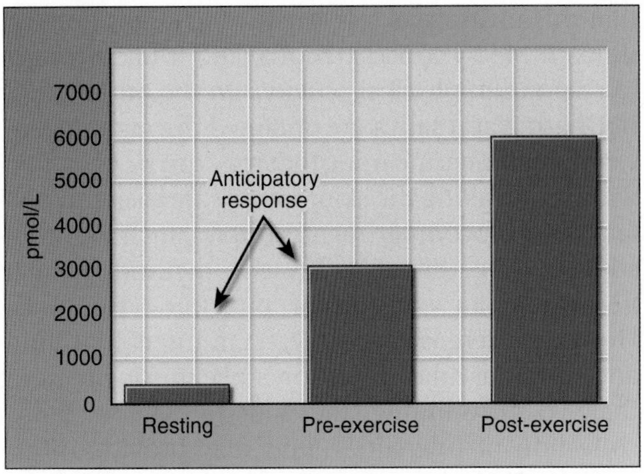

FIGURE 6.8 Example of the anticipatory response of epinephrine to a stressful lifting task. The difference between resting and preexercise concentrations represents the anticipatory response for the impending exercise. (Reproduced with permission from Fry AC, Kraemer WJ, van Borselen F, et al. Catecholamine responses to short-term high-intensity resistance exercise overtraining. *J Appl Physiol*. 1994;77(2):941–946.)

Hormone concentrations are influenced by the time of day and by anticipation of an impending stressor, such as exercise or competition.

ANTICIPATORY RESPONSES

The hormonal response occurring in anticipation of impending exercise or sport is termed the anticipatory response (10). The body possesses a number of hormones collectively called **stress hormones**. These hormones help the body to get ready for a stressful experience, whether it involves physical activity, cognitive stress, or both. They are part of the **fight-or-flight response** (20). All biological systems have methods of responding and dealing with stressful situations, whether they involve fighting the threat or fleeing from it. Experienced athletes are very familiar with the "pregame jitters" they encounter prior to an important competition. Similar feelings are also common in other scenarios, such as taking exams, public speaking, and musical recitals. In examining the hormonal responses to physical activity, it is important to separate the responses due to stressful anticipation from those due to the actual physical activity. The catecholamine (Epi) that is particularly sensitive to an anticipatory response is illustrated in Figure 6.8, although cortisol can also exhibit an anticipatory response. Blood sampling must be performed prior to the anticipatory response to determine the actual resting baseline value. It should be noted that some individuals will exhibit an anticipatory response to the actual process of taking a blood sample with a needle. In these cases, the sample must be taken when the needle has previously been inserted (i.e., via an intravenous catheter), after the individual has had time to relax and return to baseline.

BIOCOMPARTMENTS

The typical method of measuring hormonal concentrations involves venous blood sampling. Most hormones of interest are released directly into the circulation; thus, this is often the most sensitive way to measure the endocrine responses. Information on hormonal activity, however, can be collected from other sites, or **biocompartments**, in the body (21). Since hormones are ultimately degraded to their metabolic by-products, urine may be sampled to indirectly determine the quantity of hormone produced over a period of time. For example, when true baseline or resting levels are of interest, **nocturnal urine measures** are analyzed for the hormonal by-products. In this manner, the total amount of hormone produced during the sleep hours (when one is most at rest) can be estimated. Another common biocompartment is saliva, which may also be analyzed to determine hormonal concentrations, since **salivary concentrations** are related to blood concentrations. A limitation with salivary samples is that this measure is less sensitive to slight fluctuations in blood concentrations, and it takes longer to respond to physical activity. On the other hand, both urine and saliva are obtained through noninvasive methods, meaning that they can be obtained without breaking the skin, so they are easier to collect than biocompartment samples such as interstitial fluid gathered by invasive methods, which necessitate an incision or puncture (Fig. 6.9). However, there is some interest in interstitial fluid and intramuscular collection since this is the fluid that is surrounding the muscle. Theoretically, collection of interstitial fluid may provide information about the transport of hormones from circulation to the tissue (22).

RECEPTORS AND CELL SIGNALING

When a hormone molecule arrives at its target tissue, it interacts with the tissue by binding at a protein receptor. Receptors come in many different configurations, each hormone having a receptor specific to it. This is known as **receptor specificity** (8,14). This specificity has been described as being analogous to a lock and key. Just as the lock can be opened with only one particular key, one hormone can bind to only one type of receptor, resulting in the optimal desired response. In some cases, however, other similar hormones can also bind to the receptor, although the results may be slightly different or smaller in magnitude. This **cross-reactivity** exists when more than one hormone can bind at a particular receptor. Cellular receptors are a favorite site of action for many of the pharmaceutical drugs in use today. These drugs act as **analogues** to the natural chemicals of the body, meaning they are similar enough that they are able to bind to their respective receptors. Since they are not identical to the body's endogenous hormones, neurohormones, and neurotransmitters, they can result in a number of unwanted side effects. Regardless, modern science has been able to constantly improve on the specificity of these drugs, resulting in their amazing effectiveness. Receptors are often located in the cell membrane, where the circulating hormones have ready access for binding (Fig. 6.10). Steroid receptors, however, are located within the cell nucleus, since steroids can easily enter the cell due to their lipophilic nature. Regardless of the location of the receptor, as soon as a hormone binds to its receptor, the activity of the cell is modified in some manner.

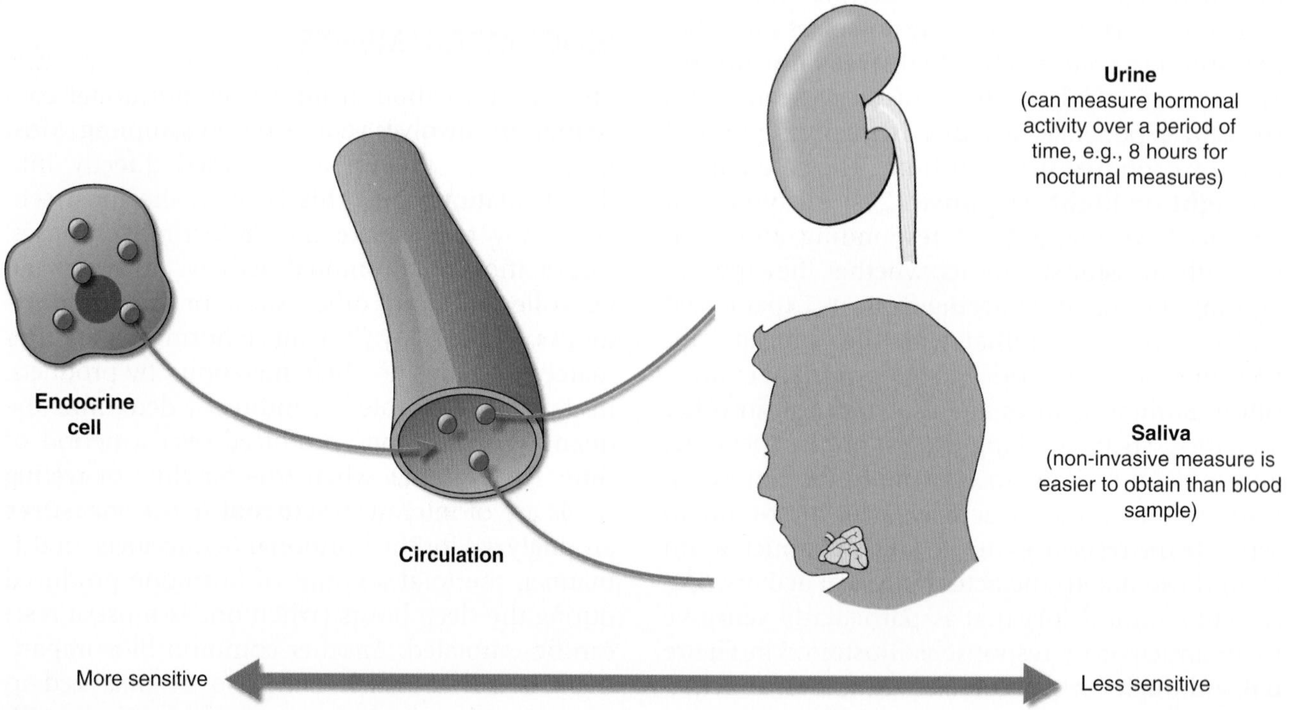

FIGURE 6.9 Hormonal levels can be determined by sampling from blood (whole, serum, or plasma) or urinary or salivary biocompartments. Sensitivity of the sample to hormonal fluctuations decreases when not taken from the circulation.

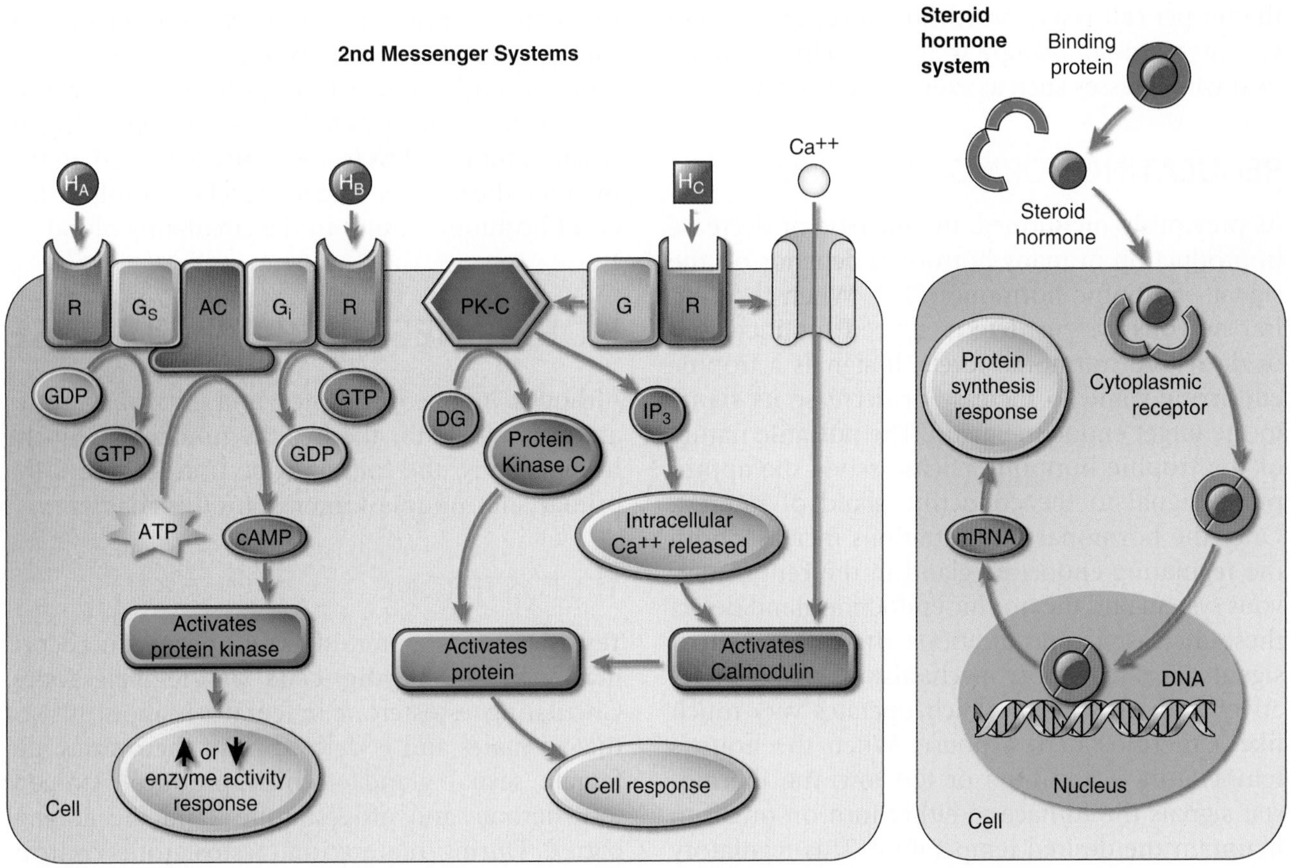

FIGURE 6.10 Hormonal intracellular signaling systems. H_{abc}, different hormones; R, receptor; G_s, stimulating G protein; G_i, inhibiting G protein; AC, adenylate cyclase; GDP, guanosine diphosphate; GTP, guanosine triphosphate; ATP, adenosine triphosphate; cAMP, cyclic adenosine monophosphate; PK-C, protein kinase C; DG, diacylglycerol; IP_3, inositol triphosphate.

Second-Messenger Systems

Figure 6.10 illustrates several of the second-messenger systems used by membrane-bound receptors. We see in this figure that several different types of hormones can interact with the **adenylate cyclase–cyclic adenosine monophosphate (cAMP) system** (14,23). When hormone A (H_a) binds to its receptor, the **stimulating G protein (G_s)** activates adenylate cyclase to produce cAMP from adenosine triphosphate (ATP). This, in turn, causes a kinase to modify an enzyme in the cell to either increase or decrease its activity. Other hormones, on the other hand, work in an opposite manner by activating an **inhibiting G protein (G_i)**, which turns off the adenylate cyclase activity. Other hormones (H_c) bind to receptors associated with a different second-messenger system, the **Diacylglycerol (DAG)-inositol triphosphate (IP_3) system** (14,24). Activation of DG results in a protein-activated cell response, while production of IP_3 releases calcium from storage sites within the cell. This calcium activates **calmodulin**, which, in turn, results in a protein-activated cell response. An alternative mechanism of action is a receptor-activated **influx** of calcium from outside the cell. As with IP_3, this activates calmodulin, which ultimately produces the desired cell response.

Nuclear Interactions

Steroid hormones work in a completely different manner (8,25,26). Since they can readily pass through the cell membrane, they are able to enter the **cytosol**, where they are bound to a **chaperone protein**, sometimes called a **cytoplasmic receptor**. This protein escorts the steroid to the cell nucleus, where it can bind to a site on the cell DNA. This initiates a process called **transcription**, which results in the coded signal for the production on a cellular protein. This signal leaves the nucleus in the form of mRNA. At the ribosomes, the protein is assembled from the various amino acids, resulting in the desired cell response. Regardless of which system is used, each hormone binds to its target receptor, which activates a cascade of events resulting in the proper cell response. Although complex, these systems work amazingly well and help our body deal with stresses such as exercise and sport.

REGULATING HORMONAL LEVELS

As previously mentioned, the increase or decrease in production of many hormones depends on the signal of trophic hormones (15). When the central nervous system detects a need for increased or decreased hormonal levels, it signals a trophic endocrine gland to increase or decrease its signal to the target endocrine gland. The pulsatile nature of the trophic hormone release sends the appropriate signal to the endocrine gland of interest. Once the hormonal concentrations increase, both the regulating endocrine gland in the central nervous system and the trophic endocrine gland detect these increased concentrations and decrease their signals. This regulatory mechanism is called a negative-feedback system, which operates very much like a thermostat in a house. When the house's temperature is too high or too low, the thermostat signals the furnace to either turn on or off to maintain the desired temperature. This regulatory mechanism is also known as **cybernetic regulation** (Fig. 6.11). The previously described system for regulating testosterone in males is a good example of negative-feedback regulation. Circulating concentrations of testosterone are detected by both the hypothalamus, which produces LH-RH, and the anterior pituitary, which produces LH. This causes the signal to the testes to be altered, depending on whether more or less testosterone is needed. In this manner, the body is able to closely control the levels of hormones found in the circulating blood.

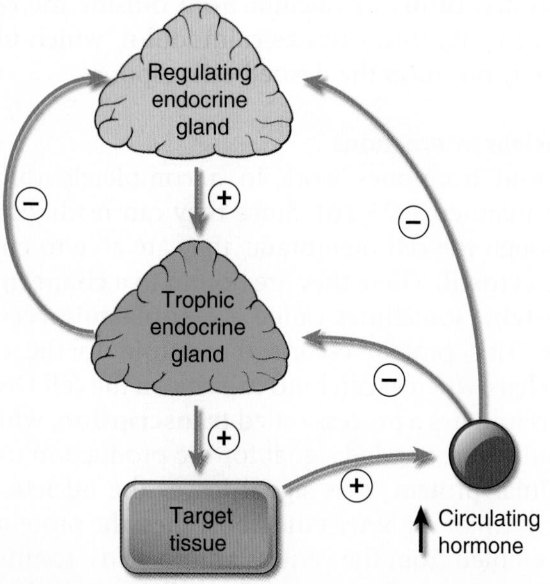

FIGURE 6.11 Example of negative-feedback regulation of circulating hormones. +, up-regulation; –, down-regulation; ↑, increased.

HORMONES VITAL TO EXERCISE

Although many hormones and neurohormones are responsible for the healthy functioning of the human body, the following section identifies the primary hormones of interest for this chapter.

TESTOSTERONE

Testosterone is a steroid hormone produced primarily by the **Leydig cells** in the male testes. Circulating testosterone in females is about 10% of that in males and is derived from the ovaries, the female sexual glands—which produce estrogen, testosterone, and progesterone—and the adrenal cortex. During maturation, testosterone contributes to many of the male sexual characteristics associated with development. Testosterone is regulated by the **hypothalamic–pituitary axis**. In this regulatory structure, the hypothalamus detects circulating concentrations of testosterone and secretes LH-RH. This, in turn, stimulates release of LH from the anterior pituitary, which functions as the primary stimulus for the release of testosterone from the testes. This process takes up to 15 minutes to occur, so faster responses are probably due to direct innervation of the testes or to sympathetic nervous activity via circulating Epi or NE. Once released, testosterone is bound to **sex hormone–binding globulin (SHBG)**, its binding protein.

CORTISOL

Cortisol is a steroid hormone secreted by the outer layer of the adrenal glands (**adrenal cortex**). It is sometimes called a **stress hormone**, since it is released when the individual experiences either physical or psychological stresses. Cortisol's principal role is to ensure the availability of energy. In this role, cortisol increases the production of glucose from either fat or protein in the liver, a process called gluconeogenesis; decreases glucose uptake; increases glycogen production in skeletal muscle;

and causes amino acids to be mobilized from skeletal muscle. Because of this breakdown of protein into amino acids, cortisol is often termed a **catabolic hormone**. Circulating levels of cortisol are detected by the hypothalamus, which secretes **corticotropin-releasing hormone (CRH)**, a polypeptide hormone involved in the stress response. CRH then stimulates the anterior pituitary to release **adrenocorticotropic hormone (ACTH)**, which in turn signals the adrenal cortex to produce and release cortisol.

TESTOSTERONE/CORTISOL RATIO

The ratio between testosterone, an **anabolic hormone** that causes the synthesis of molecules into more complex molecules, and cortisol, a catabolic hormone, has been used as a hormonal indicator of training stress (27). This can be considered for both a single aerobic training session and for a long-term training phase. With a single stressful exercise session, testosterone either increases initially or decreases. On the other hand, cortisol increases to a greater extent. The net result is that the ratio decreases. The more stressful the session, the more the ratio decreases. The ratio will also decrease over time in performing a stressful phase of training involving multiple sessions. As the individual tapers or backs off the training, the ratio returns to initial levels. As such, this ratio has been used as a marker of training stresses, and some have advocated its use to monitor recovery. Some have also advocated using the ratio between **free testosterone**, the portion of circulating testosterone not bound to SHBG, and cortisol as a more sensitive indicator. This idea is based on the fact that free testosterone is the actual hormone that is biologically available to exert its actions at the target tissue.

GROWTH HORMONE

GH is a polypeptide hormone consisting of 191 amino acids and two disulfide bonds. It is produced and secreted from the anterior pituitary gland in a pulsatile fashion. Concentrations of GH are increased by its trophic hormone, GH-RH, and decreased by **GH-inhibiting hormone (GH-IH)**, both from the hypothalamus. Many variations of GH appear to exist, because various forms of the original peptide are produced. This makes growth-hormone data difficult to interpret at times. Many of the actions of GH occur because of its effect on IGFs. Although GH is often most associated with its growth properties (including skeletal muscle), it also exerts tremendous influence on the metabolic system and energy availability. It increases muscle uptake of amino acids as well as the breakdown of lipids via **lipolysis**. The net result is that amino acids are preferentially used for anabolic purposes by muscle, and glycolytic energy sources are spared in favor of lipid energy sources.

Insulin-Like Growth Factor-I

The IGF-I system is composed of the IGF-I ligand (a 7.6-kD 70 amino acid polypeptide secreted from the liver), 6 binding proteins, an acid labile subunit, and 2 receptors. The synthesis of IGF-I has been reported to be under the regulation of GH release, but exercise-related IGF-I responses, especially at the local tissue level, appear to be independent of GH (28,29). Similar to GH, IGF-I has multiple metabolic and hypertrophic actions, including insulin-like activity and direct stimulation of protein synthesis pathways.

INSULIN AND GLUCAGONS

Insulin and glucagons are considered together, since their actions are so closely associated. Insulin is a 51 amino acid peptide hormone produced by the **beta cells** of the **pancreas**, the organ that secrets both insulin and glucagon. Insulin consists of a 21 amino acid A chain and a 30 amino acid B chain connected by two disulfide bonds. Glucagon is also a polypeptide chain but is only 29 amino acids long. It is produced by the **alpha cells** of the pancreas. Insulin and glucagons are released in response to increasing or decreasing blood glucose levels, respectively. Increasing concentrations of insulin prompt circulating glucose to be taken up by the following:

1. Adipose cells for conversion to triglycerides
2. Liver cells for conversion to glycogen
3. Skeletal muscle cells for conversion to glycogen.

The net result is control of rising blood glucose levels and storage of energy for future use. On the other hand, glucagon results in the exact opposite responses. Triglycerides are metabolized in adipose tissue, and amino acids and glycogen are metabolized in the liver. These collectively increase circulating glucose during times of high energy needs, such as exercise and sport. Both insulin and glucagon are also under control by Epi and NE from the sympathetic nervous system, causing insulin to decrease and glucagon to increase.

EPINEPHRINE

Epi, sometimes called adrenaline, is an amine neurohormone. Although it serves as a **neurotransmitter** in the central nervous system and transmits signals between the synapses of nerve cells, our interest is in its role in the circulation. Blood-borne Epi comes from chromaffin cells in the center portion (medulla) of the adrenal glands. Upon neural stimulation, the adrenal medulla dumps its contents into the renal vein, resulting in a very rapid Epi response. Furthermore, the adrenal medulla is completely surrounded by the adrenal cortex; thus, the medulla is constantly exposed to cortisol. This interaction with cortisol is critical for maintaining resting levels of Epi. When it is released into the circulation, Epi interacts with a variety of **alpha and beta receptors** in many different tissues of the body. Epi is responsible for many of the "fight-or-flight" responses previously discussed. These physiological responses to stress prepare the body to either fight or flee from an impending threat and include increased arousal and cardiac output, altered blood flow patterns, enhanced muscle contractions, and greater energy availability.

NOREPINEPHRINE

NE, also known as noradrenaline, is also an amine neurohormone. Unlike Epi, which is derived primarily from the adrenal medulla, most of the circulating NE comes from **spillover** from sympathetic nervous system synapses. In this manner, NE is sometimes considered an indicator of sympathetic nervous system activity. The adrenal medulla also produces some NE, but this is usually <20% of the Epi released.

ALDOSTERONE

Aldosterone is a steroid hormone secreted by the adrenal cortex. It is a key player in fluid regulation, responding to decreased blood pressures due to lowered blood fluid volumes. To counter this problem, aldosterone acts at the kidneys to keep sodium from being excreted. When sodium is retained, fluid is also retained, thus helping to counter the previously detected fluid loss. This response is not rapid and requires 30 minutes or more to go into effect. Small amounts of fluid loss are termed *hypohydration,* while larger losses are called *dehydration*. This can occur due to lowered fluid intakes and/or exercise in a hot environment.

ANTIDIURETIC HORMONE

Antidiuretic hormone (ADH) is a peptide hormone secreted by the posterior pituitary under hypothalamic control. Also known as arginine vasopressin, ADH responds to hydration status as does aldosterone; however, the mechanisms behind ADH are somewhat different. The concentration of proteins in the blood is known as the blood's osmolality, and this increases when fluid leaves the plasma portion of blood. This change in osmolality is readily detected in the arterial and venous circulation, resulting in a rapid ADH response. With ADH stimulation, the kidneys more readily take up fluid that would normally have been excreted. ADH is also a strong vasoconstrictor. In this manner, blood pressures are maintained even when blood fluid levels are depressed.

THYROID HORMONES

The thyroid hormones thyroxine (T_4) and triiodothyronine (T_3) are secreted by the thyroid gland. They are derived from tyrosine and contain either four or three iodine molecules respectively. They are regulated by thyrotropin, also known as thyroid-stimulating hormone (TSH) from the pituitary gland. T_4 is secreted in greater quantities than T_3, but much of T_4 is converted throughout the body to the more potent T_3. The thyroid hormones are basically responsible for increasing the body's metabolic rate and enhancing the action of other hormones.

CALCIUM-REGULATING HORMONES

Two hormones are essential for regulating calcium concentrations in the circulation. These are calcitonin from the thyroid gland and parathyroid hormone from the parathyroid gland. As calcium levels in the blood are detected, calcitonin is released to stop calcium from being taken from bone and to increase the excretion of calcium in the kidneys. Conversely, parathyroid hormone works in an opposite fashion. When blood calcium levels are low, release of parathyroid hormone stimulates bone to release calcium and inhibits excretion of calcium in the kidneys. Since the largest pool of calcium in the body is found in the skeletal system, it has been speculated that alterations of these hormones may be critical for the skeletal adaptations to physical exercise.

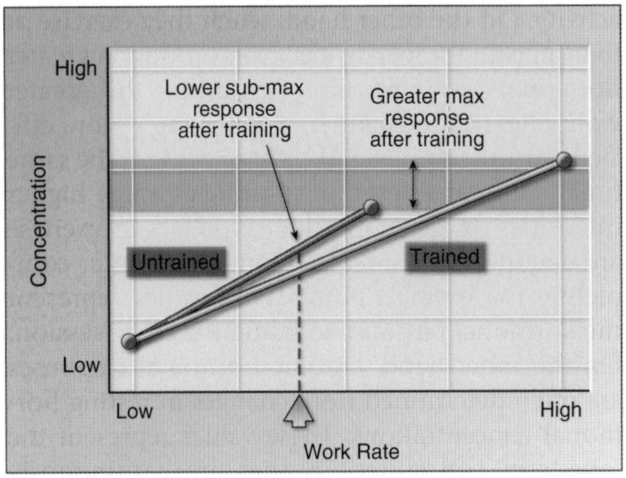

FIGURE 6.12 Common long-term training adaptations for hormonal responses to an exercise session. Note the decreased hormonal response at an absolute submaximal work rate after long-term training (indicated by the *large arrow*) but the increased hormonal response at maximal work rates. The trained individual is capable of exercising at higher work rates.

EFFECTS OF EXERCISE ON THE ENDOCRINE SYSTEM

As with any other system of the body, the endocrine system responds and adapts to the stresses placed on it. This includes sport training and other forms of exercise and physical activity. In this manner, the body adapts to the stress and ultimately produces enhanced performances or at least a tolerance for current activity levels (30). Although the hormonal response is not the only adaptation the body makes to exercise, it is certainly critical, since these hormones interact with so many other tissues and systems of the body. Our task now is to see exactly how these hormones respond and adapt and how this influences the training prescription we administer.

ACUTE AND CHRONIC TRAINING ADAPTATIONS

Regular training and physical activity result in an adaptation of the body to accommodate the stress. Hormonally, this can lead to the up-regulation or down-regulation of different hormones, depending on the types of physical activity and the physiological system involved. **Up-regulation** refers to an increase in the number of receptors on the surface of target cells, making the cells more sensitive to a hormone or other molecule; **down-regulation** is a decrease in the number of receptors on the surface of target cells, making the cells less sensitive to a hormone or other molecule. On one hand, these changes can be quite simple—they either increase or decrease the circulating concentrations found in the blood—although the changes can be more complex. Figure 6.12 illustrates an example of how some hormones can both increase and decrease in response to chronic (long-term) training (31,32). Prior to training, individuals can exercise only up to a certain work rate owing to their untrained status. As they increase their exercise intensity, the hormonal response increases accordingly. After long-term training has resulted in an increased capacity to exercise, they can exercise at a higher work rate. Now, when they exercise at the same absolute work rate as they did before training, they require less hormonal response to do the same

REAL-WORLD APPLICATION

Maximizing Your Endocrine Response

Athletes perform resistance training for a variety of reasons. One of the most common goals is skeletal muscle hypertrophy. To optimize anabolic hormone responses, the training program must be designed to do so. A resistance training session with the goal of increasing anabolic hormones responses, and in turn, inducing muscle hypertrophy, should meet the following criteria:

1. Target large muscle groups
2. Be comprised of complex, multijoint movements
3. Intensity of effort should be high
4. Volume should be high with intensity of load being moderate-to-heavy
5. Rest period should be low (~60 seconds)

activity. On the other hand, when they exercise at their maximal capacity, they can produce a greater hormonal response, thus permitting the greater work rate. In this manner, one becomes more efficient during submaximal exercise while at the same time being capable of functioning at much higher intensities. In general, acute responses to exercise are determined immediately or shortly after completing the exercise bout. These values represent the hormonal response to a single exercise session. On the other hand, chronic hormonal responses are often determined from changes in resting hormonal concentrations. These values represent the long-term concentrations that are continuously exposed to the target tissue. Of course, as shown in Figure 6.12, chronic adaptations can sometimes also alter the acute response to exercise.

RESPONSES AND ADAPTATIONS OF HORMONES TO ENDURANCE EXERCISE

The following section addresses the primary hormones of interest for this chapter and how they acutely respond to different intensities and durations of aerobic exercise. Where available, the chronic responses to long-term training are also included. Please note that the figures for each hormone indicate representative values and responses, which may vary between individuals and with different testing conditions.

During aerobic activities, most hormones increase as intensity and duration increase. Some important exceptions, however, should be noted.

Testosterone and Endurance Exercise

Acute Responses to Endurance Exercise During aerobic exercise, testosterone increases in an intensity-dependent manner. Low intensities of exercise elicit little or no response and maximum or near-maximum intensities result in a significant elevation (Fig. 6.13). During prolonged aerobic exercise, testosterone exhibits a biphasic response (35). Provided that the intensity is great enough, testosterone concentrations increase initially. If the duration of the exercise is long enough, concentrations decrease, suggesting that declining glucose levels may blunt testosterone response. Examples of this are the depressed testosterone levels reported after events such as a marathon. Because the amounts of testosterone in females are small, little or no response is observed (36).

Chronic Responses to Endurance Exercise Sometimes long-term endurance training has been associated with lower concentrations of testosterone, but this may be simply due to the effects of the huge volumes of training reported for these individuals. Testosterone is inversely related to training stress; as training stress increases, testosterone levels are lowered. However, the observed lower concentrations are not enough to be medically significant.

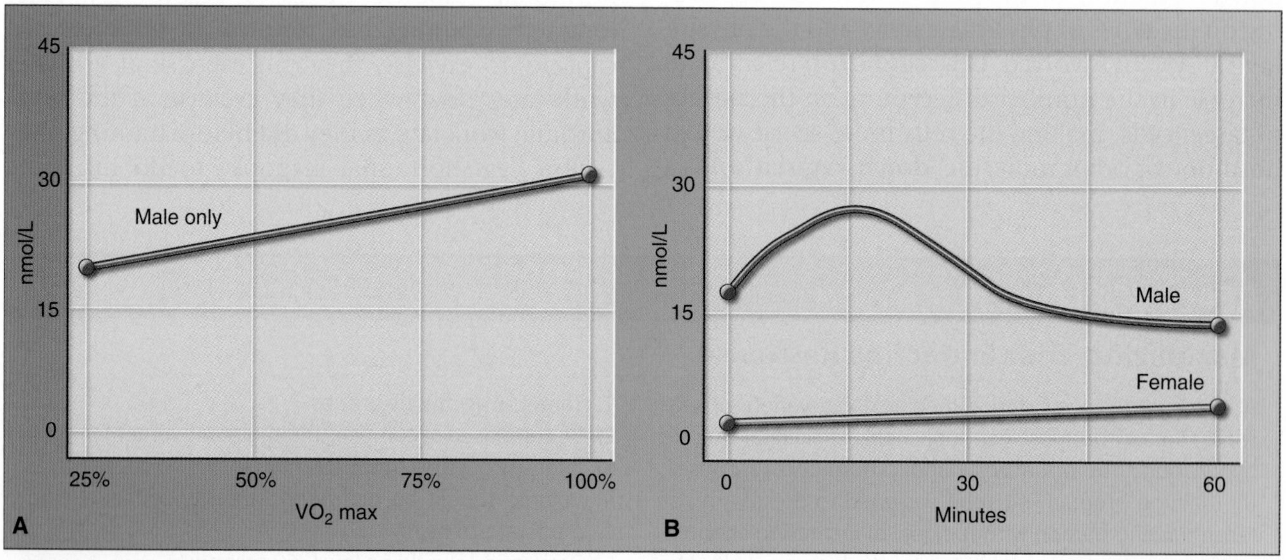

FIGURE 6.13 Responses of circulating concentrations of total testosterone to aerobic activities (33,34). **A.** Typical responses for men at different aerobic intensities (% $\dot{V}O_2$ max). **B.** Testosterone concentrations during 60 minutes of high-intensity endurance exercise for both men and women.

In addition, the fraction of testosterone measured in the blood and its other physiological roles may affect concentrations. Testosterone can be measured as a bound fraction (bound to SHBG), free, or total. Some researchers will only report the free testosterone concentrations, theorizing that it is the only one that is biologically available to the individual. Testosterone also has a potent chronic metabolic role, increasing the production of red bloods cells and thus the oxygen carrying capacity. Given these many roles of testosterone, the differential results with chronic training cannot be further explained

Gender Differences

In women, instead of testosterone, the primary sex-related hormones of interest are progesterone and the estrogens (estradiol, estrone, and estriol). As with testosterone, these hormones increase somewhat in an intensity-dependent manner (37). The phase of the menstrual cycle and energy balance can influence the acute and chronic responses. Likewise, the use of hormonally based oral contraceptives can alter these responses. Given these factors, it is hard to determine the sole effects of endurance exercise on sex-related hormones.

Cortisol and Endurance Exercise

Acute Responses to Endurance Exercise During aerobic exercise, cortisol increases, for the most part, in an intensity-dependent manner (38,39). At very low intensities, cortisol is not increased and may actually decrease slightly due to the very low stress on the metabolic systems at these intensities. Intensities >50% of $\dot{V}O_{2max}$ result in elevations of cortisol due to the energy requirements needed to perform at these levels (Fig. 6.14). A similar response is observed for prolonged aerobic exercise, with cortisol levels increasing with the duration of exercise (43).

Chronic Responses to Endurance Exercise The long-term training response includes lower cortisol concentrations (32), reflecting the body's ability to more effectively utilize the energy substrate available. However, no long-term differences and transient increases have also been reported (14). Short-term high-intensity training may temporarily increase resting levels. Similar to testosterone, this may be indicative of the stress of training.

Testosterone/Cortisol Ratio and Endurance Exercise

Because of the extremely high volumes of training that endurance athletes often perform, this hormonal ratio is often depressed among endurance athletes (45–47). This does not have to be the case, however, since this ratio can rebound when training volume decreases.

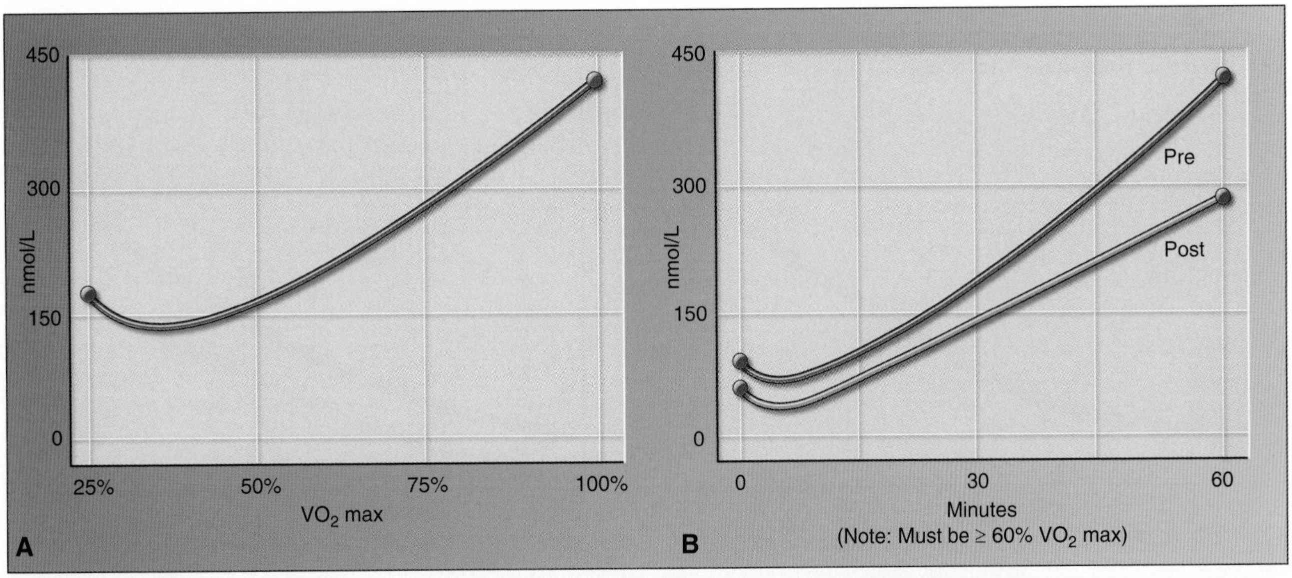

FIGURE 6.14 Responses of circulating concentrations of cortisol to aerobic activities (25,40,41,42). **A.** Typical responses at different aerobic intensities (% $\dot{V}O_2$ max). **B.** Cortisol concentrations during 60 minutes of endurance exercise at ≥60% <adV>o_{2max}. *Pre* and *post* refer to before and after long-term training.

The ratio between testosterone and cortisol is extremely important for strength adaptations. When cortisol levels are greater than testosterone levels, the body is in a catabolic state. However, when testosterone levels are higher, the body is in an anabolic state, encouraging strength adaptations.

Growth Hormone and Endurance Exercise

Acute Responses to Endurance Exercise Since GH is closely tied to energy availability, circulating concentrations are positively related to exercise intensity and is highly correlated with lactate response (38,39). Very large increases in GH levels are observed at maximal intensities of aerobic exercise. In a similar manner, the levels of GH increase with increasing durations of aerobic exercise (Fig. 6.15) (49).

Chronic Responses to Endurance Exercise Few data exist describing the chronic resting adaptations of GH to endurance exercise, but it appears that chronic training has no effect on resting GH concentrations. Women exhibit higher resting concentrations compared to men, but this is regardless of training status.

During exercise, long-term training results in lesser acute response to a given submaximal workload, suggesting a more efficient metabolic system in trained individuals (50). However, maximal exercise efforts result in a greater GH response in trained individuals (38).

Gender Differences Very little data exist concerning gender differences in GH in response to endurance training. A study in trained endurance runners reported that GH concentrations increased in men but not in women after prolonged moderate intensity running (51). However, other studies have reported no differences (52,53).

Insulin-Like Growth Factor and Endurance Exercise

Acute Responses to Endurance Exercise Increases, decreases, and no change in IGF-I concentrations during exercise have been reported. Most studies suggest a transient increase in an intensity-dependent fashion but then drop to resting values within 30 minutes of exercise (44). As previously indicated, exercising IGF-I levels are not under the control of GH and increases may be due to the release of a muscle isoform of IGF-I (29). In addition, IGF-I is highly dependent on nutritional status, which may account for the disparate results.

Chronic Responses to Endurance Exercise Chronic training produces a biphasic response of IGF-I, decreasing in the initial few weeks of training, followed by an increase that is above pretraining values (52). In addition, cross-sectional studies have suggested that IGF-I is highly correlated with $\dot{V}O_{2max}$ values, making it a possible biomarker for fitness status (54). More research is needed concerning the role IGF-I may play on endurance training adaptations.

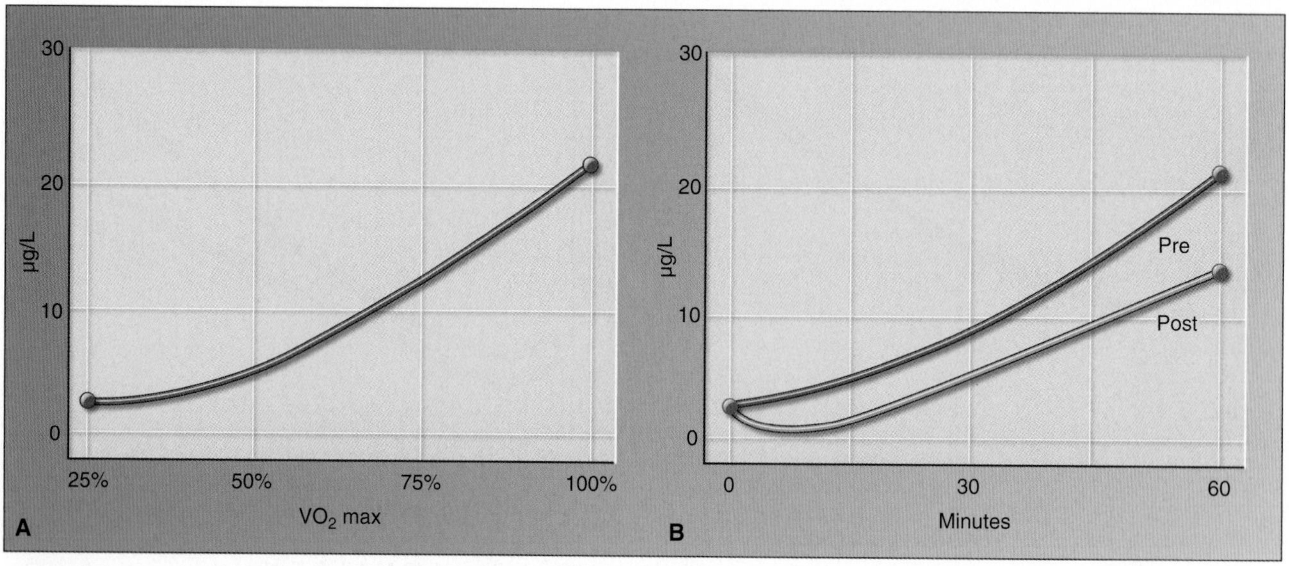

FIGURE 6.15 Responses of circulating concentrations of GH to aerobic activities (40,41,48). **A.** Typical responses at different aerobic intensities (% $\dot{V}O_2$ max). **B.** GH concentrations during 60 minutes of high-intensity endurance exercise. *Pre* and *post* refer to before and after long-term training.

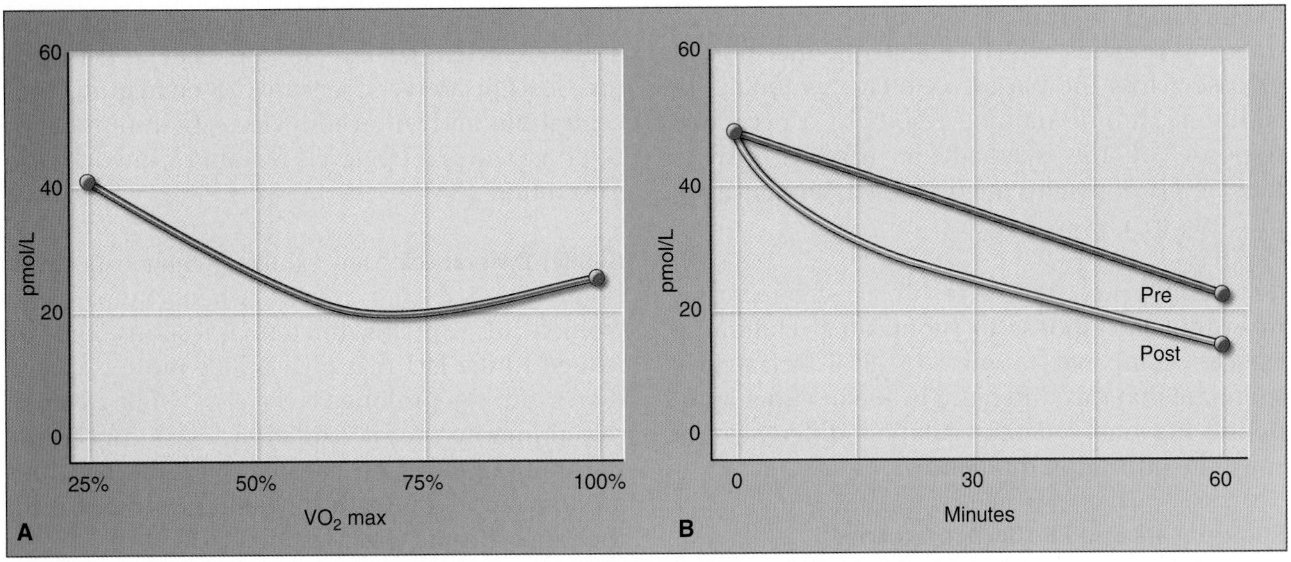

FIGURE 6.16 Responses of circulating concentrations of insulin to aerobic activities (23,57). **A.** Typical responses at different aerobic intensities (% $\dot{V}O_2$ max). **B.** Insulin concentrations during 60 minutes of high-intensity endurance exercise. *Pre* and *post* refer to before and after long-term training.

Gender Differences Similar to GH responses, gender differences in IGF-I response to endurance exercise are conflicting, with few differences being reported (51).

Insulin, Glucagon, and Endurance Exercise

Acute Responses to Endurance Exercise During aerobic exercise, insulin decreases, thus minimizing the uptake of blood glucose when it is needed for energy. Glucagon increases, however, permitting glucose to become available for energy. In this manner, these two hormones work in concert to properly regulate glucose availability during physical activity (38,39). Figure 6.16 shows the responses of insulin to aerobic activities; Figure 6.17 shows the responses of glucagon to aerobic activities.

Chronic Responses to Endurance Exercise After long-term training, the decrease in insulin is less pronounced, most likely due to the almost nonexistent change in glucagon. Glucose uptake becomes less dependent on insulin, since chronic training results

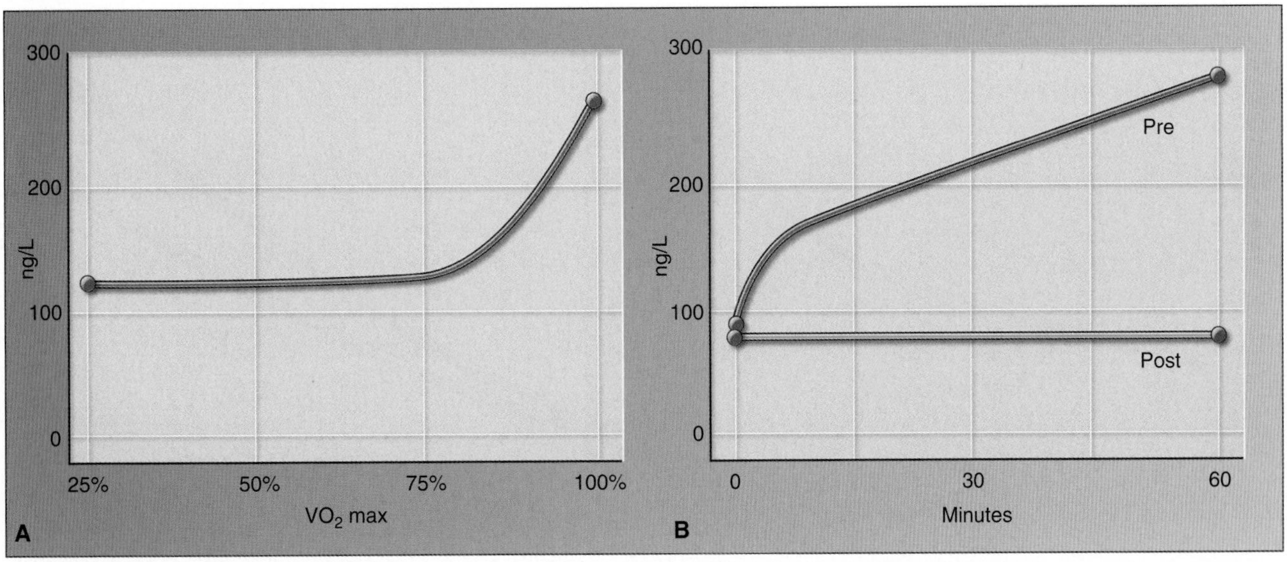

FIGURE 6.17 Responses of circulating concentrations of glucagon to aerobic activities (40,41). **A.** Typical responses at different aerobic intensities (% $\dot{V}O_2$ max). **B.** Glucagon concentrations during 60 minutes of high-intensity endurance exercise. *Pre* and *post* refer to before and after long-term training.

in increased activation of membrane glucose transport proteins, which regulate the transport of glucose across the plasma cellular membrane. In addition, chronic training results in a decreased response of the sympathetic nervous system; thus, levels of insulin are decreased and glucagon increases to a lesser extent.

Gender Differences Women exhibit greater increases in insulin in response to submaximal endurance exercise compared to men (51,55). Researchers speculate that this difference is due to either autonomic nervous system regulation differences or substrate utilization differences.

Epinephrine and Endurance Exercise

Acute Responses to Endurance Exercise Compared to other hormones, the catecholamines exhibit extremely large responses to physical exercise. Epi is particularly susceptible to an anticipatory response (56,57). In response to aerobic exercise, concentrations of Epi increase in an intensity-dependent manner (41,58) (Fig. 6.18), although the responses at low intensities are sometimes minimal. Furthermore, concentrations increase with increasing duration of aerobic exercise (38,60).

Chronic Responses to Endurance Exercise Long-term aerobic training results in an increased ability to secrete Epi at maximal intensities. On the other hand, absolute submaximal intensities result in lower concentrations after training, indicative of a more efficient system (see Fig. 6.12). The receptors for Epi are very sensitive to circulating concentrations and will readily decrease in number or responsiveness if Epi levels remain elevated for too long a time (33).

Gender Differences Men exhibit greater concentrations of Epi during exercise when compared to women (61,62). This differential response may be related to the fact that men utilize more carbohydrates during prolonged exercise, while women rely primarily on fat oxidation. Data concerning the training effect on chronic Epi concentrations are scarce, and it is unclear whether women exhibit the same chronic effects as men (63).

Norepinephrine and Endurance Exercise

Acute Responses to Endurance Exercise Although Epi and NE appear to respond similarly, they are primarily derived from different sources and their responses to exercise are not absolutely identical. As such, they represent different physiological phenomena. NE increases in an aerobic intensity-dependent manner, with greater intensities eliciting larger responses (41,58). Similar to Epi, NE increases with longer duration aerobic exercise (38,60) (Fig. 6.19).

Chronic Responses to Endurance Exercise Long-term training will result in greater NE concentrations

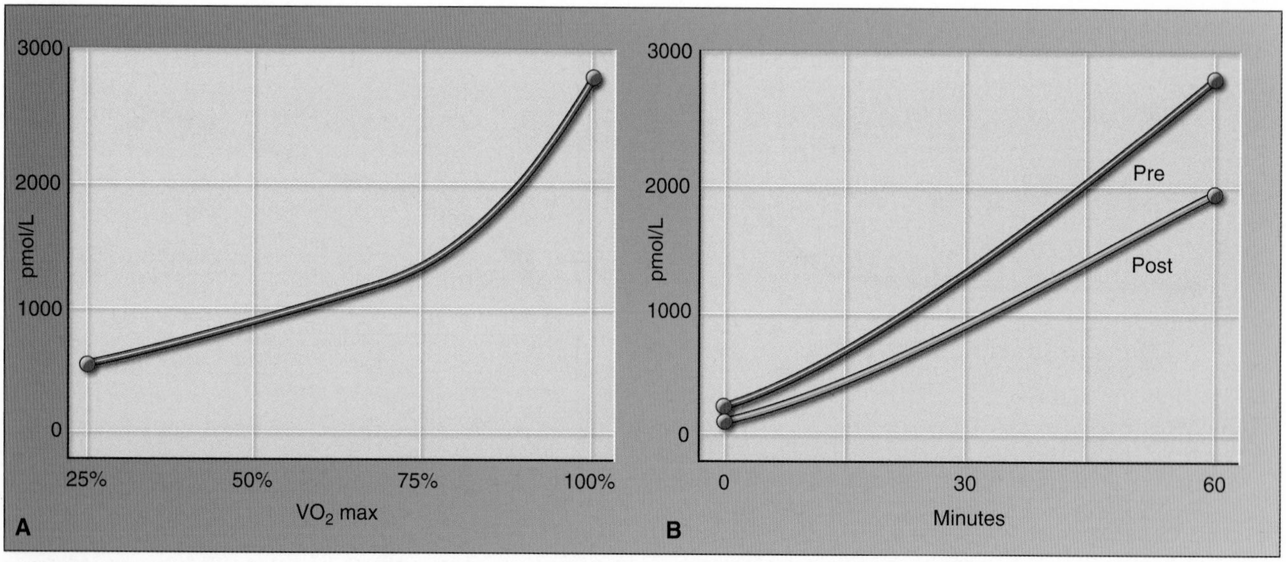

FIGURE 6.18 Responses of circulating concentrations of epinephrine to aerobic activities (18,40,43,59). **A.** Typical responses at different aerobic intensities (% $\dot{V}O_2$ max). **B.** Epinephrine concentrations during 60 minutes of high-intensity endurance exercise. *Pre* and *post* refer to before and after long-term training.

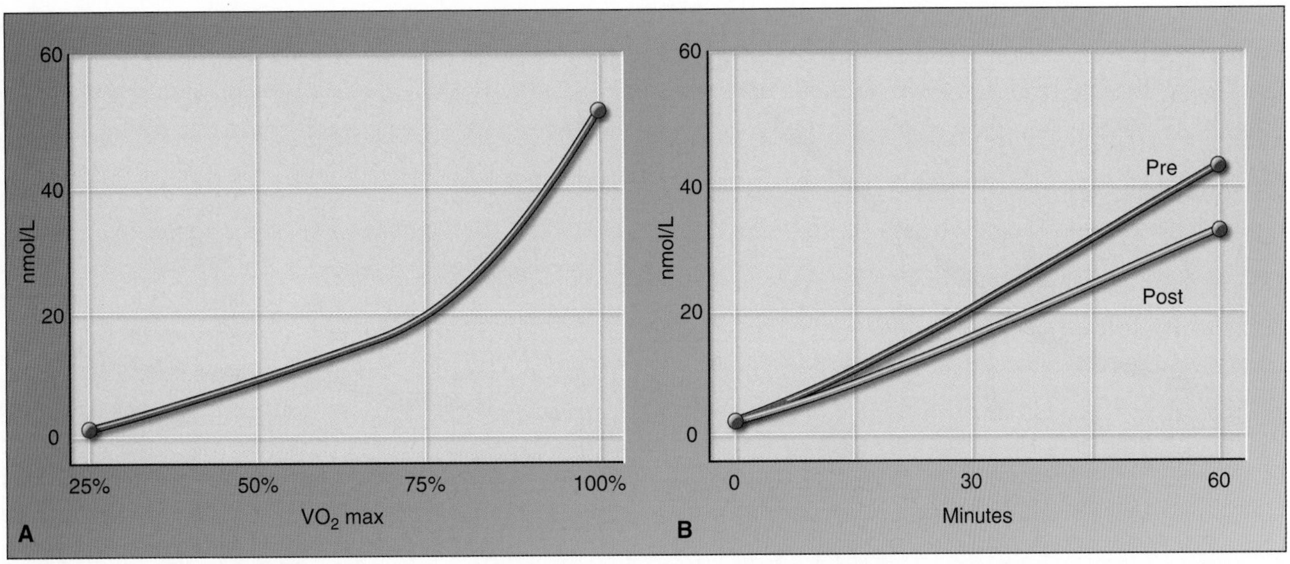

FIGURE 6.19 Responses of circulating concentrations of norepinephrine to aerobic activities (18,40,43,59). **A.** Typical responses at different aerobic intensities (% $\dot{V}O_2$ max). **B.** Norepinephrine concentrations during 60 minutes of high-intensity endurance exercise. *Pre* and *post* refer to before and after long-term training.

with maximal exercise; absolute submaximal exercise will produce smaller concentrations, again indicative of a more efficient system (see Fig. 6.12). If exercise results in excessive elevation of the catecholamines for extended periods of time, the physiological system responsible (sympathetic nervous system) can become exhausted, resulting in impaired performances (27). This has implications for overtraining, discussed further on.

Gender Differences The gender difference of NE in response to exercise is mixed, with increased responses in men reported (61) and no differences reported (53,55).

Aldosterone and Endurance Exercise

Acute Responses to Endurance Exercise As with many hormones, aldosterone increases during aerobic exercise in an intensity-dependent manner (64). Although aldosterone will increase during long-duration aerobic exercise, the extent of this increase is highly dependent on the environmental conditions (40). For example, conditions where sweat rates are high will eventually result in lowered plasma fluid levels and a concomitant decrease in blood pressure. In extreme conditions, the aldosterone response can be quite large (Fig. 6.20).

Chronic Responses to Endurance Exercise Chronic endurance training may enhance aldosterone response and sensitivity during exercise, resulting in expanded plasma volume. This in turn may explain the greater stroke volumes and lower heart rates with a given exercise intensity observed in trained athletes (66).

Antidiuretic Hormone and Endurance Exercise

Acute Responses to Endurance Exercise At low aerobic exercise intensities, ADH exhibits little or no response, but at greater intensities, ADH increases quite markedly (64).

Chronic Responses to Endurance Exercise As with aldosterone, long-duration aerobic exercise increases ADH, but again, these responses are very dependent on the environmental conditions present (40). As shown in Figure 6.21, long-term aerobic training results in lowered ADH responses at the same absolute exercise intensity, while the response increases at the same relative intensity.

Thyroid Hormones and Endurance Exercise

Acute Responses to Endurance Exercise Although the thyroid hormones are undoubtedly critical for health, their responses to exercise are reportedly quite variable (67), and little is known concerning their responses and adaptations to acute and chronic exercise. However, a recent study suggested that exhaustive endurance exercise decreases thyroid hormones for 24 hours into recovery and that cortisol responses are inversely related to the reduction, suggesting the important role thyroid hormones play in energy balance during and after exercise (68).

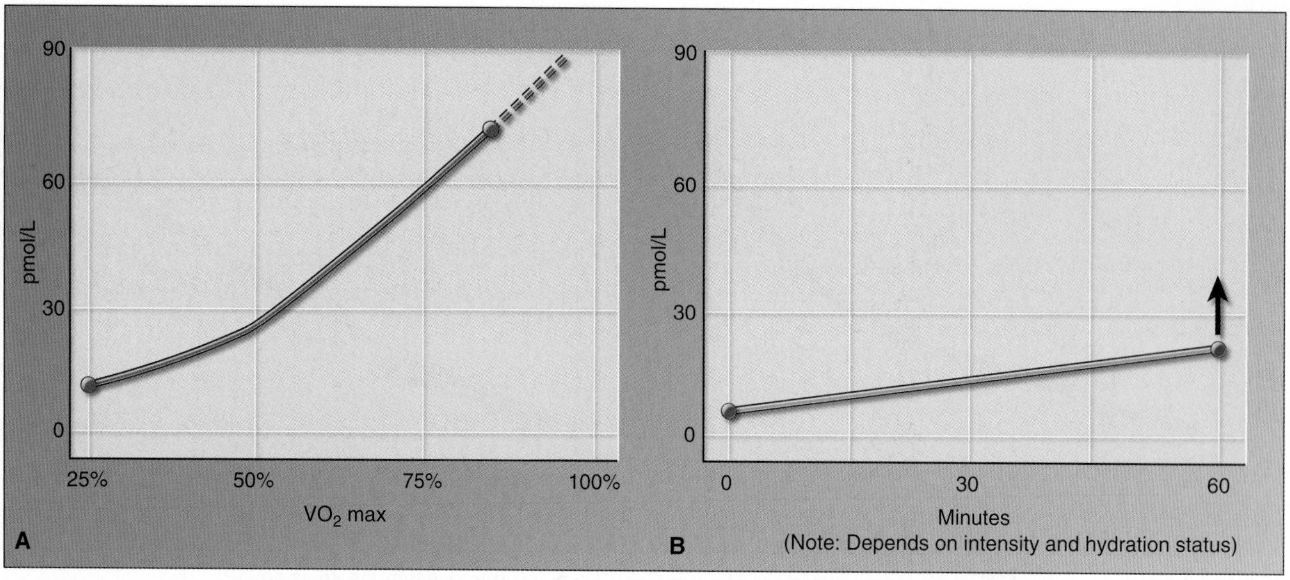

FIGURE 6.20 Responses of circulating concentrations of aldosterone to aerobic activities (35,65). **A.** Typical responses at different aerobic intensities up to 80% $\dot{V}O_2$ max. The *dotted line* indicates expected values for greater intensities. **B.** Aldosterone concentrations during 60 minutes of high-intensity endurance exercise. Note that the aldosterone response is highly dependent on the exercise intensity and the existing hydration status of the individual.

Chronic Responses to Endurance Exercise Some evidence exists that the thyroid hormones decrease chronically during stressful phases of training, but these data are not definitive. Given the acute data, it is possible that chronic decreases would result from lower hypothalamic–pituitary signaling and may be indicative of energy conservation in athletes undergoing high-intensity training (69,70).

Calcium-Regulating Hormones and Endurance Exercise

To date, it has been difficult to tie these calcium-regulating hormones in with the exercise-induced responses of the skeletal system. Although acute exercise can increase circulating concentrations of these hormones, no definitive pattern has been identified concerning acute or chronic exercise responses (67).

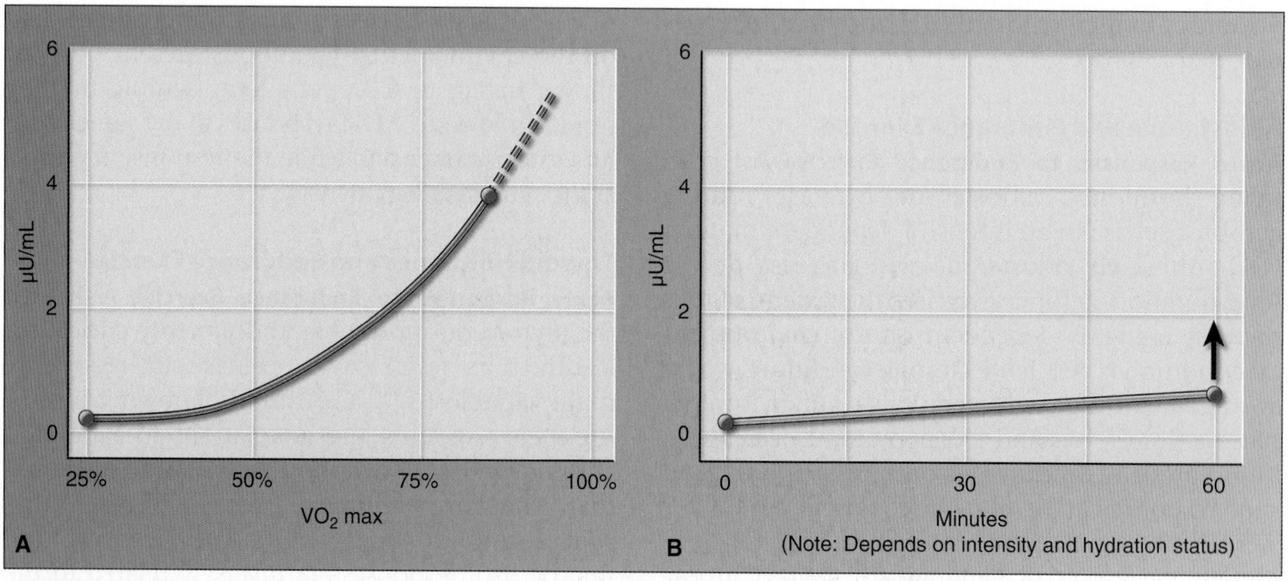

FIGURE 6.21 Responses of circulating concentrations of antidiuretic hormone to aerobic activities (35,65). **A.** Typical responses at different aerobic intensities up to 80% $\dot{V}O_2$ max. The *dotted line* indicates expected values for greater intensities. **B.** ADH concentrations during 60 minutes of high-intensity endurance exercise. Note that the aldosterone response is highly dependent on the exercise intensity and the existing hydration status of the individual.

RESPONSES AND ADAPTATIONS OF HORMONES TO RESISTANCE EXERCISE

One of the problems with studying the endocrine responses to RE is the tremendous variety possible with this training stimulus. This is best illustrated by the five acute training variables for RE (71,72). They are:

1. Choice of exercise
2. Order of exercise
3. Volume of exercise
4. Intensity (or load) of exercise
5. Interset rest intervals

These five variables represent all of the possible variables for a single weight-training session. Needless to say, each of the variables includes many options. When all five variables are considered, the number of possible combinations becomes extremely large, thus representing the huge number of stimuli RE can present. When the long-term program is added to this, the characteristics of the training program can almost be overwhelming. Regardless, much progress has been made concerning the effect of the acute training variables on the subsequent hormonal responses. Unfortunately, many questions remain unanswered concerning the hormonal responses to each of these acute training variables. For example, little is known about how changing the order of exercise influences the hormonal responses and adaptations. Furthermore, little is known about how numerous hormones respond to RE. Nevertheless, Table 6.3 summarizes much of the research on several hormonal responses to a single RE training session and the roles of the acute training variables.

> ***During heavy RE, the specific hormonal response is dependent in large part on the acute training variables: choice of exercise, order of exercise, total repetitions (volume), load or intensity, and interset rest.***

Testosterone and Resistance Exercise

Acute Responses to Resistance Exercise Testosterone readily increases during a weight-training session but requires at least a moderate training volume as measured in total repetitions (79–82). Sessions that utilize large muscle mass multijoint exercises appear to elicit larger responses than those using just small muscle mass exercises (83,84). Additionally, exercise sessions that incorporate high-power exercises such as the Olympic weightlifting movements

TABLE 6.3 ● KNOWN EFFECTS OF THE ACUTE WEIGHT-TRAINING VARIABLES ON SEVERAL HORMONAL RESPONSES TO A SINGLE EXERCISE SESSION (8,29,31,48,56,73–79)

ACUTE TRAINING VARIABLE	TESTOSTERONE	CORTISOL	GROWTH HORMONE	LACTATE
Choice of exercise	↑ With large muscle mass exercises and high-power exercises, moderately high volumes necessary	↑ With large muscle mass exercises and high-power exercises, ↑ usually with full body training session	↑ With large muscle mass exercises and high-power exercises, ↑ with free weights > ↑ with machines	↑ With large muscle mass exercises and high-power exercises
Volume of exercises	Variable responses, depends on other factors	↑ With increasing volume. Note: volume can be low if intensity is high enough	↑ With increasing volume. Note: GH response related to total work	↑ With increasing volume
Intensity of exercise	↑ With increasing relative intensity (% of 1 RM)	↑ With increasing relative intensity (% of 1 RM). Note: cortisol ↑ > testosterone ↑	↑ With increasing relative intensity (% of 1 RM). Note: volume must be high enough	Too high an intensity → smaller HLa response
Interset rest intervals	↓ Rest may ↑ testosterone (responses are variable)	↑ With decreasing rest intervals	↑ With decreasing rest intervals	↑ With decreasing rest intervals

↑, increases; ↓, decreases; RM, repetition maximum, >, greater than.

Q & A from the Field

Q ***Hormonal responses to RE seem to be very specific to the type and intensity of exercise. Can this specific hormonal response be planned based on specific goals and periods of a periodized conditioning program?***

A Yes. Specific hormonal responses help to determine the training effect on muscle tissue. In a hypertrophy phase of training, the male athlete would want to stimulate the body's own production of testosterone. This can best be accomplished by large muscle mass exercises, heavy resistance, and a moderate to high volume with short (about 60-second) rest intervals. The testosterone response in male athletes is greatest with two or more years of resistance training experience.

When constructing a training program, it is important to understand the specific goal of training. If the goal is inducing muscle hypertrophy, use exercises that will stimulate testosterone. In contrast, if muscle hypertrophy is not the goal of training, exercise routines stimulating anabolic hormones may be contraindicated.

To stimulate the body's production of GH, use resistance training protocols that stimulate high lactic acid production (high-intensity, 10-RM, short rest periods). The appropriate use of carbohydrate and protein supplements before and after the workout can also help with endogenous production of GH.

To optimize the adrenal response to resistance training, the athlete should use high-volume, large muscle mass exercises with short rest periods. Exposing the athlete to a variety of resistance training stimuli at a high intensity allows the adrenal response to take an active role in recovery. In a high-intensity protocol such as this, always monitor the athlete for signs of overtraining.

(snatch and clean and jerk) can also produce considerable increases in testosterone (84). These types of exercises (e.g., squats, bench presses, cleans, dead lifts) have large energy requirements and activate the body's endocrine and neuroendocrine systems to a greater extent than other types of REs (e.g., arm curls, leg extensions, leg curls). The relative intensity (percent of one repetition maximum (RM), or % of 1 RM) is critical, with greater relative intensities producing the largest increases (79). It must be pointed out, though, that the intensity may be so high (e.g., 100% of 1 RM) that an adequate training volume cannot be performed. The net result is little or no testosterone response (77). When very low relative intensities are used, such as 40% of 1 RM, acute responses of testosterone are also minimal (83). Some evidence also exists that decreasing the rest between sets may increase the testosterone response slightly (79). Again, it should be pointed out that too short a rest interval may mean that the loads have to be decreased below the critical level for a significant testosterone response.

Chronic Responses to Resistance Exercise Observations in resting testosterone concentrations during resistance training are inconsistent in both men and women with elevations, no differences, and reductions reported (85). Further, resting levels may depend on the current volume and intensity of training (85). In a study where resting elevations were reported during short-term high-volume training, subsequent reductions were observed when volume was reduced and intensity was increased over 7 weeks (86). Thus, substantial changes in volume and intensity may elicit transient changes in resting testosterone concentrations and values, which then return to baseline during normal training.

Cortisol and Resistance Exercise

Acute Responses to Resistance Exercise Compared to testosterone, cortisol tends to exhibit a larger acute response to RE (79). As with testosterone, cortisol responds most when large muscle mass, multijoint exercises are performed and when high-power exercises are used (84). Owing to the metabolic requirements, cortisol levels will increase when total-body training sessions are performed. Cortisol responds in a relative intensity- and volume-dependent manner (79). When interset rest intervals are decreased, cortisol responses are also increased, again most likely due to the metabolic requirements of the session (79). It should be noted that some dietary supplements have been promoted with claims that they decrease the cortisol response to exercise. Although cortisol is a catabolic hormone, it also serves an important role in the remodeling of muscle tissue. As such, decreasing or eliminating the cortisol response may not be desirable.

Chronic Responses to Resistance Exercise However, despite the role cortisol has in remodeling muscle, chronically elevated levels can be deleterious. Chronic resistance training produces inconsistent patterns of cortisol secretion as no change (18,48,87,88) reductions (42,89,90), and elevations (59) have been reported in men and women during training and short-term overreaching. Further, when compared to untrained individuals, highly resistance trained individuals appear to have less of a cortisol response to intense resistance training. This adaptation may be of little importance, as trained individuals may not be undergoing the same extreme muscular adaptations as an untrained individual.

Growth Hormone and Resistance Exercise

Acute Responses to Resistance Exercise The fact that acute RE stimulates a potent GH release in both men and women is well documented (1). However, the magnitude of acute release in response to RE depends upon several variables, including rest time between sets, volume, load, exercise selection, training status, muscle actions used, amount of muscle mass recruited, time of day, and total work. Thus, it is extremely difficult to isolate the individual variable effects on GH release. The use of large muscle mass, multijoint exercises as well as high-power exercises is critical for a large GH response (1,79). Some evidence exists that free weights may produce a larger response than machine exercises, but this may simply be related to the muscle mass involvement (91). The relative intensity and the volume of exercise are positively related to the GH response as well (79,92). The interset rest interval is extremely important, with very short rest intervals eliciting extremely large acute GH responses (79).

Chronic Responses to Resistance Exercise Chronic training may increase the GH response to acute exercise in both men and women (93). However, this response is likely due to their ability to perform more work and utilize heavier loads, as resting values do not change.

Gender Differences Women have higher resting values when compared to men. However, the data are conflicting as to whether there are differences in the acute exercise response, with no differences being reported most consistently (78). A heavy loading protocol has been reported to elicit a GH response in men, but not in women, while both genders have an equal response to a higher rep, lower rest interval protocol (42). These data suggest that factors such as lean body mass, total body mass, fat mass, nutritional intake, training status, and the menstrual cycle may all play a role in the RE-induced GH response.

Insulin-Like Growth Factor-I and Resistance Exercise

Acute Responses to Resistance Exercise The response of circulating IGF-I to an acute RE bout is variable, with some investigations showing no change (20,65) and some reporting increases (78,90,92). These reported differences may be due to the differences in protocols, subjects' trained state, and age, gender, and nutritional status. In 1991, Kraemer et al. (78) compared the responses of eight men and eight women to two different full body acute RE protocols. Protocol one utilized a 5-RM load, 3-minute rest period. Protocol two utilized a 10-RM load, 1-minute rest periods and had a higher total work than the first protocol. Both protocols were designed to control for load, rest period length, and total work (each protocol contained a secondary workout surrounding the primary protocol to equalize total work). IGF-I increased in response to both exercise protocols in both genders, but there were no significant differences between men and women.

Chronic Responses to Resistance Exercise Well-trained men are reported to have higher concentrations of IGF-I at rest compared to untrained men, despite no differences between these two groups in circulating concentrations of GH (92). Temporal changes in IGF-I levels were reported in both men and women in response to different exercise protocols that differed in volume and rest periods (94). In addition, increased resting levels of IGF-I were reported after the supplementation period, suggesting that dietary manipulation played a role in IGF-I dynamics (2).

Gender Differences Similar to GH, women have significantly higher resting values of IGF-I. The higher values at rest are reflective of the GH-mediated control of IGF-I. However, some researchers speculate that the significant increases at rest in women give further support to the concept that women may rely upon the IGF/GH axis to a greater extent than men as an anabolic signaler for strength gains, while men probably rely more on testosterone.

Lactate: Acute Response to Resistance Exercise

Although not a hormone, lactate provides insight on the metabolic characteristics of different weight-training sessions. In general, protocols that use large muscle mass, multijoint, and high-power exercises, with large training volumes and short interset rest intervals, produce the largest lactate responses (79,84,95). If the relative intensity is too great, however, the volume that can be performed becomes too low, thus compromising the lactate response.

LONG-TERM ADAPTATIONS TO RESISTANCE EXERCISE

Table 6.4 lists the long-term (chronic) responses to heavy RE (18,89,97,98). In general, resting concentrations of these hormones are not always altered, but differences in the acute responses to a resistance-training session can occur. In some cases, the response increases, indicating an enhanced capacity of the involved endocrine glands. In other cases, the response decreases, indicating greater efficiency of those hormones. At present, the responses of a number of hormones are not known.

Long-term hormonal adaptations to training are more subtle than the acute response to a single session, but they can provide an important training adaptation.

OVERTRAINING AND THE ENDOCRINE SYSTEM

Although a properly designed training program is desirable for optimal results, sometimes the exercise program is improperly prescribed, resulting in maladaptations or overtraining. Overtraining occurs when training volume and/or intensity is excessive and results in prolonged decreases in performance (27,72). Short-term performance decrements are sometimes referred to as overreaching and are often part of a planned

TABLE 6.4 ● HORMONAL EFFECTS OF LONG-TERM NORMAL RE TRAINING (15,23,38,57,69,87,95,96)

HORMONE	EFFECTS
Testosterone	Slight increase
Cortisol	Slight decrease
Growth hormone	Slight decrease
Insulin	Increase
Glucagon	Decrease
Epinephrine	Max intensity: increase
	Submax intensity: decrease
Norepinephrine	Max intensity: increase
	Submax intensity: decrease
Antidiuretic hormone	Slight decrease (depends on the environmental conditions)
Aldosterone	Slight decrease (depends on the environmental conditions)
Thyroxine	No known change
Triiodothyronine	No known change
Calcitonin	No known change
Parathyroid hormone	No known change

training program (e.g., two-a-day training sessions for many sports). As might be expected, the endocrine system has been implicated in the maladaptations occurring during overtraining. It has been suggested that monitoring certain hormones may permit monitoring of the training stresses, thus avoiding the onset of an overtrained state (73). What is not often appreciated is that different types of overtraining appear to elicit different hormonal responses (27).

Overtraining occurring from activities that emphasize aerobic endurance is often characterized by very high training volumes (45–47). Table 6.5 indicates that, except for the stress hormone cortisol, most hormonal responses eventually decrease. The decrease in catecholamines appears to be reflective of exhaustion of the sympathetic nervous system. High volumes of RE exhibit many of the same endocrine characteristics (27,72,96). Perhaps the most commonly cited variable for monitoring overtraining is the testosterone/cortisol ratio (73). In general, this appears to be indicative of the collective training stresses, although changes in this ratio can often occur when overtraining is not present. Therefore, one cannot diagnose overtraining using this variable alone. It appears that subsequent exposures to high-volume resistance exercise overtraining may permit the body to adapt to the stress, resulting in avoidance of overtraining (57,96).

Contrary to many of the common characteristics of aerobic overtraining or high-volume RE, high-intensity resistance exercise overtraining exhibits a much different endocrine profile. In general, the steroid hormones and GH are often unaffected. In fact, some studies have shown an increase in testosterone, the exact opposite of other types of overtraining (74). The catecholamines actually exhibit increased responses to exercise (56,57). It is believed that the sympathetic nervous system is still attempting to preserve performance and has not yet reached a state of exhaustion as previously described for other types of overtraining.

Although many factors can contribute to overtraining and the accompanying decreases in performance, several easily administered training variables can help (72). When training volumes and volume loads have been high, small but critical decreases in either volume or relative intensity can result in the avoidance of overtraining. Although not always the case, high volumes of RE typically depress resting testosterone and the testosterone/cortisol ratio. Simply providing a day of recovery each week, or at least a sharp decrease in volume (and usually intensity), may avoid such a problem. Such an alteration in training volume is easy to administer but often ignored.

Much like skeletal muscle adaptations, hormonal adaptations occur as a result of short- and long-term training. As training continues, the amount of hormones needed will either increase or decrease.

USING THE ENDOCRINE SYSTEM TO MONITOR TRAINING

A critical issue for many coaches and athletes is monitoring the physiological effects of the training program. This can be relevant for either the individual training session or the longer term effects of a phase of the training cycle. Obviously, obtaining blood samples from an athlete is often easier said than done, and having the blood analyzed may be

TABLE 6.5 ● ENDOCRINE RESPONSES TO OVERTRAINING (17,24,28,61,73,99)

HORMONE	AEROBIC OVERTRAINING	HIGH-VOLUME RE OVERTRAINING	HIGH-INTENSITY RE OVERTRAINING
Testosterone	Decrease	Decrease	NC or slight increase
Cortisol	Increase	Increase	NC
Tes/Cort	Decrease	Decrease	NC
Growth hormone	Increase → decrease	NC	NC
Epinephrine	Decrease	Decrease?	Increase
Norepinephrine	Decrease	Decrease?	Increase

RE, resistance exercise.

even more difficult. An alternative might be to collect salivary or urine samples, but the analyses are still time-consuming and expensive. Regardless, much valuable information may be attainable if this information is accessed.

It has been proposed that levels of fatigue, recovery, and overtraining may sometimes be monitored by tracking hormonal responses and adaptations to training.

Training Effect of a Single Session

The hormonal response to a single training session can help the coach determine whether the desired training stimulus is being applied (21). The responses of testosterone, cortisol, and GH can help determine the anabolic characteristics of the training stimulus. It has even been suggested that the thyroid hormones and insulin be also monitored for this reason, since they have also been associated with anabolic responses of muscle.

Training Intensity of a Single Session

It has been suggested that supporting information on whether proper training intensities have been applied can be deduced from the acute hormonal profiles. If hormonal responses are typically monitored, then it may be possible to evaluate whether the prescribed intensity is appropriate based on the responses of intensity-dependent hormones (21).

A training session may be designed that optimizes or minimizes the anabolic hormonal responses.

Diagnosing Fatigue

All coaches and athletes would like to know how well the training program is being tolerated (21,27,72). When the training becomes excessive, it is critical to detect this problem before it turns into a long-term overtraining syndrome. To properly do this, hormonal variables must be measured on a regular basis to determine normal values for each individual. Possible variables to monitor include testosterone, cortisol, testosterone/cortisol ratio, and catecholamines. It is important to remember that just because some of the endocrine variables change, this does not mean that overtraining has occurred or that excessive fatigue exists. It may, however, serve as a warning of impending problems.

Monitoring Recovery

Once normal hormonal levels have been determined for an individual, it is possible to find out when a fatigued individual returns to prefatigue states (21). Any hormone or neurohormone that responds to training stress may have to return to normal levels for that individual before physiological recovery is considered complete. This may be a critical step in assessing whether a periodized training program has been designed to adequately permit recovery during certain phases of the training.

OPTIMIZING THE TRAINING PROGRAM

The ultimate challenge for the reader of this chapter is to utilize the information provided in designing a strength and conditioning program. Such a program will, of course, depend on the desired goals determined for the specific purpose of the training. Although numerous physiological systems of the body must be considered, insight on the development of training programs can be deduced from the endocrine data available.

GOAL: MUSCLE HYPERTROPHY

In designing a program where muscle hypertrophy is a primary objective, it will be important to design the training stimulus to optimize the anabolic hormone response. For example, growth hormone responses are optimized when large muscle mass exercises are used with approximately 10-RM loads, while rest intervals are kept fairly short (1 minute or less). In addition, some work with relatively heavy loads is necessary to optimize the acute testosterone response.

GOAL: NO MUSCLE HYPERTROPHY

Some sports may require an individual to maintain a certain body weight (e.g., weight-class sports, activities where a large body mass is not desired). In designing a program for such individuals, it may be wise to minimize the anabolic hormone response. For example, avoiding large muscle mass exercises may minimize some of the growth hormone responses to a training session. Of course, this is also dependent on the intensities and rest intervals prescribed. In some cases, large muscle mass, multijoint exercises are necessary for the purposes of the training. In such instances, allowing longer rest intervals will definitely minimize the growth hormone response.

GOAL: HIGH-POWER PERFORMANCE

It has been suggested that optimal power performances occur when resting testosterone concentrations are relatively high (100). If this is the case, the training program must permit a long-term elevation in resting testosterone levels. One method of doing this is by decreasing the training stresses (i.e., decreasing volume and/or intensity) during the taper phase (76). In addition, chronic utilization of high relative intensities using high-power, large muscle mass exercises may contribute to slight elevations of long-term resting levels of testosterone (98).

GOAL: PEAK PERFORMANCE

If a performance peak is desired, the preceding training taper must permit the resting concentrations of certain hormones to be adequately recovered. In this case, decreasing the volume load (reps times weight) can result in elevations of resting testosterone and increases in the testosterone/cortisol ratio (76).

GOAL: AVOIDING OVERTRAINING

Although many factors can contribute to overtraining and the accompanying decreases in performance, several easily administered training variables can help (72). When training volumes and volume loads have been high, small but critical decreases in either volume or relative intensity can result in the avoidance of overtraining. Although not always the case, high volumes of RE typically depress resting testosterone and the testosterone/cortisol ratio. Simply providing a day of recovery each week, or at least a sharp decrease in volume (and usually intensity), may avoid such a problem. Such an alteration in training volume is easy to administer but often ignored.

Summary

The endocrine system comprises complex interactions of hormones and neurohormones with each other and other physiological systems. Proper responses of the endocrine system are essential for optimal adaptations to a training program. Although you may not have the ability to measure and analyze these variables, a thorough understanding of how the body responds and adapts to the stresses applied is imperative for developing truly effective programs and understanding why they are effective. Last, understanding how the endocrine system responds to the various acute training variables makes it possible to design a training prescription that provides an optimal hormonal environment for the desired results.

Maxing Out

1. Using this text and other resources, review the hormonal response to resistance training in both men and women and explain how they differ.
2. Using this text and other resources, explain the hormonal response to prolonged endurance exercise.
3. Use this text and other resources to discuss overtraining relative to hormone levels in the body. Can monitoring of hormonal levels be used to predict overtraining?

REFERENCES

1. Kraemer WJ, Ratamess NA. Hormonal responses and adaptations to resistance exercise and training. *Sports Med.* 2005;35:339–361.
2. Kraemer WJ, Volek JS, Bush JA, et al. Hormonal responses to consecutive days of heavy-resistance exercise with or without nutritional supplementation. *J Appl Physiol.* 1998;85(4):1544–1555.
3. Wilson JD, Foster DW, eds. *Williams Textbook of Endocrinology.* Philadelphia, PA: Saunders; 1992:inside front cover.
4. Young DS. Implementation of SI units for clinical laboratory data. *Ann Intern Med.* 1987;106:114–128.
5. Sporn MB, Todaro GJ. Autocrine secretion and malignant transformation of cells. *N Engl J Med.* 1980;303: 878–880.
6. Feyrter F. Ueber die These von den peripheren endokrinen Druesen. *Wien Z Inn Med.* 1946;27:9–38.
7. Ojeda SR, Griffin JE. Organization of the endocrine system. In: Ojeda SR, Griffin JE, eds. *Textbook of Endocrine Physiology.* New York: Oxford University Press; 1988:3–16.
8. Clark JH, Schrader WT, O'Malley BW. Mechanisms of action of steroid hormones. In: Wilson JD, Foster DW, eds. *Williams Textbook of Endocrinology.* 8th ed. Philadelphia, PA: Saunders; 1992:35–90.
9. Hebener JF. Genetic control of hormone function. In: Wilson JD, Foster DW, eds. *Williams Textbook of Endocrinology.* 8th ed. Philadelphia, PA: Saunders; 1992:9–34.
10. Landsberg L, Young JB. Catecholamines and the adrenal medulla. In: Wilson JD, Foster DW, eds. *Williams Textbook of Endocrinology.* 8th ed. Philadelphia, PA: Saunders; 1992:621–705.

11. Mendel CM. The free hormone hypothesis: a physiologically based mathematical model. *Endocr Rev.* 1989;10:232–274.
12. Kraemer WJ. Endocrine responses and adaptations to strength training. In: Komi PV, ed. *Strength and Power in Sport.* Oxford, UK: Blackwell; 1992:291–304.
13. Wilkerson JE, Gutin B, Horvath SM. Exercise-induced changes in blood, red cell, and plasma volumes in man. *Med Sci Sports.* 1977;9:155–158.
14. Kahn CR, Smith RJ, Chin WW. Mechanism of action of hormones that act at the cell surface. In: Wilson JD, Foster DW, eds. *Williams Textbook of Endocrinology.* 8th ed. Philadelphia, PA: Saunders; 1992:91–134.
15. Houk JC. Control strategies in physiological systems. *FASEB J.* 1988;2:97–107.
16. Veldhuis JD, Johnson LM. Cluster analysis: a simple, versatile, and robust algorithm for endocrine pulse detection. *Am J Physiol.* 1988;250:E486–E493.
17. Czeisler CA, Klerman EB. Circadian and sleep-dependent regulation of hormone release in humans. *Rec Progr Horm Res.* 1999;54:97–130.
18. Hakkinen K, Pakarinen A, Alen M, et al. Daily hormonal and neuromuscular responses to intensive strength training in 1 week. *Int J Sports Med.* 1988;9:422–428.
19. Thuma JR, Gilders R, Verdun J, et al. Circadian rhythm of cortisol confounds cortisol responses to exercise: implications for future research. *J Appl Physiol.* 1995;78(5):1657–1664.
20. Cannon WB. Bodily changes in pain, hunger, fear, and rage. New York: Appleton; 1922.
21. Viru A, Viru M. *Biochemical Monitoring of Sport Training.* Champaign, IL: Human Kinetics; 2001:61–65.
22. Nindl BC, Pierce JR. Insulin-like growth factor I as a biomarker of health, fitness, and training status. *Med Sci Sports Exerc.* 2010;42:39–49.
23. Gilman AG. G-proteins and regulation of adenyl cyclase. *JAMA.* 1989;262:1819–1825.
24. Hokin LE. Receptors and phosphoinositide-generated second messengers. *Annu Rev Biochem.* 1985;54:202–235.
25. Borer K. *Exercise Endocrinology.* Champaign, IL: Human Kinetics; 2003:45.
26. Glass CK. Differential recognition of target genes by nuclear receptor monomers, dimers, and heterodimers. *Endocrinol Rev.* 1994;15:391–407.
27. Fry AC, Kraemer WJ. Resistance exercise overtraining and overreaching: neuroendocrine responses. *Sports Med.* 1997;23(2):106–129.
28. Eliakim A, Nemet D, Cooper DM. Exercise, training, and the GH-IGF-I axis. In: Kraemer WJ, Rogol AD, eds. *The Endocrine System in Sports and Exercise.* Malden, MA: Blackwell Publishing Ltd; 2005:165–179.
29. Goldspink G, Yang SY, Hameed M, et al. The role of MGF and other IGF-I splice variants in muscle maintenance and hypertrophy. In: Kraemer WJ, Rogol AD, eds. *The Endocrine System in Sports and Exercise.* Malden, MA: Blackwell Publishing Ltd; 2005:180–193.
30. Selye H. *The Stress of Life.* New York: McGraw-Hill; 1956.
31. Kjaer M, Galbo H. Effect of physical training on the capacity to secrete epinephrine. *J Appl Physiol.* 1988;64:11–16.
32. Winder, WW, Hickson RC, Hagberg JM, et al. Training-induced changes in hormonal and metabolic responses to submaximal exercise. *J Appl Physiol.* 1979;46:766–771.
33. Atgie C, D'Allaire F, Bukowiecki LJ. Role of beta1 and beta3 adrenoceptors in the regulation of lipolysis and thermogenesis in rat brown adipocytes. *Am J Physiol.* 1997;273:C1136–C1142.
34. Chandler RM, Byrne HK, Patterson JG, et al. Dietary supplements affect the anabolic hormones after weight-training exercise. *J Appl Physiol.* 1994;76:839–845.
35. Cumming DC, Brunsting LA III, Strich G, et al. Reproductive hormone increases in response to acute exercise in men. *Med Sci Sports Exerc.* 1986;18:369–373.
36. Baker ER, Mathur RS, Kirk RF, et al. Plasma gonadotropins, prolactin, and steroid hormone concentrations in female runners immediately after a long-distance run. *Fertil Steril.* 1984;38:38–41.
37. Bonen A, Ling WYU, MacIntyre KP, et al. Effects of exercise on the serum concentrations of FSH, LH, progesterone, and estradiol. *Eur J Appl Physiol.* 1979;42:15–23.
38. Galbo H. *Hormonal and Metabolic Adaptation to Exercise.* New York: Thieme-Stratton; 1983.
39. Sutton JR, Farrell PA, Harber VJ. Hormonal adaptations to physical activity. In: Bouchard C, Shephard RJ, Stephens T, et al., eds. *Exercise, Fitness, and Health.* Champaign, IL: Human Kinetics; 1990:217–257.
40. Francesconi RP, Sawka MN, Pandolf KB, et al. Plasma hormonal responses at graded hypohydration levels during exercise-heat stress. *J Appl Physiol.* 1985;59:1855–1860.
41. Kotchen TA, Hartley LH, Rice TW, et al. Renin, norepinephrine, and epinephrine responses to graded exercise. *J Appl Physiol.* 1971;31:178–184.
42. Kraemer WJ, Staron RS, Hagerman FC, et al. The effects of short-term resistance training on endocrine function in men and women. *Eur J Appl Physiol Occup Physiol.* 1998;78:69–76.
43. Brandenberger G, Follenius M. Influence of timing and intensity of muscle exercise on temporal patterns of plasma cortisol levels. *J Clin Endocrinol Metab.* 1975;40:845–849.
44. Consitt LA, Copeland JL, Tremblay MS. Hormone responses to resistance vs. endurance exercise in premenopausal females. *Can J Appl Physiol.* 2001;26:574–587.
45. Lehmann M, Foster C, Netzer N, et al. Physiological responses to short- and long-term overtraining in endurance athletes. In: Kreider RB, Fry AC, O'Toole ML, eds. *Overtraining in Sport.* Champaign, IL: Human Kinetics; 1998:19–46.
46. Lehmann, M, Gastmann U, Petersen KG, et al. Training-overtraining: performance, and hormone levels, after a defined increase in training volume vs. training intensity in experienced middle- and long-distance runners. *Br J Sports Med.* 1992;26:233–242.
47. Lehmann M, Gastmann U, Baur S, et al. Selected parameters and mechanisms of peripheral and central fatigue and regeneration in overtrained athletes. In: Lehmann M, Foster C, Gastmann U, et al., eds. *Overload, Performance Incompetence, and Regeneration in Sport.* New York: Kluwer Academic/Plenum; 1999:7–26.
48. Häkkinen K, Pakarinen A, Kyrolainen H, et al. Neuromuscular adaptations and serum hormones in

females during prolonged power training. *Int J Sports Med.* 1990;11:91–98.
49. Lassare C, Girard F, Durand J, et al. Kinetics of human growth hormone during submaximal exercise. *J Appl Physiol.* 1974;37:826–830.
50. Wideman L, Weltman JY, Hartman ML, et al. Growth hormone release during acute and chronic aerobic and resistance exercise: recent findings. *Sports Med.* 2002;32(15):987–1004.
51. Vislocky LM, Gaine PC, Pikosky MA, et al. Gender impacts the post-exercise substrate and endocrine response in trained runners. *J Int Soc Sports Nutr.* 2008;5:7.
52. Eliakim A, Portal S, Zadik Z, et al. The effect of a volleyball practice on anabolic hormones and inflammatory markers in elite male and female adolescent players. *J Strength Cond Res.* 2009;23(5):1553–1559.
53. Friedmann B, Kindermann W. Energy metabolism and regulatory hormones in women and men during endurance exercise. *Eur J Appl Physiol Occup Physiol.* 1989;59(1–2):1–9.
54. Nindl BC. Insulin-like growth factor-I as a candidate metabolic biomarker: military relevance and future directions for measurement. *J Diabetes Sci Technol.* 2009;3(2): 371–376.
55. Tarnopolsky LJ, MacDougall JD, Atkinson SA, et al. Gender differences in substrate for endurance exercise. *J Appl Physiol.* 1990;68(1):302–308.
56. Fry AC, Kraemer WJ, van Borselen F, et al. Catecholamine responses to short-term high-intensity resistance exercise overtraining. *J Appl Physiol.* 1994;77(2):941–946.
57. Fry AC, Kraemer WJ, Stone MH, et al. Endocrine responses to over-reaching before and after 1 year of weightlifting training. *Can J Appl Physiol.* 1994;19(4):400–410.
58. Christensen NJ, Galbo H, Hansen JF, et al. Catecholamines and exercise. *Diabetes.* 1979;28:58–62.
59. Häkkinen K, Pakarinen A. Serum hormones in male strength athletes during intensive short term strength training. *Eur J Appl Physiol.* 1991;63:191–199.
60. Kinderman W, Schnabel A, Schmitt WM, et al. Catecholamines, growth hormone, cortisol, insulin, and sex hormones in anaerobic and aerobic exercise. *Eur J Appl Physiol.* 1982;49:389–399.
61. Horton TJ, Pagliassotti MJ, Hobbs K, et al. Fuel metabolism in men and women during and after long-duration exercise. *J Appl Physiol.* 1998;85(5):1823–1832.
62. Mendenhall LA, Sial S, Coggan AR. Gender differences in substrate metabolism during moderate intensity cycling (Abstract). *Med Sci Sports Exerc.* 1996;27:S213.
63. Zouhal H, Jacob C, Delamarche P, et al. Catecholamines and the effects of exercise, training and gender. *Sports Med.* 2008;38(5):401–423.
64. Tidgren B, Hjemdal P, Theodorsson E, et al. Renal neurohormonal and vascular responses to dynamic exercise in humans. *J Appl Physiol.* 1991;70:2279–2286.
65. Kraemer WJ, Aguilera BA, Terada M, et al. Responses of IGF-I to endogenous increases in growth hormone after heavy-resistance exercise. *J Appl Physiol.* 1995;79:1310–1315.
66. Convertino VA. Blood volume: its adaptation to endurance training. *Med Sci Sports Exerc.* 1991;12:1338–1348.
67. McMurray RG, Hackney AC. Endocrine responses to exercise and training. In: Garrett WE, Kirkendall DT, eds. *Exercise and Sport Science.* Philadelphia, PA: Lippincott, Williams & Wilkins; 2000:135–164.
68. Hackney AC, Dobridge JD. Thyroid hormones and the interrelationship of cortisol and prolactin: influence of prolonged, exhaustive exercise. *Endokrynol Pol.* 2009;60:252–257.
69. Baylor LS, Hackney AC. Resting thyroid and leptin hormone changes in women following intense, prolonged exercise training. *Eur J Appl Physiol.* 2003;88(4–5):480–484.
70. Simsch C, Lormes W, Petersen KG, et al. Training intensity influences leptin and thyroid hormones in highly trained rowers. *Int J Sports Med.* 200;23:422–427.
71. Fleck SJ, Kraemer WJ. *Designing Resistance Exercise Programs.* 2nd ed. Champaign, IL: Human Kinetics; 1997.
72. Fry AC. Overload and regeneration during resistance exercise. In: Lehmann M, Foster C, Gastmann U, et al., eds. *Overload, Performance Incompetence, and Regeneration in Sport.* New York: Kluwer Academic/Plenum; 1999.
73. Adlercreutz H, Harkonen M, Kuoppasalmi K, et al. Effect of training on plasma anabolic and catabolic steroid hormones and their response during physical exercise. *Int J Sports Med.* 1986;7;S27–S28.
74. Fry AC, Kraemer WJ, Ramsey LT. Pituitary-adrenal-gonadal responses to high-intensity resistance exercise overtraining. *J Appl Physiol.* 1998;85(6):2352–2359.
75. Goodman HM. *Basic Medical Endocrinology.* New York: Raven Press; 1988:103.
76. Hakkinen K, Pakarinen A, Alen M, et al. Relationships between training volume, physical performance capacity and serum hormone concentrations during prolonged training in elite weight lifters. *Int J Sports Med.* 1987;8(suppl):61–65.
77. Hakkinen K, Pakarinen A. Acute hormonal responses to two different fatiguing heavy-resistance protocols in male athletes. *J Appl Physiol.* 1993;74(2):882–887.
78. Kraemer WJ, Gordon SE, Fleck SJ, et al. Endogenous anabolic hormonal and growth factor responses to heavy resistance exercise in males and females. *Int J Sports Med.* 1991;12:228–235.
79. Kraemer WJ, Marchitelli L, McCurry R, et al. Hormonal and growth factor responses to heavy resistance exercise. *J Appl Physiol.* 1990;69(4):1442–1450.
80. Fahey TD, Rolph R, Moungmee P, et al. Serum testosterone, body composition, and strength of young adults. *Med Sci Sports.* 1976;8:31–34.
81. Gotschalk LA, Loetbel DD, Nindl BC, et al. Hormonal responses of multi-set versus single-set heavy resistance exercise protocols. *Can J Appl Physiol.* 1997;22(3):244–255.
82. Weiss LW, Cureton KJ, Thompson FN. Comparison of serum testosterone and androstenedione responses to weightlifting in men and women. *Eur J Appl Physiol.* 1983;50(3):413–419.
83. Harber MP, Fry AC, Rubin JC, et al. Skeletal muscle and hormonal adaptations to circuit weight training. *Scand J Med Sci Sports.* 2004;14(3):176–185.
84. Kraemer WJ, Fry AD, Warren BJ, et al. Acute hormonal responses in elite junior weightlifters. *Int J Sports Med.* 1992;13(2):103–109.
85. Kraemer WJ, Ratamess NJ, Hatfield DL, et al. The endocrinology of resistance exercise and training. In: Antonio J, ed.

Essentials of Sports Nutrition and Supplements. Totowa, NJ: Humana Press; 2008.

86. Ahtiainen JP, Pakarinen A, Alen M, et al. Short vs. long rest period between the sets in hypertrophic resistance training: influence on muscle strength, size, and hormonal adaptations in trained men. *J Strength Cond Res*. 2005;19(3):572–582.
87. Häkkinen K, Pakarinen A, Kraemer WJ, et al. Basal concentrations and acute responses of serum hormones and strength development during heavy resistance training in middle-aged and elderly men and women. *J Gerontol A Biol Sci Med Sci*. 2000;55:B95–B105.
88. Potteiger JA, Judge LW, Cerny JA, et al. Effects of altering training volume and intensity on body mass, performance, and hormonal concentrations in weight-event athletes. *J Strength Cond Res*. 1995;9:55–58.
89. Hakkinen K, Pakarinen A, Alen M, et al. Serum hormones during prolonged training of neuromuscular performance. *Eur J Appl Physiol*. 1985;53:287–293.
90. Marx JO, Ratamess NA, Nindl BC, et al. Low-volume circuit versus high-volume periodized resistance training in women. *Med Sci Sports Exerc*. 2001;33(4):635–643.
91. Schilling BK, Fry AC, Ferkin MH, et al. Hormonal responses to free-weight and machine exercise [abstract]. *Med Sci Sports Exerc*. 2001;33(5, suppl):S270.
92. Rubin MR, Kraemer WJ, Maresh CM, et al. High-affinity growth hormone binding protein and acute heavy resistance exercise. *Med Sci Sports Exerc*. 2005;37:395–403.
93. Taylor JM, Thompson HS, Clarkson PM, et al. Growth hormone response to an acute bout of resistance exercise in weight-trained and non-weight-trained women. *J Strength Cond Res*. 2000;14:220–227.
94. Kraemer WJ, Fleck SJ, Dziados JE, et al. Changes in hormonal concentrations after different heavy-resistance exercise protocols in women. *J Appl Physiol*. 1993;75(2):594–604.
95. Guezennec Y, Leger L, Lhoste F, et al. Hormone and metabolite response to weight-lifting training sessions. *Int J Sports Med*. 1986;7:100–105.
96. Fry AC, Kraemer WJ, Stone MH, et al. Endocrine and performance responses to high volume training and amino acid supplementation in elite junior weightlifters. *Int J Sport Nutr*. 1993;3(3):306–322.
97. Hakkinen K. Neuromuscular and hormonal adaptations during strength and power training. *J Sports Med Phys Fit*. 1989;29:9–24.
98. Hakkinen K, Pakarinen A, Alen M, et al. Neuromuscular and hormonal adaptations in athletes to strength training in two years. *J Appl Physiol*. 1988;65(6):2406–2412.
99. Hoffman J. *Physiological Aspects of Sport Training and Performance*. Champaign, IL: Human Kinetics; 2002:15–26.
100. Bosco C, Tihanyi J, Viru A. Relationship between field fitness test and basal serum testosterone and cortisol levels in soccer players. *Clin Physiol*. 1996;16:317–322.

CHAPTER 7

Nutrition

COLIN WILBORN • LEM TAYLOR • ABBIE SMITH • JOSÉ ANTONIO

OBJECTIVES

After reading this chapter, you will be able to:

- Provide dietary recommendations to a variety of athletic populations.
- Draw your own conclusions about commercially available diets.
- Determine whether or not an athlete's diet appropriately corresponds to his or her training.
- Understand the importance of timing the intake of nutrients.
- Identify the composition and quality of nutrients within different foods.

KEY TERMS

Carbohydrates
Empty Calorie
Energy Balance
Essential
Fatty Acids
Glycemic Load
Glycemic Index
Macronutrient
Magnesium
Nutrient Density
Nutrient Timing
Overtraining
Protein
Trans Fats
Triglycerides (Triacylglycerol)
Vitamin C
Vitamin E
Zinc

Introduction

Nutritional intake is essential for optimizing the performance adaptations initiated in the gym, on the track, or on the field. Of the modifiable factors contributing to optimal exercise performance, nutritional intake is one of the most easily adaptable and often overlooked. There are many important facets of proper dietary regulation of athletes including energy balance, macronutrient type, and timing of ingestion. Consistent consumption of appropriate macro- and micronutrients during periods of heavy training can improve muscle protein turnover (the breakdown of old tissue and the rebuilding of new, more functionally adapted tissue) (1,2) as well as augment the function and recovery of the nervous system (3), immune system (4), and musculoskeletal system (5). Strength and conditioning professionals must impress on their athletes the importance of understanding how to appropriately fuel the body for the demands of specific training. Coaches who neglect the nutrition component of training limit their own efficacy in terms of helping their athlete and team to improve.

ENERGY BALANCE

Energy balance is the relationship between energy ingested and energy expended. It is an important determinant of exercise performance, body composition, training adaptation, and optimal physiological functioning in athletes. Unfortunately, many hold a simplistic view of energy balance suggesting it is as simple as the equation: calories in = calories out. It is often incorrectly assumed that total energy intake is predominantly related to weight gain or loss, ignoring macronutrient composition and timing. Our body absorbs 90% to 95% of the calories taken in, so caloric intake is not 100% efficient. More so, many factors relate to energy expenditure, some of which are not affected by diet and exercise. For example, if an athlete wants to lose body fat or overall mass, eating less will produce a negative energy balance; however, the athlete may not experience the changes that he or she is expecting. Figure 7.1 lists the details regarding glycemic index (GI), one aspect concerning caloric intake.

Figure 7.2 demonstrates the relationship between energy intake and energy consumption, comparing common diets which modify macronutrient ratios. This relationship between macronutrients and energy demands determines how

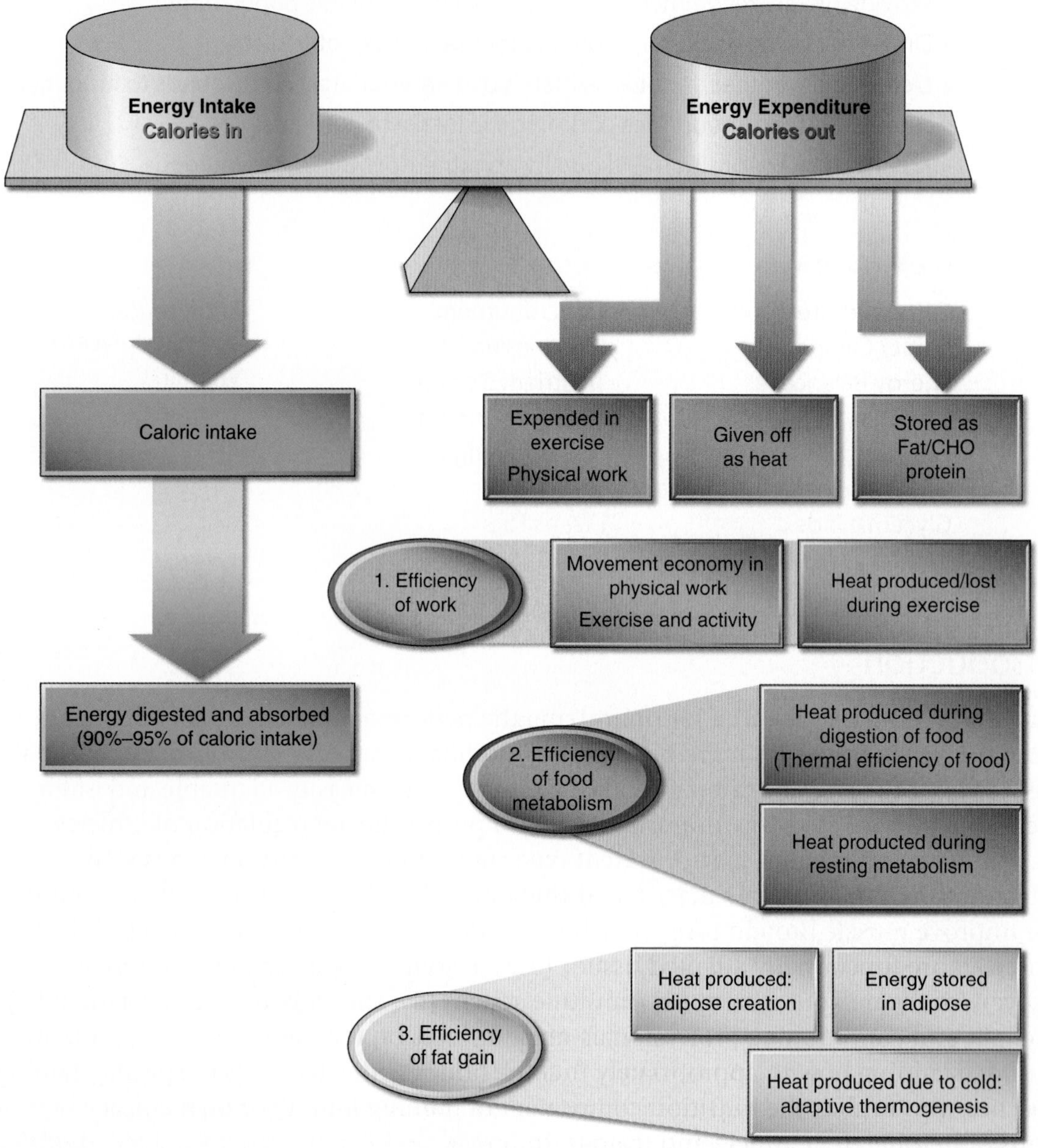

FIGURE 7.1 Factors related to the efficiency of energy intake and expenditure. (Reproduced with permission from Rampone AJ, Reynolds PJ. Obesity: thermodynamic principles in perspective. *Life Sci.* 1988;43:93–110.)

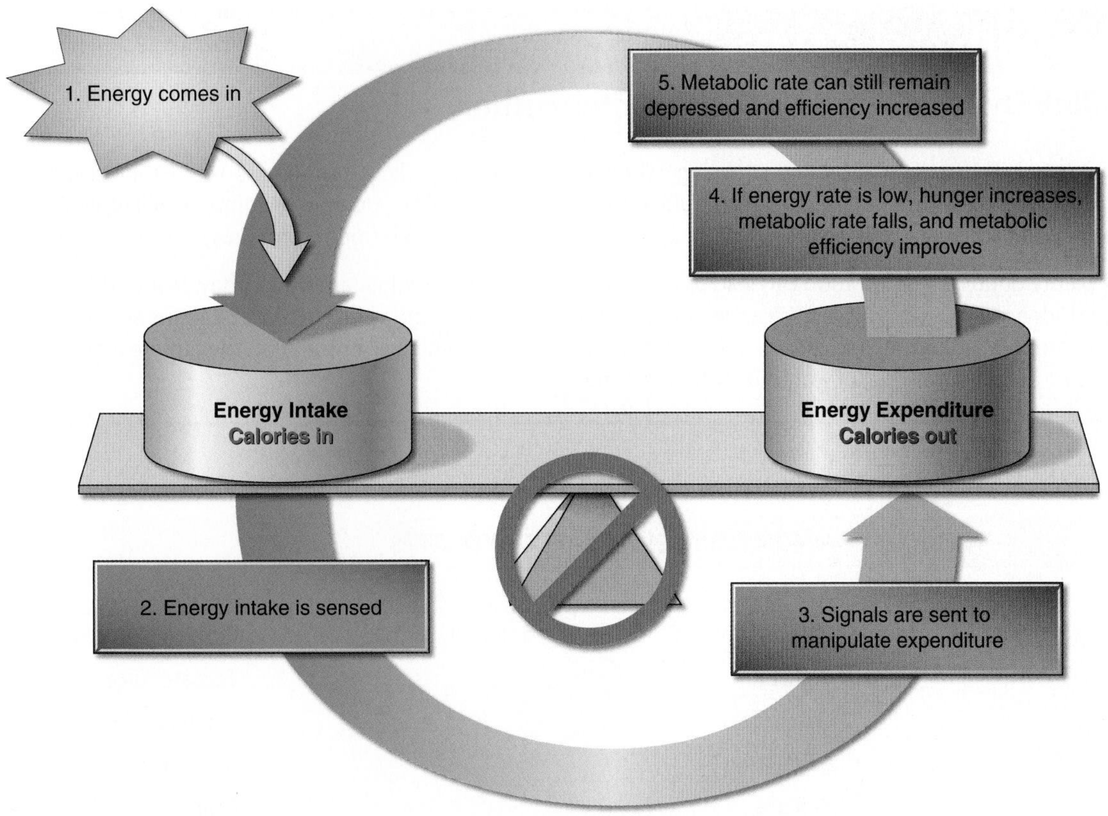

FIGURE 7.2 The relationship between energy intake and expenditure. This relationship determines how energy intake will affect body mass and composition.

energy intake will affect body mass and composition. Creating a hypocaloric intake will cause the athlete's metabolic rate to slow and muscle mass will be compromised, resulting in a negative effect on performance. Optimal performance and health are related to total energy intake, metabolic rate, tissue turnover, and muscle mass.

Since the micronutrient content of the diet is closely related to energy intake, decreases in energy consumption may lead to nutrient deficiencies. Nutrient deficiencies can lead to impaired performance through fatigue, immune suppression, lethargy, and potentially lead to overtraining. **Overtraining** is a physiological and psychological condition that occurs when the volume and intensity of an individual's training exceeds his or her recovery capacity. Dietary factors play a large role in the body's ability to recover from intense training and avoid overtraining.

The timing of nutrient ingestion plays a large role in recovery from resistance and sport training.

Athletes should eat nutrient-dense foods to increase the ratio of nutrients ingested to energy ingested. **Nutrient density** is the amount of nutrients (carbohydrate, protein, fat, vitamins, minerals) per unit of energy (kcal) in a given food. For example, athletes who habitually eat sugary breakfast cereals in an attempt to increase carbohydrate intake would benefit from exchanging these cereals for a combination of fruits, vegetables, and a whole grain like oatmeal, increasing the nutrient composition of their meal. These latter foods are not only more nutrient dense but they also have more fiber and a lower GI, which means that they cause less of an increase in blood sugar than more refined carbohydrates.

Glycemic index is a term that describes how rapidly and how long a specific carbohydrate increases blood glucose. Foods with a GI >100 raise blood glucose levels more rapidly, whereas foods with a GI of <100 raise blood glucose more slowly. In addition, high-fiber and low-glycemic carbohydrates play a role in improving health and body composition. In recent years, sports nutritionists have begun to rely on the glycemic load of food as opposed to the GI alone. The **glycemic load** takes into account the amount of carbohydrate eaten multiplied by the GI. So a large volume of carbohydrate that has a moderate GI may in fact be worse for the athlete than a food that is high on the GI but low in grams of carbohydrate. Table 7.1 lists the GIs of common sources of carbohydrates.

REAL-WORLD APPLICATION

Avoiding Overtraining with Dietary Intervention

1. Eat nutrient-dense foods. Calories are king when it comes to training intensely. Athletes should ensure they have an adequate calorie intake.
2. Get plenty of fluids. Dehydration can lead to a number of performance-related issues. This can lead to fatigue and contribute to overtraining. Athletes should strive to consume at minimum 1 Gal of water · d^{-1} when training.
3. Post workout nutrition is key. Eating a meal immediately after you train or compete will replenish glycogen stores and support protein synthesis.
4. Take a multivitamin every day. Many athletes are known to be slightly low in some vitamins and minerals. A multivitamin will ensure that the athlete is not deficient.

TABLE 7.1 ● THE GI OF COMMON SOURCES OF CARBOHYDRATES

GI	SOURCE	GI	SOURCE
Extremely high (>100)	Cake, doughnut	Moderately high (60–80)	Cranberry juice cocktail
	Waffles		Tomato juice
	Gatorade		Vanilla ice cream
	Bagel		Banana
	Pretzels		Grapes
	Corn flakes cereal		Orange
	Cheerios		Baked beans
	Rice Chex cereal		Chicken nuggets
	Rice Krispies cereal		Spaghetti
	Watermelon		Chocolate milk
	Popcorn		Power bar
	Jellybeans		
Glycemic standard = 100%	Bread, white	Moderate (40–60)	Apple
High (80–100)	Angel food cake		Apple juice
	Pound cake		Super supreme pizza (Pizza Hut)
	Bran muffin		All-bran cereal
	Pastry		Skim milk
	Coca-Cola (250 mL)		Yogurt
	Orange juice		Peanut M&Ms
	Pineapple juice		Butter beans
	Corn chips		Split peas
	Oat bread		
	Pita bread		
	Special K cereal	Low (<40)	Chickpeas
	Pineapple		Kidney beans
	White rice		Peanuts

Source: Adapted with permission from Foster-Powell K, Holt SHA, Brand-Miller JC. International table of glycemic index and glycemic load values: 2002 [Special Article]. *Am J Clin Nutr.* 2002;76:5–56.

The GI tells us which carbohydrates will have the greatest impact on blood sugar. Avoid or limit foods high on the GI. However, keep in mind that high GI carbohydrates may be warranted pre-, during, and/or postexercise.

Athletes must find ways to consume more calories from food while maintaining an optimal body composition and body mass for their specific activity. Although it may seem counterintuitive to suggest that an individual can lose fat mass while eating more food, taking advantage of appropriate food selection and strategic nutrient timing can accomplish both goals (6). Examining each **macronutrient** (i.e., carbohydrate, protein, and fat) and how to optimize times of feeding will allow individuals to develop a better understanding of how these strategies affect strength athletes.

Total energy intake combined with appropriate timing is the most important dietary factor governing the adaptive response of strength–power athletes to exercise training.

CARBOHYDRATE INTAKE

Carbohydrates are foods that are commonly referred to as sugars, starches, cellulose (fiber), and gums. Carbohydrates are converted to glucose, which is the primary source of energy for physical activity, and are the only source of energy for the brain and nervous system. Structurally, they can be classified as mono-, di-, tri-, and polysaccharides. The smallest carbohydrates are the single-unit monosaccharides, like glucose and sucrose (e.g., table sugar). Polysaccharides such as starch, cellulose, and glycogen are long chains of saccharide molecules and can be quite large.

Dietary carbohydrate intake has become a controversial topic. Carbohydrates have been demonized in the media, with some challenging the paradigm set forth by the U.S. Food Guide Pyramid (FGP) and the Canadian Food Guide and instead suggesting low-carbohydrate diets as a better option. Some short-term studies have demonstrated that a lower carbohydrate intake leads to better overall weight loss, losses in body fat, and better preservation of muscle mass. Moreover, favorable changes in triglycerides and high-density lipoprotein cholesterol typically occur when carbohydrate intakes are decreased. Very low carbohydrate diets (i.e., ketogenic diets), however, will reduce an athlete's total energy intake, impair intense exercise performance, reduce work capacity, suppress immune function, and increase perception of effort during normal exercise tasks. Although athletes could potentially benefit from a slight reduction in carbohydrate intake during rest periods and training periods of low volume/intensity, it is generally not recommended that strength–power athletes restrict carbohydrate to <10% of total energy intake.

Diets that place severe restrictions on a specific energy source, such as those in many commercial diets, should not be advised for athletes.

Although some authors recommend that as much as 70% of the diet come from carbohydrates, this amount may displace dietary protein and fat and also make fat loss more difficult, particularly if more refined carbohydrates are chosen rather than whole grains. Instead of a chronic high-carbohydrate diet, a better strategy might be to emphasize carbohydrate type (e.g., whole grain vs. refined carbohydrates) and timing (before, during, and after a workout).

The data are clear that carbohydrates are important in an athletic population. Higher carbohydrate diets can lead to increased concentrations of muscle glycogen and may therefore delay fatigue, prevent exercise-stress–induced immunosuppression (7), and—when combined with protein during the exercise and postexercise periods—stimulate an increase in muscle protein synthesis and glycogen resynthesis (8). Athletes, however, often consume the wrong types of carbohydrates at the wrong times. Rather than simply ingesting large amounts of "empty" calories during the day, athletes should replace their high glycemic index, nutrient-devoid carbohydrate choices with lower glycemic, high-fiber carbohydrate choices. The term **empty calorie** refers to a food that offers no nutritional value other than energy itself. Foods such as legumes; whole grains; minimally processed breads, pastas, and other grains; fruits; and vegetables are digested more slowly and provide more continuous energy throughout the day acting as better carbohydrate choices. By substituting lower glycemic, high-fiber foods and timing carbohydrates appropriately, athletes will be better able to manage daily energy fluctuations, ingest their daily recommendation of fiber, lose fat while preserving muscle mass, and reduce the chances of developing the micronutrient deficiencies that are common in athletic populations. On the contrary, higher glycemic carbohydrates can be ingested after exercise to promote recovery and glycogen storage—a source of rapid energy when it is most needed (during training and competition). This is the time when the large insulin response that accompanies the ingestion of high-glycemic carbohydrates may lead to an improvement in muscle recovery. By following these recommendations, athletes may be better able to manage body composition while enhancing recovery.

Different types of carbohydrates confer different physiological responses. The majority of one's caloric intake should be derived from the consumption of unprocessed, high-fiber carbohydrates.

PROTEIN INTAKE

Protein is composed of individual amino acids, which join together to form peptide chains. Although the structure of each peptide chain is unique, the overall peptide structures collectively are known as proteins. Of the 20 common amino acids, 9 are indispensable or **essential** (the term *essential* as it relates to nutrition describes nutrients that you must consume, because your body does not make them endogenously); that is, they must come from the diet. As a result of the essentiality of these amino acids, protein, unlike carbohydrate, must be present in the diet. The recommended dietary allowance (RDA) for dietary protein in sedentary individuals is 0.8 g protein $\cdot$ kg body mass^{-1}. Very few athletes are at risk for a true protein deficiency; however, it is likely that 0.8 g $\cdot$ kg^{-1} is not sufficient to offset the oxidation of amino acids with exercise and provide enough amino acids for lean tissue accretion (9). Thus, many sports nutrition scientists have suggested that athletes may need more protein than their sedentary counterparts (1.5 to 2.0 g $\cdot$ kg body mass^{-1}) (10).

Other populations will have higher protein needs as well: young athletes who are still growing, athletes training for strength and muscle mass, athletes in contact sports, endurance athletes, and women who are pregnant. At times, more than one of these situations may be present in the same athlete, thus further increasing his or her protein needs.

Different athletic populations warrant different dietary needs and recommendations. For example, an endurance athlete will have different energy requirements than a strength athlete.

Athletes will often self-select a protein intake that is higher than conventionally recommended. In seeking to optimize an athlete's protein intake, a simple rule of thumb is to plan the athlete's diet from the foundation of 1 g protein $\cdot$ lb body mass^{-1} (2.2 g $\cdot$ kg body mass^{-1}). This is easier for the athlete to understand and monitor and provides a small safety factor to ensure adequate protein intake. Once the protein intake is fixed, carbohydrate and fat intakes must be added to meet total daily energy needs. The best way to optimize an athlete's protein intake would be to experiment with a variety of levels of dietary protein and assess outcomes in terms of personal performance and body composition to determine which intake leads to the best response. Nutritional strategies should always be evaluated using an outcome-based approach.

In addition to experimenting with overall protein intake, it is important to make sure that a large percentage of daily protein comes from complete protein sources (proteins that contain all the essential amino acids [EAAs]). Even if an adequate total daily protein intake is ingested, if the protein is from an incomplete protein source (e.g., rice, grains, and other plant sources), the athlete may experience suboptimal adaptations to training. This situation can be improved by either ensuring that most of the dietary protein is from complete protein sources (e.g., animal proteins, including eggs and dairy products) or consuming enough total energy with sufficient amounts of incomplete proteins. Animal proteins are important not only as sources of complete protein but also because they provide a number of highly bioavailable nutrients, such as B vitamins, zinc, and iron, of which deficiency is more prevalent in an athletic population. While it has often been argued that increased protein intake may have harmful side effects, no current evidence shows that healthy individuals would experience harm due to a higher protein diet (11).

A complete food source such as eggs, chicken, fish, and lean beef is a preferred source of protein;

however, there are many dietary supplements (discussed in more detail in Chapter 18) that may be added to the diet. The two most common types of supplementary protein are whey and casein. While both protein types are derived from milk, casein is a slower acting protein better utilized in the evening, and whey is a faster acting protein better utilized in the morning or postworkout.

The International Society of Sports Nutrition has adopted a position stand on protein that highlights the following points (9):

1. Exercising individuals need approximately 1.4 to 2.0 g protein · kg bodyweight^{-1} · d^{-1}.
2. Concerns that protein intake within this range is unhealthy are unfounded in healthy, exercising individuals.
3. An attempt should be made to obtain protein requirements from whole foods, but supplemental protein is a safe and convenient method of ingesting high-quality dietary protein.
4. The timing of protein intake in the time period encompassing the exercise session has several benefits including improved recovery and greater gains in fat-free mass (FFM).
5. Exercising individuals need more dietary protein than their sedentary counterparts.

Strength–power athletes need more protein (1.5 to 2.0 g · kg^{-1} · d^{-1}) than the RDA (0.8 g · kg^{-1} · d^{-1}). Moreover, no evidence exists that the consumption of protein at levels two to three times the RDA is harmful to otherwise healthy individuals.

FAT INTAKE

It has become increasingly clear that dietary fat is essential to the athlete's nutrition program. The three main types of dietary fatty acids are saturated, monounsaturated, and polyunsaturated fatty acids (omega-3 and omega-6 fats are both types of polyunsaturated fatty acids). **Triglycerides** are the main storage form of fat. Triglycerides are formed from a glycerol skeleton with three **fatty acids** attached. Each of the three types of fats offers unique benefits. In the past, a simplistic view of fat was adopted because coaches and athletes believed that dietary fat made you fat; however, research has demonstrated this to be false. In fact, some fats (known as essential fatty acids) are absolutely necessary for survival. In addition, the right kinds of dietary fat can improve body composition by promoting fat loss (12). Furthermore, certain fats can improve training hormonal status (13), increase the body's ability to store glycogen, increase the body's ability to burn fat (12), and improve overall health by providing anti-inflammatory, anticarcinogenic, antioxidant, and antithrombotic effects (14). Although the American Dietetic Association recommends that <30% of the diet of a sedentary individual should come from fat, research suggests that athletes should ingest approximately 30% of the diet as fat as long as the individual proportions of fatty acids are distributed appropriately. For optimal health and performance, a balanced approach toward fat consumption is warranted; approximately 10% of dietary energy should come from saturated sources (e.g., whole-fat dairy, animal fats), approximately 10% from monounsaturated sources (many vegetable fats, especially olive oil), and approximately 10% from polyunsaturated sources (predominantly vegetable fats, especially flaxseed and fish oils). Of the polyunsaturated fats, approximately 50% should come from omega-6 fatty acids and approximately 50% from omega-3 fatty acids. It is important to realize that the distribution of fatty acids in the diet is as important as the absolute amount of fat. Therefore, athletes should pay attention to both.

A final consideration related to fat consumption is trans fat. **Trans fats** are artificial fats created when polyunsaturated vegetable oils (high in omega-6 fatty acids) are combined with hydrogen molecules to increase shelf life and stabilize the polyunsaturated oil. This process makes nonhydrogenated fat similar to saturated fat (which is naturally saturated with hydrogen), which can produce "bad" low-density lipoprotein cholesterol and potentially lead to heart disease. Consumption of trans fats leads to the inhibition of several critical enzymatic processes in the body, blood lipid abnormalities, and an increased risk of cardiovascular disease (CVD). Unfortunately, trans fats are found in many processed foods. Any food that lists hydrogenated or partially hydrogenated fats on the ingredient list contains trans fats.

It is important that athletes consume predominantly unsaturated fats. Both athletes and the general population should limit (but not eliminate) saturated fats in their diets.

TRAINING NUTRITION

During and after training and competition, the energy demands of the body are high, fluid needs increase (15), insulin sensitivity and glucose tolerance are dramatically improved (16), and skeletal muscle is primed for anabolism as long as amino acids are provided (2,17,18). Nutrition during and after exercise should focus on providing carbohydrate energy, preventing dehydration, stimulating glycogen resynthesis, and stimulating increases in skeletal muscle protein synthesis. As indicated, during the workout and postworkout periods, insulin sensitivity and glucose tolerance are improved and the efficiency of glycogen storage is highest. This makes the postworkout period the best time to ingest a larger amount of carbohydrate. In addition, since a large increase in insulin can facilitate greater glycogen resynthesis and muscle protein synthesis, higher glycemic index carbohydrates (i.e., sports drinks containing glucose or glucose polymers) should be ingested during these times. By providing a large amount of carbohydrate during this critical period, fewer carbohydrates should be ingested during the remainder of the day in order to achieve better control of body composition and to promote maximal recovery. As a starting point, athletes could begin by ingesting liquid carbohydrate–protein supplements immediately before (18) or during exercise (15) as well as immediately after exercise (8,18) so as to promote recovery. To facilitate fluid replacement as well as rapid energy delivery, the two beverages should be diluted to 8% to 12% concentrations (80 to 120 g of substrate [carbohydrate] per 1,000 mL of water) and should provide approximately 0.8 g of carbohydrate and 0.4 g protein · kg body mass^{-1}. It is important to experiment with differing amounts of energy to determine the best composition for each individual athlete.

Consumption of carbohydrate combined with protein and/or EAAs after a workout is critical in enhancing the adaptive response to exercise (i.e., greater gains in lean body mass (LBM), greater loss of fat mass, improved performance, etc.).

NUTRIENT TIMING

An exciting avenue of research is the area of **nutrient timing**, the specific time at which you consume certain nutrients to enhance the adaptive response to exercise. Certainly, we know that the composition of the food you ingest is important for promoting gains in muscle protein; however, the timing of nutrient consumption may be just as important.

In a 2007 study by Willoughby et al. (19), researchers examined the effects of pre- and postworkout protein supplementation on markers of strength, mass, and anabolism. Researchers found that 20 g of protein taken before and after resistance training workouts resulted in greater gains in FFM and strength than the placebo group that consumed 20 g of dextrose. In addition, the subjects consuming protein had a significantly greater expression of muscle-specific proteins.

In another study, subjects cycled intensely for 2.5 hours to fully deplete the muscle glycogen levels in their thigh muscles (5). Subjects supplemented immediately and 2 hours postexercise with the following:

- Group 1: carb–pro–fat (80 g carb, 28 g pro, 6 g fat)
- Group 2: carb–fat (108 g carb, 6 g fat)
- Group 3: carb–fat (80 g carb, 6 g fat)

Note that the beverages groups 1 and 2 consumed were isocaloric, meaning they contained the same number of calories. After 4 hours of recovery, the investigators found that the greatest amount of muscle glycogen was replenished in group 1. Thus, the replacement of some carbohydrate with protein may expedite muscle glycogen repletion postexercise.

Other investigations have yielded similarly interesting results. Postexercise supplementation with added protein improved time to exhaustion during a test of endurance (6). Older men who consumed a protein supplement (10 g protein, 7 g carbohydrate, 3 g fat) immediately after training (12-week resistance training program, 3 d · wk^{-1}) had greater gains in strength, muscle fiber size, and LBM compared to the group who ingested the supplement 2 hours after training (20). It has been suggested that the availability of amino acids is more important than the availability of energy immediately postexercise to promote the repair and synthesis of muscle protein.

Other health benefits may accompany the ingestion of protein immediately postexercise. In a study of healthy male recruits in the U.S. Marine Corps, subjects received a postexercise supplement during their 54-day basic training period, which was a placebo (0 g carbohydrate, 0 g protein, 0 g fat), control, or protein supplement (21). The protein-supplemented group had an average of 33% fewer total medical visits, 28% fewer visits due to bacterial/viral infections, 37% fewer visits due to muscle/joint problems, and 83% fewer visits due to heat exhaustion compared with the placebo and control groups. Muscle soreness immediately postexercise was significantly reduced on both days 34 and 54 by protein supplementation but not by the placebo or control supplements.

Some evidence suggests that nutrient timing affects body composition (22). In one study, 17 slightly overweight men were put on a 12-week program consisting of mild caloric restriction (17% reduction) and a light resistance-exercise training program utilizing dumbbells. One group ingested a protein supplement (10 g protein, 7 g carbohydrate, 3.3 g fat, and 33% of the RDA for vitamins and minerals) immediately after exercise. The other group did not consume a supplement. Protein and energy intake were the same for both groups, and protein intake met the RDA. Both groups lost an equal amount of fat; however, the protein-supplemented group maintained FFM, while the group that did not supplement lost FFM.

Although most studies have examined postworkout nutrition, some data are available that compare preworkout supplementation as well (2). Researchers compared the anabolic response of consuming a combination of an EAA (6 g) plus carbohydrate (35 g sucrose) before versus after heavy resistance exercise. Phenylalanine uptake across the leg (a measure of muscle protein anabolism) over a 3-hour period was 160% greater when the amino acid/carbohydrate supplement was taken before versus after a workout. A 2007 study (23) by the same group found that if the pre- versus postingestion was an intact protein such as whey, there does not appear to be a differential effect. Thus, consuming the proper nutrients before exercise may be more anabolic and facilitate recovery better than a postexercise consumption strategy.

A 2008 Position Stand (JISSN) by Kerksick et al. (24) found the following in regard to nutrient timing:

1. Prolonged exercise of moderate to high intensity exercise will deplete stores of energy, and prudent timing of nutrient delivery can help offset these changes.
2. Ingestion of 6 to 20 g of EAAs and 30 to 40 g of high-glycemic carbohydrate (CHO) within 3 hours after an exercise bout and immediately before exercise has been shown to significantly stimulate muscle protein (PRO) synthesis.
3. Daily postexercise ingestion of a CHO + PRO supplement promotes greater increases in strength and improvements in lean tissue and body fat percentage during regular resistance training.
4. Dietary focus should center on adequate availability and delivery of CHO and PRO. However, including small amounts of fat does not appear to be harmful and may help to control glycemic responses during exercise.
5. Irrespective of timing, regular ingestion of snacks or meals providing both CHO and PRO (3:1 CHO:PRO ratio) helps to promote recovery and replenishment of muscle glycogen.

To optimize the adaptive response to exercise, all strength–power athletes should consume a carbohydrate–protein postworkout beverage. This strategy would also be helpful for the recreational athlete or fitness enthusiast seeking to improve his or her body composition.

CARBOHYDRATE/PROTEIN RATIO

Controversy exists as to the correct or ideal combination of carbohydrate- and protein-consumed postworkout. It is difficult to make direct comparisons between investigations due to differences in subject population, treatment duration, the type of exercise performed, and nutrients ingested, etc. One can extrapolate from these studies, however, to suggest that timing may be as important (if not more so) as nutrient composition. For instance, you will find a carbohydrate-to-protein ratio of about 3:1 (approximately three times more carbohydrate than protein) and as low as 0.7:1 (30% less carbohydrate than protein) comparable for promoting recovery. Furthermore, the energy content of recovery supplements varies from 500 kcal to as little as 100 kcal. Therefore, sports nutritionists should consider each athlete individually to determine the most effective nutrient combinations for that person.

VITAMIN AND MINERAL INTAKE

Few studies have examined the micronutrient (vitamins and minerals) intakes of strength–power athletes. Clearly, however, suboptimal consumption of certain vitamins and minerals may predispose the individual to a number of diseases. For instance, according to one study, suboptimal folic acid levels, along with suboptimal levels of vitamins B_6 and B_{12}, are a risk factor for CVD, neural tube defects, and colon and breast cancer; low levels of vitamin D contribute to osteopenia and fractures; and low levels of the antioxidant vitamins (vitamins A, E, and C) may increase risk for several chronic diseases. Many people do not consume an optimal amount of all vitamins by diet alone. Subsequently, it appears prudent for all adults to take vitamin supplements.

At this moment, it is not clear that consuming extra or supplemental vitamins can improve athletic performance. Some intriguing data on nutrient intakes in strength–power athletes, however, suggest a potential benefit of supplementing with specific micronutrients. Some research has suggested that strength and power athletes are deficient on basic nutrient requirements (25,26). Furthermore, deficiencies in basic nutrient requirements can lead to illness, injury, and detriments in performance (27). There is currently a lack of conclusive evidence that exercise performance or recovery would benefit in any significant way from vitamin or mineral supplementation, unless of course a deficiency exists.

Regardless of what the composite data may be regarding the average macro- or micronutrient intakes of athletes, one could certainly argue that these data are unimportant in counseling individual athletes. To assess whether an individual athlete is meeting his or her dietary needs, it is of no utility to draw conclusions based on the scientific literature. This is because each individual must have his or her food intake separately analyzed to determine whether alterations in a particular nutrition program may be of benefit.

> ***It is impossible to determine an individual's macro- or micronutrient needs based on a composite picture derived from survey studies in the scientific literature.***

VITAMIN E

Vitamin E is a fat-soluble vitamin that may have beneficial effects in athletes. For example, in one study, 12 weight-trained men were divided into two groups: One group received 1,200 IU of vitamin E once per day for 2 weeks, while the control group received a cellulose-based placebo pill (28). Plasma creatine kinase (CK) levels (an indirect marker of muscle fiber injury) increased significantly in both groups after 24 and 48 hours; at 24 hours, however, the increase in CK was less in the vitamin E–supplemented group than in the placebo group. Plasma malondialdehyde (MDA), an indicator of free-radical interaction with cellular membranes, was elevated in both groups; however, MDA levels remained higher for a longer time in the placebo group. Thus, vitamin E may lessen the injury sustained by skeletal muscle fibers as a result of heavy resistance exercises; moreover, its antioxidant effects may be of potential benefit to athletes.

Alternatively, no effects of vitamin E supplementation (1,200 IU for 3 weeks in non–resistance-trained men) were found on recovery responses to repeated bouts of resistance exercises. According to the investigators, "vitamin E supplementation was not effective at attenuating putative markers of membrane damage, oxidative stress, and performance decrements after repeated bouts of whole-body concentric/eccentric resistance exercise" (29).

VITAMIN C

Vitamin C is a water-soluble vitamin that is needed for collagen formation and may have beneficial effects for active individuals through its effects on cortisol and via an antioxidant effect.

Twenty-four physically active young subjects who ingested vitamin C (400 mg), vitamin E (400 mg), or a placebo for 21 days before and 7 days after performing 60 minutes of box-stepping exercise were examined (30). The investigators tested the function of the triceps surae muscles and found that, compared to the placebo group, no significant alterations in maximal voluntary contraction (MVC) were found immediately after exercise; however, the recovery of MVC was superior in the vitamin C group during the first 24 hours after exercise. According to the study's authors, "... prior vitamin C supplementation may exert a protective effect against eccentric exercise-induced muscle damage." No effects were observed in the vitamin E–supplemented group.

One study had 16 male subjects randomized to a placebo or vitamin C group (31). These subjects performed a prolonged 90-minute intermittent shuttle-running test, and supplementation commenced after the cessation of exercise. That is, immediately after exercise, the subjects drank a 500-mL beverage containing 200 mg of vitamin C (or placebo) dissolved in solution. Later that same day and for the next 2 days, the subjects again consumed their treatment drinks. As a result, vitamin C supplementation had no effect on postexercise CK concentrations, muscle soreness, or muscle function of the leg extensors and flexors. Certainly, longer or prolonged consumption of vitamin C must be further examined. In one study, 16 male subjects consumed either vitamin C (200 mg twice daily for 2 weeks) or placebo. Subjects performed 90 minutes of intermittent shuttle running 14 days after supplementation commenced. As a result, it was found that vitamin C did have beneficial effects on muscle soreness, muscle function, and plasma concentrations of serum MDA (32).

Based on the very limited data on vitamins C and E, one can reasonably conclude that supplementation may have beneficial effects on a subset of individuals that have dietary or exercise-induced deficiencies. There appear to be no deleterious effects on any of the parameters measured in published studies.

MINERALS

Magnesium is an essential mineral that regulates neuromuscular, cardiovascular, immune, and hormonal function (35). Exercise may deplete magnesium, which—combined with inadequate intake—may impair energy metabolism. In a study investigating the effects of magnesium supplementation on strength development during a double-blind, 7-week strength-training program, both groups involved gained strength; however, the magnesium-supplemented group demonstrated significantly better performance compared to the

Q & A from the Field

Q ***How does dehydration affect the strength–power athlete and what recommendations would you give to prevent the harm caused by fluid loss?***

A *Dehydration* refers to both hypohydration (being dehydrated prior to exercise) and exercise-induced dehydration (i.e., that which develops during exercise). Inadequate fluid intake can adversely affect muscle metabolism, the regulation of body temperature, cardiovascular function (increased heart rate), and perceived exertion (more rapid development of fatigue).

Negative effects on performance have been demonstrated with modest (<2% of body weight) dehydration. In one investigation, college wrestlers were actively dehydrated (4.9% of body weight), after which their upper body isokinetic performance was measured (33). There was a decrease in strength of 7.6% for lat pulldowns, 6.6% in chest push, and 12% in shoulder-press repetitions. In contrast, lower body musculature was not significantly affected by the 4.9% loss.

Many athletes are reluctant drinkers during exercise and do not ingest fluid at rates equal to their fluid loss. To promote proper hydration for athletes' optimal health and performance, follow these recommendations (34):

1. Athletes are advised to drink 14 to 22 oz of fluid 2 hours prior to exercise to promote adequate hydration and allow time for the excretion of excess ingested water.
2. During exercise, athletes should start drinking early into the workout and at regular intervals. If training continues for over 1 hour, a carbohydrate-containing beverage should be ingested at a rate of 30 to 60 g $\cdot$ h^{-1} to maintain oxidation of carbohydrates and delay fatigue.
3. Immediately after exercise, athletes should consume 16 to 24 oz of fluid for every pound of body weight lost during exercise. All athletes (strength, power, or endurance) need to maximize their fluid intake and employ behavioral strategies before, during, and after exercise to enhance their training and competitive performances. (Courtesy of Jennifer Hofheins, MS, RD, LD, of the Center for Applied Health Sciences.)

control group in absolute torque, relative torque adjusted for body weight, and relative torque adjusted for LBM when "before" values were used as the covariate.

Zinc is a mineral required for the activity of more than 300 enzymes. Recently, it has been recognized that zinc may play an important role in thyroid hormone metabolism. The effects of zinc supplementation in athletes have been studied previously. Moreover, chronic exercise can have long-term effects on zinc metabolism (36). It has been reported that runners have lower plasma zinc levels than controls. One consequence of low serum zinc levels could be a reduction in muscle zinc concentrations, possibly resulting in a reduction in endurance capacity. Zinc may also be acting directly at the membrane level; changes in extracellular zinc levels have been reported to influence the twitch tension relationship in muscle. If one consumes an adequate diet rich in zinc, it is likely that zinc supplementation may be of no consequence to skeletal muscle or hormonal function. If one's diet is inadequate (e.g., vegetarians or individuals on low-energy diets), however, zinc supplementation may be considered. A 2004 study (37) found that the combination of zinc and magnesium had no effect in resistance-trained subjects.

An examination of the scientific literature shows that vitamin and mineral supplementation has either a neutral or positive effect on various health and performance indexes in exercising individuals. As a strategy, it would make sense to consume a multivitamin as an "insurance policy" against poor eating habits. Eating a diet rich in unprocessed, high-fiber carbohydrates, lean meats, and other high-quality protein sources should form the basis of one's energy intake.

DIETS

Little research is available regarding dietary manipulation to improve performance relative to strength and size in comparison to improving performance in the endurance athlete. A number of different theories, beliefs, and recommendations from health professionals are available regarding the proper way to fuel the body for better performance. Although an infinite number of dietary prescriptions are available, essentially they fall into four overall categories: diets very high in carbohydrate and very low in fat (e.g., Pritikin and Ornish); high in carbohydrate and low in fat (e.g., the U.S. Department of Agriculture (USDA) MyPyramid food guide system, Fig. 7.3);

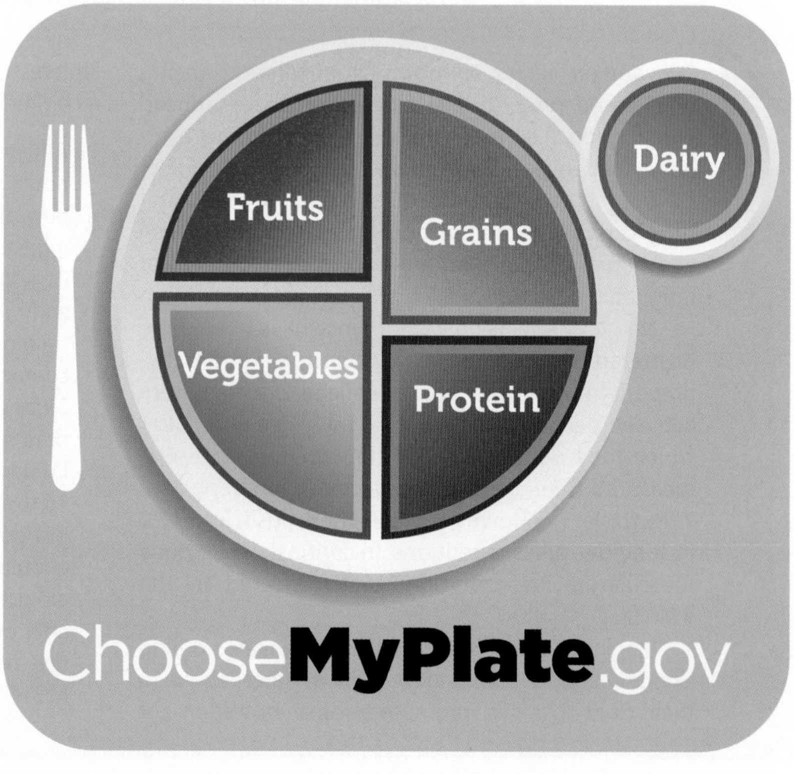

FIGURE 7.3 The USDA MyPlate food guide system.

very low in carbohydrate and high in protein and fat (e.g., Atkins or South Beach diets); and moderate in carbohydrate and higher in protein (e.g., Zone diet). Table 7.2 compares these approaches. Most people have their own dietary beliefs that may have worked for them or the athletes they train; significant scientific support exists, however, for each of the approaches mentioned above.

Eating disorders are a major concern with athletic and exercising populations. As exercise professionals, we must be aware of these disorders and be able to address the issue appropriately. This includes a basic understanding of the disorders and of the team approach to treatment (Box 7.1).

VERY HIGH-CARBOHYDRATE, VERY LOW-FAT DIETS

Carbohydrates are primarily sugars and starches and represent the primary macronutrient consumed by Americans. When we consider the dietary needs of a strength athlete, carbohydrates should be the base of a sound nutritional program. Carbohydrates provide the major source of energy for the athlete through the breakdown of glycogen (the storage form of carbohydrate) during exercise (38). Moreover, increased carbohydrate intake may delay fatigue and can enhance postexercise protein synthesis alone (39) (though not to the same extent as amino acids) or synergistically when combined with protein during

TABLE 7.2 ● COMPARISON OF POPULAR DIETS

MEAL PLAN	DIETARY RECOMMENDATIONS	COMMENTS
Ornish and Pritikin plans	≥80% Carbohydrate 10% Protein ≤10% Fat	Strength athletes do not need such a high carbohydrate intake. Fortunately there is at least a distinction made and high-quality carbohydrates are recommended with these two plans. Both the protein intake and fat intake are too low to elicit the positive benefits that these two macronutrients provide, which has been demonstrated through various research studies.
The FGP	55% –60% Carbohydrates 12%–15% Protein <30% Fat	Also a bit too high in carbohydrates for the strength athlete. Without the guidance of a nutrition professional, one mightw assume that all carbohydrates are created equal and therefore overconsume refined carbohydrates by following the FGP. The FGP also places fat in the limited category, when we know that different types of fats are clearly linked to health benefits and positive changes for the strength athlete. Another problem with the FGP is that it does not differentiate between protein sources high in saturated fat (e.g., ground beef) vs. those that are lean (e.g., whey protein powders) or contain healthy fat (e.g., salmon).
Zone diet	40% Carbohydrate 30% Protein 30% Fat	Following this diet will not provide the strength athlete with adequate energy to build LBM. This diet was not originally intended for strength–power athletes. However, if the energy intake is increased following a 40:30:30 plan, it should provide adequate protein, healthy carbohydrate, and unsaturated fat.
Atkins diet	Low-carbohydrate (25–90 $g \cdot d^{-1}$; the typical recommendation is 35–40 g) Fat and protein make up the rest of the diet. No types of fat are out of the question.	Strength athletes do not have the same macronutrient needs as endurance athletes; however, performance will be shortchanged by almost eliminating regular consumption of carbohydrates, particularly the high-fiber, low-glycemic variety. In addition, although consensus exists in much of the scientific community about strength athletes' increased protein needs above the RDA, increasing protein at the expense of unprocessed carbohydrates is not warranted. Unprocessed carbohydrates should make up the bulk of one's nutrition program.

BOX 7.1

Eating Disorders

Eating disorders are often related to disorders of self-image, self-concept, and self-esteem. They are not uncommon among athletic and exercising populations. Disordered eating is one component in the female athletic triad (discussed in Chapter 4). Additionally, compulsive exercise can be a component of some eating disorders. Three eating disorders are discussed briefly below.

Compulsive Overeating

Compulsive overeating is an "addiction" to food. Compulsive overeaters use food and eating to help with daily stresses and problem solving. Individuals who are compulsive overeaters tend to be overweight. They are aware of their inability to control their eating and may be particularly sensitive to comments about their weight or diet. Because obesity is a major health concern in today's society, we should be aware of the potential role compulsive overeating may play in this disorder.

Anorexia Nervosa

The person with anorexia may perceive himself or herself as fat or may be afraid of becoming fat. This individual probably has an emotional disorder and reacts by controlling his or her eating behaviors.

Signs of anorexia may include obsessive exercise; calorie counting or fat-gram counting; self-induced vomiting and the use of diet pills, laxatives, or diuretics; and a persistent concern with body image. Individuals with anorexia may go through periods of bulimia and their body weight is generally below average.

Bulimia Nervosa

The primary symptoms of bulimia are episodes of binging and purging. The individual will eat a large quantity of food in a relatively short time and then induce vomiting or take laxatives, often related to the guilt of overeating. The episodes of binging and purging may be related to feelings of anger, depression, stress, or anxiety. Individuals suffering bulimia may be aware of their eating disorder and usually enjoy discussing food and diet. They may also be overweight, or their weight may fluctuate greatly.

Summary

Similarities can be found among various eating disorders, the most common being some form of emotional disorder. With anorexia and bulimia, it may seem to be nothing but an obsessive concern over body image. For many of these individuals, deeper emotional issues may need to be resolved.

Young female athletes in sports such as gymnastics are considered to be at high risk for eating disorders, specifically anorexia or bulimia. Rather than causing the disorder, it may be that some sports attract anorexic/bulimic athletes, enabling them to hide their condition. A team approach to treatment should be considered that potentially involves the coach/exercise professional, the parents, a physician, a nutritionist, a psychologist, and perhaps others. This is not a disorder the exercise professional can or should try to handle alone.

recovery (8). Although carbohydrates are a crucial part of a sound nutritional program for the strength athlete, they do not play the same role with the endurance athlete who uses up glycogen stores more rapidly through lower intensity, continuous aerobic activities. Some scientific evidence suggests that carbohydrate supplementation prior to and during high-volume resistance training results in the maintenance of muscle glycogen concentration, which potentially could result in the maintenance or increase of performance during a training bout (40). Additionally, the ingestion of carbohydrates following resistance exercise may enhance muscle glycogen resynthesis, which may result in a faster time of recovery from resistance training, thus possibly allowing for a greater training volume. It is unlikely that resistance training depletes muscle glycogen to the same extent as endurance training.

As seen in Table 7.2, very high-carbohydrate, very low-fat diets, such as those developed by Pritikin and Ornish, recommend a macronutrient composition of approximately 80% carbohydrate and 10% protein while advocating <10% fat. Both of these approaches are supported by a number of scientific studies in terms of positively modulating health outcomes (e.g., heart disease, lipid values, blood pressure); no direct research, however, supports their applicability to strength athletes. In fact, these diets may be contraindicated if the goal is to cause hypertrophy or increase speed or another variable that an athlete participating in a high-intensity sport may desire, since these diets are low in both protein and fat. It has been posited that diets very high in carbohydrate and low in both protein and fat may suit the needs of a patient with heart disease; owing to the increased intake of fibrous carbohydrates and reduced intake of saturated fat, the limited amounts of protein and fat recommended will not benefit the strength athlete. However, recent work published in the American Journal of Clinical Nutrition states that "there is no significant evidence for concluding that dietary saturated fat is associated with an increased risk of CHD or CVD" (41).

Macronutrient manipulation is commonly used by strength athletes to positively influence the hormonal milieu (testosterone, growth hormone, insulin, etc.), with the intention of favoring hypertrophy. As discussed earlier, dietary fat has been shown by a number of studies to correlate with serum sex hormones (13,42), improve body composition by promoting fat loss (12), improve overall health by providing anti-inflammatory effects (14), and even increase the body's ability to store glycogen. These facts, together with the known health benefits and increases in hormone concentrations from resistance training itself, demonstrate the importance of consuming adequate amounts of dietary fat (i.e., >10% recommended with these plans).

Let's use the example of a 150-lb strength-trained athlete who needs 2,500 kcal · d^{-1}. Using the 80%/10%/10% (carbohydrate/protein/fat, respectively) model of Ornish or Pritikin, this individual would be getting approximately 500 g carbohydrate · d^{-1} or about 7.3 g carbohydrate · kg^{-1} · d^{-1} and about 63 g protein and fat · d^{-1} (i.e., about 0.9% of protein and 0.4% fat · kg^{-1} · d^{-1}). Obviously consuming a diet that replaces much of the dietary fat and protein with carbohydrate makes it impossible to obtain adequate levels of either fat or protein. As discussed earlier, the strength-trained athlete needs more than the RDA for protein each day (from 1.5 to 2.0 g · kg^{-1} · d^{-1} [3]), which is clearly much higher than the 0.9 g · kg^{-1} · d^{-1} the individual in our example would consume. Similarly, considering that glycogen is not depleted to the same extent in a strength athlete as it is in an endurance athlete, such a high intake of carbohydrate on a regular basis is unnecessary. Consequently, such a diet is not recommended for the otherwise healthy strength-training athlete.

HIGH-CARBOHYDRATE, LOW-FAT DIETS

Coming on the heels of the very high-carbohydrate plans described above, high-carbohydrate, low-fat diets, such as that of the FGP, recommend a macronutrient composition of approximately 55% to 60% carbohydrates, 12% to 15% protein, and <30% fat. Table 7.3 lists recommended

TABLE 7.3 ● RECOMMENDED SELECTIONS FOR EACH MACRONUTRIENT

CARBOHYDRATE	PROTEIN	FAT
Oatmeal	Lean red meat	Fish oil
Oat bran	Poultry (skinless, white meat)	Olive oil
Brown rice	All seafood	Flax oil
Whole-wheat pasta	Low-fat/fat-free cottage cheese	Nuts (e.g., almonds, peanuts)
Yams/sweet potatoes	Eggs	Peanut butter
Red potatoes	Protein powders composed of whey, casein, or combinations thereof	Avocado
All vegetables		
All fruits		
Quinoa		
Legumes		
Lentils		
Whole-grain bread(e.g., pumpernickel, rye)		
Low-fat/fat-free dairy		
Buckwheat		

Note: Some foods, such as legumes, lentils, dairy, and peanut butter, cross over into other categories (i.e., lentils also have protein). They are placed in the category of the macronutrient that is most abundant.

foods that contain each macronutrient. The quantity of foods recommended from each block of the FGP is dependent on the activity level of an individual; however, again, no specific energy recommendation is provided. Using the FGP model, the same 150-lb athlete from above who needs 2,500 kcal · d^{-1} would have to consume approximately 340 to 375 g of carbohydrate (~5 to 5.5 g CHO · kg^{-1} · d^{-1}), 75 to 90 g of protein (about 1.1 to 1.3 g · kg^{-1} · d^{-1}), and 83 g of fat (~1.2 g · kg^{-1} · d^{-1}).

Like the diet prescriptions described earlier, one shortcoming with the USDA FGP is that we have an individual in this example who would find it difficult to obtain adequate levels of protein (1.5 to 2.0 g · kg $protein^{-1}$ · d^{-1} for most strength-training athletes) by following the USDA's guidelines. Another limitation of the FGP is its lack of specificity when it comes to carbohydrate and fat recommendations. There is no argument that carbohydrates are used as a form of energy. In fact, they are the primary source of energy of your brain and skeletal muscles. Not all carbohydrates are alike, however. Although the FGP does emphasize a carbohydrate-based diet, it stops short of differentiating among the various types of carbohydrates. Processed carbohydrates such as white rice and pasta should be limited (not eliminated). Knowing the benefits of the other macronutrients during strength training, namely protein and fat, it would be wise to replace the refined carbohydrates in the diet with lean proteins and healthful fats. Separating the various types of proteins (e.g., red meat vs. salmon) and fat (e.g., butter vs. olive oil) is the best approach to developing a sound nutritional program for athletes.

LOW-CARBOHYDRATE, HIGH-PROTEIN DIETS

A number of diets fall into this category. The one most commonly discussed and researched is the Zone. Barry Sears, its originator, recommends a 40:30:30 ratio (carbohydrates:protein:fat, respectively), which he states will support even the most competitive athletic endeavors. The intention of this specific ratio of macronutrients is to control the body's ratio of insulin to glucagon, ultimately enhancing performance and the ability to mobilize body fat. Although no specific studies used this particular diet with strength athletes, one review (43) and one short-term study measured endurance performance utilizing the Zone diet (44). Both publications came to similar conclusions: Athletes should not implement the Zone diet in their practices.

Energy intake is the most important component of any dietary strategy. Without adequate energy, the body cannot rebuild, repair, or recuperate from training. One study demonstrated, through diet records, that at the end of the 7-week study period, subjects following the Zone diet consumed 1,994 ± 438 kcal · d^{-1} (45). Considering that these were active male subjects with a mean age of 26 years, this energy intake is much too low to support any type of athletic endeavor. It is impossible to enhance strength and performance if the body is not being fed what it needs. Going back to our previous example of the 150-lb athlete needing 2,500 kcal · d^{-1}, he would take in 250 g carbohydrate · d^{-1} (3.7 g CHO · kg^{-1} · d^{-1}), about 188 g protein · d^{-1} (about 2.75 g protein · kg^{-1} · d^{-1}), and about 83 g fat · d^{-1} (about 1.2 g fat · kg^{-1} · d^{-1}).

One positive aspect of this plan is that it provides a bit more protein than the previously mentioned diets. With this low-energy diet, the protein is particularly important so as to prevent the loss of muscle tissue. In addition, the Zone recommends consuming most carbohydrates as whole-grain carbohydrates to reduce the insulin surge associated with refined carbohydrates. Finally, Sears also separates fats into their various components and recommends increasing the intake of more healthful fats over saturated fats. This macronutrient model is closer to what we would recommend on a daily basis for strength athletes; energy needs, however, must be met first to optimize the training adaptations of the strength–power athlete.

LOW-CARBOHYDRATE, HIGH-FAT, HIGH-PROTEIN (KETOGENIC) DIETS

Carbohydrates were recently demonized with a resurgence of books on low-carbohydrate diets. These types of diets are essentially intended for weight loss; they are, however, increasing in popularity in athletics as well. Looking at the Atkins diet (one of the most popular low-carbohydrate plans) as a model, it recommends that one consumes 25 to 90 g of carbohydrate each day, with the low end of the scale as the "induction phase" when someone first begins the program and then working up to the higher end of the scale as time progresses and the individual ultimately reaches his or her goal. With this plan, both fat and protein make up the remaining energy, meaning that intakes of both macronutrients are unlimited and rather high. Our previously mentioned 150-lb athlete who consumed 2,500 kcal $\cdot$ d^{-1} in the induction phase would have an intake of 25 g of carbohydrate. By dividing protein and fat equally to meet the remaining energy needs in this example, we would provide 300 g of protein (about 4.5 g $\cdot$ kg^{-1} $\cdot$ d^{-1}) and about 133 g of fat (about 1.95 g $\cdot$ kg^{-1} $\cdot$ d^{-1}). This amount of protein is not only extremely high but unnecessary. The amount of fat in this diet plan is relatively high (e.g., no limit on intake), particularly since Atkins claims that saturated fats are no more hazardous to your health than unsaturated and polyunsaturated fats.

Scientists have begun to measure the effects of low-carbohydrate, high-fat diets on exercise performance (46). The assumption here is that although glycogen is the storage form of dietary carbohydrates, drastically reducing carbohydrates will cause only a transient negative effect on energy levels, since fat and protein metabolites can ultimately be used as sources of energy. All of the research in this area has been conducted on endurance athletes, because carbohydrates and glycogen are more crucial in terms of endurance performance. Eliminating or drastically reducing carbohydrates is more likely to be detrimental to endurance activity than it is to strength activities.

With strength training, the ultimate goal is typically hypertrophy, speed, and/or power. As discussed, protein is necessary for building muscle mass, and dietary fat is correlated to the production of serum sex hormones. It is obvious that the Atkins diet will provide an abundant amount of both protein and dietary fat. Unfortunately, with this diet, the purpose of high intakes of protein and fat is to displace dietary carbohydrate. Although not as important in short-duration, high-intensity activities, the drastic reduction of dietary carbohydrate and subsequently glycogen stores will hinder performance. Furthermore, the Atkins diet, and other similar diets, are low in total energy. No matter what the macronutrient ratio or combination, total energy is ultimately the most important factor in an athlete's diet.

Another consideration for many strength trainers is the effect of the diet on body composition, whether with regard to esthetics and/or performance. Research has demonstrated that a diet lower

REAL-WORLD APPLICATION

Nine Simple Tips for Achieving Good Nutrition for Athletes

1. Eat about six meals each day. For instance, this would include breakfast, a mid-morning meal, lunch, a mid-afternoon meal, a postworkout meal, dinner, and another meal before bedtime.
2. The bulk of your food should come from unprocessed carbohydrate foods and whole grains (e.g., vegetables of all kinds, oatmeal, brown rice, yams, sweet potatoes).
3. Protein should be consumed, approximately 2 g protein $\cdot$ kg body weight^{-1}; a more practical and easy-to-remember method is 1 g protein $\cdot$ lb body weight^{-1}.
4. The majority of dietary protein should come from lean sources such as chicken, fish, and turkey. Supplementing with whey or casein can also be beneficial.
5. Unsaturated fats such as fish fat, fats from nuts and legumes, and olive oil are to be emphasized, but you still need to consume saturated fat (e.g., from beef, eggs) on occasion.
6. Always consume a postworkout carbohydrate–protein shake that consists of a high-glycemic carbohydrate and fast-absorbing protein (e.g., whey).
7. Limit your intake of processed carbohydrate. Simple or high-glycemic carbohydrates, however, should be consumed as part of your pre-, during-, and/or postworkout beverage.
8. Not including the window before, during, and after a workout, try limiting your consumption of liquid calories (e.g., soda, beer).
9. Avoid fast food and excessive condiments. Fast food is typically high in sugar and fat and lacking in nutrient value.

in carbohydrate and higher in protein and fat may in fact have positive effects on body composition stimulating greater changes in weight loss while maintaining LBM. Supporters of the low-carb strategy suggest that this positive change (e.g., loss of body fat) is due the elimination of gross changes in plasma insulin concentrations caused by the excessive consumption of dietary carbohydrates. As yet, no long-term data demonstrate the superiority of one diet of this type over another, and the studies to date supporting high-fat diets were all of short duration (aside from one 12-month study, which showed no significant changes in body weight vs. the higher carbohydrate diet at the completion of the 12 months). It should be noted that it is virtually impossible to scientifically study the effects of a diet in the long term (i.e., more than 1 year). Thus, comparisons between and among diets are relegated to short-term studies that represent small windows of time.

Since all foods do not have identical nutrient values (i.e., whole wheat bread vs. processed white bread and lean meats vs. plant-based proteins), it is important to find high-quality sources of each nutrient.

Another limiting factor to regularly displacing dietary carbohydrate with fat and protein is the lack of variety in the foods allowed, making a low-carbohydrate lifestyle difficult to follow for a long time. The lack of variety also limits the intake of micronutrients, phytochemicals, antioxidants, and other beneficial components of food, which are all correlated with a lower incidence of various diseases. A healthy athlete is an athlete who can continually train harder and ultimately perform better. Also consider the previously discussed studies demonstrating that carbohydrates at specific times before, during, and after workouts may enhance protein synthesis, recovery, and ultimately growth (2,5,20). Drastic reductions in carbohydrate intake will not allow athletes to take advantage of this window of opportunity, when insulin levels are high from resistance exercise and muscle cells are in exact need of the nutrients that are shuttled in more rapidly with the ingestion of high-glycemic carbohydrates. Consequently, the suggestion that a low-carbohydrate, high-fat diet can enhance performance is unsound and not based on science.

It is virtually impossible to make blanket dietary recommendations for high-performance athletes without first determining their current food intake. The placement of severe restrictions on certain macronutrients, however, is probably not the best approach.

Summary

Various experts on sports nutrition may provide different answers to the same question based partly on science, anecdote, and personal experience. Blanket dietary recommendations are difficult to make because so many factors affect the optimal diet. Not only is resistance training itself important, but training history, performance goals (e.g., hypertrophy vs. power vs. changes in body composition), program design, individual responses to training and diet, and acute versus chronic adaptations to training will all play a role in nutritional recommendations.

A few basic nutritional principles can apply to all athletes. First, athletes must try to ingest as much energy as possible while achieving optimal body mass and composition for their respective sports. To do so, they should focus on ingesting approximately 1 g protein · lb body weight^{-1}. This recommendation simplifies the calculations necessary to determine needs, and the value can be adjusted based on established outcome measures. Dietary carbohydrate and fat energy should balance out the remainder of the diet with a higher proportion of carbohydrate than fat. The primary sources of carbohydrates should be primarily unprocessed low glycemic index carbohydrates that provide sufficient fiber and abundant nutrients. The intake of high glycemic index carbohydrates should be limited to the periods before, during, and after exercise. Fat intake should be substantial (~30% of total energy), with special attention to balancing saturated, monounsaturated, and polyunsaturated fats. Finally, nutrient timing through the consumption of energy (preferably in liquid form to facilitate absorption and ease of use) during and after exercise is critical to improving training response and recovery.

Dietary recommendations should be specific to the current training modality and should be regularly adjusted to meet an athlete's changing needs. Seeking the assistance of a qualified registered dietitian or sports nutritionist will allow the athlete to achieve the desired goals in a healthful but timely manner.

Maxing Out

1. A two-sport female athlete coming out of basketball season goes straight into golf season. The athlete is having trouble getting her energy levels up. She complains to you of trouble sleeping, lack of appetite, lethargy, and poor performance. You fear the athlete is suffering from overtraining. What type of nutritional advice would you give this athlete?
2. A coach at your school has been telling athletes that high protein content in the diet will cause liver failure and that athletes should limit their intake. In addition, he tells them that there is no benefit to increased intake of protein. How will you approach this issue with the coach and the athletes?
3. Being the strength coach at a small school, you are often approached by faculty and staff about diet and exercise advice. Knowing that most faculty and staff would have different energy requirements than the athletes you normally deal with, what advice would you give them? Give the faculty and staff three nutrition keys that will help them obtain their general health goals.
4. A novice long-distance runner who has participated in three half-marathons and one marathon (26.2 mi) asks for your advice regarding her nutrition program. She currently eats two to three meals per day with an emphasis on proteins, healthy fats, and low carbohydrate. What questions would you ask her and what nutrition advice might she need that is simple yet effective?
5. An 18-year-old collegiate strength athlete who is 5 ft 11 in and 198 lbs has come to you for some nutrition advice. The athlete is consuming about 4,000 kcal · d^{-1}, but he is on a meal plan at school and can only eat twice a day at the cafeteria. He feels like he is gaining weight, but fat weight. His funds are limited but needs dietary help. What advice would you give this athlete? How can his diet help him gain the lean muscle that he wants within his limited budget?

REFERENCES

1. Phillips SM, Tipton KD, Aarsland A, et al. Mixed muscle protein synthesis and breakdown after resistance exercise in humans. *Am J Physiol*. 1997;273:E99–E107.
2. Tipton KD, Rasmussen BB, Miller SL, et al. Timing of amino acid–carbohydrate ingestion alters anabolic response of muscle to resistance exercise. *Am J Physiol Endocrinol Metab*. 2001;281:E197–E206.
3. Davis JM, Alderson NL, Welsh RS. Serotonin and central nervous system fatigue: nutritional considerations. *Am J Clin Nutr*. 2000;72:573S–578S.
4. Nieman DC. Exercise immunology: nutritional countermeasures. *Can J Appl Physiol*. 2001;26(suppl):S45–S55.
5. Ivy JL, Goforth HW Jr, Damon BM, et al. Early postexercise muscle glycogen recovery is enhanced with a carbohydrate–protein supplement. *J Appl Physiol*. 2002;93:1337–1344.
6. Roy BD, Luttmer K, Bosman MJ, et al. The influence of post-exercise macronutrient intake on energy balance and protein metabolism in active females participating in endurance training. *Int J Sport Nutr Exerc Metab*. 2002;12:172–188.
7. Bishop NC, Blannin AK, Walsh NP, et al. Nutritional aspects of immunosuppression in athletes. *Sports Med*. 1999;28:151–176.
8. Rasmussen BB, Tipton KD, Miller SL, et al. An oral essential amino acid–carbohydrate supplement enhances muscle protein anabolism after resistance exercise. *J Appl Physiol*. 2002;88:386–392.
9. Campbell B, Kreider RB, Ziegenfuss T, et al. International Society of Sports Nutrition position stand: protein and exercise. *J Int Soc Sport Nutr*. 2007;4:8
10. Lemon PW, Berardi JM, Noreen EE. The role of protein and amino acid supplements in the athlete's diet: does type or timing of ingestion matter? *Curr Sports Med Rep*. 2002;1:214–221.
11. Lowery LM, Devia L. Dietary protein and resistance exercise: what do we really know? *J Int Soci Sport Nutr*. 2009;6:3
12. Terpstra AH. Effect of conjugated linoleic acid on body composition and plasma lipids in humans: an overview of the literature. *Am J Clin Nutr*. 2004;79:352–361.
13. Dorgan JF, Judd JT, Longcope C, et al. Effects of dietary fat and fiber on plasma and urine androgens and estrogens in men: a controlled feeding study. *Am J Clin Nutr*. 1996;64(6):850–855.
14. Stark AH, Madar Z. Olive oil as a functional food: epidemiology and nutritional approaches. *Nutr Rev*. 2002;60:170–176.
15. Noakes TD. Fluid replacement during exercise. *Exerc Sport Sci Rev*. 1993;21:297–330.
16. Ivy JL. Glycogen resynthesis after exercise: effect of carbohydrate intake. *Int J Sports Med*. 1998;19 (suppl 2):S142–S145.
17. Rennie MJ, Tipton KD. Protein and amino acid metabolism during and after exercise and the effects of nutrition. *Annu Rev Nutr*. 2000;20:457–483.
18. Tipton KD, Borsheim E, Wolf SE, et al. Acute response of net muscle protein balance reflects 24-h balance after exercise and amino acid ingestion. *Am J Physiol Endocrinol Metab*. 2003;284:E76–E89.
19. Willoughby DS, Stout JR, Wilborn CD. Effects of resistance training and protein plus amino acid supplementation on muscle anabolism, mass, and strength. *Amino Acids*. 2007:32(4):467–477
20. Esmarck B, Andersen JL, Olsen S, et al. Timing of postexercise protein intake is important for muscle hypertrophy with resistance training in elderly humans. *J Physiol*. 2001;535:301–311.
21. Flakoll PJ, Judy T, Flinn K, et al. Postexercise protein supplementation improves health and muscle soreness during basic military training in marine recruits. *J Appl Physiol*. 2004;96:951–956.
22. Doi T, Matsuo T, Sugawara M, et al. New approach for weight reduction by a combination of diet, light resistance exercise and the timing of ingesting a protein supplement. *Asia Pac J Clin Nutr*. 2001;10:226–232.

23. Tipton KD, Elliott TA, Cree MG, et al. Stimulation of net protein synthesis by whey protein ingestion before and after exercise. *Am J Physiol Endocrinol Metab*. 2006;292(1):E71–E76.
24. Kerksick C, Harvey T, Stout J, et al. International Society of Sports Nutrition position stand: nutrient timing. *Int J Sport Nutr*. 2008;5:18.
25. Bazzarre TL, Kleiner SM, Ainsworth BE. Vitamin C intake and lipid profiles in competitive male and female body-builders. *Int J Sport Nutr*. 1992;2(3):260–271.
26. Rokitzki L, Sagredos, AN, Reuss F, et al. Assessment of vitamin B6 status of strength and speedpower athletes. *J Am Coll Nutr*. 1994;13(1):87–94.
27. Lukaski H. Vitamin and mineral status: effects on physical performance. *Nutrition*. 2004;20(7):632–644
28. McBride JM, Kraemer WJ, Triplett-McBride T, et al. Effect of resistance exercise on free radical production. *Med Sci Sports Exerc*. 1998;30:67–72.
29. Avery NG, Kaiser JL, Sharman MJ, et al. Effects of vitamin E supplementation on recovery from repeated bouts of resistance exercise. *J Strength Cond Res*. 2003;17(4):801–809.
30. Jakeman P, Maxwell S. Effect of antioxidant vitamin supplementation on muscle function after eccentric exercise. *Eur J Appl Physiol*. 1993;67(5):426–430.
31. Thompson D, Williams C, Garcia-Roves P, et al. Post-exercise vitamin C supplementation and recovery from demanding exercise. *Eur J Appl Physiol*. 2003;89:393–400.
32. Thompson D, Williams C, McGregor SJ, et al. Prolonged vitamin C supplementation and recovery from demanding exercise. *Int J Sport Nutr Exerc Metab*. 2001;11(4):466–481.
33. Webster S, et al. Physiological effects of a weight loss regimen practiced by college wrestlers. *Med Sci Sports Exerc*. 1990;22(2):229–234.
34. Convertino VA, et al. American College of Sports Medicine position stand. Exercise and fluid replacement. *Med Sci Sports Exerc*. 1996;1:i–vii.
35. Bohl CH, Volpe SL. Magnesium and exercise. *Crit Rev Food Sci Nutr*. 2002;42:533–563.
36. Cordova A, Alvarez-Mon M. Behaviour of zinc in physical exercise: a special reference to immunity and fatigue. *Neurosci Biobehav Rev*. 1995;19:439–445.
37. Wilborn CD, Kerksick CM, Campbell BI, et al. Effects of zinc magnesium aspartate (ZMA) supplementation on training adaptations and markers of anabolism and catabolism. *J Int Soc Sport Nutr*. 2004;1(2):12–20.
38. Bergstrom J, et al. Diet, muscle glycogen and physical performance. *Acta Physiol Scand*. 1967;71:140–150.
39. Borsheim E, Cree MG, Tipton KD, et al. Effect of carbohydrate intake on net muscle protein synthesis during recovery from resistance exercise. *J Appl Physiol*. 2004;96:674–678.
40. Haff GG, Lehmkuhl MJ, McCoy LB, et al. Carbohydrate supplementation and resistance training. *J Strength Cond Res*. 2003;17:187–196.
41. Siri-Tarino PW, Sun Q, Hu FB, et al. Meta-analysis of prospective cohort studies evaluating the association of saturated fat with cardiovascular disease. *Am J Clin Nutr*. 2010;91(3):535–546.
42. Volek JS, Kraemer WJ, Bush JA, et al. Testosterone and cortisol in relationship to dietary nutrients and resistance exercise. *J App Physiol*. 1997;82(1):49–54.
43. Cheuvront SN. The zone diet and athletic performance. *Sports Med*. 1999;29(4):213–228.
44. Jarvis M, Seddon A, McNaughton L, et al. The acute 1-weed effects of the zinc diet on body composition, blood lipid levels, and performance in recreational endurance athletes. *J Strength Cond Res*. 2002;16(1):50–57.
45. Fleming J, Sharman MJ, Avery NG, et al. Endurance capacity and high-intensity exercise performance responses to a high fat diet. *Int J Sport Nutr Exerc Metab*. 2003;13(4):466–478.
46. Burke LM, Kiens B, Ivy JL. Carbohydrates and fat for training and recovery. *J Sports Sci*. 2004;22(1):15–30.
47. Rampone AJ, Reynolds PJ. Obesity: thermodynamic principles in perspective. *Life Sci*. 1988;43:93–110.

PART

onetwothreefour

Organization and Administration

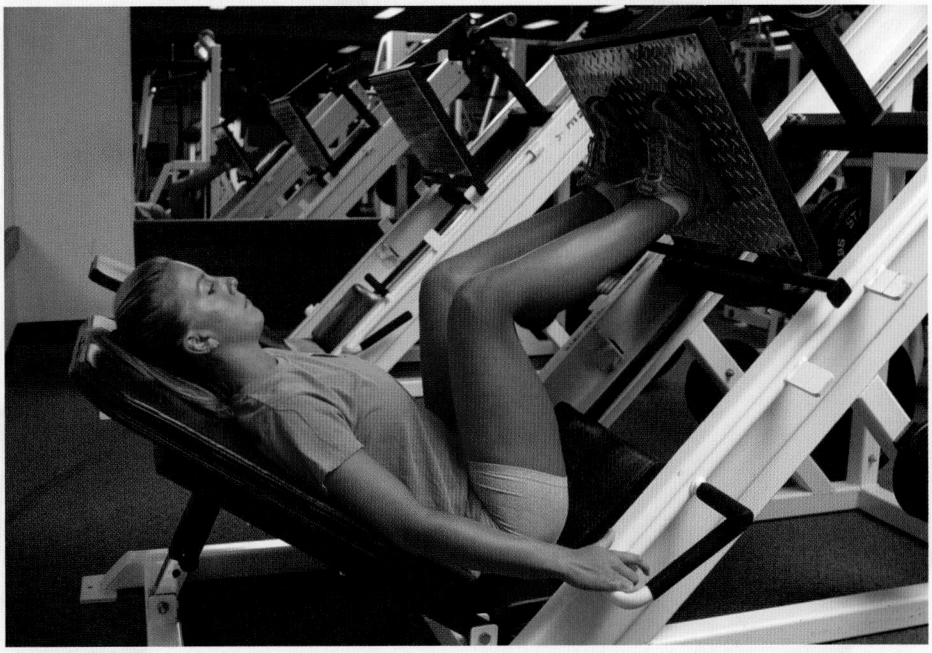

CHAPTER 8

Test Administration and Interpretation

LEE E. BROWN ● ANDY V. KHAMOUI ● EDWARD JO

OBJECTIVES

After completing this chapter, you will be able to:

- Understand the purpose of testing.
- Differentiate between validity and reliability.
- Perform a needs analysis.
- Determine appropriate testing protocols for specific performance variables.
- Familiarize yourself with statistical measures.

KEY TERMS

Assessment
Bimodal Curve
Central Tendency
Concurrent Validity
Construct Validity
Content Validity
Criterion
Evaluation
Face Validity
Interval Scores
Intraclass Correlation Coefficient (ICC)
Maximum
Mean
Measurement
Median
Minimum
Mode
N
Negatively Skewed
Normative
Ordinal
Population
Positively Skewed
Predictive Validity
Range
Ratio Scores
Reliability
Subpopulation
Sum
Standard Deviation (SD)
Standardized Scores
Test
T-Score
Validity
Variance
Z-Score

Introduction

Test and measurement is at the heart of any resistance-training program. This is the point where initial decisions are made regarding the exercise prescription and involving such topics as frequency, intensity, and volume. However, testing is not a one-time task but rather an ongoing method of evaluation throughout the prescribed program. In this sense, it is the beginning, the middle, and the end of a true individual periodized regime. The results can be used to evaluate performance and make decisions regarding the future of a program or individual. They may also be used to predict future performance in much the same way that college entrance exam scores are used to predict an individual's probability of graduating. Lastly, test scores may be used in a research environment as part of an in-depth analysis of an important question. Ultimately, the outcome of this entire process is the individualized exercise prescription that will best serve each athlete or client.

Physical testing is an ongoing task to assess the status of both the athlete and the program.

PURPOSE OF TESTING

The main reason test and measurement is at the heart of resistance training is that it determines where an individual currently stands regarding his or her training status and, more importantly, where he or she is headed. The final outcome of any training program is to arrive at a peak level of performance or to achieve some predetermined goal (1). Therefore, having goals is of no consequence if neither the exerciser nor the strength and conditioning professional knows the present state of the athlete. In short, before we can plan for a trip to go somewhere, we must first know where we currently are. In this way, a cogent strategy can be designed and implemented based on the individual and unique demands of the athlete that have been determined through test and measurement.

Using the results of a properly designed and implemented test and measurement protocol will enable the tester or coach to make objective rather than subjective decisions regarding their client's or athlete's program. The ultimate assessment will be based on hard data collected through judicious use of appropriate tests gathered under the scrutiny of a well-prepared tester. In this way individual bias can be reduced and the tester's prejudice can be eliminated when measuring an attribute on a test. There is, however, still a place for subjective reasoning during an evaluation process, but it is better utilized in the overall synergy of how the athlete's skills may be able to coordinate with the sport requirements rather than on the independent collection of raw data.

One purpose of testing is to determine the athlete's current level of performance.

The purpose of this chapter is to lay the framework for a neat and concise assessment procedure when evaluating clients or athletes. Before proceeding, it is important to understand the nomenclature used during this process.

Population: an entire group of individuals sharing some common characteristic. This might be all third graders in America or all NCAA Division I female pole-vaulters. This group is nearly always too large in number to test every member so a smaller sample is chosen as representative.

Subpopulation: the sample group mentioned above, which contains a manageable number of people in which to obtain performance measures. The results of this subpopulation will be used to infer the total population.

Test: a tool used to measure performance. This may take the form of a vertical jump test, a one-repetition maximum (1RM) strength test, or a timed muscular endurance test. The test is just a tool used to collect data in the course of the assessment procedure.

Measurement: the quantitative score derived from the test. It will be in the units described by the individual test such as inches or feet or pounds. Alone it has very little meaning since different tests have different scales, making comparisons difficult if not impossible.

Evaluation: placing a value on the measurement derived from the test. This is the point where the score must be compared to a scale and given worth. This part of the procedure requires a professional trained to choose the proper ranking scale and mindful of the intricacies involved in making decisions in the face of extraneous variables as well as individual differences associated with age, gender, and training status.

Assessment: putting all three of the aforementioned events together. Choose a test, measure the score, and then make an evaluation based on a scale comparison.

Normative: a postmeasurement scale derived from the scores of a peer group. When comparing within a subpopulation, placing the greatest score at the top and then listing the descending scores in order of magnitude generally determines this scale. In other words, if scores on a vertical jump test ranged between 28 and 12 inches, then all the other scores would be ranked between them and some value placed on each performance. Breaks in the scale can be established according to statistical rules such as central tendency, standard deviation (SD), or natural breaks.

Criterion: an a priori scale whereby the break points are known prior to testing and each person must meet an established level of performance to achieve that value level. It is important to understand that this scale is usually derived from many bouts of normative testing. When a considerable number of data are collected on enough subpopulations to constitute a logical inference of the results to the total population, then a criterion scale can be established and used for the evaluation of subsequent scores. This scale requires participants to perform at a standard level of achievement. It may be reaching a specific height during the vertical jump for a basketball team or lifting a specific amount of weight as in a preemployment screening exam or attaining a particular height before being allowed to enjoy an amusement park ride.

Testing data can be useful in justifying a program or a training method.

TEST SELECTION

To accurately evaluate athletes, proper tests must be chosen, which allow an in-depth view of an individual's performance level. This is best accomplished by choosing specific tests designed to measure only one aspect of human performance (2,3). Often many separate tests will be required to precisely measure an athlete's state of training and each test should be chosen with risks and outcomes in mind. Sport coaches sometimes make choices based on anecdotal evidence or use insensitive tests that are incapable of discriminating variable human performance. The proper procedure is to first determine what the desired outcome is and then design a test and measurement protocol around those outcomes (4).

Tests chosen should be specific to the sport and to the population being tested.

Physical tests include measurements of cardiovascular and respiratory function, strength, power, endurance, and anthropometry just to name a few. Each of these categories consists of a myriad of choices, every one of which is intended to measure a single factor of that performance characteristic within specific and detailed guidelines (5). Violation of these guidelines will result in spurious data, which are of no use whatsoever.

By understanding statistical measures, you will be able to analyze and interpret data from performance tests.

Making decisions about an individual's physical state of being is not a trivial task and carries with it severe consequences for both the evaluator and the client. The utilization of spurious data will ultimately result in drawing erroneous conclusions. The severity of prescribing exercise for an individual that is beyond his or her capacity or returning an athlete to play prior to his or her being able to participate without undue risk of danger cannot be overemphasized. Remember that bad data are worse than no data at all because they may offer an unstable foundation on which to build further training.

REAL-WORLD APPLICATION

Calculating Average Velocity during Sprint Running

The example is an athlete completing a 40-m sprint. We have electronic timing lights at 10, 20, and 30 m from the starting light gate. The average speed over the last 10 m might be used as an indication of maximum running speed. Let us assume the times and distances are as follows:

Distance	10	20	30
Time	1.741	2.890	3.995

Velocity is change in distance over change in time. Therefore:

$$\text{velocity} = (30-20)/(3.995-2.890) = 10/1.105$$
$$= 9.05\ \text{m} \cdot \text{s}^{-1}.$$

VALIDITY

Validity is the most important aspect of any assessment procedure. In order for a test to be valid it must test what it purports to test (6). That is, if one wishes to measure leg strength, then a valid test might be the squat, leg press, or dead lift. Each test would result in different scores and care would need to be exercised when choosing the proper test for a unique subpopulation, but each is a valid test of leg strength. In contrast, the vertical jump test includes leg strength as a component but is a test of leg power. Therefore, the vertical jump test is not a valid test of leg strength because it measures an individual's ability to produce power. However related strength and power might be, they are still distinct mechanisms of physical performance. Again, this is the sensitive nature of test selection.

Validity is historically measured against a "gold standard" of performance. For instance, if someone has designed a new device to test leg strength, then the procedure would be to obtain measures using the new device and compare those with the "gold standard" method (7). Using statistical techniques, it is possible to determine whether the two tests are conceptually similar and to what degree their results differ. A correlation analysis such as the Pearson product moment (r) may answer the conceptual question by determining the association of the two scores while an analysis of variance (ANOVA) may answer the degree to which the tests scores differ. These techniques are beyond the scope of this chapter but the concept should not be lost on the reader. The concept is that a test must measure what it has been designed to measure in order for the results to be a valid quantification of that physical component.

There are five major types of validity:

1. **Face validity** states that the test is logical on the surface, as when having a person lift a weight to measure strength.
2. **Content validity** states that the test includes material that has been taught or covered, for instance, testing speed after training for speed.
3. **Predictive validity** states that test scores can accurately predict future performance. An example would be the NFL measuring college football players prior to the draft to determine their potential.
4. **Concurrent validity** states that the test is a measure of the individual's current performance level. This happens when the test occurs shortly after training is completed.
5. **Construct validity** states that the test measures some part of the whole skill, such as measuring bench press strength for football linemen.

RELIABILITY

Reliability is loosely defined as repeatability. That is, the ability of a test to arrive at or near the same score upon repeated measurements in the absence of any intervention strategy. A reliable test should result in consistent scores. To accomplish this (using the new device scenario stated previously), the procedure would be to measure individuals using the new device and then allow a time delay of approximately 48 to 72 hours so no significant training effects could interfere with the results and then measure each person a second time using the identical procedures as the first measurement. If reliability is high, then people scoring well on the first test should also score well on subsequent tests (8,9).

REAL-WORLD APPLICATION

Reproducing Physical Test Results in Training and Conditioning

Reproducing test results of physical tests is important to maintain the validity and reliability of a test. Testing athletes in the weight room or on the field presents special challenges in terms of reproducing test data.

Why is reproducibility important in training and conditioning? It is important for a number of reasons, even though the data may not be used for research purposes.

You will make a decision about the type of program you use based on the results you obtain. If your results are not accurate, then you may be making the wrong decision, choosing a program that is not producing the results you seek. Pretesting and posttesting must use reproducible testing procedures so you can accurately make that decision.

Conditioning programs should focus on specific areas of weakness in a particular athlete. Those areas of weakness must be monitored on a regular basis using reproducible tests. If the tests used are not reproducible, then once again, the incorrect decision will be made.

Inconsistent test results may not motivate the athlete to improve. We know that hard work pays off with improved scores, but if the scoring is inconsistent, we are providing bad information to the athlete.

> ***A valid test measures what the test is actually trying to measure, whereas a reliable test yields consistent results.***

Documenting improvement in the athletes you train is an indication that you as a conditioning coach are doing your job. Providing your administrators with accurate testing records obtained using reproducible tests is an important step in justifying your position.

Are there steps the conditioning professional can take to improve the reproducibility of the test results? Of course!

- Standardize the testing procedures for every test. Have the procedures in writing, and provide a copy to each data collector.
- Train the data collectors to collect the test results accurately and consistently.
- Use the same data collectors as much as possible.
- Allow the same number of trials for each test.
- Test in the same environmental conditions as much as possible. Environmental conditions are best controlled indoors, so test indoors as much as possible and practical.
- Standardize the amount and type of external motivation provided to the athlete, and keep it consistent from one testing session to the next.
- Test the same time of day if possible.
- Always test after a day of rest if possible. Strenuous training of specific muscle groups may decrease performance on some tests.
- Maintain the same order of testing.

Control diet as much as possible. You may not be able to control diet to a great extent; but remember that it can have an effect on performance, both positive and negative.

The rank order of participants should remain relatively constant as in back-to-back days of handgrip strength testing. A perfect rank order between tests would mean that each person kept his or her spot in the ordinal sequence relative to all others. This almost never occurs with human testing. Employing the statistical techniques of Pearson r would establish this rank order of the two measurements and establish reliability on a continuum ranging between 1.0 and −1.0. Reliability is not an either/or proposition but rather a floating scale of different levels.

Table 8.1 depicts one strategy to use to categorize the level of reliability between two measurements taken at two different times using the same population. Remember that a negative correlation still represents reliability but simply states that as one score increases another score decreases, thereby inverting the rank order of participants. This may occur when comparing two different tests such as vertical jump height and percent body fat. Figure 8.1 shows graphical representations of the

TABLE 8.1 ● CATEGORY SYSTEM TO DETERMINE LEVEL OF RELIABILITY

R-VALUE	RELATIONSHIP
1.0–0.8	Very high
0.79–0.6	High
0.59–0.4	Moderate
0.39–0.2	Low
0.19–0	Very low

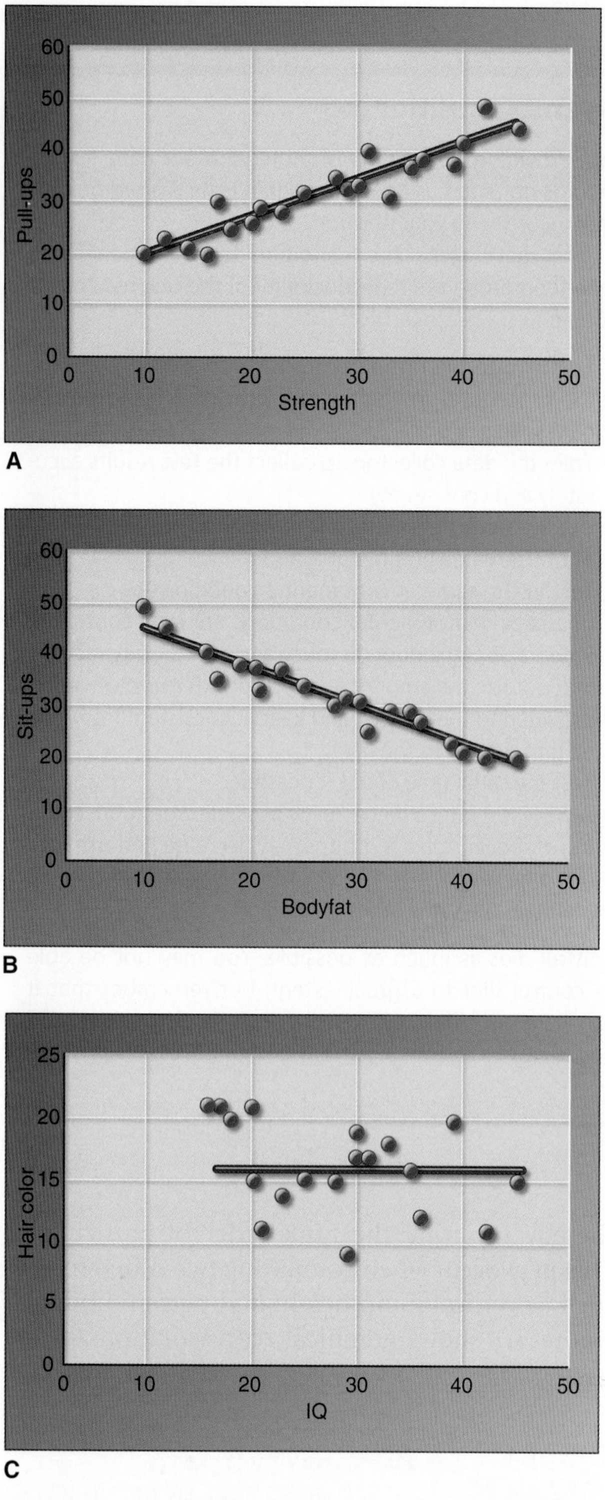

FIGURE 8.1 Graphical representation of scores when scatter-plotted. **A.** Positive relationship between strength and number of pull-ups. **B.** Negative relationship between body fat and number of sit-ups. **C.** No relationship between IQ and hair color.

scores as they appear when scatter plotted. The trend line (sometimes referred to as the "line of best fit") has been added to illustrate positive, negative, and null relationships, respectively.

Although the Pearson r correlation can be used to determine the relationship between subsequent tests in our new device scenario, it is no longer the gold standard when determining reliability. Instead, an **intraclass correlation coefficient (ICC)** can be used to better establish reliability. A Pearson r score close to 1 or −1 will denote that an individual has scored similarly with respect to his/her peers, but does not take into account any changes in the mean test score. What would happen if the group of athletes we tested on our new device all finished in the same rank order on the second test, but each scored several points higher? This would be a case in which Pearson r correlation would be high, because all of the athletes performed similarly with respect to their peers, on both tests. The test would not be reliable, however, because the mean score was higher on the second test. Therefore, the results are not repeatable. The ICC takes into account any difference that may be present, not only in the rank of each athlete, but the overall difference in the value of the scores (10). It is important to remember that the ICC, like the Pearson r, does not determine the reliability of a test in a yes or no fashion, but rather places the reliability on a theoretical continuum, which allows us to state the degree to which a test is reliable.

It should be evident then that a test may be reliable but not valid while a valid test must always be reliable. It is always important to remember that each of these procedures assumes complete cooperation of the athlete and 100% maximum effort during every test session. That is not always the case and should be carefully monitored by the individual responsible for test administration or submaximal testing should be performed (11).

Tests chosen must be valid and reliable, and must be administered using a reliable protocol.

ASSESSMENT

The first thing that should be done is a full assessment, including a medical and exercise history, obtaining a physician release if necessary, performing physiological testing, determining baseline nutritional status (to determine if referral to an RD/LD is necessary), and determining program goals. The objective of the assessment is to provide a comprehensive view of the athlete, what they are capable of, what their limitations are, and any special needs that may need to be addressed. This initial assessment may be done the first time you meet, but will be ongoing as you work with and learn about the person's needs.

MEDICAL HISTORY AND PAR-Q

The medical history should begin with a few basic questions, such as those found on the PAR-Q form. The PAR-Q is a limited tool that should not be considered to encompass all the information that you will need to know. It is a quick and easy way to determine whether a potential client is at risk for any major complications during low to moderate, but not vigorous, exercise. In addition to the PAR-Q, it is appropriate to determine the following:

- Is the person diabetic? If so, is the person able to control his or her blood glucose levels, and how does the person monitor blood glucose? Additionally, has the person ever been on a regular exercise program while diabetic?
- Does the person have asthma? If so, is the asthma exercise induced, and at what levels? Does the person use a fast-acting inhaler or other medication to control attacks?
- Does the person smoke? If so, how much and how often?
- Is there a family history of heart attack, coronary artery bypass surgery, or sudden death before age 55 in men, or age 65 in women?
- Does the person have a history of hypertension (systolic pressure $\geq$ 140, or diastolic pressure $\geq$ 90), or is he or she on antihypertensive medications?
- Does the person have a total cholesterol level >200 mg $\cdot$ dL^{-1}?
- Is the person obese, defined as a body mass index of $\geq$30, confirmed with a waist measurement of >100 cm?

You will also need to know about any previous injuries that might interfere with their ability to perform certain exercises. Ask about such things as sprains and strains, arthritis, athletic injuries, unusual pain or swelling in any of the joints, and any tightness that limits their ability to move with ease.

> *Understanding an individual's medical and exercise history will help you make an informed decision regarding exercise prescription, or whether referral to a medical professional for additional testing is indicated.*

PHYSICIAN RELEASE

The words "please consult with your physician before beginning an exercise program" are often found on the control panels of cardiovascular equipment. No matter how thorough a medical history you obtain, a physician will be better able to assess the medical ability of a person to begin an exercise program, and may have information that can help you to determine the best course of action for that person. It is a good idea to have a medical release form that describes each of the exercise components, including the levels of intensity and duration.

NUTRITION

It is important to get a basic understanding of the person's nutritional status. Nutritional programming should only be performed by a registered or licensed dietitian. However, you can obtain basic information, such as choice of foods, quantity, and timing of meals from a simple 3-day recall. Having the client recall everything ingested for the past three days will allow you to decide if more specific dietary interventions are necessary, in which case a referral to an RD/LD is necessary.

NEEDS ANALYSIS

Two main concerns when choosing proper tests to be administered to athletes are the needs of the individual and the needs of the activity. Each of these brings specific requirements to the task of test selection and should be treated with equal diligence.

> *A needs analysis should be performed to evaluate the needs of the athlete and the demands of the sport.*

First, individual needs may be assessed through traditional physiological methods such as body fat, cardiovascular, muscular strength/power, and flexibility testing. These tests are designed to evaluate the individual's present state of readiness to participate in the activity of choice. Not all tests will be required for each person as not all physiological variables are equally required across sporting activities. Furthermore, each category may compel the investigator to pick appropriate ways to measure the individual.

Second, the needs of the particular sport or activity are unique and require different physiological performance levels of the athlete or client. Some sports require maximal isometric upper body movements such as wrestling while others require submaximal continuous lower body movements such as cycling or running. Once again, the need to be specific with a test and measurement scheme is vital for the success of the program.

Testing needs to be specific to the movements and muscle groups used by the athlete during their sport.

In short, preparation for a comprehensive test and measurement system requires time and diligence of the tester at the onset of the program in order to choose tests that measure the requisite needs of both the participant and the activity. These needs should consider all aspects of human performance including, but not limited to, energy systems, duration of each repetition, duration of the entire event, muscle used, muscle actions used, range of motion involved, and speed of movement (12,13).

Table 8.2 displays a myriad of tests designed to measure strength, power, muscular endurance, and agility; yet each is unique in that it requires different muscles, muscle actions, time limits, kinetic chain limitations, and energy systems. The tests presented in this chapter are by no means the only available methods of evaluating strength, power, muscular endurance, and agility. Instead, they have

TABLE 8.2 ● VARIOUS STRENGTH, POWER, ENDURANCE, AND AGILITY TESTS

TESTS	MUSCLE GROUPS AND JOINTS USED	MUSCLE ACTIONS	TIME LIMITS	KINETIC CHAIN	ENERGY SYSTEM
Wingate anaerobic cycle	Hips, quads, ankles	Concentric	30-s	Closed	Anaerobic
Margaria-Kalamen stair climb	Hips, quads, ankles	Concentric and eccentric	2-s	Closed	ATP-PC
Isokinetic velocity spectrum	Each one individually	Concentric and eccentric	5- to 60-s	Open	ATP-PC and anaerobic
Overhead medicine ball throw	Entire body	Concentric and eccentric	2-s	Closed	ATP-PC
Counter movement vertical jump	Hips and ankles	Concentric and eccentric	2-s	Closed	ATP-PC
1RM power clean	Arms, shoulders, back, hips, quads, ankles	Isometric and Concentric and eccentric	5-s	Closed	ATP-PC
1RM squat	Entire lower body	Isometric and Concentric and eccentric	5-s	Closed	ATP-PC
1RM bench press	Entire upper body	Isometric and Concentric and eccentric	5-s	Closed	ATP-PC
Bench press body weight for total reps	Entire upper body	Isometric and Concentric and eccentric	30- to 60-s	Closed	Anaerobic
Push-up test	Upper body	Concentric and eccentric	30- to 60-s	Closed	Anaerobic
40-yd dash	Entire lower body	Concentric and eccentric	5-s	Closed	ATP-PC
T-test	Entire body	Isometric and Concentric and eccentric	10-s	Closed	ATP-PC and anaerobic
5–10–5 shuttle	Entire body	Isometric and Concentric and eccentric	5-s	Closed	ATP-PC and anaerobic
Standing long jump	Entire lower body	Concentric and eccentric	2-s	Closed	ATP-PC
Sit-up test	Abdominals	Concentric and eccentric	1 minute	Closed	Anaerobic

TABLE 8.3 ● CALCULATED RATIOS FOR FEMALE/MALE COMPARISONS OF ABSOLUTE (N · m) AND RELATIVE (N · m · kg⁻¹) PEAK TORQUE FOR KNEE EXTENSION AND FLEXION

		FEMALE/MALE RATIO FOR TORQUE VALUES							
		60 DEGREES · S^{-1}		180 DEGREES · S^{-1}		300 DEGREES · S^{-1}		AVERAGE	
	JOINT MOTION	ABS	REL	ABS	REL	ABS	REL	ABS	REL
Men	Knee extension	0.77	0.81	0.84	0.88	0.83	0.87	0.81	0.85
	Knee flexion	0.88	0.93	0.93	0.99	0.86	0.91	0.89	0.94
Women	Knee extension	0.76	0.77	0.85	0.86	0.83	0.85	0.81	0.83
	Knee flexion	0.88	0.88	0.95	0.96	0.86	0.86	0.9	0.9

Sources: Beam WC, Bartels RL, Ward RW, et al. Multiple comparisons of isokinetic leg strength in male and female collegiate athletic teams. *Med Sci Sports Exer.* 17(2), Abstract #20, 269; Wyatt MP, Edwards AM. Comparison of quadriceps and hamstring torque values during isokinetic exercise. *J Orthop Sports Phys Ther.* 3:48–56.

been selected as a representation of the vast array of choices one has in assessing an athlete's training needs. Tables 8.3-8.6 present normative data for many of these tests.

Wingate Anaerobic Cycle Test

The Wingate Anaerobic Cycle Test was designed as a means to measure overall anaerobic lower extremity power. The athlete is made to cycle as fast as possible for 30 seconds with a predetermined resistance (Fig. 8.2). This resistance is derived by multiplying the athlete's body weight (kg) by the constant 0.075 (14,15).

Specialized cycle ergometers will record the athlete's peak power and mean power during the 30-second test. This test is a good overall assessment of lower extremity power as it requires contributions from all major muscle groups of the lower extremities. Also, it can be used to measure not only peak power, but mean power over a 30-second period as well. For this reason, it is a good test to include with sports that require maximal effort for bouts that last longer than just a few seconds. One negative aspect of this test is the need for a specialized cycle ergometer that will derive the athlete's peak and mean power. These ergometers are costly and are used primarily for research purposes.

Margaria-Kalamen Stair Climb Test

This test of lower extremity power is easy and quick to perform. It is performed on a staircase and is a good measure of lower body power and explosiveness, which is important to athletes requiring speed, agility, and quickness. First, measure the subject's body weight and calculate the height of each step. The test is performed by beginning in front of a flight of at least a dozen stairs. Each step height is approximately 17.5 cm (7 in) high. Timing mats are placed on the third and ninth steps, which are connected to a timing device and are activated by the subject's body weight. The subject begins 6 m from the first step

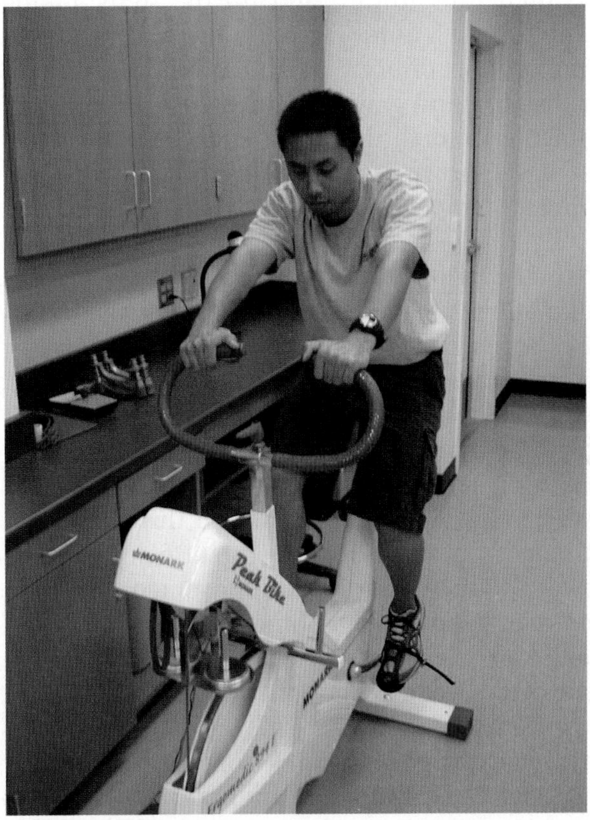

FIGURE 8.2 Wingate anaerobic cycle test. This test is a good indicator of overall anaerobic lower extremity power.

TABLE 8.4 ● COMPARATIVE DATA FOR WINGATE ANAEROBIC CYCLE TEST

	COMPARATIVE DATA FOR THE WINGATE ANAEROBIC TEST					
	PEAK ANAEROBIC POWER			MEAN ANAEROBIC POWER		
GROUP	FORCE (%WT)	ABSOLUTE (W)	RELATIVE ($W \cdot kg^{-1}$)	WORK (kJ)	ABSOLUTE (W)	RELATIVE ($W \cdot kg^{-1}$)
Men						
Non-Athletes (18–28 y)	7.5	700	9.2	16.9	563	7.3
Non-Athletes (18–24 y)	7.5	540	8.2	13.5	450	7.0
Non-Athletes (25–34 y)	7.5	700	9.2	16.2	540	7.2
Non-Athletes (35–44 y)	7.5	660	8.6	15.0	500	6.6
Cyclists (Category I–II)	10.0	1125	14.7	27.1	903	11.8
Cyclists (Category II–IV)	9.5	963	13.3	23.5	783	10.8
Women						
Non-Athletes (18–28 y)	7.5	454	454.0	11.4	381	6.3
Active Women	7.5	561	561.0	13.6	453	7.2

Sources: Inbar O, Dotan R, Baro-Or O. Anaerobic characteristics in male children and adolescents. *Med Sci Sports Exer.* 1986;18:264–269; Jacobs I. The effects of thermal dehydration on performance of the Wingate Anaerobic Test. *Int J Sports Med.* 1980;1:21–24; Maud PJ, Schultz BB. Norms for the Wingate Anaerobic Test with comparison to another similar test. *Res Q Exer Sport.* 1980;60(2):144–151; Tanaka H, Bassett DR, Swensen TC, et al. Aerobic and anaerobic characteristics of competitive cyclists in the United State Cycling Federation. *Int J Sports Med.* 1993;14:334–338.

and then runs toward and up the steps, taking them three at a time (Fig. 8.3). The result (power) is the product of body weight and the step's vertical distance and gravity divided by the total time from the third to the ninth step. Results of this test have shown a moderate correlation to the Wingate Cycle Test (16).

Isokinetic Velocity Spectrum

Isokinetic testing involves controlling the velocity of a given movement rather than the force or power with which it is performed. A computerized dynamometer is set to a specified velocity at which the lever arm of the machine can be moved (Fig. 8.4). The athlete then attempts to move the lever arm as fast as he or she can through a preset range of motion. Torque (rotational force) and power produced during the movement are then recorded by the dynamometer. These measurements can be expressed as maximal values or averaged over several repetitions to derive the mean torque and power values. This testing is often performed at a range of velocities, or spectrum, so that the tester can get a better indication of whether potential deficits exist during slow or fast velocity movements.

Isokinetic dynamometers can be used to test a variety of joints in either seated or reclined positions. These machines can only test each joint in isolation, and not as part of a dynamic movement. Therefore, they are limited in their application to the movement patterns specific to an individual sport. They do, however, provide precise, highly reliable data that can easily be compared between athletes, injured and uninjured limbs, or agonist and antagonist muscle groups (9,18,23).

Overhead Medicine Ball Throw

This test requires explosive total body movement to throw a medicine ball for maximum distance. The overhead medicine ball throw test is suitable specifically for athletes involved in sports where total body power is important. This test requires a 2- or 3-kg rubber medicine ball (men use 3 kg, women use 2 kg), tape measure, and clear open area.

The athlete begins by facing their back toward the direction they are throwing (Fig. 8.5). Feet must be shoulder width apart with heels on the start line (zero distance mark). The athlete will then start with the ball in both hands held extended over their head. While keeping the arms extended, the athlete will swing the ball down between the legs while

TABLE 8.5 ● CATEGORY FOR ABSOLUTE AND RELATIVE PEAK AND MEAN ANAEROBIC POWER AND FATIGUE INDEX BY GENDER

		PEAK ANAEROBIC POWER				MEAN ANAEROBIC POWER				FATIGUE INDEX	
CATEGORY	%ILE	ABSOLUTE (W)	RELATIVE ($W \cdot kg^{-1}$)	ABSOLUTE (W)	RELATIVE ($W \cdot kg^{-1}$)	ABSOLUTE (W)	RELATIVE ($W \cdot kg^{-1}$)	ABSOLUTE (W)	RELATIVE ($W \cdot kg^{-1}$)	MEN (%)	WOMEN (%)
Well Above Avg	95	867	11.1	602	9.3	677	8.6	483	7.5	21	20
	90	822	10.9	560	9.0	662	8.2	470	7.3	23	25
	85	807	10.6	530	8.9	631	8.1	437	7.1	27	25
	80	777	10.4	527	8.8	618	8.0	419	7.0	30	26
Above Avg	75	768	10.4	518	8.6	604	8.0	414	6.9	30	28
Average	70	757	10.2	505	8.5	600	7.9	410	6.8	31	29
	60	721	9.8	480	8.1	577	7.6	391	6.6	35	34
	50	689	9.2	449	7.6	565	7.4	381	6.4	38	35
	40	671	8.9	432	7.0	548	7.1	367	6.2	40	38
	30	656	8.5	399	6.9	530	7.0	353	6.0	43	40
	25	646	8.3	396	6.8	521	6.8	347	5.9	45	42
	20	618	8.3	376	6.6	496	6.6	337	5.7	47	44
	15	594	7.4	362	6.4	485	6.4	320	5.6	47	44
Below Avg	10	570	7.1	353	6.0	471	6.0	306	5.3	52	47
Well Below Avg	5	530	6.6	329	5.7	453	5.6	287	5.1	55	48

Sources: Maud PJ, Shultz BB. Norms for the Wingate Anaerobic Test with comparison to another similar test. *Res Q Exer Sport.* 60(2):144–151.

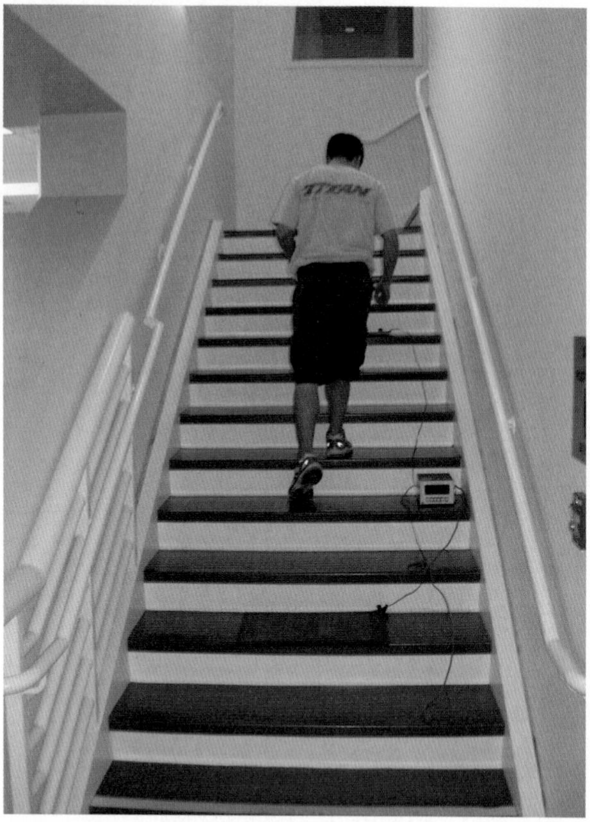

FIGURE 8.3 Margaria-Kalamen stair climb Test. This test is a good indicator of lower extremity power.

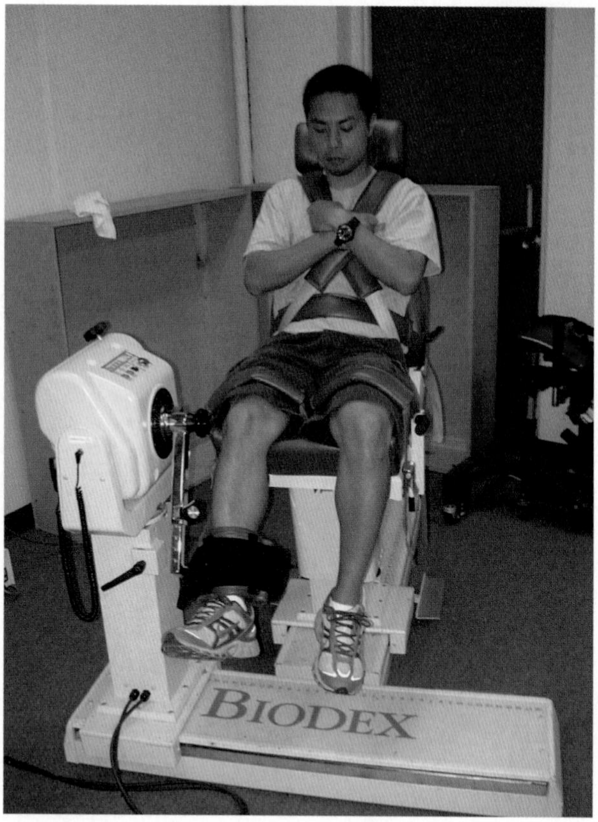

FIGURE 8.4 Isokinetic testing. Using a computerized dynamometer, this test measures torque and power at various velocities.

TABLE 8.6 ● MARGARIA-KALAMEN STAIR SPRINT TEST NORMATIVE RANGES

	MEN'S AGE GROUPS (YEARS)				
CLASSIFICATION	15–20	20–30	30–40	40–50	50+
Excellent	2,197+	2,059+	1,648+	1,226+	961+
Good	1,844–2,197	1,726–2,059	1,383–1,648	1,040–1,226	814–961
Average	1,471–1,824	1,373–1,716	1098–1,373	834–1,030	647–804
Fair	1,108–1,461	1,040–1,363	834–1,088	637–824	490–637
Poor	Under 1,108	Under 1,040	Under 834	Under 637	Under 490
	WOMEN'S AGE GROUPS (YEARS)				
CLASSIFICATION	15–20	20–30	30–40	40–50	50+
Excellent	1,785+	1,648+	1,226+	961+	736+
Good	1,491–1,785	1,383–1,648	1,040–1,226	814–961	608–736
Average	1,187–1,481	1,098–1,373	834–1,030	647–801	481–598
Fair	902–1,177	834–1,089	637–824	490–637	373–471
Poor	Under 902	Under 834	Under 637	Under 490	Under 373

Sources: Fox EL, Bowers RW, Foss ML. *The Physiological Basis of Physical Education and Athletics.* 5th ed. Dubuque, IA: Wm. C. Brown, 1993.

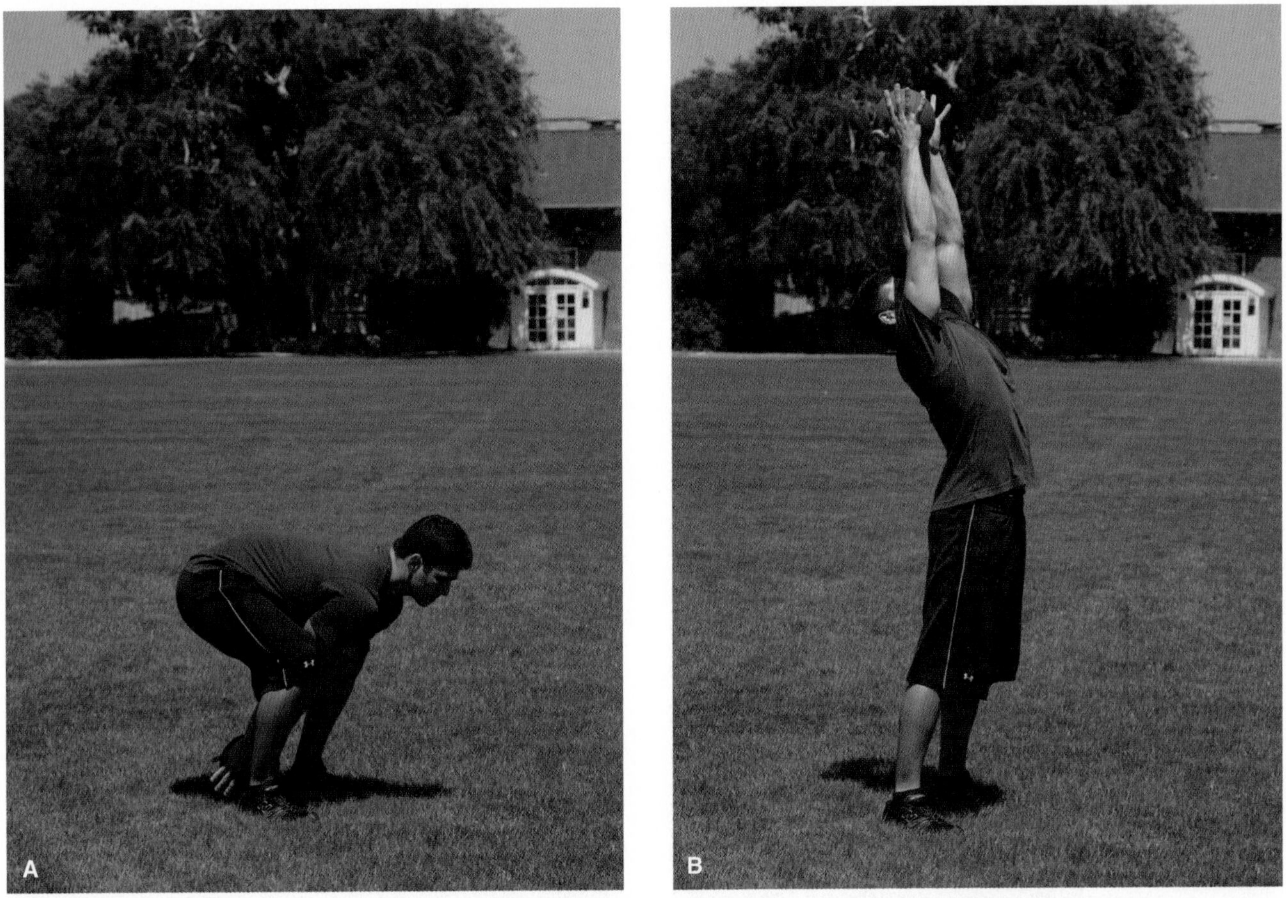

FIGURE 8.5 Overhead medicine ball throw. **A.** Starting position. **B.** Final position

flexing the knees, hips, and trunk. This serves as the countermovement. After the countermovement, the athlete will thrust the hips forward, extend the knees and trunk, flex the shoulders, while in one motion, throwing the ball back overhead. At the end of the throw, the feet can leave the ground as in a vertical jump to minimize any deceleration in the movement. These procedures should allow the muscles involved to generate power similar to the countermovement vertical jump test. The examiner is encouraged to allow the athlete several warm-up throws prior to the test.

Displacemant of the medicine ball during this test strongly correlates with the power index for the countermovement vertical jump test, which has been shown to be a reliable test for muscular power. This suggests that the overhead medicine ball throw test is reliable for assessing the total body muscular power (11).

Countermovement Vertical Jump

The vertical jump is performed, primarily, utilizing the hip extensor and ankle plantar flexor muscle groups. The athlete is instructed to jump as high as he or she can following a quick downward squatting movement. The athlete's jump height can be recorded simply by measuring the difference between chalk markings placed on a wall while standing on the ground and reaching, and at the highest point that athlete can reach while performing the countermovement jump. Commercial products involving a series of plastic sticks that rotate about a vertical axis when touched are also available to measure vertical jump height (Fig. 8.6).

This test is often a good choice with athletes as it is an essential skill in many sports. Therefore, the movement pattern and metabolic demands are similar to what the athlete might encounter in a game situation. Furthermore, improvement on a test such as this may have a direct effect on sport performance. One limitation of the countermovement vertical jump test is the fact that the technique often differs between athletes. Thus, the examiner must be careful that differences in scores on subsequent tests are due to training and not variations in the athlete's jumping technique.

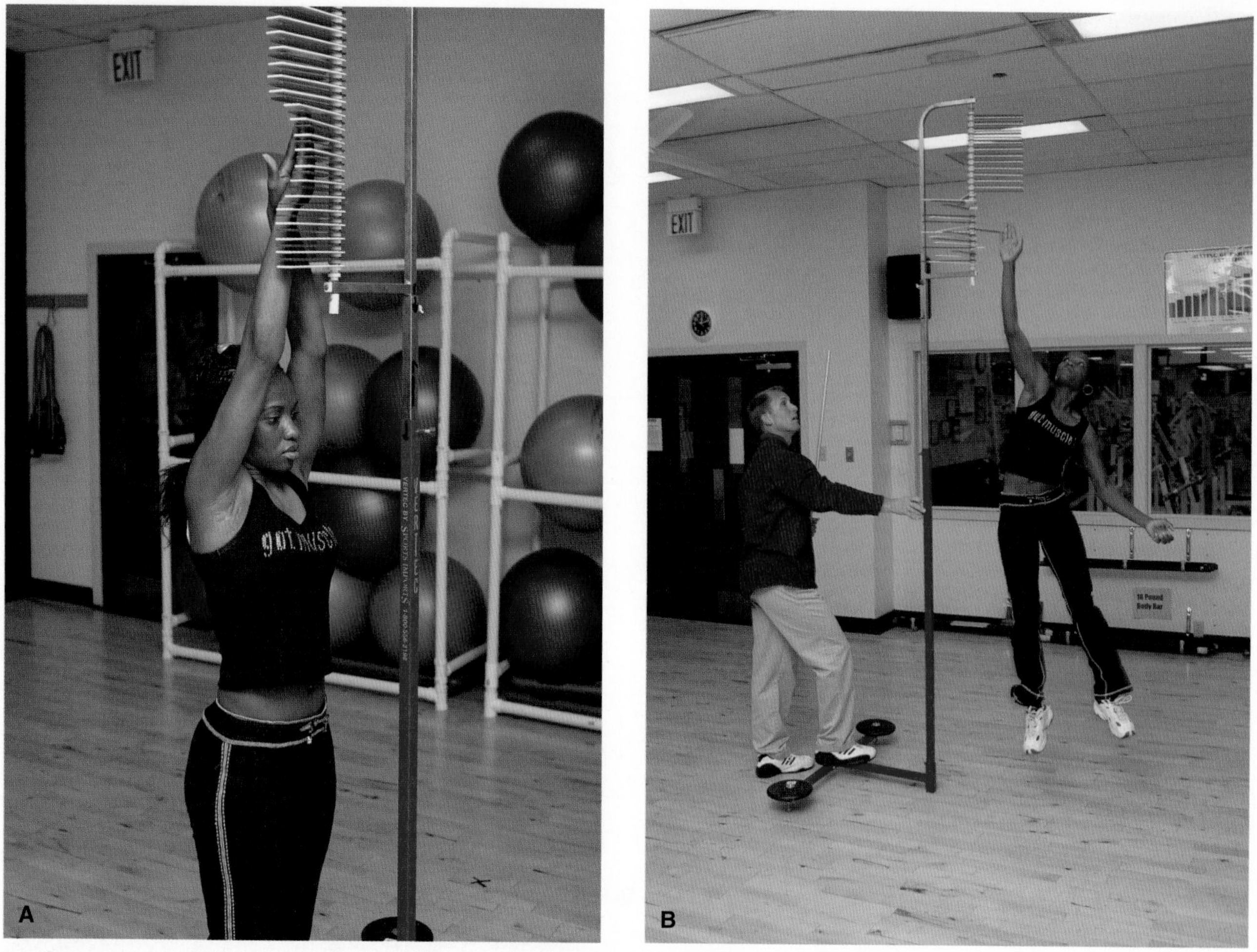

FIGURE 8.6 Countermovement vertical jump. **A.** First, determine the athlete's reach while standing on the floor. **B.** Then, have the athlete jump to determine maximum height.

One Repetition Maximum Power Clean

The power clean is an exercise performed using several upper extremity, lower extremity and core muscle groups (Fig. 8.7). Because the exercise is designed for the athlete to lift the weight as quickly as possible it is a good indication of ballistic strength. The repetition maximum power clean is considered to be the greatest load with which the athlete can perform one repetition of the movement with proper form. This test is useful for power athletes who are required to move explosively for short durations.

One-Repetition Maximum Squat

The one repetition maximum squat is considered the greatest load with which an athlete can perform the exercise in good form (Fig. 8.8). This test is a good indication of overall lower body strength as the movement requires contributions from all of the major muscle groups of the lower body. It is an important test for athletes whose sports require high amounts of lower extremity strength such as basketball and volleyball.

One-Repetition Maximum Bench Press

Like the squat test for the lower body, the 1RM bench press is often used to estimate an athlete's overall upper body strength (Fig. 8.9). Again, this value is obtain by determining the greatest load with which the athlete can perform the movement with good form. It is a particularly useful test for sports requiring upper body strength such as football. Since all athletes can benefit from improving their overall strength base a general upper body test such as this is good to include for all athletes.

Finding a true 1RM may be both difficult and unnecessary in some cases. As with other repetition maximum tests, the bench press test can be time-consuming to conduct (19). Long periods of rest are required between trials and several trials are

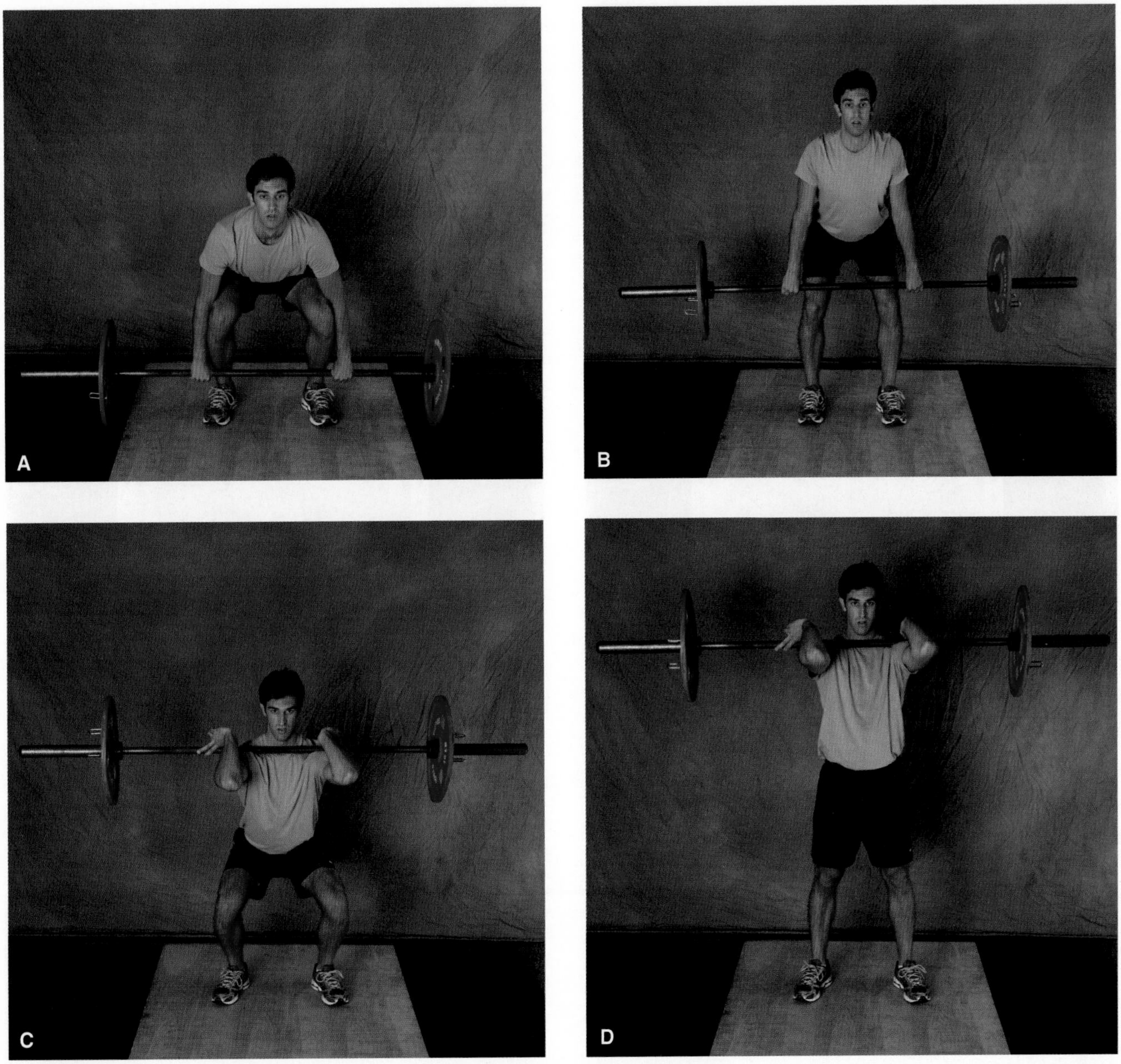

FIGURE 8.7 Power clean. **A.** Starting position. **B.** First pull. **C.** Catch. **D.** Final position.

necessary for each test. Therefore, repetition maximums are often derived using prediction equations. Many prediction equations exist and are based on the mass lifted and the amount of repetitions performed.

Bench Press Body Weight for Total Reps

This test is another good indicator of general upper body strength and muscular endurance. It may be a more valid measure than the 1RM test, because it takes into consideration individual differences in mass. Using this test would allow the strength coach to compare an athlete to his or her peers more appropriately.

Although this test provides for variations in strength due to mass, it does not consider differences in training age. Athletes who have greater training ages may be able to bench press their body weight several times without much difficulty. As such, this test may provide a base line of strength for some and muscular endurance for others. Deciding on an appropriate test for the upper body strength should take both differences in mass and training age into account.

Push-Up Test

The push-up test aims to assess an athlete's general upper body muscular endurance (Fig. 8.10). This

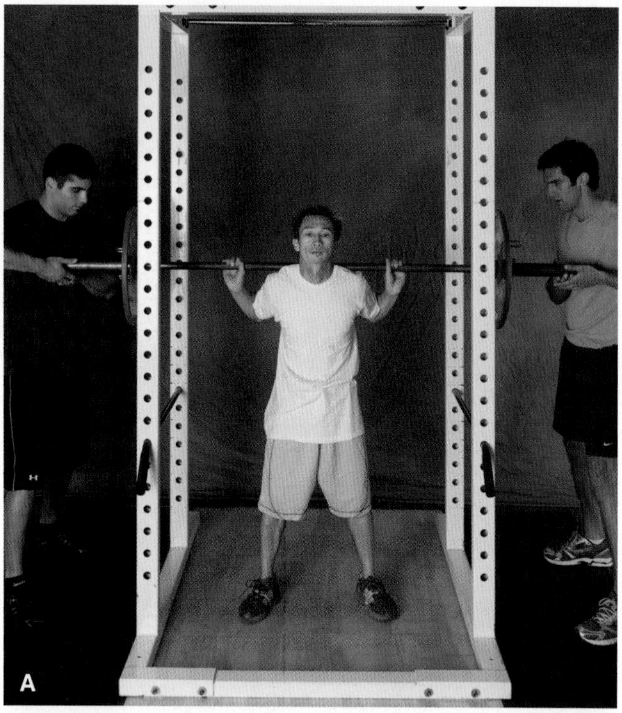

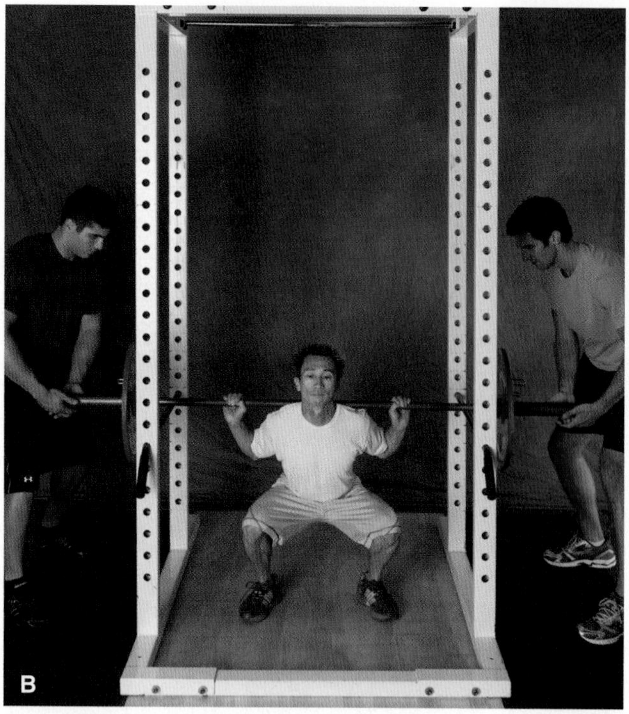

FIGURE 8.8 Squat. **A.** Starting position. **B.** Downward movement.

test is suitable for athletes whose sport requires them to endure repeated muscular contractions. To perform this test, a flat surface, optional mat, and an assistant is required. To start this test, the athlete will lie face down on the mat with hands shoulder width apart with fully extended arms. The athlete will lower their body until the elbow reaches 90 degrees and subsequently return to the starting position. The push-ups are to be continuous with no rest between repetitions. The athlete will

BOX 8.1

One-Repetition Maximum Testing Guidelines

Prior to prescribing a resistance training program, baseline performance values must be obtained for each exercise. One-repetition maximum (1RM) tests are frequently employed by strength and conditioning professionals to assess an athlete's initial strength level. This information is then used to prescribe training intensity for a given exercise as a percentage of 1RM. The following are guidelines for conducting a 1RM test.

1. Ensure that the athlete is proficient in the exercise to be assessed for 1RM.
2. Ensure that pretesting precautionary issues have been addressed (e.g., appropriate number of spotters, correct spotting technique).
3. Instruct the athlete to perform a general warm-up (low intensity aerobic exercise) to raise the core body temperature and reduce the risk for injury.
4. Instruct the athlete to perform a specific warm-up [one set of —five to ten repetitions of the exercise to be assessed using a light to moderate load (50% estimated 1RM), followed by one additional heavier but submaximal set (~70% 1RM)].
5. Instruct the athlete to lift a weight corresponding to approximately 3RM.
6. Provide 3 to 5 minutes of recovery.
7. Instruct the athlete to attempt the first 1RM trial.
8. Based on trial outcome, make load adjustments based on athlete feedback and the following guidelines:
   a. If the trial was successful, add 5 to 20 lb for upper body exercises and 10 to 30 lb for lower body exercises.
   b. If the trial was unsuccessful, remove 5 to 10 lb for upper body exercises and 10 to 20 lb for lower body exercises.
9. Provide 3 to 5 minutes of recovery between trials.
10. Repeat steps 8 and 9 until 1RM is achieved.

Source: Brown LE, Weir JP. ASEP procedures recommendation I: Accurate assessment of muscular strength and power. *J Exer Physiol.* 2001:4(3).

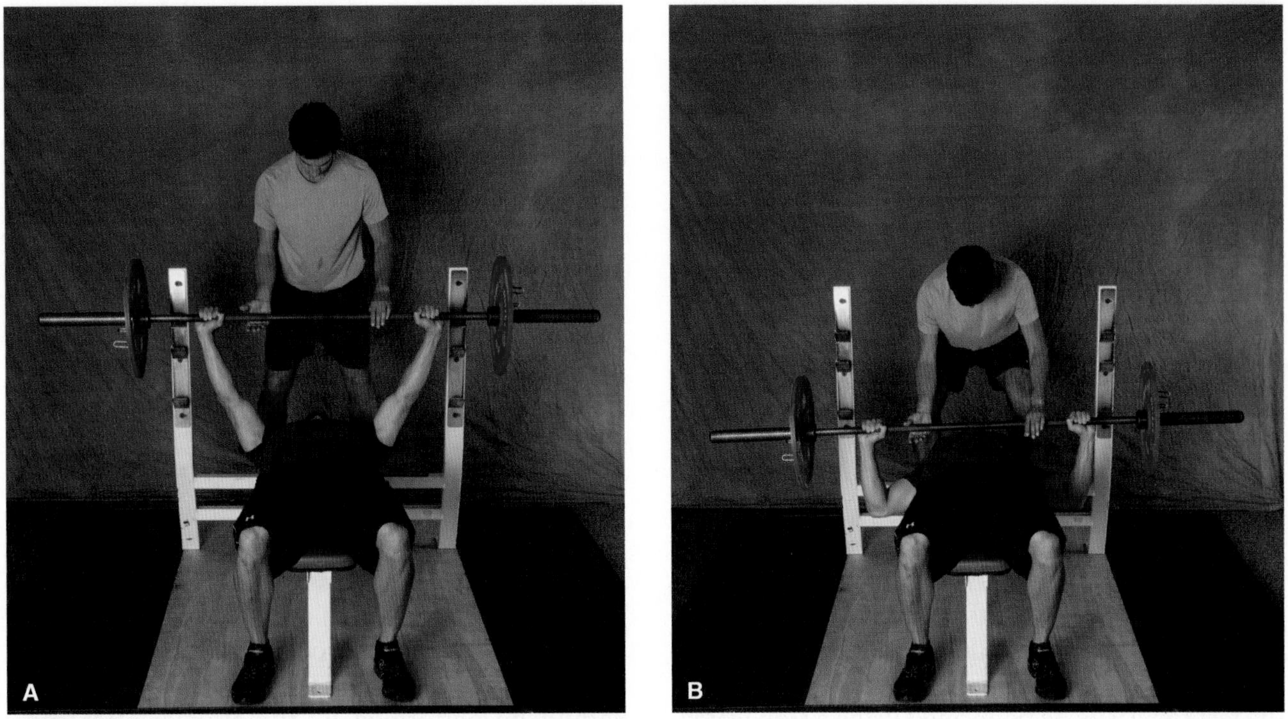

FIGURE 8.9 Bench press. **A.** Starting position. **B.** Downward movement.

complete as many successful push-ups as possible. The examiner will record the total number of successful repetitions.

Sit-Up Test

Whereas the push-up test assesses upper body muscular endurance, the sit-up test evaluates local endurance of the abdominal musculature. This test will require an assistant to secure the athlete's feet during testing in addition to an examiner who will monitor both the elapsed time and the number of repetitions performed. To begin the assessment, the athlete should be instructed to lay supine on a flat, nonslip surface with the knees positioned at a 90-degree angle. A successful repetition entails crossing of the arms over the chest, contraction of the abdominal musculature to flex the trunk into a full upright position, and a controlled return to the initial starting position (Fig. 8.11). Upon issuing a verbal command to indicate that the test has begun, the examiner will count the number of successful repetitions performed in 1 minute.

Forty-Yard Sprint

The 40-yd sprint is another highly functional test to gauge total lower body power (Fig. 8.12).

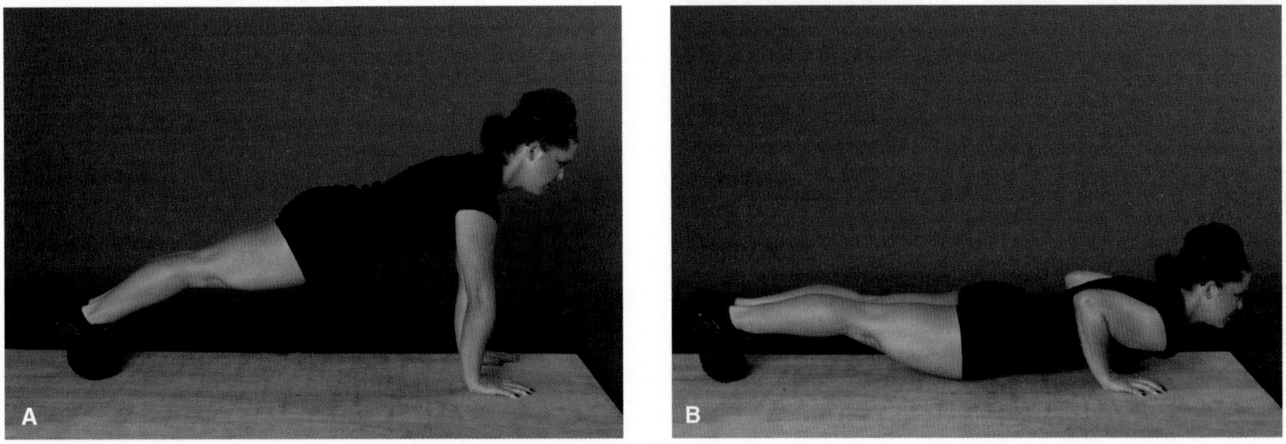

FIGURE 8.10 Push-up test. **A.** Starting position. **B.** Downward movement.

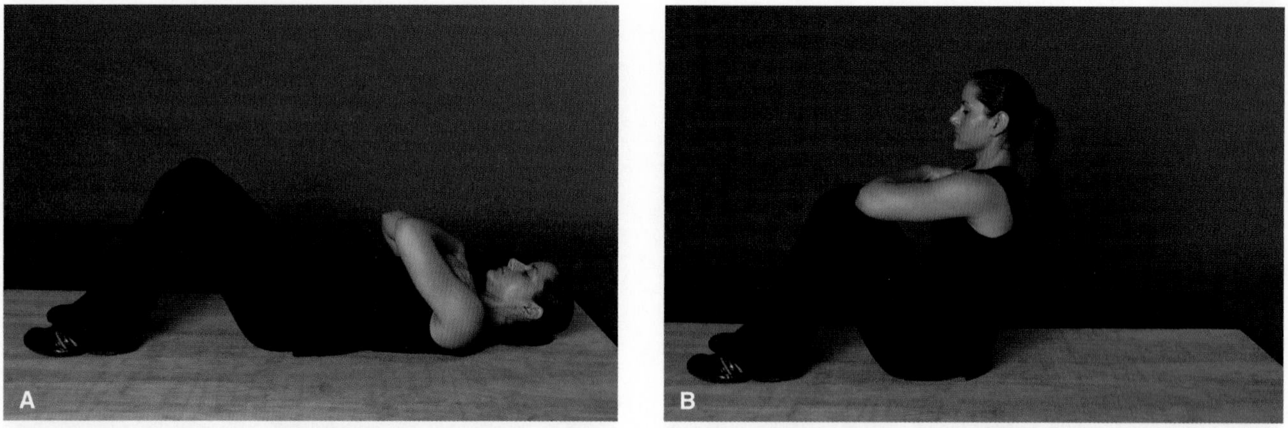

FIGURE 8.11 Sit-up test.

Sprinting at top speed is a skill required in many sports. Therefore, the 40-yd sprint is often a good test to include, as its performance may have direct application to many athletes' sports. Although many highly accurate timing devices are available, the test can easily be performed using a stop watch.

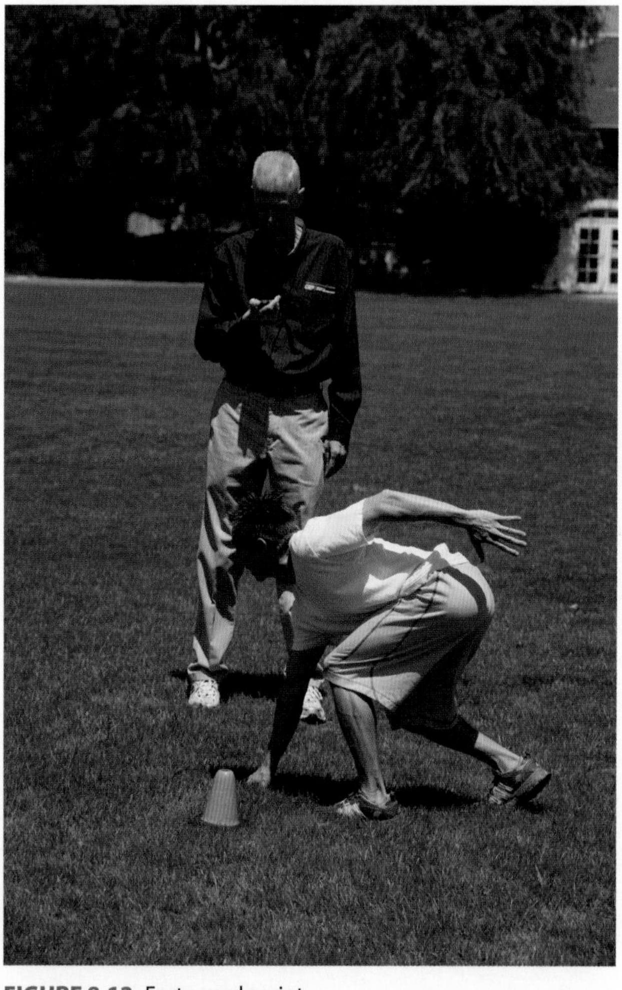

FIGURE 8.12 Forty-yard sprint.

To assess a 40-yd sprint speed, obtain the appropriate space necessary to perform the test (e.g., a straight section of track). As usual, a general and specific warm-up consisting of light aerobic activity and a few submaximal trials, respectively, should be performed by the athlete. After completing the trial runs, have the athlete get into the starting position by assuming a 4-point stance. On the tester's cue or following some other auditory stimulus, the athlete will sprint the premarked 40-yd distance, with the best of two trials recorded for later assessment.

One negative aspect of this test, however, is its potential to be overemphasized. In fact, such importance is placed on this test that highly competitive athletes often spend a great deal of time and effort practicing form drills in the hopes of running a few tenths of a second faster. Although this is a very functional and useful test, its results should be used in conjunction with other tests to identify an athlete's strengths and weaknesses. It should not be used as a direct predictor of how he or she will perform on the field.

T-Test

The T-test assesses change of direction ability in the forward and lateral planes (Fig. 8.13). This test requires four cones placed in the shape of a "T." The athlete will begin the test at the base of the 'T' in the standing position. The athlete will then sprint 10 yd forward to the first cone, shuffle laterally 5 yd to the left cone without crossing his or her feet, shuffle laterally 10 yd to the far right cone, shuffle 5 yd left back toward the center cone, and end with a 10-yd backpedal to the starting point.

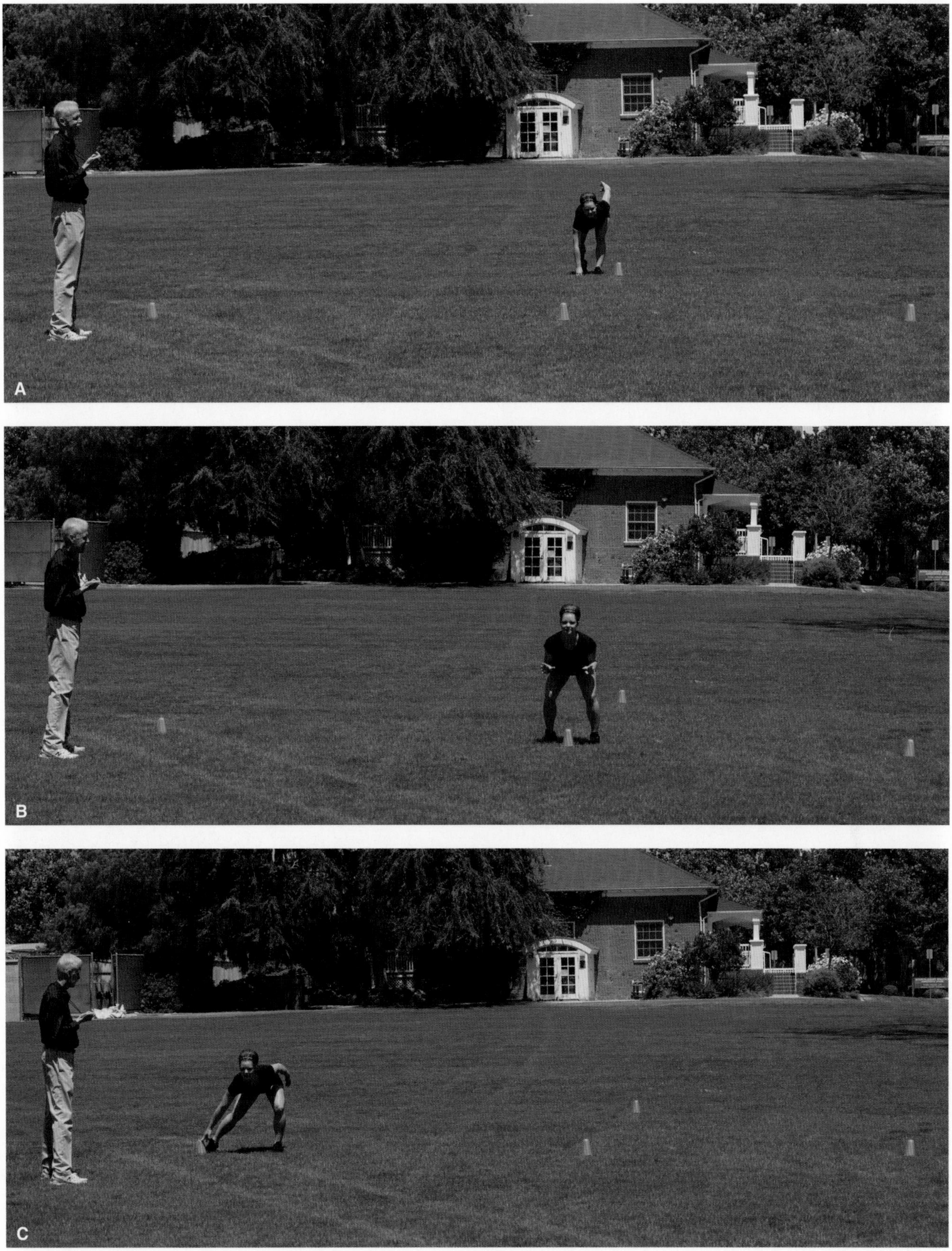

FIGURE 8.13 T-test. A. Starting position. B. Sprint forward. C. Shuffle right.

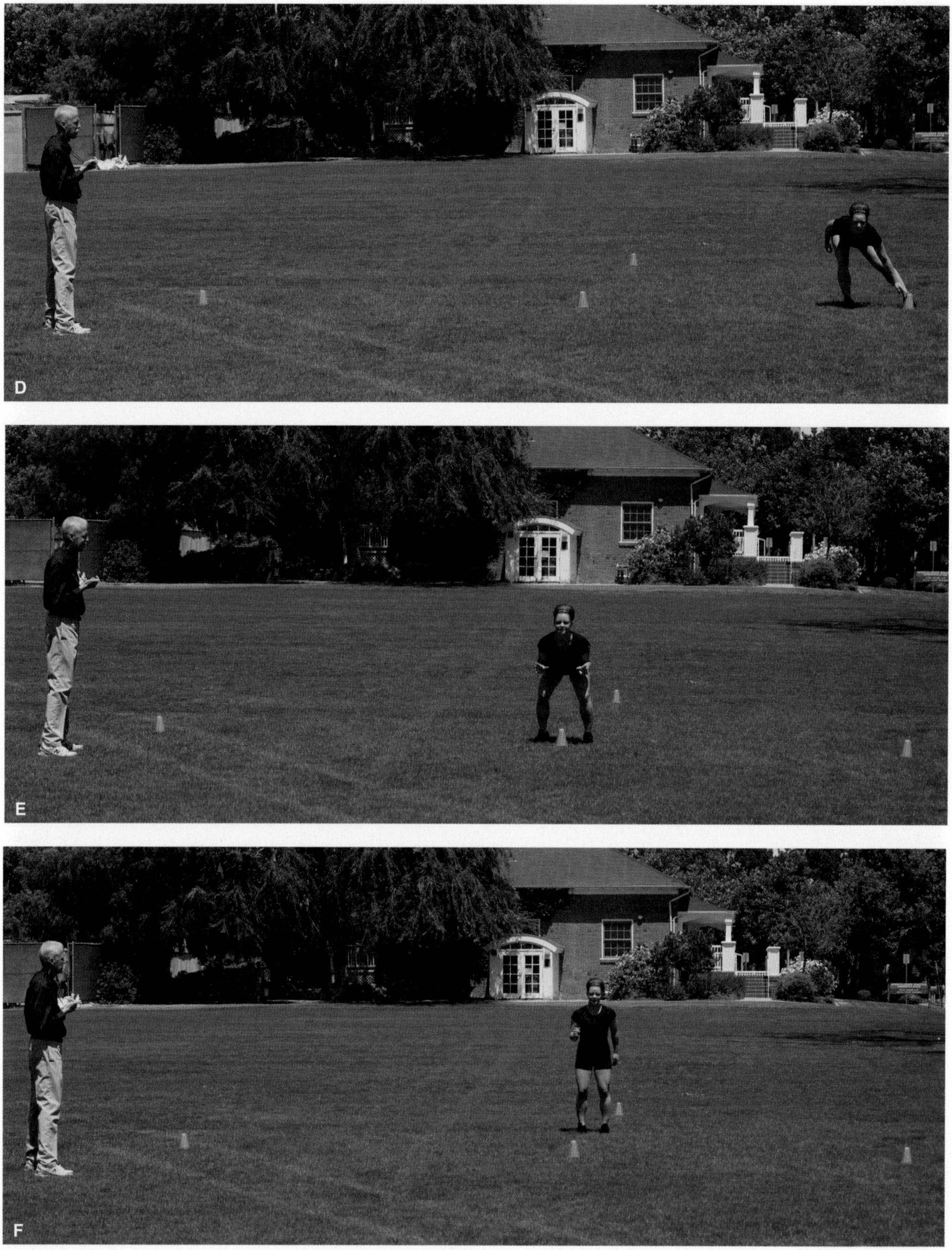

FIGURE 8.13 *(continued)* **D.** Shuffle left to far cone. **E.** Shuffle right to center cone. **F.** Backpedal to starting position.

Five—Ten–Five Shuttle

The 5–10–5 shuttle, or proagility test, is another frequently employed agility test (Fig. 8.14). The NFL combine administers the 5–10–5 shuttle as part of its test battery to assess potential draftees. This test assesses change-of-direction ability in a linear plane and it only requires three cones placed in a straight line 5 yd apart. The athlete will begin the test behind the center cone in a two point stance. The test begins when the athlete initiates movement on his or her own and sprints 5 yd to the left, touches the cone, 10 yd to the right, touches the cone, and finally 5 yd left across the starting position.

Standing Long Jump

The standing long jump is also a good functional test that measures the total lower body power (Fig. 8.15). Although the vertical jump is used to measure vertical power, the long jump is used to measure horizontal power. Being another test of lower body power, it too is a good choice for athletes requiring speed, agility, and quickness. The test is very easy to conduct; a tape measure and an open space with a flat surface are the primary requirements. First, place a piece of masking tape or other heavy-duty tape on the testing surface to serve as a starting line. Then have the athlete get into the starting position by standing with their

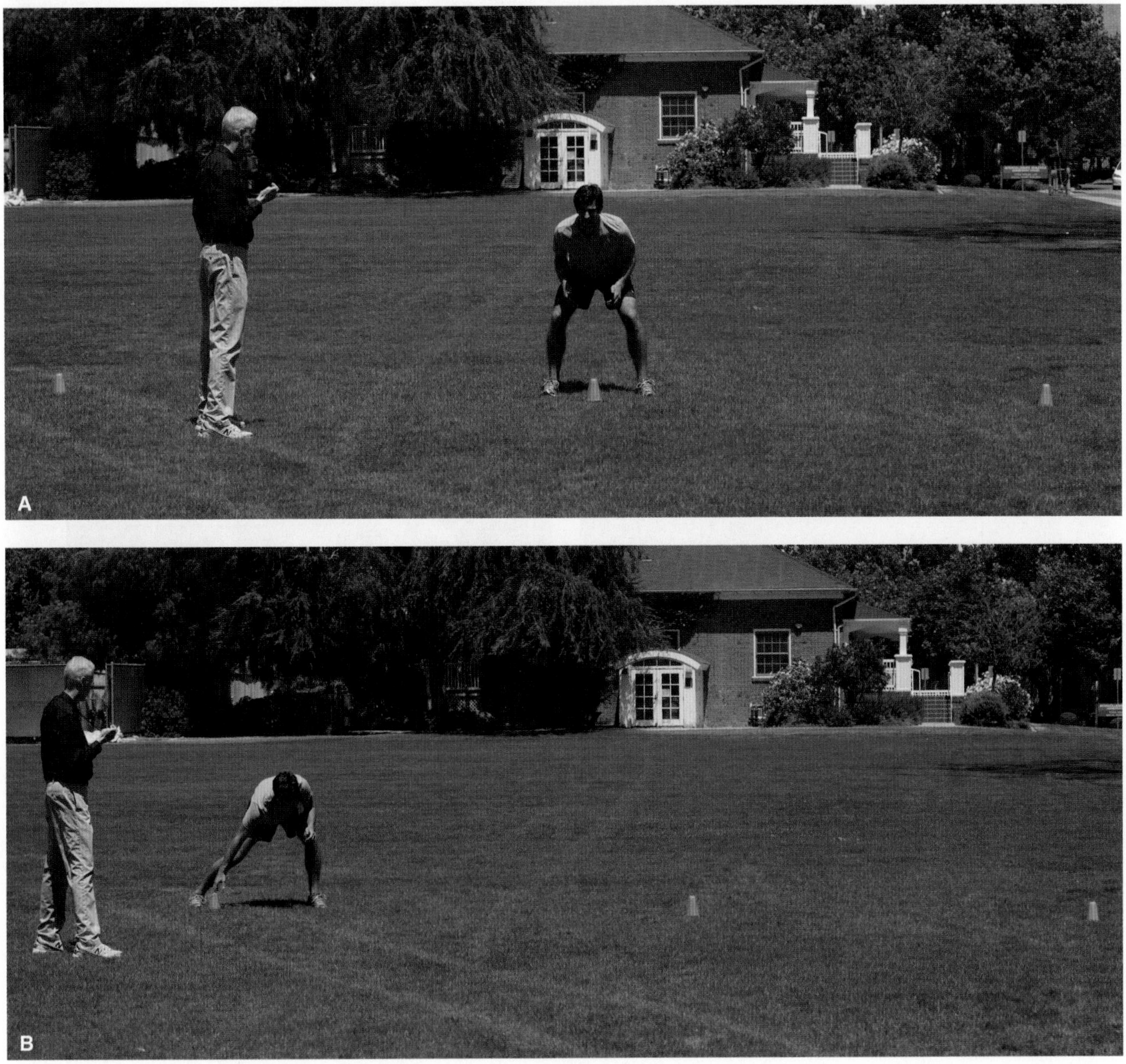

FIGURE 8.14 Five—ten–five shuttle. **A.** Starting position. **B.** Sprint right.

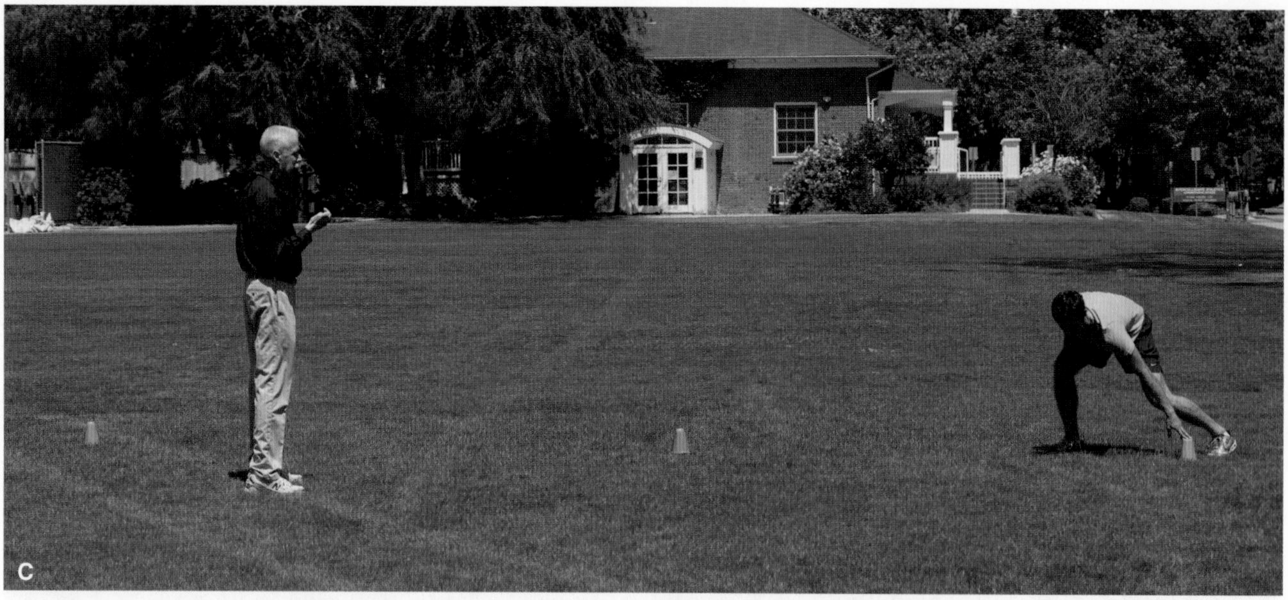

FIGURE 8.14 *(continued)* **C.** Sprint left, then back past the center cone.

toes behind the line. Instruct the athlete to jump as far as possible using a single countermovement. For the jump to be considered successful, the athlete must land with both feet without any disturbances to his or her balance. If the jump is deemed successful, the distance between the starting line and the point behind the athlete's heels constitute the jump distance. Have the athlete complete three trials with the best score recorded for later assessment.

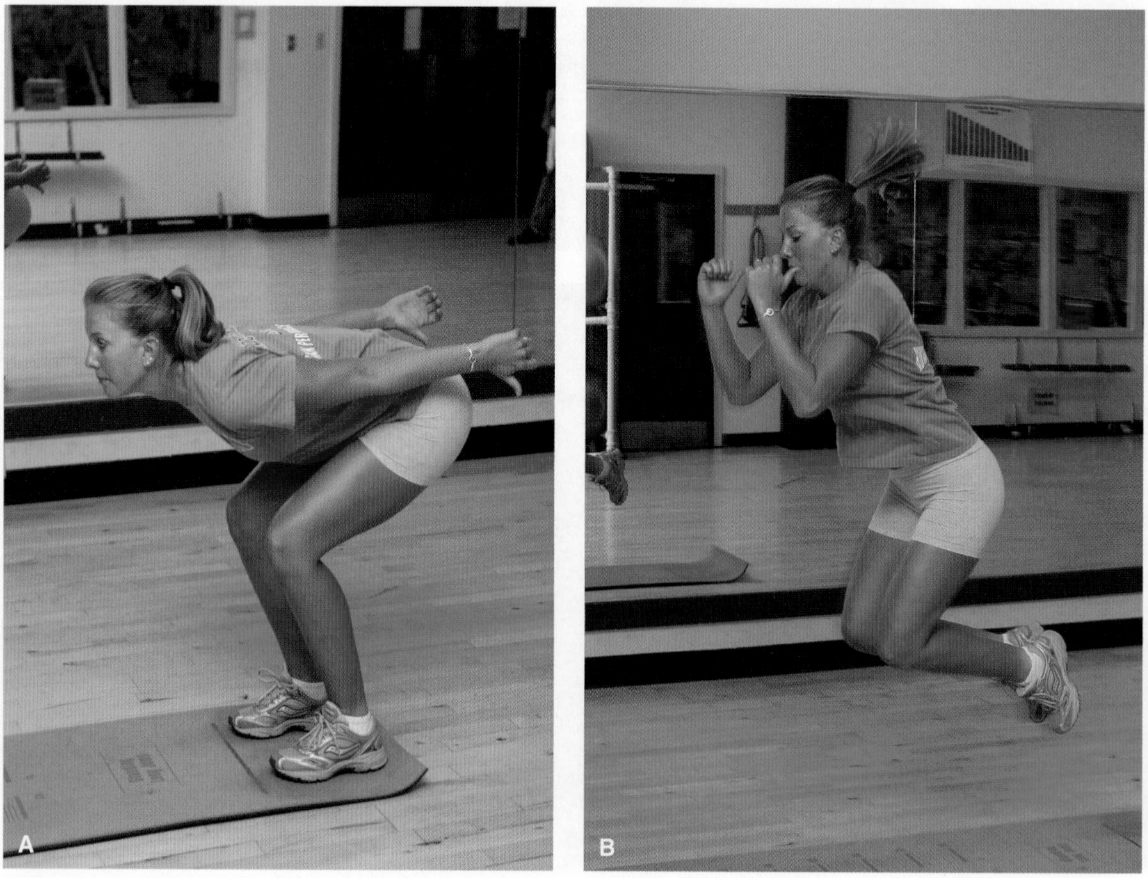

FIGURE 8.15 Standing long jump. **A.** Starting position. **B.** Jump.

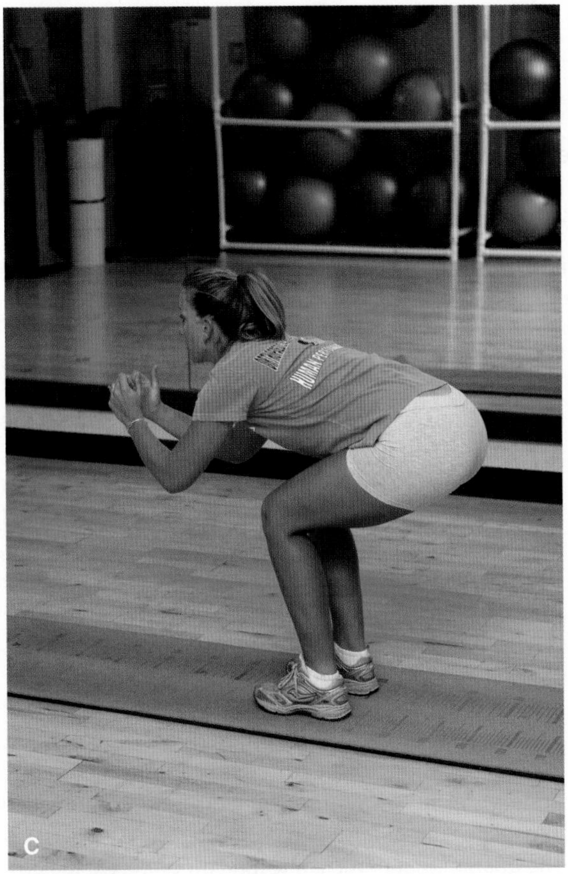

FIGURE 8.15 *(continued)* **C.** Landing.

Although this is a valid measure of lower body power, the standing long jump is a movement pattern that is not specific to many sports. Therefore, other field tests, such as the 40-yd sprint test and vertical jump may have more specific applications for many athletes.

TEST INTERPRETATION

Administering a test and recording a measurement are the simple portions of any assessment routine. The final and most complicated portion is making an evaluation of those scores. This involves placing a value on the recorded score so it may be used to help design a program of training specific to the individual. In order to accomplish this, the scores must be put into a logical order and analyzed for practical significance. Once the scores have been collected they must be compared to a proper criterion or normative scale based on the subpopulation (20–22). The scope of this book does not allow an in-depth discussion of statistical significance and therefore this discourse will focus on practical uses of test scores.

Once the test data are collected, they should be accurately interpreted to the coach and the athlete in terms of norms and expected improvement.

ORDER SCALES

Test scores fall into three main categories. Nominal scores are those that are coded for entry into a spreadsheet or statistical computer program. They represent the "real" item through the use of numbers. An example is coding gender as one for men and two for women or vice versa. One might also use a code for positional differences on an athletic team such as one for outside hitters and two for setters and three for middle blockers on a volleyball team. This procedure allows the tester to add up the number of participants who possess similar characteristics but not to perform mathematical calculations on those values.

Interval scores are those that do not possess an absolute zero, meaning that zero does not represent the absence of that variable, but that it sometimes contains negative scores and there is no standard unit of difference between scores. The most popular form of interval scoring is temperature expressed in Fahrenheit degrees. Freezing is expressed as 32 degrees; zero does not constitute no temperature, negative numbers are used to express colder temperatures, and 66 degrees is not twice as warm as 33 degrees.

Ratio scores possess all the traits not held by interval. They have an absolute zero, meaning a zero score is an absence of that variable, as in an elderly person's vertical jump score of 0 in. They contain no negative numbers and there is an absolute scale of measurement between scores, such that lifting 50 lb is exactly half as much as lifting 100 lb. This is the most popular form of physiological measurement and is predominantly used in physical activity literature and testing.

Sometimes a fourth form of scoring order is expressed as **ordinal**, which is more accurately described as a ranking system rather than a scoring scale. An ordinal system ranks scores from top to bottom or highest to lowest or greatest to least. All the other scales of measurements can be listed in ordinal rank but it does not change them from their original scaling form.

MATHEMATICAL MEASURES

There are a few variables associated with central tendency that need to be discussed so the investigator

Q & A from the Field

Q ***The head S and C coach for the football team at our university only uses four tests for the players: the 40-yd dash, vertical jump, 1RM squat, and 1RM bench press. We had such a great season last year, winning our conference championship, so the tests seem adequate, but should we be doing more?***

—graduate student intern

A Certainly we must take many things into consideration when designing a testing program. A mature, well-trained group of players might be able to continue to perform well with minimal testing. In order to determine the appropriate tests, we need to review the basic rationale for testing athletes. Remember the primary reasons for testing:

1. To determine the fitness base of the athlete
2. To determine the performance characteristics of the better players in the sport, and
3. To motivate the athletes to continue to train hard

There are other possible reasons for testing. One reason might be that the S and C coach is in the process of justifying his position on the coaching staff. Good solid data demonstrating improvement in a number of performance characteristics in the teams he trains would provide solid evidence that he is performing an important service for those athletes.

To get a total picture of the fitness base of the athlete, you will likely need tests in a number of areas of performance. These areas might include

1. Upper body strength
2. Lower body strength
3. Upper body endurance
4. Lower body endurance
5. Upper body power
6. Lower body power
7. Aerobic capacity
8. Speed
9. Speed endurance
10. Maximal anaerobic capacity

You may choose some tests that overlap two of these characteristics, or you may determine that a test is not appropriate for a particular sport. Maximal anaerobic capacity tests that cause a dramatic rise in lactic acid production might not be appropriate for a golfer, for example. Do recall, however, that aerobic capacity is used in recovery, even in anaerobic sports.

Remember also that we base our decisions about the type of training program needed on the testing results. In a mature, highly performing group of athletes, it is possible that the training protocols are well established and the testing data will not greatly affect the program. Thus, a minimal testing program might work in some specific situations. Spending less time testing allows more time for conditioning or practice of the sport, which might be an advantage in some situations.

In summary, there are several reasons to consider adding tests to the testing program described above. It is also possible to spend too much time and energy testing, taking away from training time and practice time. The correct answer to your question depends on the goals of that particular testing program. Do the athletes need more motivation to train hard? Additional tests may provide the additional motivation the athletes need. Is it important for the S snd C coach to provide data to justify his value to the team? Additional tests may prove his importance. Do the chosen tests adequately represent the physical requirements of the sport? If not, additional tests may provide the missing data. Are the tests position-specific? In football, physical demands of different positions can vary. A 40-yd dash may be appropriate for backs, while a 10- or 20-yd dash may be more appropriate for lineman. Matching testing to position-specific physical requirements will provide useful information. The training program should provide position-specific benefits to the individual athlete.

Every group of athletes will be different to some extent, and the philosophy of conditioning programs will vary from school to school as well. An S and C coach is constantly thinking about what he can do to keep the motivation high, to keep the athletes working hard, and to keep a positive attitude toward the training. The testing program should evaluate improvement in performance that is specific to the sport of football as well as to the athlete's position. A properly designed testing program can be a key component of the program!

may draw conclusions from the collected data. They are fundamental in nature and require little mathematical skill but will provide the tester with valuable information regarding the data as a whole and each individual's relationship to the overall group.

Minimum and **maximum** refer to the least score and the greatest score, respectively.

Range is the difference between the minimum and maximum and represents the overall spread of scores as a whole number. The formula is max – min.

Sum is the total of all scores combined and added together. The formula is $x_1 + x_2 + x_3 + x_4$, etc.

N is the symbol used to denote the number of people in the test group and is used in conjunction with the sum to arrive at other important variables.

Mean is simply the arithmetic average derived from the sum divided by N. It is the most sensitive of all measures of central tendency and is also used most often. It considers every score in the group and is pulled away from the middle by extreme scores. The formula is sum/N.

Median is the exact middle of the total number of scores. It is not affected by outliers, shows a position only and is rarely used for any statistical calculations. To find the median, the scores should first be placed in an ordinal ranking, and then if there is an odd number of scores, the median will be the middle score (e.g., if 11 scores then median is score #6 since 5 scores are greater and 5 scores are less). If there is an even number of scores, then the median will be an average of the two middle scores (e.g., if 12 scores then median is the average of score 6 and 7).

Mode is the score that occurs most frequently. There may be multiple modes or there may not be a mode at all. It is also not affected by extreme scores, nor is it used frequently in statistical calculations.

DISTRIBUTION OF SCORES

Once all the scores have been collected, it is beneficial to determine their measures of central tendency. **Central tendency** is the measure of the middle of a distribution of scores. The measurement community relies on scores following a few basic rules, which causes them to take familiar shapes when presented graphically. The scores can then be analyzed using basic statistical assumptions. Figure 8.16 displays a normal bell curve, the basic element and starting point of many statistical techniques. The bell curve is a frequency histogram that plots the number of times a score occurs on the vertical, or Y axis, against the raw number itself on the horizontal or X axis where scores increase as they move from left to right. The conventional hump in the middle demonstrates that the greatest number of scores fall in the middle range with fewer and fewer scores out to either side. Most tests will produce a graph that is, at least in part, similar to a bell curve. In other words, there will be a few very low and very high scores with the majority of scores being very similar. It is of paramount importance to remember that while many statistical calculations are based on the bell curve, *it almost never occurs in real-life data*. Therefore, there is a bit of error built into all statistics, and they should always be read with this in mind. The only true bell curve is when the mean, median, and mode are exactly the same number.

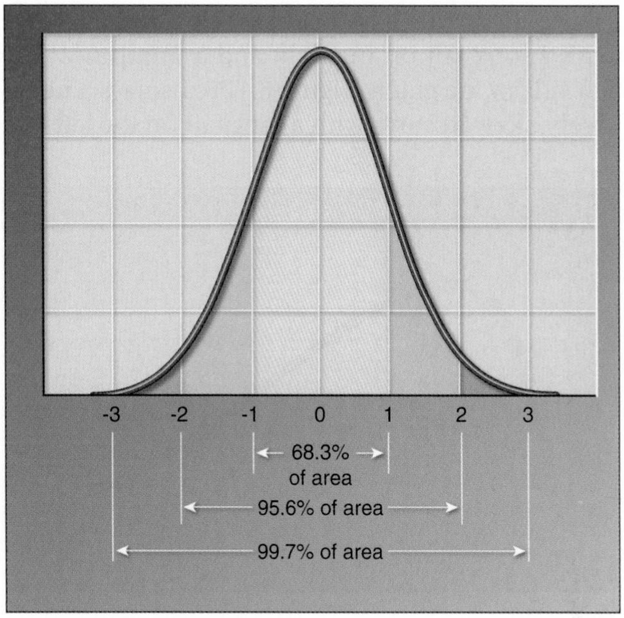

FIGURE 8.16 Normal bell curve. This commonly occurring frequency histogram demonstrates that the greatest number of scores falls in the middle range, with fewer scores at the extremes.

The hump in the bell curve shows the likeness of scores. If many of the athletes scored similarly, then the hump will be tall and thin, whereas a group with many varied scores will be short and flat. In some instances the curve does not follow such a symmetrical shape as that of the bell curve.

Figure 8.17A displays a **positively skewed** curve with a long tail on the right and a hump near the left side of the graph. Figure 8.17B displays a **negatively skewed** curve with a long tail on the left and a hump near the right side of the graph. There are even times when a group of scores may produce multiple humps. Figure 8.17C displays a **bimodal curve** where the frequency of scores was greatest in two different portions of the final outcome. Since the hump exhibits similarity of scores, a bimodal curve may reveal that the group contains two like groups of people (e.g., two genders, two athletic teams, etc.).

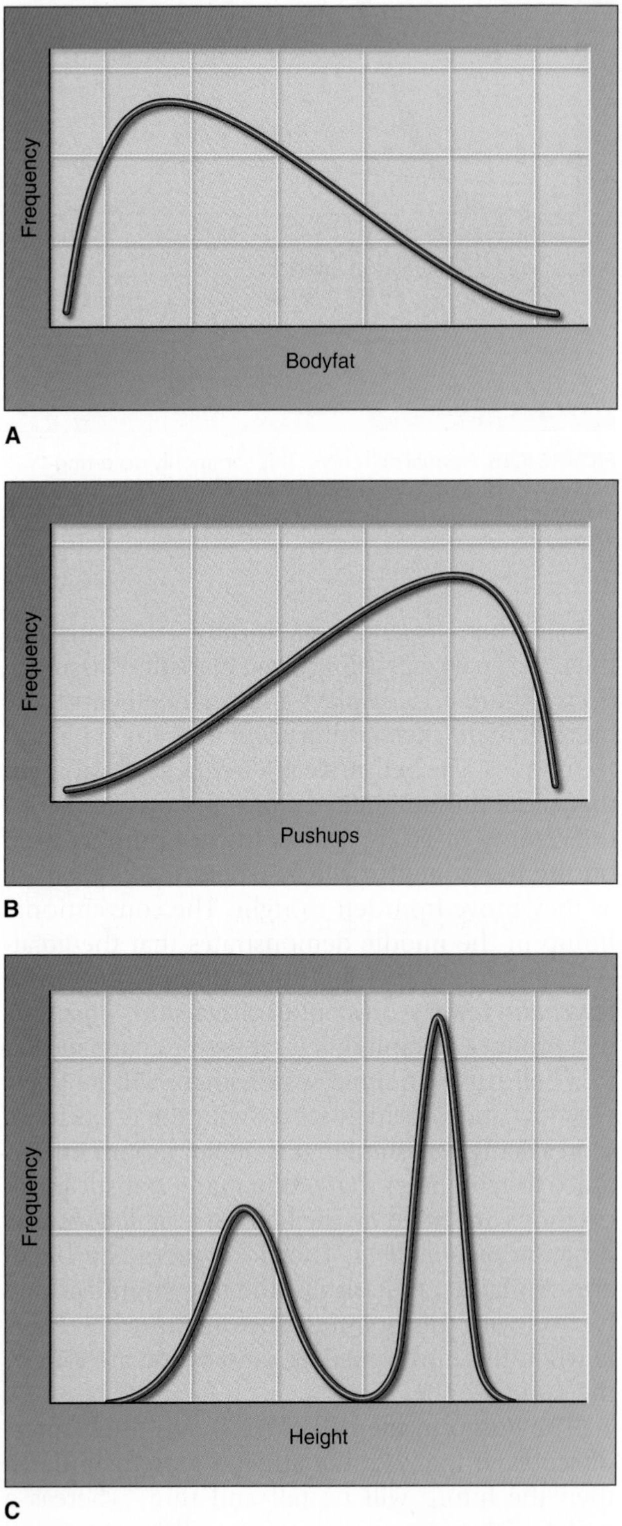

FIGURE 8.17 Likeness of scores shown by humps on graphs. **A.** Positively skewed curve. **B.** Negatively skewed curve. **C.** Bimodal curve.

VARIABILITY

The most commonly used measure of variability in scores is the **standard deviation (SD)**. It describes the scatter of scores about the mean and is used to show inclusion of scores for different percentages of the population and can be used as a measure of homogeneity when compared to the mean. It is derived through a few simple mathematical steps.

1. Calculate the deviation of each score from the mean by subtracting the mean from each raw score. Half of the deviation scores will be negative since half the scores will fall below the mean. Do not let this concern you as it will be remedied in the next step.
2. Square each deviation score by multiplying it by itself. This will convert all negative scores to positive scores.
3. Add all the squared deviations together to arrive at a sum.
4. Divide the sum of the squared deviations by $N - 1$ (e.g., if $N = 11$, then divide by 10) the answer is termed the **variance**. By eliminating one participant from the group it will better assist the tester in using the resultant data to predict the performance of other similar groups that were not tested.
5. Take the square root of the variance to counterbalance the squaring process performed earlier in the Step 2. The answer is the SD.

Now the SD can be used to explain the variability of scores previously displayed in the bell curve. Figure 8.16 shows how the mean and SD can be used to calculate group inclusion numbers. Simply stated, the mean plus or minus 1-SD includes approximately 68% of the total group population. In other words, if following a test the scores revealed a mean of 25 and an SD of 10, then it could be stated that approximately 68% of the group population had scores between 15 and 35 (e.g., 25–10 = 15 and 25 + 10 = 35). If $N = 75$, then 68% of that population would be 51 (e.g., 75 × 0.68). Likewise, the mean plus or minus 2-SD includes approximately 95% of the population while the mean plus or minus 3-SD includes approximately 99% or almost everyone in the test population. Remember that, since the bell curve almost never occurs (mean, median, and mode must be exactly the same number), there is always some error in the system. Therefore, the percentages rarely fall directly on those numbers but are most often close.

STANDARDIZED SCORES

Another important use for the SD is to calculate **standardized scores**. These are scores that express each individual score as an SD making it easier to determine each score's standard distance from the mean. This procedure allows tests with different units of measurement to be compared without confusion (e.g., vertical jump in inches vs. 1RM in pounds). They are, therefore, very popularly used with standardized tests of knowledge or for large population groups following administration of a test battery.

Standardized scores are divided into two types. First are **Z-scores**, which range between −3 and +3 and are expressed out to two decimal places. They are calculated by subtracting the mean from the raw score and then dividing by the SD. If a raw score was 35 and the mean was 25 with an SD of 10, then the equation would be (35 − 25)/10 = 1. The resultant Z-score of 1 means that the raw score of 35 is exactly 1 SD greater than the mean. Consequently, the average Z-score is zero and all positive Z-scores are raw scores greater than the mean while all negative Z-scores are raw scores that are less than the mean.

Second, **T-scores**, which range from 30 to 80 are almost identical to Z-scores. They are the same because they are derived from Z-scores. The procedure for T-scores is to multiply the Z-score by 10 and then add 50. T-scores are always positive whole numbers (i.e., no decimal places). Consequently, the average T-score is 50 and all T-scores greater than 50 are raw scores greater than the mean while all T-scores less than 50 are raw scores that are less than the mean. T-scores are used because the resultant value is always positive and easy to understand by the lay person.

Summary

A valid and reliable evaluation and assessment program begins with a careful needs analysis of both the client/athlete and the activity/sport. Appropriate tests are then chosen based on the individual needs of the situation and the results are carefully analyzed using the basic mathematical calculations of central tendency and variability. By performing these simple calculations, assumptions can be made regarding the value of each score for each participant. Scores can then be compared to population specific normative values or a criterion scale developed from those norms. In the final analysis the well-prepared and knowledgeable tester will be able to evaluate each individual's needs and subsequently prescribe an appropriate training program to meet the derived client-specific goals.

Maxing Out

1. A graduate student wanted to know something about the vertical jump of her classmates. She tested each one in the class and came up with the data set below: 19.5, 20, 21.5, 18, 17.5, 16, 22.5, 25, 24.5, 17.5. Find the mean, median, and mode of the data set and explain how to use these numbers to describe a team to a coach.
2. The basketball coach comes to you and wants an assessment of the team. You plan to do a "needs analysis" looking at both the individual player and the game of basketball. List the tests you will need to perform to answer the coach's query regarding the state of his team.
3. A colleague of yours has just developed a new assessment tool and has come to you in order for you to establish the validity and reliability of the new tool. What would you do to establish both validity and reliability of this tool? How are the two different?

CASE EXAMPLE

Designing a Performance Testing Program for an Elite Junior Tennis Athlete

BACKGROUND

You are employed in a major, well-equipped sports facility with all testing equipment available to you. You are told to prepare for a complete fitness evaluation of a 16-year-old, nationally ranked male tennis player preparing to turn pro. The player is the current national champion in the 16-and-under age group. He was first runner-up in the Junior US Open this year.

The athlete is experienced in all areas of training and conditioning. He uses free weight resistance training regularly in his program, and performs a variety of multijoint and Olympic-style lifts. He participates in a variety of speed and agility training exercises.

The athlete does participate in clay court tournaments from time to time, but his primary surface, and the surface his game is expected to excel on is a hard court surface.

Using needs analysis of the sport of tennis and a typical tennis athlete, design a complete fitness testing session to evaluate this athlete.

RECOMMENDATIONS/CONSIDERATIONS

Begin with a needs analysis of the sport of tennis. Professional tennis is an explosive fast game, particularly on hard court surfaces. The tennis athlete is required to change directions rapidly several times in a point. The ability to generate ground reaction force and transfer that force to the upper body is a key component of success in tennis. The testing program for this athlete will likely include tests for the following: muscular endurance, lower extremity muscular strength, lower extremity power, upper extremity muscular strength, upper extremity power, speed, agility, cardiorespiratory endurance, and joint range of motion. Injuries should be noted, and the musculoskeletal adaptations to those injuries should be considered.

IMPLEMENTATION

Maximal treadmill test with metabolic cart. Although tennis is primarily an anaerobic sport, recovery between points is aerobic. Moderate to moderately high levels of oxygen consumption are desirable in the tennis athlete. This test will provide information on the athlete's ability to work aerobically, and to recover between points.

Bench press. Since the athlete trains using free weights, the bench press is a good measure of upper body strength.

Squat. Again, since the athlete trains with free weights, the squat is a good choice for measuring overall lower extremity strength. The ability of a tennis player to generate ground reaction force is a key component of tennis performance.

Vertical jump. The vertical jump is an excellent choice to measure lower body power. Performance on this test is relevant to tennis as it is an indicator of the ability of the athlete to get a quick start, and may also be an indicator of the athlete's ability to generate power in the service motion.

Seated medicine ball push. This test is a measure of general upper body power.

Twenty-yard dash. Speed in tennis is limited to short distances, and 20 yd would be the maximum a player would have to run all out without stopping or changing direction.

Hexagon. This test is used to measure footwork and agility.

"T" test. This test measures lateral, backward, and forward movement over a short distance and the ability to transition among each form of locomotion.

Five-point agility run. This test measures the ability of the athlete to move in diagonal patterns, changing direction, gaining speed, decelerating, and stopping.

Underwater weighing. Measuring body composition using underwater-weighing techniques is an accurate way to determine body composition.

Push-ups in 60 seconds. In this athlete, push-ups are a test of upper body muscular endurance. In the athlete who can only perform a few push-ups, it becomes a test of muscular strength.

Sit-ups in 60 seconds. Sit-ups are a general measure of core body strength and endurance. The trunk is very important in tennis as it transfers forces from the ground to the upper extremity.

CASE EXAMPLE (*Continued*)

Designing a Performance Testing Program for an Elite Junior Tennis Athlete

RESULTS

Results are reported by percentile rank using a database of over 100 16-year-old male tennis athletes.

Maximal treadmill test with metabolic cart: 90th percentile
Bench press: 96th percentile
Squat: 91st percentile
Vertical jump: 60th percentile
Seated medicine ball push: 88th percentile
Twenty-yd dash: 88th percentile
Hexagon: 85th percentile
"T" test: 89th percentile
Five-point agility run: 87th percentile
Underwater weighing: 90th percentile

These results should be reported to the athlete, the coach, and/or the parents of the player. The one area of athletic fitness that obviously needs the most work is lower body power. Remember when conveying results to the player to point needed areas of improvement and prescribe appropriate exercise regimens to correct the identified deficits.

REFERENCES

1. Dolezal BA, Thompson CJ, Schroeder CA, et al. Laboratory testing to improve athletic performance. *Strength Cond.* 1997;19(6):20–24.
2. Enoka RM. *Neuromechanical Basis of Kinesiology.* Champaign, IL: Human Kinetics; 1988.
3. Magill RA. *Motor learning: Concepts and Applications.* 5th ed. Madison, WI: Brown & Benchmark Publishers; 1998.
4. Brown LE, Weir JP. ASEP procedures recommendations for the accurate assessment of muscular strength and power. *J Exer Physiol.* [serial online] 2001;4(3): 1–21. Available at: http://faculty.css.edu/tboone2/asep/August2001JEPonline.html. Accessed October 16, 2003.
5. Conway DP, Decker AS. Utilizing a computerized strength and conditioning testing index for assessment of collegiate football players. *Natl Strength Cond Assoc J.* 1992;14(5):13–16.
6. Graham J. Guidelines for providing valid testing of athletes' fitness levels. *Strength Cond.* 1994;16(6):7–14.
7. Brown LE, Whitehurst M, Bryant JR. A comparison of the LIDO sliding cuff and the tibial control system in isokinetic strength parameters. *Isokinet Exer Sci.* 1992;2(3):101–109.
8. Brown LE, Whitehurst M, Bryant JR. Reliability of the LIDO active isokinetic dynamometer concentric mode. *Isokinet Exer Sci.* 1992;2(4):191–194.
9. Brown LE, Whitehurst M, Bryant JR, et al. Reliability of the Biodex system 2 isokinetic dynamometer concentric mode. *Isokinet Exer Sci.* 1993;3(3):160–163.
10. Chinn S, Burney PGJ. On measuring repeatability of data from self-administered questionnaires. *Int J Epidemiol.* 1987;16:121–127.
11. Stockbrugger BA, Haennel RG. Validity and reliability of a medicine ball explosive power test. *J Strength Cond Res.* 2001;15(4):431–438.
12. Plisk SS. Anaerobic metabolic conditioning: A brief review of theory, strategy and practical application. *J Strength Cond Res.* 1991;5(1):22–34.
13. Plisk SS, Gambetta V. Tactical metabolic training: Part 1. *Strength Cond.* 1997;19(2):44–53.
14. Bar-Or O. The Wingate test: an update on methodology, reliability and validity. *Sports Med.* 1987;4:381–394.
15. Maud PJ, Shultz BB. Norms for the Wingate anaerobic test with comparison to another similar test. *Res Quart Exer Sport.* 1989;60:144–151.
16. Patton JF, Duggan A. An evaluation of tests of anaerobic power. *Aviation Space Environ Med.* 1987;58:237–242.
17. Swank AM, Adams K, Serapiglia L, et al. Submaximal testing for the strength and conditioning professional. *Strength Cond J.* 1999;21(6):9–15.
18. Taylor NAS, Sanders RH, Howick EI, et al. Static and dynamic assessment of the Biodex dynamometer. *Eur J Appl Physiol.* 1991;62:180–188.
19. Chapman PP, Whitehead JR, Binkert RH. The 225-lb reps-to-fatigue test as a submaximal estimate of 1-RM bench press performance in college football players. *J Strength Cond Res.* 1998;12:258–261.
20. Mayhew JL, Ware JR, Prinster JL. Using lift repetitions to predict muscular strength in adolescent males. *Natl Strength Cond Assoc J.* 1993;15(6):35–38.
21. Schweigert D. Normative values for common preseason testing protocols: NCAA division II women's basketball. *Strength Cond.* 1996;18(6):7–10.
22. Semenick D, Connors J, Carter M, et al. Rationale, protocols, testing/reporting forms and instructions for wrestling. *Natl Strength Cond Assoc J.* 1992;14(3):54–59.
23. Timm KE, Fyke D. The effect of test speed sequence on the concentric isokinetic performance of the knee extensor muscle group. *Isok Exerc Sci.* 1993;3(2):123–128.

CHAPTER 9

Warm-Up and Flexibility

DUANE V. KNUDSON

OBJECTIVES

After reading this chapter, you will be able to:

- Explain the difference between warm-up and stretching.
- Identify different kinds of warm-up protocols.
- Define flexibility and several mechanical variables that describe it.
- Recall the ways to measure flexibility.
- Describe ways to increase flexibility by using various stretches and understand their benefits.
- Recall the recommended exercise prescription for stretching.

KEY TERMS

Active Warm-Up
Ankylosis
Ballistic Stretching
Dynamic Stretching
Elasticity
Flexibility
Golgi Tendon Organs
Hypermobility
Hysteresis
Mechanical Strength
Muscle Spindles
Passive Stretching
Passive Warm-Up
Static Flexibility
Static Stretching
Stiffness
Stress Relaxation
Thixotropy
Viscoelastic
Warm-Up

Introduction

Athletes looking to improve sport performance or lengthen their athletic careers by reducing the risk of injury—as well as the exercising public—often focus on warm-up and flexibility routines in their training. Considerable research has been conducted on both of these issues, and with a rapid expansion in the number of studies in the last 20 years, a new picture is emerging on these important fitness issues. The consensus of the current research is supportive of training and injury-prevention beliefs related to warm-up. Tradition hypotheses about flexibility and stretching, however, are changing. This chapter summarizes what is known about the performance and injury-prevention benefits of warm-up and flexibility. These two important fitness concepts have complex relationships to performance and the risk of musculoskeletal injury. The chapter concludes with general recommendations for prescribing stretching exercises and programs.

WARM-UP

It is important to realize that warm-up and stretching are two different activities. Warm-up is designed to elevate core body temperature and stretching is primarily performed to increase the range of motion (ROM) at a joint or group of joints. It is well accepted that generalized warm-up movements are important to maximizing sport performance and reducing injury risk in physical activity. **Warm-up** consists of active or passive warming of body tissues in preparation for physical activity. **Active warm-up** consists of low-intensity movements that are effective in elevating body temperature, warming tissue, and producing a variety of improvements in physiological function. **Passive warm-up** includes external heat sources like heating pads, whirlpools, or ultrasound. Prior to vigorous exertion, athletes should perform several minutes of general body movements (general warm-up) of progressively increasing intensity. These movements should emulate the actual movements of the sport or exercise to follow. Low-intensity movement specific to the sport or activity of interest is called specific warm-up.

Warm-up benefits performance through thermal, neuromuscular, and psychological effects. In some people, warm-up may also decrease the occurrence of dangerous cardiac responses from sudden strenuous exercise. Active warm-up activities mobilize metabolic resources and increase tissue temperature. Much of the benefit of warm-up comes from the increased body temperature. Moderate-intensity active warm-up (general movements) and passive warm-up (e.g., diathermy, heating pads, whirlpool) can increase muscular performance between 3% and 9% (1,2). Large muscle group motor tasks benefit from warm-up more than fine motor tasks.

Another reason for warm-up is to prepare the tissues for the greater stresses of vigorous physical activity and thus to lower the risk of muscle–tendon injury. Biomechanical evidence supports this "injury-protective" hypothesis, since warmed-up muscle in animal models has been found to elongate more, absorbing more energy before failure compared to no warm-up. This, combined with prospective studies of warm-up, supports the theory that general warm-up prior to vigorous activity may decrease the risk of musculotendinous injury compared to no warm-up. More direct evidence of this relationship would be helpful (3,4), but it is not possible to design studies that put subjects at risk of injury.

Warm-up activities are important to prepare the body for vigorous physical activity because they increase performance and may decrease the risk of muscular injury.

Athletes and other exercisers should therefore warm-up prior to competition, practice, and physical conditioning. Recommendations for effective warm-up routines vary depending on the nature and duration of the exercise to be performed. In general, warm-up routines should use general, whole-body movements up to 40% to 60% of aerobic capacity for 5 to 10 minutes followed by 5 minutes of recovery (2). The American College of Sports Medicine recommends 5 to 10 minutes of calisthenic-type exercises and 5 to 10 minutes of progressive aerobic activity in warm-up (5). For example, tennis players may perform several minutes of light jogging and several minutes of side lunges and trunk twists, followed by the traditional 5-minute warm-up of ground strokes and serves prior to a match. Future research might be able to define conditions of optimal warm-up protocols for specific activities and there is promising work in this area. Preliminary work to optimize intensity of warm-ups for individual athletes (6) and improve jumping performance beyond traditional warm-up with the use of weighted vests (7) has been reported.

Most warm-up sessions should begin with general body movements of gradually increasing intensity, focusing on the muscles and joints to be used in training or competition. Movement and muscular contractions commonly used in active warm-up also create decreases in passive tension (8,9) and increases in ROM as large as or larger than those due to passive stretching (10,11). Recent active warm-up protocols have been sometimes called **dynamic stretching**. This terminology should be avoided because it creates confusion with well-defined terminology like **ballistic stretching** and **static stretching** that are not beneficial as warm-up activities. Static stretching currently is not recommended during warm-up routines (12,13). The reasons for this change from traditional practice are explored in the following sections on flexibility and stretching.

FLEXIBILITY

Flexibility is an important component of fitness and physical performance. Inconsistent use of terminology related to the term *flexibility* by a variety of health and exercise science professionals has led to confusion. There is a distinct difference between flexibility and joint laxity. **Flexibility** is "the intrinsic property of body tissues which determines the ROM achievable without injury at a joint or series of joints" (14). The ability to move a joint without causing injury usually refers to the major anatomical rotations at joints rather than the joint laxity or accessory motion tests that orthopedists, physical therapists, and athletic trainers often evaluate to test joint and/or ligament integrity. Flexibility can be measured in a variety of ways, and several variables of interest have emerged.

One variable is the common clinical measure of the limits of rotation through an ROM referred to as **static flexibility**. This is estimated by linear or angular measurements of the limits of motion in a joint or joint complex. For example, it might be of clinical interest to know the static flexibility of areas of the body that tend to lose ROM with inactivity, like the lower (lumbar region) back or hamstring muscle group. Many professionals employ a sit-and-reach test (Fig. 9.1), using a linear measurement that provides a good field measure of hamstring static flexibility. These tests are limited by the rise in passive tension as the muscle and connective tissue are stretched.

Tests of static flexibility, although easy to administer, have several limitations. A major weakness of these tests is that the measures obtained are subjective and largely related to the subject's stretch tolerance (15), as well as the way in which the end point of the ROM is determined. Accurate measurements also depend on strict adherence to testing methodology. Variations in instruments, body positioning, instructions, or the protocol used all heavily influence results. Another problem is the variety of conditions in which the measurements are made. For example, physical therapy uses both active ROM (unassisted) and passive ROM (therapist-assisted) tests. The ROM achievable with the assistance of the tester (passive) is usually greater than that obtained with unassisted ROM. A great deal of information must be known about testing conditions to interpret data on static flexibility.

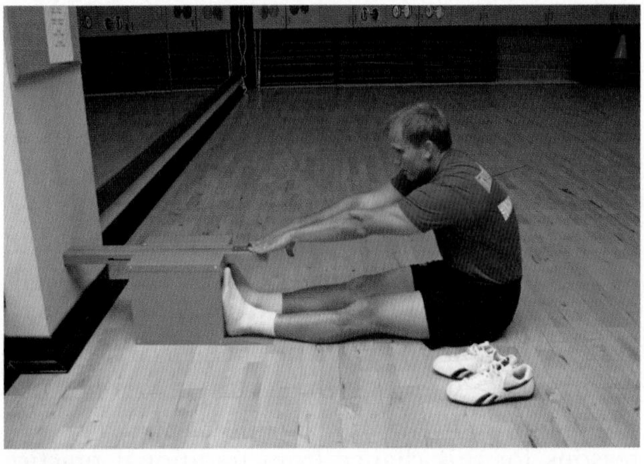

FIGURE 9.1 Since its development in the 1950s, the sit-and-reach test and several variations have become popular field tests of hamstring static flexibility.

In a research setting, we have the ability to measure mechanical properties of the muscle groups in addition to the clinical measurements of ROM. Research laboratory measurements of flexibility using computerized dynamometers have allowed the measurement of new biomechanical variables related to the mechanical properties of muscle and tendon. Two of these variables that may be related to performance and injury risk are stiffness and hysteresis. These terms are used in physics to describe properties of materials. Since the human body is composed of living materials that react to external forces in a similar fashion, the terms are also applicable to the human body.

The term **stiffness**, sometimes referred to as dynamic flexibility, refers to how quickly tissue resistance rises during a movement requiring the muscle–tendon unit to stretch. With passive stretching, the stiffness of the muscle–tendon unit measures how quickly the passive tension rises right before damage occurs. Studies show that the rise in tissue resistance (stiffness) shares only about 44% to 66% of common variance with static flexibility (15,16). Therefore, these variables are related but probably represent different functional properties of the musculature.

One problem in discussing the stiffness of muscles and tendons is the difference in the scientific and lay meaning of *stiffness* and *elasticity*. In biomechanics, stiffness and **elasticity** are synonymous, so a muscle with a quick rise in tension during stretch will tend to recover rapidly when the stretch is released. This conflicts with the colloquial meaning of the term *elasticity*, which some people relate with a low resistance to elongation.

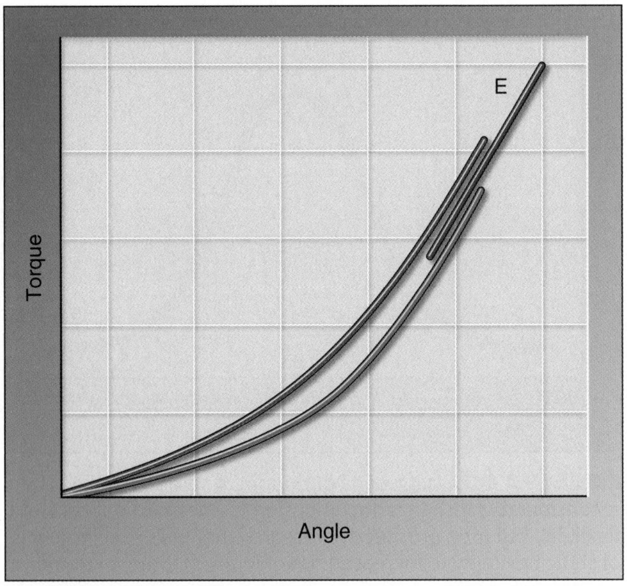

FIGURE 9.2 Schematic of a torque–joint angle plot during repeated passive stretches of a muscle group. Stress relaxation makes the passive torque at a given joint angle in subsequent stretches (*blue line*) less than in the first stretch (*purple line*). The stiffness (*E*) of the muscle group in these stretches, however, is not different.

Figure 9.2 illustrates a schematic of a torque–angle curve of the elongation phase of repeated passive stretches of a muscle group. These angular variables approximate well the load–deformation (linear) curve of the muscle and provide an in vivo (in the living animal) functional estimate of the passive stiffness of muscle groups (17). Scientists normally use linear measurements of load and deformation to define the mechanical properties of materials. Note in Figure 9.2 the torque, and therefore the tension in the muscle, rises in a complex (not linear) fashion, slowly at first and then more rapidly. Also note that the stiffness (*E*) of the muscle group does not change with repeated static stretching. Sometimes the initial response of tissues (short-range stiffness) is of interest, so the slope of the curve early in the ROM is used, but the term stiffness is usually reserved for the rise in tension late in a stretch, just before permanent damage. Short-range stiffness is that tightness in muscles when sitting in a fixed position for a long time; this stiffness is quickly reduced with just a few movements. More on the immediate and long-term biomechanical responses to stretching are covered later in the chapter.

Biological tissues have other complex behaviors that influence their function. The muscle–tendon unit resistance to stretch is **viscoelastic**. This means that tension developed during a stretch depends both on the amount of deformation and on the rate of deformation. A slow stretch of muscle will result in lower tension in the muscle and tendon for a particular joint angle compared to a fast stretch. A faster stretch would have a similar load–deformation shape curve but will have a higher stiffness because of viscoelasticity.

Although the application of materials science to the human body may seem complex, it is important to realize that the human body is a living material that responds to stress in a predictable manner. Materials science defines stiffness as the slope of the stress–strain curve in the elastic (linear) region, which is how quickly the tension rises late in elongation before the elastic limit. The elastic limit is the point on the graph depicting the lengthening of the muscle–tendon unit just before the material begins to fail or the beginning of permanent damage. Beyond the elastic limit is the plastic region, so called because this is where the deformation is not immediately recoverable in materials. Fortunately, normal vigorous physical activity rarely gets near the elastic limit for muscles or tendons, and small stretches near the elastic limit may be repaired by the body if it is given enough rest. An unusually severe or unexpected elongation can, however, cause rupture or complete failure of the tissue. Materials scientists call the maximum force or energy absorbed before complete failure the **mechanical strength** of the material.

When a muscle is stretched, but not beyond its elastic limit, it will return to resting length and recover some of the energy stored in it as it was stretched. Some of the energy, however, is lost as heat. The energy lost in the return to normal length from a deformed material is termed **hysteresis**. This represents the energy lost and can be visualized as the area (loop) between the loading (elongation) and the unloading (restitution) phases in Figure 9.3. This figure illustrates a schematic of a torque–angle curve of the elongation phase (*purple line*) and the restitution phase (*blue line*) of a static stretch.

From Figure 9.3, note that in static stretching exercises, about 40% to 50% of the energy stored in the stretch is lost as the muscle returns to normal length (18). Much of this energy loss is in the contractile and connective tissue components within the muscle. To the contrary, studies of long tendons in normal vigorous physical activity show that they recover most (80% to 90%) of the energy stored in them in the quick stretch-shortening actions common in movement (19).

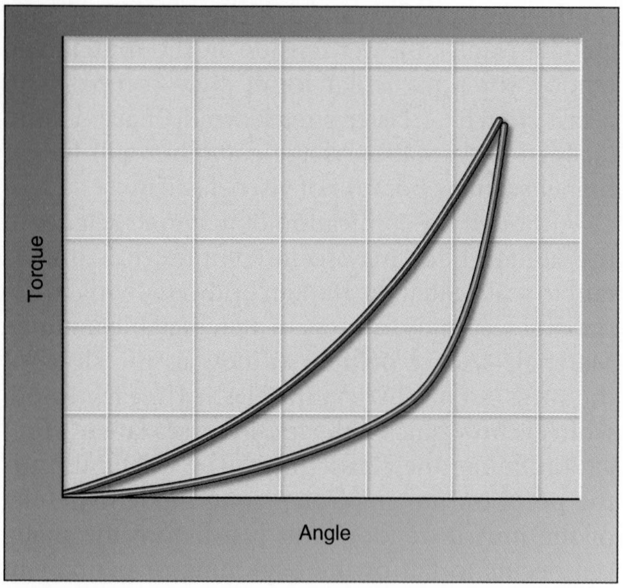

FIGURE 9.3 Schematic of a torque–joint angle plot of the elongation (*purple*) and restitution (*blue*) phases of a passive stretch of a muscle group. The energy lost (hysteresis) is the area of the loop between the loading and the unloading phases.

Measuring energy or other biomechanical variables may be better for examining the effect of stretching on muscle performance, as opposed to stiffness, because muscle tissue often does not reach the elastic region of the stress–strain curve in typical hamstring stretches (17). Stretching and other passive movement can have a greater effect on hysteresis than on the stiffness of muscle. Research on the biomechanical effects of warm-up movements and stretching is important because it could result in practical application in improving muscular performance.

The ability to move the joints of the body freely without injury is known as flexibility, and several mechanical properties and variables can be used to document important aspects of flexibility.

NORMAL STATIC FLEXIBILITY

The wealth of research on static flexibility measurements provides a general picture of what is normal static flexibility for most joints and populations. Normal static flexibility is the typical joint movement allowed between two extremes (Fig. 9.4): ankylosis and hypermobility. **Ankylosis** is pathological loss of ROM, whereas **hypermobility** is excessive ROM. Static flexibility is not a whole-body characteristic but, like fitness, is specific to joints

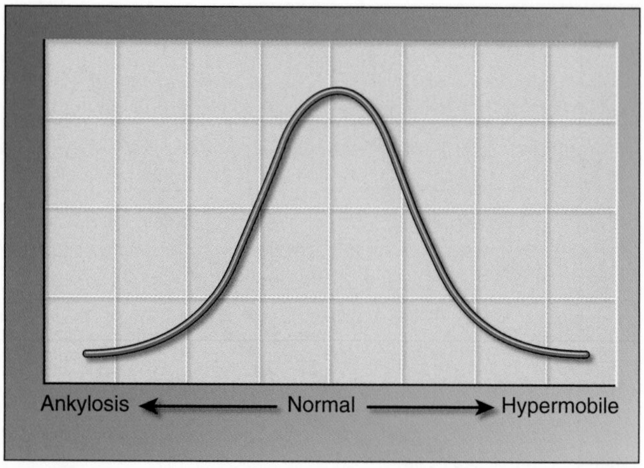

FIGURE 9.4 Schematic of a continuum of static flexibility. There is considerable research documenting the normal limits of static flexibility but little prospective research that links specific levels of static flexibility to increased risk of injury at either extreme.

and directions of movement. People may tend to have low static flexibility in one part of the body and normal or high flexibility in another. It is also clear that, in general, females have greater static flexibility than males (20), and some of these differences are related to anthropometric differences.

Fitness professionals can access data on normal ranges of static flexibility for most joints from several professional sources (see online references). Several recent reviews of flexibility have been published (see online references) and provide more information on static flexibility. It is unclear, however, whether an "optimal" level of static flexibility for muscle groups or areas of the body exists. If this is the case, it is likely that different sports would require different optimal levels of static flexibility. Future research studies should be designed to focus on determining "normative" static ranges of motion at joints in athletes participating in specific sports, as well as documenting anomalies in athletes and active people who are outside of this normative range. It is too early to make a definitive statement, but it is possible that an athlete or active person whose muscles are too tight is more prone to *muscle* injuries and that one whose muscles are too loose is more prone to *joint* injuries as well as decreased performance in strength and power activities.

Common deviations from normal static flexibility are present in many joint(s). Some people lose ROM from physical inactivity. People may also lose static flexibility with aging, from workplace or sport-specific positions, and/or repetitive movements. For example, the repetitive motion

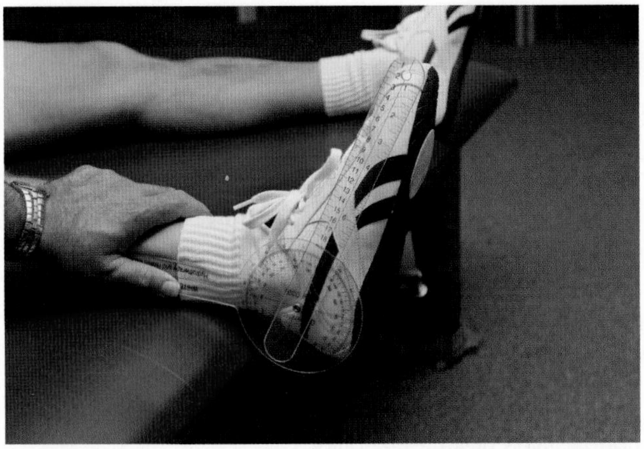

FIGURE 9.5 Repetitive work or body positions (like wearing high heels) can create tight muscles and decrease ankle static flexibility.

in several sports with overhead throwing patterns (baseball, tennis, etc.) without specific stretching intervention can result in glenohumeral internal rotation deficit. Persistent wearing of high heels can decrease ankle dorsiflexion ROM (Fig. 9.5).

Several resources provide normative data on the typical static flexibility of most major joints of the body, but current research does not identify an optimal level of static flexibility.

FLEXIBILITY AND INJURY RISK

The literature on clinical and basic science provides a very different view of the role of flexibility in injury risk and performance than what is commonly believed and practiced. What appears to be desirable, based on data on the incidence of muscle–tendon injuries, is to avoid the extremes in static flexibility. Athletes and exercisers at both extremes of static flexibility may be at a higher risk for musculoskeletal injuries (21,22). This section focuses on the association between flexibility and injury risk: The sections on stretching, further on, discuss the association between stretching and changes in muscular performance and injury risk.

Low levels of hamstring flexibility have been related to a higher risk of muscular injury in soccer (23). The common belief that greater static flexibility will always decrease the risk of muscular injury, however, appears not to be valid. This may be explained by the stability–mobility paradox. The mechanical stability and ROM at a joint or joints are inversely related. It is possible that as static flexibility increases beyond the normal range, the potential benefits of greater motion and less tissue resistance are offset by the greater instability of the joint. More research is needed to begin to define the ranges of motion for various joints, so that the best compromise of stability and mobility may be provided, along with a lower risk of injury.

A good example of the lack of an association between high levels of static flexibility and lower injury risk is provided by low back fitness testing. Although it seems logical that less flexible back or hamstring muscles would be related to the incidence of low back pain, little evidence supports this association. Despite a large body of the research, there is limited support (mixed results) for an association between lumbar/hamstring flexibility and the occurrence of low back pain. One of the largest prospective studies on this topic found no relationship between static flexibility and subsequent low back pain in adults. Therefore, the field tests of hamstring static flexibility commonly used in fitness test batteries may not be useful in predicting future low back injury.

People also commonly believe that less "stiff" muscles result in greater flexibility and a lower risk of injury. Unfortunately, little research is available on the association between muscle stiffness and injury risk. Less stiff muscles may be less susceptible to muscle strain injury (24), but few studies have been conducted in this area (25). It appears that muscle with greater stiffness is more susceptible to eccentrically induced muscle damage. Currently, the evidence is insufficient to conclude that decreased muscle stiffness will provide an injury-protective benefit. Combined with the unclear nature of the exact levels of static flexibility that decrease injury risk, this means that strength and conditioning professionals must educate athletes on the complexity of flexibility and injury risk.

A complex relationship exists between static flexibility and risk of muscular injury. Higher injury rates seem to be related to very flexible or very inflexible muscles.

ASSESSING FLEXIBILITY

Exercise prescriptions to modify flexibility should be based on valid measurements using standardized testing procedures. Static flexibility tests are based on both linear and angular measurements of the motion of a joint or group of joints. These tests

REAL-WORLD APPLICATION

The Stability–Mobility Paradox

Static flexibility is like exercise in that more is not always better. Joint motion (mobility) is inversely proportional to the stability of the joint. Decreasing muscle passive tension around a joint increases the joint's ROM but also makes it easier for the joint to be pulled out of normal position. This presents the fitness professional with a paradox. What is the right amount of static flexibility? How much motion is necessary for normal and safe movement without adversely affecting the joint or ligaments? It is not possible to give easy answers to these questions. The amount of motion depends on the joint, the requirements of the sport/activity a person engages in, and other factors. Given that the lowest injury rates seem to correspond to normal flexibility and higher injury rates with the extremes in flexibility (inflexible and hypermobile), maintenance of normal or moderate amounts of static flexibility should be the goal for most people. Unless a person participates in an activity requiring extreme flexibility (dance, gymnastics, diving), most exercise prescriptions should focus on maintaining normal levels of static flexibility.

can focus on single joints or compound movements of many body segments and joints.

Single-joint static flexibility tests are commonly used clinically in the medical professions; they often involve angular measurements (with goniometers or inclinometers) rather than linear measurements. Single-joint tests are considered better measurements of static flexibility than compound tests because they better isolate specific muscles and are less affected by anthropometric differences (26). The straight-leg-raise and active-knee-extension tests are the common hamstring flexibility tests used in physical therapy. The many variations of the sit-and-reach test are compound flexibility tests and are often validated with the straight leg raise or active knee extension.

Sit-and-reach scores are primarily associated with hamstring flexibility, but not with low back flexibility (27). Although the sit-and-reach test has been shown to be a moderately valid measure of hamstring flexibility that is only slightly affected by anthropometric variations, the prescriptive value of these measurements is limited. One study reported that 6% of children falsely passed and 12% falsely failed the sit-and-reach test relative to the straight-leg-raise test (26). If these data are consistent across all ages, people failing the sit-and-reach test should be retested with the straight-leg-raise or active-knee-extension test to make sure that they have limited hamstring static flexibility.

Current health-related norms for sit-and-reach or other static flexibility tests should be used only to identify individuals at the extremes who may be at higher risk for muscle injuries. Not enough data are available to provide specific static flexibility goals beyond the maintenance of normal flexibility. Fitness professionals must also remember that in measuring flexibility, exacting attention to testing details is necessary. Static flexibility scores are subjective and highly dependent on the subject's tolerance of the high muscle tension (discomfort) during testing. The clinical measurement of dynamic flexibility is not ordinarily practicable; it is limited to research settings because of problems related to expensive equipment, insufficient standardization, and the lack of normative data.

DEVELOPMENT OF FLEXIBILITY

Normal levels of flexibility can be maintained by regular physical activity and through specific programs of stretching and strengthening exercises. Kinesiology professionals should assess a client's flexibility and, based on these data and the client's history, develop a program to improve flexibility. Although poor flexibility can be treated with a combination of stretching and strengthening exercises (28), this section focuses on general recommendations for stretching in mass exercise prescription. Regular stretching exercises are usually recommended for most people because of their often limited physical activity and also because regular participation in some activities is associated with sport-specific flexibility imbalances. In general, stretching recommendations should be limited to the maintenance of normal levels of static flexibility because of the complex nature of flexibility and the lack of data linking specific levels of flexibility to lower injury risk. This section concludes with recent evidence on the effect of stretching on muscular performance, which has implications for the placement of stretching in the training cycle.

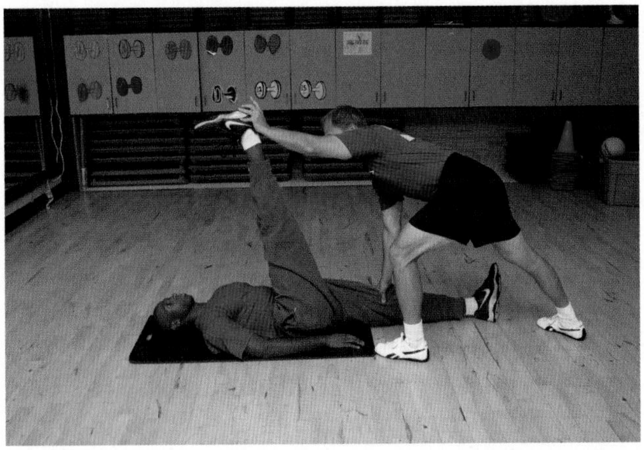

FIGURE 9.6 Passive stretching often uses external force from another person to produce a greater stretch of a muscle group.

Stretching exercises are usually classified into four types: passive, static, ballistic (dynamic), and proprioceptive neuromuscular facilitation, or PNF. **Passive stretching** uses an external force, usually another person, to stretch muscle groups (Fig. 9.6). Static stretching involves a slow increase in muscle group length and holding the stretched position at that length for a short time (usually 15 to 30 seconds). Ballistic stretching traditionally has meant fast, momentum-assisted, and bouncing stretching movements. These stretches are generally avoided because of the viscoelastic nature of muscle. For a given elongation, a fast stretch results in a higher force in the tissue and a greater risk of injury. Some refer to the active warm-up movements mentioned earlier as dynamic stretching. These stretches may be acceptable if they are performed in a relatively slow manner to create muscle elongation without imposing high levels of force on the tissue. This is probably how regular physical activity can maintain static flexibility.

The last group of stretching exercises focuses on PNF. PNF stretch routines use a specific series of movements and contractions to use neuromuscular reflexes to relax the muscles being stretched. PNF stretches can be performed with or without assistance. A simple PNF procedure is a "contract–relax" stretch where a person performs an isometric contraction of a muscle to be stretched, which is immediately followed by a static stretch of that muscle. This strategy takes advantage of the inhibitory effects of **Golgi tendon organs** as the muscle is slowly stretched. Assisted stretching procedures like PNF should be performed with care by trained subjects or sports medicine personnel. The practice of having athletes passively stretch partners should be used with caution until the athletes have been carefully trained in correct procedures and understand the risks of incorrect or high-force stretches.

The recommendations for stretching procedures are based on reviews of the basic science studies of the viscoelastic response of muscle to stretching. These recommendations (Table 9.1) are designed for group exercise prescription with normal subjects. Static or PNF stretching should be performed at least three times per week, preferably daily and after moderate or vigorous physical activity (in the cooldown phase of training). Exacting technique in stretching is recommended to safely focus tension on a muscle group or groups without systematic stress on other joint stability structures (ligaments, joint capsules, cartilage). Some experts have hypothesized, based on functional anatomy, that some stretching exercises are contraindicated because of potentially dangerous ligament and tissue loading (29).

Stretching programs should include up to four or five stretches for each major muscle group, with

TABLE 9.1 ● STRETCHING RECOMMENDATIONS FOR GROUP EXERCISE PRESCRIPTION

FITNESS VARIABLE	RECOMMENDATION
Frequency	At least three times per week, preferable daily and after moderate or vigorous physical activity
Intensity	Slowly elongate muscle and hold with low level of force to the person's perception of tightness without discomfort
Time	Up to four to five stretches held from 15–30 s. Stretch normally during the cooldown phase. Be sure to stretch only muscles that have been thoroughly warmed-up from physical activity. Warning: Stretching in the warm-up prior to physical activity may weaken muscles and decrease performance.
Type	Static or PNF stretches for all major muscle groups

Source: Adapted with permission from Knudson D, Magnusson P, McHugh M. Current issues in flexibility fitness. *PCPFS Res Digest*. 2000;3(10):1–8.

each stretch held for 15 to 30 seconds. The intensity (force) of each stretch should be minimized, slowly elongating and holding the stretched position just before the point of discomfort. The American College of Sports Medicine recommends four or more static stretches held for 15 to 60 seconds for a minimum of 2 to 3 d · wk^{-1} for each major muscle group (5). Slow elongation of muscles creates less reflex contraction through the action of **muscle spindles**. These sense muscle length and are responsible for the contraction of a stretched muscle (myotatic reflex). This reflex contraction is most sensitive to fast stretches, so slow muscle elongation in stretching exercises helps maintain relaxation in the muscle groups being stretched.

Static stretching will create a short-term increase in ROM and a decrease in passive tension in the muscle at a particular joint angle due to **stress relaxation**, which is the gradual decrease in stress (force per unit area) in a material stretched and held at a constant length. Most people can feel the decrease in passive tension in a muscle group held in a stretched position. This stress relaxation following stretching provides an immediate 10% to 30% decrease in passive tension (8,30,31), but the effect will have dissipated after 30 minutes to an hour (32,39). Holding stretches for 15 to 30 seconds is a good guideline, because most of the stress relaxation in passive stretches occurs in the first 20 seconds (17,33).

Stretching to increase static flexibility in a muscle group should normally use four to five static stretches held for 15 to 30 seconds.

Stretching should normally be performed during the cooldown period because of four lines of evidence:

1. Warmed-up tissues are less likely to be injured.
2. The placement of stretching within the workout does not affect gains in static flexibility.
3. Stretching creates immediate decrements in muscle strength expression.
4. Stretching likely has no effect of the immediate risk of muscle–tendon injury.

Programming static stretching during the cooldown period is also logical because stretching tends to relax or inhibit muscle activation (34,35). For example, static stretching is commonly used for the acute relief from muscle cramps or delayed-onset muscle soreness (DOMS). The former is indicated, but research on the latter indicates no effect of stretching before or after activity (36) on the DOMS that occurs after unaccustomed exercise. Static stretching routines in the cooldown period primarily serve to help maintain normal levels of static flexibility.

Q & A from the Field

Q ***Our high school track-and-field athletes often want to stretch before their events. I know that flexibility is an important component of performance, but I have heard rumblings in the running community for years that stretching before racing is a bad idea. Is it true that stretching prior to high-intensity track-and-field events is a bad idea?***

—high school track coach

A Athletes stretch in the warm-up for track events because they believe that it decreases their risk of injury and improves their performance. Unfortunately, research has shown that this practice is probably not justified for most athletes. Unless an athlete has a major deficit in ROM, stretching prior to vigorous exertion actually decreases most forms of maximal muscular performance for about 30 minutes to an hour. In addition, stretching prior to vigorous activity has also been shown to have no effect on the risk of muscular injury. The most important thing a coach can do is teach athletes that proper warm-up is essential for maximum performance and decreasing the risk of injury. Focus their precompetition routine around a progressive and specific active warm-up with movements related to their event. Most athletes with normal flexibility should perform their stretching routines after practice or competition.

BIOMECHANICAL EFFECTS OF STRETCHING

Stretching exercises are prescribed routinely to increase static flexibility. Considerable research has reported that stretch training can increase ROM (28), although much of this increase may be also due to stretch tolerance (3). Stretch tolerance is an analgesic effect that allows a person to accept higher tensions associated with a greater stretch of a muscle group. What is also less well known is that these long-term/training effects can be different than the short-term/immediate effects (37). This section summarizes the short-term effects of stretching on the muscular performance variables, stiffness, and hysteresis.

Passive stretching can create large tensile loads in the muscle, so it is possible to weaken and injure muscle with vigorous stretching programs. Stretching exercise is like any other training stimulus in that it results in temporary weakening before the body recovers and supercompensates for that activity. This decreased muscular performance following stretching has been reported in dozens of studies in all kinds of athletes. Decreased performance of 4% to 30% has been observed in maximal strength tests, running, and jumping. Stretch-induced decrements in muscular performance appear to be equally related to neuromuscular inhibition and decreased contractile force and can last 30 to 60 minutes (38,39). The minimum dose of static stretching to create a physiologically meaningful decrease (5%) in strength is 20 to 30 seconds (40). This is why most stretching should be performed in the cooldown phase of training and avoided in the warm-up period for athletic competition. Only athletes who require extreme static flexibility for performance (dancers, gymnasts, divers) might need to stretch at the end of the warm-up phase.

> ***Stretching should normally be performed in the cooldown phase of conditioning because stretching before activity decreases muscular performance for about 30 minutes.***

Stretching can create a short-term increase in ROM, but this improvement quickly disappears (41). This greater static flexibility is a result of lower passive tension (stress relaxation) at equivalent joint angles and increased stretch tolerance. This lower passive tension and greater ROM that people feel, however, is not the same as stiffness.

Studies of the immediate effect of stretching on muscle group stiffness have reported both no effects and small reductions. Even research using different theoretical models of stiffness over the whole ROM predicts different responses to stretching. This lack of consensus is compounded when some researchers incorrectly defined stiffness as the change in tension over the change in angle at the beginning of the load–deformation curve, not as the true mechanical stiffness of the tissue (the slope in linear region). Because we do not clearly know the immediate effects of stretching on muscle stiffness, strength and conditioning professionals should instruct athletes and other exercisers that the primary benefits of stretching are maintenance of ROM and a decrease in the passive tension of the muscles at similar joint angles.

While the evidence is mixed that static stretching immediately affects muscle stiffness, passive motion exercise can create significant reductions in muscle stiffness (8). Cyclic movements that create a slow stretch of muscle groups, just like the active warm-up described earlier, also decrease the energy lost (hysteresis) in subsequent stretches (42). Static stretching has also been observed to significantly reduce hysteresis (42–44). More research is needed on muscle hysteresis, but currently it appears that active or passive movement is an effective strategy to make muscles more compliant and recover more energy following a stretch. These properties likely have immediate benefits to many kinds of performance and should help reduce the risk of injury.

The relationship between stretching performance is complex for many reasons. Stretch training can have different effects on the various fiber and connective tissue components of the muscle–tendon complex (43,45). Second, muscles have history-dependent or a **thixotropic** response, where differences in previous muscle status (rest, concentric, active or passive stretch) have an immediate effect on the mechanical response of subsequent muscle actions. Overall performance of a multisegment biomechanical system will even be more difficult to predict because of the different kinds of performance variables, as well as the interaction of technique, neuromuscular, muscle, and tendon effects. For example, lower levels of static flexibility have been associated with better running economy (46,47); however, less stiff musculature may be more effective in utilizing elastic energy in stretch-shortening cycle movements (48–52). It is likely that the effects of stretching and flexibility on muscular performance are complex and activity specific (53). Considerable future research is needed to outline the best matching of the immediate and training effects of stretching to the many kinds of muscular performance in sport and exercise.

PROPHYLACTIC EFFECTS OF STRETCHING

The other traditional rationale for prescribing preactivity stretching is a hypothesized reduction in the risk of injury. The logic was that if there were greater static flexibility from stretching, the chance that stretching the muscle beyond this point might lead to injury would be reduced. In the case of flexibility, this logic has not been supported by scientific evidence. Muscle strains (pulls) occur more often in eccentric muscle actions rather than in passive elongation.

The larger and better-designed prospective studies have shown little or no effect of stretching on injury rate (54–57). The studies with larger samples and better controls (55,56) support the conclusion that flexibility and stretching may be unrelated to injury risk. Currently the data are insufficient to support the common prescription of stretching programs to modify flexibility based on the hypothesis of reducing the risk of muscle injury. Much more research on the effects of stretching and the associations between various flexibility levels and injury rates are needed before specific guidelines on stretching will be available.

> *Research has not confirmed the belief that stretching decreases the risk of muscular injury, so general stretching prior to physical activity probably confers no protective effect.*

Summary

Both active and passive warm-ups are common preparatory activities before exercise and athletic competition. Several lines of research have supported the beneficial effects of warm-up on improving performance and reducing injury risk. A typical warm-up should consist of general and future activity-specific movements of gradually increasing intensity. The intensity of warm-up should be moderate (up to 40% to 60% of aerobic capacity) and sustained (5 to 10 minutes) to increase the tissue temperature. Flexibility is an important property of the musculoskeletal system that determines the ROM and resistance to motion at a joint or group of joints. This property can be examined by measuring the limits of the achievable motion (static flexibility) or several other biomechanical variables of passively stretched muscle group. Normal ranges of static flexibility are well documented for most joints through a variety of tests. There is some evidence that extremes in static flexibility (top or bottom 20% of the distribution) may be associated with a higher incidence of muscle injury. Sport science research and prospective studies of flexibility and stretching indicate that stretching should not normally be performed in warm-ups. Stretching prior to physical activity decreases muscular performance and does not reduce the risk of musculoskeletal injury. Currently, little scientific evidence is available on which to base precise, individualized prescriptions of stretching development beyond the maintenance of normal levels of static flexibility. Static or PNF stretching should normally be performed during the cooldown phase of physical activity. Stretches should slowly elongate and hold muscles with low levels of force for 15 to 30 seconds. Four to five stretches per muscle group or area of the body are usually recommended.

Maxing Out

1. Dancer—A dancer/cheerleader requests your help in increasing hip flexion and abduction ROM to facilitate the split position for a variety of stunts. What stretching program would you recommend?
2. Personal training client—A manager seeks relief from neck and shoulder pain from long days on an office computer. What stretching and strengthening exercises would you recommend?
3. Athlete—An athlete who has undergone acute rehab wants to return to play and increase plantar flexion ROM following an ankle sprain. What assessments would you use to document progress and what stretching program would you employ?

CASE EXAMPLE

Postmatch Flexibility Routine in Tennis

BACKGROUND

You are a strength coach working with the university medical staff and a 20-year-old male collegiate tennis player. The player has limited internal shoulder rotation ROM in the dominant shoulder, which is common in repetitive overarm sports like tennis.

RECOMMENDATIONS/CONSIDERATIONS

Following matches, practice, and conditioning sessions, the cooldown phase will consist of a static stretching routine. This will be a typical whole-body routine but will focus extra stretching on sport-specific imbalances common in tennis players: reduced shoulder internal rotation and flexibility of the lower back and hamstrings.

IMPLEMENTATION

Three 20-second wrist flexor and extensor stretches

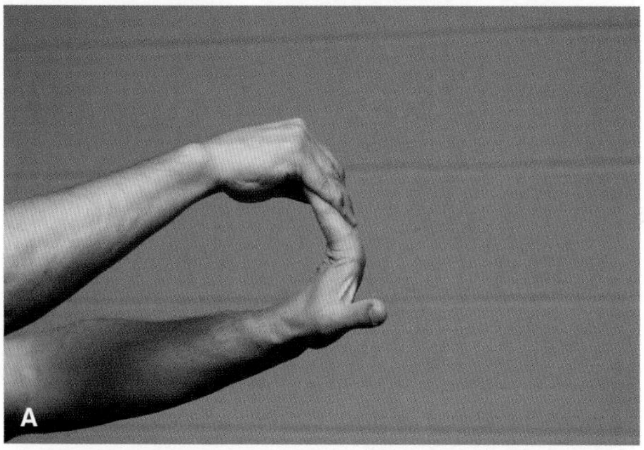

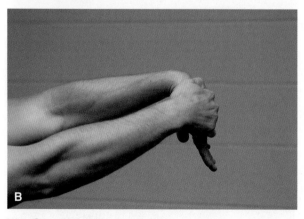

Wrist flexor and extensor stretches.

Four 20-second standing pectoralis major stretches

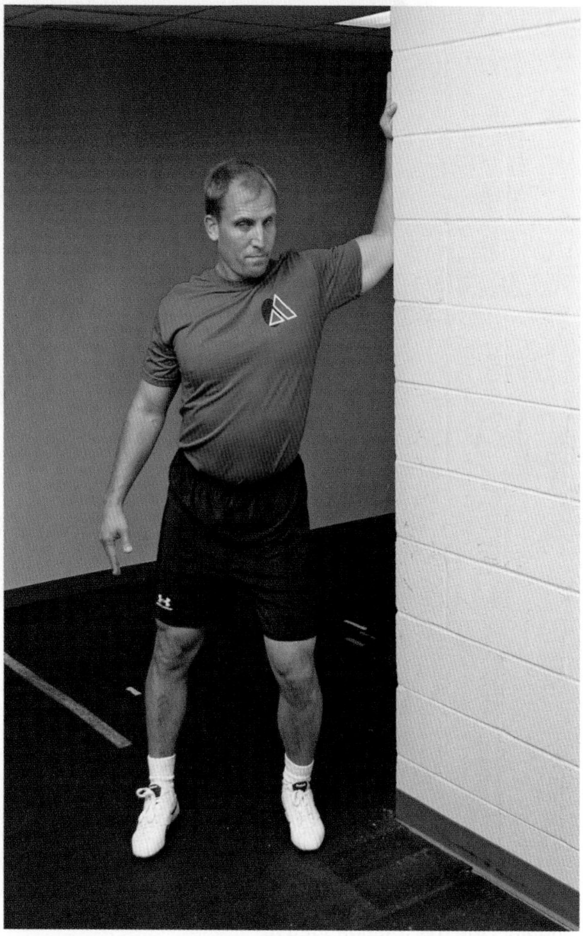

Standing pectoralis major stretch.

CASE EXAMPLE *(Continued)*

Postmatch Flexibility Routine in Tennis

Four 20-second shoulder internal rotation stretches

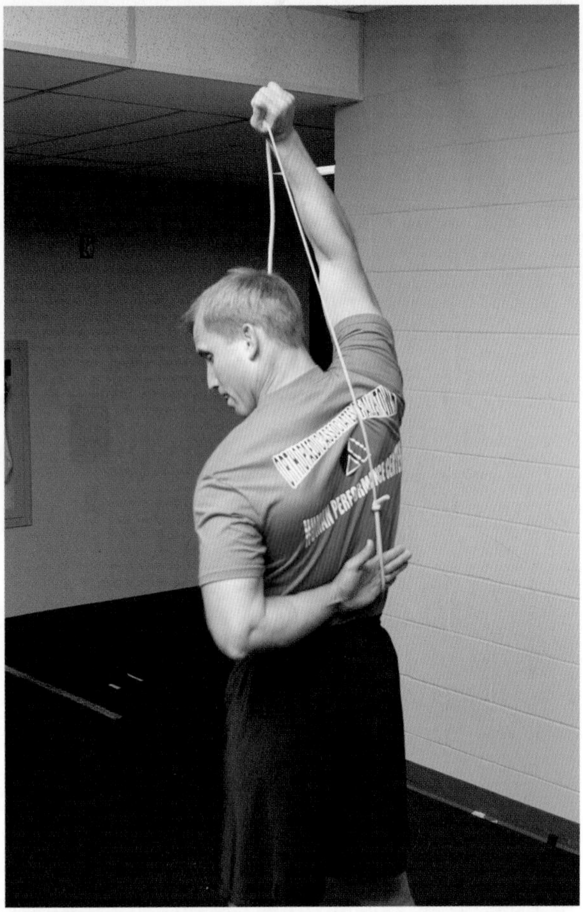

Shoulder internal rotation stretch.

Four 20-second knees to chest low back stretches

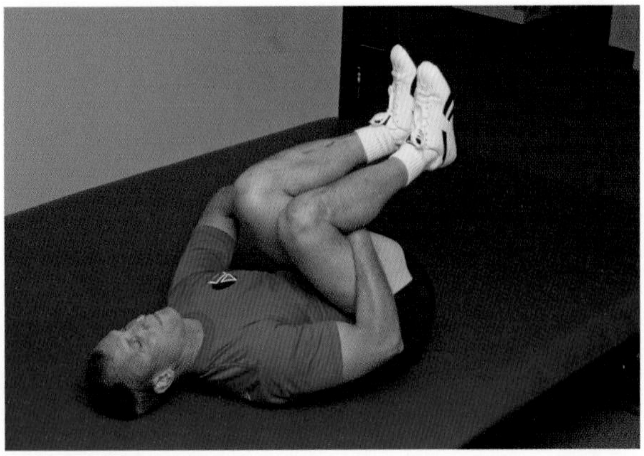

Knees to chest low back stretch.

Three 20-second trunk twists both directions

Three 20-second butterfly hip internal rotator stretches

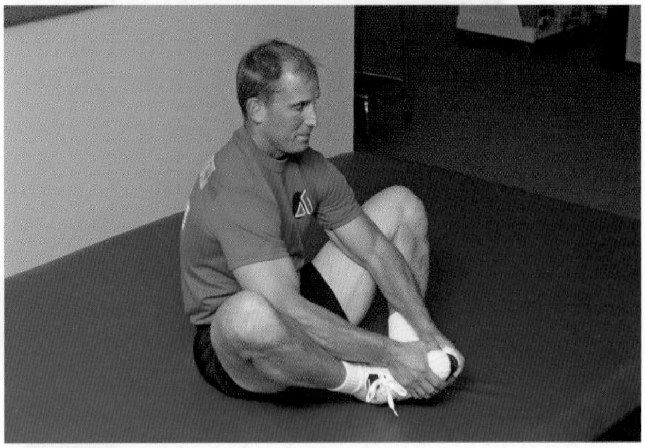

Butterfly hip internal rotators stretch.

Four 20-second seated hamstring stretches

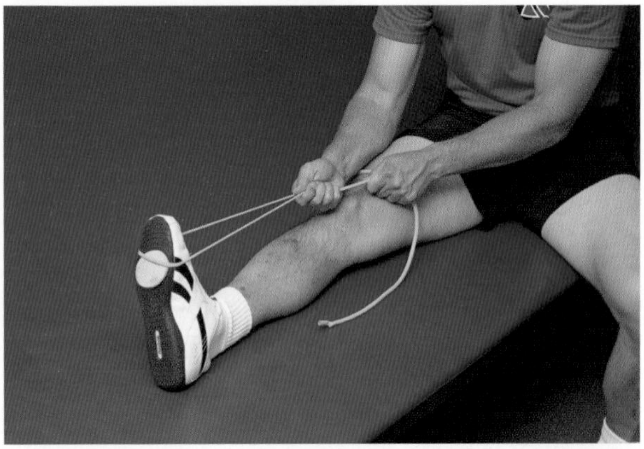

Seated calf stretch.

Three 20-second seated calf stretches

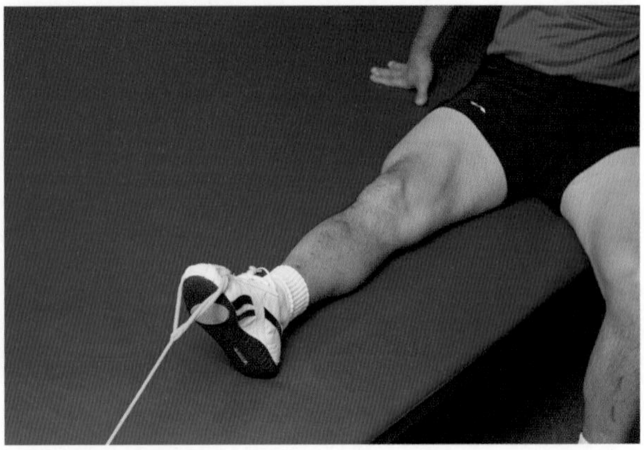

Seated dorsiflexor stretch.

(Continued)

CASE EXAMPLE *(Continued)*

Postmatch Flexibility Routine in Tennis

Three 20-second seated dorsiflexor stretches

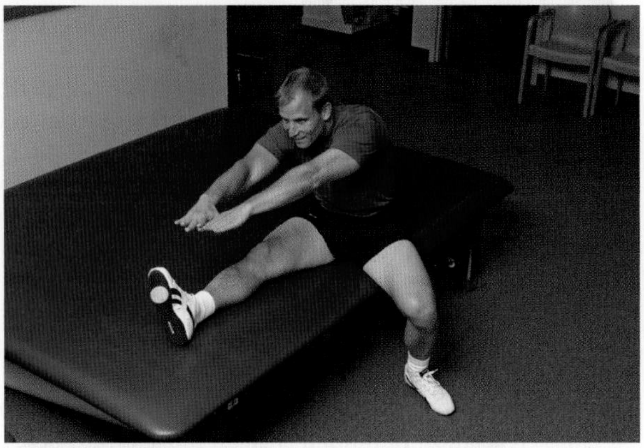

Seated hamstring stretch.

RESULTS

Results before and after (a 10-week flexibility program) indicate an improvement in ROM over the period of the training program in specific movements. Tests included shoulder internal rotation ROM, hip flexion ROM, and sit and reach.

Shoulder internal rotation ROM

Initial: dominant, 33 degrees; nondominant, 66 degrees

After training: dominant, 48 degrees; nondominant, 70 degrees.

As is typical with overhead throwing athletes, shoulder internal rotation was decreased in the dominant extremity. The prescribed program caused a change in the ROM of the dominant arm in internal rotation in the direction of normal. Because of the demands of the sport, it is unlikely that the dominant arm would ever reach the same ROM as the nondominant arm.

Hip flexion ROM with knee extended

Initial: dominant, 40 degrees; nondominant, 39 degrees

After training: dominant, 51 degrees; nondominant 50 degrees

In hip flexion, a dominant-to-nondominant difference is not as pronounced as it is in the upper extremity. Both extremities demonstrated a small increase in ROM related to hamstring extensibility from the prescribed flexibility program.

CASE EXAMPLE

Sit-and-reach flexibility

Initial: + 1 cm

After training: + 3 cm

The flexibility program resulted in a slight increase in ROM in trunk flexion. These increases in ROM related to hamstring extensibility could, in theory, maintain this athlete in a lower injury risk to hamstring and lower back compared to players with reduced or excessive flexibility. These tests support the efficacy of the training program and should be maintained and monitored in this athlete. Progression could include 30-second stretches or an addtional repetition.

REFERENCES

1. Bishop D. Warm up I: potential mechanisms and the effects of passive warm up on exercise performance. *Sports Med*. 2003;33:439–454.
2. Bishop D. Warm up II: performance changes following active warm up and how to structure the warm up. *Sports Med*. 2003;33:483–498.
3. Flopp H, Deall S, Harvey LA, et al. Can apparent increase in muscle extensibility with regular stretch be explained by changes in tolerance to stretch? *Aust J Physiother*. 2006;52:45–50.
4. Fradkin AJ, Gabbe BJ, Cameron PA. Does warming up prevent injury in sport: the evidence from randomized controlled trials. *J Sci Med Sport*. 2006;9:214–220.
5. American College of Sports Medicine. *ACSM's Guidelines for Exercise Testing and Prescription*. 8th ed. Philadelphia, PA: Lippincott Williams & Wilkins; 2010.
6. Mandengue SH, Miladi I, Bishop D, et al. Methodological approach for determining optimal active warm-up intensity: predictive equations. *Sci Sports*. 2009;24:9–14.
7. Thompsen AG, Kakley T, Palumbo MA, et al. Acute effects of different warm-up protocols with and without weighted

vest on jumping performance in athletic women. *J Strength Cond Res*. 2007;21:52–56.
8. McNair PJ, Dombroski EW, Hewson DJ, et al. Stretching at the ankle joint: viscoelastic responses to holds and continuous passive motion. *Med Sci Sports Exerc*. 2000;33:354–358.
9. Taylor DC, Brooks DE, Ryan JB. Viscoelastic characteristics of muscle: passive stretching versus muscular contractions. *Med Sci Sports Exerc*. 1997;29:1619–1624.
10. Hubley CL, Kozey JW, Stanish WD. The effects of static stretching exercises and stationary cycling on range of motion at the hip joint. *J Orthop Sports Phys Ther*. 1984;6:104–109.
11. Medeiros JM, Smidt GL, Burmeister LF, et al. The influence of isometric exercise and passive stretch on hip joint motion. *Phys Ther*. 1977;57:518–523.
12. Knudson D, Magnusson P, McHugh M. Current issues in flexibility fitness. *PCPFS Res Dig*. 2000;3(10):1–8.
13. Magnusson P, Renstrom P. The European College of Sports Sciences Position statement: the role of stretching exercises in sports. *Eur J Sport Sci*. 2006;6:87–91.
14. Holt J, Holt LE, Pelham TW. Flexibility redefined. In: Bauer T, ed. *Biomechanics in Sports XIII*. Thunder Bay, ON: Lakehead University; 1996:170–174.
15. Magnusson SP, Simonsen EB, Aagaard P, et al. Determinants of musculoskeletal flexibility: viscoelastic properties, cross-sectional area, EMG and stretch tolerance. *Scand J Med Sci Sports*. 1997;7:195–202.
16. McHugh MP, Kremenic IJ, Fox MB, et al. The role of mechanical and neural restrains to joint range of motion during passive stretch. *Med Sci Sports Exerc*. 1998;30: 928–932.
17. Magnusson SP, Aagaard P, Simonsen EB, et al. Passive tensile stress and energy of the human hamstring muscles in vivo. *Scand J Med Sci Sports*. 2000;10:351–359.
18. Magnusson SP. Passive properties of human skeletal muscle during stretch maneuvers: a review. *Scand J Med Sci Sports*. 1998;8:65–77.
19. Kubo K, Kanehisa H, Fukunaga T. Gender differences in the viscoelastic properties of tendon structures. *Eur J Appl Physiol*. 2003;88:520–526.
20. Harris ML. Flexibility. *Phys Ther*. 1969;49:591–601.
21. Jones BH, Knapik JJ. Physical training and exercise-related injuries. *Sports Med*. 1999;27:111–125.
22. Knapik JJ, Jones BH, Bauman CL, et al. Strength, flexibility, and athletic injuries. *Sports Med*. 1992;14:277–288.
23. Witvrouw E, Danneels L, Asselman P, et al. Muscle flexibility as a risk factor for developing muscle injuries in male professional soccer players: a prospective study. *Am J Sports Med*. 2003;31:41–46.
24. Wilson GJ, Wood GA, Elliott BC. The relationship between stiffness of the musculature and static flexibility: an alternative explanation for the occurrence of muscular injury. *Int J Sports Med*. 1991;12:403–407.
25. McHugh MP, Connolly DAJ, Eston RG, et al. The role of passive muscle stiffness in symptoms of exercise-induced muscle damage. *Am J Sports Med*. 1999;27:594–599.
26. Cornbleet SL, Woolsey NB. Assessment of hamstring muscle length in school-aged children using the sit-and-reach test and the inclinometer measure of hip joint angle. *Phys Ther*. 1996;76:850–855.
27. Martin SB, Jackson AW, Morrow JR, et al. The rationale for the sit and reach test revisited. *Meas Phys Ed Exerc Sci*. 1998;2:85–92.
28. Aquino CF, Fonseca ST, Goncalves GGP, et al. Stretching versus strength training in lengthened position in subjects with tight hamstring muscles: a randomized controlled trial. *Man Ther*. 2010;15:26–31.
29. Liemohn W, Haydu T, Phillips D. Questionable exercises. *PCPFS Res Digest*. 1999;3(8):1–8.
30. Magnusson SP, Aagaard P, Nielson JJ. Passive energy return after repeated stretches of the hamstring muscle-tendon unit. *Med Sci Sports Exerc*. 2000;32:1160–1164.
31. Magnusson SP, Simonsen EB, Aagaard P, et al. Visocoelastic response to repeated static stretching in human skeletal muscle. *Scand J Med Sci Sport*. 1995;5:342–347.
32. Kay AD, Blazevich AJ. Moderate-duration static stretch reduces active and passive plantar flexor moment but not Achilles tendon stiffness or active muscle length. *J Appl Physiol*. 2009;106:1249–1256.
33. McHugh MP, Magnusson SP, Gleim GW, et al. Viscoelastic stress relaxation in human skeletal muscle. *Med Sci Sports Exerc*. 1992;24:1375–1382.
34. Avela J, Kyrolainen H, Komi PV. Altered reflex sensitivity after repeated and prolonged passive muscle stretching. *J Appl Physiol*. 1999;86:1283–1291.
35. Vujnovich AL, Dawson NJ. The effect of therapeutic muscle stretch on neural processing. *J Orthop Sports Phys Ther*. 1994;20:145–153.
36. Wessel J. Wan A. Effect of stretching on the intensity of delayed-onset muscle soreness. *Clin J Sports Med*. 1994;4:83–87.
37. Shrier I. Does stretching improve performance? A systematic and critical review of the literature. *Clin J Sport Med*. 2004;14:267–273.
38. Fowles JR, Sale DG, MacDougall JD. Reduced strength after passive stretch of the human plantar flexors. *J Appl Physiol*. 2000;89:1179–1188.
39. Magnusson SP, Simonsen EB, Aagaard P, et al. Biomechanical responses to repeated stretches in human hamstring muscle in vivo. *Am J Sports Med*. 1996;24:622–628.
40. Knudson D, Noffal G. Time course of stretch-induced isometric strength deficits. *Eur J Appl Physiol*. 2005;94: 348–351.
41. Whatman C, Knappstein A, Hume P. Acute changes in passive stiffness and range of motion post-stretching. *Phys Ther Sport*. 2006;7:195–200.
42. Magnusson SP, Aagard P, Simonsen E, et al. A biomechanical evaluation of cyclic and static stretch in human skeletal muscle. *Int J Sports Med*. 1998;19:310–316.
43. Kubo K, Kanehisa H, Fukunaga T. Effect of stretching on the viscoelastic properties of human tendon structures in vivo. *J Appl Physiol*. 2002;92:595–601.
44. Kubo K, Kanehisa H, Fukunaga T. Effect of transient muscle contractions and stretching on the tendon structures in vivo. *Acta Physiol Scand*. 2002;175:157–164.
45. Mahieu NN, McNair P, De Muynck M, et al. Effect of static and ballistic stretching on muscle-tendon tissue properties. *Med Sci Sports Exerc*. 2007;39:494–501.
46. Craib MW, Mitchell VA. The association between flexibility and running economy in sub-elite male distance runners. *Med Sci Sports Exerc*. 1996;28:737–743.

47. Gleim GW, Stachenfeld NS, Nicholas JA. The influence of flexibility on the economy of walking and jogging. *J Orthop Res*. 1990;8:814–823.
48. Kubo K, Kanehisa H, Kawakami Y, et al. Elastic properties of muscle-tendon complex in long-distance runners. *Eur J Appl Physiol*. 2000;81:181–187.
49. Kubo K, Kawakami Y, Fukunaga T. Influence of elastic properties of tendon structures on jump performance in humans. *J Appl Physiol*. 1999;87:2090–2096.
50. Walshe AD, Wilson GJ, Murphy AJ. The validity and reliability of a test of lower body musculotendinous stiffness. *Eur J Appl Physiol*. 1996;73:332–339.
51. Wilson GJ, Elliott BC, Wood GA. Stretch shorten cycle performance enhancement through flexibility training. *Med Sci Sports Exerc*. 1992;24:116–123.
52. Wilson GJ, Wood GA, Elliott BC. Optimal stiffness of series elastic component in a stretch-shorten cycle activity. *J Appl Physiol*. 1991;70:825–833.
53. Gleim GW, McHugh MP. Flexibility and its effects on sports injury and performance. *Sports Med*. 1997;24:289–299.
54. Amako M, Oda T, Masuoka K, et al. Effect of static stretching on prevention of injuries for military recruits. *Mil Med*. 2003;168:442–446.
55. Pope RP, Herbert RD, Kirwan JD. Effects of flexibility and stretching on injury risk in army recruits. *Aust J Physiother*. 1998;44:165–172.
56. Pope RP, Herbert RD, Kirwan JD, et al. A randomized trial of preexercise stretching for prevention of lower-limb injury. *Med Sci Sports Exerc*. 2000;32:271–277.
57. Weldon SM, Hill RH. The efficacy of stretching for prevention of exercise-related injury: a systematic review of the literature. *Man Ther*. 2003;8:141–150.

CHAPTER 10

Resistance Exercise Techniques and Spotting

JOHN F. GRAHAM

OBJECTIVES

After reading this chapter, you will be able to:

- Recall the general adaptations to resistance training.
- Safely and effectively provide assistance during exercises by spotting.
- Understand the importance of wearing proper clothing and footwear in the weight room.
- Demonstrate the eight basic components of resistance training.
- Identify certain exercises that can have carryover to other activities.

KEY TERMS

Absolute Muscular Strength
Alternated Grip
Common
Energy Intake
Hook Grip
Hyperplasia
Hypertrophy
Intermuscular Adaptation
Intramuscular Adaptation
Muscle Recruitment
Narrow
Neutral Grip
Osteopenia
Osteoporosis
Overload
Overtraining
Pronated Grip
Relative Muscular Strength
Spotter
Sticking Point
Supinated Grip
Valsalva Maneuver
Wide

Introduction

Enclosed in this chapter is an explanation of the benefits and physiological aspects, safety, equipment, and techniques of resistance training. It also includes detailed descriptions of 22 free-weight, 8 machine-resistance-training, and 3 trunk exercises in the following classes: total-body (power/explosive), multijoint lower-body, single-joint lower-body, upper-body multijoint, and upper-body single-joint exercises. Total-body exercises emphasize loading the spine directly or indirectly in an explosive manner. Multijoint exercises involve two or more joints that change angles during the movement of a repetition. Single-joint exercises involve only one joint changing its angle during the completion of a repetition. Each exercise described in this chapter is accompanied by a detailed explanation of the type of exercise, muscles utilized, body and limb alignment, ascending and descending movement, safety points, and variations of exercise technique.

Compound, multijoint exercises can be broken down into simple, single-joint movements. For example, dead lifts and front squats can benefit the power clean. Different exercises can also activate the same muscle groups as other exercises, providing a large carryover between them. Dumbbell flies and the incline bench press activate the same muscles that are being used during the barbell bench press, thereby assisting the bench press.

BENEFITS OF RESISTANCE TRAINING

Muscles adapt to resistance training by strengthening and growing. This process, called **hypertrophy** (1–3), involves an increase in the cross-sectional area of muscle fibers, not the splitting of the muscle into additional muscle fibers, which is called **hyperplasia**. Hypertrophy has been demonstrated to occur as a result of an increase in the thickness and number of myofibrils (1–4). It is believed to be the primary mechanism governing muscle growth. A number of factors generally are responsible for muscle hypertrophy (1–4):

- **Overload**. The resistance should be greater than the muscle's previous level of adaptation.
- **Muscle recruitment**. The maximal numbers of muscle fibers should be recruited.
- **Energy intake**. An adequate amount of carbohydrate and protein should be consumed.

Resistance training can enhance absolute and relative muscle strength (1–5). **Absolute muscular strength** is the strength an individual can develop regardless of body weight. **Relative muscular strength** is defined by absolute muscular strength divided by body weight in either kilograms or pounds. Increases in muscle and explosive strength are generally tied to inter- and intramuscular adaptations and muscle hypertrophy. The term **intermuscular adaptation** refers to the proper execution of exercise technique for exercises performed at both slow and explosive speeds. As an individual acquires the proper exercise technique, less energy is required to perform the exercise; therefore, the resistance utilized can be increased. **Intramuscular adaptation** refers to how many motor units are recruited during the effort, how quickly they are recruited, and whether antagonistic motor units interfere with the movement (1–5). By undergoing resistance training, individuals can expect an increased number of motor units to be recruited at an accelerated speed along with an increased inhibition of antagonistic muscle(s). As a muscle increases in cross-sectional area (hypertrophy), it will develop more force and power than will muscles with a smaller cross-sectional area.

Increases in strength from resistance training are due to both hypertrophic and neurological adaptations.

Other benefits of resistance training include improvements in bone density and energy utilization and storage. The lack of weight-bearing activity with aging has often been linked to **osteopenia** (lowering of bone mineral mass to 1 standard deviation below young-normal levels) and **osteoporosis** (lowering of bone mineral mass to more than 2.5 standard deviations below young-normal levels). As discussed in Chapter 4, bone adapts to resistance training by increasing mineralization in a particular region of the bone to increase its strength and its ability to handle the stress due to resistance training (6). This may be accomplished through exercises using loads at greater than 75% of an individual's 3-RM (the maximum weight an individual can utilize for three repetitions) that are weight bearing in nature (multijoint, closed-chain-kinetic exercises, such as leg presses, squats, and straight-leg dead lift). If the resistance training includes light to moderate loads (40% to 60% of 1-RM), higher repetitions (12 to 25), and shorter rest periods (30 to 60 seconds), moderate increases of 5% in VO_2 (oxygen uptake) may be expected (2,7). With resistance training, individuals will utilize and store energy more efficiently. This will result in the muscle's ability to train at higher resistances and for longer periods of time. Resistance training performed with good technique through a full range of motion (ROM) can enhance muscle flexibility and reduce the likelihood of injury (2,7).

> ***The effects of a resistance-training program depend on training variables such as repetitions, intensities, and rest periods.***

Although it is not surprising that males are typically stronger than females, the differences in muscle strength are not tied to the quality of the muscle tissue or its ability to produce force or power, since in these respects no difference exists between genders. A significant difference does exist, however, in the quantity of muscle tissue in the average male (40%) versus female (23%), which is largely responsible for the male strength advantage. It is this difference that also helps to explain why women are typically 43% to 63% weaker in upper-body strength and 25% to 30% weaker in lower-body strength (2,7). Conditioning programs for male and female athletes for the same sport should be essentially the same, as the physiological demands of the sport are the same.

> ***Males generally have a greater absolute strength than females, but males and females are very similar in relative strength.***

Overtraining is characterized by a decline in performance over a time. This occurs when an individual's body is not given enough time to recuperate from training prior to the next training session (1–5,7). Symptoms of overtraining include but are not limited to the following:

- An increase in morning resting heart rate
- An unintentional decrease in body weight
- Inability to perform in a training session at the same level of strength, power, or endurance as had been achieved earlier
- An increase in muscle soreness from one training session to the next
- Extreme muscle soreness and stiffness on the day immediately following a training session
- A decrease in appetite

Once an individual becomes overtrained—that is, by exhibiting two or more of the warning signs listed above—the frequency, intensity, and duration of activity should be reduced until the symptoms dissipate. Obviously, it is more effective to prevent overtraining than to recover from it. Guidelines for preventing overtraining include increasing training intensity and duration gradually (<5%), utilizing periodized training (gradual cycling of specificity, intensity, and volume of training to achieve peak levels of performance and/or fitness at a designated time), following sound nutritional guidelines, and devoting adequate time to sleep and recovery. The risk of overtraining may be increased in training the multisport athlete (see the case study further on).

> ***Proper planning using a periodized resistance-training program will help prevent overtraining.***

SAFETY

Training equipment and facilities can provide a safe environment for exercise as long as basic safety guidelines are utilized.

SPOTTING

Probably the most critical aspect of safe training once the facility and equipment utilized have been inspected is the use of a spotter or spotters, particularly with free-weight exercises. A **spotter** is a knowledgeable individual who assists in the proper

REAL-WORLD APPLICATION

Training Male and Female Athletes for the Same Sport

You are asked to evaluate the conditioning program for both the boys and girls on your high school's basketball teams. You are asked to make recommendations to the coaches as to changes that they could consider.

Observed: After observing the training program you note that the girls' team uses only body-weight exercises while the boys' team is using only machines.

Recommendations: The boys' and girls' teams should not be using separate programs, since they are training for the same sport. It is recommended that both teams use free-weight exercises that focus on lower-body power. Machines can be used to train areas of muscular weakness or imbalance.

execution of an exercise (2,7,8). His or her responsibility is to ensure that the exerciser completes all repetitions with good technique, to assist the exerciser with completion of a repetition when needed, and to summon help when necessary (2,7,8). This responsibility should be taken very seriously, as failure to do so may result in serious injury not only to the exerciser but to the spotter as well. Exercises that involve the use of free weights over the head (standing barbell press), with the barbell resting on the back (barbell lunge or back squat), racked at the front of the upper shoulders (barbell front squat), or over the face (barbell bench press or supine triceps extension) will require the use of one or more spotters who are skilled at safely spotting, since these maneuvers are the most potentially harmful to the athlete. Exercises involving raising the barbell or dumbbell to the side or front of the body below shoulder level and power exercises generally do not require a spotter.

Barbells should always be loaded evenly on both sides and the weights secured with collars.

Exercises performed overhead and with the barbell on the front or back of the shoulders should be performed inside a power rack with the safety bars placed at an appropriate height. Individuals who are not spotting or performing the exercise should remain at a safe distance from the power rack. Because the loads utilized in these exercises can be substantial, spotters ideally should be nearly as strong and as tall as the exerciser. All additional barbells, collars, plates, weight trees, and other equipment should be outside the area immediately surrounding the immediate exercise area. Collars should be utilized regardless of the level of the load being used so as to prevent weight plates from sliding off the barbell. For maximum safety, three spotters (one directly behind the exerciser and one on each side of the barbell) should be present. All three should assist with removing the load from the rack as well as returning the load to the rack on completion of the repetitions.

Spotting must be taken seriously to ensure safe lifting practices. The focus of the spotter must be solely on the lifter throughout the entire exercise. Communication between the lifter and the spotter is a necessity. For example, the spotter must know the intentions of the lifter (i.e., repetition goals and when to provide aid).

For exercises performed over the face, the spotter should hold the barbell with an alternated grip inside the exerciser's grip to ensure that the barbell does not leave the exerciser's hands and land on the exerciser's face, neck, or chest. In the case of an exercise where the athlete's grip is narrow, the spotter may grasp the barbell immediately outside the exerciser's grip. Spotters should be conscious of body alignment (flat back, feet shoulder-width apart in a solid base, and a bent-knee position), as they may be called on quickly to help the exerciser by catching the barbell or by helping to lift the load. Dumbbell exercises may pose a different challenge to the spotter, as they require more skill to assist in exercises. For the safety of the exerciser, it is important for spotters to spot by standing as close to the dumbbells as possible and spotting near the wrists, so that the spotter can quickly support the exerciser if his or her elbows collapse, thus preventing the dumbbells from falling inward toward the exerciser's chest or face. For exercises in which one dumbbell is used, such as seated overhead triceps extension or supine dumbbell pull-over, it is

Q & A from the Field

Q ***You notice that a particular exerciser in your program looks fatigued. What questions might you ask him? What possible causes of the fatigue should you consider?***

A How much sleep is he getting? What are his eating habits? Is he getting enough recovery between training sessions? Is there enough variety in his exercises? You should consider overtraining, drug use, disease, psychological problems, and normal emotional stresses as possible causes.

important to spot with the hands directly on or slightly below the dumbbell.

In selecting the number of spotters for a given exercise, an exerciser should consider the load being lifted, the physical strength and height of the spotters, and the experience level of both the exerciser and spotters. The heavier the load, the greater the risk for injury and the severity of injury to both the exerciser and the spotter should the exerciser fail to complete a repetition and an inadequate spot be provided. For most exercises that involve overhead lifting with a barbell, a barbell on the back or shoulders with heavier loads, and over-the-face exercises with heavier loads, a lead spotter should be placed immediately behind the lifter to direct the other spotters placed on each side of the barbell. As the number of spotters increases, so does the potential for errors in timing. Prior to the first lift, the exerciser should tell the spotter(s) how the barbell will be lifted from the rack, how many repetitions will be performed, and how the barbell will be returned to the rack. This ensures that the exercise can be performed safely and that the spotters do not disrupt the exercise.

By varying exercises, volumes, and intensities, safe and well-planned resistance training can have positive effects on skeletal muscle growth, neuromuscular coordination, and bone mineral density in both, men and women.

Exercises that require explosive power should not utilize a spotter. Spotting these exercisers places both the exerciser and the spotter at increased risk for injury. Exercisers performing these explosive lifts should be taught the proper technique for missing a lift. To miss a lift when the barbell is in front of the body, the proper technique is to push the barbell forward and release it as the lifter moves backward. To miss a lift with the barbell behind the body, the lifter should release the barbell and jump forward. For the safety of not only the exerciser but also other exercisers in the surrounding area, power exercises should be performed on a segregated power platform clear of other exercisers and equipment.

EXERCISE APPAREL

Proper clothing when exercising with resistance equipment is critical for two major reasons: safety and etiquette. It is important to wear a workout shirt that covers the chest, upper back, and shoulders to avoid losing control of a barbell on exercises where the barbell rests on the upper shoulders (e.g., barbell back squats). Without a shirt that covers those areas, a barbell may slip off the body, putting the exerciser, spotters, and other exercisers nearby at risk for injury. Covering the upper body with a T-shirt is also important on exercises that require the exerciser to lie prone or supine on a bench. Not doing so is poor etiquette and may also cause damage to the equipment's upholstery.

Clothing provides a layer of protection from exercise equipment and also provides friction between the lifter and the bar. For example, the bar does not slide off of the back during a squat as easily while clothed as it would on a bare back. Shoes protect the feet from foreign objects lining the floor and also provide a stable base, encouraging proper lifting technique.

Footwear is also important in resistance training. Closed-toe training shoes that provide a solid, stable base should be used at all times. The proper shoes will ensure that the exerciser has a stable lifting base, which is critical for all explosive lower-body, squatting, overhead-lift, or lifting-from-the-floor exercises. Closed-toe shoes also provide some protection against dropped plates, barbells, and dumbbells. Sandals and bare feet should never be permitted in the resistance-training area for reasons of safety and hygiene.

Safety is extremely important in a resistance-training program, and proper precautions should be taken at all times.

RESISTANCE-TRAINING TECHNIQUE

If benefits are to be maximized, every resistance-training exercise will provide its own unique challenges. Many exercisers have similarities as well as differences. Understanding similarities and differences is essential for the proper selection of exercises in the design of a resistance-training prescription. The proper execution of a resistance-training exercise has eight basic components:

1. Objective for exercise selection
2. Equipment alignment
3. Body alignment
4. Stabilization of body
5. Movement of body during exercise
6. Speed of movement
7. Breathing
8. Initiation and return of exercise equipment

In selecting an exercise, it is essential to ensure that the exercise matches the objective of the resistance-training program. For example, exercisers often perform numerous sets of chest exercises while not balancing them with an appropriate number of upper back exercises or failing to perform leg exercises. Spot enhancement or reduction of a given section of the body is not achievable (2,3,9). It is important for exercisers to recognize the importance of balance in a resistance-training exercise prescription. You are only as good as your weakest link.

To choose appropriate exercises, the lifter or coach must understand how to select the proper exercises. Selection of exercises, proper alignment, movement, and speed of movement are all components of resistance training.

Equipment alignment means setting the equipment up properly so that the exercise can be performed safely and with maximum benefit. The proper resistance should be set on a machine exercise, the barbell should have equal resistance on each side, or dumbbells of identical resistance should be selected. Collars should be placed securely on each side of the barbell to make sure that weights do not slide or fall off the barbell, causing the barbell to tip. Hooks for barbell exercises in which the barbell is placed on the shoulder should be set 3 to 4 in. below shoulder level so that the exerciser can drop under the barbell to remove it from the rack to initiate the set and then return it to the rack above the hooks before sliding it back down on the hooks at the completion of the set. Safety bars on the power rack should be set slightly below the end ROM on squat or power exercises performed within the rack. Cams, seats, and arm and leg lengths on machines should be adjusted to the exerciser's optimal safe ROM.

As a general rule, select exercises that work opposing muscle groups.

In positioning the body during resistance training, the axial skeleton and its immediate attachments are of the highest priority (2,3,9). This means that particular attention should continuously be paid to the positioning of the pelvis, spinal column, and shoulder girdle before and during any resistance-training exercise. The spinal column is in its most stable and therefore strongest position when it and the pelvis are all in neutral positions with a slight thoracic kyphosis and lumbar lordosis. To place the torso in an ideal resistance-training position, the athlete should pull the shoulder blades back slightly and down, lift the sternum slightly out and up, and pull the chin slightly back and down, creating or maintaining the natural arch in the thoracic and lumbar regions of the spine (2,3,9). Once the body is positioned correctly, the positioning of the hands is important. The two primary handgrip positions are the **pronated grip** (palms down and knuckles up) and **supinated grip** (palms up and knuckles down). A variation of either grip is the **neutral grip** (knuckles point laterally). Other grips include the **alternated grip** (one hand supinated and the other pronated). In performing exercises that require a stronger grip (Olympic-style lifts), a **hook grip** (wrapping the index and middle fingers around the thumb, which is placed against the bar first, the ring and little fingers holding the bar rather loosely) designed to add at least 10% to any pulling motion is used (10). Along with the handgrip, grip width must be considered. The three grip widths are **common** (shoulder width), **wide** (outside of shoulder width), and **narrow** (inside shoulder width).

Before performing any exercise, it is important to know the correct grip and grip width.

Regardless of whether the exercise is performed utilizing a barbell, dumbbell, or machine, stabilization of the body is critical. A stable position enables an exerciser to maintain proper body alignment during an exercise, which in turn ensures that the appropriate stress is placed on the intended muscles and joints. Exercises that call for a standing position require the feet to be positioned at shoulder width, with the feet securely in contact with the floor. Whether the exerciser is seated, prone (lying face down), or supine (lying face up), his or her head, shoulders (front or back), chest or upper back, lower back, and buttocks or pelvis should be in contact with the bench or machine. The feet must remain in contact with the floor unless the height of the machine does not permit or require the feet to be in contact with the floor or the exercise is a lower-body open-chain exercise.

The movement of the body during an exercise does not have a definitive set point. Although exercises generally have a maximum ROM, the ideal ROM will depend on variations in the exerciser's musculoskeletal, neurological, and biomechanical systems. Modern exercise machines are often designed with a range of controls for both the eccentric and concentric muscle actions. Additionally, power racks allow the exerciser to control ROM in barbell exercises when necessary owing to considerations of safety, injury reconditioning, or technique.

Speed of motion with exercises depends on the type of exercise being performed. With the exception of power or explosive lifts, exercises should be performed in a slow, controlled manner to increase the likelihood that a full ROM can be achieved. The eccentric muscle action should be performed over a 4-second period with a 1-second hold at completion before initiating the concentric movement. The concentric movement should be performed over a 2- to 4-second period with a 1-second hold at the completion before initiating the eccentric muscle action. When exercises are performed quickly, momentum will increase, negatively impacting body alignment, stabilization of the body, and movement.

In instructing exercisers on breathing during resistance training, the most important point to stress is to breathe at some point during every repetition. The most strenuous portion of a repetition, typically where the lifter is most likely to fail, is referred to as the **sticking point** (2). This is the point in the ROM of any joint where the mechanical advantage of the lever system is the lowest. The exact angle of the sticking point will depend on the mechanical properties of a specific joint. A general rule of thumb is for exercisers to inhale before initiating an exercise or at the less stressful phase of the repetition and to exhale upon passing the sticking point or the most stressful phase of a repetition. For more advanced exercisers, utilizing heavier resistances, such as those exercises that load the vertebral column and place stress on it, the use of the **Valsalva maneuver** (expiring against a closed glottis, which when combined with contracting the abdomen and rib cage muscles, creates rigid compartments of fluid in the lower torso and air in the upper torso) may be warranted in maintaining proper vertebral alignment and support (2,8). The Valsalva maneuver, however, should be utilized only through the sticking point of a lift. Periods that exceed 1 to 2 seconds of breath holding while working against a resistance may cause dizziness, disorientation, excessively high blood pressure, and blackouts.

As a final aspect of resistance-training technique, it is very important for exercisers to recognize the importance of properly lifting a resistance to initiate a set and returning the resistance to its starting position at the completion of a set. In using a barbell with a power rack or bench to perform exercises that require loading of the vertebral column or overhead or over-the-face exercises, at least one spotter should be used to guide the exerciser in removing the resistance from its starting position and then returning it at the completion of the set to ensure that the barbell is safely removed and returned. For the safety of the exerciser and others in the immediate area as well as for equipment maintenance, exercise should be initiated with the resistance being lifted from its resting position and returned to its starting position slowly.

RESISTANCE-TRAINING EXERCISES

Power Exercises (2,8,10–14)
Power clean
Power snatch
Power jerk

Hip/Thigh Exercises (2,8,15,12,13,16–21)
Back squat
Front squat
Dead lift
Barbell lunge
Stiff-leg dead lift
Leg press
Leg extension
Leg curl
Standing heel raise

Chest Exercises (2,12,22–26)
Bench press, dumbbell
Bench press, barbell
Incline press, dumbbell
Incline press, barbell
Dumbbell fly

Upper Back Exercises (2,12,21,27,28)
Dumbbell one-arm row
Lat pull-down
Seated cable row

Shoulder Exercises (2,12,21,29,30)
Dumbbell seated shoulder press
Machine shoulder press
Barbell upright row
Dumbbell prone posterior raise

Triceps Exercises (2,12,21)
Supine triceps extension
Triceps pushdown

Biceps Exercises (2,12,21)
Barbell bicep curl
Dumbbell seated alternate-arm bicep curl

Forearm Exercises (2,12,21)
Wrist curl
Reverse wrist curl

Abdominal and Lower Back Exercises (2,12,31)
Abdominal crunch
Back extension

Power Exercises

Power Clean

Type of Exercise

Total body/power (explosive) exercise

Muscles Used

Gluteus maximus, hamstrings (semimembranosus, semitendinosus, biceps femoris), quadriceps (vastus lateralis, vastus intermedius, vastus medialis, rectus femoris), soleus, gastrocnemius, trapezius, and deltoids (anterior, medial, and posterior)

Starting Position

Use a standard barbell. The lifting position is identical to that for the power snatch except for the hand position. The feet are between hip- and shoulder-width apart and pointing forward or just slightly outward. Squat and grasp the barbell with a shoulder-width or slightly wider pronated hand position using a closed or hook grip. Arms are outside the knees, elbows extended and pointing outward. Stand so that the barbell is over the balls of the feet and close to the shins. Back is rigid and flat or slightly arched. Head is up or slightly hyperextended. Chest is held up and out. Shoulder blades should be squeezed together. Trapezius and upper back should be relaxed and in a slight state of stretch. With the heels always remaining in contact

(continued)

Power Clean *(continued)*

with the floor, the body weight should be balanced between the balls and middles of the feet. Shoulders are slightly in front of or over the barbell (Fig. 10.1A,B).

Upward Motion: First Pull

Initiate the power clean by taking in a deep breath and holding it. Lift the barbell off the floor through forceful hip and knee extension. Maintain a constant position of the torso in relation to the floor throughout the first pull. In other words, make sure that the hips do not rise faster or before the shoulders, and keep the back flat or slightly arched. The head should remain in a neutral position in relation to the spine. The shoulders should remain slightly in front of or over the barbell. The elbows should still be fully extended. During the first pull, keep the barbell as close to the shins as possible. Continue to hold your breath (Fig. 10.1C,D).

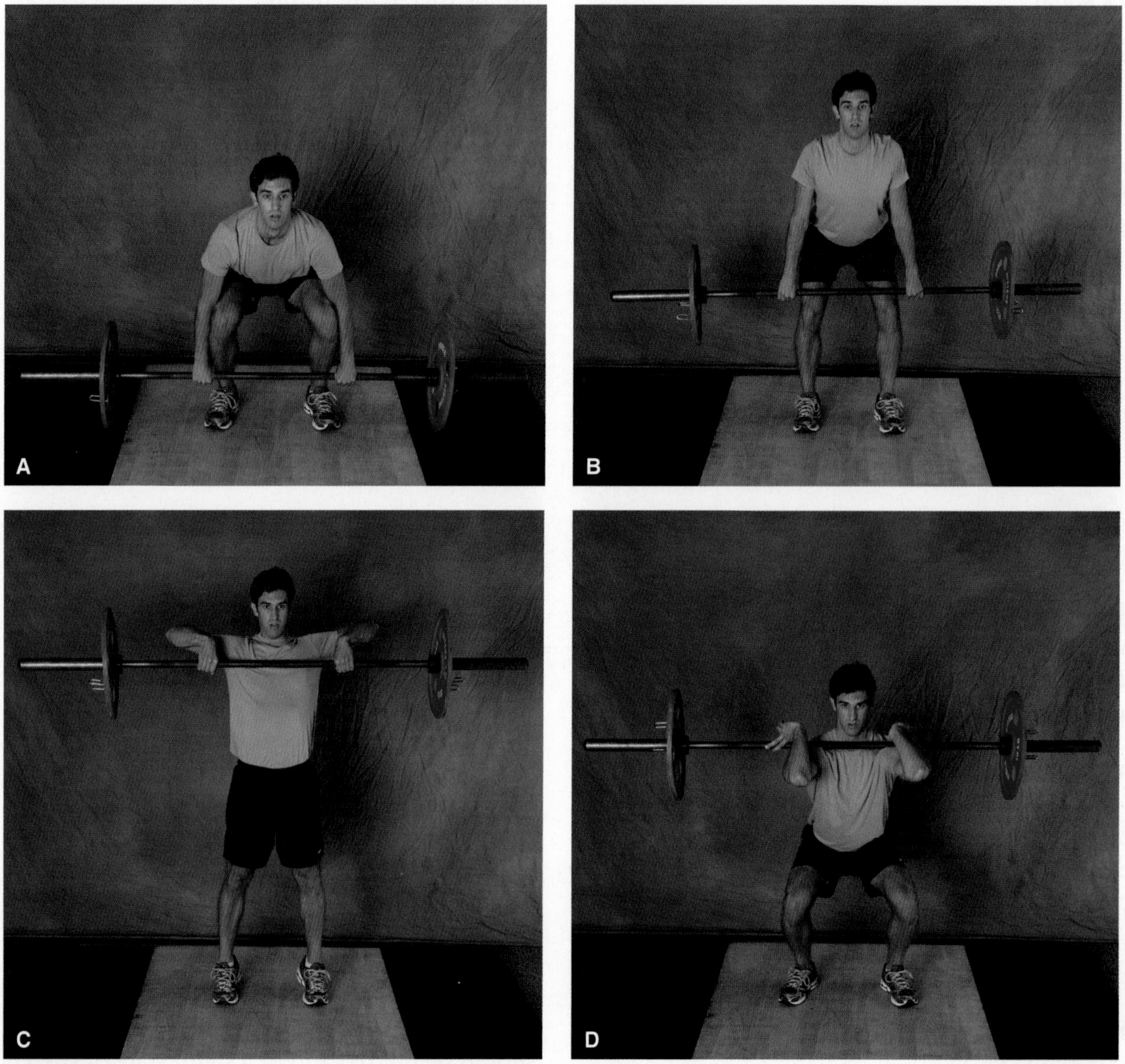

FIGURE 10.1 Power clean. **A.** Starting position. **B.** First pull. **C.** Second pull. **D.** Catch position.

Power Clean *(continued)*

Upward Motion: Transition (Scoop)

Explosively drive the hips forward and slightly increase the knee bend to enable the knees to move under and the thighs to move against the barbell. As the knee bend is increased, shift the body's weight forward toward the front half of the feet while still keeping the heels in contact with the floor. The back should remain slightly arched or flat. The shoulders should remain over or ahead of the barbell. The head should remain in line with the spine. Keep the elbows fully extended and pointing out. Continue holding the initial breath. At the completion of the scoop, the body should be in position for the initiation of the second pull.

Upward Motion: Second Pull (Power Phase)

With the barbell touching the body between the knees and midthigh, initiate the second pull by explosively extending the hips, knees, and ankles. Keep the shoulders over the barbell. Maintain a straight elbow position as long as possible while the hips, knees, and ankles are extending. Simultaneously, fully extend the lower extremity joints and rapidly shrug the shoulders upward. The elbows should continue to remain extended and pointing out during the shrugging movement. Upon fully elevating the shoulders, rapidly flex the elbows to begin pulling the body under the barbell. With the elbows moving up and out to the sides, pull with the arms as high as possible. The powerful upward acceleration from the second pull will result in an erect torso and head. The feet will come off the floor.

Upward Motion: Catch

After the lower body has fully extended and the barbell reaches near maximal height, pull the body under the bar by rotating the arms and hands around then under the barbell. Rapidly bend the knees and hips to a half-squat position. The feet should return to the floor pointing straight ahead or slightly outward at a width slightly wider than that at the starting position. The barbell should be caught at the clavicles and anterior deltoids with the head facing forward; neck neutral; feet flat on the floor pointing straight ahead or slightly outward; body weight over the front half of the foot with the heels in contact with the floor; knees and hips flexed to a half-squat position to absorb the impact of the weight; back flat; upper arms parallel to the floor; elbows fully flexed; and the wrists extended. The barbell is caught with the torso almost fully erect and the shoulders slightly in front of the buttocks. The position is similar to the midposition of the front squat, enabling the barbell to be directly over the body's center of gravity. If the torso is too erect, however, the momentum of the barbell will push the shoulders backward and possibly hyperextend the lower back, resulting in a potential risk of injury. Upon catching the barbell and establishing control and balance, complete the catch by standing to a fully erect position. Exhale and return to normal breathing pattern (Fig. 10.1E).

Downward Motion

Unless maximal or near-maximal loads are used, the barbell should be returned to the floor in a controlled manner. Lower the barbell in two separate movements. While maintaining a flat back, slowly flex the hips and knees and lower the barbell to the thighs while keeping the barbell close to the body. Continue to maintain the flat back while continuing to flex the hips and knees as the barbell is lowered to the floor. Keep the barbell close to the thighs and shins during the descent. A rapid drop or release of the barbell should be avoided with any resistance below maximal or near-maximal level. Once the barbell has reached the floor, reposition it and the body for the next repetition. In utilizing submaximal loads, the barbell should be lowered to the floor without relaxing or releasing tension; touch the plates to the floor, and then immediately (without a pause, provided that the body is in the correct starting position) and explosively lift the barbell for the next repetition.

(continued)

Power Clean *(continued)*

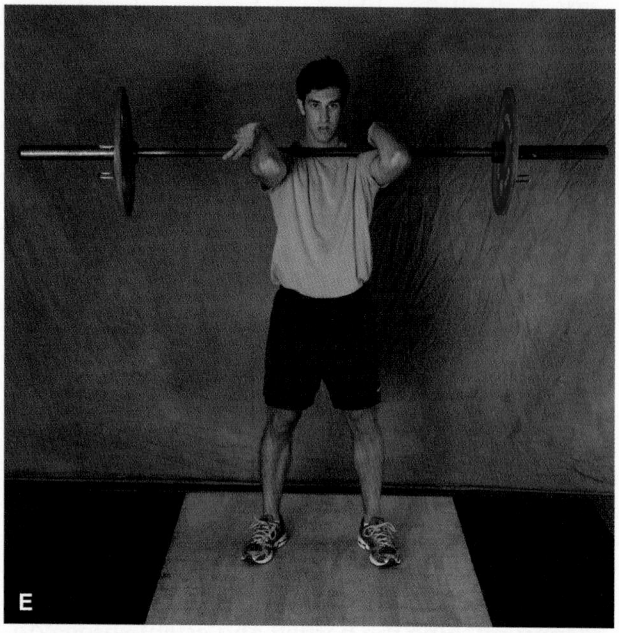

FIGURE 10.1 *(Continued)* **E.** First position.

Power Snatch

Type of Exercise

Total-body/power (explosive) exercise

Muscles Used

Gluteus maximus, hamstrings (semimembranosus, semitendinosus, biceps femoris), quadriceps (vastus lateralis, vastus intermedius, vastus medialis, rectus femoris), soleus, gastrocnemius, trapezius (upper portion), deltoids (anterior, medial, and posterior), and triceps brachii

Starting Position

Use a standard barbell. The lifting position is identical to the power clean except for the hand position. The feet are between hip- and shoulder-width apart and pointing forward or just slightly outward. Squat and grasp the barbell with a wider-than-shoulder-width grip (measured by measuring the distance from the knuckle edge of the clenched fist of an arm extended out to the side and parallel to the floor, across the back of the upper arm/upper back, to the outside edge of the opposite shoulder) and pronated hand position using a closed or hook grip. Arms are outside the knees, elbows extended and pointing outward. Stand so that the barbell is over the balls of the feet and close to the shins. Back is rigid and flat or slightly arched. Head is up or slightly hyperextended. Chest is held up and out. Shoulder blades should be squeezed together. Trapezius and upper back should be relaxed and in a slight state of stretch. With the heels always remaining in contact with the floor, the body weight should be balanced between the balls and middles of the feet. Shoulders are slightly in front of or over the barbell (Fig. 10.2A,B).

Upward Motion: First Pull

Initiate the power snatch by taking a deep breath and holding it. Lift the barbell off the floor through forceful hip, knee, and ankle

Power Snatch *(continued)*

extension. Maintain a constant position of the torso in relation to the floor throughout the first pull. Make sure that the hips do not rise faster or before the shoulders, and keep the back flat or slightly arched. The head should remain in a neutral position in relation to the spine. The shoulders should remain slightly in front of or over the barbell. The elbows should still be fully extended. During the first pull, keep the barbell as close to the shins as possible. Continue to hold your breath (Fig. 10.2C,D).

Upward Motion: Transition (Scoop)

Explosively drive the hips forward and slightly increase the knee bend to enable the knees to move under and the thighs against the barbell.

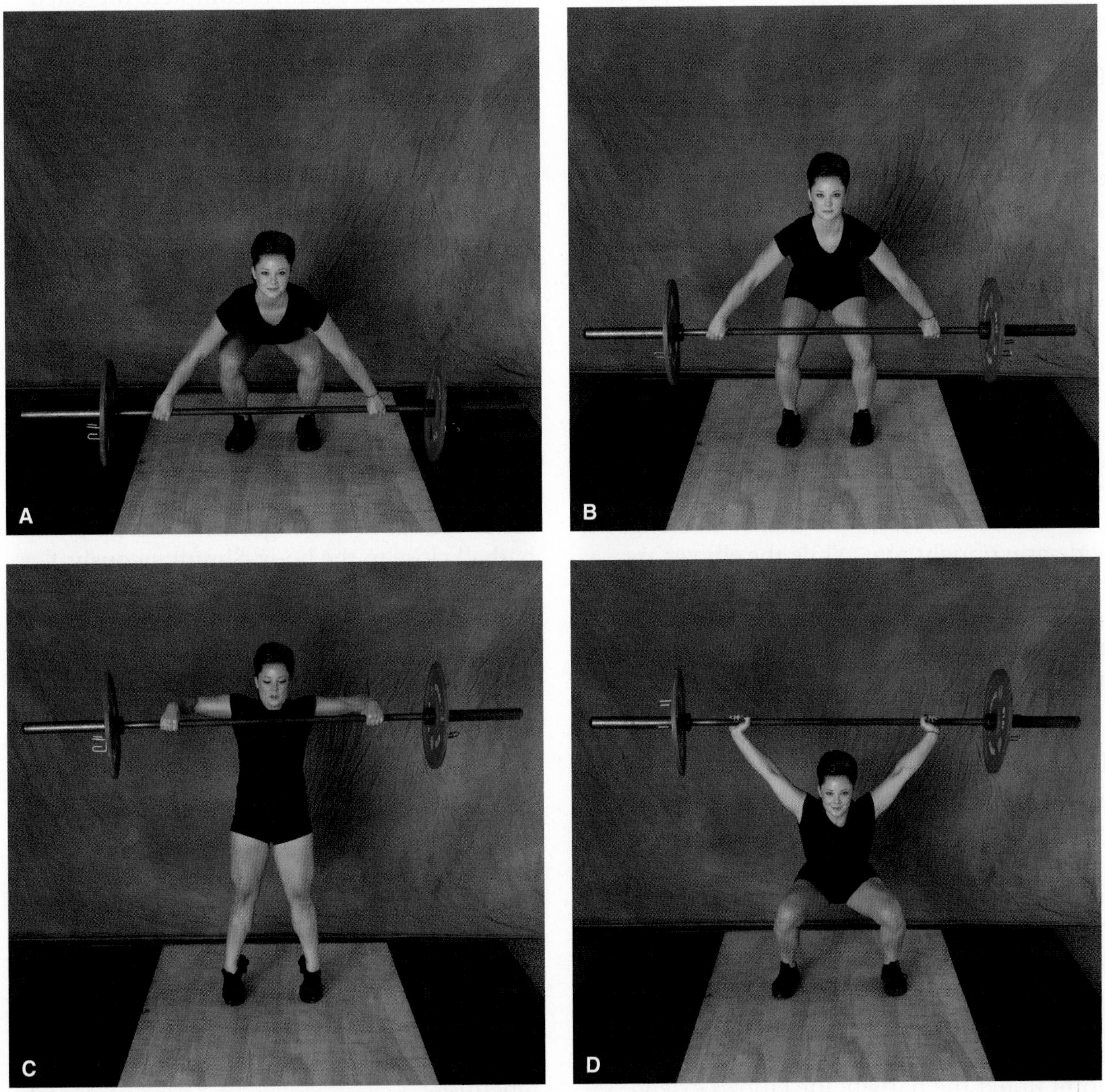

FIGURE 10.2 Power snatch. **A.** Starting position. **B.** First pull. **C.** Second pull. **D.** Catch position.

(continued)

Power Snatch *(continued)*

As the knee bend is increased, shift the body's weight forward toward the front half of the feet while still keeping the heels in contact with the floor. The back should remain slightly arched or flat. The shoulders should remain over or ahead of the barbell. The head should remain in line with the spine. Keep the elbows fully extended and pointing out to the sides. At the completion of the scoop, the body should be in position for initiation of the second pull.

Upward Motion: Second Pull (Power Phase)

With the barbell touching the body between the knees and midthigh, initiate the second pull by explosively extending the hips, knees, and ankles. Keep the shoulders over the barbell. Maintain a straight elbow position as long as possible while the hips, knees, and ankles are extending. Simultaneously fully extend the lower extremity joints and rapidly shrug the shoulders upward. The elbows should continue to remain extended and pointing out during the shrugging movement. Upon fully elevating the shoulders, rapidly flex the elbows to begin pulling the body under the barbell. The upper-body movement resembles that of an elongated wide-grip upright row. While the elbows are moving up and out to the sides, pull with the arms as high as possible. The powerful upward acceleration from the second pull will result in an erect torso and head. The feet will come off the floor.

Upward Motion: Catch

After the lower body has fully extended and the barbell reaches near-maximal height, pull the body under the barbell by rotating the arms and hands around and then under the barbell. Rapidly bend the knees and hips to a half-squat position. The feet should return to the floor pointing straight ahead or slightly outward at a width slightly wider than that of the starting position. As the arms reach a point under the barbell, the elbows extend rapidly to push the barbell up and the body downward under the barbell. The bar should be caught overhead with fully extended elbows, an erect/tight torso, the head in a neutral position in relation to the spine, knees flexed moderately, feet flat on the floor, the body weight over the center of gravity, and the barbell slightly behind or directly above the head. Upon catching the barbell and establishing control and balance, complete the catch by standing to a fully erect position. Exhale and return to a normal breathing pattern (Fig. 10.2E).

Downward Motion

If rubber bumper plates are used, the barbell may be returned to the floor by a controlled forward drop to the floor. The bounce of the bar should be controlled with the hands on or near the bar. Unless maximal or near maximal loads are used, however, the barbell should be returned to the floor in a controlled manner. Lower the barbell in two separate movements. While maintaining a flat back, slowly flex the hips and knees while simultaneously reducing the tension of the upper body musculature and lower the bar to the thighs while keeping the barbell close to the body. Simultaneously, flex the knees and hips to cushion the impact of the barbell on the thighs. Continue to maintain the flat back while continuing to flex the hips and knees as the barbell is lowered to the floor. Keep the barbell close to the thighs and shins during the descent. A rapid drop or release of the barbell should be avoided, with any resistance below maximal or near maximal level. Once the barbell has reached the floor, reposition it and the body for the next repetition. In utilizing submaximal loads, the barbell should be lowered to the floor without relaxing or releasing tension. Touch the plates to the floor and then immediately (without a pause, providing the body is in the correct starting position) explosively lift the barbell for the next repetition.

Power Snatch *(continued)*

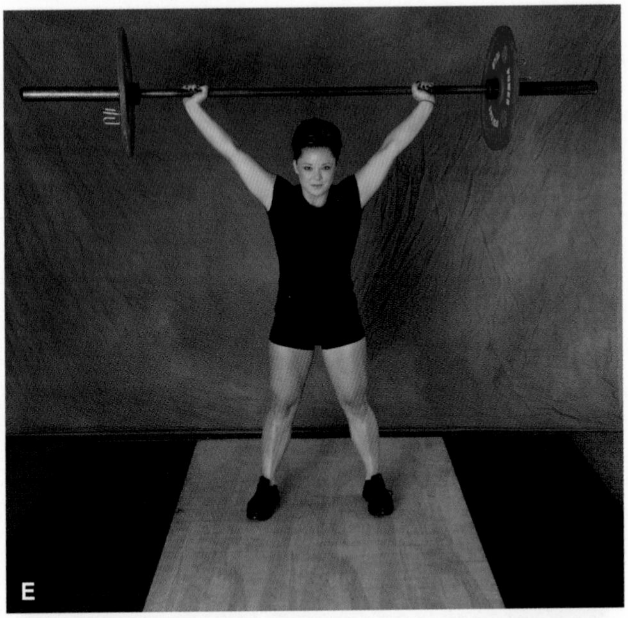

FIGURE 10.2 *(Continued)* **E.** Finish position.

Power Jerk

Type of Exercise

Total-body/power (explosive) exercise

Muscles Used

Gluteus maximus, hamstrings (semimembranosus, semitendinosus, biceps femoris), quadriceps (vastus lateralis, vastus intermedius, vastus medialis, rectus femoris), soleus, gastrocnemius, erector spinae, trapezius, and deltoids (anterior, medial, and posterior)

Starting Position

Position a standard barbell at chest level in a squat or power rack. Use a closed, pronated grip, slightly wider than the shoulders. Lift the barbell from its supports. If it is placed in front of the body, keep head slightly back with chin tucked in; shoulders elevated with elbows high/in front of barbell. If barbell is placed behind the head, keep head in neutral position or tilted forward slightly. Assume a natural stance (heels at shoulder width, toes pointing slightly outward). Feet should be firmly on training platform with weight distributed between heel and forefoot. The torso is rigid and upright (Fig. 10.3A,B).

Upward Motion

Dip 6 to 8 in (10% of body height) by flexing hips and knees, achieving a "power position" while maintaining complete foot contact with the platform. Immediately reverse direction with explosive extension of hips, knees, and ankles; weight may shift to forefoot. Jumping and pushing explosively enough to completely extend the body and lift the feet off the platform, complete upward drive. Drive barbell overhead with powerful leg action (not pressed with shoulders/arms) (Fig. 10.3C).

Downward Motion

Unless maximal or near-maximal loads are used, the barbell should be lowered to the shoulders and then replaced on the rack (or platform) in a controlled manner (a rapid drop or release should be avoided with a submaximal resistance).

(continued)

Power Jerk *(continued)*

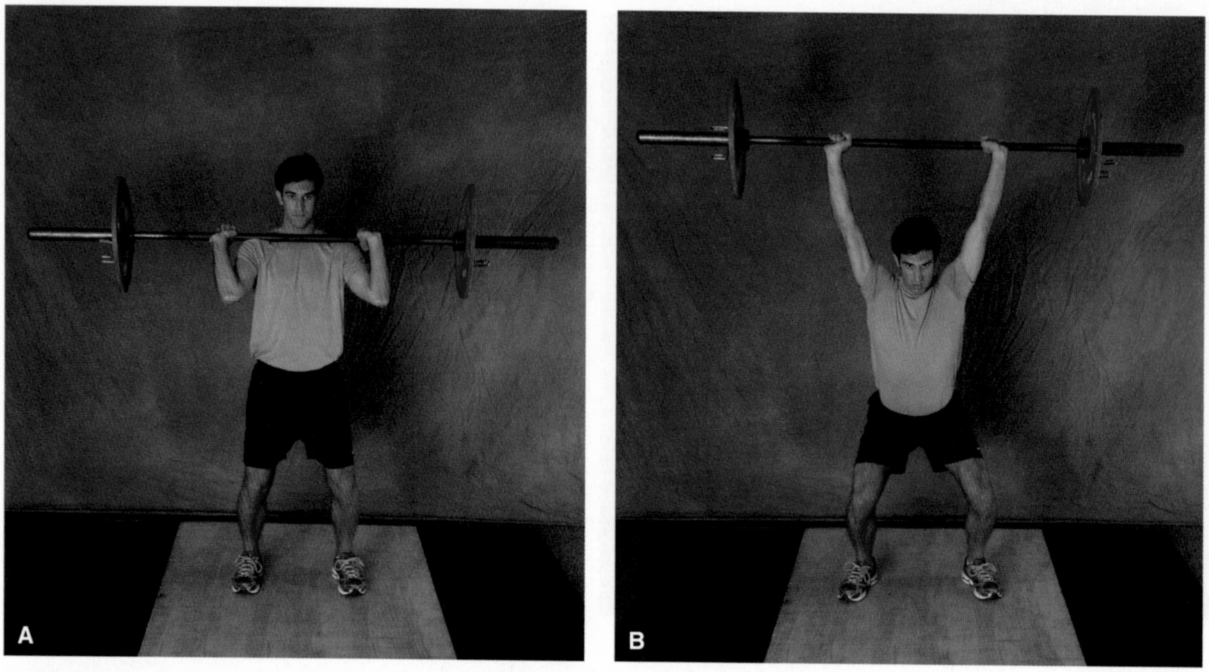

FIGURE 10.3 Power jerk. **A.** Starting position. **B.** Catch position.

Variation in Upward Motion: Split Jerk

Athlete explosively splits legs front/back as barbell leaves torso and feet lift off platform. Key is dynamic placement of front foot one to two foot lengths ahead of hips (complete foot contact with platform is maintained). Shins are vertical. Back foot is placed two to three foot lengths behind hips; supported on forefoot (heel off platform); knee is slightly flexed. Hip-width stance should be maintained to maintain stable base. Athlete pushes himself or herself under the barbell, then straightens arms and locks barbell overhead. Head shifts to neutral position; barbell is caught directly above hips, shoulders, and elbows. Note: Once the basic mechanics of the lift are mastered, the split allows the athlete to receive the barbell in a lower overhead position. Athlete pushes off front leg first, bringing it back under hips. Rear leg is brought forward under hips. Final position (barbell, elbows, shoulders, hips, knees, and ankles) in same vertical plane. Assume a natural stance (heels at shoulder width, toes pointing slightly outward). Feet should be firmly on training platform with weight distributed between heel and forefoot. Hips and knees fully extended. The torso is rigid and upright. Shoulders elevated, arms fully extended and locked, supporting barbell overhead. Head in neutral position. Eyes focused straight ahead, not looking up at barbell. Barbell is under control.

! *Safety:* ***Technique on How to Miss***

If athlete loses control of the barbell or cannot complete a rep for any reason, he or she should quickly get out from underneath and let it drop (without trying to save it on the way down). Use the barbell's downward momentum to move out of the way (the athlete is told to "keep your grip and push yourself away from the barbell as it falls"). Stay between the plates (this does not mean that the athlete should remain under a falling barbell but rather should move backward or forward, not sideways, to escape).

Power Jerk *(continued)*

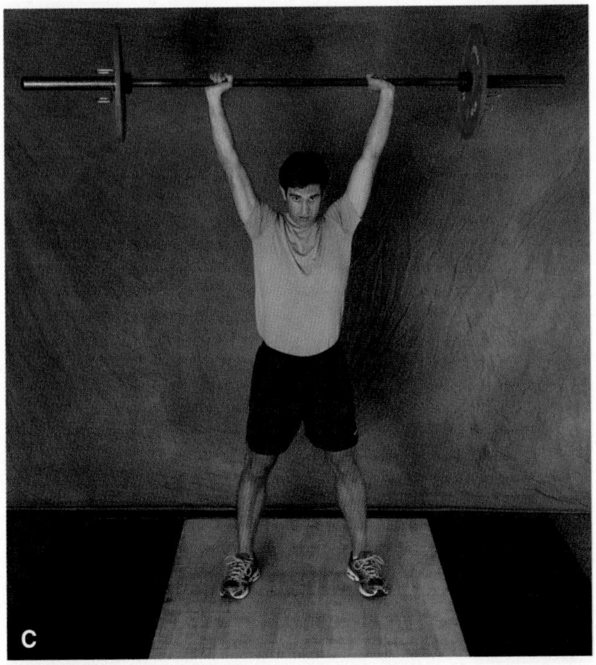

FIGURE 10.3 *(Continued)* **C.** Finish position.

Hip/Thigh Exercises

Back Squat

Type of Exercise

Lower body/multijoint

Muscles Used

Gluteus maximus, quadriceps (vastus lateralis, vastus intermedius, vastus medialis, rectus femoris), hamstrings (semimembranosus, semitendinosus, biceps femoris)

Starting Position

Position a standard barbell at chest level in a squat or power rack. Step underneath the barbell and position the base of the neck/upper middle back and the hips and feet directly under the barbell. Grasp the barbell using a pronated grip slightly wider than shoulder width. Place the barbell evenly above the posterior deltoids at the base of the neck (high barbell placement). Raise the elbows upward to provide a secure location for the barbell to rest on and prevent the bar from sliding down the back during the execution of the lift. To lift the barbell from the rack, extend the hips and knees and take a step backward. Feet are between hip- and shoulder-width apart and pointing forward or just slightly outward. Torso should remain erect. Keep chest out and up. Shoulders are back. Keep head and neck straight with eyes looking straight ahead. Before beginning the initial descent, take a breath and hold it (Fig. 10.4A).

Downward Motion

Initiate the exercise by slowly flexing the knees and hips. Descend with control. Maintain a flat back with a high elbow position. Avoid leaning forward or rounding the upper back during the descent phase. Keep the eyes focused straight ahead with the head erect. Keep the body weight centered over the heels and midfoot portions of both feet. The heels of both feet should remain in contact with the floor at all times throughout

(continued)

Back Squat *(continued)*

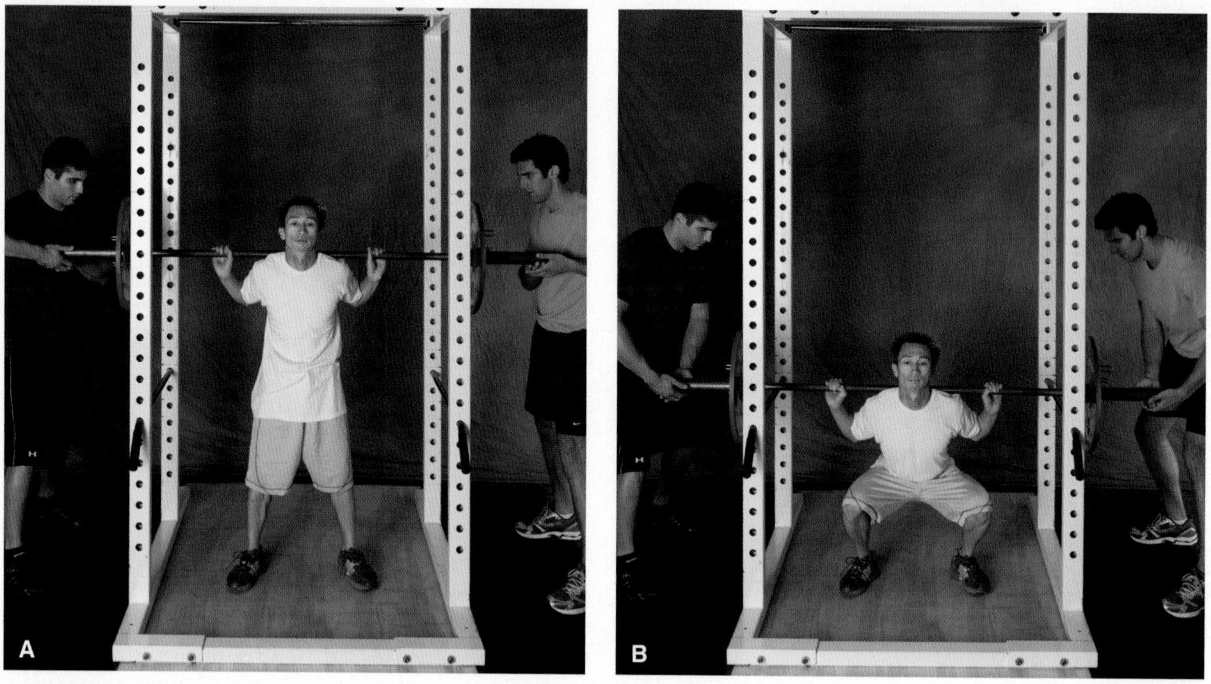

FIGURE 10.4 Back squat. **A.** Starting position. **B.** Finish position.

the descent. Keep the knees above or slightly in front of the ankles. Do not allow the knees to move in front of the feet. Continue the descent until the backs of the thighs are parallel to the floor, heels begin to lift off the floor, or the trunk begins to round or flex in a forward direction. The flexibility of the lower body will determine the actual depth of the descent. At the bottom position of the descent, avoid bouncing or increasing the rate of descent before beginning the ascent. Continue to hold your breath from the beginning of the descent (Fig. 10.4B).

Upward Motion

Lift the barbell forcefully and with control by extending the knees and hips. Keep the back flat. Do not round the upper back or lean forward during the ascent. Arms should remain tight and head erect with eyes looking straight ahead. Push through the entire foot on both feet with weight evenly distributed from the heels to the toes to make sure that the entire foot remains in contact with the floor. Keep the hips directly under the barbell. Avoid having the body weight move toward the toes. Keep the knees positioned above to

Q & A from the Field

Q ***In observing an exerciser in the squat, you note that she has too much forward trunk lean during the descent. Additionally, you notice that she has her heels on blocks of wood to raise them off of the floor. What advice would you consider for this athlete?***

A This athlete should lower the bar position and focus on keeping her head up during the lift. She should also work on gastrocnemius ROM so as to allow the heels to be flat during the lift.

Back Squat *(continued)*

slightly in front of the ankles. Continue the ascent by extending the lower body joints at a consistent rate until the initial standing position is reached. Continue holding your breath from the beginning of the descent through the midpoint of the ascent, then exhale and breathe normally before beginning the descent of the next repetition.

Returning the Weight to the Rack

At the completion of the set, return the barbell to the rack by slowly walking forward and returning the barbell to the support hooks of the rack.

Variation: Back Squat with Low Barbell Placement

Place the barbell evenly on the posterior deltoids at the middle of the trapezius. Grasp the barbell with an overhand closed grip wider than shoulder-width grip. The handgrip is generally wider than in the high barbell position to adjust for the lower barbell position.

Front Squat

Type of Exercise

Lower body/multijoint

Muscles Used

Gluteus maximus, quadriceps (vastus lateralis, vastus intermedius, vastus medialis, rectus femoris), hamstrings (semimembranosus, semitendinosus, biceps femoris)

Starting Position

Position a standard barbell at chest level in a squat or power rack. Grasp the barbell using a pronated grip slightly wider than shoulder width. Rotate the arms such that the barbell can be evenly placed across anterior deltoids/clavicles. The backs of the hands should be slightly outside the shoulders, located next to the barbell resting on the deltoids. Lift the elbows up and forward (upper arms should be parallel or as close as possible to the floor) to increase the stability of the barbell on the shoulders. Wrists should be hyperextended and elbows fully flexed. To lift the barbell from the rack, extend the hips and knees and take one to two steps backward. Feet are between hip- and shoulder-width apart and pointing forward or just slightly outward. The torso should remain erect. Keep chest out and up. Shoulders are back. Keep head and neck straight with eyes looking straight ahead. Before beginning the initial descent, inhale (Fig. 10.5A).

Downward Motion

Initiate the exercise by slowly flexing the knees and hips. Descend with control. Maintain a flat back with a high elbow position. Avoid leaning forward or rounding the upper back during the descent phase. Keep the eyes focused straight ahead with the head erect. Keep the body weight centered over the heel and midfoot portion of both feet. The heels of both feet should remain in contact with the floor at all times throughout the descent. Keep the knees above or slightly in front of the ankles during the descent. Do not allow the knees to move in front of the feet. Continue the descent until the backs of the thighs are parallel to the floor, heels begin to lift off the floor or the trunk begins to round or flex in a forward direction. The flexibility of the lower body will determine the actual depth of the descent. At the bottom position of the descent, avoid bouncing or increasing the rate of descent before beginning the ascent (Fig. 10.5B).

(continued)

Front Squat *(continued)*

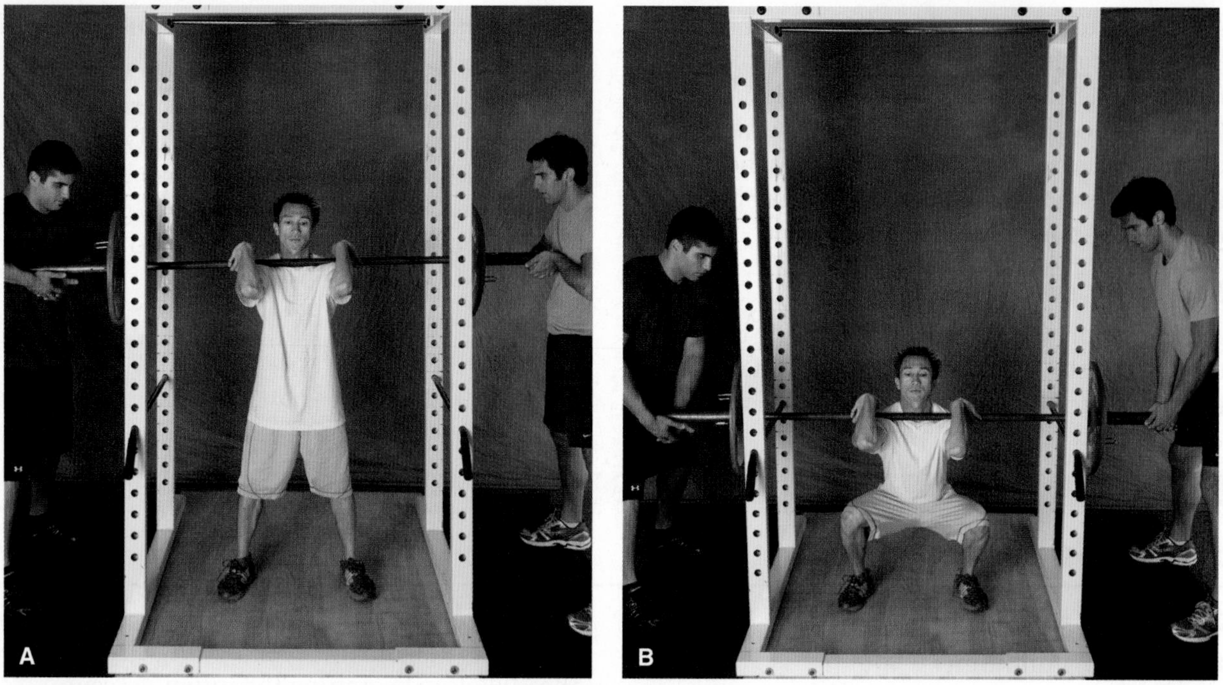

FIGURE 10.5 Front squat. **A.** Starting position. **B.** Finish position.

Upward Motion

Lift the barbell forcefully and with control by extending the knees and hips. Keep the back flat. Do not round the upper back or lean forward during the descent. Arms should remain tight and head erect with eyes looking straight ahead. Push through the entire foot on both feet with weight evenly distributed from the heels to the toes to ensure the entire foot remains in contact with the floor. Keep the hips directly under the barbell. Avoid having the body weight move toward the toes. Keep the knees positioned above to slightly in front of the ankles. Continue the ascent by extending the lower body joints at a consistent rate until the initial standing position is reached. Continue holding the breath from the beginning of the descent through the midpoint of the ascent, then exhale and breathe normally before beginning the descent of the next repetition.

Returning the Weight to the Rack

At the completion of the set, return the barbell to the rack by slowly walking forward and returning the barbell to the support hooks of the rack.

Variation: Front Squat with Closed-Arm Grip

Flex the elbows and cross the forearms in front of the chest. Position the barbell evenly on the anterior deltoids without touching it with the hands. Once the barbell is correctly placed, put both hands on top of the barbell and utilize pressure from the fingers to keep it in position. This is an open grip, since the thumb will not be able to encircle the barbell because of the shoulders being in the way.

Dead Lift

Type of Exercise

Lower body/multijoint

Muscles Used

Gluteus maximus, erector spinae, hamstrings (semimembranosus, semitendinosus, biceps femoris), quadriceps (vastus lateralis, vastus intermedius, vastus medialis, rectus femoris), trapezius, rhomboids, deltoids, and finger flexors

Starting Position

Use a standard barbell. The lifting position is identical to the power snatch and power clean except for the hand position. The feet are between hip- and shoulder-width apart and pointing forward or just slightly outward. Squat and grasp the barbell with an alternated grip (one palm supinated [facing forward] and one palm pronated [facing backward]) and hands slightly wider than shoulder-width apart. Arms are outside the knees, elbows extended and pointing outward. Stand so that the barbell is over the balls of the feet and close to the shins. Back is rigid and flat or slightly arched. Head is up or slightly hyperextended. Chest is held up and out. Shoulder blades should be squeezed together. Trapezius and upper back should be relaxed and in a slight state of stretch. With the heels always remaining in contact with the floor, the body weight should be balanced between the balls and middles of the feet. Shoulders are slightly in front of or over the barbell (Fig. 10.6A).

Upward Motion

Initiate the dead lift by extending the hips and knees at the same rate, maintaining a constant angle of the torso in relation to the floor. While keeping the body weight over the middle of the feet, ensure that the hips do not rise faster than the shoulders, and keep the back rigid and flat or slightly arched. Shoulders should remain slightly in front of or over the barbell, and elbows should be fully extended. Keep the barbell as close to the shins as possible during the ascent and slightly shift the body weight back toward the heels. As soon as the barbell reaches the knees, shift the body weight slightly forward toward the balls of the feet while keeping the heels on the floor. The back should remain rigid and flat or slightly arched, shoulders should remain slightly in front of or over the barbell, elbows should remain fully extended, and head is up or slightly hyperextended. Continue to simultaneously extend the hips and knees until the body reaches a fully erect torso position. The elbows should remain fully extended, like two steel rods, throughout the execution of the ascent. During the ascent the breath should be held until the barbell reaches

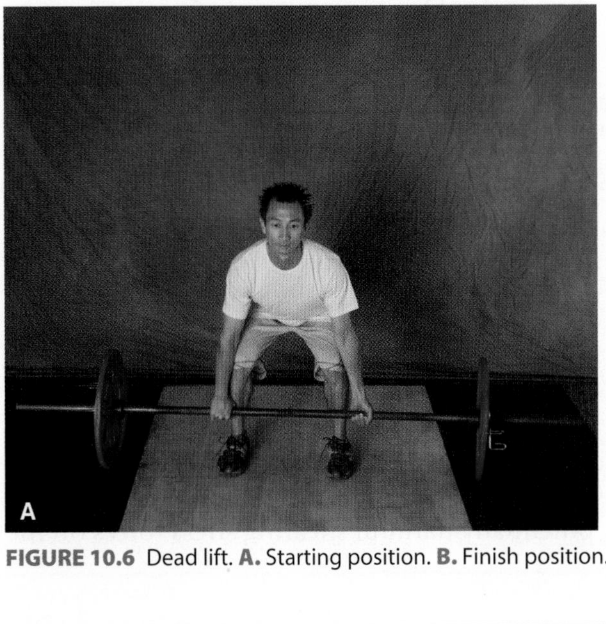

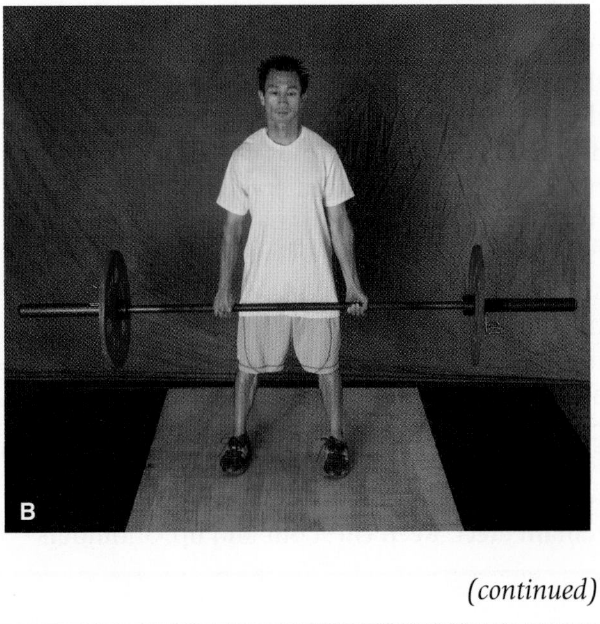

FIGURE 10.6 Dead lift. **A.** Starting position. **B.** Finish position.

(continued)

Dead Lift *(continued)*

the knees before exhaling and then breathing normally (Fig. 10.6B).

Downward Motion

Keeping a rigid and flat or slightly arched back, flex the hips and knees and lower the barbell back to the floor with control. The barbell should remain close to the body (knees and shins) throughout descent. Lightly touch the plates on the barbell to the floor and come to stop without releasing the tension on the barbell. Inhale during descent. Begin the ascent for the next repetition.

Variation

The dead lift may be performed with a shoulder-width grip, with both hands pronated to simulate the starting position utilized on a power clean. With this grip position, wrist straps may be utilized to improve grasp on the barbell.

Barbell Lunge

Type of Exercise

Lower-body/multijoint

Muscles Used

Gluteus maximus, iliopsoas, quadriceps (vastus lateralis, vastus intermedius, vastus medialis, rectus femoris), hamstrings (semimembranosus, semitendinosus, biceps femoris), soleus, and gastrocnemius

Starting Position

Position a standard barbell at chest level in a squat or power rack. Load the barbell evenly on both sides and secure weights with collars. Step underneath the barbell and position the base of the neck/upper middle back and the hips and feet directly under the barbell. Grasp the barbell using a pronated grip slightly wider than shoulder width. Place the barbell evenly above the posterior deltoids at the base of the neck (high barbell placement). Raise the elbows upward to provide a secure location for the barbell to rest on and prevent the barbell from sliding down the back during the execution of the lift. To lift the barbell from the rack, extend the hips and knees to lift the barbell off the rack and take a few (two or three) steps backward to clear the rack and allow adequate room to lunge forward. Feet are between hip- and shoulder-width apart and pointing forward. Torso should remain erect. Keep chest out and up. Shoulders are back. Keep head and neck straight with eyes looking straight ahead. Before stepping forward, inhale (Fig. 10.7A).

Downward Motion

Take an elongated step straight forward with one leg (lead leg). Keep the arms firm and the torso in an erect position as the lead foot goes forward and comes in contact with the floor. The rear leg (trail leg) remains constant in the starting position, but as the lead leg moves forward, balance should shift to the ball of the foot of the trail leg as the trail leg begins to flex. Place the lead foot flat on the floor with the foot pointing straight forward. To maintain balance, ensure that the lead leg moves directly forward from its original starting position and the lead ankle, knee, and hip remain in the same vertical plane. Avoid stepping to the right or left or allowing the knee to shift to one side or the other. Once balance is established on both feet, flex the lead knee to enable the trail leg to bend toward the floor. The trail leg should flex slightly less than the lead leg. The torso should remain erect with the shoulders kept directly above the hips and the head erect, facing forward. The lowest finish position of the ascent should occur when the trail leg is 1 to 2 in from the floor, the lead leg is flexed to 90 degrees, and the knee is directly above or slightly in front of the ankle. To avoid potentially harmful shearing stress forces on the

Barbell Lunge *(continued)*

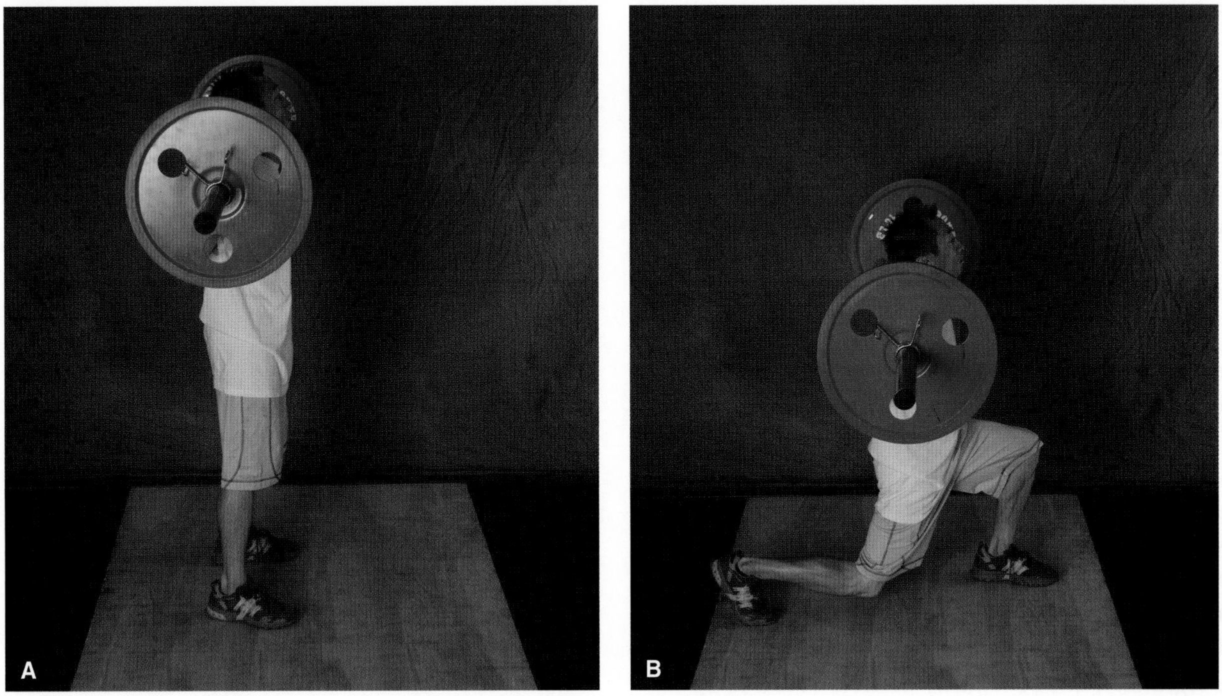

FIGURE 10.7 Barbell lunge. **A.** Starting position. **B.** Finish position.

lead leg's knee joint, it is critical that the lead knee should not extend past the lead foot. At the completion of the descent, a concentrated effort to "sit back" on the trailing leg should be made, as if sitting on the front edge of a bench in the strength-training facility. The depth of the barbell lunge depends on the athlete's hip joint flexibility, particularly the iliopsoas muscles. The lead foot should remain flat on the floor as the toes of the trail foot are extended and the ankle is dorsiflexed (Fig. 10.7B).

Upward Motion

While maintaining an erect torso, shift the balance forward to the lead foot and forcefully push off the floor with the lead foot by plantar flexing it while extending the lead knee and hip joints. As the lead foot returns to the starting position, balance should shift to the trail foot, so that the trail foot regains full contact with the floor. The lead foot should be lifted back to its original starting position with the feet between hip- and shoulder-width apart and pointing forward. Avoid touching the lead foot to the floor until it is returned to the finish position (unless balance is lost). Once the lead foot is returned to the starting position, divide the body weight equally over both feet. Torso should remain erect, as in the beginning position. Exhale at the completion of the ascent. Pause momentarily to fully gain balance, switch lead legs, and repeat the procedure.

Returning the Weight to the Rack

At the completion of the set, return the barbell to the rack by slowly walking forward and returning the barbell to the support hooks of the rack.

Variation (Lunges with Dumbbells)

If balancing a barbell is too difficult for the exerciser, dumbbells held at the sides may be substituted as an alternative.

(continued)

Stiff-Leg Dead Lift

Type of Exercise

Lower-body/single-joint

Muscles Used

Gluteus maximus, erector spinae, hamstrings (semimembranosus, semitendinosus, and biceps femoris)

Starting Position

Use a standard barbell. The lifting position is identical to that used in the power clean. The feet are between hip- and shoulder-width apart and pointing forward or just slightly outward. Squat and grasp the barbell with a pronated or alternated closed grip and hands at or slightly wider than shoulder-width apart. Arms are outside the knees, elbows extended and pointing outward. Stand so that the barbell is over the balls of the feet and close to the shins. Back is rigid and flat or slightly arched. Head is up or slightly hyperextended. Chest is held up and out. Shoulder blades should be squeezed together. Trapezius and upper back should be relaxed and in a slight state of stretch. With heels always remaining in contact with the floor, the body weight should be balanced between the balls and middles of the feet. Shoulders are slightly in front of or over the barbell. Lift the barbell off the floor by performing a dead-lift exercise. The body alignment and barbell position at the completion of the dead-lift ascent (hips and knees extended, torso erect, barbell touching the front of the thighs, and elbows extended) is the starting position for the stiff-leg dead lift (Fig. 10.8A).

Downward Motion

Inhale before beginning the descent. Slightly flex the knees to reduce stress on the knee joint before initiating the descent. While keeping the back flat and the knees slightly flexed, gradually reduce the stress on the lower back, gluteals, and hamstrings to allow the hips and torso to flex forward and the barbell to be lowered slowly and with complete control toward the floor. Continue flexing the hips and torso until the trunk begins to round or the heels begin to lift off the floor (this is the endpoint of the descent). Keep the barbell close to the thighs and shins throughout the descent. Do not release or rapidly drop the barbell during the descent. Always lower the barbell without relaxing or releasing tension, keeping the knees in a slightly flexed position (Fig. 10.8B).

Upward Motion

Slowly extend the hips and torso, and raise the barbell upward while keeping the knees stationary and slightly flexed. Maintain the flat back and extended elbow position. Do not flex the

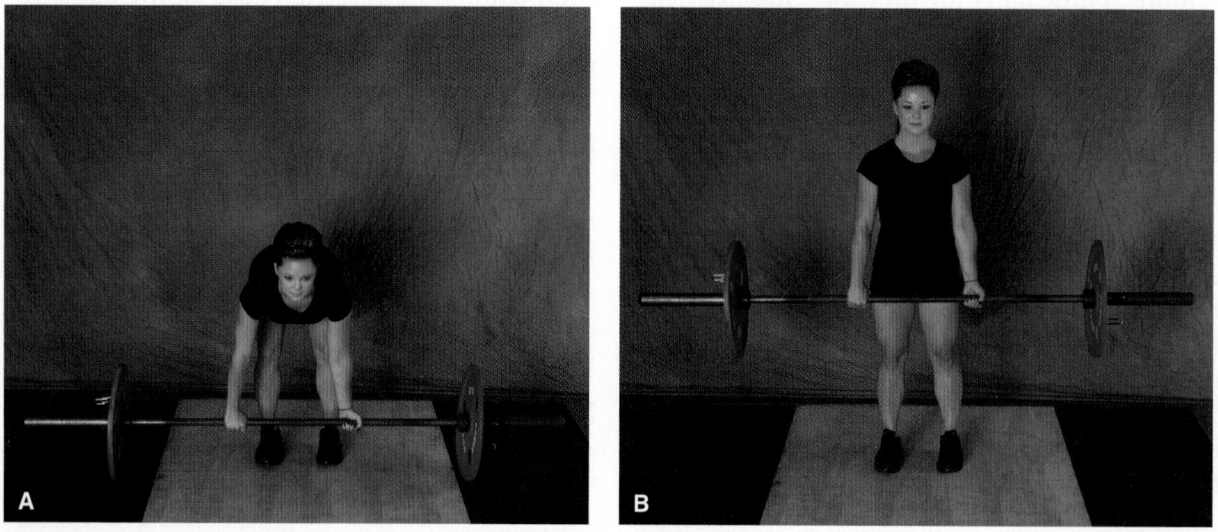

FIGURE 10.8 Stiff-legged dead lift. **A.** Starting position. **B.** Finish position.

Stiff-Leg Dead Lift *(continued)*

elbows to assist in the upward movement of the barbell. Once full hip extension has been reached, stand erect. Exhale at the completion of the ascent.

Variation

This movement may also be performed with a pair of dumbbells of equal weight or specially designated plate-loaded equipment.

Leg Press

Type of Exercise

Lower body/multijoint

Muscles Used

Gluteus maximus, quadriceps (vastus lateralis, vastus intermedius, vastus medialis, rectus femoris), hamstrings (semimembranosus, semitendinosus, biceps femoris)

Starting Position

Load the machine with the appropriate weights. Set the machine seat and/or back pad at the appropriate position (hips and torso should form a 90-degree angle). Sit in the machine, positioning the lower back, with hips and buttocks pressed evenly and in the center of the pads. All body segments other than the legs must be firmly positioned and secured against any movement during the exercise so as to provide maximal support to the spine and lower back. Place the feet shoulder- and hip-width apart with the toes pointing straight up the footplate. It is important that both feet be in the same position vertically and horizontally on each side. Position both upper and lower legs parallel to each other. Grasp the handles on each side of the frame and extend the hips and knees to full extension without locking the knees. Keep the hips securely positioned on the seat and the back against the back pad as the platform is raised. Remove the support mechanism from the platform. The lower body should remain stationary as it absorbs the weight of the platform. When the platform is free of its supports, regrasp the handles on each side of the machine frame to help keep the body firmly in place. All subsequent repetitions should be initiated from this position. Just prior to the descent, take a deep breath and hold it (Fig. 10.9A).

Downward Motion

Begin the descent by flexing the knees and hips with control. Do not allow the platform to accelerate as it is lowered. Ensure that the upper and lower legs remain parallel to each other throughout the descent; departures from this position could place undue stress on the lower back, hips, or knees. The hips and buttocks should remain stationary against the seat pad while the back remains flat against the back pad. Avoid shifting the hips or allowing the buttocks to lose contact with the seat. Avoid releasing the handgrips during the descent. Maintaining a firm grip on the handles is essential to a stationary body position. Continue the descent by flexing the knees and hips until one of the following occurs: the thighs become parallel to the platform, the hips lift off the back pad, the buttocks lose contact with the seat pad, or the heels come off the footplate (Fig. 10.9B).

Note: The point where one of these four events occurs should be considered the end ROM or the completion of the descent. The extent of the exercise ROM is dependent upon the individual's magnitude of spinal, hip, knee, and ankle flexibility as well as the machine's individual setup and adjustment capabilities. At the completion of the descent, avoid bouncing the platform, releasing the handgrip, or relaxing the torso to initiate the ascent.

(continued)

Leg Press *(continued)*

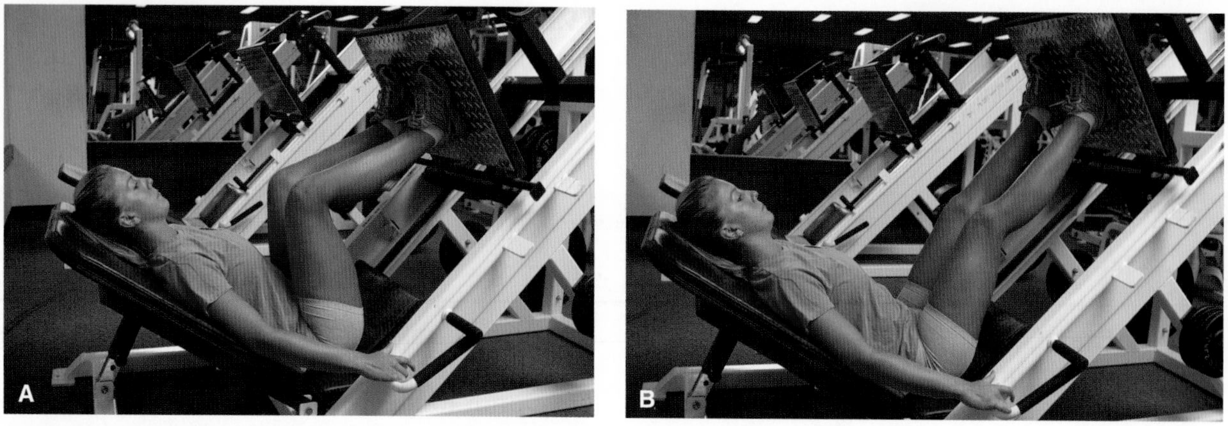

FIGURE 10.9 Leg press. **A.** Starting position. **B.** Finish position.

Upward Motion

Press the platform up forcefully under control through the heels by extending the knees and hips. Keep the upper and lower legs parallel; do not allow the knees to move in or out. Avoid shifting the hips or allowing the buttocks to move off the seat pad. Continue pressing the platform upward until the knees are fully extended but not locked. Exhale as the platform passes the midpoint of the ROM. At the completion of the set, move the supports back into place and exit the machine.

Leg Extension

Type of Exercise

Lower body/single joint

Muscles Used

Quadriceps (vastus lateralis, vastus intermedius, vastus medialis, rectus femoris)

Starting Position

Adjust the seat so that the back of the knee touches the front of the seat pad and the knee joint lines up with the axis of the lever arm. Sit upright on the seat with the back and hips pressed evenly against their pads. Hook the feet under the ankle pad such that the insteps of the feet touch the pad when the ankles are dorsiflexed. The thighs, lower legs, and feet should be parallel to each other. Grasp either the side handles or the edges of the seating platform to steady the body throughout the movement. Inhale prior to beginning the exercise (Fig. 10.10A).

Upward Motion

Keeping the thighs, lower legs, and feet parallel to each other, extend the knees with control until the tops of the toes line up with knee height. Avoid rapidly lifting the resistance or accelerating the weight past the top position. To avoid upper and lower extremity movement, maintain contact with the machine pads throughout the upward motion while keeping a firm grasp on the side handles or the edges of the seating platform during the upward motion. Exhale once the resistance has passed the sticking point (Fig. 10.10B).

Downward Motion

Slowly allow the knees to flex back to the initial starting position. Avoid lowering the resistance quickly during the descent. Keep the back and thighs in contact with their respective pads. Keep the thighs, lower legs, and feet parallel to each other throughout the descent. Stop the descent just before the resistance comes in contact with the remainder of the plates and begin the upward motion. Inhale as the resistance is lowered.

Leg Extension *(continued)*

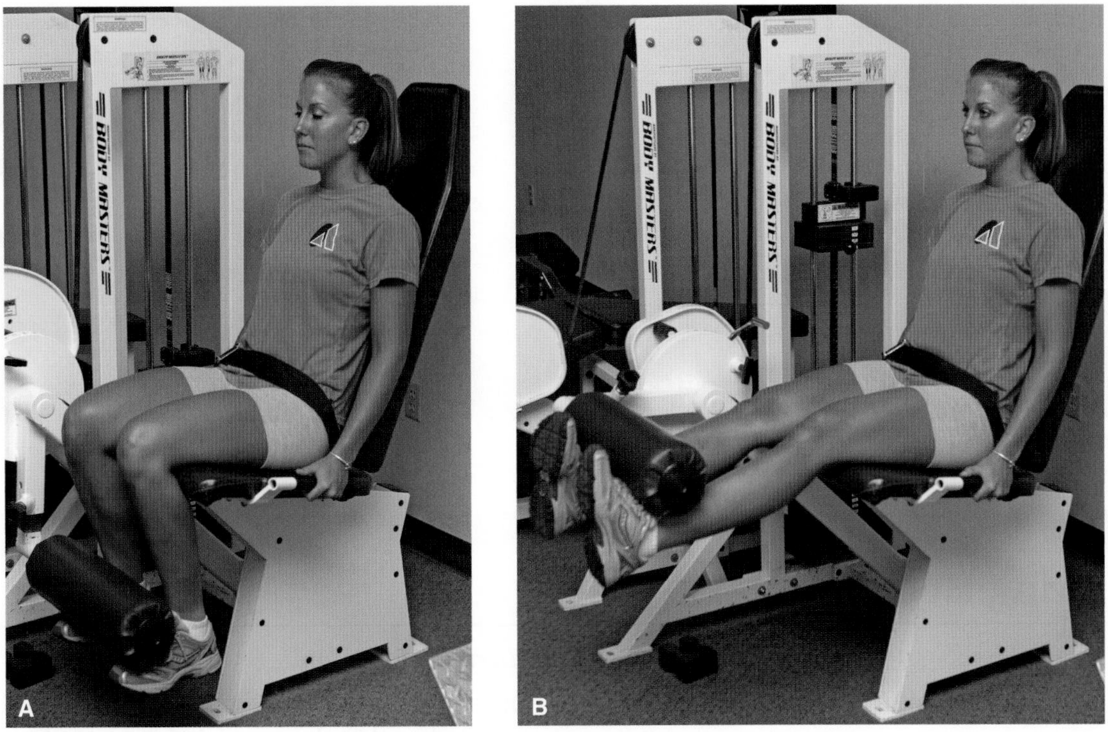

FIGURE 10.10 Leg extension. **A.** Starting position. **B.** End position.

Leg Curl

Type of Exercise

Lower body/single joint

Muscles Used

Hamstrings (semimembranosus, semitendinosus, biceps femoris)

Starting Position

Lie prone on the machine with the hips, thighs, and torso resting on the padded surface. Place the tops of the kneecaps slightly over the edge of the padded surface of the machine with the knees lining up with axis of the lever arm. Adjust the position of the ankle pads such that the bottoms of the pads are 3 in above the heels (just above the tops of the shoes). Position the feet, lower legs, and thighs parallel to each other. Grasp onto the side handles or padded surface of the machine (Fig. 10.11A).

Upward Motion

Inhale prior to initiating the ascent. Flex the knees with control and lift the resistance until the ankle pads nearly reach the buttocks, depending on the level of quadriceps flexibility and limb length. To minimize the use of hip and upper-body movement, maintain contact with the padded surface and keep a firm grip on the handles or torso pad throughout the upward motion. Avoid rapidly lifting the resistance or kicking with the legs to raise the resistance. Also avoid rapidly lifting the resistance through the sticking point before exhaling (Fig. 10.11B).

Downward Motion

Slowly allow the knees to extend back to the initial starting position. Avoid lowering the resistance quickly during the descent. Keep the thighs, lower legs, and feet parallel to each other throughout the descent. Stop the descent just before the resistance comes in contact with the remainder of the plates and begin the upward motion. Inhale prior to beginning the upward motion.

(continued)

Leg Curl *(continued)*

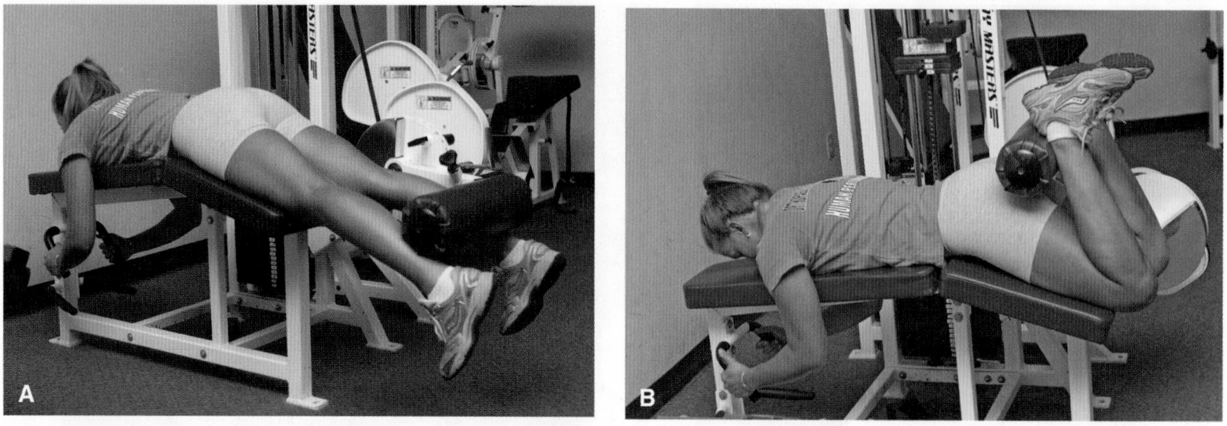

FIGURE 10.11 Leg curl. A. Starting position. B. End position.

Standing Heel Raise

Type of Exercise

Lower body/single joint

Muscles Used

Gastrocnemius, soleus

Starting Position

The shoulder pads on the machine should be adjusted so that the exerciser is required to flex his or her knees to get under the pads. The body should be positioned evenly under the shoulder

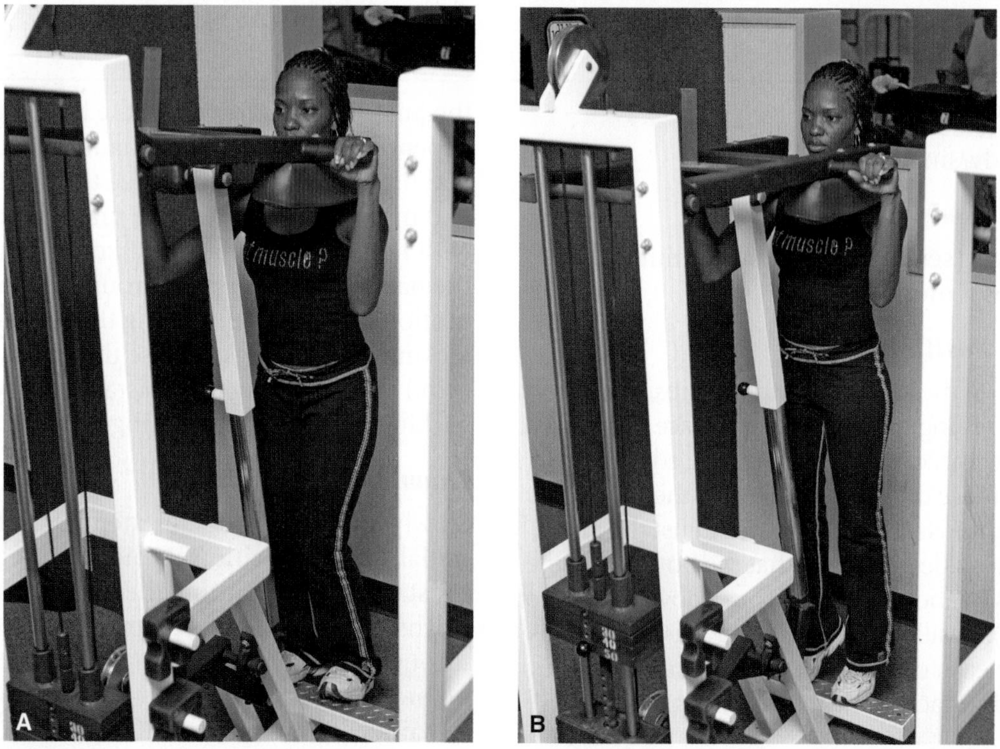

FIGURE 10.12 Standing heel raise. A. Starting position. B. End position.

Standing Heel Raise *(continued)*

pads. The feet should be positioned so that the heels hang over the back edge and slightly below the step with the arches and balls of the feet on the outside edge of the step. The legs and feet should be parallel to each other. The exerciser then stands erect, raising the resistance off the weight stack. The hips should be directly under the shoulders with the knees extended but not locked (Fig. 10.12A).

Upward Motion

Inhale prior to initiating the upward motion. Plantar flex the ankle through a full ROM while keeping the head up, torso erect, and legs and feet parallel to each other. Place equal pressure on the balls of both feet throughout the upward motion. Do not slightly invert or evert the ankles. Keep the legs straight but not locked throughout the upward motion. Avoid rapidly lifting the resistance through the sticking point before exhaling (Fig. 10.12B).

Downward Motion

Slowly allow the ankles to dorsiflex back to the initial starting position with the heels slightly below the step. Inhale as the heels lower back to the starting position. Stop at the bottom position before slowly reinitiating the upward motion for the next repetition.

Chest Exercises

Bench Press, Dumbbell

Type of Exercise

Upper body/multijoint

Muscles Used

Pectoralis major, pectoralis minor, deltoid (anterior), serratus anterior, triceps brachii

Starting Position

Select two dumbbells of equal weight with a closed grip. Place the dumbbells on the floor next to the lower end of an adjustable bench. Lift the dumbbells up from the floor by using the legs. Align the dumbbells such that the end closest to the little finger is against the front of the thighs (hands are facing in, and handles are parallel to each other) Sit down on the lower end of the adjustable bench with the dumbbells resting on the top of the thighs. Recline to the supine position such that the dumbbells are moved to the lateral aspect of the chest near the armpit even with the midchest level while reclining. Position the feet flat on the floor with the head, shoulders, and buttocks evenly and firmly on the bench. Dumbbells should be rotated to place the thumb side of the dumbbell against the lateral portion of the chest such that both handles are in line with one another, simulating a barbell running through both dumbbell handles. Another option is to perform the exercise with the dumbbell kept in the neutral position (with the handles of the dumbbells parallel to each other). Each repetition will begin from this same position (Fig. 10.13A).

Upward Motion

Press the dumbbells upward and together with control. Keep the head, body, and feet in their original position. Do not arch the lower back or lift the buttocks off the bench. The wrists should remain firm and straight, the forearms almost perpendicular to the floor, and the hands aligned with each other. Do not allow the

(continued)

Bench Press, Dumbbell *(continued)*

dumbbells to move out of control as they are being raised. Press the dumbbells upward until the elbows are fully extended but not locked. Bring the dumbbells together with control at the completion of the movement; do not bang the dumbbells together. Exhale as the dumbbells are lifted (Fig. 10.13B).

Downward Motion

Lower and separate the dumbbells with control toward the midchest. To maintain a stable position on the bench, lower both dumbbells at the same rate. Keep the wrists firm and straight, the forearms almost perpendicular to the floor, and the hands aligned with each other. Avoid movements forward and backward or side to side. Lower the dumbbells to a lateral portion of the chest near the armpit at midchest level. Dumbbells should be lowered to a lateral portion of the chest such that both handles are in line with one another where a barbell would touch the chest. Dumbbells should not be bounced off the chest at the bottom position or arch the back to lift the chest upward. Maintain a stable position with the feet flat on the floor and the head, shoulders, and buttocks evenly and firmly on the bench. Inhale as the dumbbells are lowered.

Completion of the Set

After lowering the dumbbells to the lateral chest on the last repetition, rotate the dumbbells to the abdominal area. Sit up slowly and return the dumbbells to the thigh before standing up and returning the dumbbells to the dumbbell rack or floor.

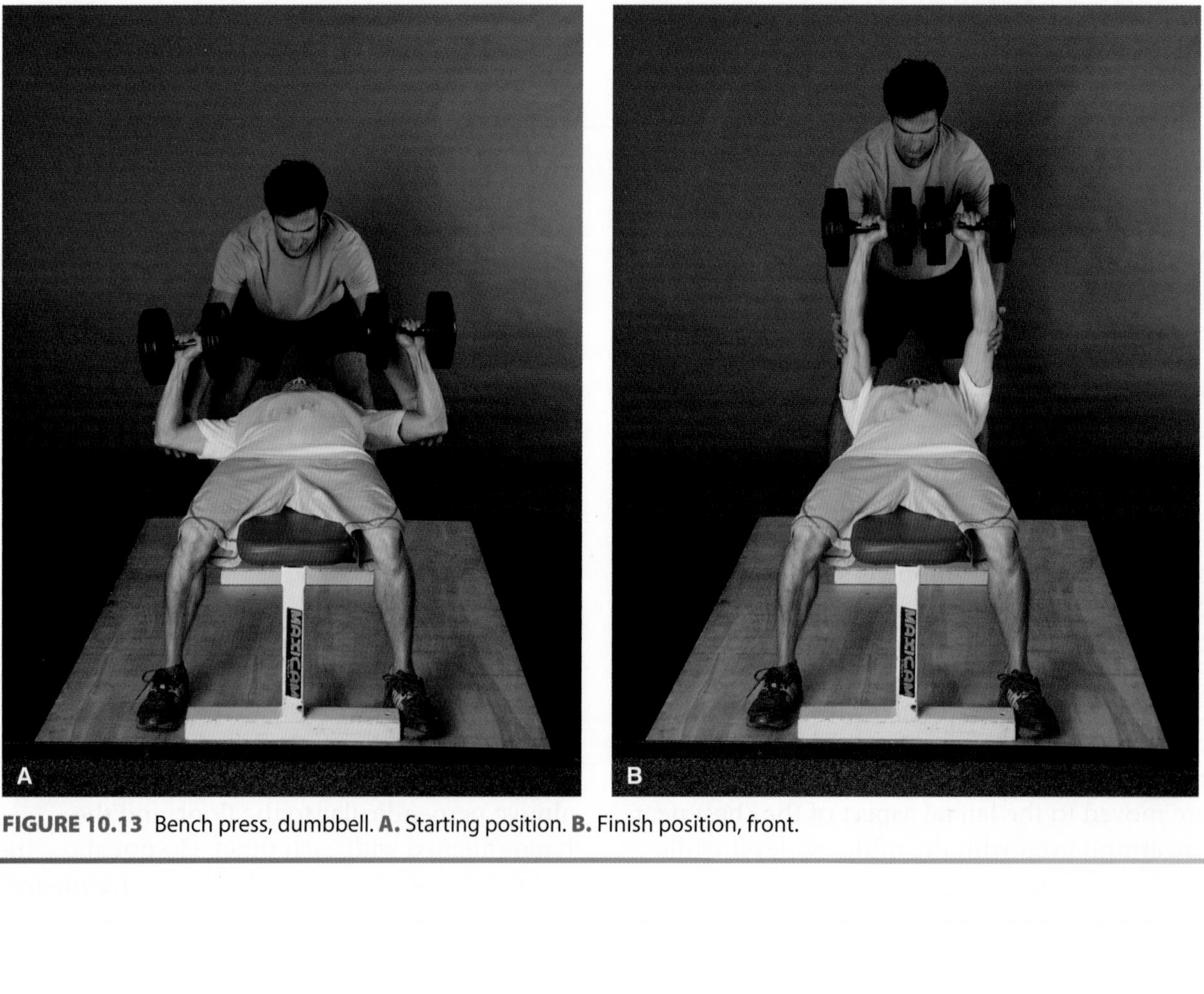

FIGURE 10.13 Bench press, dumbbell. **A.** Starting position. **B.** Finish position, front.

Bench Press, Barbell

Type of Exercise

Upper body/multijoint

Muscles Used

Pectoralis major, pectoralis minor, deltoid (anterior), serratus anterior, triceps brachii

Starting Position

Position a barbell on two equal standards of a bench or two equal hooks of a power rack with an adjustable bench. The two standards or hooks should be set such that the elbow is bent slightly (10 degrees) when grasping the barbell. Load barbell evenly on both sides, and secure weights with collars. Lie supine on the bench and slide up or down until the eyes are directly under the barbell. The head, shoulders/upper back area, and buttocks should be firmly and evenly placed on the bench and both feet securely placed on the floor on either side of the bench. Both scapulae should be retracted, and the pelvis should be tilted posteriorly. Once this position is established, it should be maintained throughout the set. Grasp the barbell with a closed pronated grip slightly wider than shoulder width. Grip should be wide enough that the hand is over the elbow. Lift the barbell off the standards or hooks to a position directly above the chest with the elbows fully extended. All subsequent repetitions begin from this position (Fig. 10.14A).

Downward Motion

Inhale and begin the descent by lowering the barbell in a slow, controlled manner toward the chest. The elbows will move down past the torso and slightly away from the body. Wrists should be kept firm and rigid, ensuring that the barbell remains over the longitudinal axis of the ulna and not in the distal portion of the hand. Forearms are parallel to each other and perpendicular to the floor. Lower the barbell to lightly touch the midchest; avoid bouncing the barbell off the chest or lifting the buttocks off the bench to raise the barbell. Keep the head, shoulders/upper back area, and buttocks in contact with the bench and both feet securely on the floor. Keep the body rigid throughout the descent (Fig. 10.14B).

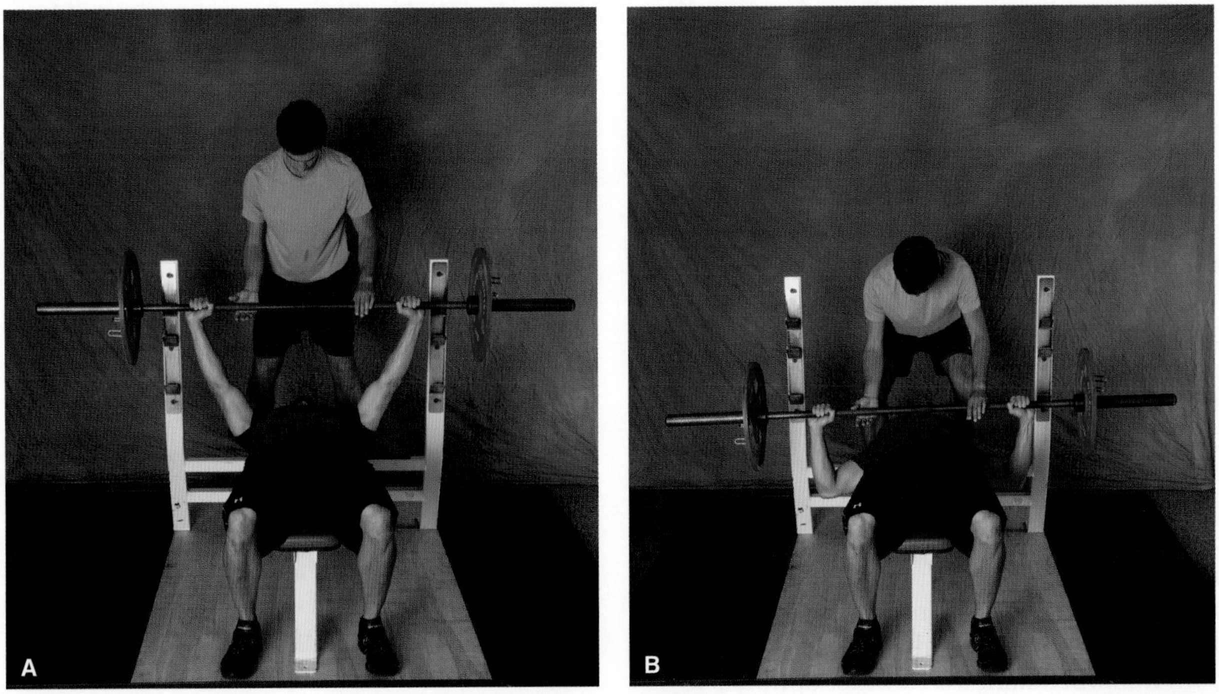

FIGURE 10.14 Bench press, barbell. **A.** Starting position. **B.** Finish position.

(continued)

Bench Press, Barbell *(continued)*

Upward Motion

Press the barbell up and slightly backward forcefully. Begin exhaling at the midpoint of the ascent. Avoid arching the lower back or lifting the feet or buttocks from their position. Keep the wrists rigid and the forearms perpendicular to the floor and parallel to each other. Continue pressing the barbell upward until the elbows are fully extended but not forcefully locked. At the completion of the lift, the barbell should be in line with the supporting joints (i.e., wrist, elbow, shoulder). At the completion of the set, return the barbell to the rack. Do not release the grip on the barbell until both ends of the barbell are securely on the standards or hooks. Keep the body rigid throughout the ascent.

Incline Press, Dumbbell

Type of Exercise

Upper body/multijoint

Muscles Used

Pectoralis major, pectoralis minor, deltoid (anterior), serratus anterior, triceps brachii

Starting Position

Select two dumbbells of equal weight and hold with a closed grip. Place the dumbbells on the floor next to the lower end of an adjustable bench. Adjust the bench such that the upper end of the bench is set at a 45-degree upward angle and the base of the bench is tilted upward to prevent the lifter from sliding. Lift the dumbbells up from the floor by using the legs. Align the dumbbells such that the end closest to the little finger is against the front of the thighs (hands are facing in and handles are parallel to each other). Sit down on the lower end of the adjustable bench with the dumbbells resting on the top of the thighs. Lean back to the incline position such that the dumbbells are moved to the lateral aspect of the chest slightly above the armpit and midchest level while in the incline position. Position the feet flat on the floor with the head, shoulders, and buttocks evenly and firmly on the bench. Dumbbells should be rotated to place the thumb side of the dumbbell against the upper lateral portion of the chest such that both handles are in line with one another, simulating a barbell running through both dumbbell handles. Another option is to perform the exercise with the dumbbells kept in the neutral position (parallel to each other). Each repetition will begin from this same position (Fig. 10.15A).

Upward Motion

Press the dumbbells upward and together with control. Keep the head, body, and feet in their original position. Do not arch the lower back. The wrists should remain firm and straight, the forearms almost perpendicular to the floor, and the hands aligned with each other. Do not allow the dumbbells to move out of control as they are being raised. Press the dumbbells upward until the elbows are fully extended but not locked. Bring the dumbbells together with control at the completion of the movement directly above the eyes; do not bang the dumbbells together. Exhale as the dumbbells are lifted (Fig. 10.15B).

Downward Motion

Lower and separate the dumbbells with control toward the upper chest. To maintain a stable position on the incline bench, lower both dumbbells at the same rate. Keep the wrists firm and straight, the forearms almost perpendicular to the floor, and the hands aligned with each other. Avoid movements forward and backward or side to side. Lower the dumbbells to a lateral portion of the chest slightly above the armpit and midchest level. Dumbbells should be lowered to a lateral portion of the chest such that both handles are in line with one another where a barbell would touch the upper chest.

Incline Press, Dumbbell *(continued)*

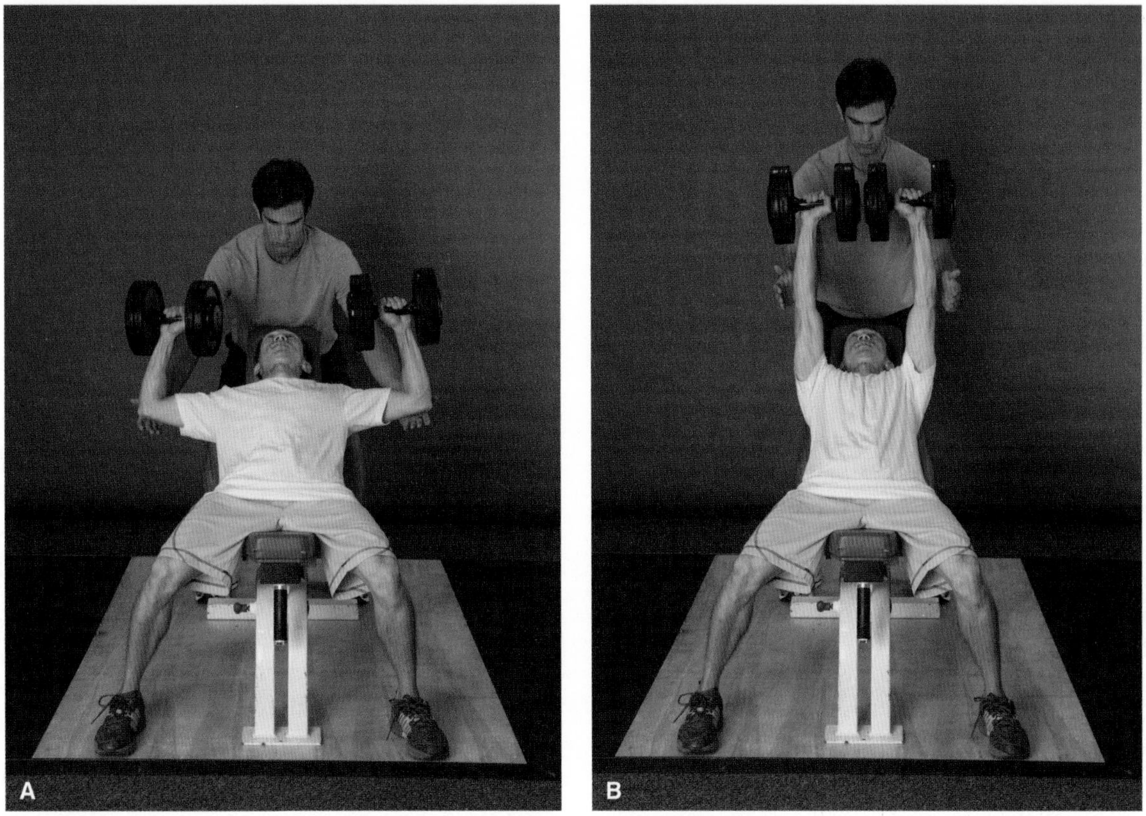

FIGURE 10.15 Incline press, dumbbell. **A.** Starting position. **B.** Finish position.

Dumbbells should not be bounced off the chest at the bottom position. Avoid arching the back to lift the chest upward. Maintain a stable position with the feet flat on the floor and the head, shoulders, and buttocks evenly and firmly on the bench. Inhale as the dumbbells are lowered.

Completion of the Set

After lowering the dumbbells to the upper lateral chest on the last repetition, rotate the dumbbells toward the midline of the body and lower them to the thigh. Sit up completely and return the dumbbells to the dumbbell rack or floor.

Q & A from the Field

Q *An exerciser states that she has reached a plateau in the bench press and is unable to increase in weight. What variations can you suggest to the program to help break this plateau?*

A Alternate exercises such as flies, incline press, or decline press can be used to add variety. Dumbbells can be used to require the athlete to balance the load, and lighter weights can be used explosively to increase power. The athlete may be overtraining, and some time off or a period of active rest may be necessary.

(continued)

Incline Press, Barbell

Type of Exercise

Upper body/multijoint

Muscles Used

Pectoralis major, pectoralis minor, deltoid (anterior), serratus anterior, triceps brachii

Starting Position

Position a barbell on two equal standards of an incline bench or two equal hooks of a power rack with an adjustable bench. The two standards or hooks should be set such that the elbow is bent slightly (10 degrees) when grasping the barbell. Load barbell evenly on both sides and secure weights with collars. Lie supine on the bench and slide up or down until the eyes are directly under the barbell. The head, shoulders/upper back area, and buttocks should be firmly and evenly placed on the bench, and both feet should be securely placed on the floor on either side of the bench. Once this position is established, it should be maintained throughout the set. Grasp the barbell with a closed pronated grip, slightly wider than shoulder width. Grip should be wide enough that the hand is over the elbow. Lift the barbell off the standards or hooks to a position directly above the chest with the elbows fully extended. All subsequent repetitions begin from this position (Fig. 10.16A).

Downward Motion

Inhale and hold the breath throughout the descent and the change of direction. Begin the descent by lowering the barbell in a slow, controlled manner toward the chest. The elbows will move down past the torso and slightly away from the body. Wrists should be kept firm and rigid, making sure that the barbell remains over the longitudinal axis of the ulna and not in the distal portion of the hand. Forearms are parallel to each other and perpendicular to the floor. Lower the barbell to lightly touch the upper third of the chest, between the clavicles and the midchest; avoid bouncing the barbell off the chest or lifting the buttocks off the bench

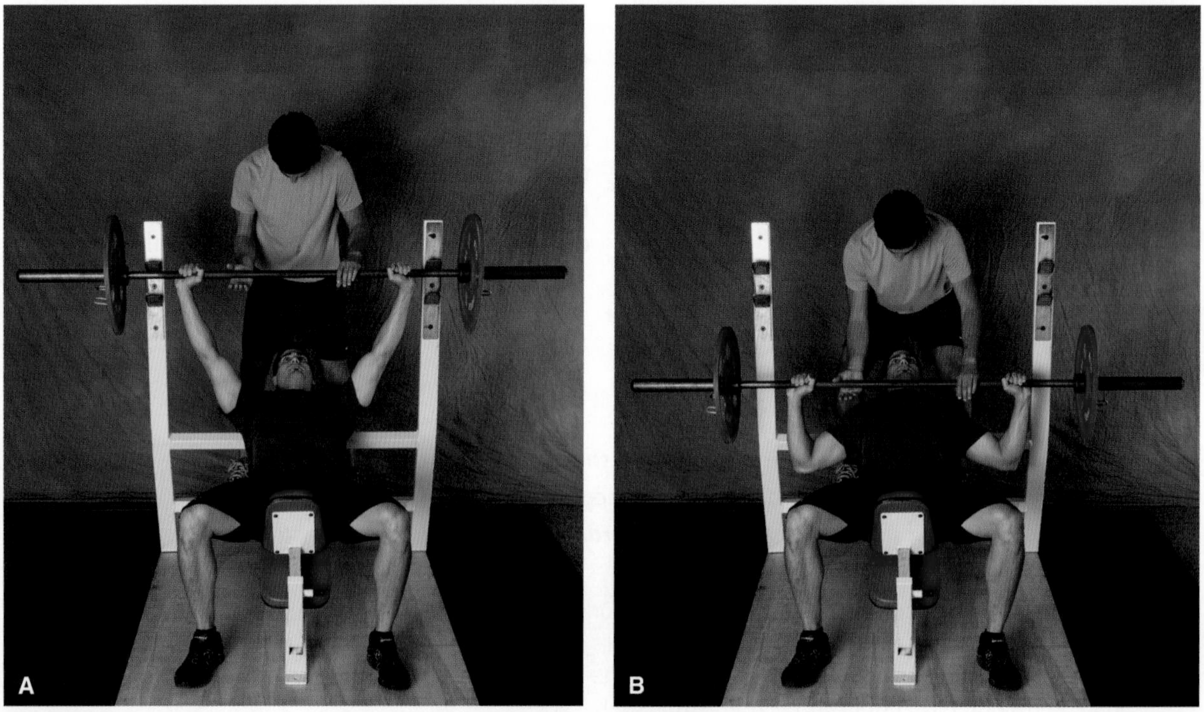

FIGURE 10.16 Incline press, barbell. **A.** Starting position. **B.** Finish position.

Incline Press, Barbell *(continued)*

to raise the barbell. Keep the head, shoulders/upper back area, and buttocks in contact with the bench and both feet securely on the floor. Keep the body rigid throughout the descent (Fig. 10.16B).

Upward Motion

Press the barbell up and slightly backward forcefully. Begin exhaling at the midpoint of the ascent. Avoid arching the lower back or lifting the feet or buttocks from their position. Keep the wrists rigid and the forearms perpendicular to the floor and parallel to each other. Continue pressing the barbell upward until the elbows are fully extended but not forcefully locked. At the completion of the lift, the bar should be in line with the supporting joints (i.e., wrist, elbow, shoulder). At the completion of the set, return the barbell to the rack. Do not release the grip on the barbell until both ends of the barbell are securely on the standards or hooks. Keep the body rigid throughout the ascent.

Dumbbell Fly

Type of Exercise

Upper body/single joint

Muscles Used

Pectoralis major, pectoralis minor, deltoid (anterior), serratus anterior

Starting Position

Select two dumbbells of equal weight and hold with a closed grip. Place the dumbbells on the floor next to the lower end of an adjustable bench. Lift the dumbbells up from the floor by using the legs. Align the dumbbells such that the end closest to the little finger is against the front of the thighs (hands are facing in and handles are parallel to each other). Sit down on the lower end of the adjustable bench with the dumbbells resting on the top of the thighs. Recline to the supine position such that the dumbbells are moved to the lateral aspect of the chest near the armpit even with the midchest level while reclining. Press the dumbbells up to an extended position of the elbows directly above the chest. Position the feet flat on the floor with the head, shoulders, and buttocks evenly and firmly on the bench. Dumbbells should be rotated to place them in a neutral position (parallel to each other) with the elbows rotating out. Flex the elbows slightly before beginning the downward motion. Each repetition will begin from this same position (Fig. 10.17A).

Downward Motion

With a controlled motion, slowly lower the dumbbells with a wide arc. No movement should occur at the elbow joint, only at the shoulders. Inhale as the dumbbells are lowered. As the downward motion continues, the elbows will go from pointing out to the side to pointing toward the floor. Keep the shoulders, upper arm, elbow, lower arm, wrists, and hands in a nearly vertical plane parallel to the floor. The elbows and wrists should remain in a slightly flexed position throughout the downward motion. Continue the downward motion until they are level with the chest and parallel to each other. Avoid lifting the buttocks off the bench at the end of the downward motion (Fig. 10.17B).

Upward Motion

With a controlled motion, raise the dumbbells in an arc, simulate hugging a large pillar with the arms. Keep the feet flat on the floor and the head, shoulders, and buttocks evenly and firmly on the bench; avoid arching the lower back or elevating the shoulders to assist with the upward motion. Keep the shoulders, upper arm, elbow, lower arm, wrists, and hands in a nearly vertical plane parallel to the floor as in the downward motion. The elbows and wrists should remain in a slightly flexed position throughout the upward motion. Exhale once the dumbbells pass the sticking point. Continue the slow, controlled, wide arc

(continued)

Dumbbell Fly *(continued)*

with the dumbbells until they are repositioned over the chest in the starting position.

Completion of the Set

After lowering the dumbbells to the lateral chest on the last repetition, rotate the dumbbells to the abdominal area. Sit up slowly and return the dumbbells to the thigh before standing up and returning the dumbbells to the dumbbell rack or floor.

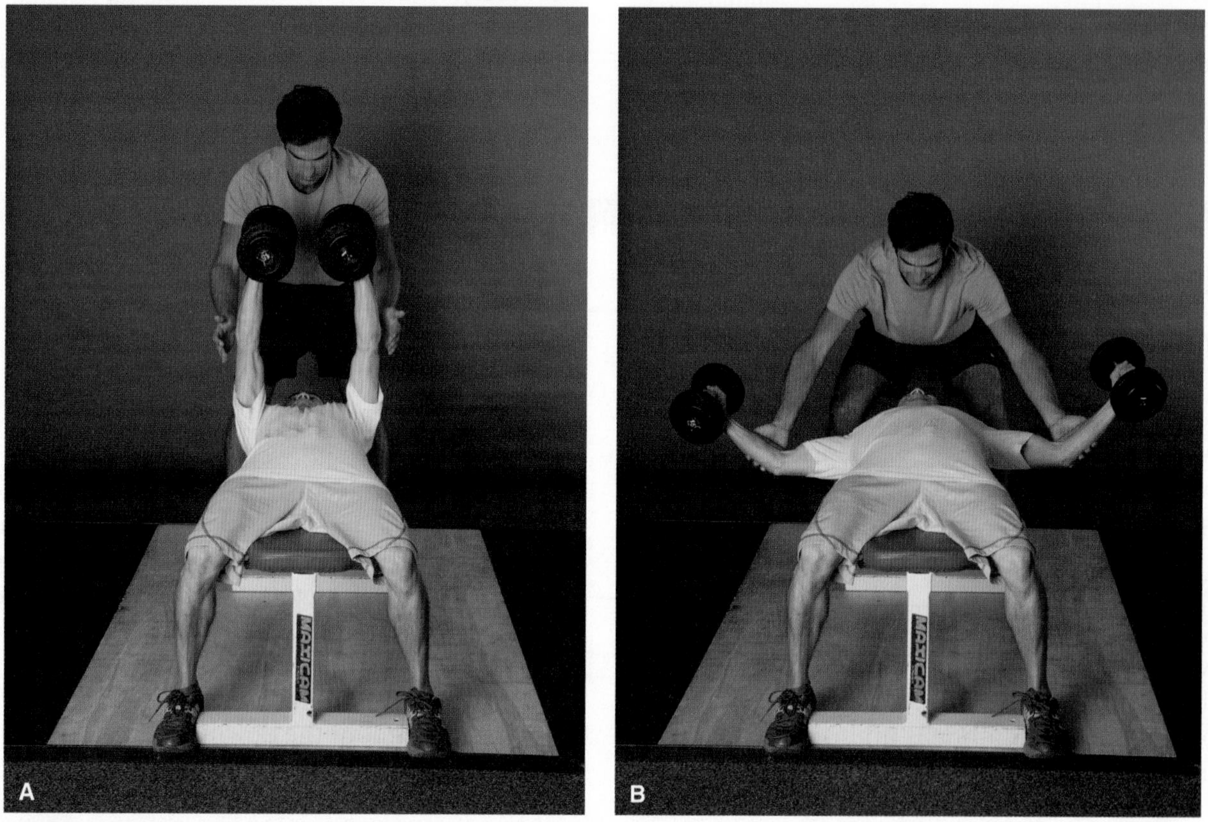

FIGURE 10.17 Dumbbell fly. **A.** Starting position. **B.** Finish position.

Upper Back Exercises

Dumbbell One-Arm Row

Type of Exercise

Upper body/multijoint

Muscles Used

Latissimus dorsi, middle trapezius, rhomboids, teres major, posterior deltoid, biceps brachii, brachialis, brachioradialis

Starting Position

Select a dumbbell of appropriate weight. Place the dumbbell on the floor next to the left upper end of an adjustable bench. Stand to the left of a bench that is elevated 30 degrees at the upper end of the bench. Kneel on the bench with the right leg on the bench and the left foot flat on

Dumbbell One-Arm Row *(continued)*

the floor. Place the right hand at the upper end of the bench. Keep the body weight back toward the right heel with a minimum amount of stress placed on the right hand. Position the slightly flexed left leg on the left side of the bench behind the back end of the bench with the toes pointing forward. The left leg should remain in a slightly flexed position throughout the exercise. The upper extremity should remain parallel to the elevated bench. Reach down and grasp the dumbbell with a closed, neutral grip (palm of the hand facing in) of the left hand. Position both hips, left knee, and right elbow so that the torso is at a 30-degree angle to the floor (parallel to the bench). Hang the dumbbell (at a slightly upward angle) down at full elbow extension on the left side of the body while keeping the shoulders parallel. Keep the back flat and the eyes focused straight ahead. Inhale just before raising the dumbbell (Fig. 10.18A).

Upward Motion

Begin by pulling the dumbbell up toward the torso. Keep the upper left arm and elbow next to the side of the body as the dumbbell is raised. Keep the wrist straight; do not curl the wrist upward. The left elbow should be pulled past the side to enable the dumbbell to be pulled to the rib cage midway between the shoulder and hip. Maintain the flat back at a 30-degree upward angle and stationary head, shoulder, elbow, hand, knee, and foot position throughout the ascent. Do not swing or jerk the upper body upward in an attempt to help raise the dumbbell. Continue pulling the dumbbell until it reaches the left rib cage midway between the shoulder and hip. Exhale as the dumbbell is lifted (Fig. 10.18B).

Downward Motion

Lower the dumbbell slowly and under control until the elbow is fully extended while

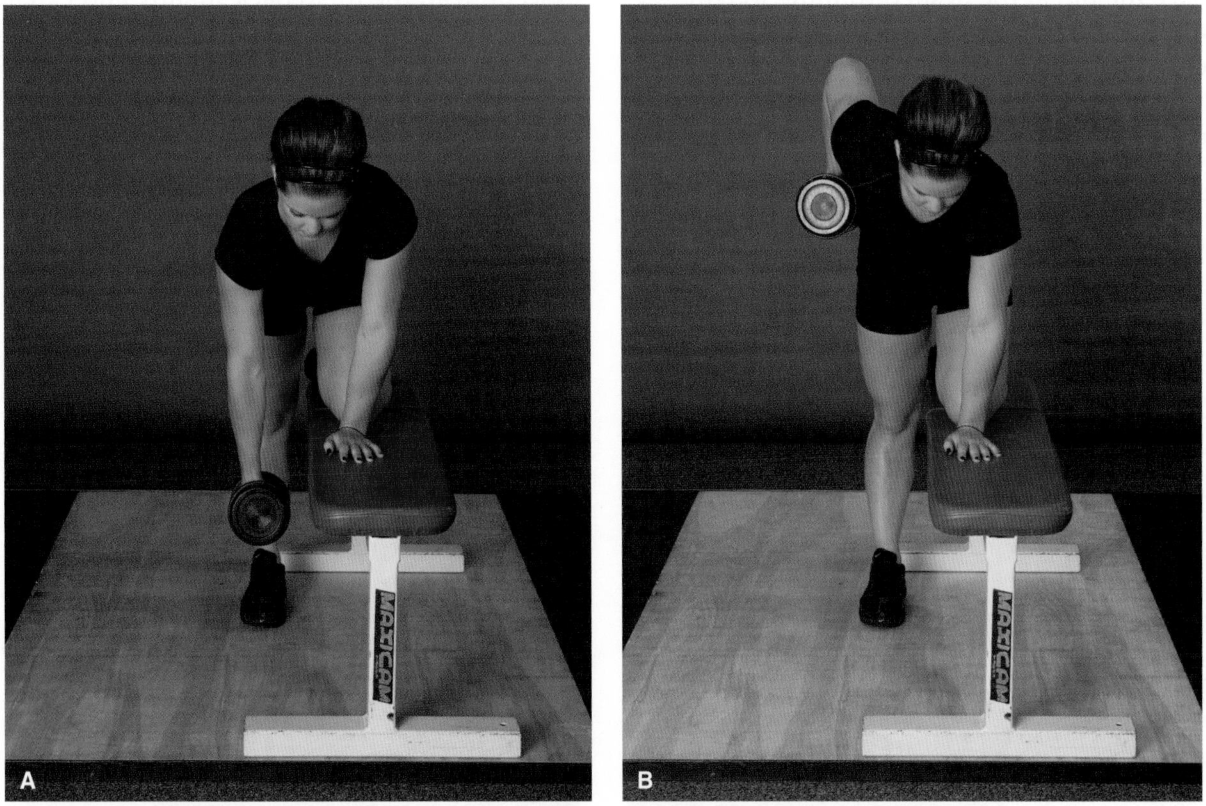

FIGURE 10.18 Dumbbell one-arm row. **A.** Starting position. **B.** Finish position.

(continued)

Dumbbell One-Arm Row *(continued)*

keeping the shoulders parallel to each other. Maintain the flat back at a 30-degree upward angle and maintain stationary head, shoulder, elbow, hand, knee, and foot positions throughout the exercise. Keep the left knee slightly flexed and the left foot flat on the floor throughout the descent. Inhale as the dumbbell is returned to the starting position. After completing the set with the left arm, release the dumbbell, stand on the right side of the bench, and repeat the procedure using the right arm.

Lat Pull-Down

Type of Exercise

Upper body/multijoint

Muscles Used

Latissimus dorsi, middle trapezius, rhomboids, teres major, posterior deltoid, biceps brachii, brachialis, brachioradialis

Starting Position

Place the pin at the desired training weight in the selectorized weight stack attached to the machine. Grasp the long bar with a closed, pronated grip. The grip width should be slightly wider than shoulder width on a straight bar or on the downward bend of a bent bar. Pull the bar downward and move into a seated position. If the seat is attached to the machine, sit down facing the weight stack with the legs under the thigh pads. The seat should be adjusted to enable the thighs to be parallel to the floor with the feet flat on the floor. The elbows should be fully extended with the selected load suspended above the remainder of the weight stack. Before initiating the descent, lean the torso back slightly and extend the neck to enable the bar to pass by the face as it is pulled down. This position will also decrease the impingement stress on the shoulder joints (Fig. 10.19A).

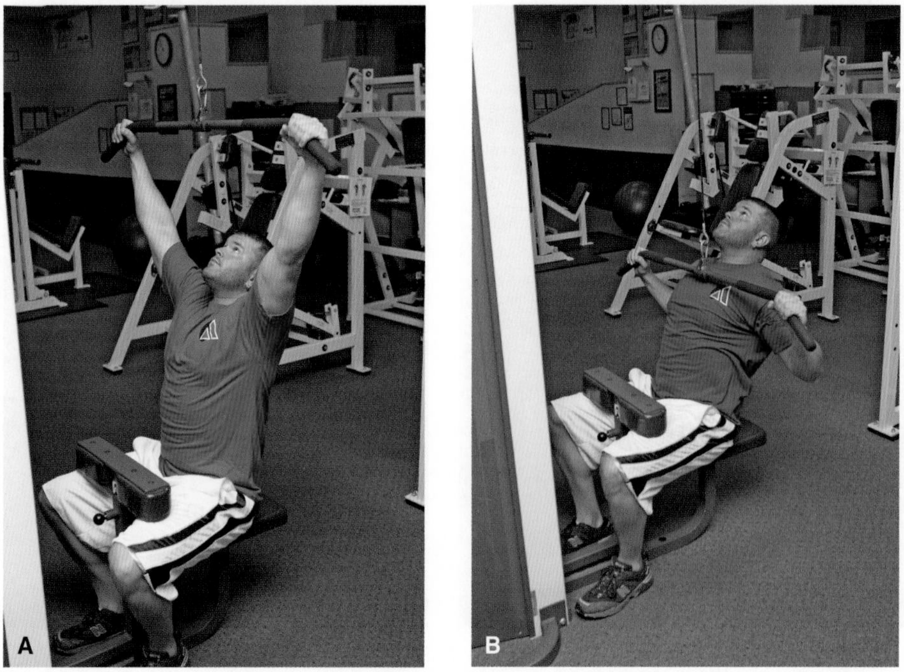

FIGURE 10.19 Lat pull-down. **A.** Starting position. **B.** Finish position.

Lat Pull-Down *(continued)*

Downward Motion

Inhale to initiate the descent. Begin the descent by adducting the scapulae and upper arms. The elbows should move down and back as the chest simultaneously moves up and out while the bar is lowered. Continue pulling the bar down and back until the bar lightly touches the upper chest near the clavicles. The torso should be leaning back slightly at the completion of the descent. The lower body should remain fixed throughout the descent. Avoid quickly leaning back farther or jerking the torso to help pull the bar down. Exhale at the completion of the descent (Fig. 10.19B).

Upward Motion

Return the bar back under control to the starting position. Avoid allowing the arms to return upward rapidly during the ascent. Maintain the same backward torso lean and position of the lower body throughout the ascent. Inhale as the bar rises to the start of the descent. The completion of the ascent is reached when the elbows reach full extension.

Seated Cable Row

Type of Exercise

Upper body/multijoint

Muscles Used

Latissimus dorsi, middle trapezius, rhomboids, teres major, posterior deltoid, biceps brachii, brachialis, brachioradialis

Starting Position

Place the pin at the desired training weight in the selectorized weight stack attached to the machine. Sit erect with a flat back on the bench facing the handle and the pulley. Grasp the handles with a closed neutral grip (palms facing each other) and the elbows

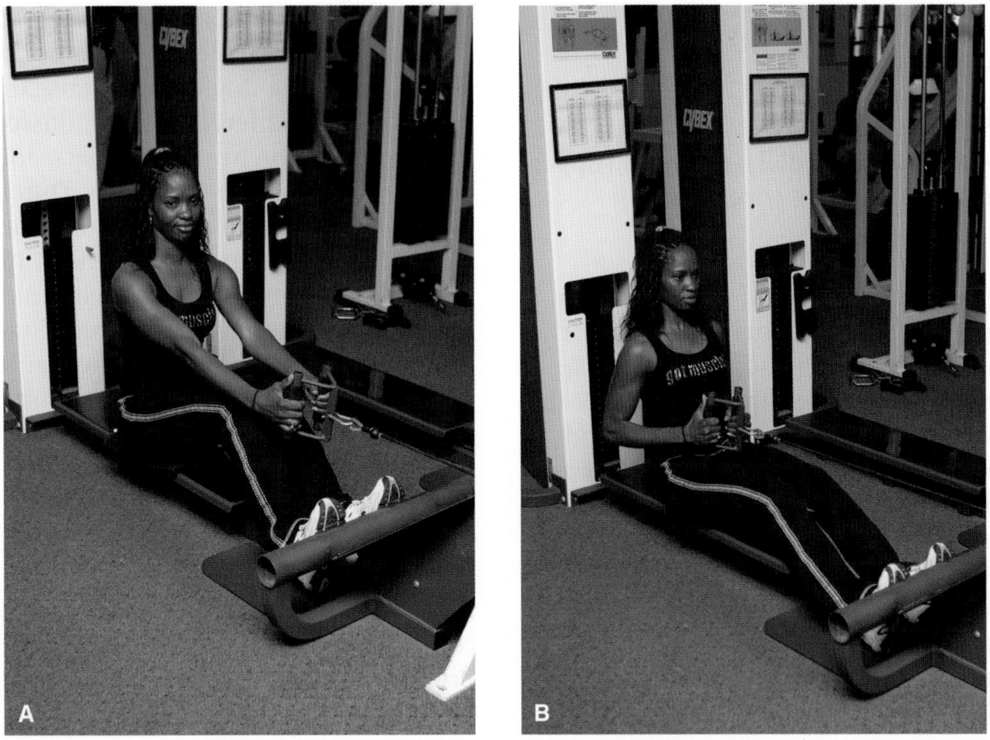

FIGURE 10.20 Seated cable row. **A.** Starting position. **B.** Finish position.

(continued)

Seated Cable Row *(continued)*

fully extended. Place the feet against the foot stops with a bent knee position. Keeping a flat back, slide back on the bench until the knees are bent slightly, keeping the elbows fully extended. Inhale prior to initiating the movement (Fig. 10.20A).

Backward Motion

Pull the handles toward the upper abdomen in a controlled motion. Maintain an erect torso throughout the backward motion. Keep the elbows close to the body as the handles are pulled back to the upper abdomen. Do not pull the handles quickly or arch the back to move the resistance. Exhale as the resistance is pulled through the sticking point (Fig. 10.20B).

Forward Motion

Keeping the torso erect and upright, elbows pointing down, allow the arms with control to fully extend back returning the resistance to the starting position. Inhale as the resistance is returned to the starting position.

Completion of the Set

Keeping a flat back slide forward on the bench allowing the knees to flex keeping the elbows fully extended until the resistance reaches the weight stack. Avoid rounding your back to return the resistance to the weight stack.

Shoulder Exercises

Dumbbell Seated Shoulder Press

Type of Exercise

Upper body/multijoint

Muscles Used

Deltoid (anterior and medial), trapezius (upper portion), serratus anterior, triceps brachii

Starting Position

Select two dumbbells of equal weight using a closed grip. Place the dumbbells on the floor next to the lower end of an adjustable bench. Adjust the bench such that the upper end of the bench is set at a 90-degree upward angle and the base of the bench is parallel to the floor to prevent sliding. Lift the dumbbells up from the floor by using the legs. Align the dumbbells such that the end closest to the little finger is against the front of the thighs (hands are facing in and handles are parallel to each other). Sit down on the lower end of the adjustable bench with the dumbbells resting on the top of the thighs. Lift the dumbbells into their starting position by quickly flexing the hips one hip at a time, using the thigh to help raise the dumbbells to shoulder level. Position the feet flat on the floor with the head, shoulders, and buttocks evenly and firmly on the bench. Dumbbells should be rotated to place the thumb side of the dumbbell against the outside of the shoulder such that both handles are in line with one another, simulating a barbell running through both dumbbell handles. Another option is to perform the exercise with the dumbbells kept in the neutral position (parallel to each other). Each repetition will begin from this same position (Fig. 10.21A).

Upward Motion

Press the dumbbells upward and together with control. Keep the head, body, and feet in their original position. Do not arch the lower back. The wrists should remain firm and straight, the

Dumbbell Seated Shoulder Press *(continued)*

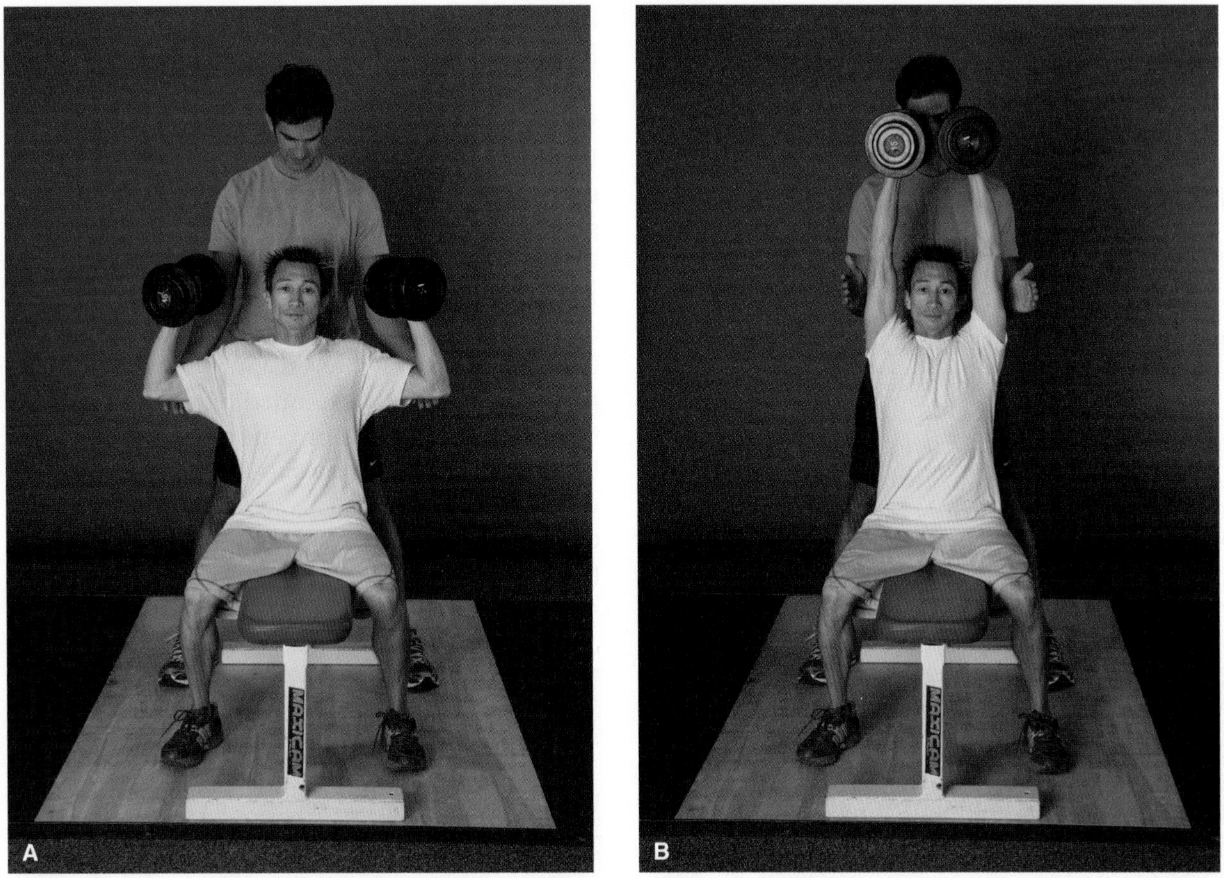

FIGURE 10.21 Dumbbell seated shoulder press. **A.** Starting position. **B.** Finish position.

forearms almost perpendicular to the floor, and the hands aligned with each other. Do not allow the dumbbells to move out of control as they are being raised. Press the dumbbells upward until the elbows are fully extended but not locked. Bring the dumbbells together with control at the completion of the movement directly above the middle of the head; do not bang the dumbbells together. Exhale as the dumbbells are lifted past the sticking point (Fig. 10.21B).

Downward Motion

Lower and separate the dumbbells with control toward the outer shoulder. To maintain a stable position on the bench, lower both dumbbells at the same rate. Keep the wrists firm and straight, the forearms almost perpendicular to the floor, and the hands aligned with each other. Avoid movements forward and backward or side to side. Lower the dumbbells to the outer portion of the shoulder such that both handles are in line with one another where a barbell would touch the upper shoulders. Dumbbells should not be bounced off the shoulder at the bottom position. Avoid arching the back. Maintain a stable position with the feet flat on the floor and the head, shoulders, and buttocks evenly and firmly on the bench. Inhale as the dumbbells are lowered.

Completion of the Set

After lowering the dumbbells to the outer shoulder on the last repetition, rotate the dumbbells toward the midline of the body and lower them to the thigh. Return the dumbbells to the dumbbell rack or floor.

(continued)

Machine Shoulder Press

Type of Exercise

Upper body/multijoint

Muscles Used

Deltoid (anterior and medial), trapezius (upper portion), serratus anterior, triceps brachii

Starting Position

Place the pin at the desired training weight in the selectorized weight stack attached to the machine. Adjust the seat height such that the handgrips are in line with the tops of the shoulders and the base of the neck. Position the feet flat on the floor with the head, shoulders, and buttocks evenly and firmly on the machine. The head, shoulders, and upper back should be pressed against the vertical pad. Grasp both handles with a closed pronated or neutral (optional) grip (Fig. 10.22A).

Upward Motion

Begin the motion by pushing the handles upward. Exhale as the resistance passes the sticking point. Avoid arching the lower back or lifting the feet or buttocks from their position. Keep the wrists rigid and the forearms perpendicular to the floor and parallel to each other. Continue pressing the resistance upward until the elbows are fully extended but not forcefully locked. At the completion of the lift, the handles of the machine should be in line with the supporting joints (i.e., wrist, elbow, shoulder). Keep the body rigid throughout the ascent (Fig. 10.22B).

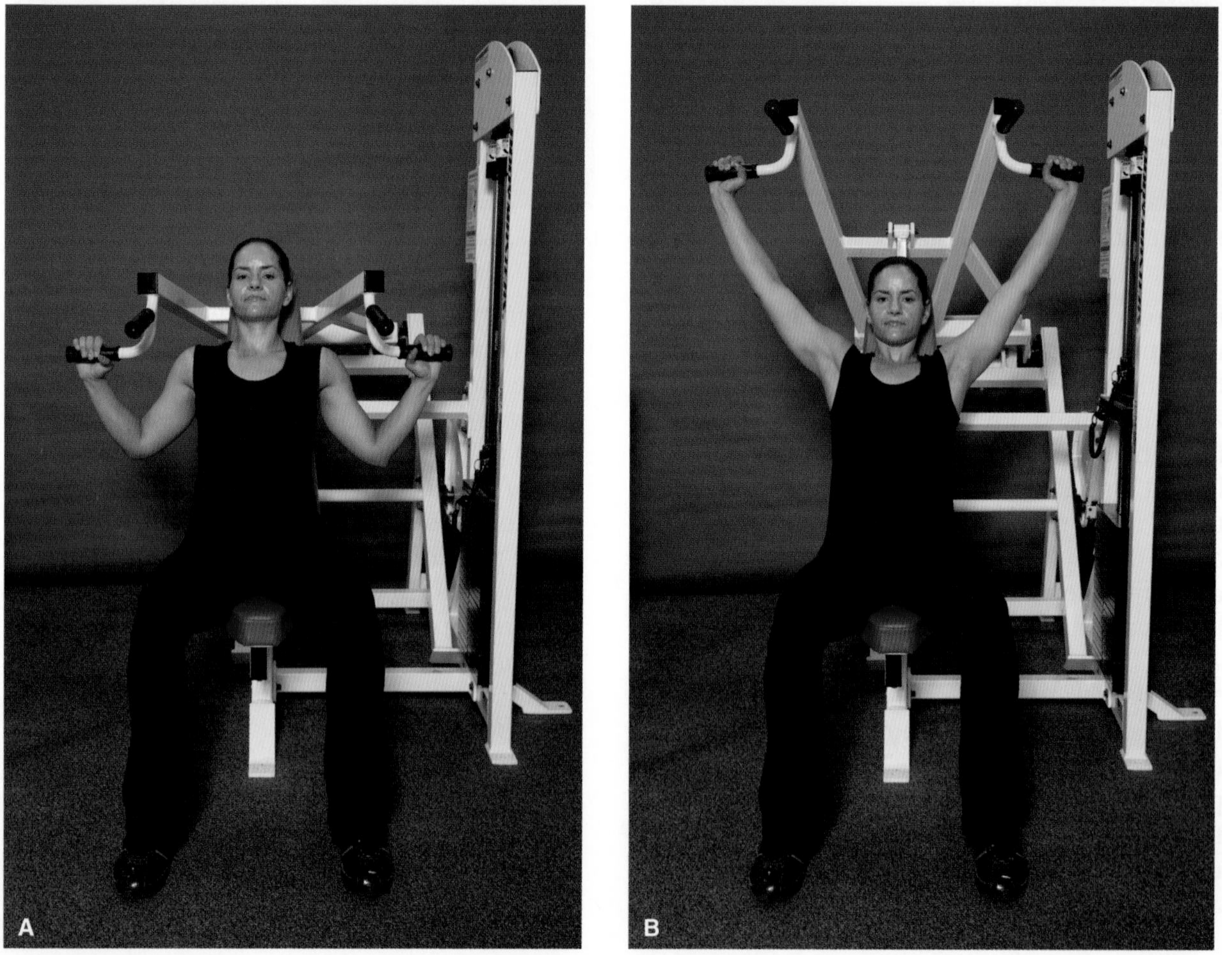

FIGURE 10.22 Machine shoulder press. **A.** Starting position. **B.** Finish position.

Machine Shoulder Press *(continued)*

Downward Motion

Begin the descent by lowering the resistance in a slow, controlled manner toward the chest. The elbows will move down past the shoulder and slightly away from the body. Wrists should be kept firm and rigid, ensuring that the barbell remains over the longitudinal axis of the ulna and not in the distal portion of the hand. Forearms are parallel to each other and perpendicular to the floor. Lower the resistance to shoulder height; avoid bouncing the resistance off the weight stack, lifting the buttocks off the bench, or arching the back. Keep the head, shoulders/upper back area, and buttocks in contact with the bench and both feet securely on the floor. Keep the body rigid throughout the descent.

Barbell Upright Row

Type of Exercise

Upper body/multijoint

Muscles Used

Anterior, medial and posterior deltoid, trapezius, serratus anterior, brachialis, biceps brachii, brachioradialis

Starting Position

Load barbell evenly on both sides and secure weights with collars. Grasp the barbell evenly with a closed, pronated grip narrower than shoulder width but not closer than thumb width apart from each other. Hold the barbell against the front of the thighs with the elbows fully extended. Position the feet flat on the floor shoulder width apart, knees flexed slightly, torso erect, shoulders back, and eyes looking straight ahead (Fig. 10.23A).

Upward Motion

Begin the upward motion by lifting the barbell vertically along the front of the body past the abdomen and chest by flexing the elbows and abducting the shoulders. Maintain an erect upper torso while keeping the knees still slightly flexed and feet flat on the floor. The

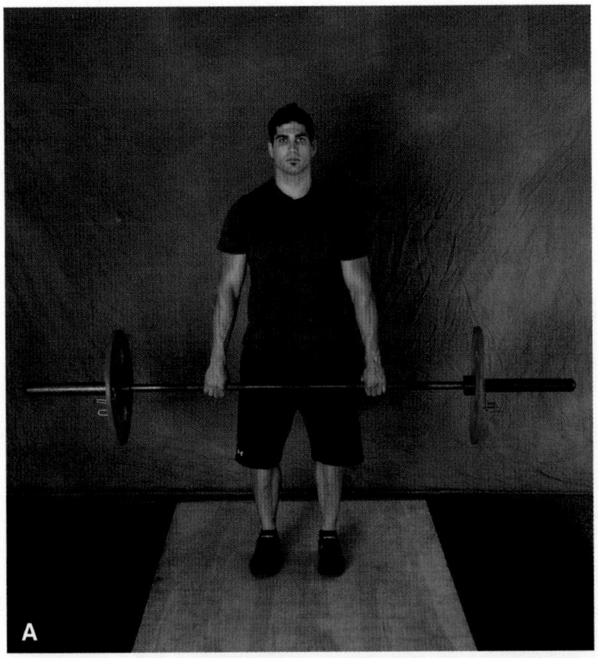

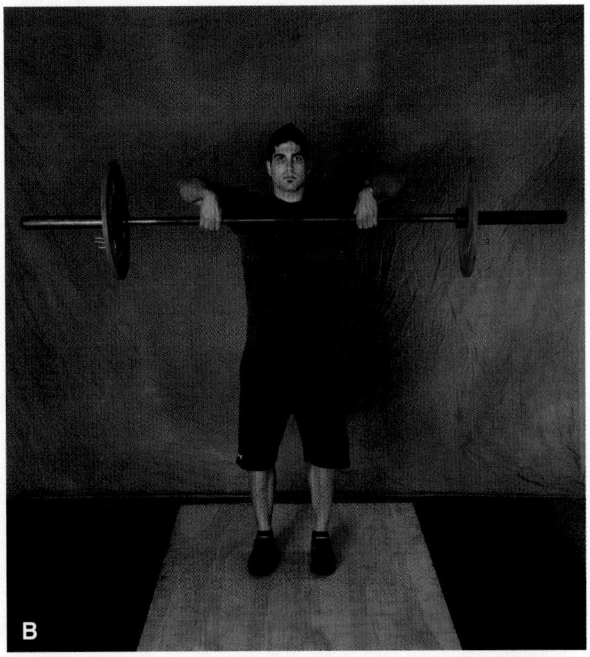

FIGURE 10.23 Barbell upright row. **A.** Starting position. **B.** Finish position.

(continued)

Barbell Upright Row *(continued)*

barbell should not swing away from the body or upward in an uncontrolled manner. Avoid rising up on the toes, extending the knees, or shrugging the shoulders to assist in the ascent of the barbell. Keep the wrists rigid throughout the ascent. Continue with the upward pull of the barbell until the elbows are slightly higher than the shoulders and wrists (the barbell should be elevated to a point between the sternum and the chin depending upon the individual's arm length and shoulder flexibility). Exhale at the completion of the ascent (Fig. 10.23B).

Downward Motion

Slowly lower the barbell under control, keeping the barbell close to the body throughout the descent until the elbows are fully extended and the barbell is against the front of the thighs. Avoid bouncing the barbell against the thighs, rapidly extending the elbows, leaning forward with the torso, or shifting the body weight to the balls of the feet. Maintain an erect upper torso, knees slightly flexed, and the feet flat on the floor shoulder width apart. Inhale as the barbell is lowered during the descent.

Dumbbell Prone Posterior Raise

Type of Exercise

Upper body/single joint

Muscles Used

Infraspinatus, teres minor, trapezius, deltoids (anterior, medial, and posterior)

Starting Position

Select two dumbbells of equal weight. Place the dumbbells on the floor next to the upper end of a slightly elevated adjustable bench. Lie prone on the weight bench with the hips, thighs, and torso resting on the padded surface. Slide up the bench so that the chin rests over the top edge of the bench. Grasp the dumbbells with a closed grip, and rotate them to a neutral hand position with the handles parallel to each other and with the elbows pointing out to the side. The arms extend straight down from the shoulders with a slight flex in the elbows (Fig. 10.24A,B).

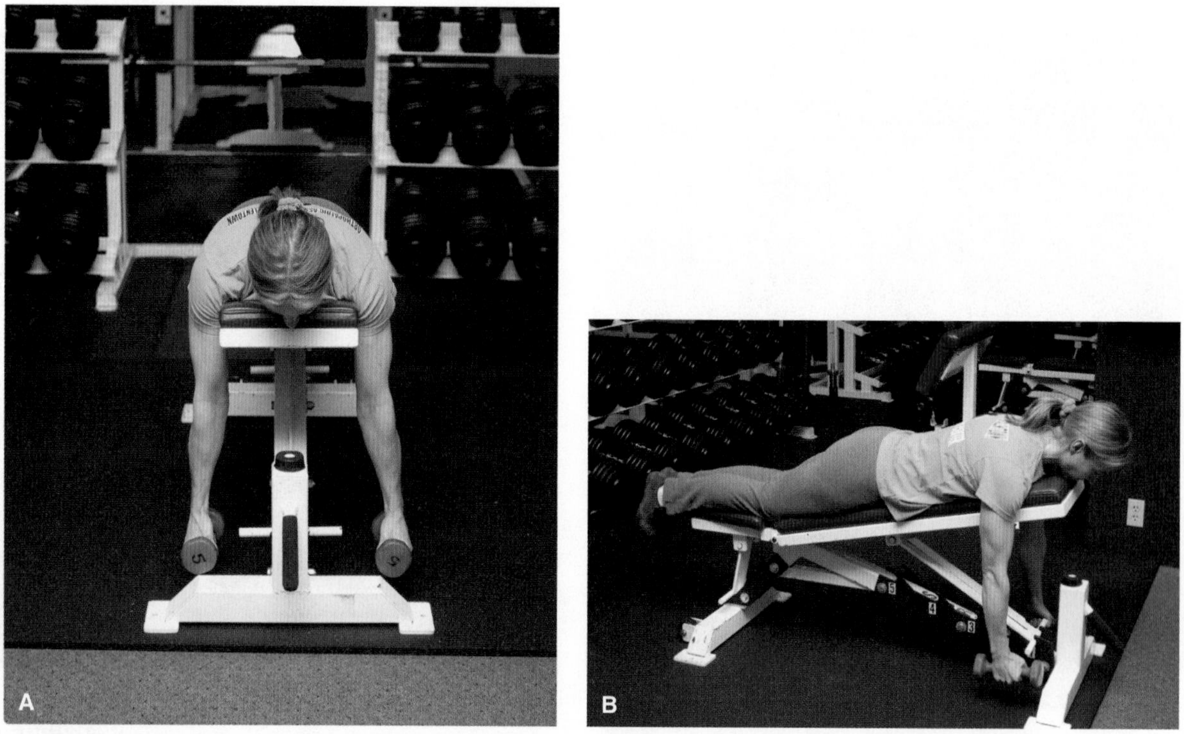

FIGURE 10.24 Dumbbell prone posterior raise. **A.** Starting position, front view. **B.** Starting position, side view.

Dumbbell Prone Posterior Raise *(continued)*

Upward Motion

Inhale and raise the dumbbells with control simultaneously out to the sides while maintaining the slight bend in the elbows; movement should not occur at the elbow joints, only at the shoulders. Throughout the upward motion, the upper arms and elbows should rise together, before and slightly higher than the lower arm and hands. Avoid lifting the weight rapidly. Keep the head, neck, or upper torso in contact with the bench throughout the upward motion. Exhale as the resistance is lifted through the sticking point. Continue lifting the resistance until the arms are approximately parallel to the floor or nearly level with the shoulder height (Fig. 10.24C,D).

Downward Motion

Lower the dumbbells with control while keeping the head, neck, or upper torso in contact with the bench throughout the downward motion. Allow the dumbbells to continue to descend, keeping the dumbbells parallel to each other until they return to their hanging starting position. Inhale as the dumbbells return to the starting position.

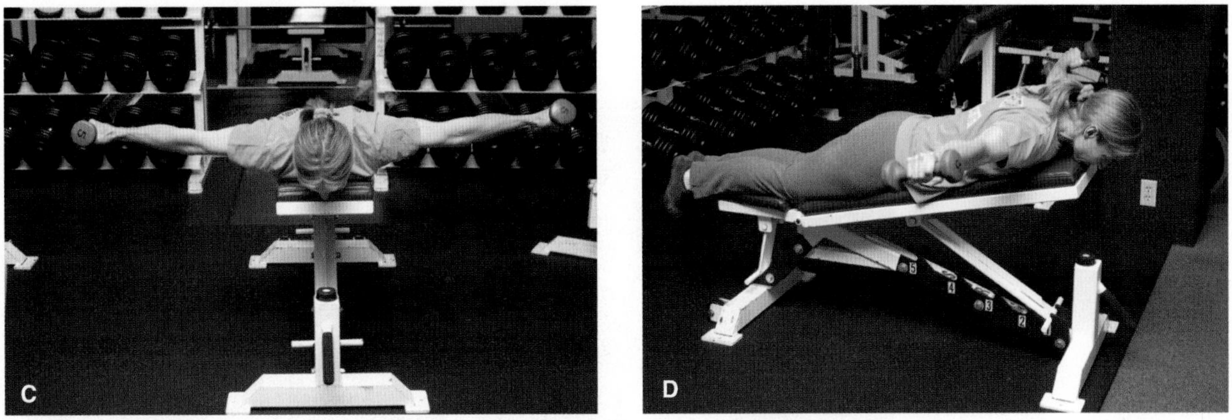

FIGURE 10.24 *(Continued)* **C.** Finish position, front view. **D.** Finish position, side view.

Triceps Exercises

Supine Triceps Extension

Type of Exercise

Upper body/single joint

Muscles Used

Triceps brachii

Starting Position

Load an EZ curl barbell evenly on both sides and secure weights with collars. Sit at one end of an adjustable flat bench, and then lie back so the head rests on the other end of the bench. The head, shoulders/upper back area, and buttocks should be firmly and evenly placed on the bench, and both feet should be securely placed on the floor on either side of the bench. Have a spotter lift the barbell so it can be grasped with a closed, pronated grip at either the inside or outside hand position of the barbell. Move the barbell to a position where the arms are parallel to each other and perpendicular to the floor; this requires the barbell to be held with the elbows extended over the eyes. The upper arms should be externally rotated so that the elbows point toward the feet (Fig. 10.25A).

(continued)

Supine Triceps Extension *(continued)*

Downward Motion

Lower the barbell with control toward the top of the forehead. The elbows should point toward the feet as they begin to flex. The upper arms should remain parallel to each other and perpendicular to the floor. Keep the head, shoulders/upper back area, and buttocks firmly and evenly placed on the bench with both feet securely placed on the floor on either side of the bench. Avoid arching the back during the downward motion. The barbell should nearly touch the forehead at its lowest position. Caution should be taken to control the speed of the descent so that the barbell does not strike the face. Inhale during the downward motion (Fig. 10.25B).

Upward Motion

Lift the barbell upward with control by extending the elbows while keeping the elbow and upper arms stationary. Keep the head, shoulders/upper back area, and buttocks firmly and evenly placed on the bench with both feet securely placed on the floor on either side of the bench. Continue pressing the barbell until the elbows are fully extended with the barbell directly above the eyes. Exhale as the resistance is lifted through the sticking point.

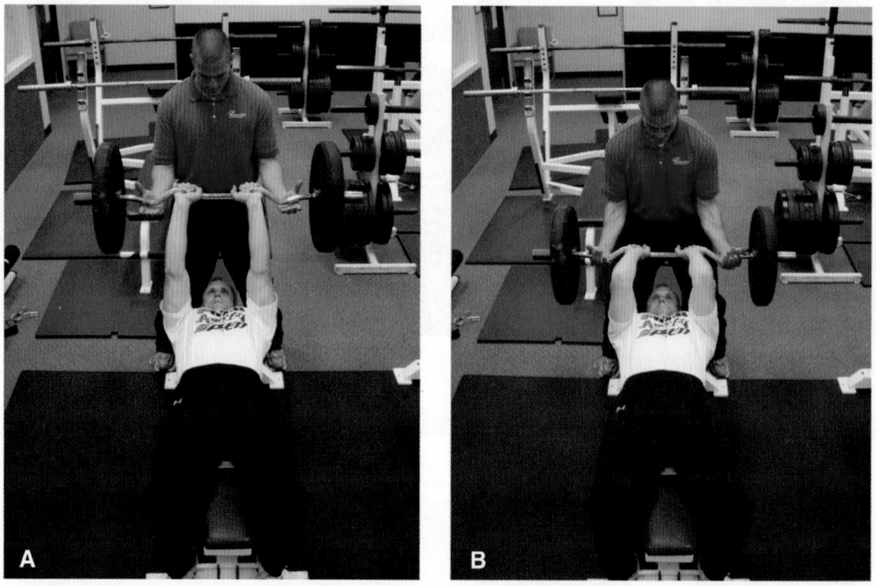

FIGURE 10.25 Supine triceps extension. **A.** Starting position. **B.** Finish position.

Triceps Pushdown

Type of Exercise

Upper body/single joint

Muscles Used

Triceps brachii

Starting Position

Place the pin at the desired training weight in the selectorized weight stack attached to the machine. Grasp a Tri-V bar or rope with a closed pronated grip. Hands will be approximately 8

Triceps Pushdown *(continued)*

to 10 in apart. Place the feet shoulder or hip width apart with the torso erect and the knees slightly flexed. Position the body so that the cable is positioned at a perpendicular angle in the starting position. Move the Tri-V bar down from its stationary position to a position where the elbows are next to the anterior portion of the torso touching the lower rib cage; the lower arm is straight out from the body with the wrists straight and hands even with chest level. Keep the head in a neutral position with the cable directly in front of the nose, with shoulders back and abdominal muscles slightly contracted. Avoid leaning forward or positioning the head to the side of the cable. Inhale prior to initiating the downward motion. All subsequent repetitions should begin from this position (Fig. 10.26A).

Downward Motion

While maintaining an erect posture, push the Tri-V bar down with control from the chest level toward the upper thigh. Keep the elbows tight to the anterior portion of the torso, touching the lower rib cage. Keep the body centered with the cable in front of the middle of the face. Maintain a slight flex in the knees throughout the downward motion. Exhale as the resistance is lifted through the sticking point. Avoid locking the elbows at the bottom position (Fig. 10.26B).

Upward Motion

Extend the elbows with control to allow the Tri-V bar to return to the initial starting position. The initial starting position is a position where the elbows are next to the anterior portion of the torso touching the lower rib cage; the lower arm is straight out from the body with the wrists straight and hands even with chest level. It is critical throughout the upward motion to ensure that the elbows are next to the anterior portion of the torso touching the lower rib cage. Inhale as the bar returns to the starting position.

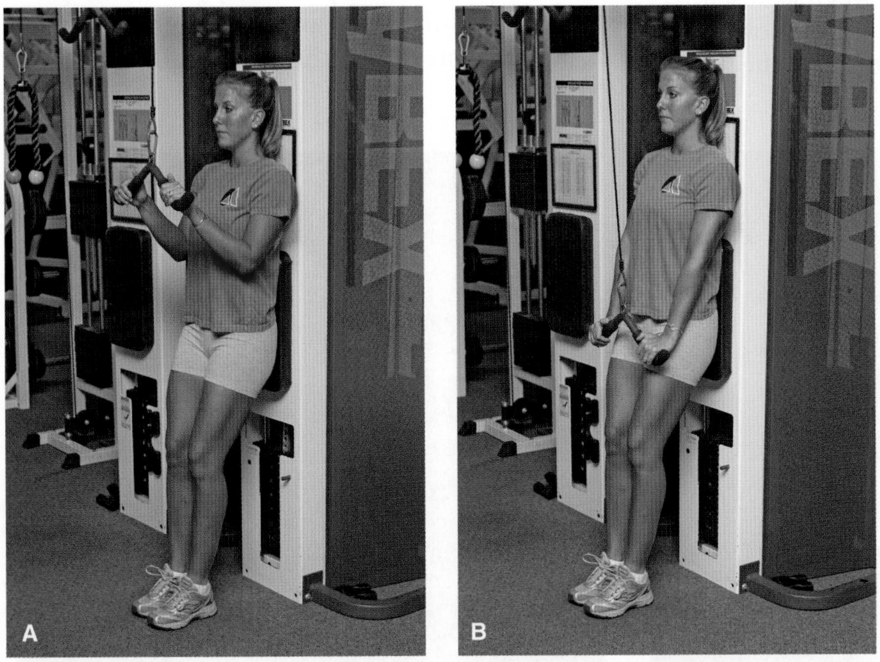

FIGURE 10.26 Triceps pushdown. **A.** Starting position. **B.** Finish position.

Biceps Exercises

Barbell Bicep Curl

Type of Exercise

Upper body/single joint

Muscles Used

Biceps brachii, brachialis, brachioradialis

Starting Position

Load barbell evenly on both sides and secure weights with collars. Grasp the barbell evenly with a closed, supinated grip shoulder-width apart. Hold the bar against the front of the thighs with the elbows fully extended. Position the feet flat on the floor shoulder-width apart, knees flexed slightly, torso erect, shoulders back, and eyes looking straight ahead. Inhale prior to initiating the upward motion (Fig. 10.27A).

Upward Motion

Flex the arms at the elbows raising the barbell in an arc pattern with control. Keep the elbows tight to the anterior portion of the torso touching the lower rib cage as the barbell is raised. The movement should occur at the elbows, not at the shoulders. Keep the feet flat on the floor shoulder-width apart, knees flexed slightly, torso erect, shoulders back, and eyes looking straight ahead. Avoid swinging the barbell, arching the lower back, rising up on the toes, or shrugging the shoulders to lift the resistance. Continue flexing the elbows until the barbell reaches a point above chest level approximately 2 to 3 in from the body. Avoid moving the elbows forward at the completion of the upward motion. Exhale as the barbell passes the sticking point (Fig. 10.27B).

Downward Motion

Lower the barbell with control until the elbows are fully extended. Avoid bouncing the barbell on the thighs at the bottom position. Flexing the torso forward, rise up on the toes, or forcefully extend the elbows during the downward motion. Keep the elbows tight to the anterior portion of the torso touching the lower rib cage as the barbell is lowered. Maintain an erect upper body posture with the knees slightly flexed and the feet flat on the floor. Inhale during the downward motion.

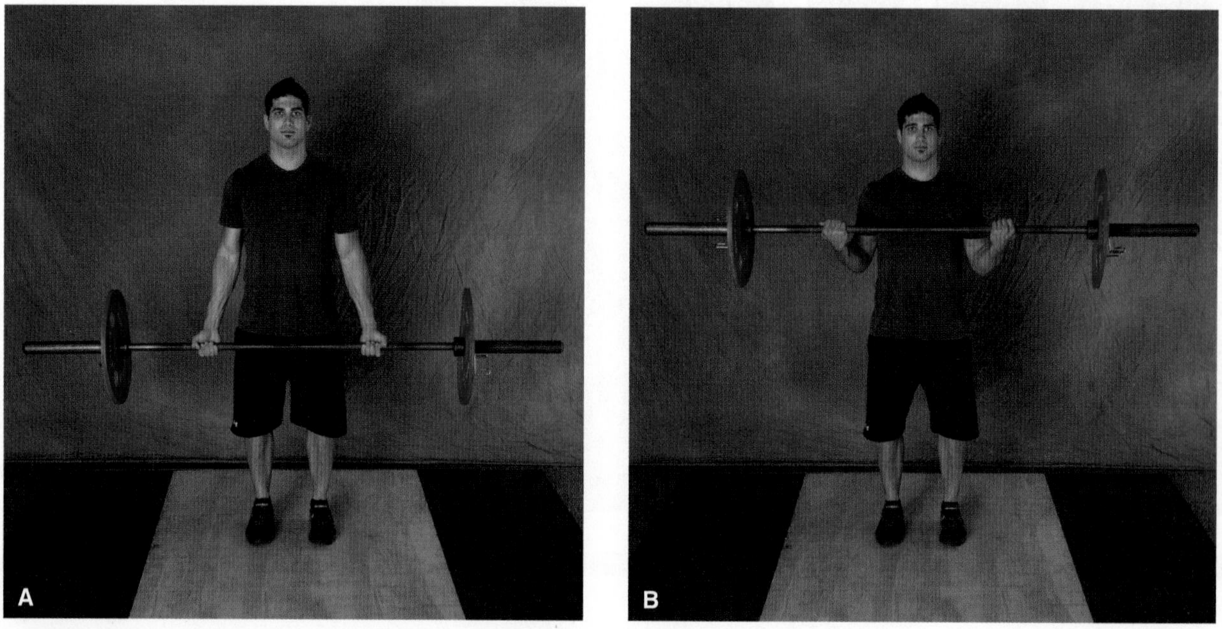

FIGURE 10.27 Barbell bicep curl. **A.** Starting position. **B.** Finish position.

Dumbbell Seated Alternate-Arm Bicep Curl

Type of Exercise

Upper body/single joint

Muscles Used

Biceps brachii, brachialis, brachioradialis

Starting Position

Select two dumbbells of equal weight with a closed grip. Place the dumbbells on the floor next to the lower end of an adjustable bench. Adjust the bench such that the upper end of the bench is set at a 75-degree upward angle and the base of the bench is parallel to the floor to prevent sliding. Lift the dumbbells up from the floor by using the legs. Sit down on the lower end of the adjustable bench with the dumbbells resting on the top of the thighs. Allow the dumbbells to hang at the side with the elbows fully extended and the hands supinated (palms facing forward). Inhale just before lifting the first dumbbell (Fig. 10.28A).

Upward Motion

Initiate the exercise by raising one dumbbell upward with control in an arc by flexing the arm at the elbow. Keep the elbows tight to the anterior portion of the torso, touching the lower rib cage as the barbell is raised. The movement should occur at the elbow, not at the shoulders. Keep the feet flat on the floor, torso erect, shoulders back, and eyes looking straight ahead. Avoid swinging the dumbbell, arching the lower back, rising up on the toes, or shrugging the shoulders to lift the dumbbell. Continue flexing the elbow until the dumbbell reaches a point above chest level approximately 2 to 3 in from the body. Avoid moving the elbow forward at the completion of the upward motion. Exhale as the dumbbell passes the sticking point. Keep the opposite arm still at the side of the body (Fig. 10.28B).

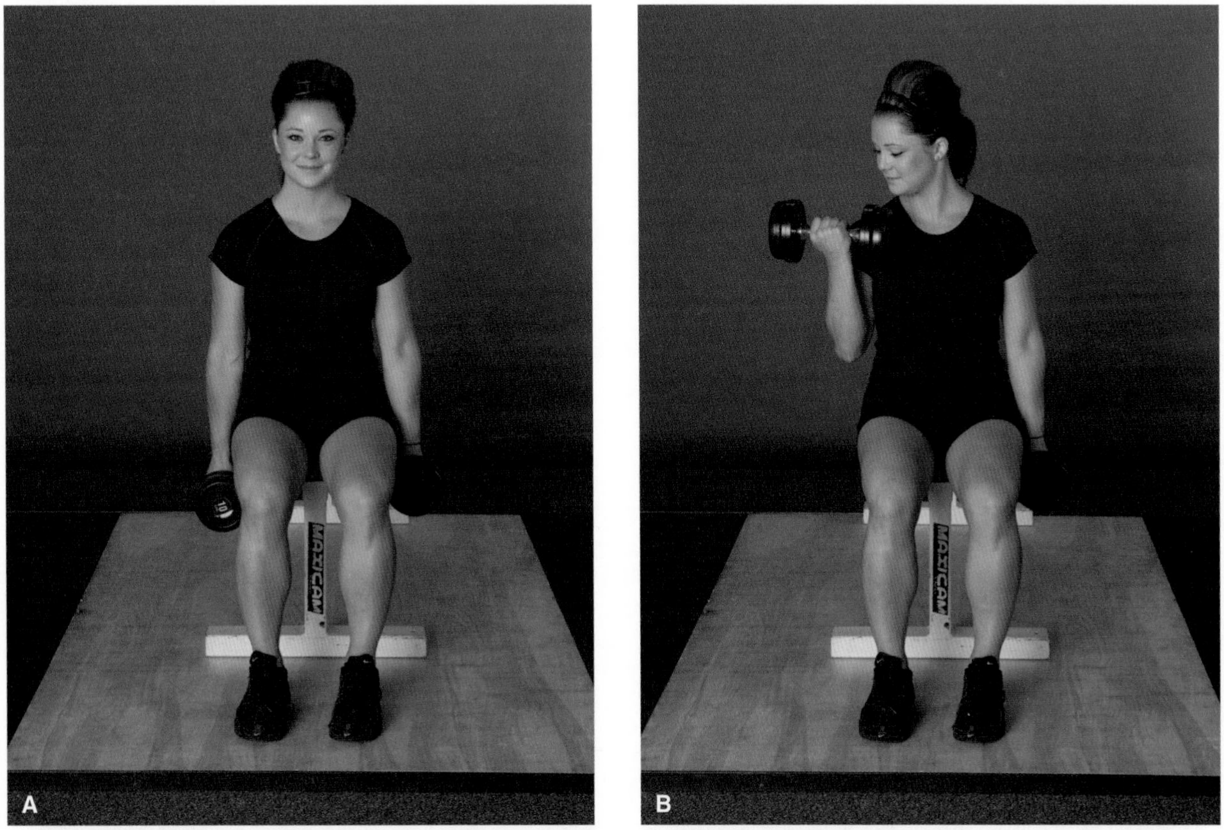

FIGURE 10.28 Dumbbell seated alternate arm bicep curl. **A.** Starting position. **B.** Finish position.

(continued)

Dumbbell Seated Alternate-Arm Bicep Curl *(continued)*

Downward Motion

Lower the dumbbell with control until the elbow is fully extended. Avoid forcefully extending the elbow during the downward motion. Keep the elbow tight to the anterior portion of the torso, touching the lower rib cage as the dumbbell is lowered. Maintain an erect upper body posture with the feet flat on the floor. Inhale during the downward motion. Keep the opposite arm still at the side of the body until the repetition is completed and then repeat the upward and downward movements with the opposite arm.

Forearm Exercises

Wrist Curl

Type of Exercise

Upper body/single joint

Muscles Used

Flexor carpi radialis, flexor carpi ulnaris, palmaris longus, flexor digitorum superficialis, flexor digitorum profundus

Starting Position

Grasp two even weight dumbbells with closed supinated grips, shoulder-width apart. Sit on the end of a bench. Position the legs at 90 degrees with the feet and legs parallel to each other and the toes pointing straight ahead. Place the forearms and elbows on top of the thighs

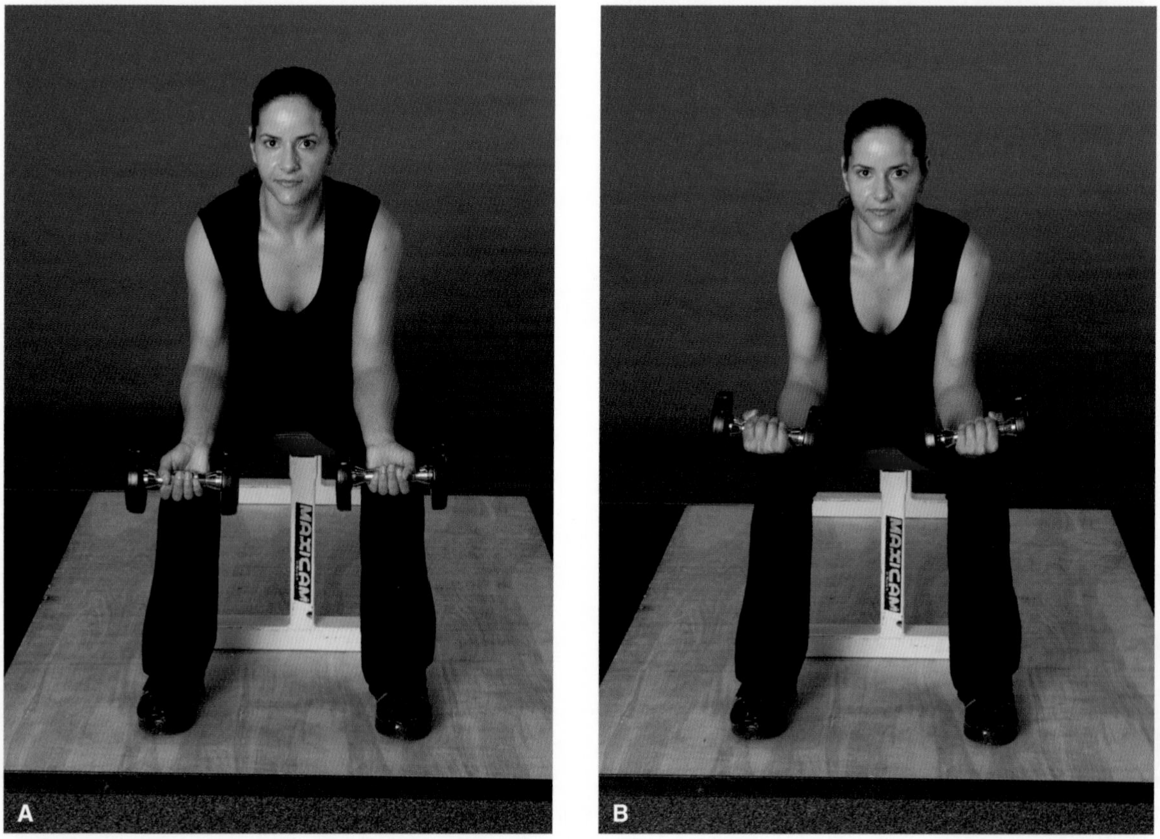

FIGURE 10.29 Wrist curl. **A.** Starting position. **B.** Finish position.

Wrist Curl *(continued)*

and lean forward slightly. The wrists should extend slightly past the front of the knee. Extend the wrists with control toward the floor and open the fingers so the dumbbells rest on the fingertips. Inhale before initiating the upward motion (Fig. 10.29A).

Upward Motion

Lift the dumbbells with control by flexing the fingers and then the wrists through a full ROM without moving the forearms or elbows. Do not jerk or rapidly move upward. Exhale as the dumbbells pass the sticking point (Fig. 10.29B).

Downward Motion

Return the dumbbells with control to the starting position by first extending the wrists and then the fingers. Avoid rapidly dropping the dumbbells during the downward motion. Inhale at the completion of the downward motion.

Reverse Wrist Curl

Type of Exercise

Upper body/single joint

Muscles Used

Extensor carpi radialis longus, extensor carpi radialis brevis, extensor carpi ulnaris, extensor digitorum, extensor digiti minimi, extensor indicis

Starting Position

Grasp two even weight dumbbells with closed pronated grips, shoulder-width apart. Sit on the

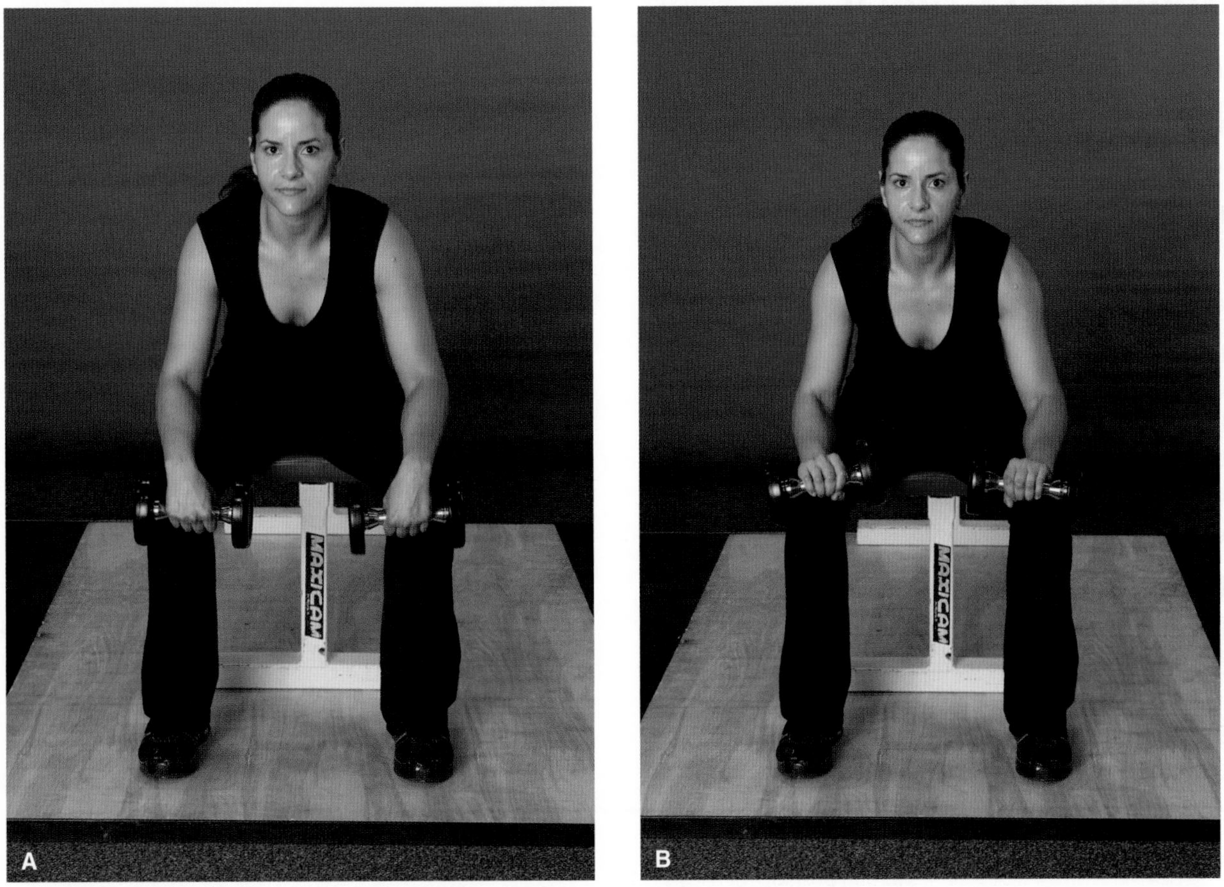

FIGURE 10.30 Reverse wrist curl. **A.** Starting position. **B.** Finish position.

(continued)

Reverse Wrist Curl *(continued)*

end of a bench. Position the legs at a 90-degree angle with the feet and legs parallel to each other and the toes pointing straight ahead. Place the forearms and elbows on top of the thighs, and lean forward slightly. The wrists should extend slightly past the front of the knee. Flex the wrists with control toward the floor while keeping the fingers closed. Inhale before initiating the upward motion (Fig. 10.30A).

Upward Motion

Lift the dumbbells with control by extending the wrists through a full range of motion without moving the forearms or elbows. Do not jerk or rapidly move upward. Exhale as the dumbbells pass the sticking point.

Downward Motion

Lower the dumbbells with control toward the floor by flexing the wrists. Avoid rapidly dropping the dumbbells during the downward motion. Inhale at the completion of the downward motion (Fig. 10.30B).

Abdominal and Lower Back Exercises

Abdominal Crunch

Type of Exercise

Trunk

Muscles Used

Rectus abdominis, obliques externus abdominis, tensor fascia latae, rectus femoris

Starting Position

Lie supine on an exercise mat or padded floor. Place hands behind the head with fingers interlaced and elbows out to the side. Bend the knees to a 90-degree angle, and place the feet flat on the floor. Inhale prior to initiating the exercise (Fig. 10.31A).

Upward Motion

Keeping the neck straight cradled in the hands, the lower back and buttocks flat on the floor, and the knees at a 90-degree angle with feet on the floor, curl the torso upward with control until the upper back is lifted off the floor or exercise mat. Keep the fingers interlaced behind the head. Exhale as the sticking point is passed (Fig. 10.31B).

Downward Motion

With control, keeping the neck straight and cradled in the hands, the lower back and buttocks flat on the floor, and the knees at a 90-degree angle with feet on the floor, allow the torso to uncurl back to the starting position when the upper back reaches the floor or exercise mat. Keep the fingers interlaced behind the head. Inhale at the completion of the downward motion.

Variation of the Exercise

For more experienced exercisers, the lower legs may be lifted parallel to the floor or placed on an exercise bench with the lower back and buttocks flat on the floor and the knees at a 90-degree angle perpendicular to the floor.

Abdominal Crunch *(continued)*

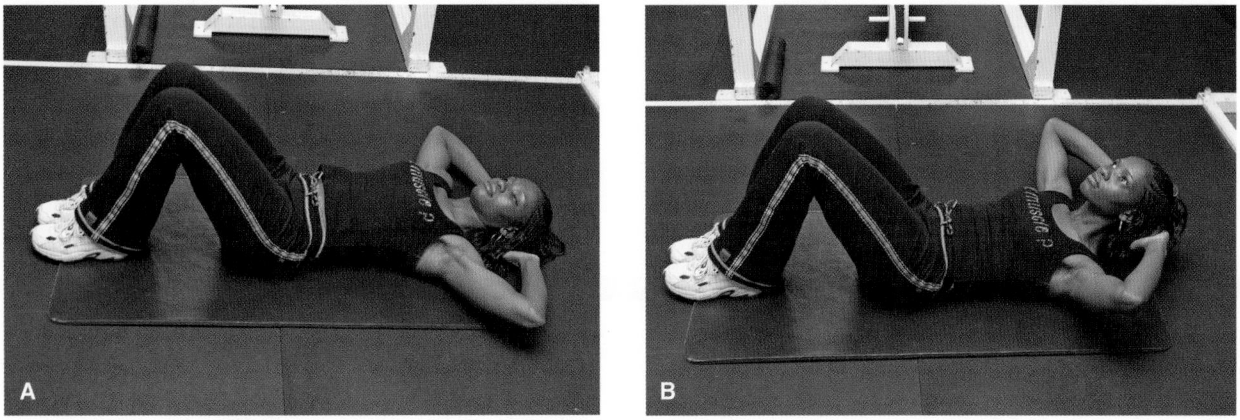

FIGURE 10.31 Abdominal crunch. A. Starting position. B. Finish position.

Back Extension

Type of Exercise

Trunk

Muscles Used

Longissimus thoracis, quadratus lumborum, iliocostalis lumborum,, iliocostalis thoracis, intertransversarii laterales lumborum, gluteus maximus, hamstrings (semimembranosus, semitendinosus, biceps femoris)

Starting Position

Sit on the machine in an upright posture with your feet on the footplate so your knees are slightly bent and the back of your legs are in firm contact with

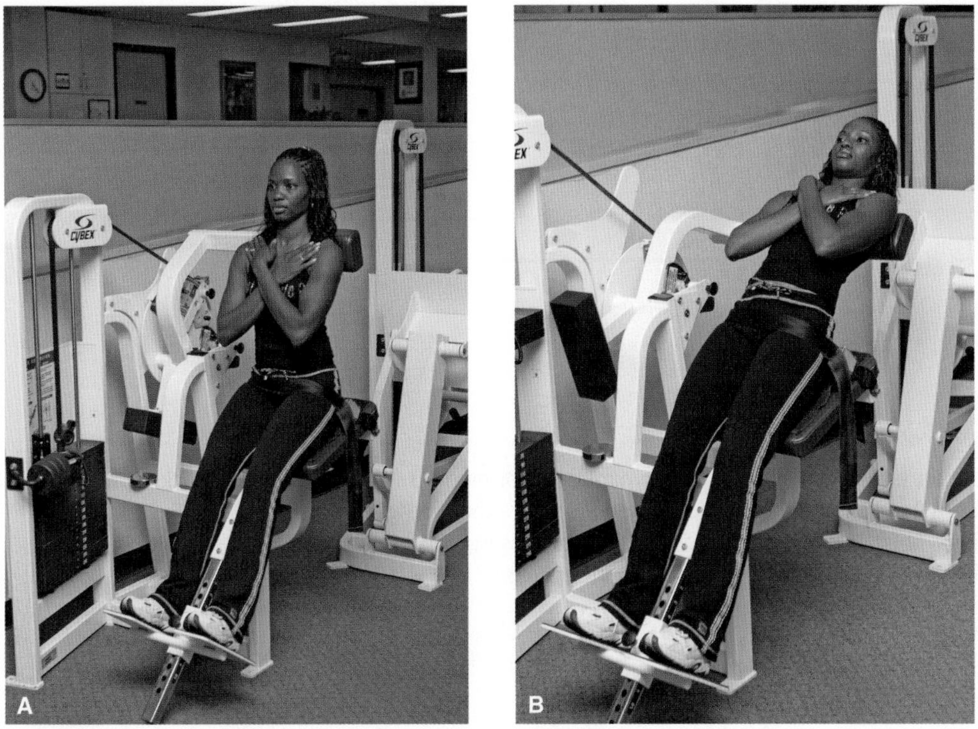

FIGURE 10.32 Back extension. A. Starting position. B. Finish position.

(continued)

Back Extension *(continued)*

the seat. Make sure the back pad is in contact with your shoulder blades, and then place your hands, overlapped, across your chest (Fig. 10.32A).

Back Motion

Keep your head and neck in a neutral position and slowly begin to extend your torso backward until you reach a position that is straight from your feet to your head (Fig. 10.32B).

Forward Motion

Reverse your position while performing a slow trunk flexion movement until you return to the upright sitting posture.

Summary

Resistance training has numerous benefits, including hypertrophy and increased bone mineral density. Prior to beginning a resistance-training program, an exerciser should be familiar with proper attire, spotting techniques, and breathing techniques. Prior to performing a specific exercise, an exerciser should know the proper movement of the exercise as described in this chapter.

TABLE 10.1 ● UPPER-BODY EXERCISES

EXERCISE	BENCH PRESS, BARBELL	BARBELL UPRIGHT ROW	SUPINE TRICEPS EXTENSION
Type of exercise			
Muscles used			
Grip type			
Grip width			
Number of spotters			

TABLE 10.2 ● LOWER-BODY EXERCISES

EXERCISE	POWER CLEAN	BACK SQUAT	DEAD LIFT
Type of exercise			
Muscles used			
Grip type			
Grip width			
Feet width			
Number of spotters			

Maxing Out

1. An experienced strength-training participant is performing a 3-RM exercise in the back squat. How many spotters are required? Where should they be positioned? What are their responsibilities?
2. Complete Table 10.1 for the listed upper-body exercises.
3. Complete Table 10.2 for the listed lower-body exercises.

CASE EXAMPLE

Designing a Resistance-Training Program for a Young Multisport Athlete

BACKGROUND

You are a strength coach who is working with a 14-year-old male athlete who participates in multiple sports. He has been trained using weight machines for the past year. He wants to increase his sport-specific strength.

RECOMMENDATIONS/CONSIDERATIONS

After performing a needs analysis and on the basis of your client's potential, you decide to begin using free weights for squats and bench press. Free weights are chosen because of their increased specificity to sports.

IMPLEMENTATION

The free-weight squat and bench press are going to be implemented into the strength training program over a 10-week period.

Weeks 1 and 2. The first 2 weeks are used to introduce the free-weight exercises. Light weights are used, and proper form is stressed. Half the sets performed will use the traditional machines, and half will use the free-weight exercises.

Weeks 3 to 6. Once the athlete has learned proper form, moderate resistance can be used in weeks 3 to 6. Most of the sets are performed using free weights, but 1 to 2 sets a week may still be performed with machines.

Weeks 7 to 10. At this point, the athlete should be comfortable with the free weights and be performing all of the sets with free weights using moderate resistance.

RESULTS

At the end of the 10-week period, the athlete was successfully incorporating the free-weight bench press and free-weight squat into his program. Testing after the program found the following results:

- Increased body weight
- No increase in percentage of body fat
- Increased vertical jump
- Increased push-ups in 1 minute

REFERENCES

1. Brooks GA, Fahey TD, White TP. *Exercise Physiology: Human Bioenergetics and Its Applications*. 2nd ed. Mountain View, CA: Mayfield, 1996.
2. Earle RW, Baechle TR, Wathen D. Resistance training. In: Baechle TR, Earle RW, eds. *Essentials of Strength Training and Conditioning*. 3rd ed. Champaign, IL: Human Kinetics; 2008.
3. Hoffman JR, Ratamess NA. *A Practical Guide to Developing Resistance Training Programs*. Monterey, CA: Coaches Choice; 2006.
4. Zatsiorsky VM. *The Science and Practice of Strength Training*. Champaign, IL: Human Kinetics; 1995.
5. Cissik JM. *The Basics of Strength Training*. New York: McGraw-Hill; 2001:17–21.
6. Nutter J. Physical activity increases bone density. *NSCA J*. 1986;8(3);67–69.
7. Baechle TR, Groves BR. *Weight Training: Steps to Success*. 2nd ed. Champaign, IL: Human Kinetics; 1998:6–10.
8. Fleck SR, Kraemer WJ. *Designing Resistance Training Programs*. 3rd ed. Champaign, IL: Human Kinetics, 2004.
9. Aaberg E. *Resistance Training Instruction*. Champaign, IL: Human Kinetics; 1999:35–48.
10. Newton H. *Explosive Lifting For Sports*. Champaign, IL: Human Kinetics; 2002.
11. Barnes M, Cinea KE. Explosive movements. In: Brown LE, ed. *Strength Training*. Champaign, IL: Human Kinetics; 2007.
12. Frederic D. *Strength Training Anatomy*. Champaign, IL: Human Kinetics; 2006.
13. Graham JF. Exercise technique: power clean. *Strength Cond J*. 2000;22(6):63–65.
14. Graham JF. Exercise technique: power snatch. *Strength Cond J*. 2001;23(1):57–59.
15. Barnes M, Cinea KE. Lower body exercises. In: Brown LE, ed. *Strength Training*. Champaign, IL: Human Kinetics; 2007.
16. Graham JF. Exercise technique: deadlift. *Strength Cond J*. 2000; 22(5):18–20.
17. Graham JF. Exercise technique: back squat. *Strength Cond J*. 2001;23(5):28–29.
18. Graham JF. Exercise technique: barbell Lunge. *Strength Cond J*. 2002;24(5):30–32.
19. Graham JF. Exercise technique: front squat. *Strength Cond J*. 2002;24(3):75–76.
20. Graham JF. Exercise technique: leg press. *Strength Cond J*. 2004;26(3):53–54.
21. Graham JF. Exercise technique: leg curl. *Strength Cond J*. 2005;27(1):59–60.
22. Barnes M, Cinea KE. Upper body exercises. In: Brown LE, ed. *Strength Training*. Champaign, IL: Human Kinetics; 2007.

23. Graham JF. Exercise technique: dumbbell bench press. *Strength Cond J.* 2000;22(4):71–72.
24. Graham JF. Exercise technique: barbell bench press. *Strength Cond J.* 2003;25(3):50–51.
25. Graham JF. Exercise technique: barbell incline press. *Strength Cond J.* 2005;27(6):22–23.
26. Graham JF. Exercise technique: dumbbell incline press. *Strength Cond J.* 2007;29(6):35–36.
27. Graham JF. Exercise technique: dumbbell one-arm row. *Strength Cond J.* 2001;23(2):59–68.
28. Graham JF. Exercise Technique: front lat pulldown. *Strength Condition J.* 2003;25(5):42–43.
29. Graham JF. Exercise technique: barbell overhead press. *Strength Cond J.* 2008;30(3):70–71.
30. Graham JF. Exercise technique: dumbbell shoulder press. *Strength Cond J.* 2008;30(3):54–55.
31. Barnes M, Cinea KE. Torso exercises. In: Brown LE, ed. *Strength Training*. Champaign, IL: Human Kinetics; 2007.
32. Faigenbaum A, Westcott W. *Strength & Power for Young Athletes.* Champaign, IL: Human Kinetics; 2000.
33. Graham JF. Exercise technique: barbell upright row. *Strength Cond J.* 2004;26(5):60–61.
34. Graham JF. Resistance exercise techniques and spotting. In: Chandler TJ, Brown LE, eds. *Conditioning for Strength and Human Performance.* Philadelphia, PA: Lippincott Williams & Wilkins.
35. Harman EA, Rosenstein RM, Frykman PN, et al. Effects of a belt on intra-abdominal pressure during weightlifting. *Med Sci Sports Exer.* 1989;21(2):186–190.
36. Lander JE, Hundley JR, Simonton RL. The effectiveness of weight-belts during multiple repetitions of the squat exercise. *Med Sci Sports Exer.* 1990;24(5):603–609.
37. Lander JE, Simonton RL, Giacobbe JKF. The effectiveness of weight-belts during the squat exercise. *Med Sci Sports Exer.* 1990;22(1):117–126.
38. NSCA Certification Commission. *Exercise Technique Checklist Manual.* Lincoln, NE: NSCA Certification Commission; 2008.

CHAPTER 11

Facility Administration and Design

N. TRAVIS TRIPLETT

OBJECTIVES

After reading this chapter, you will be able to:

- Recognize the phases of design and planning of a strength and conditioning facility.
- Identify the primary duties involved in strength and conditioning facility maintenance and safety.
- Recognize the main programming and scheduling needs of the various athletic groups that utilize the strength and conditioning facility.
- Determine the primary concepts in assessing space requirements for the users and the equipment within the strength and conditioning facility.
- Identify the most common areas of possible litigation in a strength and conditioning facility.

KEY TERMS

Assumption of Risk
Dynamic Correspondence
Liability
Negligence
Product Liability
Risk Management
Standard of Care

Introduction

Strength and conditioning professionals are not only expected to design and implement sound training programs but also to manage the strength and conditioning facility. Some of the major administrative issues include the number of athletes and availability of competent coaches, equipment, space, and time (1). This chapter discusses these topics in the larger context of facilities and equipment, legal duties and concepts, liability exposure, and policies and procedures.

The strength and conditioning profession involves the combined competencies of sport/exercise science, administration, management, teaching, and coaching. Practitioners must also comply with various laws and regulations. Collectively, this creates remarkable challenges in terms of facility administration and design, in turn requiring considerable experience, expertise, and resources. Practitioners and their employers are jointly responsible for addressing these challenges and, in turn, fulfilling the standard of care involved in providing safe and effective programs and services to athletes.

A safe training environment requires that employees avoid any negligent supervision with a client and/or while setting up a facility, understand the standard care that is required, and recognize the risks that may occur.

FACILITIES AND EQUIPMENT

Most architects design facilities based on the principle that form follows function, meaning that the design of a structure should be determined by its purpose. Although this concept seems straightforward, the reality is that many facilities were originally designed for another purpose. Furthermore, they often contain obsolete equipment. Even in state-of-the-art facilities, periodic upgrades may be desirable because the equipment manufacturing industry is dynamic, regularly offering new features and innovations based on practitioners' input. Since facility design and program administration are interrelated, equipment content and arrangement should allow other practitioners with sound philosophies to implement their programs there without requiring significant changes. This concept also seems simple enough, but actually requires careful planning.

Administer your programs in such a way that you would be proud to let a qualified visitor observe your normal operations.

LAYOUT AND SCHEDULING

The first step in planning and designing a new facility is to form a committee. This overall process can be subdivided into predesign, design, construction, and preoperation phases (2).

The practitioner should assess existing equipment based on the program needs of all athletic teams using the facility (2). This step should involve several issues, including number of athletes using the facility, specific types of training required by each group, age groups, and training experience (i.e., developmental needs) of athletes using the facility, when training fits into each team's schedule, as well as any repairs or adaptations that must be made to meet special needs.

The design of the facility should be considered in arranging existing equipment (2). Issues to consider include location, access, supervision location, ceiling height, flooring, environmental factors, electrical, mirrors, and other considerations (e.g., drinking fountains, rest rooms, telephones, signs, bulletin boards, storage, and repair areas).

In arranging equipment, safety is a key concern, along with the purpose and function of each individual piece (2). Issues to address include placement, spacing, and traffic flow. Figure 11.1 shows an example of a properly designed strength/power area. Specific concerns for particular areas (e.g., stretching/warm-up, circuit training, free weight, Olympic lifting, metabolic) should be considered in calculating space needs. For example (3):

- For performing standing exercises from a rack, consider the bar length plus a double-wide

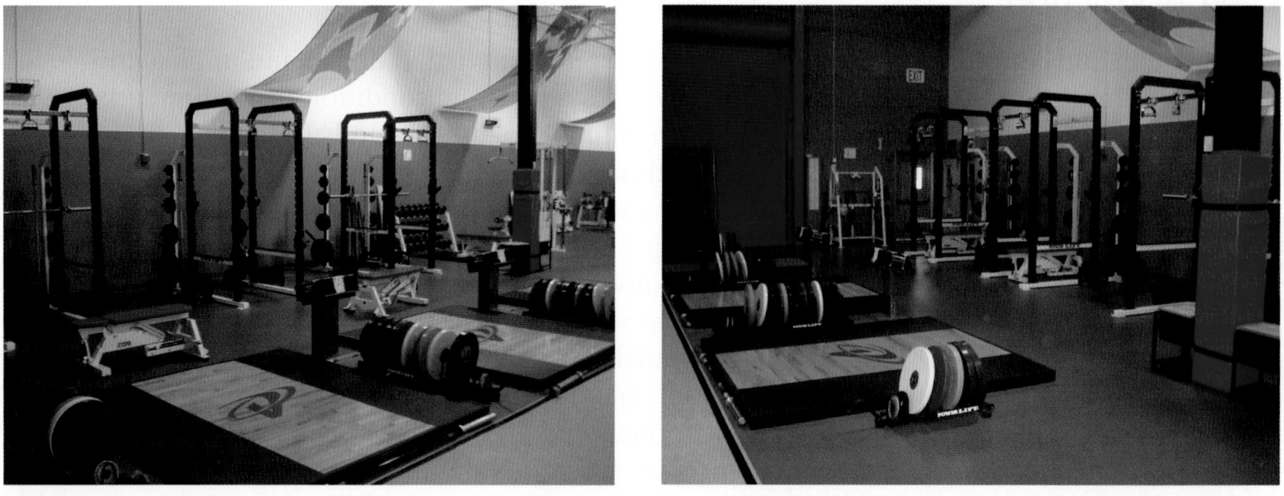

FIGURE 11.1 A strength/power area must be designed with regard to facility layout and arrangement as well as equipment safety and function.

(6-ft) safety space cushion, and multiply this by a suggested user space width of 8 to 10 ft [e.g., if using a 7-ft Olympic bar for the back squat exercise, (7 ft + 6 ft) × (10 ft) = 130 ft^2].
- For performing Olympic-style weightlifting exercises, consider the platform length plus a 4-ft perimeter walkway safety space and multiply this by the platform width plus another 4-ft perimeter walkway safety space [e.g., (8 ft + 4 ft) × (8 ft + 4 ft) = 144 ft^2].

When scheduling the facility, consider seasonal athletic priorities with regard to peak hours (specific recommendations are provided below under "Duties and Responsibilities: Liability Exposure"). Other issues to consider include staff-to-athlete ratios and equipment availability relative to group size.

Regardless of the training strategies used, a basic objective of facility design and layout is to optimize visibility and accessibility. In many cases, this must be achieved in spite of limited staff, high athlete volume, and time pressure. Depending on how various training methods and movements are prioritized, the challenge is to equip and arrange the facility for maximum capacity without compromising effectiveness, efficiency, or safety.

Although the specific content of each facility is a matter of discretion, some basic guidelines can be inferred from available evidence and practical experience. Practitioners should critically evaluate the pros and cons of various equipment choices rather than making decisions based on dogmatic beliefs about "free weights versus machines," "functional versus traditional training," and so on.

On one hand, training apparatus should be chosen according to transfer of training effect. This issue can be approached on several fronts, including mechanical specificity or **dynamic correspondence** (the basic mechanics of training movements being specific to the demands of competitive activity), metabolic effects (such as the influence of energy costs and endocrine responses on training adaptations), and coordination/skill acquisition. On the other hand, consideration should be given to practical issues, including the following:

- Versatility
- Coaching/teaching requirements (and corresponding staffing/spotting responsibilities)
- Safety
- Cost, space/time efficiency

In terms of strength/power training, the consensus emerging from the literature is that unguided-resistance equipment is superior in most regards, particularly when used with qualified instruction and supervision (4–7). There seem to be multiple reasons for this, which in turn provide useful criteria for selecting equipment. In general, the facility should be designed and equipped for a variety of training tasks consistent with the program's goals and objectives, enabling athletes to perform various multijoint, multiplane movements that challenge their coordinative abilities. Although certain stations are likely to get higher priority than others, most should be suitable for exercises, where range of motion is an acceleration path involving high-power levels and rates of force development as well as different regimes of muscular work (concentric, eccentric, isometric, and stretch-shortening cycle where appropriate). Additional criteria are discussed below under "Duties and Responsibilities: Liability Exposure," but those outlined above can be used as a starting point in most settings.

MAINTENANCE AND SAFETY

The practitioner's primary responsibility is to provide a safe training environment for all athletes, while performance enhancement and injury prevention typically get high priority as well (2). Specialized activities and responsibilities can be delegated among staff members who, in turn, should work cooperatively as a team.

Practitioners have a responsibility to maintain and clean the facility and equipment (2). Establishing frequent maintenance and cleaning schedules, and keeping the required supplies, tools, and other items on hand, helps ensure safety, protect investments, and maintain appearance, cleanliness, and functionality.

Environmental factors are also important for participants' health and safety. Some specific issues to consider include (2,8)

- Control of sound/video systems by the facility coordinator and qualified supervisors (e.g., volume low enough to allow clear communication between the spotter and lifter at all times)
- Air temperature kept constant at 72°F to 78°F (22°C to 26°C).
- Ventilation systems working properly (optimum 12 to 15 air exchanges · h^{-1}; minimum 8 to 10 air exchanges · h^{-1}); no detectable strong odors in the room

- Equipment and floor not slick due to humidity
- Facility well lit and free of dark areas; bulbs changed regularly
- Exit sign well lit
- Extension cords large enough for electrical load; properly routed, secured, and grounded
- Safety, regulation, and policy signs posted in clear view

In keeping with these areas of responsibility, it is imperative to understand litigation issues (3,9–15). In so doing, practitioners can effectively manage, but not totally eliminate, participants' risk of injury. It is also important to understand the concept of **product liability**, which is defined as a manufacturer's and/or vendor's legal responsibilities if someone sustains injury or damage due primarily to a defect or deficiency in design or production (9), as well as actions that can place one at risk for litigation. These issues are discussed in detail in the following sections. Box 11.1 provides basic guidelines for planning and designing a new facility.

An important consideration relative to facility planning is to evaluating the needs of the athletes and teams who will be using the facility.

LEGAL DUTIES AND CONCEPTS

Practitioners and their employers share legal duties to provide an appropriate level of supervision and instruction to do the following: meet a reasonable standard of care, provide and maintain a safe environment for athletes, inform users of the risks inherent in and related to their activities, and prevent unreasonable risk or harm resulting from negligent instruction or supervision (10–13). In fact, these legal duties and concepts define the organizational and administrative tasks of the profession.

BOX 11.1

Facilities and Equipment

Form a committee of professionals to do the following:

- Assess existing equipment based on the needs of all athletic teams using the facility.
- Consider the design of the facility and arrange existing equipment. Safety and function are top priorities in determining equipment arrangement.
- Consider seasonal athletic priorities, staff-to-athlete ratios, and equipment availability relative to group size.
- Establish frequent maintenance and cleaning schedules to ensure safety, protect investments, and maintain the facility's appearance, cleanliness, and functionality.

The practitioner's primary responsibility is to provide a safe training environment for all athletes.

A strength and conditioning professional should have an understanding of the following legal terms (2):

- **Assumption of risk**. Voluntary participation in activity with knowledge of the inherent risk(s). Practitioners must thoroughly inform participants of the risks involved in athletic and conditioning activities. Ideally, athletes should be required to sign a statement indicating their understanding and acceptance of the risk.
- **Liability**. A legal responsibility. Practitioners must take reasonable steps to ensure safe participation in conditioning activities, prevent injury, and act prudently when an injury occurs (9).
- **Negligence**. Failure to exercise the care a prudent person would under similar circumstances. For a practitioner to be guilty of negligence, there must be duty, breach of duty, proximate cause, and damages (15). He or she is negligent if proven to have a duty to act and to have failed to act with the appropriate standard of care, proximately causing injury or damages to another person.
- **Standard of care**. What a prudent and reasonable person would do under similar circumstances. A practitioner is expected to act according to his or her education, training, and certification status.

Practitioners and their employers share a legal duty to provide an appropriate level of supervision and instruction.

TYPES OF STANDARDS

In addition to standards for desired operational practices published by professional organizations such as the National Strength and Conditioning

Q & A from the Field

Q ***I just accepted the position of strength and conditioning coordinator at a small university. The varsity weight room is filled with obsolete and nonfunctional equipment, and the budget is too small to afford all the items we will need to reequip the facility this year. What should I do?***

A This is a common situation and can be a big challenge as well as an opportunity. Some suggestions are provided here.

Create a priority list of the equipment you plan to replace or upgrade. Be specific in terms of how many of each item you will need and how much they will cost, keeping in mind that many equipment vendors provide discount incentives for buying multiple pieces of equipment. Plan on upgrading in phases, being as objective as possible so your personal preferences do not influence your choices. Start with the "need to have" items, no matter how badly you want the "nice to have" ones. If it is ugly but functional, defer replacing it until later. For example, old/rusted barbells and plates may not be pretty but will be adequate temporarily. Spend the available money on high-priority equipment that cannot be donated or built on site.

Once you have compiled your upgrade plan, coordinate your efforts with your athletic director. Consider several issues here. Ask permission to approach local boosters or businesses for "gifts in kind." Most universities have a comprehensive incentive program for such donations, and many boosters are happy to exchange services and/or materials for tickets or other credits. The key is to be careful not to undermine your athletic director's fund-raising efforts since he or she may already be planning to approach some of the same people you have in mind. Many athletic directors set aside some reserve budget money until late in the fiscal year in case there should be any unforeseen expenses. Ask him or her to consider directing a portion of that to the weight-room upgrade, being sure to emphasize how it can benefit every team's performance as well as recruiting.

If you have a particular vendor in mind for the majority of your upgrade, inquire about that company's computerized design capabilities. They may be able to offer floor plans, elevations, or other drawings that will help everyone involved in the project to visualize the end result.

Assuming your athletic director gives his or her approval, approach the athletic department's fund-raising/development coordinator. Ask for referrals to specific boosters who can offer useful products or services, such as building-supply centers that might donate lumber for platforms, welders who might fabricate equipment, etc. Do your homework before contacting them. Boosters are usually gratified to know that you are giving them first consideration and have seen their advertisements in media guides, game-day programs, stadium signage, and so on.

One caveat: in recruiting the services of welders, carpenters, or other contractors, work with them to make sure that everything they build or modify meets industry specifications. If the equipment should fail at some point, the university will be liable for any resulting injuries or damages.

Association (NSCA), standards for technical/physical specifications have been published by independent organizations. In a negligence lawsuit, established standards of care can be used to gauge a practitioner's professional competence by comparing his or her actual conduct with written benchmarks of expected behavior. In addition to standards and guidelines established by allied organizations such as the American College of Sports Medicine (ACSM) (16,17), American Heart Association (AHA) (16,18), and National Athletic Trainer's Association (NATA), other associations have also delineated standards of practice (Aerobics and Fitness Association of America, American Physical Therapy Association, National Association for Sport and Physical Education). Moreover, relevant technical/physical specifications have been published by the U.S. Consumer Product Safety Commission and the American Society for Testing and Materials (19,20).

Policies of a facility may require employees to have specific experiences and/or certifications. Also, as an employee, understanding the safety procedures of the facility are of utmost importance.

APPLYING STANDARDS OF PRACTICE TO RISK MANAGEMENT

Risk management is a proactive administrative process that helps minimize legal liability and also minimizes the frequency and severity of injuries and subsequent claims and lawsuits (10,21). It may not be possible to eliminate risk of injury and liability exposure, but these can be effectively minimized with risk-management strategies. Although the coordinator is ultimately responsible for risk management, all practitioners should be involved in various aspects of the process. Eickhoff-Shemek (22) proposes a four-step procedure (adapted from Head and Horn [23]) for applying standards of practice to the risk management process:

1. *Identify and select standards of practice as well as all applicable laws.* Because so many standards of practice are published by various organizations, it is challenging for the practitioner to be aware of all of them and to determine which ones are appropriate in implementing the risk-management plan. In terms of participant safety, the most conservative or stringent standards in a given industry should generally be used.
2. *Develop risk-management strategies reflecting standards of practice and all applicable laws.* This step involves writing procedures describing specific responsibilities and/or duties that staff would carry out in particular situations. The procedures should be written clearly, succinctly, and without excessive detail. Once the written procedures are finalized, they should be included in the staff policies and procedures manual.
3. *Implement the risk-management plan.* Implementation of the risk-management plan primarily involves staff training to ensure that the practitioner's daily conduct will be consistent with written policies and procedures and selected laws and standards of practice. The policies and procedures manual should be used in conjunction with initial training of new employees as well as during regular in-service training where all employees practice a particular procedure. From a legal perspective, it is also important to explain to staff why it is essential to carry out such duties appropriately.
4. *Evaluate the risk-management plan.* Like the law, standards of practice are not static and need to be updated periodically to reflect change. The risk-management plan should be formally evaluated at least annually as well as after each incident of accident or injury to determine whether emergency procedures were performed correctly and what could be done to prevent a similar incident in the future.

Application of standards of practice to the risk-management process involves a four-step process: identify and select standards of practice as well as all applicable laws; develop risk-management strategies reflecting standards of practice and all applicable laws; implement the risk-management plan; and evaluate the risk-management plan.

REAL-WORLD APPLICATION

Policies and Procedures

Here is a sample policy for a strength and conditioning facility: *"Work with an attentive spotter and use appropriate safety equipment (e.g., power racks) for performing movements where free weights are supported on the trunk or moved over the head/face. Olympic lifts are an exception to the spotter rule and should be performed on an 8-ft by 8-ft platform that is clear of people and equipment."*

Remember that when you write a policy, you have to think about how it can be enforced. To carry out this policy and to make sure it is enforced, several steps should be taken: (a) The staff must be trained on what is expected of them both in terms of teaching spotting and dealing with athletes who fail to use a spotter. (b) The athletes must be trained in spotting, what lifts need a spotter, and the number of spotters needed. It is a necessity to train incoming athletes as they enter the program, and you may find that it is necessary to reinforce this training each year. (c) Decide in advance on the consequences for not following the policy. Be fair, but if you let some break the policy and not others, consider the legal implications if the athlete who has not followed the policy is injured.

DUTIES AND RESPONSIBILITIES: LIABILITY EXPOSURE

Although every program and facility is unique, it is instructive to examine the practitioner's duties and responsibilities in terms of common areas of liability exposure (14). These are interrelated. For example, proper instruction and supervision are associated with personnel qualifications as well as facility layout and scheduling. Noncompliance in one area can affect others, thereby compounding the risk of negligence and potential litigation. Practitioners and their employers share the corresponding duties and responsibilities.

The NSCA's *Strength and Conditioning Professional Standards and Guidelines* (14) identifies nine areas of liability exposure: preparticipation screening and clearance; personnel qualifications; program supervision and instruction; facility and equipment setup, inspection, maintenance, repair, and signage; emergency planning and response; records and record keeping; equal opportunity and access; participation by children; and supplements, ergogenic aids, and drugs. Within these areas of liability exposure, a total of 11 standards ("must dos") and 13 guidelines ("should dos") are proposed. These further define the tasks involved in facility organization and administration.

Preparticipation Screening and Clearance

A physical examination (preferably conducted by a licensed physician) is imperative for all athletes prior to participating in a program. This should include a comprehensive health and immunization history (as defined by current guidelines from the Centers for Disease Control and Prevention) as well as relevant physical exam, including an orthopedic evaluation. Cardiovascular screening, as discussed below, is also recommended. The practitioner does not need a copy of the results but must require a signed statement verifying proof of medical clearance to participate. Athletes who are returning from an injury or illness or have special needs must be required to show proof of medical clearance before beginning or returning to participation.

Currently, no universally accepted standards are available for screening athletes, nor are there approved certification procedures for healthcare professionals who perform such examinations. The joint Pre-Participation Physical Evaluation Task Force of five organizations has published a widely accepted monograph, including detailed instructions on performing a preparticipation history and physical exam and determining clearance for participation, and a medical evaluation form to copy and use for each examination (24). The AHA and ACSM have also published statements on preparticipation screening for those involved in fitness-related activities (16,18,25). Relevant issues can be summarized as follows:

Educational institutions have ethical, medical, and possible legal obligations to implement cost-efficient preparticipation screening strategies (including a complete medical history and physical examination), thereby ensuring that high school and college athletes are not subject to unacceptable risks. Support for such efforts, especially in large athletic populations, is mitigated by cost-efficiency considerations, practical limitations, and awareness that it is not possible to achieve zero risk in competitive sports.

A properly qualified healthcare provider (with requisite training, medical skills, and background to reliably perform a physical examination, obtain a detailed cardiovascular history, and recognize heart disease) should perform the preparticipation athletic screening. A licensed physician is preferable, but an appropriately trained registered nurse or physician assistant may be acceptable under certain circumstances in states where nonphysician healthcare workers are permitted to perform preparticipation screening. In the latter situation, a formal certification process should be established to demonstrate the examiner's expertise in performing cardiovascular examinations.

To ensure proper medical care is given, it is important to obtain consent to treat as well as a record of any previous medical history of the client prior to any physical activity within a facility.

The best available and most practical approach to screening populations of competitive sports participants is a complete and careful personal and family medical history and physical examination designed to identify (or raise suspicion of) cardiovascular risk factors known to cause sudden death or disease progression. Such screening is an obtainable objective and should be mandatory for all athletes. Initially, a complete medical history and physical examination should be performed before participation in organized high school athletics (grades 9 to 12). An interim history should be obtained in intervening years.

For collegiate athletes, a comprehensive personal/family history and physical examination should be performed by a qualified examiner initially upon entering the institution, before beginning training and competition. Screening should be repeated every 2 years thereafter unless more frequent examinations are indicated. An interim history and blood pressure measurement should be obtained each subsequent year to determine whether another physical examination and possible further testing is required (e.g., due to abnormalities or changes in medical status).

To initially classify participants by risk for triage and preliminary decision making, health appraisal questionnaires should be used before exercise testing and/or training. Participants can be further classified for exercise training on the basis of individual characteristics after the initial health appraisal (and medical consultation and/or supervised exercise test if indicated). Written and active communication between facility staff and the participant's personal physician or healthcare provider is strongly recommended when a medical evaluation/recommendation is advised or required. Participants should also be educated about the importance of the preparticipation health appraisal and medical evaluation/recommendation (if indicated) as well as potential risks incurred without them.

PERSONNEL QUALIFICATIONS

To properly supervise and instruct athletes utilizing facilities and equipment, qualified and knowledgeable personnel must be hired. A three-pronged approach is recommended:

1. *The practitioner should acquire expertise, and have a degree from a regionally accredited college/university in one or more of the topics comprising the "scientific foundations" domain identified in the Certified Strength and Conditioning Specialist (CSCS) Examination Content Description* (26) *or a relevant subject.* He or she should also make an ongoing effort to acquire knowledge and competence in the content areas outside his or her primary area of expertise.
2. *Professional organizations offer certifications with continuing education requirements as well as a code of ethics for practitioners interested in acquiring the necessary competencies.* Depending on one's specific duties, responsibilities, and interests, relevant certifications offered by other governing bodies may also be appropriate.
3. *The "performance team" model, which involves aligning a staff composed of qualified professionals with interdependent expertise and shared leadership roles, can enhance practitioners' knowledge and skill development* (27,28). The profession's scope of practice has expanded and diversified to the point where it is very challenging and often not possible for one individual to acquire proficiency in all areas. The team model can also improve a hierarchical (single-leader) work group's productivity as well as each individual's learning and skill acquisition (27).

It is difficult to overemphasize the importance of qualified staffing in fulfilling the institution's and practitioners' shared legal duties for safety, supervision, and standard of care. Lack of qualified instruction and supervision can be identified, either directly or indirectly, as a causative factor in the available information on injuries and litigations associated with weight training. In some cases this is clearly documented (29–31), while in others it can be inferred. For example, despite the technical and athletic nature of Olympic-style weightlifting, the relatively high coach-to-athlete ratio and corresponding standard of care are likely reasons for its low incidence of injury (32,33).

PROGRAM SUPERVISION AND INSTRUCTION

About 80% of all court cases concerning athletic injuries deal with some aspect of supervision (9). Although serious accidents are rare in supervised exercise programs, the liability costs associated with inadequate or lax supervision are high; plaintiffs' recovery rate in such negligence lawsuits is almost 56% (34). Poor facility maintenance, defective equipment, and inadequate instruction and/or supervision are the main causes of these incidents. The importance of staffing is readily apparent in each circumstance. For example, in a review of 32 litigations arising from negligent weight-training supervision, three issues were raised by the plaintiff's attorneys in each case (35): poor instruction or instructor qualifications; lax/poor supervision; and failure to warn of inherent dangers in the equipment, facility, or exercise. The issue of professional instructors' qualifications, as discussed in the previous section, is a prevalent trend in such litigations.

Athletes must be properly supervised and instructed at all times to ensure maximum safety. Bucher and Krotee (36) recommend the following principles:

- Always be there.
- Be active and hands-on.
- Be prudent, careful, and prepared.
- Be qualified.
- Be vigilant.
- Inform athletes of safety and emergency procedures.
- Know athletes' health status.
- Monitor and enforce rules and regulations.
- Monitor and scrutinize the environment.

In addition to the physical presence of qualified practitioners, effective instruction and supervision involves several practical considerations (13,34,37,38).

- A clear view of all areas of the facility, or at least the zone being supervised by each practitioner, and the athletes in it. This issue is related to facility design and layout; including equipment placement with respect to visibility, versatility, and accessibility.
- A practitioner's proximity to the group of athletes under his or her care, which involves the ability to see and communicate clearly with one another and quick access to athletes in need of immediate assistance or spotting.
- Number and grouping of athletes to make optimal use of available equipment, space, and time.
- Athletes' age(s), experience level(s), and need(s)
- The type of program being conducted (i.e., skillful/explosive free-weight movements versus guided-resistance exercises) and corresponding need for coaching and spotting.

In theory, practitioners should promote an optimal training environment by distributing activities throughout the day. Even with careful planning, however, most facilities have times of peak usage as a result of team practices and athletes' class schedules. Beyond a certain point, it is impractical to simply schedule activities over a wider range of times in order to maintain an acceptable professional-to-athlete ratio. The central issue is to provide adequate facilities and qualified staff such that all athletes are properly instructed and supervised during peak usage times (17,39,40). Likewise, practitioners should emphasize proper techniques, movement mechanics, and safety, and utilize instructional methods, procedures, and progressions consistent with accepted professional practices to minimize injury risk and liability exposure.

Even when reasonable steps are taken to make optimal use of facility and staff, a potential mismatch exists between available resources and demand for programs and services in many settings. The combined effects of explosive growth in collegiate/scholastic athlete participation (especially among women), corresponding liability exposures, and equal opportunity/access laws create a remarkable standard-of-care load and liability challenge for practitioners and their employers. A two-pronged approach can thus be recommended:

1. *During peak usage times, activities should be planned, and required number of qualified staff should be present such that recommended guidelines are achieved.* These guidelines include the minimum average floor space allowance per athlete (100 ft^2), professional-to-athlete ratios (1:10 junior high school, 1:15 high school, 1:20 college), and number of athletes (≤3) per barbell or training station (33,37,39,41). Ideally, this corresponds to one practitioner per three to four training stations and/or 1,000-ft^2 area (junior high school); five training stations and/or 1,500-ft^2 area (high school); or six to seven training stations and/or 2,000-ft^2 area (college), respectively. Professional discretion can be used to adjust these guidelines with respect to the practical considerations discussed above.
2. *Practitioners and their employers should work together toward a long-term goal of matching the professional-to-athlete ratio in the facility to each sport's respective coach-to-athlete ratio.* This is relatively straightforward in collegiate settings, where the NCAA limits the number of coaches per sport and compiles sports participation data. In the absence of similar information in other settings, such determinations can be made on an individual-institution basis (or possibly according to trends within a district, division, or state).

FACILITY AND EQUIPMENT SETUP, INSPECTION, MAINTENANCE, REPAIR, AND SIGNAGE

In some cases, practitioners are involved in all phases of facility design and layout. Perhaps more commonly, they assume responsibility for an existing facility, in which case the opportunities to plan or modify it may be limited. In either case, the practitioner and his or her employer are jointly responsible for maximizing the facility's safety, effectiveness, and efficiency such that allotted space and time can be put to optimal use.

Practitioners should establish written policies and procedures for equipment/facility selection, purchase, installation, setup, inspection, maintenance, and repair. These should be included in the overall policies-and-procedures manual (as discussed in the next section). Safety audits and periodic inspections of equipment, maintenance, and repair should be conducted and status reports issued. Manufacturer-provided user's manuals, warranties, operating guides, and other relevant records regarding equipment operation and maintenance (e.g., selection, purchase, installation, setup, inspection, maintenance, and repair) should be kept on file and followed (36).

As mentioned previously, practitioners must understand the concept of product liability. Although this issue applies to manufacturers and vendors, certain actions and/or behaviors can increase the practitioner's responsibility, consequently putting him or her at risk for claims or lawsuits. The following steps can minimize equipment-related liability exposure (9,36):

- Buy equipment exclusively from reputable manufacturers and be certain that it meets existing standards and guidelines for professional/commercial (not home) use.
- Use equipment only for the purpose intended by the manufacturer. Do not modify it from the condition in which it was originally sold unless such adaptations are clearly designated and instructions for doing so are included in the product information.
- Post any signage provided by the manufacturer on or in close proximity to the equipment.
- Do not allow unsupervised athletes to utilize equipment.
- Regularly inspect equipment for damage and wear that may place athletes at risk for injury.

EMERGENCY PLANNING AND RESPONSE

An emergency response plan is a written document delineating the proper procedures of caring for injuries that may occur to participants during activity. All facilities should have such a document, but the document itself does not save lives. In fact, it may offer a false sense of security if not supported with appropriate training and preparedness by astute, professional staff. Therefore, practitioners must:

- Know the emergency response plan and the proper procedures for dealing with an emergency (i.e., location of phones, activating emergency medical services, designated personnel to care for injuries, ambulance access, and location of emergency supplies) (42,43).
- Regularly review and practice emergency policies and procedures (i.e., at least quarterly).
- Maintain current certification in guidelines for cardiopulmonary resuscitation (CPR). First-aid training and certification may also be necessary if sports medicine personnel (e.g., certified athletic trainer [ATC], physician) are not immediately available.
- Adhere to universal precautions for preventing exposure to and transmission of blood-borne pathogens (44,45).

RECORDS AND RECORD KEEPING

Documentation is fundamental to program and facility management. A variety of records should be kept on file (36,46–48).

- Policies and procedures manual (as discussed in the next section)
- Manufacturer-provided user's manuals, warranties, and operating guides as well as equipment selection, purchase, installation, setup, inspection, maintenance, and repair records
- Personnel credentials
- Professional standards and guidelines
- Safety policies and procedures, including a written emergency response plan

Training logs, progress entries, and/or activity instruction/supervision notes.

- Injury/incident reports, preparticipation medical clearance, and return to participation clearance documents (after the occurrence of an injury, illness, change in health status or an extended period of absence) for each participant under the practitioner's care

- In collegiate and scholastic settings, athletes may already be required to sign protective legal documents covering all athletically related activities; whereas in other settings, the practitioner should consider having participants sign such legal documents.

Legal and medical records should be kept on file as long as possible in the event of an injury claim or lawsuit. It is good practice to maintain files indefinitely or consult with a legal authority, because statutes of limitations vary from state to state (48). As is the case with other organizational and administrative tasks, adequate staff are necessary to properly keep and maintain such records.

EQUAL OPPORTUNITY AND ACCESS

In most organizations, institutions, and professions, discrimination or unequal treatment (e.g., according to race, creed, national origin, gender, religion, age, handicap/disability, or other such legal classifications) are prohibited by federal, state, and possibly local laws and regulations. For example, practitioners employed in federally funded educational settings must comply with civil rights statutes, including Title IX of the Education Amendments of 1972, which mandates gender equity in providing opportunity and access to athletic facilities, programs, and services. Practitioners must obey the letter and spirit of these laws when working with athletes and staff.

PARTICIPATION IN STRENGTH AND CONDITIONING ACTIVITIES BY CHILDREN

Resistance training can be an important component of youth fitness, health promotion, and injury prevention. When properly designed and supervised, such programs are safe and can increase children's strength, motor fitness skills, sports performance, psychosocial well-being, and overall health (49,50). Many of the benefits associated with adult activities are attainable by prepubescent and adolescent athletes who participate in age-specific training, but it is important for the practitioner to take certain precautions.

Despite children's physical ability to train, they must be supervised at all times.

An alarming incidence of injuries to young children was observed in a 20-year retrospective review of weight-training injuries evaluated and/or treated in US hospital emergency departments (29). Children under 7 years of age are almost six times more likely to be injured than those above 15 years of age, with most of such injuries (80%) resulting from playing with or around weight-training equipment in the home. According to the U.S. Consumer Product Safety Commission ("Prevent Injuries to Children from Exercise Equipment"; CPSC document #5028), about 8,700 children below 5 years of age are injured each year with exercise equipment, with an additional 16,500 injuries per year to children 5 to 14 years of age. This has clear implications regarding exposing children in these age groups to such equipment or facilities and the importance of supervision.

SUPPLEMENTS, ERGOGENIC AIDS, AND DRUGS

The issue of nutritional supplement and drug use is complicated by several factors. According to the Dietary Supplement Health and Education Act of 1994, supplements are regulated as foods rather than drugs. This raises concerns about quality control/assurance and possible consequences for consumers.

Practitioners are often approached for advice on nutrition and supplementation and should be aware of the following: The Federal Trade Commission has primary responsibility for advertising claims. Simply stated, advertising for any product, including dietary supplements, must be truthful, substantiated, and not misleading. The U.S. Food and Drug Administration has primary responsibility for product labeling claims. The legislation enforced by this agency includes "Current Good Manufacturing Practices" and selected portions of the Federal Food, Drug and Cosmetic Act related to dietary supplements. Manufacturing practices for nutritional supplements established by the U.S. Pharmacopeia and National Formulary are cited as primary resources in this legislation.

The boundaries between dietary supplements, drugs, and conventional foods are not clear. This is especially challenging for competitive athletes and coaches, because such products may contain substances that are banned by one or more sport governing bodies, despite a manufacturer's or vendor's use of terms such as *herbal, legal, natural, organic, safe and effective,* etc. Furthermore, supplement manufacturers are constantly developing new products with different combinations of ingredients, making it more challenging to identify those that may be problematic.

Banned-substance policies and procedures, testing protocols, and related rules and regulations differ among sport governing bodies. A compound that is legal according to one governing body may, therefore, be illegal according to another.

Standards and guidelines can be identified across nine areas of liability exposure: preparticipation screening and clearance; personnel qualifications; program supervision and instruction; facility and equipment setup, inspection, maintenance, repair, and signage; emergency planning and response; records and record keeping; equal opportunity and access; participation by children; and supplements, ergogenic aids and drugs.

POLICIES AND PROCEDURES

Strength and conditioning professionals must develop policies and procedures that allow them to provide safe and effective programs and services and to fulfill their standard of care for athletes. This requires a working understanding of facility and equipment considerations, legal concepts, and duties and responsibilities dictated by liability exposures, as described in previous sections.

It is important that the program has a well-defined mission along with identifiable goals and objectives (47). Safety, performance enhancement, and injury prevention are fundamental goals. These should be complemented with specific objectives as part of a holistic mission statement.

Clearly define and distinguish job titles, descriptions, and duties for various positions (47). These should be developed for the director, associate(s) and/or assistant(s), facility supervisor(s), and other staff members including interns, administrative assistants, and others.

Understand pertinent staff policies and activities involved in achieving the mission, which in essence consists of the goals and the specific objectives of the program (47). Staff members should be accountable for maintaining a professional code of conduct and working cooperatively as a team. This involves a wide range of issues, including staff meetings, athlete orientation, annual planning, budgeting, staff facility use, relationships with athletes and other staff, professional goals, posted information, visitor tours, coaching and spotting procedures, testing, record keeping, athlete incentives, etc.

Understand the administrative decisions involved in the implementation of any strength and conditioning program to ensure safety and effectiveness (47). These issues are interdependent, as discussed throughout this chapter.

A written policies and procedures manual is essential to implementing a safe and effective

REAL-WORLD APPLICATION

Mission Statement

Here is an example of a mission statement for a strength and conditioning program: *"The strength and conditioning program will empower athletes and coaches to optimize their capabilities, and thereby achieve excellence through learning and applying fundamentally sound principles."*

Notice that it is broad, so it must be accompanied by goals and objectives to help professionals adhere to the mission statement. Mission statements will be different in different institutions and should be a product of the core beliefs of the administration and staff. From time to time, the mission statement should be reevaluated to make sure that it still reflects the core beliefs of the program.

BOX 11.2

Guidelines for Policies and Procedures

- Safety, performance enhancement, and injury prevention are fundamental goals in developing and clarifying the program's mission, goals, and objectives.
- Job titles, descriptions, and duties should be clearly defined and distinguished for respective positions.
- Practitioners should be accountable for maintaining a professional code of conduct and working cooperatively as a team.
- Understand the administrative decisions involved in safe and effective program implementation.
- Create a policies-and-procedures manual.

program (47). In addition to the issues itemized above, the manual should address facility access, daily operation, telephone/music system use, rules and regulations, and emergency procedures as well as equipment/facility selection, purchase, installation, setup, inspection, and maintenance, and repair. This type of documentation may seem mundane, but is fundamental to managing programs or facilities involved in serving people.

Policies and procedures should be clearly delineated to all staff and athletes using the facility. They need not be rigid or static. On the contrary, they should be compiled with insight and discretion and revised periodically as circumstances dictate. Box 11.2 provides basic guidelines for writing policies and procedures.

Sound policies and procedures should be developed to ensure the safety of the athlete and guide administrative decisions.

Summary

The issues of facility administration and design are fundamentally important in all aspects of strength and conditioning practice. Unfortunately, they often involve tasks in which the practitioner has little formal training.

Ample resources are available in some settings. In many others, however, they are not. Budgets, equipment, facilities, and staff are often limited or lacking altogether. This results in a mismatch between demand for and provision of safe and effective programs and services. Professionals and their employers share a legal duty to fulfill their standard of care for athletes. The individual practitioner is not solely responsible for fulfilling it (unless he or she is self-employed); the individual and his or her employer are jointly responsible for doing so.

The NSCA's *Strength and Conditioning Professional Standards and Guidelines* document (38) is one of the main resources cited in this chapter. Its implementation will present significant challenges and involve ambitious changes in many programs. Resistance can probably be expected from some athletic directors/employers because it will prompt them to allocate more resources to their programs. Nonetheless, the employing institution or business has a legal responsibility to help practitioners provide or obtain the resources needed to fulfill their standard of care.

Maxing Out

1. You are the strength and conditioning coordinator at a college program and a team coach approaches you with a program obtained from another university, asking you to implement it with her team in place of the one you have offered. Develop and explain your policy regarding such workouts, including how it will affect the team's programming and scheduling privileges in the varsity weight room.
2. You are the strength and conditioning coordinator at a college program, and your athletic director is expressing concern that the facility looks like a "football weight room" equipped with too many free weights. He feels that this is causing several problems such as compromising the programs and services provided to other teams, discouraging other teams' recruits from attending the school, and placing the university at risk of a Title IX lawsuit. You are subsequently directed to put together a proposal on how to reequip the weight room with more machines and fewer free weights to make it more accommodating for all sports. Develop and explain your policy regarding equipment selection with respect to performance enhancement and injury prevention.

CASE EXAMPLE

Program Scheduling, Supervision, and Instruction

BACKGROUND

You coordinate a collegiate strength and conditioning program that is responsible for programming and servicing a total of 362 student-athletes in 16 sports:

SPORT	SQUAD SIZE (MEN)	SQUAD SIZE (WOMEN)
Baseball	31	—
Basketball	16	14
Cross country	13	13
Football	96	—
Golf	10	8
Soccer	26	23
Softball	—	18
Tennis	10	10
Track and field	32	28
Volleyball	—	14
Total athletes	234	128

Including yourself, you have a three-person staff and 6,000-ft^2 weight room equipped with eight Olympic lifting platforms, eight self-contained power stations, four plyometric stations, and various secondary equipment. It is the first week of September; fall sport athletes have completed preseason camp and classes have begun. Your task is to schedule team workouts for the first 6 weeks of the fall semester such that in-season sports (cross country, football, soccer, volleyball) train 2 days per week, whereas off-season sports train 3 days per week. Your programs involve periodized multiset free-weight training, including explosive movements.

RECOMMENDATIONS AND CONSIDERATIONS

Begin by surveying team coaches regarding which days they prefer to train and whether their team is available in the morning (e.g., before 8 AM) or afternoon (usually after 3 PM). Make it clear to everyone in advance that in-season sports have scheduling priority in the weight room because their schedules are less flexible due to practices, meetings, and games. Fall sport teams often compete twice weekly (e.g., Wednesdays and Saturdays), further limiting the number of days they are available to train.

The advantage of morning training sessions is that they reduce the demand for weight room time during peak (afternoon) hours. The disadvantages are that they can conflict with athletes' sleep and/or meals and lengthen the staff's workday. The latter problem can be alleviated to an extent by allowing flex time for those staff working the early shift (e.g., leaving work after morning sessions are completed and returning in the afternoon).

Certain team coaches may allow some or all of their athletes to train during off-peak times individually or in small groups (e.g., between 8 AM and 3 PM). Likewise, in any given week, there may be athletes on various teams who have academic commitments during their team workouts and need to use this option. Once again, this reduces demand on the weight room during peak hours. Also, some coaches have no use for strength and conditioning programs and services at all, thus reducing the demand further.

Some coaches may also be willing to train varsity and junior varsity athletes on different schedules. This can be extremely useful with large teams in sports such as football. Finally, it is helpful to recruit qualified interns to assist with program implementation, especially during busy times.

IMPLEMENTATION

With a 6,000-ft^2 facility and three-person staff, there may be opportunities to schedule two or three teams concurrently during peak usage times. With smaller teams, it may be feasible to start two sessions simultaneously; in larger-group situations, it may be advisable to stagger their starting times every 20 to 30 minutes. Since

CASE EXAMPLE (*Continued*)

Program Scheduling, Supervision, and Instruction

most of these sports have common demands in terms of total-body power and rate of force development (RFD) and can benefit from the same exercises/equipment, it is helpful to designate specific training stations for each group to minimize congestion. In any case, workouts should be planned to comply with the following recommended guidelines:

- 100-ft^2 average floor space allowance per athlete = maximum capacity of 60 athletes
- 1:20 professional-to-athlete = up to three-group capacity, with each practitioner supervising one group and up to six or seven training stations (or 2,000-ft^2 area)
- ≤3 athletes per barbell or training station = equipment capacity of 60 athletes (if distributed between platforms, power stations, and plyometric stations)

RESULTS

Here is an example schedule (**boldface** indicates in-season teams).

DAY	MON	TUE	WED	THURS	FRI
Time					
7:00 AM	**M. Soccer (26)**		**M. Soccer (26)**	M. Basketball (16)	
	W. Soccer (23)		**W. Soccer (23)**	Softball (18) W. Tennis (10)	
8:00	**V. Football (10)**	**J.V. Football (10)**	**V. Football (10)**	**J.V. Football (10)**	**J.V. Football (10)**
9:00	**V. Football (10)**	**J.V. Football (10)**	**V. Football (10)**	**J.V. Football (10)**	**J.V. Football (10)**
10:00	**V. Football (10)**	**J.V. Football (10)**	**V. Football (10)**	**J.V. Football (10)**	**J.V. Football (10)**
	M. Golf (3)				
11:00	**V. Football (10)**	**J.V. Football (10)**	**V. Football (10)**	**J.V. Football (10)**	**J.V. Football (10)**
Noon	closed	closed	closed	closed	closed
1:00 PM	**V. Football (10)**	**J.V. Football (10)**	**V. Football (10)**	**J.V. Football (10)**	**J.V. Football (10)**
	M. Golf (5)				
2:00	2:45 W. Basketball (14)		2:45 W. Basketball (14)		W. Basketball (14)
					2:30 W. Golf (8)
3:00	3:30 Baseball (31)	W. Tennis (10)	3:30 Baseball (31)	M. Golf (10)	3:30 Baseball (31)
4:00	Softball (18)		Softball (18)		
5:00	Track and Field (60)	**M. X-Country (13)**	Track and Field (60)	**M. X-Country (13)**	Track and Field (60)
		W. X-Country (13)	**W. X-Country (13)**		
6:00	M. Basketball (16)	W. Golf (8) M. Tennis (10)	M. Basketball (16)	M. Tennis (10)	
			Volleyball (14)		

Keep in mind that each time the fall, winter, or spring sports' in-season phases begin or end, you need to do it all over again, which means that you have to design six different versions of the schedule every academic year.

ACKNOWLEDGMENT

The author wishes to thank Steven Plisk, the author of this chapter in the first edition of this book, and the source for the material presented within.

REFERENCES

1. Kraemer WJ, Dziados J. Medical aspects and administrative concerns in strength training. In: Kraemer WJ, Häkkinen K, eds. *Strength Training for Sport*. Oxford, UK: Blackwell Science; 2002:163–175.
2. Greenwood M, Greenwood L. Facility organization and risk management. In: Baechle TR, Earle RW, eds. National Strength and Conditioning Association. *Essentials of Strength Training and Conditioning*. 3rd ed. Champaign, IL: Human Kinetics; 2008:543–568.
3. Kroll B. Structural and functional considerations in designing the facility: part I. *NSCA J.* 1991;13(1):51–58.
4. Morrissey MC, Harman EA, Johnson MJ. Resistance training modes: specificity and effectiveness. *Med Sci Sports Exer.* 1995;27(5):648–660.
5. Nosse LJ, Hunter GR. Free weights: a review supporting their use in rehabilitation. *Athl Train.* 1985;20(4): 206–209.
6. Stone MH, Borden RA. Modes and methods of resistance training. *Strength Cond.* 1997;19(4):18–24.
7. Stone M, Plisk S, Collins D. Training principles: evaluation of modes and methods of resistance training-a coaching perspective. *Sports Biomech.* 2002;1(1):79–103.
8. Armitage-Johnson S. Providing a safe training environment: part II. *Strength Cond.* 1994;16(2):34.
9. Baley JA, Matthews DL. *Law and Liability in Athletics, Physical Education and Recreation*. Boston, MA: Allyn & Bacon; 1984.
10. Eickhoff-Shemek J. Standards of practice. In: Cotten D, Wilde J, Wlohan J, eds. *Law for Recreation and Sport Managers*. 2nd ed. Dubuque, IA: Kendall/Hunt Publishing; 2001:293–302.
11. Halling DH. Liability considerations of the strength and conditioning specialist. *NSCA J.* 1990;12(5):57–60.
12. Halling DH. Legal terminology for the strength and conditioning specialist. *NSCA J.* 1991;13(4):59–61.
13. Herbert DL. Supervision for strength and conditioning activities. *Strength Cond.* 1994;16(2):32–33.
14. National Strength and Conditioning Association. *Strength and Conditioning Professional Standards and Guidelines*. Colorado Springs CO: National Strength and Conditioning Association; 2009.
15. Rabinoff MA. Weight room litigation: what's it all about? *Strength Cond.* 1994;16(2):10–12.
16. Balady GJ, Chaitman B, Driscoll D, et al. American Heart Association and American College of Sports Medicine. Recommendations for cardiovascular screening, staffing and emergency policies at health/fitness facilities. *Circulation.* 1998;97(22):2283–2293; *Med Sci Sports Exer.* 1998;30(6):1009–1018.
17. Tharrett SJ, Peterson JA, eds., for the American College of Sports Medicine. *ACSM's Health/Fitness Facility Standards and Guidelines*. 2nd ed. Champaign, IL: Human Kinetics; 1997.
18. Maron BJ, Thompson PD, Puffer JC, et al. American Heart Association. Cardiovascular pre-participation screening of competitive athletes. *Circulation.* 1996;94(4):850–856; *Med Sci Sports Exer.* 1996;28(12):1445–1452.
19. American Society for Testing and Materials. ASTM Standard Consumer Safety Specification for Stationary Exercise Bicycles: Designation F1250-89. West Conshohocken, PA: ASTM; 1989.
20. American Society for Testing and Materials. ASTM Standard Specification for Fitness Equipment and Fitness Facility Safety Signage and Labels: Designation F1749-96. West Conshohocken, PA: ASTM; 1996.
21. Eickhoff-Shemek J. Distinguishing protective legal documents. *ACSM Health Fitness J.* 2001;5(3):27–29.
22. Eickhoff-Shemek J, Deja K. Four steps to minimize legal liability in exercise programs. *ACSM Health Fitness J.* 2000;4(4):3–18.
23. Head GL, Horn S. *Essentials of Risk Management*. 3rd ed, Vol. I. Malvern, PA: Insurance Institute of America; 1995.
24. Pre-participation Physical Evaluation Task Force. American Academy of Family Physicians, American Academy of Pediatrics, American Medical Society for Sports Medicine, American Orthopaedic Society for Sports Medicine and American Osteopathic Academy of Sports Medicine. *Pre-participation Physical Evaluation*. 2nd ed. New York: McGraw-Hill; 1996.
25. Maron BJ, Thompson PD, Puffer JC, et al. American Heart Association. Cardiovascular pre-participation screening of competitive athletes: addendum. *Circulation.* 1998;97 (22):2294.
26. NSCA Certification Commission. *Certified Strength and Conditioning Specialist (CSCS) Examination Content Description*. Lincoln, NE: NSCA Certification Commission; 2000.
27. Katzenbach JR, Smith DK. *The Wisdom of Teams*. Boston, MA: Harvard Business School; 1993.
28. Katzenbach JR, Beckett F, Dichter S, et al. *Real Change Leaders*. New York: Times Books/Random House; 1995: 217–224.
29. Jones CS, Christensen C, Young M. Weight training injury trends: a 20-year survey. *Phys Sportsmed.* 2000; 28(7): 61–72.
30. Reeves RK, Laskowski ER, Smith J. Weight training injuries: part 1. Diagnosing and managing acute conditions. *Phys Sportsmed.* 1998;26(2):67–96.
31. Reeves RK, Laskowski ER, Smith J. Weight training injuries: part 2. Diagnosing and managing chronic conditions. *Phys Sportsmed.* 1998;26(3):54–63.
32. Hamill BP. Relative safety of weightlifting and weight training. *J Strength Cond Res.* 1994;8(1):53–57.
33. Stone MH, Fry AC, Ritchie M, et al. Injury potential and safety aspects of weightlifting movements. *Strength Condition.* 1994;16(3):15–21.
34. Morris GA. Supervision-an asset to the weight room? *Strength Cond.* 1994;16(2):14–18.
35. Rabinoff MA. 32 reasons for the strength, conditioning, and exercise professional to understand the litigation process. *Strength Cond.* 1994;16(2):20–25.
36. Bucher CA, Krotee ML. *Management of Physical Education and Sport*. 11th ed. New York: McGraw-Hill; 1998.

37. Armitage-Johnson S. Providing a safe training environment: part I. *Strength Cond.* 1994;16(1):64–65.
38. Herbert DL, Herbert WG. *Legal Aspects of Preventive, Rehabilitative and Recreational Exercise Programs.* 3rd ed. Canton, OH: PRC Publishing; 1993.
39. Hillmann A, Pearson DR. Supervision: the key to strength training success. *Strength Cond.* 1995;17(5):67–71.
40. Kroll B. Liability considerations for strength training facilities. *Strength Cond.* 1995;17(6):16–17.
41. Jones L. *USWF Coaching Accreditation Course: Club Coach Manual.* Colorado Springs, CO: U.S. Weightlifting Federation; 1991.
42. Anderson JC, Courson RW, Kleiner DM, et al. National Athletic Trainers' Association Position Statement: Emergency Planning in Athletics. *J Athl Train.* 2002;37(1):99–104.
43. Schluep C, Klossner DA, eds. National Collegiate Athletic Association. *2003–04 NCAA Sports Medicine Handbook.* 16th ed. Indianapolis, IN: NCAA; 2003.
44. Centers for Disease Control and Prevention/U.S. Department of Health and Human Services. Perspectives in disease prevention and health promotion update: universal precautions for prevention of transmission of human immunodeficiency virus, hepatitis B virus, and other bloodborne pathogens in health-care settings. *MMWR. Morb Mortal Wkly Rep.* 1988;37(24):377–388.
45. Occupational Safety and Health Administration. U.S. Department of Labor. *OSHA Regulations (Standards-29 CFR) 1910.1030: Blood-Borne Pathogens.* Washington DC: OSHA; 1996.
46. Cotten DJ, Cotten MB. *Legal Aspects of Waivers in Sport, Recreation and Fitness Activities.* Canton, OH: PRC Publishing; 1997.
47. Epley B, Taylor, J. Developing a policies and procedures manual. In: Baechle TR, Earle RW, eds. National Strength and Conditioning Association. *Essentials of Strength Training and Conditioning.* 3rd ed. Champaign, IL: Human Kinetics; 2008:569–588.
48. Herbert DL. A good reason for keeping records. *Strength Cond.* 1994;16(3):64.
49. Faigenbaum AD, Kraemer WJ, Cahill B, et al. National Strength and Conditioning Association. Youth resistance training: position statement paper and literature review. *Strength Cond.* 1996;18(6):62–75.
50. Faigenbaum AD, Micheli LJ. *Current Comment from the American College of Sports Medicine: Youth Strength Training.* Indianapolis, IN: American College of Sports Medicine; 1998.

PART

onetwothreefour

Exercise Prescription

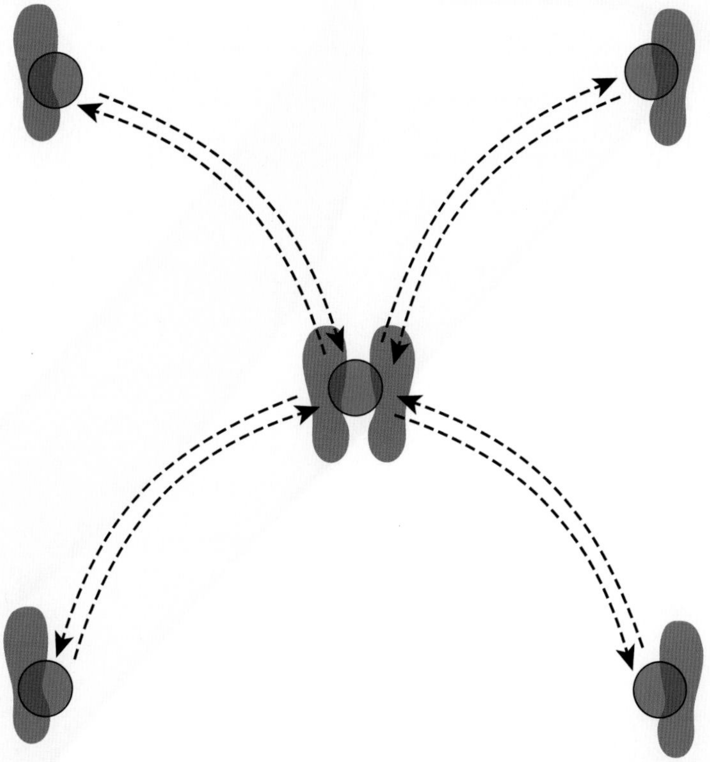

CHAPTER 12

Evidence-Based Practice in Strength and Conditioning

WILLIAM E. AMONETTE • KIRK L. ENGLISH • BARRY A. SPIERING • WILLIAM J. KRAEMER

OBJECTIVES

After reading this chapter, you will be able to:

- Determine, for yourself, what evidence is credible.
- Appreciate the dynamic nature of knowledge and the continual process.
- Work together with scientists and coaches to bridge the gap between science and application.
- Execute the six-step process of implementing evidence-based practice.
- Implement evidence-based strength and conditioning practices with colleagues and coaching staffs.

KEY TERMS

Academic Training
Background Question
Beneficiary of Knowledge
Bias
Consumer of Knowledge
Critical Appraisal of a Topic (CAT)
Data
Directed (Foreground) Question
Disseminate
Evidence-Based Practice (EBP)
Experimental Research
Google Scholar
Independent Variable
Journal Club
Levels of Evidence
Meta-Analysis
Non–Peer-Reviewed Literature
Observational Research
Peer-reviewed Literature
Practical Experience
Practitioner
Producer of Knowledge
PubMed
Randomized Controlled Trial (RCT)
Scientific Research
Systematic Review

Introduction

In the second *Rocky* movie, the main character, Rocky Balboa, is training to fight Apollo Creed for the heavyweight championship. Apollo is a quicker, more experienced fighter and thus Rocky's trainer, Mickey, implements a strategy to improve Rocky's speed. Mickey takes his boxer to a fenced area of Philadelphia, throws a chicken on the ground, and commands Rocky to chase the chicken. The reluctant fighter asks why he should do something as ridiculous as chase chickens when he is preparing to fight for the heavyweight championship. Mickey replies, "First, because I said so. And second, is because chicken chasing is how we used to train back in the old days. If you can catch this thing, you can catch greased lighting."

Unfortunately, this scenario is somewhat reflective of the answers given by some strength and conditioning coaches, sport coaches, and personal trainers when queried regarding the underlying rationale for their training programs: "it's how we've always done it." More than ever, information to evaluate training recommendations is readily available—often in vast quantity, although some areas of study lag behind due to the time and expense that they necessitate (e.g., training studies). Much of this information is credible and useful; however, there is also an abundance of "misinformation." The contemporary strength and conditioning coach must develop a systematic, objective process to evaluate information and decipher "truth" from "fad." **Evidence-based practice (EBP)** is an emerging concept in strength and conditioning that provides a systematic method of integrating research knowledge with the practical experience of the coach. Ultimately, using such a strategy can enhance the efficacy and safety of strength and conditioning programs.

THE ORIGIN OF EVIDENCE-BASED PRACTICE

EBP is a term that was born out of the "evidence-based medicine" (EBM) movement in the early 1990s, although the ancient origin of using scientific observation to substantiate practice can be traced to biblical times (The Book of Daniel) (1). Modern or contemporary EBM began in the early to mid-1990s, when David Eddy first used the term "evidence based" in a 1990 paper published in the *Journal of the American Medical Association* (2). However, David Sackett (formerly of McMaster University in Canada) created a distinct focus for EBM—the use of current evidence to make clinical decisions for an individual and is widely recognized as the founder of EBM. Sackett defined EBM as follows: "Evidence-based medicine is the conscientious, explicit, and judicious use of current best evidence in making decisions about the care of individual patients. The practice of evidence-based medicine means integrating individual clinical expertise with the best available external clinical evidence from systematic research" (3).

RELEVANCE OF EBP IN STRENGTH AND CONDITIONING

EBP is a systematic process that integrates scientific knowledge with the strength and conditioning coach's expertise to develop effective training

BOX 12.1

David Sackett's Definition of Evidence-Based Medicine

"Evidence based medicine is the conscientious, explicit, and judicious use of current best evidence in making decisions about the care of individual patients. The practice of evidence based medicine means integrating individual clinical expertise with the best available external clinical evidence from systematic research."

programs for individual athletes. Although strength and conditioning coaches do not prescribe medicine, they do prescribe exercise. Exercise, like medicine, results in expected and predictable physiologic responses, although the underlying mechanisms that mediate many of them are still under intense investigation. For example, it is well established that an increase in physical work rate prompts an increase in heart rate, oxygen consumption, and systolic blood pressure in an intensity-dependent manner. Likewise, if an athlete completes 10 sets of 10 repetitions with 75% of 1-repetition maximum, one can expect a release of certain anabolic and catabolic hormones that might affect recovery. These well-understood physiological responses can be used to prescribe exercise, but what happens when we apply unique stimuli (e.g., new exercise equipment or nutritional supplements) that are not well studied?

Our knowledge of human physiology and its relationship to strength and conditioning is incomplete and constantly evolving.

AN EXAMPLE FROM STRENGTH AND CONDITIONING

Scientific literature has documented the physiological responses to common modalities of exercise like running, cycling, and weightlifting. However, in an attempt to improve practice or gain performance advantage, new exercise devices are constantly developed that provide physiological and mechanical stimuli that differ from routine aerobic or resistance exercises. For example, in the mid to late 1990s, a novel training modality, whole body vibration (WBV), was introduced to the exercise community. Over the last decade, WBV has become a popular and trendy training tool despite the lack of substantial **levels of evidence** for some of its reported uses (e.g., hormonal stimulation, weight loss, reduction of cellulite). Although studies supporting the use of vibration to improve some aspects of health were published in the 1930s and 1940s (4,5), in the late 1990s most of what was known about vibration was its deleterious effects on the human skeleton (i.e., vibration was/is a known occupational hazard). However, a series of papers published in the late 1990s by Bosco et al. (6–8) demonstrated positive physiological responses to WBV applied vertically to the feet. They showed that standing in an isometric squat position on a vibrating plate for five sets of 2 minutes with a 30 Hz vibration with accelerations equal to approximately 4 g increased lower extremity power by 12% in 10 days compared to control subjects (6). In 2000, they demonstrated an acute increase in testosterone and growth hormone and a decrease in cortisol following a session of WBV applied during isometric squats (9). Later, in 2001, Rubin et al. (10) published a paper in *Nature* showing WBV applied to the feet of adult sheep increased trabecular bone mineral density by 34.2%. Although the plate used by Rubin vibrated vertically, it was quite different than the device used by Bosco. Rubin used a very low-magnitude (0.2 to 0.3 g) vibration stimulus applied for 20 continuous minutes, 5 d · wk^{-1}. Sometime in the early 2000s, a third type of vibration stimulus was introduced. The new vibration devices employed a "side alternating" vibration stimulus by a plate that worked like a teeter-totter. The metal plate employed in these studies rotated about a fulcrum, providing a rapidly alternating unilateral stimulus; some of the original studies with these plates showed a slightly increased metabolic stimulus during exercise (11–13).

In the early 2000s, vibration was a novel tool that certainly showed promise as a training stimulus. Soon after the publication of these studies, vibration plates were manufactured and sold commercially. They were marketed to athletes and the general public as a universal training tool to improve power, bone density, increase growth hormone concentrations, reduce fat, and increase flexibility. There was certainly a measure of truth underlying most of the claims, but the acute physiological and chronic responses were/are still poorly understood. The marketed plates ranged in frequency (10 to 65 Hz), intensity (0.2 to 4.0 g), and direction (predominantly vertical [bilateral] and rotary [side alternating]). Unlike common aerobic or resistance exercise modalities for which there are understood and predictable responses to exercise frequency, intensity, volume, etc, very little was/is known about the responses to frequency, intensity, or duration of WBV training. Yet, WBV plates are now widely available in fitness centers and many NCAA, NFL, NBA, and MLB weight rooms.

In reality, the popular use of WBV likely exceeds the level of credible evidence to support its use. Ten years later, the current evidence supports increased neuromuscular activity during vibration (14,15) and neuromuscular potentiation resulting from vibration exposure (16). It also supports training with WBV for improving strength (17) and power (18). Increases in bone mineral density may arise from WBV training (19); WBV may also attenuate bone loss in bed rest (20). There is not, however, evidence that supports sitting on the plate to perform exercise to increase activation of the "core musculature," heavy resistance training on the plate, or the use of WBV as a significant contributor to weight loss (21). Yet, some plates are marketed and routinely used for such purposes. This is not to say that one day there might not be convincing evidence to support these practices, but compelling evidence for such use currently does not exist.

The question arises: how could a tool with supporting evidence for only a limited set of applications gain such popularity and widespread use in such a short period of time? The answer is multifactorial, but a root cause is the process by which information is disseminated and interpreted. In the early 2000s, there were probably very few exercise science programs or textbooks that discussed WBV. Therefore, the three sources from which information could be derived were peer-reviewed publications, a small group of experts who studied WBV, and vibration plate manufacturers. Some plate manufacturers cited legitimate scientific findings in their marketing materials, but at times, the findings were cited without context to better support the product; needless to say, few potential users examined the actual science behind the claims.

Motivated by a sincere desire to determine the effectiveness of their products, legitimate and substantial research is frequently funded by industry or corporations. Industry grants are often awarded to independent researchers at universities for unbiased evaluation of their products; subsequently, the findings of these studies may be published in reputable peer-reviewed journals. However, marketing brochures, product labels, and other forms of advertisement that cite findings from research are incapable of disseminating study design, control, population, and the multitude of variables needed to determine the applicability or generalizability of the research. In such cases, it is essential that the consumer is properly trained to find, read, and interpret the actual published research data to assess the potential usefulness of products to their practice.

Legitimate scientific findings may be displayed in product marketing material, but it is essential for the consumer to read and interpret the science in context to establish the applicability of a product to their practice.

THE STATE OF THE INDUSTRY

WBV is just a single example, but it serves as a microcosm of the support industry within the strength and conditioning field. A plethora of devices and gadgets supported by little supporting evidence are sold as the newest tool, essential to improving human performance. The devices are manufactured and developed so fast that even the most up-to-date academic textbooks and lectures cannot keep pace with the industry.

Exercise devices are just a part of the evolving industry that supports the strength and conditioning field. The nutritional supplement industry is now a multimillion dollar enterprise constantly developing new products that may or may not be effective, safe, or legal for sports use. While most supplement companies investigate the usefulness and safety of their products, the industry is poorly regulated. Consequently, some product labels or marketing materials contain claims based on poor science or anecdote alone. Due to the lack of industry regulation, the only safeguard against misinformation is for the consumer to find and interpret the science supporting the products.

In addition to the evaluation of exercise devices and nutritional supplements, there is a need to appraise new and emerging programming strategies. Strength and conditioning coaches may train individuals with underlying health conditions or who are rehabilitating an injury. In each case, there is a need to search for and find information to evaluate the efficacy or safety of various training strategies.

EBP may be particularly important for strength and conditioning coaches evaluating (a) novel training devices, (b) programming theories, (c) nutritional supplements, and (d) exercise for populations with special needs.

KNOWLEDGE IS A DYNAMIC PHENOMENON

The entry-level requirement for most strength and conditioning positions is a bachelor's degree in human performance, exercise physiology, biomechanics, or a similar field. Additionally, many collegiate and professional strength and conditioning jobs now require a master's degree in addition to professional experience. Undoubtedly, an individual who has completed a degree at an accredited university has a basic level of knowledge. Furthermore, if he or she has obtained certification from the National Strength and Conditioning Association (NSCA) or the American College of Sports Medicine (ACSM), he or she has demonstrated competence in basic and advanced training strategies as currently understood. However, it is important to realize that the optimal training strategy in 2011 may not be so in 2021. Knowledge is a dynamic phenomenon; science and practice constantly furnish additional information that steers training strategies. Therefore, implementing strategies because "it's the way we've always done it," or it is "how we were taught in school" may not be the best approach to training. The dynamic nature of knowledge suggests that it is essential that all practicing strength and conditioning professionals must be students for life as the efficacy of old and new practices, exercise devices, and supplements may be validated over time (e.g., creatine).

For example, in the 1990s, there were few models of periodization that received scientific attention. The most researched and scientifically supported model was Matveyev's strength/power model (22–24). In this model, exercise volume was high at the beginning of the training phase and intensity was low. As the sport athlete approached the competition season, intensity gradually increased and volume decreased. Now, however, preliminary research suggests that reversing Matveyev's model (i.e., peaking with lower intensity and higher volume) may provide similar strength results for endurance athletes (25). Newer research also supports the use of undulating models of periodization in which more than one muscular quality (i.e., hypertrophy, strength, and power) is trained during a given phase (26,27). Although future research is needed to replicate these findings, validation of such models may provide unique and effective ways to help athletes achieve peak performance. In the 1990s though, these models were simply not supported by science, and **practitioners** who completed degrees in the 1990s who are not committed to reading research may be unaware of such advancements.

Three Domains of Knowledge

We generally obtain quality information and sound knowledge from three different domains: **academic training**, **practical experience**, and **scientific research**. As discussed earlier, academic training provides a sound knowledge base, but lecture materials are developed from knowledge at a single point in time. Practical experience and lessons learned in the weight room also provide a valuable source of knowledge. Interestingly, practice may at times be in advance of academic or research knowledge. Although most practitioners primarily use theory that has been generated through research, practitioners naturally experiment. For example, a strength coach may notice a positive trend in the performance of athletes using a certain combination of resistance and plyometric exercises. Such a trend suggests that this particular combination is superior to the current standard routine. Logically, the coach will continue to use the new combination despite no direct scientific evidence to support it.

> *The practice of strength and conditioning may generate information contributing to the field of knowledge in advance of scientific research.*

Finally, knowledge may be obtained by reviewing written sources of evidence. Written sources of evidence can be broadly divided into two categories: **peer-reviewed** and **non–peer-reviewed**. Peer-reviewed is simply a term to indicate that the information published in a particular journal has been critically examined by knowledgeable scientists in the field. Generally, this process insures that poor, unsubstantiated work does not end up in a discipline's body of literature. On the other hand, non–peer-reviewed literature includes the popular press, industry periodicals, and other media that transmit expert (and nonexpert) opinion; opinions are always biased.

> *Non–peer-reviewed material should be interpreted with caution because there may not be credible evidence behind the author's statements and any claims that are not rigorously evaluated.*

Such a division between peer-reviewed and non–peer-reviewed is a safeguard against the proliferation of unsubstantiated claims. It is of utmost importance that science, of which the field of strength and conditioning is a part, be founded on objective, reproducible data—and not merely on the thoughts and opinions of "experts." As a side note, individuals deserving of the title of "expert" are those that have produced large amounts of data in a particular focus area—whether those data are formal research studies or substantial practical contributions, for example, the successful training of numerous top-level athletes. It is essential to understand that the title of "expert" should not be conferred on an individual based on his or her ubiquitous presence, strong opinions, and/or commercial interests in a particular area; instead, "experts" should be acclaimed as such due to their substantial contributions to exercise science both in scientific research and practical experience. Ultimately, experts are always subservient to scientific evidence.

There are three key groups in the generation and transfer of information: **producers of knowledge** (researchers and academics), **consumers of knowledge** (practitioners), and **beneficiaries of knowledge** (athletes) (28,29). Researchers who are actively involved in studying physical and physiological phenomena generate **data** leading to a better understanding of training. Through natural experiment and trial and error, coaches may also contribute to knowledge. The data generated by researchers and academics may be used by the strength and conditioning coach to construct better training plans that eventually benefit the athlete (Fig. 12.1). The nature of the strength and conditioning industry now demands that every coach must, at a minimum, be a "consumer of research."

THE PROCESS OF EVIDENCE-BASED PRACTICE

EBP is a systematic process and an objective means of gathering, evaluating, and integrating evidence into practice. It is initiated via questions concerning the training or nutritional plan of an athlete. After conducting an initial testing session and needs analysis, it may be necessary to initiate the EBP process to formulate the most effective plan. Questions may also come from industry trends or new and innovative training strategies. Implementing EBP requires a six-step process: (step 1) develop a question, (step 2) search for evidence, (step 3) evaluate the evidence, (step 4) incorporate the evidence into practice, (step 5) consistently reevaluating the evidence, and (step 6) disseminate information.

STEP 1: DEVELOP A QUESTION

The first step in the EBP process is the development of an answerable question (30). Questions may be broadly divided into two categories: **background questions** and **direct questions**. Both types of questions may be used at different times depending on the nature of the knowledge sought.

Background Questions

Background questions are more general and deal with underlying physiological or physical

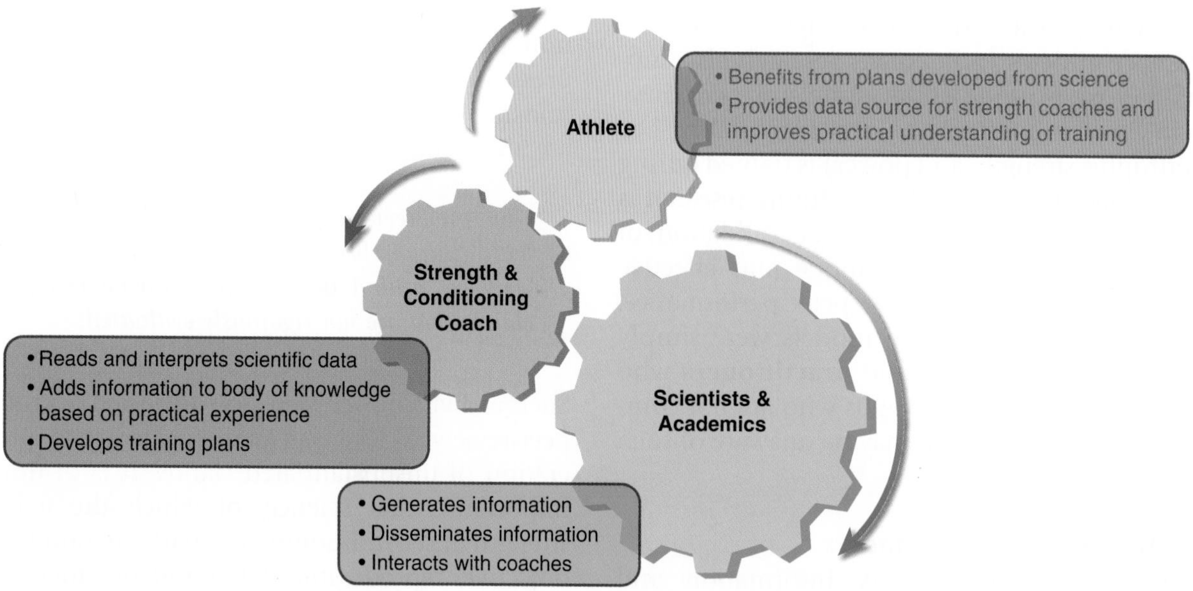

FIGURE 12.1 Pictorial description of the generation, dissemination, interpretation, and implementation of knowledge. Scientists, strength and conditioning coaches, and the athlete all play a role in the process.

mechanisms associated with training. To borrow from the fictitious example provided in the chapter introduction, if a strength coach is interested in implementing chicken chasing as a strategy to improve the foot speed of his or her athletes, he or she may ask questions like, "what is the dominant energy system employed in chicken chasing?" Or, "what muscle groups are used in chicken chasing?" Such questions may not supply evidence as to the effectiveness of chicken chasing, but would provide the coach with a better understanding of the physical and physiological demands of the activity.

Directed Questions

Directed questions (often called "foreground questions" in EBM literature) are more focused and lead to a better understanding of the effectiveness of an intervention. It has been suggested that good directed questions should include the following components: population, intervention, comparison, outcome, and time (PICOT) (31).

- **Population:** The development of appropriate directed questions first requires the determination of the sample population. In the original fictitious example, Mickey was training an adult male boxer. It is important to define the population because different populations may respond differently to the same stimulus (e.g., age or gender differences).
- **Intervention:** The experimental intervention must be determined, which in this case is chicken chasing.
- **Comparison:** To develop an effective question, we must also consider a comparison group. For example, chicken chasing may be more effective than a sedentary lifestyle for improving foot speed, but may not be as effective as jump rope or ladder drills. Generally, the comparison group should be one employing standard training methods.
- **Outcome:** Defining an appropriate outcome measurement is also essential to the development of a sound question. Generally, the gold standard measurement (e.g., vertical jump, one-repetition maximum squat strength) for a given sport or physical ability should be used as the outcome. For example, a strength coach could measure the number of foot contacts completed in a 60-s box run drill with a 24-in box as a test of determining foot speed. As such, the evidence-based (EB) practitioner should search for studies using the 60-s box run drill as the primary outcome measure.
- **Time:** In order to ask an appropriate question, the evidence-based practitioner should choose an appropriate time frame for comparison. Varying amounts of time are needed to produce measurable changes in different physiologic variables. If one asks, "is multiple-set strength training more effective than single-set training in improving 1-repetition maximum strength over a 3-week period?" the answer may be different than if the time period was defined as 16 weeks. Simply put, the effectiveness of a given program or device is dependent on the time period over which it is studied. Therefore, an appropriate directed question for chicken chasing would be, "In adult male boxers, is chicken chasing more effective than traditional foot speed training (i.e., jump rope) at improving the number of foot contacts in the 60-s box run drill over a 12-week period?"

REAL-WORLD APPLICATION

Developing a Question: Similar to a Needs Analysis

Much like the needs analysis of a sport and its athletes, developing a research question requires taking a step back and looking at the bigger picture. For example, the sport of basketball requires the ability to jump; players also need to have long limbs. A researcher must look at his question with a similar mindset. For example, boxing requires chasing an opponent around the ring with rapid changes in direction. Because of this, it seems like chicken chasing may be beneficial to a boxer because it resembles chasing an opponent around the ring. Now that a background question has been developed, it is time to develop directed questions such as: How long will the subjects chase the chicken? What type of chickens will be used? Who will the subjects be, so that the outcomes can be applied to boxing? What will foot speed be compared to? How many times will the boxer chase the chicken?

BOX 12.2

Components of a Well-Defined Directed Question Using the Acronym "PICOT"

Population
Intervention
Comparison
Outcome
Time

BOX 12.3

Sample Background and Directed Questions for Evaluating Evidence Associated with Chicken Chasing and Foot Speed

Background: What are the primary muscle groups used during chicken chasing?
Directed: In adult male boxers, is chicken chasing more effective than jump rope at improving speed in the 10-m sprint over a 12-week period?

Directed questions are more in-depth and lead to a clearer understanding of the efficacy of a device, programming technique, or supplement.

STEP 2: SEARCH FOR EVIDENCE

After formulating a question, the strength and conditioning coach should search for evidence (30). General information may be found in textbooks or by consulting experts. However, unbiased information is best obtained from peer-reviewed resources. In years past, obtaining peer-reviewed information was cumbersome. Today, however, public availability of medical databases and widespread online access to peer-reviewed journals makes it relatively easy to find quality information.

Although there are many medical and scientific databases available for search (Table 12.1), the two most widely used and publically available databases are **PubMed** (http://www.ncbi.nlm.nih.gov/PubMed/) and **Google Scholar** (http://scholar.google.com). PubMed is the public access site to the National Library of Medicine's database. It contains an abundance of abstracts and links to publically available journals. It can be searched through the general entry page or by entering more sophisticated word strings (Fig. 12.2). If searching for information on chicken chasing, we might enter in the term "chicken chasing and boxing." This would result in a number of links to article abstracts (if this were a realistic example). However, this may lead to an abundance of superfluous articles, making it necessary to add search terms to narrow

TABLE 12.1 ● COMMON DATABASES USED TO SEARCH FOR PEER-REVIEWED EVIDENCE

DATABASE	DESCRIPTION
Medline	Likely the most comprehensive database to search for medically based journals. Has robust, expanded search features to facilitate directed searches.
PubMed	Public access to the Medline database. Users can freely search and read abstracts; contains some links to online journals. Also contains specific features to allow searches for RCTs or systematic reviews.
Google Scholar	Publically available database containing peer-reviewed information. Contains links to many online journals and free abstracts. Also provides links to government reports.
Sport Discus	Database specifically for exercise and sports science. Contains many of the same articles as other medical databases, but also searches journals specific to the exercise discipline. Some articles are non–peer-reviewed.
CINAHL	Allied health sciences database that contains some unique features and journals. Is popular within the field of nursing.
Web of Science	One of the most comprehensive databases for allied health sciences. Contains links to conference proceedings; user can search for the number of times a particular article has been cited in peer-reviewed literature.
Cochrane Library	Contains links to systematic reviews for a variety of allied health sciences by discipline. Also allows users to search specifically for funded trials.

Some are publically available, while others require a subscription

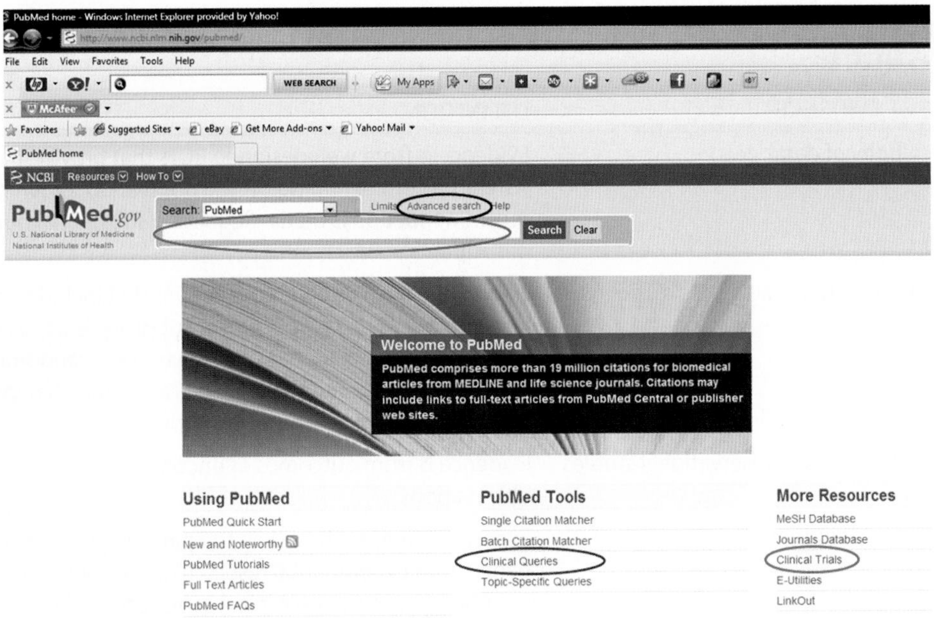

FIGURE 12.2 Screen shot from PubMed website. Highlighted in this image is the general search box, advanced search button, the tab to search for specific clinical trials, and the clinical queries button designed specifically for EBP.

the search. By clicking the "advanced search" tab, searches can be narrowed by publication date, publication type, language, and many other important journal characteristics. Interestingly, PubMed now contains built-in tools to directly assist with evidence-based searches. Clicking on the "Clinical Queries" tab redirects users to a page that permits searching directly for the highest forms of evidence (see next section). One may also narrow a search to look only for "therapeutic interventions," which would return articles focused specifically on training responses (Fig. 12.3).

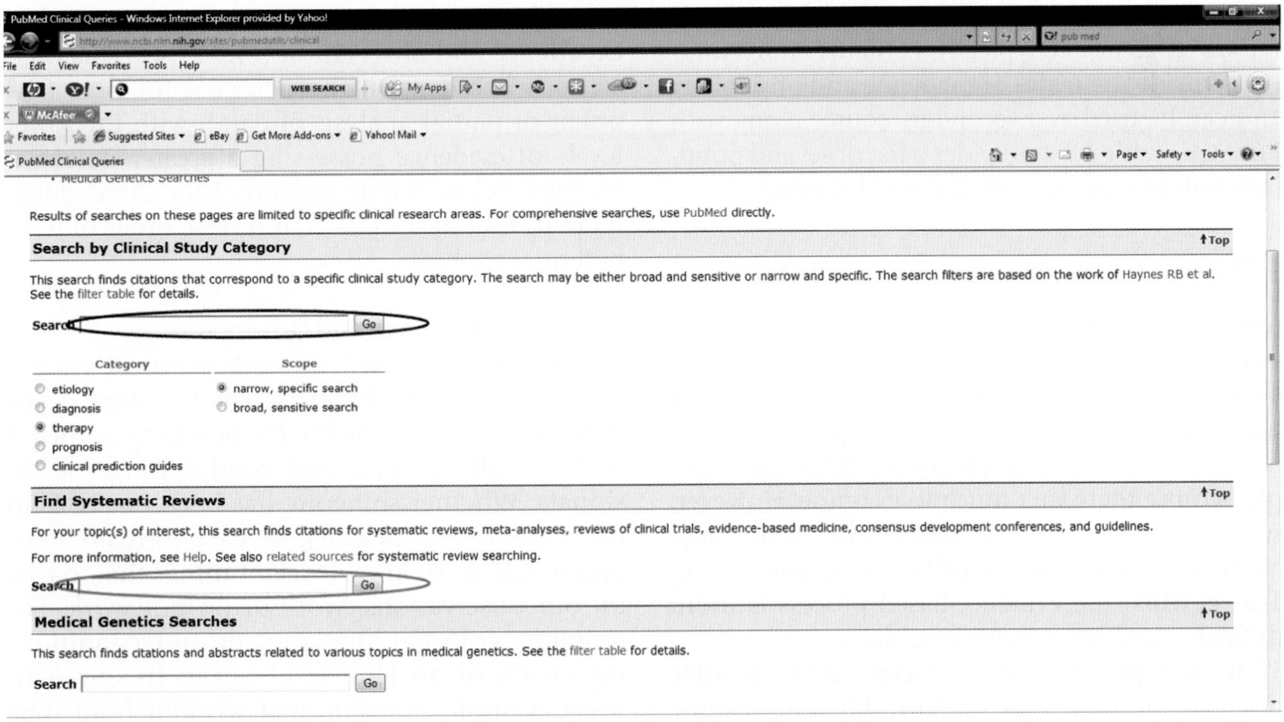

FIGURE 12.3 Screen shot from clinical queries tab within PubMed. Highlighted in this image are the search boxes for clinical study categories (RCT) and systematic reviews.

TABLE 12.2 ● LEVELS OF EVIDENCE AS SUGGESTED BY THE NATIONAL HEART, LUNG, AND BLOOD INSTITUTE

CATEGORY	SOURCE OF EVIDENCE	DEFINITION
A	RCTs (rich body of data)	Evidence is from well-designed RCTs that provide a consistent pattern of findings in the population for which the recommendation is made. Requires a substantial number of participants.
B	RCTs (limited body of data)	Evidence is from intervention studies that include only a limited number of RCTs, post hoc or subgroup analysis of RCTs, or meta-analysis of RCTs. Pertains when few randomized trials exist, they are small, and the results are somewhat inconsistent or were from a nonspecific population.
C	Nonrandomized trials, observational studies	Evidence is from outcomes of uncontrolled trials or observations.
D	Panel consensus judgment	Expert judgment is based on the panel's synthesis of evidence from experimental research or the consensus of panel members based on the clinical experience or knowledge that does not meet the above-listed criteria.

These categories of evidence have been adopted by the ACSM for their position stand on resistance exercise in healthy populations.
Source: Ratamess NA, Alvar BA, Evetoch TK, et al. Progression models in resistance training for healthy adults. *Med Sci Sport Exerc*. 2009;41:687–708; National Institutes of Health and National Heart, Lung, and Blood Institute. Clinical guidelines on the identification, evaluation, and treatment of overweight and obesity in adults: the Evidence Report. NIH Publication. *Obes Res*. 1998;6(suppl 2):51S–209S.

Google Scholar is a relatively new search engine that can be found through the advanced search buttons on the Google web page. Google Scholar, like PubMed, returns peer-reviewed articles in response to search terms. It typically contains more journals outside the realm of medicine and physiology and can be used as a secondary source along with PubMed. Table 12.2 provides a list of several popular databases for strength and conditioning.

STEP 3: EVALUATE THE EVIDENCE

After conducting a thorough search, one must examine and evaluate the evidence obtained in order to reach a final answer to the operational question (30). When evidence in a particular area is scarce, the evaluation process is rather easy, simply because there isn't much to examine. However, some questions and searches will yield large amounts of literature, which may be conflicting. This is when the evidence-based process is more difficult—and more indispensable.

If two peer-reviewed articles, using similar designs and methods, obtain different results, which one is right—which should be "believed?" In order to sift through conflicting evidence, it is vital to establish a hierarchy for different types of information. Most EBP models use the following hierarchy for ranking evidence: (a) experimental research; (b) observational research; (c) practical experience and observation (Fig. 12.4). This hierarchy is based upon the potential for **bias** (the unfair or partial analysis of data), with the lower levels of evidence possessing a greater potential for bias. Below is a discussion of the three global types of EBP information in reverse order of their potential for bias.

Practical Experience and Observation

Information obtained through practical experience or personal observation is the most basic type of evidence and is (hopefully!) gathered daily by all strength and conditioning professionals. Whether someone has been in the field for 6 months or 25 years, we each have an accumulated store of knowledge of things that, based on our observations, work or do not work. For example, consider the strength and conditioning coach of an elite level boxer. In our fictitious example, conventional wisdom (and thus practice) dictated for the character Mickey that, to develop agility, lateral movement, and quick

Q & A from the Field

Q The strength and conditioning coaches on staff at the university are evaluating the use of chains and bands for use during power training phases. I cannot find a lot of evidence to support their use over traditional training methods. Should I implement this type of training?

—Assistant Strength & Conditioning Coach

A Training using bands or chains attached to the end of the barbell is a new and popular strength and power training method. It helps to overcome some limitations associated with traditional strength training (i.e., the mismatch between the constant force requirements of lifting a weight versus the variation in force-generating capacity through the range of motion). Chains and bands apply greater resistance at the top of the range of motion, potentially allowing for improved matching of force requirements to force-generating capacity.

Because this is a relatively new training method, there are few studies evaluating this technique. At least one study has shown that following long-term training, there is no difference in power development during the bench press exercise in athletes using chains, bands, or traditional weight training methods (32). Given the lack of conclusive evidence, I certainly would not replace traditional resistance training and plyometrics with chain or band training. However, it may be used sparingly to augment traditional training programs.

reflexes, boxers need to incorporate chicken chasing into their workout regimen. Mickey likely developed his opinion on the training strategy from years of training experience and positive results observed in boxers over time.

Observational Research

Generally, research evidence can be divided into two categories: observational and experimental. **Observational research** denotes work in which exposure to the intervention occurs naturally; the researcher merely observes certain physiological or physical traits of the exposed and unexposed groups. Suppose we wanted to test the association between chicken chasing and foot speed in boxers; this could be studied retrospectively by measuring a 60-s box run on a large cohort (group) of boxers (Fig. 12.5). Then, each boxer could be interviewed about their previous training practices for foot speed. The 60-s box run scores of boxers who previously used chicken chasing for speed training could be compared to those who used conventional training methods. If the average speed (i.e., number of contacts) of the boxers who chase chicken for training was greater than those who do not, we could conclude that chicken chasing is associated with improved foot speed in boxers. The same type of association could also be determined prospectively using the experimental design provided in Figure 12.6.

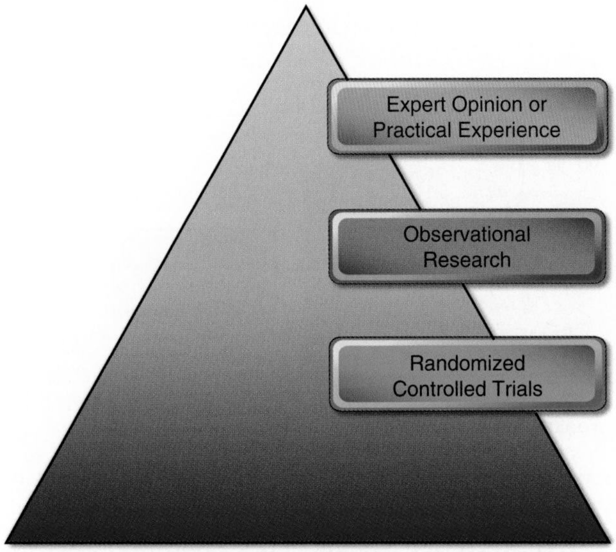

FIGURE 12.4 Model for establishing levels of evidence.

Although this association may provide some evidence that chicken chasing is an effective training method, there are many uncontrolled variables. For example, we do not know the level of exposure to chicken chasing. Some boxers may have used chicken chasing sparingly while others may have used the technique on a daily basis. Additionally, we

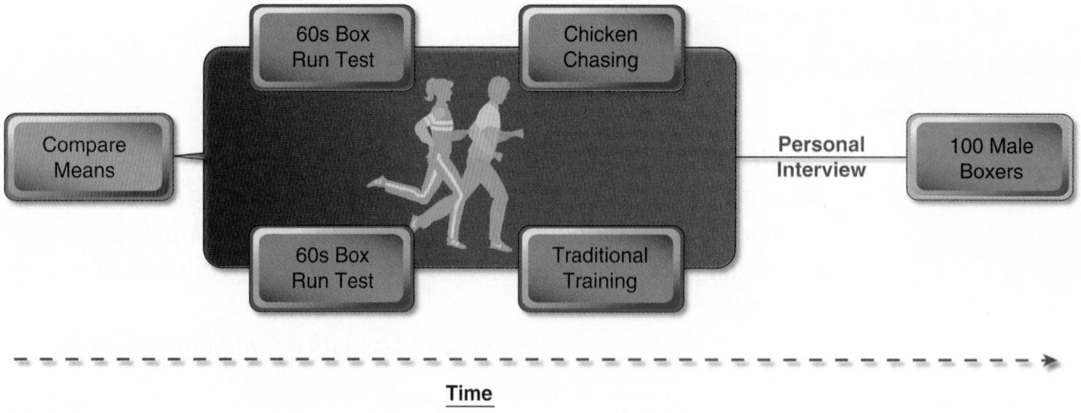

FIGURE 12.5 Retrospective cohort (observational) study design to investigate the association between chicken chasing and foot-speed.

do not know the type of chicken being chased; perhaps some chickens are faster than others, creating a greater overload stimulus for some boxers than others. Finally, we do not know what other exposures were present. It is possible the boxers incorporating chicken chasing augmented training with conventional speed training. Thus, there are many factors that may have influenced speed in an observational study. Therefore, although providing interesting data, observational research may not offer the best indication of the effectiveness of the new method.

Observational research can be either retrospective (looking backward in time) or prospective (looking forward in time). Regardless of the direction, there are many potential confounding variables in this type of research.

Experimental Research

Experimental research denotes control of exposure to the intervention or independent variable (e.g., chicken chasing) by the scientist or researcher. The study design that is most robust and least prone to bias is a **randomized controlled trial (RCT)**. To study the effectiveness of chicken chasing with an RCT, boxers would be asked to volunteer for a study to test the effectiveness of a novel training approach for speed development. Volunteers who have never been exposed to the practice of chasing chickens would be randomly assigned to one of three groups: no speed training (control group), conventional speed training, and chicken chasing. Before the study, an independent investigator who was unaware of group allocations would test the foot speed of all the boxers using a 60-s box run drill. Training would then be conducted by experienced

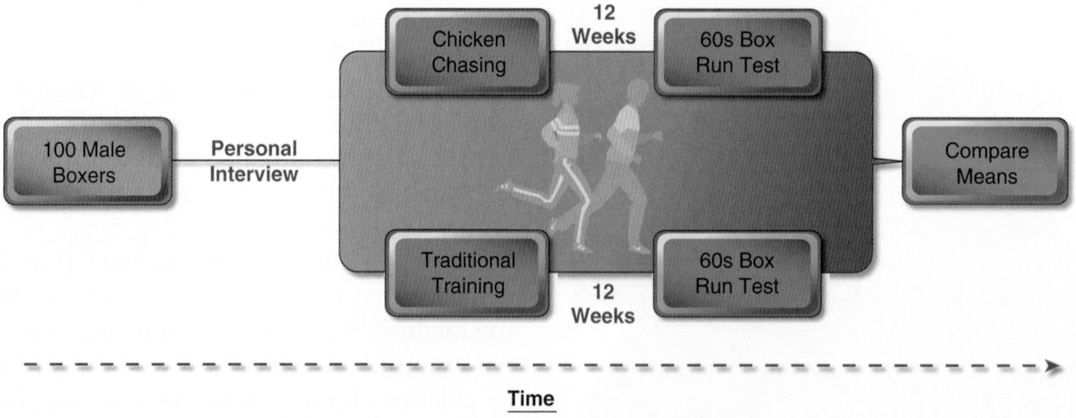

FIGURE 12.6 Prospective cohort (observational) study design to investigate the association between chicken chasing and foot speed.

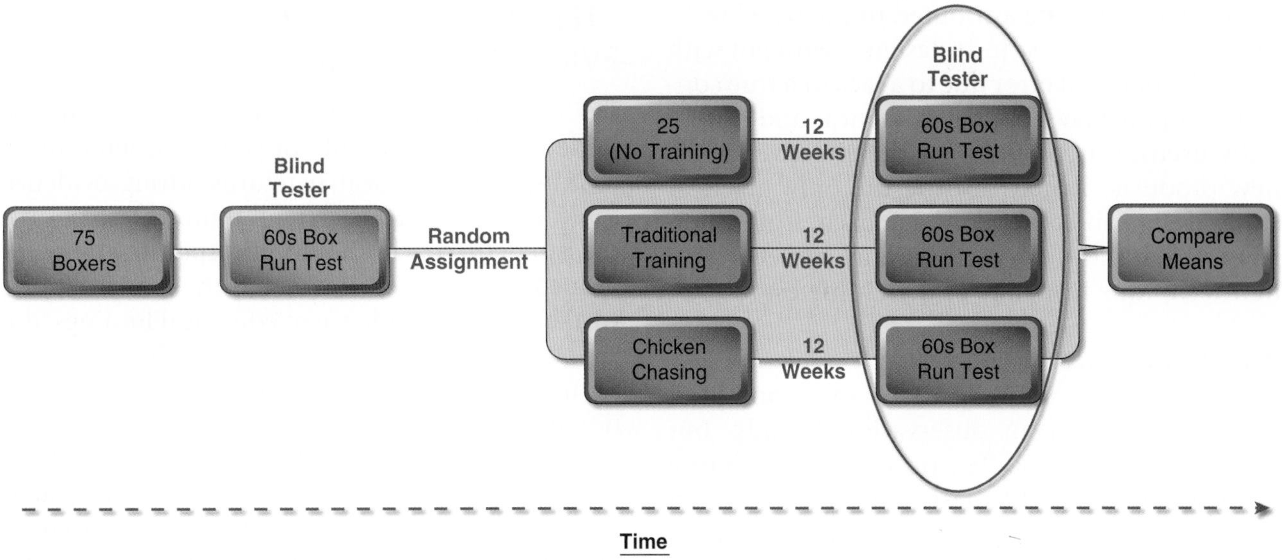

FIGURE 12.7 Randomized controlled trial (RCT; experimental) study design to investigate the association between chicken chasing and foot-speed.

trainers. At the end of the study period, the blinded investigator would measure the foot speed in all boxers using the same 60-s box run drill. Only after testing would the blinded investigator become aware of group allocations. At the end of the study period, the speed of the athletes in all three groups would be compared using appropriate statistical procedures and a determination made as to whether or not chicken chasing improves speed compared to conventional training and no training (Fig. 12.7).

Tracking Studies

In many cases, an RCT may not be feasible in athletic populations. Therefore, the best and most applicable sports science results are often provided from "tracking studies" (similar to case-series design or "outcomes research" in medicine). In tracking studies, coaches or scientist collect data in standardized ways to track the progress of their athletes. When novel techniques become available (e.g., our fictitious example of chicken chasing), the coach can augment traditional training with the innovative technique and continue to track the progress of the athletes (Fig. 12.8). Assuming the tests are performed in identical ways and there are no other changes in the preparation of the athlete (e.g., no other new training tools, changes in diet), increases in

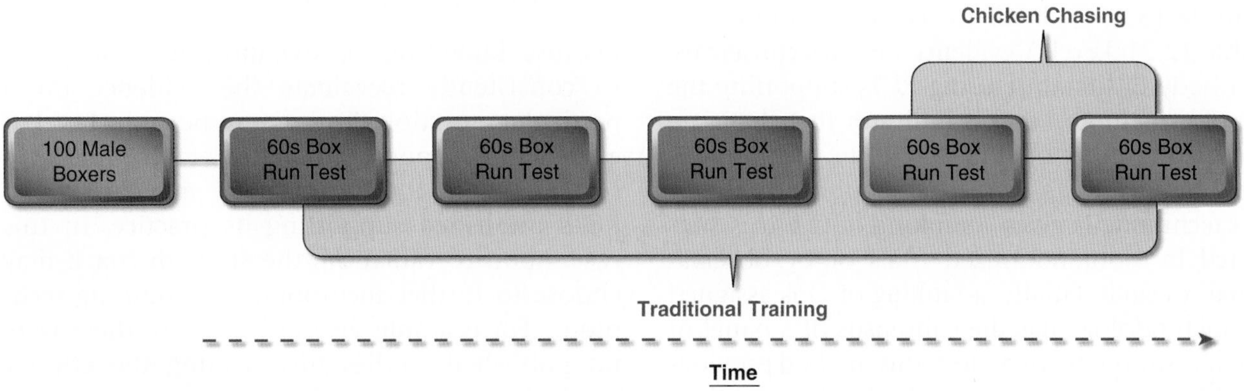

FIGURE 12.8 Tracking study design to investigate the usefulness of chicken chasing on foot speed. Although such studies lack control, they may be the most common and potentially useful for sports science purposes.

performance may be attributed to the novel technique. Although this study design is wrought with potential bias and error due to a lack of a true control group, it may provide a practical and potentially useful way of assessing the effectiveness of new products. It may also be the only practical study design in some cases as coaches are often leery of withholding the potential benefits of a new technique from any of their athletes.

Ranking evidence

An RCT affords more control over potential confounders than an observational study, but sometimes even RCTs produce conflicting evidence. One of the basic tenets of research is that results must be reproducible. If there is not a consensus within a body of literature, a coach should carefully evaluate each study to determine the group of studies with the greatest control. If there is no consensus within the literature, then there is simply not strong evidence to support the theory.

If, however, there are a large number of studies that support the use of a training methodology, such as chicken chasing, there may be a published **systematic review** or **meta-analysis**. Such reports use systematic procedures to pool and compare data from multiple articles to develop a consensus statement. A systematic review of RCTs with homogeneity of results constitutes one of the strongest forms of evidence.

Levels of Evidence

Several investigators and agencies have suggested methods for ranking evidence. Many disciplines have developed their own recommendations, but the one used by the ACSM was established originally by the National Heart Lung and Blood Institute (33,34). Evidence is ranked from A–D (Table 12.2). Level A evidence denotes consensus, or a body of literature using RCTs supporting the use of a method. Level B indicates that there are a limited number of studies, but the technique is supported by RCTs. Evidence supporting the use of a technique is given a ranking of C if it is supported by nonrandomized trials or by observational research. Finally, a ranking of D is assigned if a methodology has the consensus of a panel of experts. Although not perfect, this method provides an objective way of ranking the level of certainty that a training method is effective and useful.

STEP 4: INCORPORATE THE EVIDENCE INTO PRACTICE

The ultimate goal of the evidence-based search is to determine the validity of certain programming techniques. If the search returns strong evidence for the efficacy of a certain training technique, the strength coach should incorporate the technique into practice. However, if the search returns weaker levels of evidence or equivocal findings, the strength coach may choose to use the new technique sparingly, but not at the expense of traditional training.

To return to an earlier example, there is level B evidence to support the use of WBV as a neuromuscular potentiation tool to improve strength (17) and power (18). Therefore, if available, one may choose to incorporate WBV training into practice, but certainly should not incorporate it at the expense of traditional resistance, plyometric, or explosive weightlifting exercises that have a more substantial body of literature supporting their use. Instead, WBV should be used to augment or supplement the gold-standard training to improve power.

Some argue that the incorporation of EBP may lead to "cookie cutter" approaches to therapy, medicine, or in this case, training. The authors of this chapter do not advocate the wholesale use of protocols published in literature. Scientific protocols are designed specifically to control for outside confounders. Therefore, strength and conditioning coaches should use the principles supported by science and certainly have freedom to create programs that fit the needs of their athletes or a particular athletic scenario.

STEP 5: CONSISTENTLY REEVALUATE THE EVIDENCE

Because knowledge is dynamic, it is necessary to consistently reevaluate the evidence for a particular question. There may be only Level C evidence to support a practice at the time of a search, but in the future, there may be several RCTs published supporting its practice. In this case, upon reevaluation, the strength coach may choose to further incorporate the training technique. For example, in April of 2010, there were no published studies investigating the efficacy of chicken chasing for improving foot speed in boxers. Therefore, this technique should be used

BOX 12.4

Six-Part Process of Evidence-Based Practice

1. Develop an answerable question.
2. Search for evidence.
3. Evaluate and rank the evidence.
4. If supported, incorporate evidence into practice.
5. Consistently reevaluate the evidence.
6. Disseminate the evidence.

sparingly (if at all) when training boxers. However, if future experiments indicate that chicken chasing is indeed effective, coaches will only learn of this "emerging" training strategy if they consistently reevaluate the evidence.

Because knowledge is dynamic, EBP is a continual process. It is necessary to search and re-search on a routine basis for new evidence to support practice.

STEP 6: DISSEMINATE INFORMATION

After completing an evidence-based search, it is important for a strength and conditioning coach to **disseminate** the information to their staff and even to their athletes. This may be particularly important when the search uncovers information that is controversial or goes against common practice and conventional wisdom. In such cases, it is important to inform athletes and staff why you have chosen to use a technique that is different or unique and to reassure them that it is not without thought or supporting evidence that it is being implemented.

While completing the search, the strength and conditioning coach should document his or her search approach. Documentation should include the databases searched, key terms used, any inclusion/exclusion criteria for articles, and a list of articles used to make EBP decisions. If this information is thoroughly documented, the search can be easily repeated by the coach or a colleague in the future.

Along with sharing information with the staff and athletes, the strength and conditioning coach should consider writing and publishing the information in a peer-reviewed journal such as the *Strength & Conditioning Journal* (for professional education), *Journal of Strength and Conditioning Research* (for research findings) and/or presenting their findings at the annual meeting of the NSCA. One particularly interesting aspect to report is how scientific evidence has influenced practice and how it has been integrated with knowledge gained through practical expertise. Such information may provide guidelines to other coaches considering the same questions. It may also be helpful to scientists who are searching for topics to investigate that are relevant to practice.

Publishing results describing how scientific evidence was integrated into practice creates a useful tool that may improve other coaches' practice or influence future scientific study.

PRACTICAL IMPLEMENTATION OF EVIDENCE-BASED PRACTICE IN STRENGTH AND CONDITIONING

To this point, we have discussed the rationale for implementing EBP in strength and conditioning and the associated systematic process. However, of chief importance is how to actually put the process into practice. One of the oft-cited criticisms of EBP is that it is too time consuming and requires expertise not taught in universities. The time commitment necessary for success as a strength and conditioning coach is substantial, and it may seem burdensome to add another task to an already crowded schedule. However, advancements in technology have significantly reduced the time commitment necessary to practice evidence-based strength and conditioning. In years past, searching for peer-reviewed information may have required a practitioner to travel to a library, use a library computer to search for information, physically pull the archived journal from the shelves, and photocopy the article from the journal. Today, the widespread availability of information on the Internet has significantly reduced the time and effort required to perform EBP searches. In fact, the entire search can often be performed from an office computer that is connected to the Internet; journal articles can be stored on the hard drive of a computer or printed directly from the office computer. Depending on the expertise of a coach, the process may initially take more time. However, as the coach repeats the process of searching for evidence, it is likely that he or she will become more efficient and the process will take less time. Nevertheless, there are a few practical guidelines we suggest for incorporating EBP into practice.

COMMIT TIME TO EVIDENCE-BASED PRACTICE

The first and most important practical suggestion to incorporating EBP into strength and conditioning practice is to schedule time on a weekly basis to search for evidence. If time is not specifically scheduled for EBP, it will likely be replaced by some other activity. If the strength and conditioning coach truly desires to be an evidence-based practitioner, it must become a priority. Of course, committing time to EBP will be easier if it is supported by management and highly regarded by other staff members. If not, the strength coach may need to lead by example and commit his or her own personal time to practice. Ultimately, the benefits of better programs will outweigh the drawbacks of a small sacrifice of time.

CONSISTENTLY READ SCIENTIFIC JOURNALS

The second practical suggestion to implementing EBP is to consistently read scientific journals in one's discipline. If a coach is a member of the NSCA or ACSM, this process is easy. Members receive either monthly or bimonthly issues of the *Journal of Strength & Conditioning Research*, *Strength and Conditioning Journal*, or *Medicine and Science in Sport and Exercise*. Each of these journals is devoted to publishing articles relevant to strength and conditioning, exercise physiology, or biomechanics. Read these journals, along with other discipline-specific journals, on a routine basis. If you are not a member of these organizations, join them if for no other reason than the benefit of receiving the journals. In addition to reading these journals, it may be advantageous for the strength and conditioning coordinator to budget money to order other discipline-specific journals and make them available to the entire staff. At the collegiate level, the library may have funding to order such journals.

DEVELOP AN ACCOUNTABILITY SYSTEM WITHIN THE COACHING STAFF

It is much easier to be an evidence-based practitioner when the entire staff is committed to the process. In such a case, it may be helpful to hold each other accountable to searching for evidence. Begin to incorporate the "language" of EBP. Although it may not be possible in all cases, understand the level of evidence that supports your practices. When you see other staff members doing things that are novel, ask them "what evidence supports this new practice?" In many cases, the practice may be based on practical experience alone, which is certainly acceptable. However, asking such questions may prompt the coach to initiate his or her own evidence-based search to substantiate the practice. Of course, this search should be repeated often as science changes and evolves rapidly.

CULTIVATE PROFESSIONAL RELATIONSHIPS

Developing professional relationships with individuals outside of the coaching staff may be beneficial in implementing EBP. Strength and conditioning coaches may want to cultivate professional working groups with exercise and sport scientists actively involved in research. Such individuals may see training from a different perspective and provide insight into current scientific trends. They may also have access to sophisticated testing equipment and often are willing to assist in the assessment of athletes. The relationship would also benefit the scientist. One criticism often levied against science is that the protocols implemented in research are dissimilar to the actual programs used in the weight room. Through consistent communication, the strength and conditioning coach can provide practical recommendations to improve study protocols. Coaches may also inform scientists of current industry trends, new tools, or supplements that can be studied in the laboratory. Ultimately, this will lead to better, more timely studies that have an immediate impact on practice.

Q & A from the Field

Q ***I am an amateur cyclist training for a new competition. I've heard that because endurance athletes are not trying to build muscle and primarily utilize carbohydrates and fat for fuel, they don't need to eat much protein. How much protein do I need for performance in my sport?***

—Amateur Cyclist

A A common myth associated with sports nutrition is that protein is only important for strength–power athletes interested in building muscle. However, there is evidence that suggests protein may be just as important for you as an endurance athlete because of its ability to stimulate muscle protein synthesis to prevent muscle wasting. To answer your question, I developed an evidence-based question, "how much protein should a 35-year-old male amateur cyclist consume?" Using the PubMed search engine, I used the following search terms: "protein requirements for endurance athletes," and it turned up 59 articles. However, using the same search term under the "Clinical Queries/Systematic Review" engine yielded five papers. One of the articles was for middle-distance athletes and another characterizes nutritional status. Two were the same articles published in two different journals: a joint position stand of the American Dietetic Association (ADA), Dieticians of Canada (DC), and the ACSM (35). Position stands are excellent resources as they are inevitably rigorous, evidence-based syntheses of all existing literature on a particular topic. The 2009 ADA/DC/ACSM position stand recommends a daily protein intake of 1.2 to 1.7 g · kg^{-1}; this recommendation does not distinguish between strength and endurance athletes (35). This is clearly an excellent starting point, a foundation from which to further explore. However, this may not be as compelling as evidence that is more specific: a study (or studies) of young competitive endurance athletes. So, I scanned the titles of the original 59 articles searching the entire PubMed database. A 2004 review article by Tarnopolsky (36) looks promising; in fact, it is right on target. The review summarizes (among others) several studies that used moderate to well-trained endurance athletes that were both young and middle aged. A synthesis of these studies yielded a recommendation of 1.1 g · kg^{-1} · d^{-1} needed to maintain nitrogen balance (an index of adequate protein intake). A 2006 review by Phillips (37) comes to a similar conclusion. Fielding and Parkington (38) recommend 1.2 to 1.4 g · kg^{-1} · d^{-1} in a 2002 review paper.

These reviews and position stands, themselves based on numerous individual studies, recommend a range of 1.1 to 1.7 g · kg^{-1} of daily protein intake. Based on the breadth and recent publication of the ADA/DC/ACSM position stand, 1.2 g · kg · d^{-1} is a prudent low end point. Considered together, the other articles suggest that 1.4 g · kg · d^{-1} is a reasonable upper limit.

IMPLEMENT STAFF JOURNAL CLUBS OR CRITICAL APPRAISAL OF A TOPIC GROUPS

Finally, developing staff **journal clubs** or **critical appraisal of a topic (CAT)** groups can help in implementing EBP. At a weekly staff meeting, one staff member can be assigned the task of finding, reviewing, and presenting an article relative to practice. They can then discuss how this article supports or opposes current staff practice.

An even better approach might be to routinely assign CATs to staff members—a technique that originated in EBM (39). When performing a CAT, the EB practitioner follows the first four basic steps: (a) develop a question, (b) search for evidence, (c) evaluate or rank the evidence, and (d) develop a consensus statement for how the evidence informs practice. In a way, a CAT becomes a mini-systematic review. For the purpose of staff meetings, CAT topics could be assigned to an individual coach and he or she could be asked to find the five articles with the highest level of evidence that supports a practice used by the staff. The assigned coach could then present the topic to the staff and write a consensus statement to be circulated within the staff. This process is a bit more time-consuming than journal club, so this could be implemented on a monthly

BOX 12.5

Five Suggestions for Practically Implementing EBP in Strength and Conditioning

1. Schedule and commit time to EBP on a weekly basis.
2. Consistently read discipline-specific scientific journals.
3. Develop an accountability system within the coaching staff.
4. Cultivate professional relationships.
5. Initiate staff journal clubs or CAT groups.

or quarterly basis depending on the size of the staff. Also, if the CAT is performed in a systematic and professional manner, it is possible that the results could be submitted for publication. Such practice would aid in the professional development of the staff, add credibility and notoriety to the strength and conditioning program, and potentially assist strength and conditioning coaches at other locations who are considering the same questions.

CATs can be used to disseminate research findings to staff members or other coaches through peer-reviewed publication.

Summary

Exercise prescription will never be governed solely by research evidence; it shouldn't be. At the end of the day, a significant and important component of exercise design is creativity; hence, the "art and science of practice." However, at its foundation, exercise prescription should be directed by science. EBP is a term that originated in the medical field. It describes a systematic process of asking answerable questions, finding evidence, evaluating evidence, and incorporating that evidence into practice. Given the rapid increase in available exercise devices, gadgets, program theories, and nutritional supplements, the incorporation of EBP into strength and conditioning is now a necessity. EBP provides a defined paradigm for strength and conditioning coaches to remain on the cutting edge of science and to incorporate the latest, most effective tools in practice. It also provides a means to eliminate novel tools that may be unsafe or ineffective and training techniques that are antiquated. Ultimately, the goal of EBP is a better and more efficient product for athletes and a weight room that incorporates only proven methods.

To once again borrow from Rocky Balboa's trainer, Mickey, if chicken chasing is the most effective tool for improving the foot speed of boxers, construct a chicken pen in the weight room, buy a few chickens, and make chicken chasing a staple of your training programs. However, if the evidence suggests there is a better way, remove the chickens from the weight room and devote your time and money to techniques that are well supported by science.

Maxing Out

1. Your little brother's high school football coach is telling the team to run until they puke during summer preseason training. Your brother and his friends complained to the coach, but he responded that they must do it because that is what his coach made them do 20 years ago when they won the state championship. Is this coach's rationale of training evidence-based? Based on what you learned in this chapter, explain how his conditioning program can become more evidence-based.
2. You are a practicing strength and conditioning coach. You attend a conference where researchers are suggesting that a new type of training is superior to all others and that coaches should immediately begin implementing it into their programs. As a coach, you know that this novel training strategy is not practical in the weight room. How would you go about asking the researcher to take the information presented to you and figure out a way to use it on a day-to-day basis?
3. The researcher from the scenario above tells you that if it can be done in the laboratory, it can be done in a weight room. Where can you look for additional information related to the topic so you can draw your own conclusions by combining the information you find with the novel training method?

REFERENCES

1. Claridge JA, Fabian TC. History and development of evidence-based medicine. *World J Surg*. 2005;29:547–553.
2. Eddy DM. Practice policies: where do they come from? *JAMA*. 1990;263:1265, 1269, 1272 passim.
3. Sackett DL, Rosenberg WM, Gray JA, et al. Evidence based medicine: what it is and what it isn't. *BMJ*. 1996;312:71–72.
4. Sanders C. Cardiovascular and peripheral vascular diseases: treatment by a motorized oscillating bed. *JAMA*. 1936;106:916.

5. Whedon GD, Deitrick JE, Shorr E. Modification of the effects of immobilization upon metabolic and physiologic functions of normal men by the use of an oscillating bed. *Am J Med*. 1949;6:648–711.
6. Bosco C, Cardinale M, Tsarpela O, et al. The influence of whole body vibration on jumping performance. *Biol Sport*. 1998;15:157–164.
7. Bosco C, Colli R, Introini E, et al. Adaptive responses of human skeletal muscle to vibration exposure. *Clin Physiol*. 1999;19:183–187.
8. Bosco C, Cardinale M, Tsarpela O. Influence of vibration on mechanical power and electromyogram activity in human arm flexor muscles. *Eur J Appl Physiol*. 1999;79:306–311.
9. Bosco C, Iacovelli M, Tsarpela O, et al. Hormonal responses to whole body vibration in men. *Eur J Appl Physiol*. 2000;81:449–454.
10. Rubin C, Turner AS, Bain S, et al. Anabolism—Low mechanical signals strengthen long bones. *Nature*. 2001;412:603–604.
11. Rittweger J, Ehrig J, Just K, et al. Oxygen uptake in whole-body vibration exercise: influence of vibration frequency, amplitude, and external load. *Int J Sports Med*. 2002;23:428–432.
12. Rittweger J, Schiesel H Felsenberg D. Oxygen uptake during whole-body vibration exercise: comparison with squatting as a slow voluntary movement. *Eur J Appl Physiol*. 2001;86:169–173.
13. Rittweger J, Beller G Felsenberg D. Acute physiological effects of exhaustive whole-body vibration exercise in man. *Clin Physiol*. 2000;20:134–142.
14. Abercromby AFJ, Amonette WE, Layne CS, et al. Variation in neuromuscular responses during acute whole-body vibration exercise. *Med Sci Sports Exerc*. 2007;39:1642–1650.
15. Cardinale M, Lim J. Electromyography activity of vastus lateralis muscle during whole-body vibrations of different frequencies. *J Strength Cond Res*. 2003;17:621–624.
16. Cochrane DJ, Stannard SR, Firth EC, et al. Acute whole-body vibration elicits post-activation potentiation. *Eur J Appl Physiol*. 2010;108:311–319.
17. Marin PJ, Rhea MR. Effects of vibration training on muscle strength: a meta-analysis. *J Strength Cond Res*. 2010;24:548–556.
18. Marin PJ, Rhea MR. Effects of vibration training on muscle power: a meta-analysis. *J Strength Cond Res*. 2010;24:871–878.
19. Gilsanz V, Al Wren T, Sanchez M, et al. Low-level, high-frequency mechanical signals enhance musculoskeletal development of young women with low BMD. *J Bone Miner Res*. 2006;21:1464–1474.
20. Rittweger J, Beller G, Armbrecht G, et al. Prevention of bone loss during 56 days of strict bed rest by side-alternating resistive vibration exercise. *Bone*. 2010;46:137–147.
21. Rittweger J. Vibration as an exercise modality: how it may work, and what its potential might be. *Eur J Appl Physiol*. 2010;108:877–904.
22. Stone MH, O'Bryant H Garhammer J. Hypothetical model for strength training. *J Sports Med Phys Fitness*. 1981;21:342–351.
23. Stone MH, O'Bryant H, Garhammer J, et al. Theoretical model of strength training. *NSCA J*. 1982;4:36–39.
24. Rhea MR, Alderman BL. A meta-analysis of periodized versus nonperiodized strength and power training programs. *Res Q Exerc Sport*. 2004;75:413–422.
25. Rhea MR, Phillips WT, Burkett LN, et al. A comparison of linear and daily undulating periodized programs with equated volume and intensity for local muscular endurance. *J Strength Cond Res*. 2003;17:82–87.
26. Rhea MR, Ball SD, Phillips WT, et al. A comparison of linear and daily undulating periodized programs with equated volume and intensity for strength. *J Strength Cond Res*. 2002;16:250–255.
27. Buford TW, Rossi SJ, Smith DB, et al. A comparison of periodization models during nine weeks with equated volume and intensity for strength. *J Strength Cond Res*. 2007;21:1245–1250.
28. Ho K, Lauscher HN, Best A, et al. Dissecting technology-enabled knowledge translation: essential challenges, unprecedented opportunities. *Clin Invest Med*. 2004;27:70–78.
29. Ho K, Chockalingam A, Best A, et al. Technology-enabled knowledge translation: building a framework for collaboration. *Can Med Assoc J*. 2003;168:710–711.
30. Sackett DL, Straus SE, Richardson SW, et al. *Evidence-Based Medicine: How to Practice and Teach EBM*. Edinburgh, UK: Hancourt Publishers Limited; 2000.
31. Law M, MacDermid J. *Evidence-Based Rehabilitation: A Guide to Practice*. Thorofare, NJ: SLACK Inc.; 2008.
32. Ghigiarelli JJ, Nagle EF, Gross FL, et al. The effects of a 7-week heavy elastic band and weight chain program on upper-body strength and power in a sample of division 1-AA football players. *J Strength Cond Res*. 2009; 23:756–764.
33. Ratamess NA, Alvar BA, Evetoch TK, et al. Progression models in resistance training for healthy adults. *Med Sci Sport Exerc*. 2009;41:687–708.
34. National Institutes of Health and National Heart, Lung, and Blood Institute. Clinical guidelines on the identification, evaluation, and treatment of overweight and obesity in adults: the Evidence Report. *NIH Publication*. 1998;98–4093:288.
35. Rodriguez NR, Di Marco NM, Langley S. American College of Sports Medicine position stand. Nutrition and athletic performance. *Med Sci Sports Exerc*. 2009;41:709–731.
36. Tarnopolsky M. Protein requirements for endurance athletes. *Nutrition*. 2004;20:662–668.
37. Phillips SM. Dietary protein for athletes: from requirements to metabolic advantage. *Appl Physiol Nutr Metab*. 2006;31:647–654.
38. Fielding RA, Parkington J. What are the dietary protein requirements of physically active individuals? New evidence on the effects of exercise on protein utilization during post-exercise recovery. *Nutr Clin Care*. 2002;5: 191–196.
39. Sackett DL Parkes J. Teaching critical appraisal: no quick fixes. *Can Med Assoc J*. 1998;158:203–204.

CHAPTER 13

Improving Aerobic Performance

MARK KOVACS • MELISA LEMUS

OBJECTIVES

After reading this chapter you will be able to:

- Understand the differences between training aerobic and anaerobic athletes.
- Familiarize yourself with the seven factors that affect aerobic performance.
- Recall various modes of training that an aerobic athlete may use throughout an exercise program.
- Explain what should be included while prescribing exercise for an aerobic athlete.
- Describe how to properly manipulate variables of an exercise program: choice of exercise, intensity, volume, and rest.

KEY TERMS

Continuous Training
Fartlek Training
Interval Training
Lactate Threshold
Maximal Oxygen Consumption
Repetitions
Taper

Introduction

Aerobic exercise is important for athletes in any sport that requires training or competition over an extended period of time (i.e., >3 to 5 minutes). It is unclear, however, the extent to which traditional aerobic exercise is necessary for athletes in nonendurance sports (e.g., football, baseball, basketball). With explosive nonendurance athletes (speed, power, and strength sports), where performance is measured over a matter of a few seconds or less, the case has been made that aerobic fitness is important for recovery from competition and training (since we use the oxidative system to recover from anaerobic training) and that aerobic energy pathways may contribute to anaerobic performance (1).

As greater knowledge is gained in the area of training specificity, the usefulness of aerobic exercise for nonendurance athletes has become a major discussion point among scientists, coaches, and trainers. Although traditional aerobic training may not be appropriate for explosively trained athletes, depending on the sport, sprint/interval training may be useful in maintaining or, to some extent, improving aerobic metabolism if structured approximately.

The extent to which traditional aerobic exercise is necessary for various athletes in nonendurance sports (e.g., football, baseball, basketball) is not clear.

There are practical studies that have shown little relationship between maximal oxygen consumption ($\dot{V}O_2$) and recovery from anaerobic exercise in some nonendurance sports (10). Additionally, differences in aerobic power do not explain differences in performance during various phases of a 30-second all-out test (13). In this study, aerobic power provided only marginal contributions to anaerobic performance. Therefore, if the goal of training is improved anaerobic performance, then aerobic training may not be the most time-efficient mode of training.

Although results like these are hardly conclusive, we should pause and reconsider the role of aerobic exercise in nonendurance athletes. Also remember that the aerobic/anaerobic requirements of athletic performance span a continuum. Most athletes need both anaerobic and aerobic training, and the way this is integrated into the athlete's overall program is vital to the success of the athlete. The remainder of this chapter examines aerobic exercise prescription from an endurance athlete's perspective and considers how these programs apply to the athlete needing both anaerobic and aerobic training programs.

The importance of aerobic exercise in endurance athletes is well documented. We must reassess the role of aerobic exercise in nonendurance athletes.

FACTORS THAT INFLUENCE AEROBIC EXERCISE PERFORMANCE

Understanding those factors that influence aerobic exercise performance is important for helping both with athlete selection of and for planning endurance training programs. A number of factors influence aerobic performance. These include, but are not limited to, the following:

1. Maximal oxygen consumption
2. Lactate threshold
3. Fuel utilization
4. Fiber-type characteristics
5. Movement economy
6. Maximal aerobic power
7. Fatigue (central and peripheral)

Maximal oxygen consumption refers to the maximum rate at which an individual can consume oxygen. It is limited by cardiac output, pulmonary function, and cellular metabolism (2). Relative maximal oxygen consumption (milliliters per kilogram per minute) in elite female cyclists accounts for a significant part of bicycle racing performance (3). The results of a study like this should be interpreted with care, however, as it does not necessarily look at enough factors to determine whether other factors could make a more significant contribution to performance. For example, the only other variables studied were minute ventilation, heart rate, minute ventilation divided by maximal oxygen consumption, and heart rate divided by maximal oxygen consumption. As the next few paragraphs show, other factors may well have significant impacts on endurance performance.

Lactate threshold (seen in Fig. 13.1) is a term that has one meaning but has sometimes been interchanged with other words or phrases. From a practical as well as literal standpoint, an individual's lactate threshold is the exact point during an exercise that if greater intensity is provided there will be an exponential increase in blood lactate concentration. This is sometimes referred to as the *onset of blood lactate* (OBLA) (4). This exponential increase in lactate typically occurs around 50% to 60% of $\dot{V}O_{2max}$, while it occurs at higher work rates in trained individuals (65% to 80% of $\dot{V}O_{2max}$) (5).

In one study, two groups of cyclists were compared (6). One group (group H) had an average maximal oxygen consumption of approximately 68 $mL \cdot kg^{-1} \cdot min^{-1}$ and 5 years of cycling experience. The second group (group L) had an average maximal oxygen consumption of approximately 66 $mL \cdot kg^{-1} \cdot min^{-1}$ and almost 3 years of cycling experience. Both groups exercised at 88% of maximal oxygen consumption and their time to fatigue and lactate accumulation was measured. Investigators found that group H could exercise for more than an hour (on average), while group L could exercise for

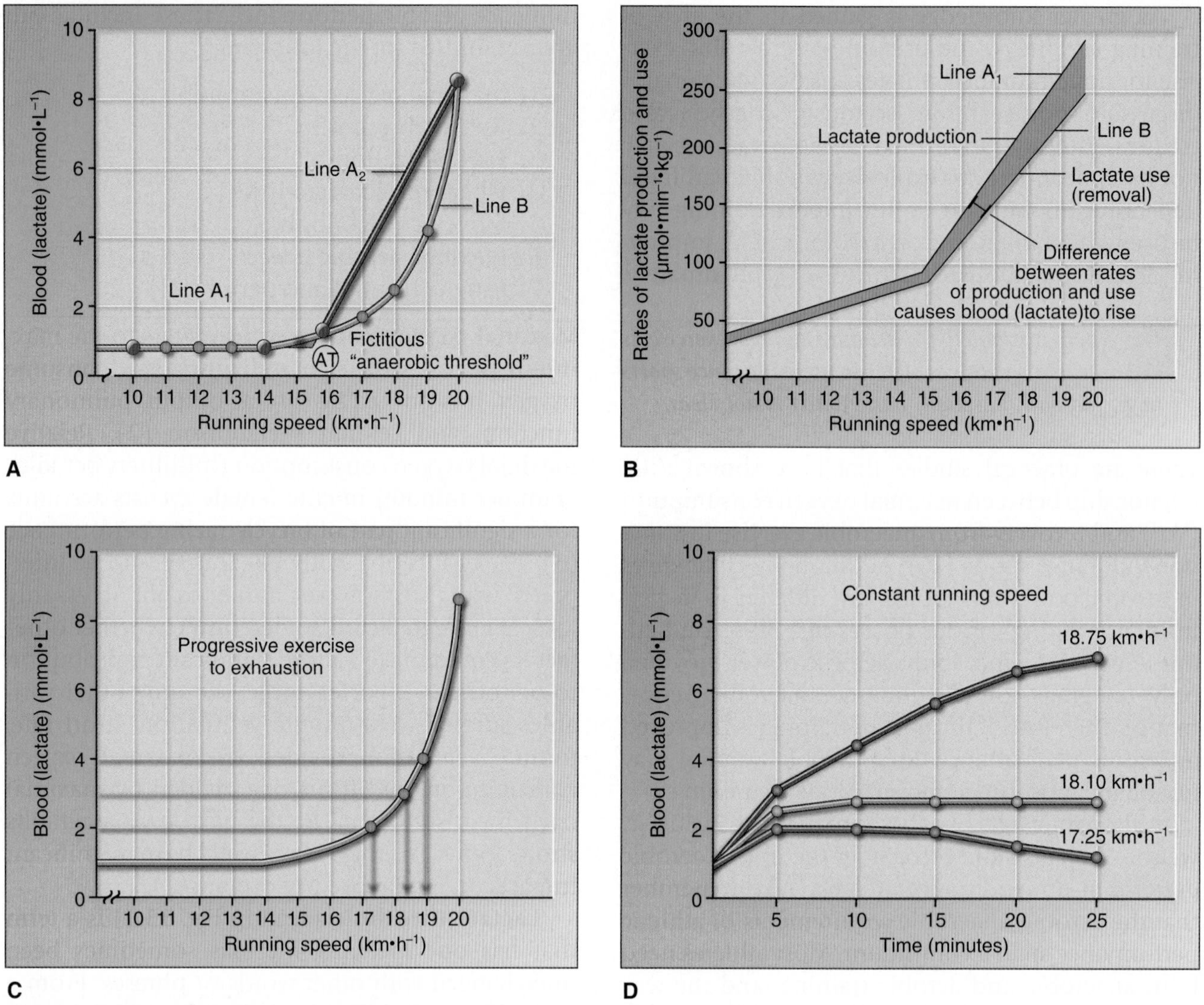

FIGURE 13.1 **A.** The relationship of blood lactate to running speed. **B.** Rates of lactate production and use as a function of running speed. **C.** The response of blood lactate to running speed to exhaustion. **D.** The response of blood lactate to a constant running speed.

an average of only about 30 minutes. Group L accumulated twice as much lactate as group H. In other words, since maximal oxygen consumption was nearly similar between the two groups, other factors, one of which may have been the accumulation of lactic acid, influenced endurance performance.

The ability to use fuel efficiently can have a large impact on endurance performance. In the same study mentioned above (6), glycogen utilization was compared by having the subjects exercise at 80% of maximal oxygen consumption. Group L oxidized almost twice as many carbohydrates as group H, and group L used more than twice as much glycogen per kilogram. In other words, the group with the better performance (group H) was able to spare its glycogen stores during exercise, enabling it to exercise longer at a greater intensity.

Muscle fiber types will also have an influence on endurance performance. Theoretically, those individuals with a higher percentage of type I muscle fibers will perform better at endurance tasks. The higher performing group (6) averaged approximately 66% type I fibers, while the lower performing group averaged approximately 47%.

When training using traditional aerobic training, type I muscle fibers are primarily being used.

Finally, the economy with which one exercises will affect one's performance. This refers to the skill

REAL-WORLD APPLICATION

Strength-Training and Endurance Athletes

Strength training, within reason, is important for endurance athletes. It can help to prevent injuries by targeting muscles and joints that are prone to injury. For example, it can help to improve strength imbalances in a runner's knee or a swimmer's shoulder. It can also help to improve an athlete's ability to apply force. Even though endurance athletes are taking many steps, strokes, or revolutions during a race, an athlete who can generate more force will still have the ability to get somewhere faster than the one who cannot.

There are a number of guidelines for strength-training and endurance athletes:

1. Keep it in perspective. Endurance athletes are not strength and power athletes. They cannot tolerate high volumes and intensities of strength training combined with their endurance training; this can lead to overtraining or injury. Overly intense strength training can also be counterproductive in another way; putting on too much muscle mass on an endurance athlete will negatively affect his or her exercise economy, thereby detracting from event performance.
2. Resistance training does not have to mean weight training. Since the focus is not on drastically increasing maximal strength or hypertrophy, resistance training can be done in a number of ways, including in the weight room, through calisthenics, and with medicine balls or other implements.
3. Keep the stresses of the athlete's endurance training in mind. If the athlete's endurance training stresses a given joint (e.g., the effect of pounding from running on the knee), then strength training should not further aggravate that.
4. Strength training is an ineffective tool for training maximal oxygen consumption; it does not effectively improve aerobic metabolism in trained athletes. However, it does an excellent job of improving one's anaerobic metabolism and one's tolerance to it. Adjusting the length of the sets and the recovery intervals can be a great way to further enhance these pathways.

part of performing endurance exercise. One who can perform the exercises more efficiently may spare energy stores and move faster than one who cannot.

Training using various modes of exercise within a training program may help increase exercise economy. Increasing an endurance athlete's exercise economy by constantly manipulating the choice of exercise is an important factor as it relates to optimal performance.

Aerobic endurance is affected by maximal oxygen consumption, lactate threshold, fuel utilization, muscle fiber type, and exercise economy.

APPROACHES TO AEROBIC TRAINING

As with other modes of exercise (e.g., strength training, plyometrics, agility training, speed training), there are many methods to train for aerobic endurance and exercises to use.

As with the other modes of exercise, this is made further confusing by a lack of standardization of terms, a lack of science to support some training approaches, and coaching prejudice. This chapter attempts to clear up some of the confusion by grouping the different approaches to endurance training into categories and explaining the advantages and disadvantages of each.

Lack of standardization of terms, lack of scientific support, and coaching prejudice can make it difficult to understand the different approaches to aerobic training.

Several broad approaches to endurance training are considered in this chapter:

1. Continuous training (long slow distance [LSD])
2. Fartlek training
3. Interval training
4. Repetitions
5. Pace/Tempo

Specific modes of exercise are selected to train specific energy systems. Once the mode of exercise is selected, intensity will be determined based on the specific exercise.

CONTINUOUS TRAINING: LSD

Continuous training is designed to increase an athlete's endurance base, maximal oxygen consumption, and tissue respiration capacity (2,7). It is also known as LSD training, overdistance training, and aerobic threshold training (7,8). Typically, continuous training is done for lengths of between 30 minutes and 2 hours at a constant pace (lower intensity than race pace), generally between 60% and 70% of maximal oxygen capacity—also described as conversation pace (8–10). Others recommend basing the training on competition distances. Overdistance training has been recommended to last between two and five times competition distances (11). This approach might be workable for an 800- to 5,000-m athlete, but it would be more difficult for a marathoner. Table 13.1 provides a 12-week sample training program for an experienced female half-marathoner. Table 13.2 provides a 12-week sample program for a 40-year-old man who is a first-time marathon runner.

Some experts recommend a slightly different approach to continuous training (8). The method includes an approach similar to that for interval training but using longer work intervals (see below for more on interval training). Repetitions lasting between 10 minutes and 2 hours are recommended. Each repetition is performed between one and six times at approximately 60% of maximal oxygen consumption, with 1- to 2-minute recovery jogs between repetitions.

There is debate on the usefulness of continuous training for an endurance athlete. In one study, 7 weeks of steady-state pace training (12) improved maximal oxygen consumption in runners by an average of nearly 5 mL · kg^{-1} · min^{-1}, improved 3.22-km run performance by an average of just over a minute, improved the 10-km time by nearly 6 minutes, and improved anaerobic power by nearly 0.5 W · kg^{-1} of body mass. Disadvantages include that this approach may lack specificity, does not develop a sense of race pace, may expose athletes to overuse injuries, and does not stimulate the correct metabolic and physiological adaptations to increase speed (2,7).

Continuous training may lack specificity to many sports and activities and may expose athletes to overuse injuries. It does appear to improve maximal oxygen consumption and performance potential in endurance athletes.

FARTLEK TRAINING

Fartlek is a Swedish word meaning "speed play," and **fartlek training** has been a major training tool of athletic development for decades. The runner alternates between fast, intense running and slower recovery jogs. For example, a runner may jog to the first hill, sprint it up, jog down, run at race pace for a few minutes, etc. Theoretically, fartlek provides the advantages of interval training without the boredom of performing laps on a track or the risks of intense work on hard surfaces (7,10). It also allows the athlete to run at "faster than race pace" for shorter differences which can improve speed and also improve lactate tolerance. One difficulty with traditional fartlek training is that it is more difficult to prescribe specific heart rates and/or exercise intensities due to the intermittent nature of training.

Fartlek training should be hard, continuous, and structured (e.g., run for 1 minute at race pace and then perform a recovery jog for 1 minute, repeat 25 times) (13). Running would be at approximately 70% of maximal oxygen consumption combined with sprints or hill work at approximately 85% to 90% of maximal oxygen consumption for short periods of time. This is usually performed once per week for between 20 and 60 minutes depending on the athlete's competition distances and goals.

INTERVAL TRAINING

Interval training allows for a greater quantity of normally exhaustive exercise to be performed (11). An increase in total work in a given time period can be accomplished as a result of a properly structured interval training program. It has a number of benefits to an endurance athlete. First, it teaches race pace or faster (2). Second, depending upon how the variables are manipulated, it can improve anaerobic metabolism (2,11,14). It can enhance maximal oxygen consumption (2,11,14) and finally it can improve muscular endurance.

Studies performed with highly trained cyclists show that interval training programs improve 40-km time-trial performance, maximal oxygen consumption, peak power output, time to exhaustion at 150% of peak power output, and buffering capacity (15–17). Interval training also improved the running velocity at maximal oxygen consumption and 3,000-m run time in middle-distance runners (18).

TABLE 13.1 ● TWELVE-WEEK SAMPLE PROGRAM FOR HALF-MARATHON ELITE FEMALE RUNNER WITH 12 YEARS OF EXPERIENCE AND A GOAL RACE PACE OF 6.35-MINUTE MILES

Age: 30 y old | Weight: 135 lb

Body Fat: 14% | Height: 5 ft 7 in

VO_{2max}: 58 mL · min^{-1} · kg^{-1}

HR_{max}: 190 bpm

Race Pace Goal: 6.35-min/mi

[a]1-mi warm-up and 1-mi cooldown

WEEK	MONDAY	TUESDAY	WEDNESDAY	THURSDAY	FRIDAY	SATURDAY	SUNDAY
1	Off	Speed work: 6 mi[a] 2 × 600 m + 4 × 800 m W:R 1:1 >52 mL· min^{-1}· kg^{-1} HR_{max}: 162–171 bpm	Recovery run or cross-training (swimming or biking) 30–45 min total: 5 mi if run at <35 mL· min^{-1}. kg^{-1} 95–115 bpm	Fartlek run: 30–45 min Total: 5 mi Easy pace: <40 mL· min^{-1}· kg^{-1} Fast pace: 49–51 mL· min^{-1}· kg^{-1}	Tempo run: 20–30 min[a] Total: 6.5 mi Lactate threshold pace 152–171 bpm	Recovery run or cross-training Total: 4 mi 95–115 bpm 35 mL· min^{-1}· kg^{-1}	LSD 7 mi 35 mL· min^{-1}· kg^{-1} 135–140 bpm
2	Off	Speed work: 6.5 mi[a] 6 × 800 m + 1 × 1,000 m W:R 1:1 >52 mL· min^{-1}· kg^{-1} 162–171 bpm	Recovery run/XT 30–45 min Total: 4–6 mi <35 mL· min^{-1}· kg^{-1} 95–115 bpm	Off	Tempo run: 20–30 min[a] Total: 6–7 mi 46 mL· min^{-1}· kg^{-1} 152–171 bpm	Recovery run/XT 30–45 min Total: 4–6 mi <35 mL· min^{-1}· kg^{-1} 95–115 bpm	LSD 9 mi 35 mL· min^{-1}· kg^{-1} 135–140 bpm
3	Off	Tempo run: 25–35 min[a] Total: 7 mi 46 mL· min^{-1}· kg^{-1} 152–171 bpm	Off	Fartlek Run: 30–45 min Total: 5 mi Easy pace: 40 mL· min^{-1}· kg^{-1} Fast pace: 49–52 mL· min^{-1}· kg^{-1}	Intervals Total: 6–8 mi[a] 3 × 2 min 3 × 2.5 min active recovery W:R 1:1 >52 mL· min^{-1}· kg^{-1} 162–171 bpm	Off	LSD 10 mi 35 mL· min^{-1}· kg^{-1} 135–140 bpm

(Continued)

TABLE 13.1 ● TWELVE-WEEK SAMPLE PROGRAM FOR HALF-MARATHON ELITE FEMALE RUNNER WITH 12 YEARS OF EXPERIENCE AND A GOAL RACE PACE OF 6.35-MINUTE MILES *(Continued)*

WEEK	MONDAY	TUESDAY	WEDNESDAY	THURSDAY	FRIDAY	SATURDAY	SUNDAY
4	Off	Fartlek run: 20–30 min Total: 3 mi Easy pace: 40 mL· min^{-1}· kg^{-1} Fast pace: 49–52 mL· min^{-1}· kg^{-1}	Recovery run/XT 20–30 min Total: 3–4 mi <35 mL· min^{-1}· kg^{-1} 95–115 bpm	Speed work: 4 mi[a] 2 × 800 m + 1 × 1,000 m W:R 1:1 >52.2 mL· min^{-1}· kg^{-1} 162–171 bpm	Off	Recovery run/XT 20–30 min Total: 3–4 mi <35 mL · min^{-1} · kg^{-1} 95–115 bpm	LSD 6 mi 35 mL · min^{-1} · kg^{-1} 135–140 bpm
5	Speed work: 5–6 mi[a] 2 × 800 m + 5 × 1,000 m W:R 1:1 >52 mL · min^{-1}· kg^{-1} 162–171 bpm	Recovery run/ XT 30–45 min Total: 4–5 mi <35 mL· min^{-1}· kg^{-1} 95–115 bpm	Off	Tempo run: 30–40 min[a] Total: 7 mi 46 mL· min^{-1}· kg^{-1} 152–171 bpm	Recovery run/XT 30–45 min Total: 4–5 mi <35 mL · min^{-1} · kg^{-1} 95–115 bpm	LSD 11 mi 35 mL · min^{-1} · kg^{-1} 135–140 bpm	Recovery run/XT 20–30 min Total: 3–4 mi <35 mL · min^{-1} · kg^{-1} 95–115 bpm
6	Off	Speed work: 6–7 mi[a] 2 × 1,000 m + 6 × 1,200 m W:R 1:0.5 >52 mL· min^{-1}· kg^{-1} 162–171 bpm	Recovery run/XT 30–45 min Total: 4–6 mi <35 mL· min^{-1}· kg^{-1} 95–115 bpm	Tempo run: 40 min[a] Total: 8 mi 46 mL· min^{-1}· kg^{-1} 152–171 bpm	Recovery run/XT 30–45 min Total: 4–5 mi <35 mL · min^{-1} · kg^{-1} 95–115 bpm	LSD 12 mi 35 mL · min^{-1} · kg^{-1} 135–140 bpm	Recovery run/XT 20–30 min Total: 3–4 mi <35 mL · min^{-1} · kg^{-1} 95–115 bpm
7	Off	Tempo run: 45 min[a] Total: 8–9 mi 46 mL· min^{-1}·kg^{-1} 152–171 bpm	Recovery run/XT 30–45 min Total: 4–6 mi <35 mL· min^{-1}· kg^{-1} 95–115 bpm	Interval[a] 2 × 2.5 min + 4 × 4 min Active recovery W:R 1:1	Recovery run/XT 30–45 min Total: 4–5 mi <35 mL · min^{-1} · kg^{-1} 95–115 bpm	Off	LSD 13 mi: race simulation 7 mi @ 135–140 bpm/35 mL · min^{-1} · kg^{-1} 6 mi @ race pace 6.35 mi / h^{-1}
8	Off	Tempo run: 20–25 min[a] Total: 4–5 mi 46 mL· min^{-1}· kg^{-1} 152–171 bpm	Recovery run 20–30 min Total: 3–4 mi <35 mL· min^{-1}· kg^{-1} 95–115 bpm	Speed work: 3–4 mi[a] 2 × 1,000 m + 1 × 1,500 m W:R 1:0.5 >52 mL· min^{-1}· kg^{-1} 162–171 bpm	Off	LSD 8 mi 35 mL · min^{-1} · kg^{-1} 135–140 bpm	Off

9	Speed work: 6–7 mi[a] 1 × 800 m + 2 × 1,000 m+ 2 × 1,200 m + 1 × 1,500 m W:R 1:1 >52 mL · min^{-1} · kg^{-1} 162–171 bpm	Recovery run/XT 30–45 min Total: 4–6 mi <35 mL · min^{-1} · kg^{-1} 95–115 bpm	Off	Tempo run: 40 min[a] Total: 8 mi 46 mL · min^{-1} · kg^{-1} 152–171 bpm	Recovery run/XT 30–45 min Total: 4–5 mi <35 mL · min^{-1} · kg^{-1} 95–115 bpm	LSD 14 mi 35 mL · min^{-1} · kg^{-1} 135–140 bpm	Recovery run 30–45 min <35 mL · min^{-1} · kg^{-1} 95–115 bpm
10	Off	Speed work: 6–7 mi[a] 2 × 800 m + 3 × 1,200 m + 1 × 1,500 m W:R 1:1 >52 mL · min^{-1} · kg^{-1} 162–171 bpm	Recovery run/XT 30–45 min Total: 4–6 mi <35 mL · min^{-1} · kg^{-1} 95–115 bpm	Tempo run: 45 min[a] Total: 8–9 mi 46 mL · min^{-1} · kg^{-1} 152–171 bpm	Recovery run/XT 30–45 min Total: 4–5 mi <35 mL · min^{-1} · kg^{-1} 95–115 bpm	LSD 15 mi 35 mL · min^{-1} · kg^{-1} 135–140 bpm	Recovery run 30–45 min <35 mL · min^{-1} · kg^{-1} 95–115 bpm
11	Off	Speed work: 5–6 mi[a] 1 × 800 m + 2 × 1,000 m + 2 × 1,500 m W:R 1:1 >52 mL · min^{-1} · kg^{-1} 162–171 bpm	Recovery run 30–45 min Total: 4–6 mi <35 mL · min^{-1} · kg^{-1} 95–115 bpm	Tempo run: 45 min[a] Total: 8–9 mi 46 mL · min^{-1} · kg^{-1} 152–171 bpm	Recovery run/XT 30–45 min Total: 4–6 mi <35 mL · min^{-1} · kg^{-1} 95–115 bpm	LSD 13 mi: race simulation 5 mi 135–140 bpm/8 mi @ 6.35 mi · h^{-1}	Off
12	Recovery run 30–45 min Total: 4–6 mi <35 mL · min^{-1} · kg^{-1} 95–115 bpm	Speed work: 3–4 mi[a] 1 × 800 m + 1 × 1,200 m W:R 1:1 >52 mL · min^{-1} · kg^{-1} 162–171 bpm	Recovery run 20–30 min Total: 3–4 mi <35 mL · min^{-1} · kg^{-1} 95–115 bpm	Tempo run: 15–20 min[a] Total: 4 mi 46 mL · min^{-1} · kg^{-1} 152–171 bpm	Easy jog 20 min <35 mL · min^{-1} · kg^{-1} 95–115 bpm	Off	Race Time !!!!!!!!!!!!!!!!!!!!!!!1

TABLE 13.2 ● TWELVE-WEEK SAMPLE PROGRAM FOR A 40-YEAR-OLD MALE FIRST-TIME MARATHON RUNNER AND A GOAL RACE PACE OF 9-MINUTE MILES.

Sex: Male
Age: 40 y old
Body fat %: 19
Height: 6 ft 1 in
Weight: 170 lb
Race pace goal: 9-min mi
VO_{2max}: 45 mL · min^{-1} · kg^{-1}
HR_{max}: 180 bpm

XT: Cross-training: swimming or biking

First-timer: this athlete has been running consistently for the past 3 mo between 10 and 15 mi · wk^{-1}

WEEK	MONDAY	TUESDAY	WEDNESDAY	THURSDAY	FRIDAY	SATURDAY	SUNDAY
1	Off	4 mi 25–30 mL · min^{-1} · kg^{-1} 120–130 bpm	XT: 30 min	4 mi 25–30 mL · min^{-1} · kg^{-1} 120–130 bpm	Off	4 mi 25–30 mL · min^{-1} · kg^{-1} 120–130 bpm	LSD 6 mi 25–30 mL · min^{-1} · kg^{-1} 120–130 bpm
2	Off	4 mi 25–30 mL · min^{-1} · kg^{-1} 120–130 bpm	XT: 30 min	Fartlek: 5 mi Easy: 90–100 bpm Hard: 145–155 bpm	Off	4 mi 25–30 mL · min^{-1} · kg^{-1} 120–130 bpm	LSD 7 mi 25–30 mL · min^{-1} · kg^{-1} 120–130 bpm
3	XT: 30 min	5 mi 25–30 mL · min^{-1} · kg^{-1} 120–130 bpm	Off	Fartlek: 5 mi Easy: 90–100 bpm Hard: 145–155 bpm	XT: 30–45 min	4 mi 25–30 mL · min^{-1} · kg^{-1} 120–130 bpm	LSD 9 mi 25–30 mL · min^{-1} · kg^{-1} 120–130 bpm
4	Off	3 mi 25–30 mL · min^{-1} · kg^{-1} 120–130 bpm	Off	Fartlek: 3 mi Easy: 90–100 bpm Hard: 145–155 bpm	Off	3 mi 25–30 mL · min^{-1} · kg^{-1} 120–130 bpm	LSD 6 mi 25–30 mL · min^{-1} · kg^{-1} 120–130 bpm
5	XT: 30–45 min	5-mi intervals[a] 2 × 1 min + 2 × 2 min @ 150–160 bpm/33–40 mL · min^{-1} · kg^{-1}	Off	Fartlek: 6 mi Same as above	XT: 30–45 min	6 mi 25–30 mL · min^{-1} · kg^{-1} 120–130 bpm	LSD 11 mi 25–30 mL · min^{-1} · kg^{-1} 120–130 bpm
6	Off	6-mi intervals[a] 2 × 2 min + 1 × 3 min @ 150–160 bpm/33–40 mL · min^{-1} · kg^{-1}	XT: 30–45 min	Tempo run: 20 min[a] + 2 mi 36 mL · min^{-1} · kg^{-1} 145–162 bpm	Off	6 mi 25–30 mL · min^{-1} · kg^{-1} 120–130 bpm	LSD 13 mi 25–30 mL · min^{-1} · kg^{-1} 120–130 bpm

7	Off	8-mi intervals[a] 3 × 2 min + 2 × 3 min @ 150–160 bpm/33–40 $mL \cdot min^{-1} \cdot kg^{-1}$	XT: 30–45 min	8 mi: 4-mi Fartlek	Off	7 mi 120–130 bpm	LSD 25–30 $mL \cdot min^{-1} \cdot kg^{-1}$ 25–30 $mL \cdot min^{-1} \cdot kg^{-1}$ 120–130 bpm
8	Off	5 mi intervals[a] 2 × 2 min + 1 × 3 min	XT: 30–45 min	6 mi 25–30 $mL \cdot min^{-1} \cdot kg^{-1}$ 120–130 bpm	Off	4 mi: 2 mi Tempo run 36 $mL \cdot min^{-1} \cdot kg^{-1}$ 145/162 bpm	LSD 11 mi 25–30 $mL \cdot min^{-1} \cdot kg^{-1}$ 120–130 bpm
9	Off	Speed work: Total: 6 mi[a] 1 × 800 + 2 × 1,000 + 1 × 1,200 34–40 $mL \cdot min^{-1} \cdot kg^{-1}$ 153–162 bpm (add 2-mi warm-up/ cooldown)	XT: 30–45 min	Tempo run: 20–30 min[a] +2 mi @ LSD intensity	8 mi 25–30 $mL \cdot min^{-1} \cdot kg^{-1}$ 120–130 bpm	Off	LSD 17 mi 25–30 $mL \cdot min^{-1} \cdot kg^{-1}$ 120–130 bpm
10	Off	Speed work: total: 7 mi[a] 1 × 800 m + 3 × 1,000 m + 1 × 1,200 m 34–40 $mL \cdot min^{-1} \cdot kg^{-1}$ 153–162 bpm (add 2.5-mi warm-up/ cooldown)	XT: 30–45 min +3 mi LSD intensity	Tempo run: 30 min[a] 25–30 $mL \cdot min^{-1} \cdot kg^{-1}$	9 mi 120–130 bpm	Off 20 mi	LSD 25–30 $mL \cdot min^{-1} \cdot kg^{-1}$ 120–130 bpm
11	Off	Speed work: total: 5 mi[a] 1 × 1,000 m + 2 × 1,200 m + 1 × 800 m 34–40 $mL \cdot min^{-1} \cdot kg^{-1}$ 153–162 bpm	Off 36 $mL \cdot min^{-1} \cdot kg^{-1}$	Tempo run: 20 min[a] 25–30 $mL \cdot min^{-1} \cdot kg^{-1}$ 145–162 bpm	6 mi 120–130 bpm	Off 14 mi	LSD 25–30 $mL \cdot min^{-1} \cdot kg^{-1}$ 120–130 bpm
12	Off	3 mi 2 × 2 min at 9-min mi pace	Off	4 mi 25–30 $mL \cdot min^{-1} \cdot kg^{-1}$ 120–130 bpm	Off	Off or run 2 mi 25–30 $mL \cdot min^{-1} \cdot kg^{-1}$ 120–130 bpm	Race day!!!!!

Several variables can be manipulated during interval training:

- The intensity of the exercise
- The duration of the exercise interval
- The length of the recovery
- The number of repetitions of the exercise–recovery interval

Intensity of the Exercise

Obviously, the intensity of the exercise interval will affect the workout's total volume. It will also affect the rest of the week's workouts (i.e., more intense exercise sessions will require more days of rest or less intense workouts). Intense interval training can result in a dramatic reduction in muscle glycogen concentration, an increase in muscle lactate concentrations, and a decrease in pH (more acidic environment). In one study, seven highly trained cyclists (mean maximal oxygen consumption of 5.14 L · min^{-1}) performed eight intervals on an ergometer (19). Each interval, lasted 5 minutes, was performed at 86% of maximal oxygen consumption and was followed by 60 seconds of active recovery. After the last interval, resting muscle glycogen concentrations had decreased by more than 50%. Muscle lactate had increased by nearly 500% and pH had dropped noticeably (19).

Recommendations for the intensity of an interval session vary. Some authors use maximal oxygen consumption as the determinant of exercise intensity. They recommend anywhere from 75% to close to 90% of maximal oxygen consumption (20,21). In addition to the wide variability of suggested exercise intensities, the other drawback to this approach is that one must know the maximal oxygen consumption (and the running, cycling, or swimming pace at which it occurs) for the athlete. Although useful, this may not be practical or possible in every athletic training situation.

The distance of the interval to be run and the athlete's best time for that interval distance represent another noninvasive way to determine interval intensity. For example, interval training guidelines are determined by one's best time running a given distance. If intervals are performed for 200 yd, one would add between 10% and 40% to the best time at that distance and run the intervals with the new time. This may be a more practical way to determine interval intensities than basing them on maximal oxygen consumption.

Duration of the Exercise Interval

The duration of the exercise interval will be dictated by the goals of the training and sometimes by the distance to be covered in the race. Interval training can be organized around targeting specific energy systems (7,22). We know that up to about the first 6 seconds of exercise will be fueled primarily by ATP and CP. Up to about 2 minutes will be primarily fueled by glycogen, and if exercise is intense enough, lactic acid will be produced. After 2 to 3 minutes of exercise, oxygen will be used to break down glycogen and other energy stores that are used as the major fuel source.

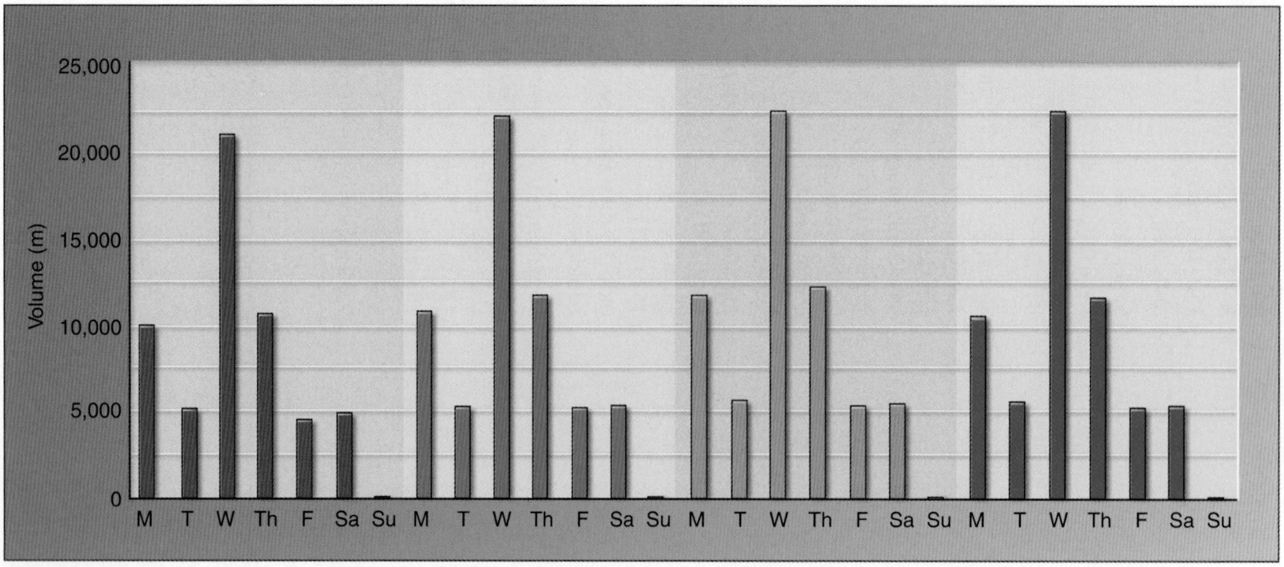

FIGURE 13.2 Preparation phase. Running volume in meters over 4 weeks. Note that the total volume gradually increases during weeks 1, 2, and 3; total volume then decreases during week 4.

Q & A from the Field

Q The university has had a successful cross-country team for the last several years. Recently I've been put in charge of designing their workouts. I understand how to incorporate the different types of endurance training, but I'm having trouble figuring out how to balance out the hard and easy days. How do I go about determining all that?

—Graduate assistant coach

A This can be a confusing topic for any strength and conditioning professional. First, determine when the competitions are; this will dictate the training calendar. The period around the competitions will be your competition phase. This period will see the most intense training. The remaining time will be divided between preparation and precompetition. The precompetition phase usually lasts 4 weeks and consists of training of increasing intensity. Preparation should ideally make up the bulk of the training; with low to moderate intensity (intensity should increase over time). Figure 3.2 shows a sample running program in the preparation phase with the volume gradually increasing in weeks 1 through 3 and decreasing slightly in week 4 to allow the athlete to recover.

Once the rough calendar has been determined, break each phase into 4-week cycles. The easiest way to do this is to have a 3:1 approach (i.e., intensity increases for the first 3 weeks, then week 4 is a recovery week). This would mean that week 2 is more difficult than week 1, week 3 is more difficult than week 2, and week 4 is less difficult than week 2 (though slightly more difficult than week 1).

Within a 4-week cycle, decide on the intensity levels for each week. They may be high-intensity (i.e., three peaks), medium-intensity (i.e., two peaks), or low-intensity (i.e., one peak) work. Remember that a race always counts as a peak. In general, the weeks in the competition phase will consist of high-intensity weeks; the rest of the training time (preparation and precompetition) will consist primarily of low- and medium-intensity weeks, with a few high-intensity weeks thrown in.

Once you've determined how many peaks a week will have, organize the training week around the peaks as described in Figure 13.3 (p. 316).

In summary, to help determine how to balance our hard and easy days may take several steps:

1. Determine when the competitions are.
2. Divide up the calendar into competition, precompetition, and preparation phases.
3. Break each phase into 4-week cycles.
4. Decide upon an intensity for each week within a 4-week cycle.
5. Distribute the peaks according to the guidelines laid out in this chapter.

Length of Recovery

If the duration of the interval can affect what energy system the interval trains, the length of the recovery can affect how that energy system is trained and how it adapts. For example, if one wants to increase an athlete's tolerance to lactic acid, then intervals would last up to 2 to 3 minutes and would limit recovery times. This would result in the lactic acid accumulating in the muscles. If, however, the goal is to perform each repetition as close to maximum as possible, the athlete's ability is enhanced to remove lactic acid; intense intervals lasting up to 2 to 3 minutes would still be used, but complete recovery between intervals would be allowed.

Recovery times should also be driven by exercise intensity. Some recommendations more than double the amount of recovery time between intervals in moving from an intensity of 80% of maximal oxygen consumption to 90% (from 90–120 seconds to 120–300 seconds) (21). Unless the goal is to get the athlete used to functioning with high levels of lactic acid, recovery times must be increased as intensity increases.

Number of Repetitions

There are a number of approaches to calculating the number of repetitions (or total volume) of the interval training sessions. Workout volume can be based on the length of the athlete's competitive

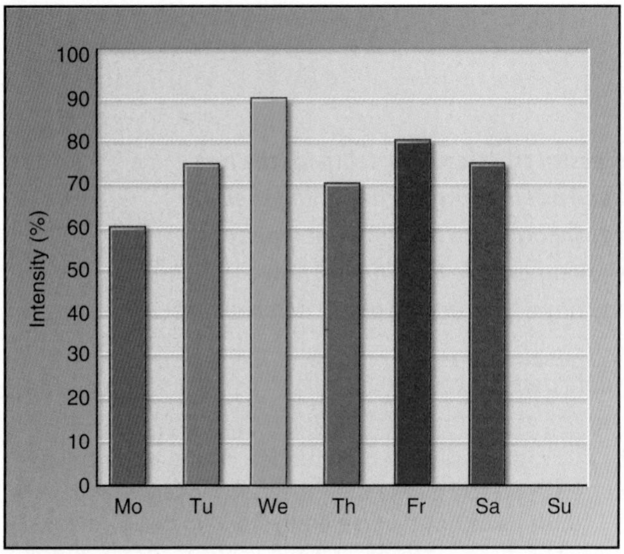

A

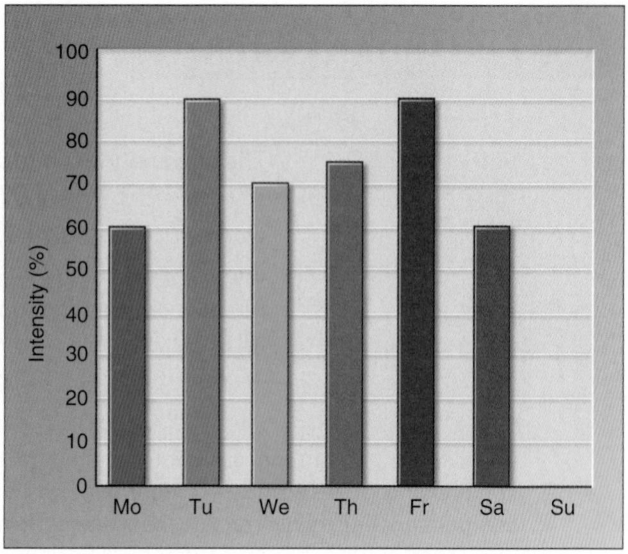

B

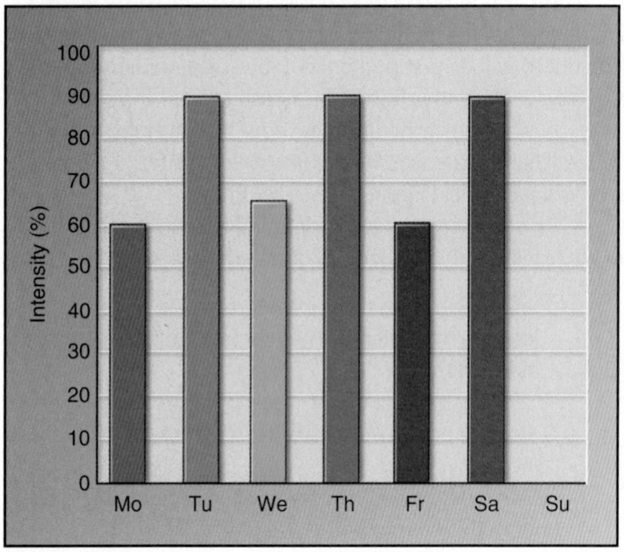

C

FIGURE 13.3 Examples of workouts with different numbers of peaks. **A.** Week with one peak. **B.** Week with two peaks. **C.** Week with three peaks.

distance, with the workout's volume equaling between one and three times the competitive distance (2). For example, an 800-m runner would perform between 800 and 2,400 m of intervals in a workout. One must be careful with a guideline like this, as it will not serve a long-distance athlete such as a marathoner well as they may require greater volume.

Intensity and volume of training are inversely related. If the intensity of the exercise is high, the volume will be lower.

A second method is to base volume on the intensity at which the intervals will be run. As intensity increases, total workout volume would decrease. For example, it has been recommended to cut the volume of 2,000-m intervals from 12,000–16,000 m to 6,000–12,000 m per workout when intensity increases from <85% to >85% (21).

A final method is to determine volume by fatigue. Using this method, it is recommended that intervals be run until the athlete's heart rate is >120 bpm after 2 minutes of recovery (20). This is a simple, "field-friendly" way to determine exercise volume, but it fails to take into account individual ages, heart rate responses to exercise, etc. However, it clearly highlights that the athlete is not recovered.

When it comes to interval training, remember that it is extremely demanding on the athlete and that the athlete is going to need a fitness base before engaging in it. Engaging in this type of training before the athlete's running form is consistent, endurance base is built up, and muscles/skeleton/connective tissue are ready will lead to a greater likelihood of injury and/or burnout.

Interval training appears to be an effective way to target an athlete's deficiencies, but it is extremely demanding and requires a solid fitness base before this training activity is initiated.

Repetitions

Repetitions are a more intense version of interval training. Repetitions are performed at a faster pace with complete recovery between bouts (7). They are designed to increase speed as well as both the capacity for and the tolerance of anaerobic metabolism. Generally, repetitions are defined in the literature as being of high intensity, 90% of maximal oxygen consumption and above, with complete recovery between repetitions (7,21).

Repetitions are generally performed for 30- to 90-second bouts, with a work:rest ratio of around 1:5. For example, if an athlete performed a 30-second bout at 90% of maximal oxygen consumption, he or she would then perform low-intensity recovery work for 150 seconds. The workout approach just described would be ideal for cyclists, swimmers, recreational endurance athletes, and other athletes looking to improve their speed.

More concrete recommendations regarding repetitions and training for distance runners can be used (21). For example, a 5-km runner should have a total volume of repetitions between 3,300 and 7,500 m per workout session. Long-distance runners should cover one-tenth, one-fifth, or one-third the total racing distance in each repetition workout. Recovery times would range from 5 to 30 minutes (21).

Tapering

Tapering is a crucial component of any training program as endurance athletes get ready for important competitions. Taper is defined as a period of decreased training volume and increased training intensity that takes place prior to a competition. It is important for the strength and conditioning coach to implement a taper into endurance athletes' programs to achieve peak performances for competitions (23).

In designing a taper, strength and conditioning coaches need to take into consideration the volume of the training program. It has been showed that those athletes who train fewer than 4 hours a week will not benefit from a 1 to 2 weeks taper; instead just 2 days of tapering prior to race will be sufficient (23). As any other program design, strength and conditioning coaches need to consider which races are important and which ones are not (training races).

1. Different types of tapers can be included into an endurance program in order to achieve peak performance. There are three broad types of taper: minor, moderate, and major. Minor tapers are used with races that are not qualifiers and allow the athlete to train as planned and will require from 1 to 5 days depending on the volume of training (24,25). Moderate tapers are used for those races that are qualifiers and will require from 3 to 14 days of taper, also depending on the volume of training (23). And last, major tapers are done only once a year for the most important event and will require from 7 to 21–30 days (23). It has been concluded that progressively decreasing the volume by 60% to 90% during a major taper will improve performance and allow the athlete to feel fresh and not burned out prior to racing (26). As a conclusion, tapering needs to be included into endurance athletes' training programs in order to improve results and prevent early fatigue during competitions.

The length of the recovery period will be determined based on the intensity and volume. If the intensity is high, the athlete will need a longer rest period to recover. If the intensity is lower, the recovery time will decrease.

Now that we've reviewed the different approaches to training used with endurance athletes, we can consider how the different approaches fit together in an athlete's personalized program design.

ORGANIZING AEROBIC EXERCISE TRAINING

The rest of this chapter provides basic principles to help with the program design process. It then offers a sample training program to illustrate the application of these principles. Table 13.3 provides a 12-week sample program for a male Olympic distance triathlon runner with 5 years of experience. Key principles include the following:

1. Warm up properly (see Chapter 9). In recent years, methods of warming up have been reassessed by conditioning professionals. In the past, an endurance athlete would start out slowly for 5 to 10 minutes, breaking a light sweat, and then stretch for another 5 to 10 minutes, and finally would ease into the workout, gradually picking up speed and intensity. Although starting out slowly for the first 5 to 10 minutes is important (it moves blood into the muscles, warms joints to be trained, and raises heart rate gradually), today the thinking is that static stretching performed before a workout session is counterproductive (27)—see Chapter 9. One option is to perform active activity-specific flexibility exercises (such as leg swings, high knee exercises) for 10 to 30 minutes before the actual workout. Drills can become gradually faster and more intense as the athlete progresses through the warm-up, allowing him or her to begin the workout at full speed (Table 13.4).
2. Balance the light, medium, and heavy days. It is highly recommended to alter hard and easy days (7,28). Obviously, races or competitions will alter training weeks. The 2 days before a competition are typically low-intensity days (28). Low-intensity training days typically take the form of lower intensity 30- to 40-minute efforts (20).
   a. One intense workout per week: This should be sc heduled toward the middle of the week (e.g., Wednesday or Thursday).
   b. Two intense workouts per week: Separate the intense workouts with 1 or 2 less intense days in between (e.g., higher intensity workouts on Tuesday and Friday, Wednesday and Saturday).
   c. Three intense workouts per week: Separate the intense workouts with low-intensity days (e.g., higher intensity workouts on Tuesday, Thursday, and Saturday).
3. Establish a fitness base first. Most endurance programs focus on continuous training and fartlek training for the first part of the training year. This is to give the athlete's muscles, joints, and skeleton a chance to adapt to training as well as to build up the athlete's cardiovascular system (8,28). Training volume should be increased by no more than 5% to 10% per week (28). Any more than such an increase could result in overuse injuries and burnout, and less might not promote maximal physiological development. For example, an athlete running a total weekly volume of 30 mi $\cdot$ wk^{-1} in the first week of training should move up to only 31.5 to 33 mi$\cdot$wk^{-1} in the second week.
4. Determine weak points and deficiencies and train them. As with every other sport, it's important to determine what is limiting an athlete's performance and target it through training. For example, intervals can be used to get an athlete used to tolerating lactic acid or recovering from it.
5. Don't neglect resistance training. Resistance training is often overlooked by endurance athletes. It's important for preventing injuries and for improving the ability to exert force. Resistance training does not have to be all weight-room training; it can take the form of calisthenics, hill running, medicine ball work, etc.

In designing an aerobic exercise training program, keep the following factors in mind: warm up properly, balance the hard and easy days, establish a fitness base first, determine weak points and then train them, and don't neglect resistance training.

Although there is research showing that each type of endurance training is effective, most of that is focused on one type of training (15–18). The effect of different types of endurance training on performance in collegiate cross-country runners has been evaluated (29). The study surveyed the training of 14 division I cross-country teams that qualified for NCAA Cross-Country Nationals and

TABLE 13.3 ● TWELVE-WEEK SAMPLE PROGRAM FOR A MALE OLYMPIC DISTANCE TRIATHLON RUNNER WITH 5 YEARS OF TRIATHLON EXPERIENCE AND A RACE GOAL TIME OF 38 MINUTES AND 45 SECONDS.

Sex: Male

Age: 35 y old

Height: 5 ft 9 in

Weight: 165 lb

Body fat %: 8

$\dot{V}O_{2max}$: 55 mL · min^{-1} · kg^{-1}

HR_{max}: 185 bpm

History: Triathlete who has 5 y of experience. This athlete was a high school cross-country team member. He continued to run until he discovered triathlons and he decided to start competing and training consistently.

Record time: 6.2 mi in Olympic triathlon race: 39 min 30 s

Race pace goal for Race A Olympic triathlon race: 38 min 45 s

[a]Workout consists of 1-mi warm-up and 1-mi cooldown

WEEK	MONDAY	TUESDAY	WEDNESDAY	THURSDAY	FRIDAY	SATURDAY	SUNDAY
1	X/T	4 mi 36–38 mL · min^{-1} · kg^{-1} 120–138 bpm	X/T	Tempo run[a]: 20 min 44–46 mL · min^{-1} · kg^{-1} 160–165 bpm 5–6 mi	X/T	LSD 6 mi 32–34 mL · min^{-1} · kg^{-1} 130–140 bpm	X/T
2	X/T	4 mi 36–38 mL · min^{-1} · kg^{-1} 120–138 bpm	X/T	Tempo run[a]: 20 min Total: 5–6 mi 44–46 mL · min^{-1} · kg^{-1} 160–165 bpm	X/T	LSD 7 mi 32–34 mL · min^{-1} · kg^{-1} 130–140 bpm	X/T
3	X/T	5 mi 36–38 mL · min^{-1} · kg^{-1} 120–138 bpm	X/T	Tempo run[a]: 20 min Total: 5–6 mi 44–46 mL · min^{-1} · kg^{-1} 160–165 bpm	X/T	LSD 8 mi 32–34 mL · min^{-1} · kg^{-1} 130–140 bpm	X/T
4	X/T	3 mi 36–38 mL · min^{-1} · kg^{-1} 120–138 bpm	X/T	Tempo run[a]: 15 min Total: 4 mi 44–46 mL · min^{-1} · kg^{-1} 160–165 bpm	X/T	LSD 5 mi 32–34 mL · min^{-1} · kg^{-1} 130–140 bpm	X/T

(Continued)

TABLE 13.3 ● TWELVE-WEEK SAMPLE PROGRAM FOR A MALE OLYMPIC DISTANCE TRIATHLON RUNNER WITH 5 YEARS OF TRIATHLON EXPERIENCE AND A RACE GOAL TIME OF 38 MINUTES AND 45 SECONDS. *(Continued)*

WEEK	MONDAY	TUESDAY	WEDNESDAY	THURSDAY	FRIDAY	SATURDAY	SUNDAY
5	X/T	Speed work[a] Total: 5 mi 1 × 400 m + 2 × 800 m + 1 × 1,000 m + 1 × 400 m W:R 1:1 41–49 $mL \cdot min^{-1} \cdot kg^{-1}$ 155–165 bpm	X/T	Tempo run[a]: 25-min Total: 6–7 mi 44–46 $mL \cdot min^{-1} \cdot kg^{-1}$ 160–165 bpm	X/T	LSD 9 mi 32–34 $mL \cdot min^{-1} \cdot kg^{-1}$ 130–140 bpm	X/T
6	X/T	Speed work[a] Total: 5 mi 2 × 400 m + 4 × 800 m + 1 × 1,000 m W:R 1:0.5 active recovery 41–49 $mL \cdot min^{-1} \cdot kg^{-1}$ 155–165 bpm	X/T	Hill repeats[a] Total: 6–7 mi 6%–8% incline 4 × 3–4 min 2 mi at LSD pace W:R 1:1 41–49 $mL \cdot min^{-1} \cdot kg^{-1}$ 155–165 bpm	X/T	Race simulation 3 mi LSD pace 4 mi at 6.20 pace 3 mi LSD pace	X/T
7	X/T	Tempo run[a]: 25–30 min Total: 6–7 mi 44–46 $mL \cdot min^{-1} \cdot kg^{-1}$ 160–165 bpm	X/T	Intervals[a] Total: 6–7 mi 4 × 4 min	Off	LSD 11 mi 32–34 $mL \cdot min^{-1} \cdot kg^{-1}$ 130–140 bpm	X/T
8	X/T	Speed work[a] Total: 4–5 mi 1 × 400 m + 2 × 800 m + 1 × 1,000 m W:R 1:0.5 41–49 $mL \cdot min^{-1} \cdot kg^{-1}$ 155–165 bpm	X/T	Tempo run[a]: 15–20 min Total: 3–4 mi 44–46 $mL \cdot min^{-1} \cdot kg^{-1}$ 160–165 bpm	Off	LSD 8 mi 32–34 $mL \cdot min^{-1} \cdot kg^{-1}$ 130–140 bpm	X/T
9	X/T	Tempo run[a]: 25–30 min Total: 6–7 mi 44–46 $mL \cdot min^{-1} \cdot kg^{-1}$ 160–165 bpm	X/T	Speed/hill run[a] Total: 6–7 mi 1 × 400 m + 1 × 800 m + 6%–8% incline hill: 4 × 4 min 2 mi easy W:R 1:1 41–49 $mL \cdot min^{-1} \cdot kg^{-1}$ 155–165 bpm	Off	LSD 12 mi 32–34 $mL \cdot min^{-1} \cdot kg^{-1}$ 130–140 bpm	X/T

10	X/T	Speed work[a] Total: 6 mi 1 × 400 m + 1 × 800 m + 3 × 1,000 m + 1 × 1,200 m W:R 1:0.5 41–49 mL · min^{-1} · kg^{-1} 160–165 bpm	X/T	Tempo run[a]: 30–35 min Total: 8–9 mi Add 3 mi easy recovery 44–46 mL · min^{-1} · kg^{-1} 160–165 bpm	Off	LSD 13 mi 32–34 mL · min^{-1} · kg^{-1} 130–140 bpm	X/T
11	X/T	Hill run[a] (6%–8% incline) Total:7–8 mi 5 × 5 min Add 3 easy recovery mi W:R 1:1 41–49 mL · min^{-1} · kg^{-1} 155–165 bpm	X/T	Interval run[a] Total: 6–7 mi 3 × 3-min race pace 3 × 2-min race pace W:R 1:0.5 active recovery Add 2 mi easy recovery 44–46 mL · min^{-1} · kg^{-1} 160–165 bpm	Off	LSD 10 mi 32–34 mL · min^{-1} · kg^{-1} 130–140 bpm	
12	X/T	Speed work[a] Total: 4 mi 1 × 800 m + 1 × 1,000 m + 1 × 1,200 m W:R 1:0.5 active recovery 41–49 mL · min^{-1} · kg^{-1} 160–165 bpm	X/T	Interval run[a] Total: 3–4 mi 3 × 2-min race pace 1 × 3-min race pace W:R 1:0.5 active recovery 44–46 mL · min^{-1} · kg^{-1} 160–165 bpm	Off	Easy run: 2 mi Bike: 5 mi Swim: 600 yd	Olympic distance triathlon time!!!

TABLE 13.4 ● EXAMPLE OF A WARM-UP FOR A RUNNER

EXERCISE	REPETITION/DURATION	SETS	REST
Jog	800 m	1	Walking recovery
Leg swings, front/back	10 each leg	2	Jog 20 m after each set
Leg swings, side/side	10 each leg	2	Jog 20 m after each set
Hip circles	10 each leg	2	Jog 20 m after each set
Eagles[a]	10 each leg	2	Jog 20 m after each set
Stomach eagles	10 each leg	2	Jog 20 m after each set
Forward lunges	20 m	2	Jog 20 m after each set
Backward lunges	20 m	2	Sprint 20 m after each set
Inchworms[b]	20 m	2	Sprint 20 m after each set
High knee walks	20 m	2	Sprint 20 m after each set
High knee skips	20 m	2	Sprint 20 m after each skip
Stride-length runs	Sprint 20 m, set sticks up at 80% of stride length beginning at the 20-m mark, perform drill for 40–60 m	2	Walking recovery

[a]Eagles are performed with the athlete lying supine, arms stretched out to the sides. Keeping the right leg straight, the athlete attempts to lift the right leg across the body until it touches the left hand. This should be repeated with the left leg. Repeat for the desired number of repetitions.
[b]Inchworms start in the push-up position. Athlete will keep the legs as straight as possible while attempting to walk the feet up to the hands. When the feet reach the hands, the athlete should walk the hands out until he or she is again in the push-up position. Repeat for the desired distance.

16 division I cross-country teams that did not qualify. Training was broken down into three phases; May to August (transition), August to October (competition), and November (peak). Nationals were in November.

Endurance training modes were divided into interval, tempo, repetition, hill, and fartlek. Note that the modes had slightly different definitions than those given in this chapter (29).

In the transition phase, those teams that qualified for the Nationals had more days of rest and used cross-training more than nonqualifiers. They also found a positive correlation between performing tempo runs, repetitions, intervals, fartlek, and twice-per-day training and team performance (i.e., the more those training modes were used, the slower the team's mean 10-km time) (29).

During the competition phase, the qualifying teams ran more speed work and had higher mileage than the nonqualifying teams. A positive correlation was found between mean team time with running intervals and mean team time with fartlek training during the competition phase. The more interval running and fartlek training were used, the slower the team's mean 10-km time (29).

During the peak phase, the more intervals a team used, the higher its placing was (29). These results may be limited because they were based on the self-reporting of the various coaches.

This study suggests a number of interesting possibilities. First, the extensive use of intervals during transition and competition phases may be too intense. Second, fartlek training may not be structured and difficult enough to produce training adaptations. Finally, twice-daily training, or at least excessive amounts of training, can result in overtraining, which could have a negative impact on performance. Its applications to other situations are limited at best. However, the study does demonstrate that this type of research is possible and could be done in other athletic situations.

Summary

Successful training and competition in aerobic activities depend on the interaction of a number of factors, including age, training status, maximal oxygen consumption, lactate threshold, fuel utilization, muscle fiber types, and exercise economy. There are many approaches to training to improve aerobic performance, each of which seeks to develop one or more of the factors that limit performance. Each of these approaches has advantages and limitations that must be carefully thought out during the planning of an athlete's training. As with all physical training, each individual athlete will need different training plans based on his or her goals, strengths, and weaknesses.

Maxing Out

1. A track coach comes to you and wants to determine the distances for continuous training sessions for 800-m runners. If you were to base those distances on the length of the race, how long should the continuous runs be?
2. A high school cross-country coach is trying to determine the duration, recovery time, and number of intervals for her high school athletes. What are the different ways presented in this chapter for determining this information? Which one would be the most appropriate for the coach's situation?
3. A recreational 5-km runner is having trouble with her warm-ups. She complains of feeling sluggish and has been having hamstring trouble during her runs. Her warm-ups currently consist of stretching for 5 minutes and then beginning her run, gradually increasing her pace over the first mile. List some things that can be modified in her warm-up to improve its effectiveness.

CASE EXAMPLE

Designing Continuous, Interval, and Repetition Training Programs for a Recreational Cyclist

BACKGROUND

You are employed as a personal trainer and hired by a recreational cyclist who wants to compete in a 20-mi race in 16 weeks. This individual has been cycling for 3 years recreationally and can easily complete the 20 mi; however, she would like to improve her speed and does not know how to go about doing so. Apply the guidelines presented in this chapter to design a 16-week-long workout program, training three times per week, to improve her performance in a 20-mi race.

RECOMMENDATIONS/CONSIDERATIONS

We have 16 weeks. Starting backward from the competition, the 4 weeks prior (which we'll designate weeks 1 through 4, week 1 being the week of competition) will be our competition phase and will consist of the most intense workouts (intervals and repetitions, some continuous work). Weeks 5 through 8 will be a peaking phase and will see the gradual integration of high-intensity workouts (continuous work and intervals). Weeks 9 through 16 will be our preparation phase and will primarily consist of low- and medium-intensity workouts, mostly continuous work.

IMPLEMENTATION

Preparation Phase Our athlete will train three times per week: Tuesdays, Thursdays, and Saturdays. Bowing to reality, the longest ride of the week will occur on Saturday (i.e., Saturdays will be the peak). On Tuesdays there will be a shorter ride at approximately 60% effort. On Thursdays there will be a moderate ride at 60% to 70% effort. On week 16 (i.e., the first week of training), the longest training session will be performed at the race distance (i.e., 20 mi); Tuesday's workout will be conducted at 50% of Saturday's distance (i.e., 10 mi); Thursday's workout will be conducted at 75% of Saturday's distance (i.e., 15 mi). Volume will be increased for the following weeks: 15, 14, 12, 11, and 10. Volume will be increased by 5% in each of these weeks. Weeks 13 and 9 will serve as recovery weeks; volume for these weeks will be equal to that for weeks 15 and 11. This means that by week 10, the distances for each day will be

CASE EXAMPLE

Designing Continuous, Interval, and Repetition Training Programs for a Recreational Cyclist

Tuesday: 12.1 mi
Thursday: 18.15 mi
Saturday: 24.2 mi

Peaking Phase Our athlete will continue training three times per week. Beginning with this phase, Thursday will become the peak and will consist of interval training. Saturday will remain the long day, with Tuesday as a recovery ride. Saturday's distances will never increase over 24.2 mi. Interval training will be designed initially to improve our athlete's ability to recover from lactic acid. As she is not an elite athlete, intensity will be 75%. Intervals will last 3 minutes. Since we're targeting recovery, she will achieve close to full recovery between intervals (i.e., 2 minutes of slow riding between each interval).

Week 8 will see long-ride volumes equal to that of week 12; this step back is being taken because of the addition of the intervals. In week 8, our athlete will perform only four intervals. The number of intervals, like the distance of the other rides, will increase over weeks 7 and 6, with week 5 being a recovery week. With this in mind, week 6 (the most difficult week) will look like this:

Tuesday: 12.1 mi
Thursday: six 3-minute intervals (with 2-minute recovery rides)
Saturday: 24.2 mi

Competition Phase With this phase, repetitions will be used on Tuesday's workouts, Thursday will remain interval training, and Saturday will remain a continuous training session. Repetitions will consist of 90 seconds of near-maximal activity, followed by 450 seconds of recovery riding (i.e., 1:5 work:rest ratio). Intervals will now focus on training her to tolerate large levels of lactic acid; they will remain 3 minutes in length but recovery will be cut in half to 1 minute. Continuous training will continue to be capped at 24.2 mi.

Week 4 will see continuous training distances equivalent to those of week 7 and the performance of only four intervals on Thursday's workout. This step back is being taken because of the addition of repetitions on Tuesday. Tuesday's workout will consist of four repetitions during week 4. Weeks 3 and 2 will see an increase in the number of repetitions, intervals, and continuous training distance (to 24.2 mi). Week 1 will be a recovery week, with the race being at the end of that week.

Week 2 (the most difficult week) will look like this:

Tuesday: six 90-second repetitions (450-second recovery rides)
Thursday: six 3-minute intervals (1-minute recovery ride)
Saturday: 24.2 mi

REFERENCES

1. Kovacs M, Chandler WB, Chandler TJ. *Tennis Training: Enhancing On-Court Performance*. Vista, CA: Racquet Tech Publishing; 2007.
2. Brooks GA, Fahey TD, White TP, et al. *Exercise Physiology: Human Bioenergetics and Its Applications*. 3rd ed. Mountain View, CA: Mayfield; 2000.
3. Pfeiffer RP, Harder BP, Landis D, et al. Correlating indices of aerobic capacity with performance in elite women road road cyclists. *J Strength Cond Res*. 1993;7(4):201–205.
4. Heck H, Mader A. Justification of the 4-mmol/l lactate threshold. *Int J Sports Med*. 1985;6:117–1130.
5. Gollnick P, Bayly W, Hodgson D. Exercise intensity, training, diet, and lactate concentration in muscle and blood. *Med Sci Sports Exerc*. 1986;18:334–340.
6. Coyle EF, Coggan AR, Hopper MK, et al. Determinants of endurance in well-trained cyclists. *J Appl Physiol*. 1988;64(6):2622–2630.
7. Bowerman WJ, Freeman WH. *High-performance Training for Track and Field*. 2nd ed. Champaign, IL: Leisure Press; 1991.
8. Bompa TO. *Periodization: Theory and Methodology of Training*. 4th ed. Champaign, IL: Human Kinetics; 1999.
9. Pfeifer H, Harre D. Fundamentals and methods of endurance training. In: Harre D, ed. *Principles of Sports Training*. Berlin, Germany: Spotverlag; 1982.
10. Dick FW. *Sports Training Principles*. 4th ed. London, UK: A&C Black; 2002.
11. McArdle WD, Katch FI, Katch VL. *Exercise Physiology: Energy, Nutrition, and Human Performance*. 6th ed. Baltimore, MD: Lippincott Williams & Wilkins; 2006.

12. Priest JW, Hagan RD. The effects of maximum steady state pace training on running performance. *Br J Sports Med.* 1987;21(1):18–21.
13. de Swart A. Cross-country methods for year 2000. *Modern Athlete Coach.* 2000;28(4):38–40.
14. Karp JR. Interval training for fitness professionals. *Strength Cond J.* 2000;22(4):64–69.
15. Weston AR, Myburgh KH, Lindsay FH, et al. Skeletal muscle buffering capacity and endurance performance after high-intensity interval training by well-trained cyclists. *Eur J Appl Physiol Occup Physiol.* 1996;75(1):7–13.
16. Laursen PB, Shing CM, Peake JM, et al. Interval training program optimization in highly trained endurance cyclists. *Med Sci Sports Exerc.* 2002;34(11):1801–1807.
17. Lindsey FH, Hawley JA, Myburgh KH, et al. Improved athletic performance in highly trained cyclists after interval training. *Med Sci Sports Exerc.* 1996;28(11):1427–1434.
18. Smith TP, McNaughton LR, Coombes JS. Effects of a 4-week interval training program using Vo_{2max} and T_{max} on performance in middle distance athletes. *Med Sci Sports Exerc.* 1999;31(5 suppl):S282.
19. Stepto NK, Martin DT, Fallon KE, et al. Metabolic demands of intense aerobic interval training in competitive cyclists. *Med Sci Sports Exerc.* 2001;33(2):303–310.
20. Freeman WH. *Peak When It Counts.* Mountain View, CA: Tafnews Press; 1996.
21. Schmolinsky G. *The East German Textbook of Athletics.* Toronto, CA: Sports Books Publishers; 1996.
22. Koziris LP, Kramer WJ, Patton JF, et al. Relationship of aerobic power to anaerobic performance indices. *J Strength Cond Res.* 1996;10(1):35–39.
23. McNeely E, Sandler D. Tapering for endurance athletes. *Strength Cond J.* 2007;29(5):18–24.
24. Maglischo E. *Swimming Fastest.* Champaign, IL: Human Kinetics; 2003.
25. Stafford I. *Coaching for Long-Term Athlete Development.* Leeds, UK: The National Coaching Foundation; 2005:27–50.
26. Smith D. A framework for understanding the training process that leads to elite performance. *Sports Med.* 2003;33:1103–1126.
27. Holdeman J. Minimizing injury and maximizing performance in fast running: warming up and warming down. *Track Coach.* 2004;167:5336–5346.
28. Daniels J. Designing periodized training programs: distance running. In: Foran B, ed. *High-performance Sports Conditioning.* Champaign, IL: Human Kinetics; 2001.
29. Kurz MJ, Berg K, Latin R, et al. The relationship of training methods in NCAA division I cross country runners and 10,000 meter performance. *Strength Cond J.* 2000;14(2):196–201.

CHAPTER 14

Periodization of Training

G. GREGORY HAFF

OBJECTIVES

After reading this chapter, you will be able to:

- Explain why periodization does not follow a true linear plan.
- Differentiate between micro-, meso-, and macrocycles.
- Characterize the different phases and subphases of periodization.
- Incorporate all factors of training into a program.
- Develop a periodized outline for athletes of various sports.

KEY TERMS

Accumulation
Annual Training Plan
Bicycle
Block Periodization
Competitive Phase
Density
Frequency
General Preparatory
Involution
Macrocycles
Mesocycles
Microcycles
Monocycle
MultiYear Training Plans
Overreaching
Overtraining
Periodization
Precompetitive Subphase
Preparatory Phase
Preparedness
Quadrennial Training Plans
Realization
Specific Preparatory
Summated Microcycle
Taper
Training Day
Long-term Training Plans
Transition Phases
Transmutation
Tricycle

Introduction

Periodization of training is a concept that is widely accepted and used by coaches and sports scientists as a method for optimizing the training process. Though this concept is widely accepted, there appears to be a large degree of confusion about what periodization is and how it is appropriately applied. This is most evident in the resistance-training literature where some believe periodization is simply the manipulation of sets, repetitions, or resistance (1–3). In reality periodization is a much more comprehensive theoretical and practical paradigm in which workloads from multiple training factors are managed in order to maximize adaptation, whilst decreasing overtraining potential. For example, an athlete may engage in a periodized training plan in which resistance training, agility and sprint training, metabolic conditioning, and tactical or technical work is undertaken at varying levels of emphasis. If these factors are mismanaged or not sequenced and integrated correctly, fatigue can become excessive and overtraining can occur, which collectively decreases the potential for optimizing athletic performance, which is the primary purpose of a periodized training plan.

CENTRAL CONCEPTS IN PERIODIZATION

While some authors suggest that the major concepts central to the appropriate application of a periodized training plan are not based upon scientific inquiry (4), the reality is that periodization is a comprehensive theoretical and practical paradigm based upon robust scientific study (5). The process of establishing a periodized training plan allows the coach or sports scientist to structure the training process in order to stimulate specific physiological and performance outcomes at appropriate times (5). To accomplish these goals, the application of the training process must allow for the integration and sequencing of the multiple training factors that are required in the preparation of athletes from various sporting backgrounds.

While the basic concepts of periodization were established over five decades ago (6), the methods of applying these concepts have been continually adapted to address the needs of the modern athlete (6–9). In an attempt to modernize the concept, several authors have misinterpreted the basic tenets of periodization and created a form of training that violates many of the core concepts associated with the construction of a periodized training plan (1,2,10–12). Because of these issues, it is essential to revisit some of the classic material on periodization and demonstrate how these methods can be adapted and applied to the training of modern athletes. Therefore, the purpose of this chapter is to discuss the core concepts of periodization and methods of applying specific models of periodization to the preparation of modern athletes.

DEFINING PERIODIZATION

Central to the confusion about **periodization** is the wide array of definitions used to describe the concept (1–3,5,13–15). For example, some authors have oversimplified the concept by simply stating that periodization is planned variation (1–3). While planned variation is an important aspect of periodization, the central tenets of periodization are more inclusive and must consider the appropriate sequencing and integration of training factors that are necessary to stimulate specific physiological and performance gains at the predetermined time points. For example, Olbrect (16) suggests that periodization is a method for structuring the training process into different sequential and mutually dependent training periods in order to optimize performance at the appropriate time. Plisk and Stone (17) further expand upon this definition by suggesting that periodization is the logical phasic manipulation of training factors in order to optimize the overall training process. While these are just example definitions, a comprehensive review of the literature clearly indicates that an accurate definition of periodization must include reference to the logical sequencing and integration of training factors in order to appropriately represent the core concepts of periodization (5,14–16,18,19).

> *A true definition of periodization must take into consideration that training must be sequenced, integrated, and applied in a logical fashion.*

Therefore, for this book chapter, periodization should be defined as the logical and systematic sequencing of multiple training factors in an integrative fashion in order to optimize specific physiological and performance outcomes at predetermined time points.

> *True linear periodization does not exist. One of the main tenets of periodization is the removal of linearity in the training process.*

GOALS OF PERIODIZATION

Conceptually a periodized training plan has several basic goals which include (a) optimizing the athlete's level of performance at predetermined time points, (b) maximizing specific physiological and performance adaptations with structured training interventions, (c) reducing the athlete's overtraining potential, and (d) developing the athlete over the long term (13,20).

The ability of periodized training models to accomplish these goals is largely dependent upon a logical multidimensional application of training variation. Too often variation in training is limited to simply modulating the intensity and volume of training (2,3,10,21–23) when in fact other factors such as the training focus, exercise selected, mode of training, and the **density** or **frequency** of training can be varied (13,24–26). While variation at the level of an individual training session or day is important, it is equally important to consider variation at all levels of the planning process (i.e., **microcycle**, **mesocycle**, **macrocycle**, **annual training plan**, and **multiyear training plan**). Additionally, variation should never be excessive or randomly applied; rather, it should be carefully crafted considering the interrelation and sequencing of each training stimulus (13). Appropriate variation is further facilitated by considering the various levels of planning central to the periodization process and the hierarchical structure typically employed in the process.

BOX 14.1

Steps in the Planning Process

STEPS	PLANNING PROCESS	ACTIVITIES	ITEM NEEDED
1	Determine the multiyear training objectives	• Establish the multiyear training objectives	• Current performance data from which to extrapolate a reasonable rate of improvement
2	Establish the annual training plan	• Break the annual training plan into macrocycles	• The athlete's multiyear plan • The athlete's past competitive results • Competitive schedule • Overall multiyear plan goals
3	Break each macrocycle into phases and subphases	• Establish when the preparatory competitive, and transition phases are • Subdivide the major phases into general, specific, precompetitive, and competitive subphases • Determine where testing will occur in order to monitor the training plan	• The athlete's individualized annual training plan • Information about the athlete's training history • Testing results to determine which characteristics need to be targeted • A test battery that has been shown to adequately monitor training status.

BOX 14.1

Steps in the Planning Process *(Continued)*

STEPS	PLANNING PROCESS	ACTIVITIES	ITEM NEEDED
4	Establish the mesocycle structures	• Based upon the macrocycles, break each subphase into mesocycle blocks • Determine the training targets for each mesocycle block based upon the athlete needs and the needs analysis for the sport • Determine the frequency of training in each block	• The macrocycle breakdown for the athlete's annual training plan • A needs analysis for the sport which establishes the training factors which need to be targeted
5	Determine the microcycle structures	• Using the mesocycle plan as a guide, design the microcycle workload variations • Determine the basic variations in the microcycle for workload and intensity	• Overall mesocycle plans • Athlete's academic or work schedule • Availability of training facilities
6	Design the individual training day	• Determine the training day's intensity and workload in context with the microcycle plan • Determine how the training factors integrate	• Information about the number of training sessions to be contained in the day and the time that is needed. • The microcycle plan that indicates the factors to be trained on each day
7	Plan the training session	• Plan the training session to target specific factors such as warm-up, main training bout, and cool down • Determine which primary factors are targeted in the session	• The microcycle plan and the individual training day plan • Information about the factors that are being trained in the microcycle and the intensity and volume fluctuations

Though variation is a key component of a periodized training program, it should never be applied randomly or excessively.

BASIC HIERARCHY OF PERIODIZED TRAINING MODELS

The creation of a periodized training model is based upon breaking the training plan into specific interrelated periods of time, which are structured to meet precise goals (Table 14.1) (5). From a hierarchical standpoint, each of these periods is interdependent and is structured based upon the multiyear training plan (Fig. 14.1) (5,6). These long-term planning structures range between 2 and 4 years and establish the broad training objectives and sequential development of specific target attributes. Most often these **long-term training plans** are 4 years in length and are termed quadrennial training plans. Generally, **quadrennial training plans** are structured for the preparation of Olympic athletes but also are used for the development of both high school and collegiate athletes (27). From a sequential standpoint, the first 3 years of the quadrennial plan serve to elevate the athlete's physiological and performance capacity so that the highest level of performance is achieved in the fourth year of the training plan. To accomplish this goal, each of the four annual training plans contained in the quadrennial plan will target specific goals and objectives that are interrelated, with the adaptations established in one annual plan serving as the foundation for the subsequent annual training plan. Therefore, the structure of each annual training plan is based upon the global objectives established by the quadrennial plan (19,27) the athlete's developmental status (5), and the athlete or team's competitive schedule (5,19,27).

A central component of a periodized training plan is the development of multiyear training plans from which individual annual training plans are created.

Typically, there are three main annual training plan constructs that include the **monocycle**, **bicycle**,

TABLE 14.1 ● TRAINING PERIODS COMMONLY USED WHEN CREATING A PERIODIZED TRAINING PLAN

PERIOD	DURATION	DESCRIPTION
Quadrennial plan	4 y	Four sequenced and interlinked annual plans. Often used with the preparation of Olympic athletes, but also useful with high school and collegiate athletes. Used to guide the long term development of the athlete.
Annual training plan	1 y	A year of training, which is structured into single or multiple macrocycles depending upon the needs of the competitive sport and the individual athlete's level of development.
Macrocycle	Several months to a year	A macrocycle typically represents an entire season of training that contains periods of preparation, competition, and transitions. Contains sequenced and interlinked mesocycles that target the specific goals established by the macrocycle structure and the objectives set forth by the annual training plan.
Mesocycle	2–6 wk	Mesocycle structures are typically 4 wk in duration but can range between 2 and 6 wk depending upon the structural needs of the macrocycle. Are also referred to as training blocks in some periodization models.
Microcycle	2 d to 2 wk	A microcycle is a small-sized training cycle that is composed of multiple training sessions that are structured in a 7-d format. Typically the microcycle has specific objects that are based upon the mesocycle, macrocycle, and annual training plan structure.
Training day	1 d	One day of training is often composed of a single or multiple training sessions. Is designed in the context of the loading structures established by the microcycle and mesocycle structure.
Training session	Several hours	Typically contains several hours of training. However, if the workout contains >30 min of rest between bouts of training, it would be classified as multiple training sessions

Note: Adapted from Issurin (6,7,30), Stone et al. (13), Siff (25), Bompa and Haff (5), and Siff and Verkoshansky (47).

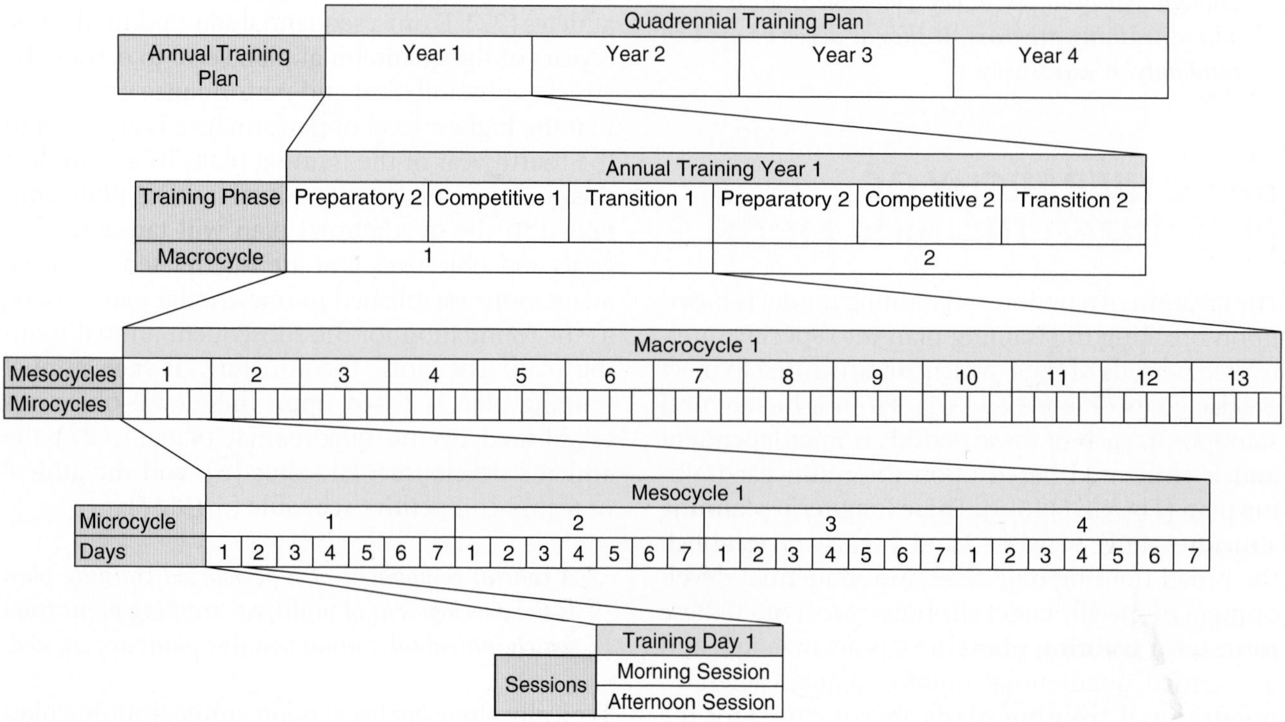

FIGURE 14.1 Training hierarchy: from quadrennial to individual training sessions.

and **tricycle** training plan structure (Fig. 14.2). While these three variants should meet the needs of most athletes, there are at least 16 additional variants that can be employed in the development of an annual training plan (28). Regardless of which variant is employed, the number of competitive periods engaged by the athlete serves as the foundation for determining how to subdivide the annual training plan. For example, sports such as American collegiate soccer contain two competitive seasons (e.g., a spring and fall season), which would require a bicycle annual training plan structure, while collegiate distance runners may employ a tricycle structure (e.g., cross country, indoor track, and outdoor track seasons). Once the number of competitive periods is established, the annual training plan can be broken into macrocycles.

Macrocycles are structured to contain an entire season of training. Frequently, the annual training plan is used interchangeably with the term macrocycle (5,6), but with sports that contain multiple seasons over the calendar year the annual training plan would contain multiple macrocycles (e.g., bicycle or tricycle annual training plan) (5). This cycle is used to establish when preparatory, competitive, and transition phases are employed based upon the competitive requirements of the athlete or sport. As a whole, the general loading paradigm across the macrocycle moves from higher volumes during the preparatory phase toward higher intensity training with an increasing emphasis on technique or tactical-based training during the competitive phase (29).

A macrocycle is best described as a season; therefore, for sports with multiple seasons, there will be multiple macrocycles contained in the annual training plan.

PREPARATORY PHASE

The global objectives of the **preparatory phase** of training is to establish the physiological, psychological, and technical adaptations necessary for competitive success (5). Typically, this phase can last between 3 and 6 months depending upon the length of the macrocycle, the individual sports requirements, or the athlete's level of development (5). When constructing the annual training plan, coaches will generally allot a greater time to the preparatory phase with less developed athletes such as those in high school. More advanced athletes, because of their greater training base, will be able to dedicate less time to this phase of training. Additionally, the allotment of preparatory training

Annual Training Plan Type	Annual Training Plan Structure								
Monocycle	Macrocycle								
	Preparatory				Competitive			Transition	
Bicycle	Macrocyle 1				Macrocycle 2				
	Preparatory		Competitive	Transition	Preparatory		Competitive	Transition	
Tricycle	Macrocyle 1			Macrocycle 2			Macrocycle 3		
	Preparatory	Competitive	Transition	Preparatory	Competitive	Transition	Preparatory	Competitive	Transition

Note: Adapted from Bompa and Haff[5], Bondarchuk[28] and Counsilman and Counsilman[19]

FIGURE 14.2 Example annual training plan structures. (Adapted from Bompa and Haff [5], Bondarchuk [28], and Counsilman and Counsilman [19]).

Q & A from the Field

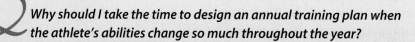

Q *Why should I take the time to design an annual training plan when the athlete's abilities change so much throughout the year?*

A The annual plan is a road map from which the remainder of your training plan is constructed. It gives the broad goals that are used to construct the training plan from. For example, the annual training plan details when the competitions are and when we would want to taper. It does not detail the exact methods used to taper, it simply outlines where we should taper. The mesocycle and microcycle plans will give more detailed methods for the training process and can be varied when issues such as injury or poor or elevated performance occur.

targeted for an individual annual training plan will be subdivided amongst the macrocycles established for that year of training. Regardless of the length of the preparatory phase, there are two general subphases that are established: (a) the general and (b) the specific preparatory subphases (5,7).

General Preparatory Subphase

The primary focus of the **general preparatory** subphase is to establish a general physical training base (5). This is accomplished by utilizing a large variety of training means that target the development of general fitness, and motor abilities or skills that are undertaken for relatively higher volumes and lower intensities (30,31) Because this subphase targets the development of a general fitness base, it is typically undertaken during the early part of the preparatory phase of the macrocycle or annual training plan (5). Generally, more advanced athletes will spend less time in this training subphase when compared to the less developed athlete (e.g., novice or high school athlete) because of their more developed fitness base.

Specific Preparatory Subphase

The **specific preparatory** subphase is used to translate the basic fitness characteristics established in the general preparatory subphase of training into more sport-specific fitness, motor abilities, and technical abilities (19). This subphase contains periods of higher volume training that is coupled with periods of high-intensity training that is specifically designed to translate the previously established fitness gains into very specific performance characteristics. This subphase strengthens the overall training base while preparing the athlete for the upcoming competitive phase of training. More advanced athletes generally dedicate more of their global preparatory work to this subphase when compared to their lesser developed counterparts.

Traditionally, the above sequence of general and specific subphases is used in the classic models of periodization, while an alternative approach suggests that these two phases should run concurrently (19,28) based upon the time frame necessary to achieve sporting form or reach a higher level of preparedness.

> *Novice athletes will dedicate more of their annual training plan to the general preparatory phase when compared to more developed athletes.*

COMPETITIVE PHASE

The **competitive phase** is used to elevate or maintain the physiological and sport-specific skills developed in the preparatory phase of training (14) while concurrently increasing the athlete's level of **preparedness** and performance at key time points established in the annual training plan. During this phase, there is a reduction in the degree of emphasis on general physical preparation as the training emphasis shifts toward more skill-based conditioning activities (32), technical or tactical preparation, and maintenance of sport-specific fitness.

Precompetitive Subphase

The **precompetitive subphase** interlinks the preparatory phase with the main competitive subphase. This subphase is marked by an increasing emphasis on technical or tactical training as well as initial competitions such as exhibition games or preseason competitions. While some competitions exist in this subphase, the emphasis is not on competitive success; rather, the competitions are used as training tools that help the coach gauge the athlete's progress toward the main competitive goals (5).

Main Competitive Subphase

The main competitive subphase is designed with the express purpose of elevating the athlete's overall levels of preparedness and optimizing competitive performance. The length of this subphase is largely dictated by the competitive schedule. As such, the training interventions will vary in order to modulate fatigue levels whilst maintaining or slightly elevating sport-specific fitness and skills developed in previous phases of training. The culmination of this subphase is the primary competition or tournament contained in the macrocycle or annual training plan. Typically, an 8- to 14-day **taper** is constructed at the end of this subphase to stimulate a super compensation of both preparedness and performance.

The competitive phase for team sports is largely dependent upon league or conference schedules. Individual sports offer more freedom in deciding competitive schedules.

TRANSITION PHASE

Transition phases are crucial linking structures that are used to bridge between macrocycles or annual training plans (5,14,33). Structurally the transition phase is designed to refresh the athlete physically and mentally while performing a significantly reduced training load that targets the maintenance of fitness and minimizes the emphasis on sport specific skills. Traditionally, these phases last between 2 and 4 weeks but can be extended to 6 weeks if needed (5,26,34). When extended for long durations (>2 to 4 weeks), a detraining effect will occur, which would require the next preparatory phase to be longer as it will be necessary to reestablish fitness level achieved in the previous macrocycle or annual training plan.

The transition phase is a period between macrocycles and annual training plans in which the athlete has the opportunity to recover from the previous training cycle.

MESOCYCLE

Once the phases of the macrocycle are established, the mesocycle structure and sequence can be determined. The mesocycle is considered a medium-duration training cycle that typically contains two to six interrelated microcycles (weeks of training) (7,13,16,24,26,30,35,36). When examining some contemporary training literature, the mesocycle is sometimes referred to as a block (6,7,30) or as a summated microcycle structure (13,17). Regardless of the terminology used, the most common mesocycle length is generally around 4 weeks in duration (17,24,35,37). Four-week mesocycle blocks are commonly used because they allow for delayed training effects to be superimposed, which allows for the exploitation of residual training effects that magnify the cumulative effects of training (6,7,13,30,35,38). Additionally, after about 4 weeks of a given mesocycle asymptotic training, effects begin to occur and are typically manifested as a stagnation or decline in physiological and/or performance gains (37). However, if at this point the training stimulus is varied and a new mesocycle structure is employed, these effects can be avoided, and continued adaptations can be stimulated.

Though there are infinite numbers of mesocycle structures that can be employed to create a training plan, there are three basic structures or blocks that can be sequenced (Fig. 14.3): (a) **accumulation**, (b) **transmutation**, and (c) **realization** (Table 14.2).

Accumulation

The accumulation (6), developmental (39), or concentrated loading block (17) is a mesocycle structure that is designed to develop an overall fitness base with the use of substantial workloads that target basic athletic abilities such as muscular strength, anaerobic endurance, or aerobic endurance (6). Generally these types of blocks range between 1 and 6 weeks in duration depending upon the time frame necessary to attain the targeted training effect, the rate of detraining, and the overall competitive schedule.

Structurally, the length of these blocks of training is proportional to the stability of the training effect (6,30). Specifically, the longer the block the greater the accumulated fatigue, the greater the training residuals, and the longer the duration before performance and preparedness are elevated (5,17). As a whole, these mesocycles are structured to target a primary and complementary training

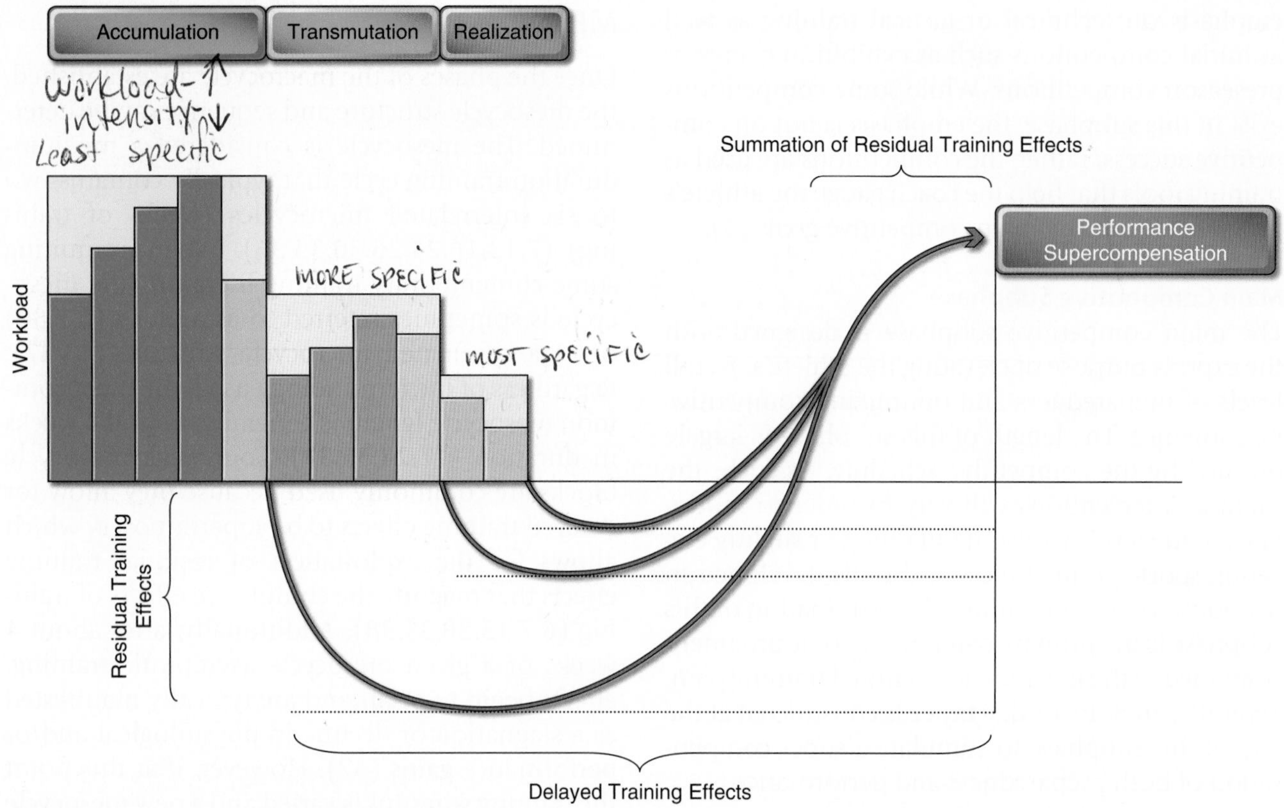

FIGURE 14.3 Interrelation of residual training effects, delayed training effects, and the mesocycle sequence.

TABLE 14.2 ● THREE BASIC MESOCYCLE BLOCK STRUCTURES

BLOCK CLASSIFICATION	ALTERNATIVE NAMES SEEN IN THE LITERATURE	DURATION	CHARACTERISTICS
Accumulation	Concentrated loading block Developmental block General block	1–6 wk	1. High training volumes and loads 2. Tends to create the longest training residuals 3. Marked by the highest levels of fatigue 4. Elevates general fitness 5. Provides the training base for subsequent blocks
Transmutation	Normal training block Competitive block Phase potentiation block Specific block	2–4 wk	1. Builds upon the foundation established in the accumulation block 2. Produces relatively short training residuals 3. Elevates preparedness 4. High intensities of training may result in cumulative fatigue
Realization	Peaking block Taper block Restoration block Competitive block	8–14 d	1. Marked by reduced training loads 2. Further elevated preparedness 3. Induces recovery 4. Elevates performance levels 5. Facilitates the convergence of training residuals established in the accumulation and transmutation blocks

Note: Adapted from Issurin (6,7), Plisk and Stone (17) and Bondarchuk (39), factors that provide the foundation from which subsequent mesocycles are used to elevate the sport-specific preparedness of the athlete.

Transmutation

The **transmutation** (6,7), competitive (39), or phase potentiating block (17) is employed after an accumulation block and is designed to translate the adaptations and skills developed in the preceding block into sport-specific characteristics that allow for the elevation of preparedness. This is accomplished by establishing training goals that are targeted by sport-specific training methods that focus on the competitive activity and utilizing higher intensities of training (7). Structurally this block is 2 to 4 weeks in duration to exploit the training residuals established in the accumulation block while minimizing the rate of **involution** (training decay) of these training residuals (6,7). If this block is extended beyond 4 weeks, the rate of involution of the training residuals established in the accumulation phase will increase resulting in a reduction of basic fitness, physiological adaptations and skills necessary to perform at a high level. If constructed and applied correctly, this block will serve as the foundation for high levels of performance.

Realization

The realization (6,7), restoration (39), peaking (5), or taper (13) block is utilized prior to a major competition and is designed to maximize the athlete's preparedness as well as increase the potential for a high level of performance. In the classic sense, a taper should last between approximately 8 and 14 days and contain a reduction in training workload, while maintaining both frequency and intensity of training (40), which results in reductions in fatigue and elevations in both preparedness and performance. Conceptually the realization block is similar to a taper except that the main goal of this block is to cause the convergence of the training residuals generated by both the accumulation and realization blocks, which allows for the maximization of the targeted training attributes and creates an optimization of performance (6,7).

MICROCYCLES

The smallest and most basic training structure is the microcycle. The microcycle targets very specific training objectives, which serves as the basis for achieving the goals set forth by the mesocycle structure. Generally, the microcycle can vary in duration from 2 days to 2 weeks depending upon the phase of training established in the annual training plan. For example, during a preparatory phase the microcycle is typically 7 days in duration, while in the competitive phase the microcycle can be condensed in order to meet the demands of the competitive schedule.

The structure of the microcycle is largely dependent upon where it falls within the overall training plan, the training requirements established, the athlete's training status or ability to tolerate training, and the time allotted for training (26). While it is difficult to give exact microcycle structures, it is widely accepted that the microcycle should contain both heavy and light training days so that recovery and adaptation can be maximized. Additionally, there are five basic structures (Table 14.3), which include ordinary, shock, precompetitive, competitive, and recovery microcycle structures.

These basic microcycle structures serve as the basic building blocks from which a mesocycle of training can be constructed. Specifically, they can be sequenced in order to target specific physiological and performance outcomes. Overall the actual sequence will be dictated by the type of mesocycle employed, the phase of training that the microcycle is contained in, and the overall needs of the athlete (Fig. 14.4).

TRAINING DAY

The smallest training unit is the individual **training day**. A individual training day can contain one or more interconnected training sessions (25) that are constructed to meet the goals and demands established by the microcycle. The density or number of training sessions contained within each day is largely dependent upon the athlete's level of development, time allotted for training, and the goals established by the training plan. It is generally accepted that training days that contain multiple smaller training sessions result in a greater training effect and allow for a greater level of training variation. Therefore, when possible, a training day should contain multiple training sessions.

Subdividing the annual training plan into macrocycles, mesocycles, and microcycles that target the specified training goals is an essential component of a periodized training plan.

TABLE 14.3 ● MICROCYCLE STRUCTURES

MICROCYCLE CLASSIFICATION	CHARACTERISTICS
Ordinary	Lower training load, typically submaximal in nature Training loads are gradually increased with each microcycle
Shock	Contains sudden increases in training load applied in conjunction with high training volumes Typically used with advanced athletes in both competitive and preparatory phases of training Has the potential to induce specific physiological and performance gains Is typically followed by ordinary microcycle structures Designed to prepare the athlete for subsequent competitive microcycles
Precompetitive	May be considered as the early part of the taper or realization block Marked by reduced training volumes and sport-specific training methods Occurs immediately before a competition Is an extension of the precompetitive microcycle
Competitive	Contains immediate training preparation, travel to competition, site preparation, warm-up, actual competition, and recovery Contains a reduced training load in order to induce recovery
Recovery	Allows the athlete to heal, rest, and prepare for subsequent training blocks

Note: Adapted from Kurz (26), Siff (25), and Stone et al. (13)

SEQUENCING AND INTEGRATION OF TRAINING

The idea that periodized training models should be sequenced and integrated is not new (41). Strong research support exists for structuring training in a sequential fashion (42–44). Central to the sequencing concept is that the physiological adaptations that are stimulated in one mesocycle are exploited by the subsequent mesocycle. For example, when attempting to promote optimal gains in power, the following sequence may be warranted (42):

Strength Endurance ⇒ strength ⇒ power and speed

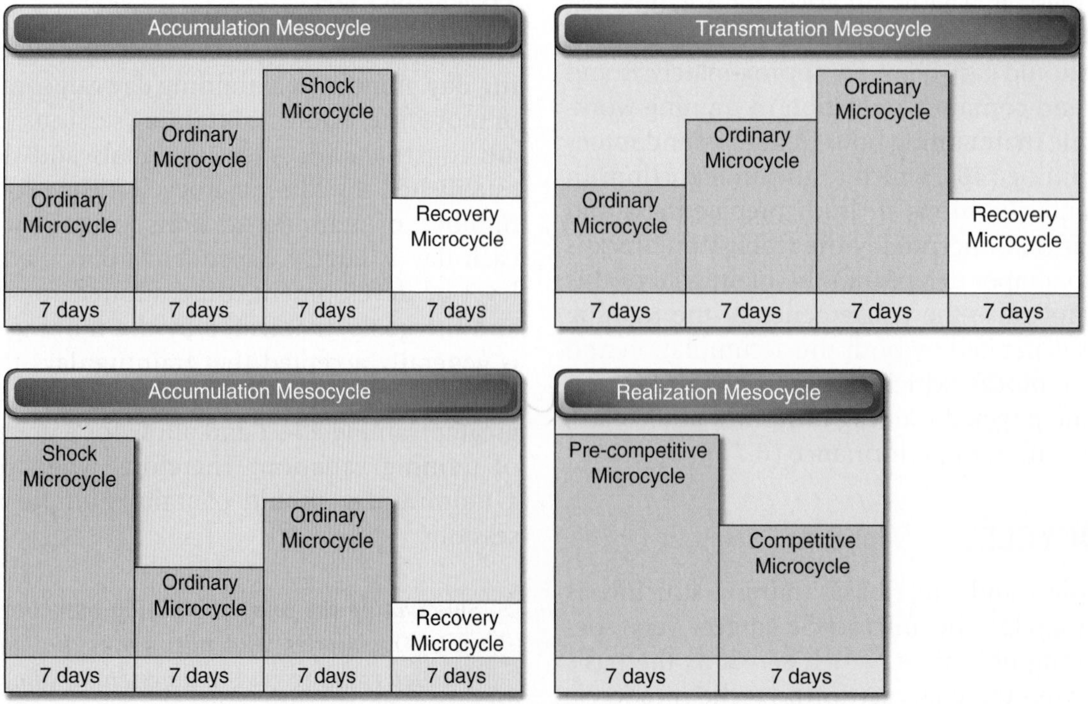

FIGURE 14.4 Potential microcycle configurations based upon mesocycle block structure

In this example, a mesocycle that focuses on strength endurance would develop the general fitness base from which strength can be maximized. Once strength is increased, the potential to develop power and speed characteristics are enhanced (45).

The second concept associated with sequencing of training is the integration of training factors as each mesocycle should contain a primary, secondary, and tertiary emphasis (5). For example, when attempting to develop speed, the training program should contain elements of maximal strength, muscular power, and speed agility. Therefore, during each mesocycle, varying degrees of emphasis would be placed on each of these elements (Fig. 14.5). Figure 14.5 gives two examples of how one may sequence and integrate a training plan. For example, Figure 14.5A is an example of how speed may be developed across three mesocycles. The primary focus of mesocycle no. 1 is the development of maximal strength while muscular power is the secondary emphasis. In mesocycle no. 2, the emphasis is shifted toward muscular power, while the maximal strength has a reduced emphasis. By mesocycle no. 3, the maximal strength emphasis is further decreased and the muscular power emphasis is decreased slightly. Across all three mesocycles, there is a progressive increase in a focus on speed and agility work. Figure 14.5B gives an example of how the training factors could be sequenced and integrated for a team sport.

Generally the success of the sequenced training plan is largely dependent upon the ordering of successive mesocycles in accordance with mechanical specificity (17,25,36,46,47), metabolic specificity (13,48,49), and the time course of the stability and involution of residual training effects (7,24,25,30,35,37,47). An additional consideration is the compatibility of the training factors contained in each mesocycle. For example, if one is trying to develop maximal strength, performing aerobic training would mute the adaptive responses required to maximize strength. Ultimately, there are an infinite number of possible sequential models that can be utilized when periodizing a training plan.

Failure to sequence the training factors can result in a reduction in the athlete's performance potential.

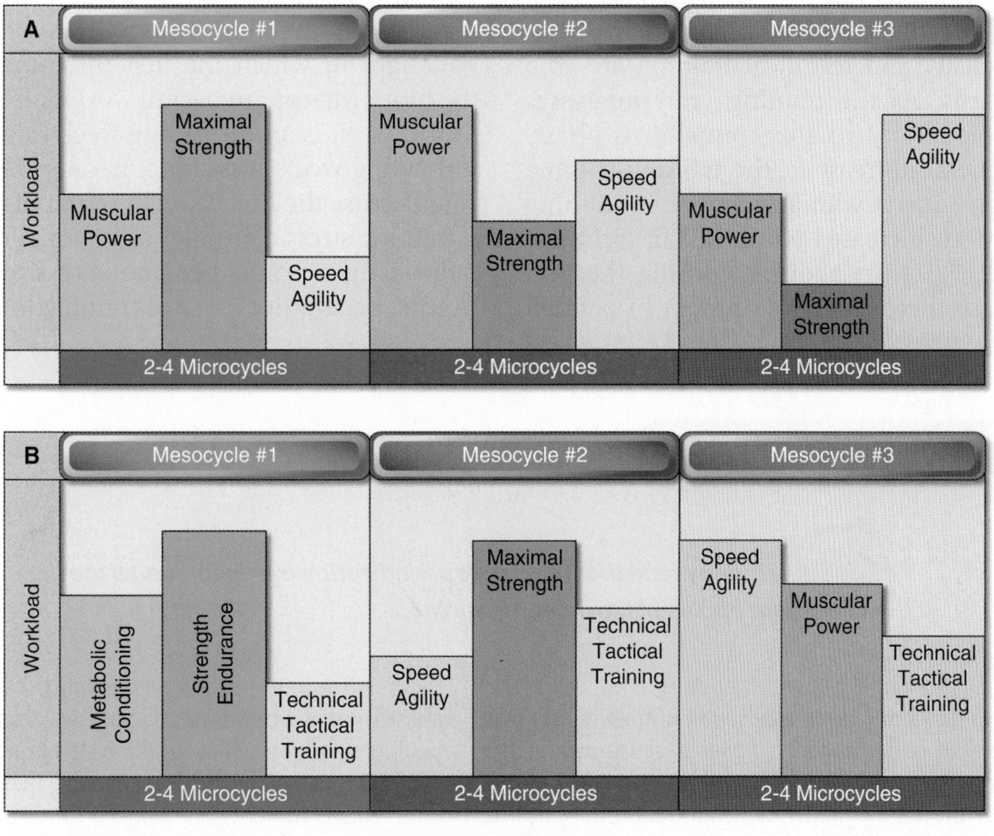

FIGURE 14.5 A,B. Example integrated training structure.

MODELS OF PERIODIZATION

When examining the literature on periodization, it is important to note that true periodization models are nonlinear because of the variations employed at each of the hierarchical levels. While there are numerous possibilities for constructing a periodized training plan, the vast majority of the structures will fall into one of three basic formats: classic, summated microcycle, or block periodization models.

CLASSIC MODELS OF PERIODIZATION

Though often misrepresented by many authors as being a linear model of periodization (2,11,22), the classic model is in fact a nonlinear application of training, which contains wave-like increases in workloads at the microcycle, mesocycle and macrocycle level (15,31,50). As a whole, the concept of linearity in a periodized training plan violates the core tenets of periodization as variation of the various training factors are applied in a sequential and integrated fashion.

The main characteristics of the classic model are centered on a sequential pattern in which training volumes are higher in the preparatory phase, whereas intensity and technical training are of a lower emphasis. As the training year progresses from the preparatory to the competitive phase, there is a general decrease in the training volume that occurs in concert with an increase in training intensity and an increased emphasis on technical training (18,19,31). In addition, during the preparatory phase there is a development of parallel abilities, specifically attempting to simultaneously develop a variety of divergent physiological functions (19,25,51). Typically, the development of these abilities is undertaken for long periods of time, which may be of particular importance for the novice athlete who must develop a physiological base. This approach may not be best for the intermediate or advanced athlete because it may not maximize the physiological and performance adaptations required by these athletes (Box 14.2) (19,25,51). Therefore, the classic approach has been suggested for beginner athletes, while intermediate and advanced athletes should consider more complex sequential periodization models such as summated microcycle or block periodization models.

SUMMATED MICROCYCLE MODELS

The **summated microcycle** model is a method of sequencing and integrating training variation into the periodized plan, which may be of particular use with more developed athletes who can tolerate greater training stress. This model allows variation to be applied in a cyclical pattern, which can magnify the adaptive response to the training plan. In this model, the mesocycle block is typically 4 weeks in duration and follows a 3:1 loading paradigm in which the first three microcycles of the block increase in overall workload, whereas the fourth week is an unloading week (Fig. 14.6). The unloading week is essential because fatigue is elevated across the first 3 weeks of the mesocycle and if training stress continues to increase, the accumulative fatigue could become excessive and result in the occurrence of overtraining. Additionally,

Q & A from the Field

Q ***I recently read that the classic periodization is a linear model that is not applicable to modern training.***

A The classic model of periodization is in no way linear; it is in fact a nonlinear application of training. No true model of periodization is linear because one of the major tenets of periodization is to remove linearity. While the classic model of periodization may not be the best for intermediate and advanced athletes, the classic model works exceptionally well with novice or beginning athletes. It allows for a stabilization of training effects as well as technical mastery that is essential for the development of beginners.

REAL-WORLD APPLICATION

Periodiozation for a Young High School Discus Athlete

A high school freshman who is planning on throwing the discus this coming spring sits with her coach to determine how to prepare for the upcoming season. She is relatively untrained and has never participated in a resistance-training program, nor has she thrown the discus before. If you were to consult with her coach, how might you design the training program?

There are numerous ways in which the training program could be constructed. The best approach would be to consider this athlete's individual needs and mold the training program to her goals and objectives. Obviously, there are several strategies that could be considered based upon the concepts of periodization.

1. The first step is to consider this athlete's development as a long-term process in which a multiyear plan should be developed, specifically a quadrennial plan in which her highest levels of performance would be targeted for her senior year.
2. When constructing the annual training plan that will be used for her freshman year, the primary factors to consider are the development of a training base in which longer general preparatory phases would be considered. In this context, targeting strength development as well as performing conditioning activities to get this individual in shape is extremely important. Additionally, this athlete will need to learn how to throw the discus, so there will be substantial time working on remedial drill work at specific time points in the year.
3. To develop the annual training plan, a detailed list of competitions that this athlete will compete in should be generated. This will serve as the foundation for establishing the competitive phase of the annual training plan.
4. To monitor the athlete's progress, consider spacing performance assessments periodically throughout the training year, which examine multiple factors such as muscular strength, muscular power, technical proficiency, and markers of throwing performance. These tests will help in the evaluation of this annual training plan's success.

It is obvious that this novice athlete will not require advanced training techniques. Consider some of the following.

1. Utilize a classic periodization model approach. This will allow the athlete to have longer periods of development, which will be the foundation for subsequent annual training plans.
2. Since she is a novice, she will require less training volume, intensity, and variation in order to get improvements. As she progresses, her program will need to be modified, specifically in subsequent annual training plans.
3. When implementing the training plan, it is important that the coach communicates with the athlete in order to garner feedback about how the athlete feels about the program as well as to educate the athlete about the training process and why things are being targeted at specific time points.
4. Because this athlete has a low training base, be careful to only target a few complementary training factors at any given time point.

after about 3 to 4 weeks of increasing workloads, training can become asymptotic, and involution or training stagnation begins to occur. Therefore, the application of an unloading week during the fourth week of the block is necessary in order to allow for recovery and adaptation before engaging in the next mesocycle of training.

Typically, in this model, training activities progress from extensive to intensive training structures. For example, in strength training the progression across the four microcycles of a block might be

Strength endurance ⇒ maximal strength ⇒ maximal strength ⇒ strength power

Strength endurance ⇒ maximal strength ⇒ strength power ⇒ peaking

These basic sequential patterns are typically used when attempting to maximize strength and power-generating capacity. From a sequential standpoint, each successive mesocycle block would have an overall increase in workload (Fig. 14.6).

To further enhance the effectiveness of the summated microcycle model intramicrocycle variation strategies can be employed in which heavy/light day paradigms can be used (Fig. 14.7) (13). By employing this microcycle strategy, the workload encountered on each day can be manipulated to better balance training stressors with both recovery and adaptation. This strategy allows for variations in the training focus across the microcycle as well as increases the potential for positive physiological and performance adaptations. For example,

BOX 14.2

Potential Problems with the Classic Model of Periodization

Though the classic model of periodization is excellent for many athletes, it may be disadvantageous when working with intermediate and advanced athletes because of the following:

1. The classic model is structured in a fashion in which only small periods of novel stimuli are presented, which are followed by long periods of monotonous training. While this is advantageous for the beginning athlete, it may handicap the intermediate and advanced athletes
2. The classic model relies upon a multifaceted training approach to developed a balanced physiological and performance base that does not allow for an optimization of any specific training factor. As a result, with advanced athletes, this model may mute or result in smaller gains in performance (36).
3. The classic model contains long preparatory periods, which are advantageous for novice athletes but do not take advantage of the advanced athletes' training base. Specifically, these long periods of preparation may do not include enough variation to allow for a maximization of performance in the advanced athlete.
4. The general progression of training may create excessive amounts of fatigue, which can impede the athlete's ability to maximize technical competency (25,52).
5. When the classic model was developed, the competitive calendar was less robust than seen in the contemporary sporting world (7,30). Because of the increased number of competitions, additional planning paradigms are warranted that allow the athlete to achieve high levels of preparedness at key time points.

The classic model is a nonlinear model, which is excellent for novice to intermediate athletes, especially when heavy/light training days are employed.

a heavy/light day structure could alter between maximal strength and speed-strength development. The overall increase in variation employed in both the microcycle and mesocycle may stimulate greater adaptations across the overall training plan.

An additional summated microcycle method is to apply periods of intentional **overreaching**, which results in symptoms similar to **overtraining** (13,17). In this application, short periods of overreaching or intensified training are utilized to saturate the system is a particular training foci, while complimentary training factors are trained at a reduced level. Generally, this increased training stimulus is applied for 1 to 4 weeks in duration depending upon the phase of training and the targeted outcomes. Stone et al. (13) suggest that the utilization of this type of summated microcycle can result in significant improvements in strength and power development when utilized by intermediate to advanced athletes. In this application, the first microcycle of the block would be designed to overreach the athlete, whereas microcycles 2 and 3 would return the athlete to normal training loads, and the fourth microcycle would be an unloading microcycle.

When constructing the training plan, various summated microcycles can be sequenced into a training plan in order to develop specific performance outcomes (Fig. 14.8). For example, in Figure 14.8, two blocks that contain a traditional summated microcycle can be followed by several training blocks that contain intentional overreaching microcycles. There are numerous possibilities for constructing these types of training structures depending upon the phase of training being targeted as well as the individual athlete's needs.

Summated microcycles are groups of interrelated microcycles that are generally structured into 4-week training blocks that allow for greater intermesocycle variation.

Block Periodization Models

Block periodization is an evolution of the classic models of periodization, specifically designed to address the demands of modern athletes (6,7,39). In particular, block periodization models structure mesocycle blocks that target a minimal number of compatible training foci. There are three main mesocycle structures that contain 2- to 4-week training blocks that are employed in a sequential fashion in order to exploit the cumulative and residual training effects of each mesocycle (6). Central to this concept is the long-term development of specific physiological adaptations and performance-based capabilities. These adaptations create training residuals which are related to the rate of involution and can be exploited to optimize performance at specific time points.

Regardless of interpretation of the block model (6,7,17,39), several key concepts are central to the model. First, each mesocycle is designed to target a minimal number of compatible training foci. Secondly, there are a small number of mesocycle structures that can be used in a sequential manner. Thirdly each mesocycle lasts between 2 and 6 weeks

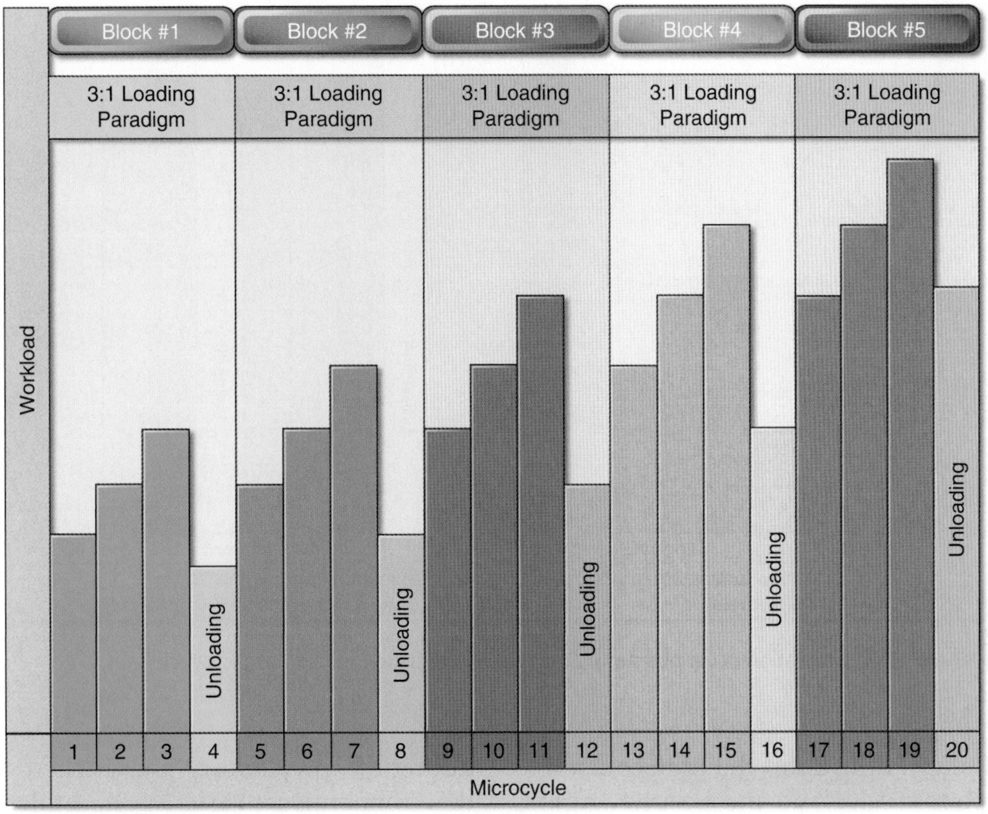

FIGURE 14.6 Example summated microcycle structure.

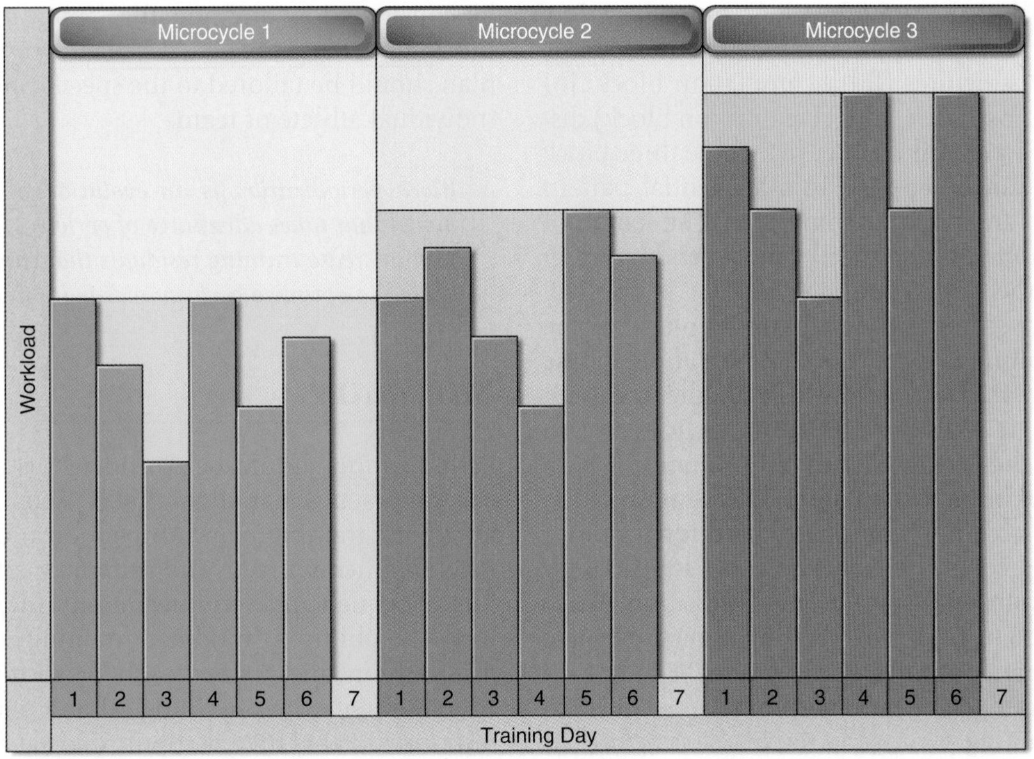

FIGURE 14.7 Example summated microcycle with heavy and light day structures.

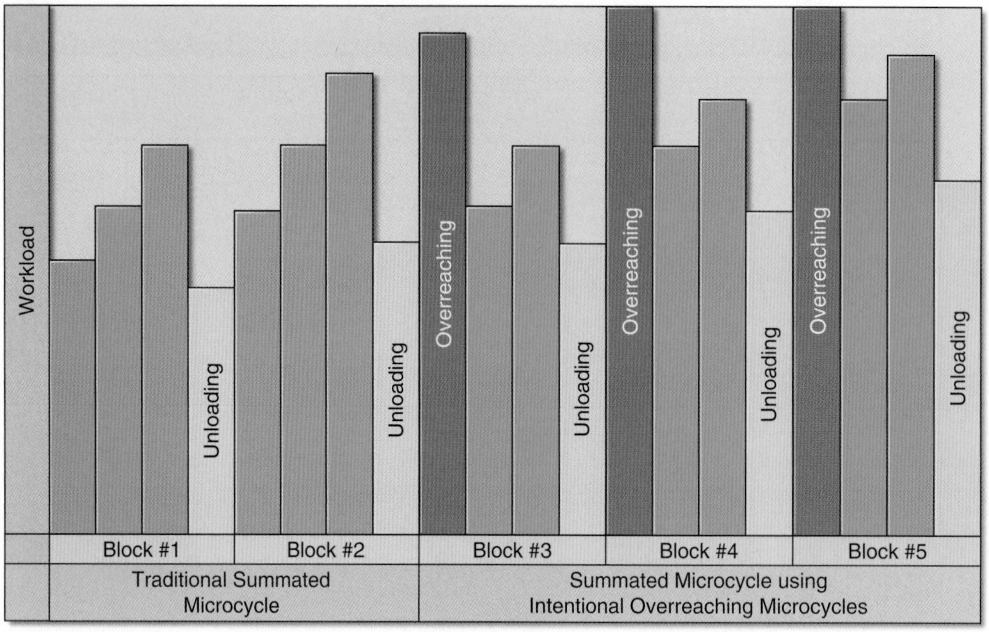

FIGURE 14.8 Integration of various summated microcycle structures into a macrocycle.

(Table 14.2), depending upon the time course for optimizing performance and the positive exploitation of the cumulative training effects and the training residuals. Finally, the sequential joining of the individual blocks serves as the foundation of macrocycle and annual training plan, thus allowing for performance to be optimized (6).

The basic structure of a block model revolves around sequential application of the three basic mesocycle structures ([a] accumulation block, [b] transmutation block, and [c] realization block) discussed earlier in this chapter (6). These three block structures can be applied in a sequential pattern to develop an annual training plan. The length of the accumulation phase will vary depending upon when in the annual training plan it is applied. For example, during the preparatory phase of the annual training plan, the accumulation phase could last 4 to 6 weeks, while in the competitive phase, it could be applied for as little as 1 to 2 weeks. The length of the transmutation phase would then be dependent upon the duration of the preceding accumulation phase, with longer times to induce recovery being needed after longer accumulation phases. Typically, the realization phase would last 8 to 14 days depending upon the degree of performance optimization required. Figure 14.9 give an example of how one might construct an annual training plan using the block structure. In this example, the accumulation phases are longer during the preparatory phase when compared to the competitive phase. As the athlete progresses across the annual plan, the level of peaking should increase with each realization block. Therefore, the lowest competitive performance should occur in microcycle 9 and the highest in microcycle 52. It is important to note that this example is only to be considered as one potential application of the block model and the actual structure of the annual plan should be tailored to the specific needs of the individual athlete or team.

Block periodization is an evolution of the classic model that takes advantage of periods of accumulation to create training residuals that can be manipulated to optimize performance more frequently.

Summary

Periodization should be considered as a theoretical and practical paradigm that is used to structure an athlete training plan. All periodization models when applied correctly are nonlinear and include logical sequencing and integration of training factors. The ability to modulate training stressors in this fashion allows the coach or sports scientist to manipulate the physiological and performance responses so that they are optimized at very distinct time points.

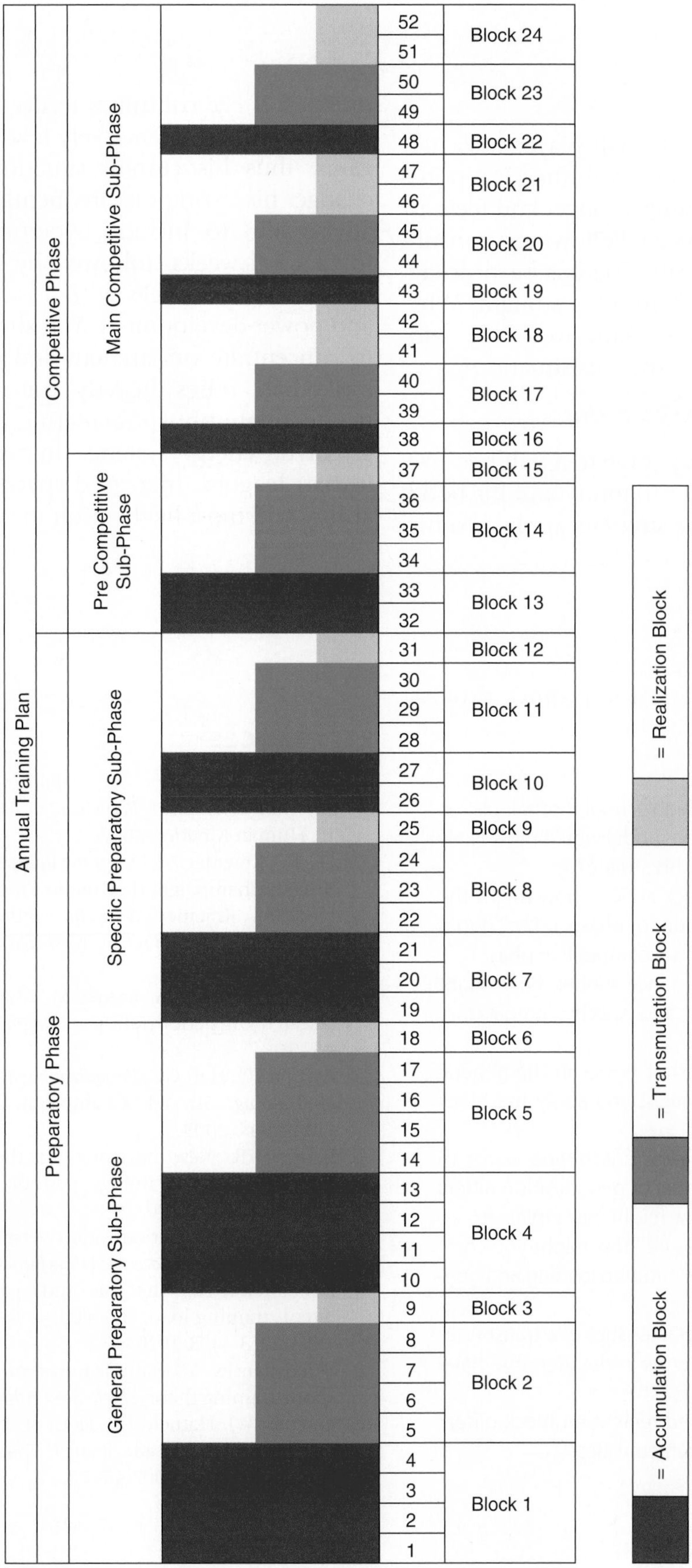

Note: Adapted from Issurin[6,7], Plisk and Stone[17] and Bondarchuk[39].

FIGURE 14.9 Example annual training plan using a block periodization model. (Adapted from Issurin [6,7], Plisk and Stone [17], and Bondarchuk [39]).

CASE EXAMPLE

Designing a Periodized Training Program for a Recreational Basketball Player

BACKGROUND

Lee is a recreational basketball player who has been resistance training for 6 months. He reports that he is no longer getting stronger and feels as though he has hit a plateau. Following a consultation with you, you realize he has been doing the same workout for 6 months straight. Why have Lee's strength gains come to a halt, and what can be done to improve his situation?

CONSIDERATIONS/RECOMMENDATIONS

Lee's strength gains have come to a halt because his program has lacked variability and his body has fully adapted to the stressors applied to his muscles. If Lee continues to do the same workouts, he will experience very few, if any, strength gains, thus his current situation. Lee should change his workouts frequently. You should advise him to include hypertrophy workouts for 4 to 6 weeks, followed by strength workouts for 4 to 6 weeks with a focus on strength and power development. You should advise Lee to concentrate on strength and power because basketball relies heavily on the adenosine triphosphate-phosphocreatine (ATP-PCr) and glycolytic energy systems. In recreational basketball leagues, increased speed and jumping ability will most likely result in success.

Maxing Out

1. You are working with a high school football player. What type of periodization model would most likely be the most effective for this athlete?
2. When working with a track athlete, how might the preparatory and competition phase differ? What determines the length of the competitive phase?
3. When working with a distance runner, how might the general preparatory and specific preparatory phase differ?
4. You are working with a shot putter in the general phase of training; how might you apply the block model of periodization?
5. You are talking with a fellow coach who wants to know how the classic model of periodization differs from the block model; how might you explain it?
6. After looking at the literature, how might you compare developmental, concentrated loading and general blocks?
7. What are the general characteristics of a transmutation block? What other terms in the literature have been used to describe these?
8. How do a competitive and realization block differ? What are their general characteristics?

REFERENCES

1. Kraemer WJ, Fleck SJ. *Optimizing Strength Training: Designing Nonlinear Periodization Workouts*. Champaign, IL: Human Kinetics; 2007.
2. Fleck S, Kraemer WJ. *Designing Resistance Training Programs*. 3rd ed. Champaign, IL: Human Kinetics; 2004.
3. Fleck SJ, Kraemer WJ. *The Ultimate Training System: Periodization Breakthrough*. New York: Advanced Research Press; 1996.
4. Cissik J, Hedrick A, Barnes M. Challenges applying the research on periodization. *Strength Cond J*. 2008;30(1): 45–51.
5. Bompa TO, Haff GG. *Periodization: Theory and Methodology of Training*. 5th ed. Champaign, IL: Human Kinetics Publishers; 2009.
6. Issurin VB. New horizons for the methodology and physiology of training periodization. *Sports Med*. 2010;40(3):189–206.
7. Issurin V. Block periodization versus traditional training theory: a review. *J Sports Med Phys Fitness*. 2008;48(1):65–75.
8. Bondarchuk AP. The role and sequence of using different training-load intensities. *Fitness Sports Rev Int*. 1994;29(3-4):202–204.
9. Verkoshansky Y. Main features of a modern scientific sports training theory. *New Stud Athlet*. 1998;13(3):9–20.
10. Kraemer WJ, Hatfield DL, Fleck SJ. Types of muscle training. In: Brown LE, ed. *Strength Training*. Champaign, IL: Human Kinetics; 2007:45–72.

11. Rhea MR, Ball SD, Phillips WT, et al. A comparison of linear and daily undulating periodized programs with equated volume and intensity for strength. *J Strength Cond Res*. 2002;16(2):250–255.
12. Baker D, Wilson G, Carlyon R. Periodization: the effect on strength of manipulating volume and intensity. *J Strength Cond Res*. 1994;8(4):235–242.
13. Stone MH, Stone ME, Sands WA. *Principles and Practice of Resistance Training*. Champaign, IL: Human Kinetics Publishers; 2007.
14. Nádori L, Granek I. *Theoretical and Methodological Basis of Training Planning with Special Considerations Within a Microcycle*. Lincoln, NE: NSCA; 1989.
15. Harre D. Principles of athletic training. In: Harre D, ed. *Principles of Sports Training: Introduction to the Theory and Methods of Training*. Berlin, Germany: Sportverlag; 1982:73–94.
16. Olbrect J. *The Science of Winning: Planning, Periodizing, and Optimizing Swim Training*. Luton, UK: Swimshop; 2000.
17. Plisk SS, Stone MH. Periodization strategies. *Strength Cond J*. 2003;25(6):19–37.
18. Matveyev L. *Periodization of Sports Training*. Moscow, Russia: Fizkultura i Sport; 1965.
19. Counsilman JE, Counsilman BE. *The New Science of Swimming*. Englewood Cliffs, NJ: Prentice Hall; 1994.
20. Smith DJ. A framework for understanding the training process leading to elite performance. *Sports Med*. 2003;33(15):1103–1126.
21. Fleck SJ, Kraemer WJ. *Designing Resistance Training Programs*. 2nd ed. Champaign, IL: Human Kinetics; 1997.
22. Kraemer WJ, Vingren JL, Hatfield DL, et al. Resistance training programs. In: Thompson WR, Baldwin KE, Pire NI, et al., eds. *ACSM's Resources for the Personal Trainer*. Baltimore, MD: Lippincott, Williams, & Wilkins; 2007:372–403.
23. Kraemer WJ, Ratamess N, Fry AC, et al. Influence of resistance training volume and periodization on physiological and performance adaptations in collegiate women tennis players. *Am J Sports Med*. 2000;28(5):626–633.
24. Zatsiorsky VM. *Science and Practice of Strength Training*. Champaign, IL: Human Kinetics; 1995.
25. Siff MC. *Supertraining*. 6th ed. Denver, CO: Supertraining Institute; 2003.
26. Kurz T. *Science of Sports Training*. 2nd ed. Island Pond, VT: Stadion Publishing Company, Inc.; 2001.
27. Jeffreys I. Quadrennial Planning for the High School Athlete. *Strength Cond J*. 2008;30(3):74–83.
28. Bondarchuk AP. Periodization of sports training. *Legkaya Atletika*. 1986;12:8–9.
29. Haff GG, Kraemer WJ, O'Bryant HS, et al. Roundtable discussion: periodization of training—part 1. *J Strength Cond Res*. 2004;26(1):50–69.
30. Issurin V. *Block Periodization: Breakthrough in Sports Training*. Michigan: Ultimate Athlete Concepts; 2008.
31. Matveyev LP. *Fundamentals of Sports Training*. Moscow, Russia: Fizkultua i Sport; 1977.
32. Gabbett T, King T, Jenkins D. Applied physiology of rugby league. *Sports Med*. 2008;38(2):119–138.
33. Rowbottom DG. Periodization of training. In: Garrett WE, Kirkendall DT, eds. *Exercise and Sport Science*. Philadelphia, PA: Lippincott, Williams, & Wilkins; 2000:499–512.
34. Dick FW. *Sports Training Principles*. 4th ed. London, UK: A and C Black; 2002.
35. Zatsiorsky VM, Kraemer WJ. *Science and Practice of Strength Training*. 2nd ed. Champaign, IL: Human Kinetics; 2006.
36. Verkhoshansky YU. *Fundamentals of Special Strength Training in Sport*. Livonia, MI: Sportivy Press; 1986.
37. Viru A. *Adaptations in Sports Training*. Boca Raton, FL: CRC Press LLC; 1995.
38. Kukushkin GI. *System of Physical Education in the USSR*. Moscow, Russia: Raduga; 1983.
39. Bondarchuk AP. Constructing a training system. *Track Tech*. 1988;102:254–269.
40. Bosquet L, Montpetit J, Arvisais D, et al. Effects of tapering on performance: a meta-analysis. *Med Sci Sports Exerc*. 2007;39(8):1358–1365.
41. Matveyev LP. *Periodisterung Des Sportlichen Trainings*. Moscow, Russia: Fizkultura i Sport; 1972.
42. Harris GR, Stone MH, O'Bryant HS, et al. Short-term performance effects of high power, high force, or combined weight-training methods. J. *Strength Cond Res*. 2000;14(1):14–20.
43. Cristea A, Korhonen MT, Hakkinen K, et al. Effects of combined strength and sprint training on regulation of muscle contraction at the whole-muscle and single-fibre levels in elite master sprinters. *Acta Physiol (Oxf)*. 2008;193(3):275–289.
44. Garcia-Pallares J, Sanchez-Medina L, Carrasco L, et al. Endurance and neuromuscular changes in world-class level kayakers during a periodized training cycle. *Eur J Appl Physiol*. 2009;106(4):629–638.
45. Cormie P, McGuigan MR, Newton RU. Adaptations in athletic performance following ballistic power vs strength training. *Med Sci Sports Exerc*. 2009;42(8):1582–1598.
46. Stone MH, Plisk S, Collins D. Training principles:evaluation of modes and methods of resistance-training—a coaching perspective. *Sport Biomech*. 2002;1(1):79–104.
47. Siff MC, Verkhoshansky YU. *Supertraining*. 4th ed. Denver, CO: Supertraining International; 1999.
48. Plisk SS, Gambetta V. Tactical metabolic training: part 1. *Strength Cond J*. 1997;19(2):44–53.
49. Conley M. Bioenergetics of exercise training. In: Baechle TR, Earle RW, eds. *Essentials of Strength Training and Conditioning*. 2nd ed. Champaign, IL: Human Kinetics; 2000:73–90.
50. Nádori L. *Training and Competition*. Budapest, Hungary: Sport; 1962.
51. Verkhoshansky YU. *Programming and Organization of Training*. Moscow, Russia: Fizkultura i Sport; 1985.
52. Verkhoshansky YU. *Osnovi Spetsialnoi Silovoi Podgotovki i Sporte (Fundamentals of Special Strength Training in Sport)*. Moscow, Russia: Fizkultura i Sport Publishers; 1977.

CHAPTER 15

Strength and Conditioning for Sport

MICHAEL H. STONE ● MEG E. STONE

OBJECTIVES

After reading this chapter, you will be able to:

- Demonstrate an understanding of the basic training principles.
- Explain the training process, including the importance of the technical, tactical, psychological, and physiological aspects of training. Demonstrate an understanding of the role of periodization in the training process.
- Incorporate various methods used in training advanced athletes.
- Explain the role of single sets versus multiple sets in a training program.
- Explain the role of training to failure in a training program.
- Demonstrate an understanding of the importance of monitoring athletes for overtraining.

KEY TERMS

Active Rest (AR)
Competition Phase (C)
Exercise Intensity
General Preparation (GP)
Macrocycles
Mesocycles
Microcycles
Overload
Overreaching
Peaking (P)
Periodization
Relative Intensity
Special or Specific Preparation (SP)
Specificity of Exercise and Training
Training Density
Training Intensity (TI)
Training Volume
Variation
Volume Load (VL)

Introduction

There are many factors concerned with the intricacies of strength/power training and subsequent adaptations. These factors include sex differences, optimum loading schemes, complex and contrast exercises, and sequenced loading. While many of the details of the factors are only just now beginning to emerge, there is strong evidence that the manner and phases in which training is presented to the athlete can make a profound difference in performance outcome.

The purpose of this chapter is to *briefly* discuss physiological and performance adaptations to periodized resistance training as well as the periodization of training modes and methods that can enhance specific adaptations. This discussion deals primarily with traditional methods of programming for resistance training. For a more detailed discussion of advanced training methods, refer to Bompa and Haff (38), Plisk and Stone (1), and Stone et al. (2).

BASIC TRAINING PRINCIPLES

There is little doubt that the training method, which includes the manipulation of reps and sets, loading, movement velocity, rest and recovery aspects, etc., can make a significant difference in the physiological and performance adaptations resulting from a resistance-training program (3–5). For example, high-volume programs generally have a greater influence on body composition and endurance factors than do low-volume programs, whereas high-intensity programs have a greater influence on maximum strength compared to low-intensity programs (5–8). It is also probable that the choice of training mode (type of equipment) can influence the adaptations to a training program (9). Evidence also indicates that the level of athlete can result in somewhat different adaptations to training. For example, among relatively weak subjects (or athletes), strength training will provide as great or greater increases in power as will power training (2,10). Additionally, there is evidence that prior strength training or having higher levels of maximum strength can potentiate power training (2,3,10).

There are three basic training principles: overload, variation, and specificity (2,8). If each of these principles is appropriately addressed as a result of logically applied exercise prescription, fatigue management is enhanced, overtraining potential will be reduced, and the potential for superior performance augmented.

The three basic training principles are overload, variation, and specificity; to optimize the training adaptations, these principles must be appropriately integrated into the training plan.

Overload involves providing an appropriate stimulus for attaining a desired level of physical, physiological, or performance adaptation. Overload can be conceptualized as an exercise and training stimulus that goes beyond normal levels of physical performance. An exercise prescription for overload could include range of motion, absolute and relative intensity (RI) levels, frequency, and duration factors. All overload stimuli will have some level of intensity, RI (percentage of maximum), and volume. The quantification of overload stimuli for various modes (weights, variable resistance devices, semi-isokinetic devices, rubber bands, etc.) of resistance training can be challenging. Quantification of some forms of overload—elastic resistance, for example—is difficult. For this discussion, the quantification of overload stimuli deals with weight training.

Intensity is an often misunderstood component of an exercise prescription. There are several aspects to the intensity component. Intensity factors are associated with the rate of performing work and the rate at which energy is expended (8). Intensity factors can be separated into two aspects: training intensity (TI) and movement, or exercise, intensity (8).

Training intensity (TI) is concerned with the rate at which a training exercise or training session proceeds; it can be estimated by the average mass (weight) lifted per exercise, per day, per week, etc. and relates to the training density. For example, within a session, the average load lifted is directly related to the time taken to complete the exercise. Typically, for a given number of repetitions, a heavier load requires more time to complete. Additionally, the greater the number of repetitions per set, the longer it takes for completion. Thus the work rate is dictated by loading and repetition number (see Tables 15.1 and 15.2).

The **relative intensity** is a percent of the one-repetition maximum (1 RM). The 1 RM is stable only in advanced strength trainers. Thus, using RI to plan training programs must be carried out with this aspect in mind.

Exercise intensity is the actual power output of a movement. Power is defined as a work rate or as the product of force and velocity. The product of force and velocity forms an inverted U, with peak power occurring at approximately 30% of the peak isometric force in single-joint exercises. Peak power has been shown to be associated with approximately 30% to 80% of the 1 RM, depending upon the type of exercise and the trained state. The exact percentage of the 1 RM at which peak power occurs appears to depend on whether the exercise involves single or multiple joints, whether the body weight is also involved in the movement, and whether or not the movement is joint-range-limited or ballistic (11). Typically, for single-joint nonballistic exercises, peak power occurs at about 30% to 40% of 1 RM; for whole-body nonballistic movements, peak power occurs at approximately 40% to 60%; and 70% to 85% for semiballistic weightlifting movements (12,13). There is some controversy over the optimum loading for jumping movements. Some data indicate that peak power occurs at 0 load (body mass) regardless of strength level (10,14); however,

TABLE 15.1 ● DAY 1: GP PHASE

	SET	REPETITIONS	LOAD	VL	TI	TIME FOR SET EXECUTION (S)	KG · S^{-1}
	1	10	60	600		40	15.0
	2	10	100	1,000		45	22.2
	3	10	140	1,400		47	29.8
	4	10	140	1,400		52	26.9
	5	10	140	1,400		55	25.5
TOTAL	5	50	580	5,800		239	119.4
Mean					116	47.8	24.3

VL = sum of load lifted (sets × mass); TI = VL/repetitions (or mean load/sets).

other data indicate that stronger subjects (particularly when strength is normalized for body mass differences) may produce similar or higher peak powers at loads between 0% and 40% of 1 RM (4,15,16).

It appears that the type of exercise, level of training and fatigue level can influence the 1-RM percentage at which maximum power occurs; with stronger or more experienced strength athletes producing maximum power at slightly higher percentages than less trained or weaker athletes (11,16,17). Thus, the RI can be used to estimate (and to manipulate) the exercise intensity, with very heavy or very light weights producing lower power outputs than those in the middle range for nonballistic, most ballistic, and semiballistic movements and lighter loads producing higher power outputs during jumps. Thus, in planning the training program, a variety of loads producing different power outputs should be used as this can produce both increases in peak power as well as alter the range over which power is produced (2,16).

Training density deals with the frequency of training per session, per day, per week, etc. For example, day 1 might contain four training sessions, each of equal volume, and day 2 might contain two training sessions of similar volume. Day 1 would have a higher training density. One week could contain 5 training sessions, while another could contain 10; the training density in week 2 would be higher.

Training volume is a measure or estimate of the total work performed and is strongly related to total energy expenditure (18–20). Although TI (and RI) can be estimated by the amount of weight lifted, the training volume is related to the number of repetitions and sets per exercise, the number and types of exercises used (large vs. small muscle mass), and the frequency (i.e., number of times per day, week, month, etc.) with which these exercises are repeated.

Volume load (VL) is a reasonable estimate of the amount of work accomplished during training and is commonly used in both research and practical settings (2,14). VL is calculated by summing the product of the load and the number of repetitions

TABLE 15.2 ● DAY 2: COMPETITION PHASE

	SET	REPETITIONS	LOAD	VL	TI	TIME FOR SET EXECUTION (S)	KG · S^{-1}
	1	5	60	300		15.0	20.0
	2	5	120	600		17.0	35.3
	3	5	165	825		25.0	33.0
	4	5	165	825		26.0	31.7
	5	5	165	825		28.0	29.4
TOTAL	5	25	525	3,375		111.0	149.4
Mean					135	22.2	30.4

VL = sum of load lifted (sets × mass); TI = VL/repetitions (or mean load/sets).

for each set. This can be done for each exercise per week, month, etc. and the summed total for the combined exercises represents an estimate of the total work accomplished. This approach works well, provided there are no major changes in the exercises performed. If the exercises are changed markedly (i.e., 1/4 squats vs. full squats), then to make better comparisons, the VL for each exercise should be multiplied times the vertical distance the bar moves (21). The application of TI and volume can be considered in terms of the training session (i.e., all of the exercises performed during a specified period) or in terms of single exercises. An understanding of overload factors can aid in the programming of training, including methods (i.e., sets and repetitions), velocity of exercise, and exercise selection.

The interaction/association of VL and TI can be illustrated by calculating these factors for two sample training sessions (using actual data from the squat as an example). Table 15.1 contains the data for day 1, the general preparation (GP) phase; Table 15.2 contains the data for day 2, the competition phase.

In this example, the VL for day 1 was larger than that for day 2 (5,800 vs. 3,375 kg); however, the TI was larger for day 2 than for day 1 (135 vs. 116). VL and TI are inversely related. Furthermore, TI is directly related to the rate at which the load is lifted (kilograms per second) and is an indication of the rate of training. Calculation of the TI, while reflecting work rate (kilograms per second), is less time-consuming than measuring and calculating kilograms per second and thus has a practical advantage. The average VL and TI can be easily calculated per week, month, or phase of training. In this manner, using these variables, a reasonable record of training progress can be made.

Variation involves appropriate manipulation in TI, speed of movement, volume, and exercise selection. Appropriate variation is a primary consideration for continued adaptation over the course of long-term training programs (22,23). Appropriate sequencing of volume, intensity, and exercise selection, including speed–strength exercises in a periodized manner, can lead to superior enhancement of a variety of performance abilities (3).

Several different levels of variation are possible in a training program (i.e., long-term, short-term, day-to-day, etc.) The level of variation in the training program is directly related to the level of the athlete.

Specificity of exercise and training is the most important consideration in selecting both methods and modes for resistance training, especially if athletic performance enhancement is a primary goal. Specificity includes both bioenergetics and mechanics of training. This discussion is concerned with the mechanical aspects of specificity.

SPECIFICITY AND TRANSFER-OF-TRAINING EFFECT

As previously noted, *mechanical specificity* refers to the kinetic and kinematic associations between a training exercise and a physical performance. Mechanical specificity includes movement patterns, peak force, rate of force development, acceleration, and velocity parameters. Mechanical specificity stems from observations of intra- and intermuscular task specificities (2). Task specificity deals with the manner in which the motor cortex organizes motor unit (MU) activation (intramuscular tasks) and whole muscle activation patterns (intermuscular tasks). There is good evidence that both intra and intermuscular task specificities play a major role in strength–power training. Basically, the greater similarity a training exercise has to the actual physical performance, the greater the probability of transfer (8,9,24,25). For example, intramuscular task specificity (25,26) suggests that for a specific task only a defined pool of MUs will be activated; evidence of this can be found from practical and research aspects. For example, bodybuilders indicate that to fully develop a muscle many different exercises for that muscle must be used. This observation of bodybuilders has support from a research aspect. Abe et al. (27) has shown that muscle hypertrophy does not occur uniformly throughout a muscle nor does it occur uniformly in each region of the body (e.g., upper vs. lower). Mechanical specificity has been extensively studied as it affects strength-training exercise. Of particular importance is explosive strength and power.

Transfer-of-training effect deals with the degree to which a training exercise promotes adaptation in performance. To maximize the potential for "transfer-of-training effect," a training exercise must use reasonable levels of movement pattern specificity and overload.

EXPLOSIVE STRENGTH AND POWER

Among untrained and moderately trained subjects, heavy weight training can produce positive performance effects in the entire force velocity curve (3,4,10,28). Indeed, evidence exists which indicates that among relatively weak athletes, increasing maximum strength will also increase rate of force development and power as much or more than power training (10). However, both observational and objective evidence indicate that among advanced strength-trained subjects, considerable high-velocity training is necessary to make additional alterations in the high-velocity end of the force velocity curve (3,10,28).

Although isometric training can result in an increased peak rate of force production and velocity of movement, especially in untrained subjects (24), the isometric training effect on dynamic explosive force production is relatively minor, particularly among well-trained athletes (28,29). Although several parameters can be affected, traditional heavy weight training primarily increases maximum strength, especially as measured by a 1 RM. In contrast, the primary effect of typical ballistic training is an increased rate of force production and velocity of movement, (3,4,28,29). Additionally, high-power training can alter a wide range of athletic performance variables to a greater extent than does traditional heavy weight training, especially in subjects with a reasonable initial level of maximum strength (3,30). Indeed, an initial high maximum strength level appears to potentiate the development of high-power outputs and increased movement velocity (9,31,32).

The type of training program (i.e., high-volume, high-intensity) can make a marked difference in the type of adaptation (i.e., body composition, strength, power, etc.) to the program.

It is also important to select modes of exercise that will have the greatest transfer-of-training effect. It is doubtful that single-joint exercises will have as much impact on performance, which is multijoint in nature, as multijoint training exercises (9,33). In selecting training modes, a number of considerations and performance criteria can be used (9,34). These criteria can maximize the transfer-of-training effect.

Movement pattern characteristics include the following (9,34):

1. The type of muscle action (e.g., concentric, eccentric, SSC)
2. Accentuated regions of force production
3. The complexity, amplitude, and direction of movement
4. Ballistic versus nonballistic movements

There also must be an overload application for successful performance adaptation. During early training (beginners), the task itself supplies sufficient overload for development. However, if overload is not continued, then sport performance will not improve beyond adaptation to simple practice of the sport. Factors to be overloaded include force production, rate of force production, and power output. In choosing exercises for training explosive athletic performance, ballistic movements and rate of force production are especially important.

THE TRAINING PROCESS

Training is a *process* which prepares an athlete, *technically, tactically, psychologically, physiologically*, and *physically* for the highest possible levels of performance (2). It is also a commitment on the coach and athlete's part. The training process involves all of the factors that provide for athlete enhancement. This includes nutrition, sleep, the training plan, sport science, the monitoring program, and sport medicine. This chapter deals with one aspect of the training process: the training plan. Whereas periodization provides the basic framework, program planning involves making decisions related to the number of sets, intensity of the exercise, volume, load, and rate of progression. In general, multiple-set periodized training programs will demonstrate greater gains in performance over the long term than single-set or nonperiodized programs.

PERIODIZATION

Conceptually, **periodization** represents the theoretical framework for planning the training program. Periodization can be defined as a logical phasic method of manipulating training variables in order to increase the potential for achieving specific performance goals (35,36). Thus, a basic tenet of periodization is training nonlinearity. The primary goals of periodization are (a) reduction of overtraining potential and (b) peaking at the appropriate time or providing a maintenance program for sports with a specific season. The goals are met by appropriately manipulating volume and intensity factors and by appropriate exercise selection. It is important to understand that variation can take place at several different levels. A brief overview of periodization is provided in Box 15.1.

Periodization represents the theoretical framework for planning training programs.

Periodization involves planned variation in volume and intensity of training to promote maximal performance at the desired time and to decrease the chance for overtraining.

Traditional periodized training can be divided into three stages or levels: the **macrocycle** (long-length cycle), the **mesocycle** (middle-length cycle), and the **microcycle** (short-length cycle, or day-to-day variation). Each macro- and mesocycle generally begins with high-volume, low-intensity training and ends with high-intensity, low-volume training. The macro- and mesocycle can contain four phases: (a) preparation (general and special), (b) competition, (c) peaking, and (d) transition or active rest (AR). Each of these phases typically has different goals and requires different degrees of variation in training variables. Figure 15.1 illustrates a traditional macrocycle for a novice athlete.

The **general preparation (GP)** is a high-volume phase, usually lasting a few weeks,

BOX 15.1

Periodization

Periodization is the framework of the cyclical manipulation of training variables to promote maximum performance at the appropriate time of the year while decreasing the chances of overtraining. Periodization principles can also be applied to seasonal sports such as rugby and American football.

In its simplest form, periodization is variation planning: both short- and long-term planning. As the competitive season approaches, training should progress from less specific to more specific. Less specific training is performed in the off-season or during periods with less emphasis on competition and then progresses to sport-specific training as the competitive season approaches.

The decisions made in programming a periodized training program should be based on scientific evidence. The science of conditioning is a process of adaptation to new information, and conditioning programs should evolve with science. One potential limiting factor in the application of training principles and programming theory is that some sports or age groups have not been well studied. In this case, we must extrapolate from the research that is available to design the best possible training programs for these athletes.

Today, periodized training programs have been applied to a variety of individual and team sports. Some of these programs are based on direct scientific evidence and some are based on logical application of scientific principles based on similar sports or activities.

The application of periodization to training programs to improve athletic performance is an evolving science.

Q & A from the Field

Q ***I have heard the terms linear and undulating periodization used lately. What do these terms mean?***

A *Linear periodization* is used to describe periodized programs that increase load and intensity in a direct linear fashion over a specific time period. The term, however, is a misnomer, as all periodized programs provide a cyclical framework in which certain characteristics of training (e.g., endurance, strength, power) are emphasized or deemphasized and should utilize variations in loading that include hard days followed by easier days or recovery days. *Undulating periodization* is also a misnomer. All periodization programs will have various degrees of undulation of volume and intensity; depending upon the framework of the periodization concept, there can be more or less variation. Beginning athletes, for example, generally respond better to programs with less variation in load and intensity. Advanced athletes can generally maintain higher loads and intensities and greater variation from 1 day to the next. All periodized programs should vary the load and intensity of training; some programs contain more variation and some less.

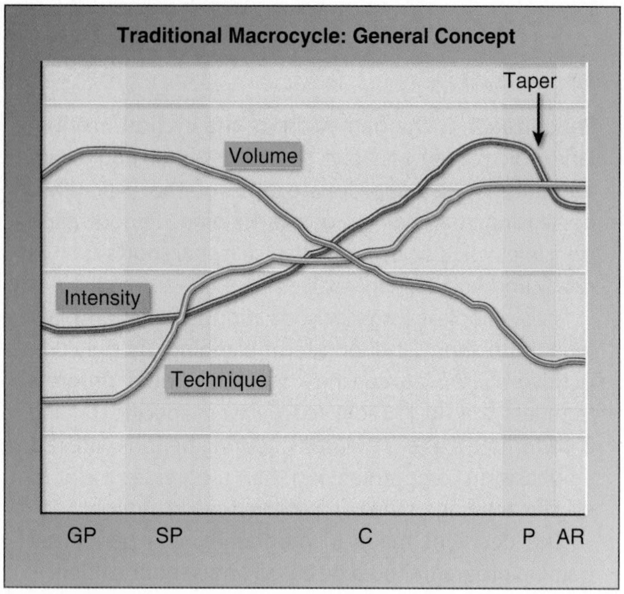

FIGURE 15.1 Traditional macrocycle for novices. GP, general preparation; SP, special preparation; C, competition; P, peaking; AR, active rest.

designed to enhance sports-specific fitness and associated physiological parameters. **Special or specific preparation (SP)** deals with relatively high-volume training in which the exercises are more specific to the activity in terms of movement pattern and velocity. It is used as a transition phase linking high-volume, less specific GP training to high-intensity, very specific training associated with competition. During the **competition phase (C)**, intensity factors are adjusted in keeping with the characteristics of the sport. For example, in a sport requiring high-power outputs, more time is spent on using high exercise intensities; for a sport in which great strength is required, a greater emphasis can be placed on high training intensities. Volume during the competition phase is decreased. The competition phase can last several months.

The competition phase is generally characterized by a low volume of training and high intensity of training. The intensity of training should match the intensity required for participation in the sport.

Peaking (P) is a phase lasting a short time (usually <4 weeks). During the early portion of peaking, volume is typically reduced as TI (or exercise intensity, depending on the sport or performance goals) is increased or maintained at relatively high levels. During the last few days before competition, intensity factors are also reduced to encourage adequate recovery. The later portion of a peaking phase, when volume is markedly reduced, is referred to as a "taper" (37).

Peaking is a short phase generally characterized by a low volume of training while maintaining sport-specific intensities. The last few days before competition, both the volume and intensity are reduced to promote recovery.

Active rest (AR) is a phase in which volume and intensity are decreased markedly to facilitate recovery from the training cycle. Recovery includes healing and rehabilitation of any injuries that may have occurred as well as recovery from the emotional rigors of competition. Complete rest allows sports-specific fitness to deteriorate to a degree from which it is difficult to recover without extensive training. Compared to complete rest, AR allows for less deterioration of fitness and a faster return to peak fitness during the next cycle. AR usually lasts about 1 week. A modification of the typical scheme can be made for sports with a definite season in which winning all contests (games) is a goal, such as basketball. A typical general modification for seasonal sports is to prolong the competition phase and remove the peaking phase.

In recent years, some sports have moved to a marked increase in competitions often coming relatively close together; for this type of sport scenario, the classic approach does not work well. Additionally, the traditional model of periodization has been criticized for two basic reasons. First, many coaches (not understanding all of the nuances of periodization) have attempted to increase the volume of several different training variables simultaneously. This approach can cause difficulty in fatigue management due to high volumes of training (2,38). Often noncompatible methods (e.g., power and endurance) were trained simultaneously (2,38). As a result, Verkoshansky developed the "conjugated successive system" (39), Stone et al. developed "phase potentiation" (2), and Issurin further developed "block periodization" (40). Essentially, all three of these "models" are very similar in their approach to obviating the criticisms. They use the basic concepts of the traditional model on a shorter time scale between competitions, do not simultaneously increase the volume of noncompatible exercises, and do not increase the volume of many different aspects to the point where volume is "unmanageable" (2,38,40,41).

These models also use the idea of linking together a series of concentrated loads. A concentrated load is *unidirectional*, meaning that one characteristic of physiological development (e.g., endurance, strength, power) is being emphasized. The training plan offered in this chapter is largely based on these models. For a more detailed discussion concerning periodization training, see Bompa and Haff (38), Plisk and Stone (1), Stone et al. (2), and Chapter 14. There are several training factors that can negatively impact the basic periodization framework. Two of the more important of these factors are the volume of work and training to failure which impacts the relative TI.

SINGLE SETS VERSUS MULTIPLE SETS

The role of volume in producing hypertrophy, strength, and power has been well documented (2,7). Although there has been controversy (42), the majority of studies and reviews that have carefully examined training with one set versus training with multiple sets, with both men and women, indicate that superior results can be obtained in a wide variety of performance and physiological variables including strength, power, and hypertrophy by using multiple sets (8,43–45). Maximum strength, power, and positive adaptations in body composition are among the variables that can be altered to a greater extent by using multiple sets. The superior effects of multiple sets are particularly apparent among advanced weight trainers (8,22,23,44). Furthermore, these effects can be enhanced by the use of periodization/variation techniques along with the multiple set protocols.

TRAINING TO FAILURE

It is commonly believed that training to failure is necessary to stimulate maximum hypertrophy, strength, or power gains; however, there is very little evidence for this belief. This belief is based on the idea that fatigue results in MUs dropping out forcing other, larger, MUs to be recruited. While this does happen, it is also true that higher intensity and ballistic exercises also recruit additional MUs (7). Although metabolite buildup and fatigue during resistance exercise may influence the result (46), they are not necessary to produce strength gains (47,48). Indeed, recent study has shown that over a 16-week training period, consistent training to failure does not produce the same degree of hypertrophy, strength, or power (49,50).

It should be noted that basing training on RM ranges promotes training to failure (51). For example, 8- to 12-RM training entails starting with a weight for which 8 repetitions can be accomplished; over time, more repetitions can be accomplished until 12 are reached at which time the load is increased reducing achieved repetitions to 8, and the process starts over. During this process, failure (or near failure) is consistently a result. This type of training represents poor fatigue management and is often counterproductive (2,48,51). Good fatigue management is particularly important when multiple types and modes of training are being integrated.

TRAINING ADVANCED ATHLETES

Most advanced and elite athletes use some form of periodization (Fig. 15.2). Advanced and elite athletes may require greater variation and more creative approaches to training compared to lower level and beginning athletes. Greater variation is necessary as a result of several factors, including the facts that (a) advanced athletes train with greater volumes and intensities than beginners and novices, thus they may be closer to an overtraining threshold, and (b) as genetic limitations are approached, greater variation and novel approaches to training may be necessary to "provoke" additional adaptation. Several creative resistance-training approaches may stimulate further strength–power adaptations.

Advanced athletes may require greater variations in volume and intensity of training compared to beginning athletes to promote continued adaptations to the training stimulus.

Sequenced Training (Phase Potentiation)

As previously noted, prior exposure to strength training and increased maximum strength levels can potentiate gains in power resulting from power training. Examination of longitudinal and cross-sectional studies (8,10,28) suggests that sequenced training, heavy weight training over a few weeks followed by speed–strength training, or combination training (heavy training plus high-power or high-speed training), can produce superior results in speed and power gains compared to heavy weight training or speed–strength training alone. More importantly, evidence indicates that this type of sequenced training (a form of phase potentiation) can beneficially alter a wide variety of athletic performance variables to a greater extent than either

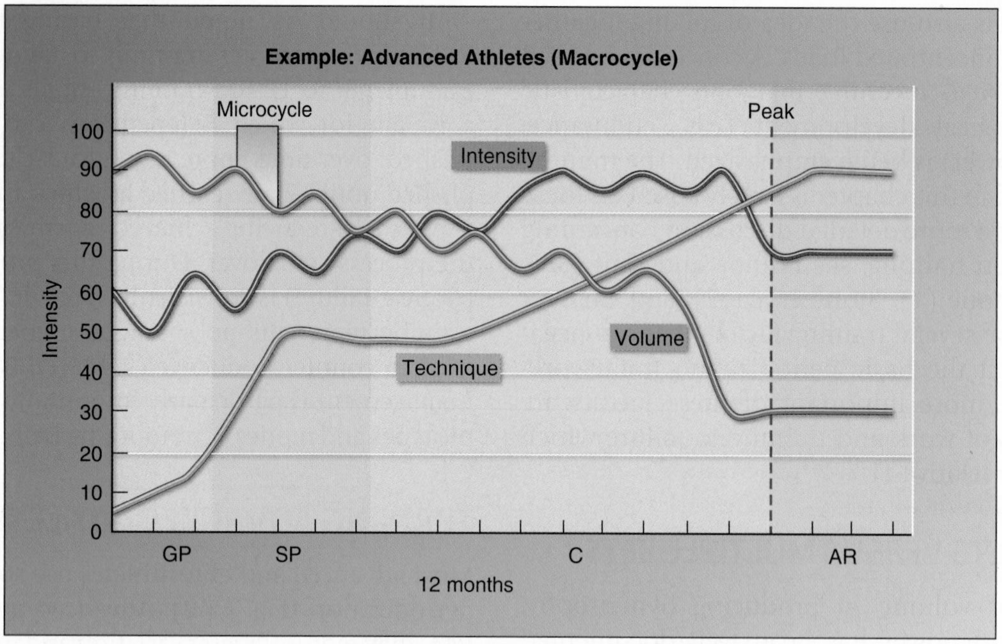

FIGURE 15.2 Typical traditional periodized approach for advanced athletes. Notice the greater variation compared to Figure 15.1. GP, general preparation; SP, special preparation; C, competition; P, peaking; AR, active rest.

heavy weight training or speed–strength training (3,52). To produce maximum gains in power, the following sequence would be reasonable (3):

Strength endurance → strength → power and speed

Each phase may last several weeks, depending on the needs of the athlete, type of sport, and placement in the overall macrocycle or annual plan.

Evidence suggests that sequenced training may produce superior results in terms of improving speed and power. For strength–power athletes, sequenced training begins with a cycle of strength–endurance training followed by a strength-training emphasis followed by speed–strength training or a combination of heavy training with high-power or high-speed training.

Q & A from the Field

Q ***I thought speed was one of those variables that really could not be improved. Can resistance training really improve the running speed of my athletes?***

A Yes, the appropriate resistance-training program can improve running speed assuming that the athlete has not reached his or her physiological peak. Here are some components you can likely modify with resistance training: (a) One factor in running speed is generating ground reaction force; the more force you apply to the ground in the appropriate direction, the faster you will move. Interestingly, there is good evidence that vertical force (i.e., stride length) is the primary limiting factor among advanced sprinters. (b) Another factor is stride rate, which involves not only the force you apply to the ground but also the speed with which you can cycle your stride. A limiting factor here is bringing the trail leg forward rapidly. Resistance training of the hip flexors and integrating this training into running form can improve speed. (c) Speed of movement is partly a function of fast-twitch muscle fibers. Appropriately designed resistance-training programs facilitate speed and power development by training and improving the capacity of fast-twitch muscle fibers.

Microcycles

The phase potentiation (block) model is built upon microcycles and summated microcycles. A microcycle is the shortest repeatable cycle and is typically defined as 1 week. Variation is accomplished by day-to-day alterations in volume and intensity factors. Variation is necessary to reduce overtraining potential; reduction of overtraining is better accomplished at the microcycle level then any other level of training. It is well known that heavy, intense training loads are necessary for ultimate athletic achievement; however, frequent heavy loads and training monotony increase "training strain" and the potential for negative training outcomes (53,54). Further, data from both human (53) and animal (55) models indicate that multiple "light" days within a microcycle can allow a given training load to be accomplished with a greater potential for positive adaptations and fewer negative outcomes (35,36,53). Some of the negative side effects of training may be associated with changes in the maximum strength available in training (T_{max}). For example, observations by the authors indicate that T_{max} can decrease across a microcycle due to accumulated fatigue, thus the 1 RM representing T_{max} on Monday may not be T_{max} on Friday. If accumulative fatigue is not taken into consideration, loads based on a percentage of T_{max} (or a contest maximum) may actually represent a much larger percentage of the true maximum strength level at the end of the microcycle. Thus, appropriate variation in volume and intensity can offset fatigue-induced alterations in T_{max}. Additionally, training variables can be altered daily to provide variation in movement, a factor, which in turn, may provide a further stimulus for both maximum strength and power development (3). Although there are several ways of producing alterations in training variables, variation can be simply and efficiently produced by using a heavy/light day system.

Appropriate variations in volume and intensity of training are important to allow adequate recovery from intense training sessions and reduce the chance of accumulated fatigue and overtraining.

Box 15.2 illustrates an example in which the emphasis of training is on development of leg and hip strength primarily using the squat. In this example, several factors must be considered.

BOX 15.2

Example of Squat Training Program

Squats: M and Th: 3 × 5 at target load
Pulls: W and S
Squat T_{max} = 200 kg
Day M T W TH F S SU
RI H R MH M R M R
RI = % of T_{max} for 3 × 5
H 80% to 85%
MH 75% to 80%
M 70% to 75%
L 65% to 70%
R Rest

The first aspect is the level of the athlete: This type of variation in intensity will not work well with beginners because of the instability of T_{max}. The second aspect is that intensity of training is altered through variations of RI; the exact percentage used will change with individual athletes, the type of exercise, the set/repetitions scheme, and fatigue (21). Because of these factors, a percentage range should be used. So, in the above example, the athlete might squat 160 kg on Monday but only 140 kg on Friday for three sets of five repetitions. On both days, maximum efforts would be made to enhance appropriate adaptations (56). RI can also be calculated based on set and repetitions rather than a 1 RM, as follows. Remember that RI is the percent of maximum for the set and repetition protocol.

VH = 100%
H = 90% to 95%
MH = 85% to 90%
M = 80% to 85%
ML = 75% to 80%
L = 70% to 75%

So, for example, if 100 kg were the maximum for 3 × 5 in the squat (i.e., 100% = VH), then on a moderate (M) lifting day, only 80 to 85 kg would be used. This method works well with advanced athletes for whom estimates of 100% for sets and reps can be predicted for various exercises with reasonable accuracy, as their T_{max} and training loads are relatively stable over long periods.

In the creation of effective microcycle variation, the effects of other training activities must also be considered. If running or other conditioning activities are also included in the overall training program, then the additional energy

REAL-WORLD APPLICATION

Fatigue and Decreased Performance

A weight lifter training for a competition is having trouble sustaining a reasonable level of training performance and is feeling quite fatigued. How would you examine her condition and what factors might you manipulate (as a coach) to remedy this problem?

Multiple factors may lead to decreased performance and fatigue in an athlete. Consider all possibilities, but focus on the factors that are most likely with the specific athlete you are working with.

1. The obvious factor to consider first is a potential imbalance between training and recovery. Evaluate the volume and intensity of training.
2. Evaluate the nutritional habits of the lifter. Is the athlete eating properly? Is the athlete getting enough total calories? Carbohydrates? Protein?
3. What is the emotional/psychological status of the athlete? Maybe the athlete is burned out or is no longer enjoying the sport. Maybe there are personal problems with family members, friends, etc.
4. Are there any medical problems that could be causing fatigue? Perhaps a physical examination from a physician is needed to rule out specific medical conditions. As the athlete in this example is a female, are there menstrual cycle disturbances?
5. Is there a possibility the athlete is using or abusing drugs? Specific drugs are related to specific behaviors, and drug use and/or abuse can certainly be related to fatigue.

Obviously some of these problems need the assistance of other professionals: a medical doctor, a sport psychologist, etc. As the coach, you can do several things to help the athlete.

1. Make sure the training program is not too intense or that there is not too much work being performed, and that the athlete is getting adequate time for recovery. Hard days of training should be followed by lighter days or recovery days. There should be variation in volume and intensity factors from one workout to the next. Adequate time should be allowed for recovery. Adequate sleep is critical to recovery. Make sure the athlete is not participating in additional physical activity that is detracting from the weightlifting performance.
2. Make sure the athlete is eating a balanced diet, eating enough calories, and adequately hydrated.
3. Monitor the athlete for common symptoms of overtraining.

demands and increased physical and emotional stress must be taken into account. In this context, planning and tracking alterations by VL can be more valuable than tracking alterations in intensity. VL can change with the type of exercises, repetitions, and intensity. Table 15.3 illustrates alterations in VL resulting from changes in repetitions.

It can be noted that even when the load is constant, the addition or deletion of repetitions can alter the VL, and therefore the total work accomplished. Importantly, the higher volume of work on day 1 will probably require more time and energy for recovery (19). On the other hand, higher intensities of training would require greater recovery time and energy if the VLs were equal.

TABLE 15.3 ● ALTERATIONS IN VL RESULTING FROM CHANGES IN REPETITIONS

	Day 1: 3 × 10 Repetitions (Target Load)				Day 2: 3 × 5 Repetitions (Target Load)			
	SET	REPETITIONS	LOAD (KG)	VL (KG)	SET	REPETITIONS	LOAD (KG)	VL (KG)
	1	10	60	600	1	5	60	300
	2	10	100	1,000	2	5	100	500
	3	10	140	1,400	3	5	140	700
	4–6	30	160	4,800	4–6	15	160	2,400
Total	6	60		7,800	6	30		3,900
Mean			130				130	

TABLE 15.4 ● ALTERATIONS IN VL RESULTING FROM CHANGES IN TI

	DAY 1: 3 × 5 REPETITIONS (TARGET LOAD)				DAY 2: 3 × 5 REPETITIONS (TARGET LOAD)			
	Set	Repetitions	Load (Kg)	Vl (Kg)	Set	Repetitions	Load (Kg)	Vl (Kg)
	1	5	60	300	1	5	60	300
	2	5	100	500	2	5	120	600
	3	5	140	700	3	5	160	800
	4–6	15	160	2,400	4–6	15	180	2,700
Total	6	30		3,900	6	30		4,400
Mean			130				147	

VL can also be strongly affected by alterations in TI, as seen in Table 15.4.

In this example, using constant sets and repetitions, an increase in loading (TI) can produce a marked increase in VL and therefore in total work and total energy expenditure (exercise plus recovery). In actual practice, combinations of intensity and repetition changes accomplish alterations in VL. Often increases in load necessitate additional "warm-up" sets. The designation of heavy and light days based on VL must take into consideration the TI, RI, number of sets, repetitions, and the trained state. Tables 15.5 and 15.6 illustrate actual data from heavy and light days within a microcycle on 2 days in which exercises were repeated.

From this example, it can be observed that a reduction in target load by 20% (with appropriate alterations in warm-up sets) can result in a reduced VL of approximately 22%.

Because total energy expenditure is related to the VL, care must be taken in "matching" the resistance-training program with the requirements for other aspects of conditioning. If one aspect is being emphasized—for example, strength adaptation—then a light day for training must remain a light day. It should be noted that increasing the amount of work performed in non–strength-training aspects, so that the day becomes a heavy-workload day, defeats the purpose of having a light day and can increase the probability of negative adaptation. So, for example, in a sport requiring strength/power training that also requires other conditioning aspects such as running and tactical training, it is imperative that the workloads for individual components complement each other and not interfere with the goals of the training period phase. Table 15.7 provides an example of a mesocycle in which improving maximum strength is the goal, where different aspects of training would be adjusted so that strength development is not reduced.

Or if tactical training were a priority, for example, during football season, then a different schedule would be appropriate, as in Table 15.8.

SUMMATED MICROCYCLES

Microcycles can be grouped together or summated into "blocks," so that each block presents a specific pattern of volume and intensity loading. The blocks can then be repeated throughout a mesocycle such that specific stimuli are "re-presented" in a cyclical

TABLE 15.5 ● DATA FROM A HEAVY DAY WITHIN A MACROCYCLE: MONDAY VL (HEAVY) SETS OF 5 (TARGET × 85)

EXERCISE	SET	1	2	3	4	5	6	7	TOTAL
Squats	(1 RM = 200)	300	500	700	850	850	850	450[a]	4,500
Push press	(1 RM = 100)	250	300	400	400	400	250[a]		2,000
Bench press	(1 RM = 140)	300	500	600	600	600	325[a]		2,925
Total									9,425

[a]Reduced load sets for optimal power output.

TABLE 15.6 ● DATA FROM A LIGHT DAY WITHIN A MACROCYCLE: THURSDAY VL (LIGHT) SETS OF 5—TARGET SETS REDUCED IN LOAD BY 20%

EXERCISE	SET	1	2	3	4	5	6	7	TOTAL
Squats	(1 RM = 200)	300	500	700	700	700	450		3,350
Push press	(1 RM = 100)	250	300	325	325	325	250[a]		1,575
Bench press	(1 RM = 140)	300	400	475	475	475	325[a]		2,450
Total									7,375

[a]Reduced load sets for optimal power output.

fashion. Generally, a block consists of 4 weeks. A typical block would be one in which volume and intensity are increased for 3 weeks followed by an "unload" week, creating a 3/1 block (2,57,58). The unload week can be used to reduce the potential for overtraining and to allow for adaptation and supercompensation (Fig. 15.3). Care should be taken in using this type of 3/1 approach because the heaviest loading takes place in the third week, and the accumulation of fatigue from microcycles 1 to 3 may preclude adaptation to speed–strength work (therefore the need for an unload week). In advanced athletes, if improved maximum strength, power, and speed are the training goals, then other strategies may be more effective. One such strategy entails planned overreaching.

Summated microcycles consist of microcycles grouped into "blocks" so that each block presents a specific pattern of volume and intensity of loading. The blocks can be repeated in a cyclical fashion with the desired result of maximizing training adaptation.

Overreaching can occur as a result of a large increase in VL. Overreaching can result in chronic fatigue and other symptoms similar to the initial stages of overtraining (54). Provided that the overreaching phase is not too extensive, a return to normal training volumes can result in a "supercompensation effect," promoting an increased performance. These supercompensation effects may be associated with the anabolic state and changes in the testosterone:cortisol ratio (59,60). By carefully planning the overreaching phase (with subsequent return to normal training and adding a taper), performance may be enhanced (Fig. 15.4). It may also be possible to incorporate a short overreaching phase into a summated block scheme, so that the overreaching phase is periodically repeated and a cumulative effect is achieved. Figure 15.5 represents this type of approach. This approach of using planned overreaching with summated blocks can be used by intermediate and advanced athletes.

Planned overreaching is an intentional increase in volume and intensity that places the athlete in a state of overreaching. If the overreaching phase is not too extensive, recovery can result in a "supercompensation effect," promoting increased performance.

Fundamental conditioning addresses fitness parameters specifically associated with a sport. Fundamental conditioning usually emphasizes

TABLE 15.7 ● MICROCYCLE WITHIN A MESOCYCLE EMPHASIZING STRENGTH IMPROVEMENT

DAY	M	T	W	TH	F	S	SU
WTVL	H	R	MH	R	L	M	R
R/AV	L	M	R	M	R	M	R
TTV	L	L	R	L	R	L	R

WTVL = weight-training volume load; R/AV = running, agility training volume; TTV = tactical training volume.

TABLE 15.8 ● MICROCYCLE WITHIN A MESOCYCLE EMPHASIZING TACTICAL IMPROVEMENT

DAY	M	T	W	TH	F	S	SU
WTVL	L	R	L	R	L	M	R
R/AV	L	M	R	M	R	M	R
TTV	H	L	M	MH	R	M	R

WTVL = weight-training volume load; R/AV = running, agility training volume; TTV = tactical training volume.

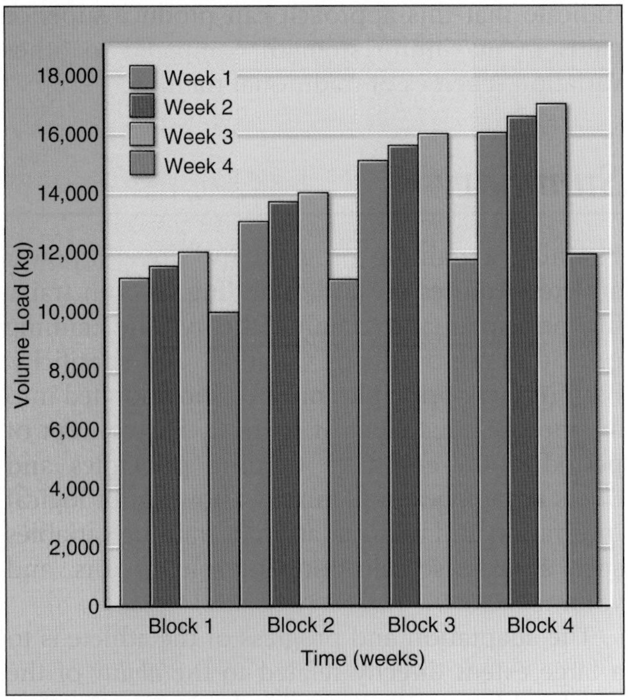

FIGURE 15.3 Summated microcycles. This graph represents a 3/1 cycle, or 3 weeks of increasing VL followed by 1 unload week.

specific endurance aspects. For example, in strength–power sports, strength endurance would be a priority. It has been the observation of the authors that advanced athletes and their coaches often reduce or completely neglect fundamental conditioning, believing that years of training

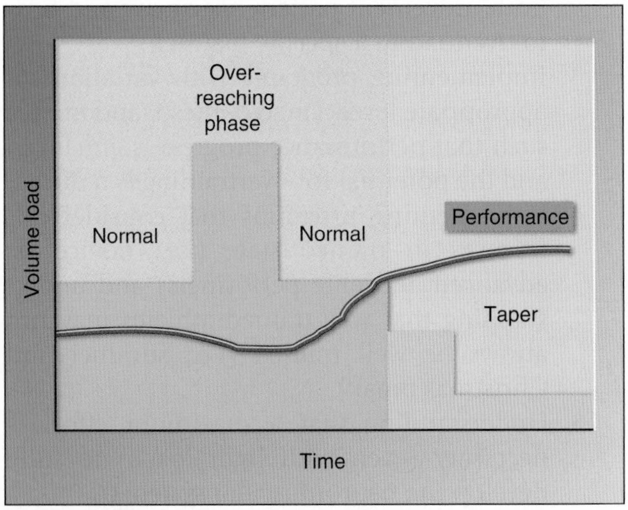

FIGURE 15.4 Planned overreaching (conceptual). Training volume is markedly increased for a short period. Performance may decline during overreaching. A return to "normal training" can result in a performance boost. A taper may further enhance the performance.

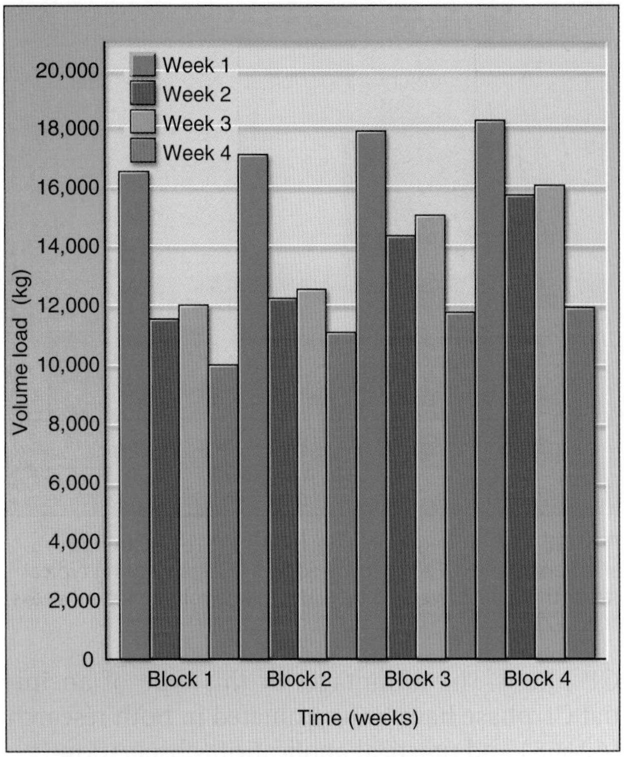

FIGURE 15.5 Planned overreaching (summated microcycles). Each block begins with an overreaching microcycle followed by a taper, producing a 1/2/1 block (1 week overreaching/2 weeks normal training/1 week taper). Taken from actual data among collegiate throwers using the squat.

obviate the need for more basic exercise or higher volume work. However, there are several reasons why fundamental conditioning phases may be of benefit:

1. All training programs require occasional or periodic decreases in training volume and intensity or periods of rest. This decrease can result in a loss of sports-specific fitness, which can include negative alterations in body composition, endurance capabilities, and recoverability.
2. Periodically reintroducing this type of training variation offers a break (both physiologically and psychologically) from higher intensity training.
3. Properly applied as a unidirectional concentrated load (61), fundamental training can enhance subsequent adaptation to higher intensity exercise.

Figure 15.6 represents a mesocycle protocol in which a strength–endurance concentrated loading (CL) lasting for 4 weeks is introduced as part of a

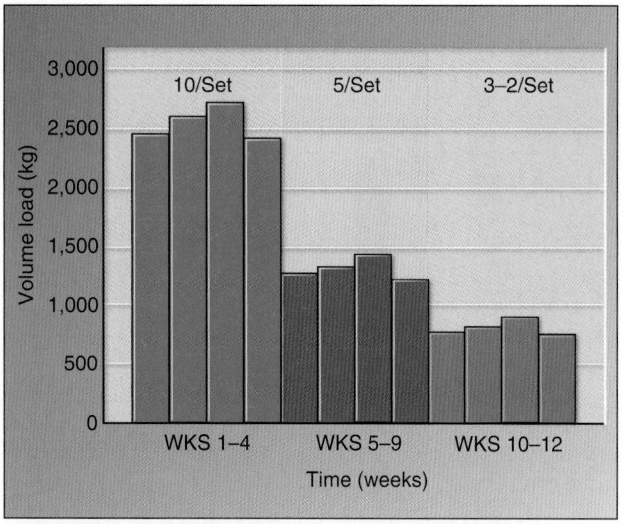

FIGURE 15.6 Strength training: model 1 (51). CL (strength–endurance weeks 1 to 4), followed by a CL representing typical strength training (weeks 5 to 9) and then a volume taper (weeks 10 to 12).

GP phase. The advantages of this type of an initial CL phase have been evaluated in both research (62–65) and practical application/observation.

The initial CL phase can also be integrated with cyclically repeated overreaching phases to produce a training protocol, which can make use of the advantages of both phases (Fig. 15.7). Objective data using advanced strength trainers (66) as well as with national- and international-level athletes indicate that this approach can produce superior gains in maximum strength compared to other variation schemes or traditional training.

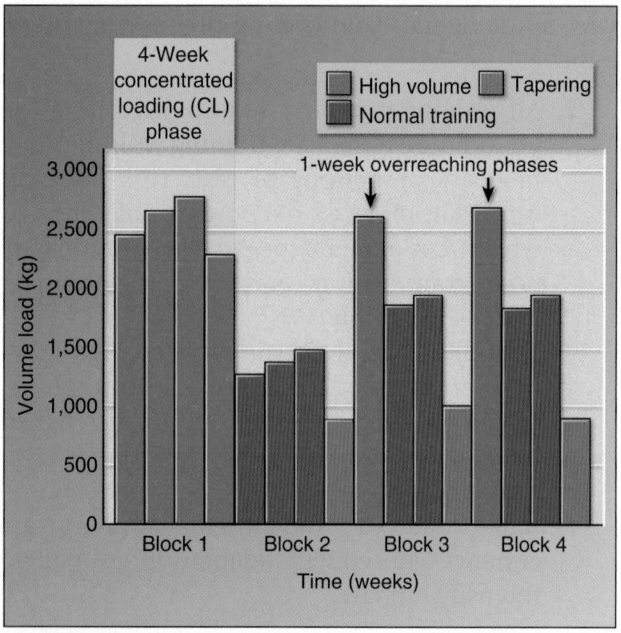

FIGURE 15.7 Strength/power training: model 2 (44). The combination of a strength–endurance CL and short-term overreaching.

Summary

Planning a training program for strength/power athletes requires an understanding of both training principles and training theory. The training principles are overload, variation, and specificity. Each of these principles must be incorporated into an appropriate system of training. The concept of periodization embraces training principles and offers advantages in planning, allowing for logical integration and manipulation of training variables such as exercise selection, intensity factors, and volume factors.

The adaptation and progress of the athlete is to a large extent directly related to the *ability* of the coach/athlete to create and carry out appropriate training plans. This ability includes

1. An understating of how different types of exercises can affect strength and strength-related variables (i.e., maximum force, rate of force development, power, etc.).
2. An understanding of the characteristics of exercises necessary for maximizing transfer-of-training effect such that training exercises have the greatest potential for carryover to performance. This understanding includes both movement pattern specificity and how to overload in a specific manner.
3. Implementing programs with variations at appropriate levels (macro, meso, and micro) such that performance progress is enhanced and the potential for overtraining is reduced.
4. Implementing programs that consider differences in trained state (i.e., novice vs. advanced and elite performers) and understanding that well-trained athletes may not always be well trained (i.e., summer and Christmas break).
5. Understanding that a maximum effort is necessary (even with light loads) to fully develop the neuromuscular system).

For the coach/athlete, development of this ability is paramount and serves to advance sport performance.

Maxing Out

1. You are strength and conditioning coach for track and field at a high school. Create a generalized plan for (a) a thrower, (b) a sprinter, (c) a distance runner, (d) a basketball player.
2. A college distance runner is training toward the conference championships; what type of strength training program should be performed during the competitive season?
3. You are coaching a college sprinter; what type of resistance-training exercises would be performed in the GP and competition phases? Would there be differences based on gender?
4. You are coaching a high school American football team. How would you manipulate volume and intensity factors for different developmental characteristics (e.g., strength–endurance, strength, power, speed) during various parts of the training program (summer vs. fall vs. in-season)?
5. How would you develop an annual plan for an elite weight lifter versus a beginner?

CASE EXAMPLE

Training Program for a Novice Shot-Putter

BACKGROUND

A novice (high school) shot-putter is in a competition phase. He comes to you for advice on his training program. Are you going to advise this athlete to work more toward speed and power or strength? Consider the long-term implications of the training program, as the athlete has the next 2 years to compete and potentially has a collegiate career ahead as well.

RECOMMENDATIONS/CONSIDERATIONS

In the novice athlete, establishing a strength base on which to build over the next 2+ years is critical. Although the resistance-training program will have variations within cycles and from one cycle to the next, a novice athlete should spend the bulk of his or her time establishing a strength base.

IMPLEMENTATION

For the first year, including the competition phase, the athlete could be advised to train throughout the year with training goals designed primarily toward strength. Cycles of speed and power or cycles that are a mixture of strength and power can be used on an occasional basis for variety. The second year, with an adequate strength base, the athlete can begin to spend more time working toward speed, power, and explosiveness.

RESULTS

Maximum strength and power should be measured on a regular basis. Results in the first year should reflect rather large gains in basic strength, especially leg and hip strength. Although strength is being emphasized in the first years, considerable gain in power and speed should also be realized. It should be remembered that at this age (high school), the gains in performance will be a combination of maturation and training adaptations. For an enthusiastic, well-motivated young athlete, the key may not be pushing him or her in the weight room but rather holding back. Although the coach does not want to dampen enthusiasm, care must be taken not to produce excessive fatigue or injuries. For example, over the first year for a 15-year-old 95-kg male novice shot-putter with good motivation, it would not be unusual to expect a 50-kg increase in the 1-RM squat, 25 kg in the bench press, and a 5- to 10-cm increase in the countermovement vertical jump.

REFERENCES

1. Plisk S, Stone MH. Periodization strategies. *Strength Cond J*. 2003;25:19–37.
2. Stone MH, Stone ME, Sands WA. *Principles and Practice of Resistance Training*. Champaign, IL: Human Kinetics; 2007.
3. Harris G, Stone MH, O'Bryant HS, et al. Short term performance effects of high speed, high force and combined weight training. *J Strength Cond Res*. 2000;14:14–20.
4. McBride JM, Triplett-McBride TT, Davie A, et al. A comparison of strength and power characteristics between power lifters, Olympic lifters and sprinters. *J Strength Cond Res*. 1999;13:58–66.
5. Stone MH, Fleck SJ, Triplett NT, et al. Health- and performance-related potential of resistance training. *Sports Med*. 1998;11:210–231.
6. Conley MS, Rozenek RR. Health aspects of resistance exercise and training. *Strength Cond J*. 2001;23:9–23.
7. Frobase I, Verdinck A, Duesberg F, et al. Auswirkungen untersheidllicher belastungs-intensitaten im rahmen eines post-operativen stationaren aufbautrainings auf leistungsdefizite des m quadriceps femoris. *Zeitschr Orthop*. 1993;131:164–167.
8. Stone MH, Plisk SS, Stone ME, et al. Athletic performance development: volume load—1 set versus multiple sets, training velocity and training variation. *Strength Cond J*. 1998;20:22–31.
9. Stone MH, Plisk S, Collins D. Training principle: evaluation of modes and methods of resistance training—a coaching perspective. *Sport Biomech*. 2002;1:79–104.
10. Cormie P, McGuigan MR, Newton RU. Adaptations in athletic performance following ballistic power vs. strength training. *Med Sci Sports Exerc*. 2010;42(8):1582–1598.
11. Newton RU, Kraemer WJ, Hakkinen K, et al. Kinematics, kinetics and muscle activation during explosive upper body movements. *J Appl Biomech*. 1996;12:31–43.
12. Garhammer JJ. A comparison of maximal power outputs between elite male and female weightlifters in competition. *Int J Sport Biomech*. 1991;7:3–11.
13. Garhammer JJ. A review of the power output studies of Olympic and powerlifting: methodology, performance prediction and evaluation tests. *J Strength Cond Res*. 1993;7:76–89.
14. Nuzzo JL, McBride JM, Dayne AM, et al. Testing of the maximal dynamic output hypothesis in trained and untrained subjects. *J Strength Cond Res*. 2010;24(5):1269–1276.
15. Driss T, Vandewalle H, Quiwevre J, et al. Effects of external loading on power output in a squat jump on a force platform: a comparison between strength and power athletes and sedentary individuals. *J Sport Sci*. 2001;19:99–105.
16. Stone MH, O'Bryant HS, McCoy L, et al. Power and maximum strength relationships during performance of dynamic and static weighted jumps. *J Strength Cond Res*. 2003;17:140–147.
17. Baker D, Nance S, Moore M. The load that maximizes mechanical power output during jump squats in power-trained athletes. *J Strength Cond Res*. 2001;15:92–97.
18. Burleson MA, O'Bryant HS, Stone MH, et al. Effect of weight training exercise and treadmill exercise on post-exercise oxygen consumption. *Med Sci Sports Exerc*. 1998;30:518–522.
19. Melby C, Scholl C, Edwards G, et al. Effect of acute resistance exercise on postexercise energy expenditure and resting metabolic rate. *J Appl Physiol*. 1993;75:1847–1853.
20. Williamson DL, Kirwan JP. A single bout of concentric resistance exercises increases BMR 48 hours after exercise in healthy 59–77 year old men. *J Gerontol*. 1997;52A:M352–M355.
21. Stone MH, O'Bryant H. *Weight Training: A Scientific Approach*. 2nd ed. Minneapolis, MN: Burgess Publishing; 1987.
22. Kraemer WJ. A series of studies: the physiological basis for strength training in American football: fact over philosophy. *J Strength Cond Res*. 1997;11:131–142.
23. Kramer J, Stone MH, O'Bryant HS, et al. Effects of single versus multiple sets of weight training: impact of volume, intensity and variation. *J Strength Cond Res*. 1997;11:143–147.
24. Behm DG. Neuromuscular implications and applications of resistance training. *J Strength Cond Res*. 1995;9:264–274.
25. Sale DG. Neural adaptations to strength training. In: Komi PV, ed. *Strength and Power in Sport*. London: Blackwell; 1992:249–265.
26. Loeb GE. Hard lessons in motor control from the mammalian spinal cord. *Trends Neurosci*. 1987;10:108–113.
27. Abe T, Kojima K, Kearna CF, et al. Whole body hypertrophy from resistance training: distribution and total mass. *Br J Sport Med*. 2003;37:543–545.
28. Hakkinen K. Neuromuscular adaptation during strength training, aging, detraining and immobilization. *Crit Rev Phys Rehabil Med*. 1994;6:161–198.
29. McDonagh MJN, Hayward CM, Davies CTM. Isometric training in human elbow flexor muscles. *J Bone Joint Surg*. 1983;64:355–358.
30. Wilson GJ, Newton RU, Murphy AJ, et al. The optimal training load for the development of dynamic athletic performance. *Med Sci Sports Exerc*. 1993;25:1279–1286.
31. Stone MH, Moir G, Glaister M, et al. How much strength is necessary? *Phys Ther Sport*. 2002;3:88–96.
32. Stone MH, Sanborn K, O'Bryant HS, et al. Maximum strength-power-performance relationships in collegiate throwers. *J Strength Cond Res*. 2003;17:739–745.
33. Zajac FE, Gordon ME. Determining muscle's force and action in multi-articular movement. *Exerc Sport Sci Rev*. 1989;17:187–230.
34. Siff M. Biomechanical foundations of strength and power training. In: Zatsiorsky V, ed. *Biomechanics in Sport*. London: Blackwell; 2001:103–139.
35. Stone MH, O'Bryant HS, Pierce KC, et al. Periodization: effects of manipulating volume and intensity. Part 1. *Strength Cond J*. 1999;21(2):56–62.
36. Stone MH, O'Bryant HS, Pierce KC, et al. Periodization: effects of manipulating volume and intensity. Part 2. *Strength Cond J*. 1999;21(3):54–60.
37. Mujika I, Padilla S. Scientific basis for precompetition tapering strategies. *Med Sci Sports Exerc*. 2003;35:1182–1187.
38. Bompa TO, Haff GG. *Periodization: Theory and Methodology of Training*. Champaign, IL: Human Kinetics; 2010.
39. Verkoshansky, Y. Organization of the training process. *N Stud Athl*. 1998;13:21–31.
40. Issurein V, Sahrobajko IV. Proportion of maximal voluntary strength values and adaptation peculiarities of muscle to strength exercises in men and women. *Human Physiology. Academy of Sciences USSR*. 1985;11(1):17–22.

41. Breil FA, Simone N, Weber SK, et al. Block training periodization in alpine skiing: effects of 1-day HIT on Vo_{2max} and performance. *Eur J Appl Physiol.* 2010;109(6):1077–1086.
42. Carpenelli RN, Otto RM. Strength training: single versus multiple sets. *Sports Med.* 1998;26:75–84.
43. Borst SE, De Hoyos DV, Garzarella L, et al. Effects of resistance training on insulin-like growth factor-I and IGF binding proteins. *Med Sci Sports Exerc.* 2001;33:648–653.
44. Marx JO, Ratames NA, Nindl BC, et al. Low-volume circuit versus high-volume periodized resistance training in women. *Med Sci Sports Exerc.* 2001;33:635–643.
45. Rhea MR, Alvar BA, Ball SD, et al. Three sets of weight training superior to 1 set with equal intensity for eliciting strength. *J Strength Cond Res.* 2002;16:525–529.
46. Rooney KJ, Herbert RD, Balnave RJ. Fatigue contributes to the strength training stimulus. *Med Sci Sports Exerc.* 1994;26:1160–1164.
47. Folland JP, Irish CS, Roberts JC, et al. Fatigue is not a necessary stimulus for strength gains during resistance training. *Br J Sports Med.* 2002;36:370–373.
48. Peterson MD, Rhea MR, Alvar BA. Applications of the dose-response for muscular strength development: a review of meta-analytic efficacy and reliability for designing training proscription. *J Strength Cond Res.* 2005;19(4):950–958.
49. Izquierdo-Gabarren M, Gonzalez de Txabarri R, Garcia-Pallares J, et al. Concurrent endurance and strength training not to failure optimizes performance gains. *Med Sci Sports Exerc.* 2010;42(6):1191–1199.
50. Izquierdo M, Ibañez J, González-Badillo JJ, et al. Differential effects of strength training leading to failure versus not to failure on hormonal responses, strength, and muscle power gains.; *J Appl Physiol.* 2006;100(5):1647–1656.
51. Stone MH, Chandler TJ, Conley MS, et al. Training to muscular failure: is it necessary. *Strength Cond J.* 1996;18(3):44–48.
52. Medvedev AS, Rodionov VF, Rogozkin VN, et al. Training content of weightlifters during the preparation period (translation: Yessis M). *Teoriya I Praktika Fizicheskoi Kultury.* 1981;12:5–7.
53. Foster C. Monitoring training in athletes with reference to overtraining syndrome. *Med Sci Sports Exerc.* 1998;30:1164–1168.
54. Stone MH, Keith R, Kearney JT, et al. Overtraining: a review of the signs and symptoms of overtraining. *J Appl Sports Sci Res.* 1991;5:35–50.
55. Bruin G, Kuipers H, Keizer HA, et al. Adaptation and overtraining in horses subjected to increasing training loads. *J Appl Physiol.* 1994;76:1908–1913.
56. McBride JM, Triplett-McBride TT, Davie A, et al. The effect of heavy- vs light-load jump squats on the development of strength, power, and speed. *J Strength Cond Res.* 2002;16:75–82.
57. Fry RW, Morton AR, Keast D. Periodisation of training stress: a review. *Can J Sports Sci.* 1992;17:234–240.
58. Matveyev LP. *Fundamentals of Sports Training.* Moscow: Progress Publishers; 1981.
59. Fry AC, Kraemer WJ, Stone MH, et al. Relationships between serum testosterone, cortisol and weightlifting performance. *J Strength Cond Res.* 2000;14(3): 338–343.
60. Stone MH, Fry AC. *Increased Training Volume in Strength/Power Athletes. Overtraining in Sport.* Champaign, IL: Human Kinetics; 1997:87–106.
61. Verkhoshansky YV. *Fundamentals of Special Strength Training in Sport.* Moscow: Fizkultura i Spovt; 1977. [English version (translation: Charniga A Jr) Livonia, MI: Sportivny Press, 1986.]
62. O'Bryant HS, Byrd R, Stone MH. Cycle ergometer and maximum leg and hip strength adaptations to two different methods of weight training. *J Appl Sports Sci Res.* 1988;2:27–30.
63. Stone MH, O'Bryant H, Garhammer J, et al. A theoretical model of strength training. *Natl Strength Cond Assoc J.* 1982;4:36–39.
64. Willoughby DS. The effects of mesocycle-length weight training programs involving periodization and partially equated volumes on upper and lower body strength. *J Strength Cond Res.* 1993;7:2–8.
65. Zatsiorsky VM. *Science and Practice of Strength Training.* Champaign, IL: Human Kinetics; 1995.
66. Stone MH, Potteiger J, Proulx CM, et al. Comparison of the effects of three different weight training programs on the 1 RM squat. *J Strength Cond Res.* 2000;14: 332–337.

CHAPTER 16

Resistance Exercise Prescription

BARRY A. SPIERING • WILLIAM E. AMONETTE • WILLIAM J. KRAEMER

OBJECTIVES

After reading this chapter, you will be able to:

- Identify key components of a "needs analysis" for a sport athlete or client.
- Discuss benefits and limitations of various resistance exercise modes.
- Understand basic biology and physics that underlie the acute resistance exercise programming variables.
- Determine appropriate exercise prescriptions for increased muscle cross-sectional area, strength, power, and endurance.

KEY TERMS

Assistance Exercises
Closed Kinetic Chain Exercise
Exercise Order
Frequency
Fundamental Exercises
Load (i.e., intensity)
Multiple-Joint Exercises
Muscular Strength
Open Kinetic Chain Exercise
Periodization
Progression
Progressive Overload
Repetition Maximum (RM)
Rest Intervals
SAID principle
Single-Joint Exercises
Split Routine
Systematic Variation
Volume

Introduction

The prescription of a resistance exercise to improve performance presents a formidable challenge to the strength and conditioning professional. One must consider numerous acute programming variables (e.g., choice of exercises, number of repetitions) while attempting to design appropriate long-term resistance training plans that meet the needs of athletes involved in a variety of sports and activities. Fortunately, however, by following sequential procedures based on scientific evidence, and not on anecdotal recommendations, the practitioner can design a resistance training program that is specific to the sport/activity, is individualized to the athlete's needs, allows for long-term progression, and provides the opportunity for athletic achievement.

NEEDS ANALYSIS

The first step in designing a resistance training program is performing a needs analysis. To ensure optimal performance, the resistance training program must be individualized in accordance with the specific needs of the sport/activity and of the athlete. These needs can be ascertained by answering the following questions:

- What are the physical needs of the sport (e.g., muscular strength, hypertrophy)?
- Which specific muscle groups or movement patterns are most important for the sport?
- What types of muscle actions are needed and used in the sport and what are the kinetics of the sport?
- What are the individual athlete's physical strengths and weaknesses (these qualities are addressed via test administration and interpretation [Chapter 8])?
- Does the athlete have any health/injury concerns?
- What are the common sites of injury for the sport/activity?

Answering these questions will provide the fundamental information necessary for designing the resistance training regimen and set the stage for the implementation and manipulation of acute program variables. Most of this information can be obtained by searching peer-reviewed literature sources, performing time–motion analyses of game film, or by talking with sport coaches, the sports medicine staff, or the athlete. For many sports, information describing the physical characteristics of elite versus nonelite athletes, physiologic or metabolic measurements of sporting movements, and/or data describing the biomechanics of sports can be obtained using databases such as "PubMed" or "Google Scholar." Data might also be available describing sports-specific injury predispositions and training strategies to prevent such injuries. The widespread availability of quality information from peer-reviewed sources creates a sound foundation for performing an appropriate needs analysis and developing an evidence-based program for virtually any sport.

Performing a needs analysis assists the strength and conditioning professional in designing a specific and individualized resistance exercise program.

ACUTE PROGRAM VARIABLES

Once the needs of the athlete/sport have been determined, the practitioner can begin designing a resistance training program. This process requires an appreciation of how to properly implement and manipulate acute program variables to ensure that the program meets the specific needs of the athlete, allows for optimal progression over time, and prevents training plateaus. Therefore, this section introduces the acute program variables and their influence on the responses and adaptations to resistance exercise.

EXERCISE SELECTION

In general, exercises commonly used in resistance training programs can be classified as (a) single-joint or multiple-joint, (b) large muscle group or small muscle group, or (c) open kinetic chain or closed kinetic chain. **Single-joint exercises** stress one joint (or muscle group). For example, the arm curl stresses elbow flexion (biceps muscle group). These exercises isolate specific muscle groups, require less skill, and consequently some believe pose less risk of injury. Alternately, **multiple-joint exercises** stress two or more joints (or muscle groups). For example, the back squat stresses hip and knee extension (gluteus, hamstrings, and quadriceps muscle groups). These exercises require more complex neural activation and coordination; however, it is believed that they are more effective for increasing functional muscular strength and power (Box 16.1).

Multiple-joint exercises that stress large muscle groups invoke a greater metabolic and hormonal stimulus than single-joint exercises that stress small muscle groups.

Larger muscle group exercises (e.g., back squat) invoke significantly greater metabolic responses than smaller muscle group exercises (e.g., arm curl). Furthermore, large muscle group exercises, especially bilateral triple (hip, knee, and ankle) extension exercises, evoke greater acute anabolic hormonal responses (1). For example, exercises such as deadlifts and squat jumps produce greater testosterone and growth hormone responses than exercises such as bench press and seated shoulder press. It has also been demonstrated that bilateral resistance exercise results in a greater anabolic response than a similar unilateral exercise.

BOX 16.1

Free Weights and Machines

Strength and conditioning professionals are often faced with the option of using free weights, machines, or both to train a specific movement or muscle group. Before making this decision, however, it is important that one is aware of the advantages and disadvantages of each. Weight machines are generally believed to be safer to use than free weights, easier to learn, and allow the athlete to perform exercises that might be difficult with free weights (e.g., leg extensions, leg curls, pull downs). On the other hand, use of free weights might necessitate muscular coordination patterns that more closely mimics movement requirements of a specific task and thus likely more beneficial for improving performance. Therefore, it is recommended that novice athletes use both free weight and machine exercises, while free weight exercises are emphasized for experienced athletes.

Therefore, the amount of muscle mass involved has direct implications on the metabolic and hormonal responses to resistance training.

An **open kinetic chain exercise** is an exercise in which the distal end of the moving segments is free or not in contact with the ground or a fixed apparatus (e.g., dumbbell biceps curl). Conversely, in a **closed kinetic chain exercise**, the distal end of the moving segment is fixed or in contact with the ground or a fixed apparatus (e.g., squat). Closed kinetic chain exercises require the activation of multiple muscle groups to stabilize the joint during movement, whereas open kinetic chain exercises result in significantly less activation of the opposing muscle groups (2). Exercises can also be classified with respect to the joint movements. Multi-joint exercises are routinely divided into three movement-based categories: (a) upper body pushing, (b) upper body pulling, or (c) lower body, triple extension exercises. Upper body pushing and pulling exercises can be further divided into subcategories of horizontal and vertical. A bench press, for example, would be classified as a horizontal pushing exercises and an overhead press as a vertical pushing exercise. Likewise, a bent-over row is classified as a horizontal pulling exercise and pull-up as a vertical pulling exercise. Triple extension exercises, as the name implies, involve the extension of three joints: the hip, knee, and ankle. They are essential because nearly all sports involve some variation of triple extension (e.g., running, jumping, tackling in football). Triple extension exercises can be described as double- or single-leg support exercises. An example of a double-leg support triple extension exercise is the front squat or deadlift; lunges or step-ups would be classified as single-leg support exercises.

An important concept to consider when designing a resistance training program is the agonist/antagonist/stabilizer relationship. By performing physical activities and sport-specific resistance training, the prime movers undergo significant adaptations to increase performance. However, as the agonist increases its capabilities, the antagonist might become increasingly susceptible to injury. Therefore, it is recommended that all major muscle groups are trained during resistance exercise programs to ensure that appropriate attention is given to both agonist and antagonist muscle groups, to prevent muscle imbalances, and to minimize the risk of injury. Classifying exercises by movement patterns might help with prescribing resistance exercise regimens that result in muscular balance. The strength and conditioning coach should ensure that a comparable volume of pushing and pulling exercises are utilized within a training cycle. This strategy might help mitigate muscular imbalances between agonist and antagonist muscle groups (Box 16.2).

All major muscle groups should be trained during a resistance exercise program to avoid muscular imbalances.

EXERCISE ORDER

Exercise order (the sequencing of specific exercises within a session) significantly affects force production, fatigue rate, and muscle recruitment patterns during a resistance exercise session (3). Over the duration of a long-term training program, performing an exercise last (as opposed to first) significantly impairs gains in maximal strength. As already discussed, multiple-joint exercises are considered more effective in increasing functional muscular strength than single-joint exercises. Therefore, these exercises should be given priority within the training session (i.e., placed early in the training sessions when fatigue is minimal). Additionally, exercises that result in significant spinal loading and support perhaps should be performed before exercises that do not require direct spinal support (e.g., back squats before leg press). The following recommendations regarding exercise order have been made (4):

When training all major muscle groups in a workout:

- Perform large muscle group exercises before small muscle group exercises.
- Perform multiple-joint exercises before single-joint exercises.
- Rotate upper and lower body exercises.
- For power training, perform total-body explosive exercises (from most to least complex) before basic exercises. For example, perform power cleans before back squats. This is especially important when teaching new exercises.
- Rotate between pushing and pulling upper body exercises.

Another important concept to consider is the sequencing of exercises sets. Most exercise sets are sequenced in a horizontal format; that is, if three sets of an exercise are prescribed, all three sets of that exercise are performed before beginning a new exercise. For example, if three sets of five repetitions are prescribed on the back squat, overhead press, and bent-over row exercises, all three sets of back squats would be performed prior to beginning the overhead press exercise. However, at times, it might be advantageous to implement a vertical sequencing format. If the previous three exercises were vertically sequenced, one set of back squats would be performed, followed by one set of overhead press and one set of bent-over row exercises. Circuit weight training is a form of vertical sequencing where an athlete moves between exercises with little or no rest periods. It is commonly used in preparation phases of training to establish a conditioning base due to the higher metabolic demands of this type of exercise.

"Super sets" are another form of vertical sequencing where one set of two different exercises (usually opposing muscle groups) is performed consecutively without rest. If a strength and conditioning coach prescribed three sets of eight on the barbell biceps curl and triceps press-down exercise, a super-set strategy could be implemented where one set of barbell curls was immediately preceded by one set of triceps press down (followed by a rest). There is no clear physiological advantage of super-setting over traditional horizontal sequencing; however, it might be used as a time-saving strategy for smaller, single-joint exercises that do not require high metabolic demands.

BOX 16.2

Forms of Resistance Training

Although resistance training typically involves barbells, dumbbells, and machines, it should be pointed out that other forms of resistance training are available. For example, a strength and conditioning practitioner might also wish to include medicine balls, plyometrics, elastic tubing, and/or partner-assisted exercises. These forms of resistance add diversity to the "choice of exercise" acute program variable. Moreover, because less resistance is applied during these exercises, high-velocity movements can be effectively trained in a sport-specific manner (e.g., plyometrics).

EXERCISE INTENSITY

Intensity (i.e., load) is the amount of weight lifted or the resistance with which one exercises and is highly dependent upon other acute program variables such as exercise order, muscle action, and rest interval length. There is an inverse relation between the **load** and the maximal number of repetitions performed; as the load increases, the number of repetitions that can be performed decreases (5). Intensity is typically prescribed as a percentage of the athlete's one-**repetition maximum** (1-RM) (e.g., 85% 1-RM) (Box 16.3) or as a weight that allows a specific number of repetitions (e.g., 6-RM). Altering training load affects hormonal, neural, and metabolic responses and adaptations to resistance training.

BOX 16.3

Protocol for Determining One-Repetition Maximum Strength

1. Ten repetitions at 50% of estimated 1-RM
   - 1 to 2 minutes rest
2. Three to five repetitions at 75% of estimated 1-RM
   - 2 to 4 minutes rest
3. One repetition at 90% of estimated 1-RM
   - 2 to 4 minutes rest
4. Increase the load by 5% to 10% and attempt another 1-RM lift
   - 2 to 4 minutes rest
5. Continue process of increasing the load by 5% to 10% and attempting 1-RM lifts until the athlete can no longer lift the weight through the full range of motion using correct technique. 1-RM should be determined within five 1-RM attempts.

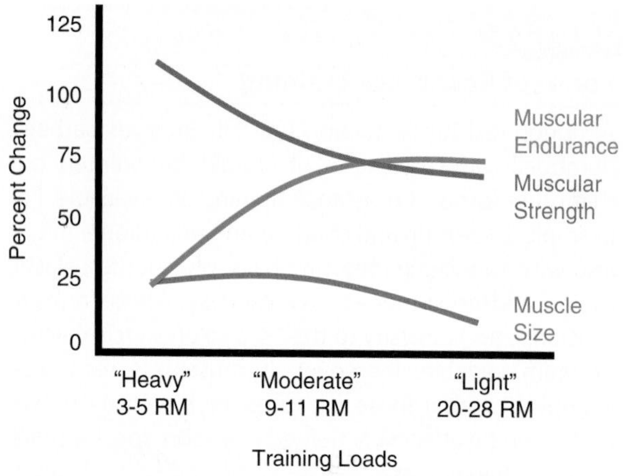

FIGURE 16.1 The RM continuum. Certain muscular characteristics are best trained using a specific RM load.

Certain muscular characteristics are best trained using specific RM loads (Fig. 16.1). It is generally believed that optimal gains in maximum strength are obtained by training at loads that are heavier than 6-RM (6). This is not to say that improvements in hypertrophy or endurance will not occur using such loads; however, these characteristics might not be optimally trained.

VOLUME

Training **volume** is typically expressed as

Volume = Sets (number) × Repetitions (number)

Volume load is a measure of total work performed and can be expressed as

Volume-Load = Sets × Repetitions × Load (weight)

Manipulation of training volume can be achieved by altering the number of exercises performed per session, the number of sets performed per exercise, or the number of repetitions performed per set. As with training intensity, changes in training volume influence neural, metabolic, and hormonal responses and adaptations to resistance exercise.

Increased metabolic and hormonal responses are associated with high training volume.

REST INTERVALS

Rest intervals between sets and exercises can significantly influence the responses and adaptations to resistance exercise. Responses to short rest intervals include elevated heart rate and subjective ratings of perceived exertion, increased lactate and growth hormone concentrations, and reduced performance during subsequent sets. Over the course of 4 weeks, short (30 to 40 seconds) rest intervals attenuated strength gains as compared to long (2 to 3 minutes) rest intervals (7,8). However, it was recently demonstrated that 2- or 4-minute rest periods do not alter strength gains during the back squat exercise over a 12-week training period (9). This indicates that rest intervals of ≥2 minutes are optimal for strength gains; however, extended rest periods do not further enhance this adaptation.

Short rest periods are associated with greater metabolic and hormonal responses; however, very short rest periods might attenuate strength gains.

FREQUENCY AND WORKOUT STRUCTURE

Training **frequency** is the number of training sessions performed during a specific period of time (e.g., 3 sessions · wk^{-1}) and is dependent upon volume, intensity, exercise selection, level of conditioning and/or training status, recovery ability, nutritional intake, and training goals. Sessions using heavy loads, intense eccentric (ECC) contractions, high training volume, and/or large muscle group or multiple-joint exercises might require increased recovery time before subsequent sessions. Furthermore, needed recovery time might differ between age groups or gender. For example, it has been shown that untrained women of various ages recovered only 90% to 94% of their strength 2 days after a leg press routine of 5 sets of 10 repetitions using a 10-RM load (10), indicating additional rest might be required for such populations before the next training bout. Additionally, research indicates that the acute hormonal response might differ between age groups (11) and training experience, indicating that older or less-trained athletes could require longer rest periods between training bouts.

Individual training sessions can be arranged into exercise groupings that stress the entire body or specific muscles/movements during a single session. Although combined workout routines are generally more efficient, it might be necessary during certain training phases to employ a **split routine**. Early in a training phase when skeletal muscle hypertrophy is a predominant training goal, high-volume training strategies might be necessary. During such periods, logistical constraints (e.g., National Collegiate Athletic Association rules

TABLE 16.1 ● EXAMPLE TRAINING FREQUENCIES AND FOUR DIFFERENT WORKOUT STRUCTURES[a]

	MONDAY	TUESDAY	WEDNESDAY	THURSDAY	FRIDAY
Workout A	1. Back squat	Off	Off	1. Back squat	Off
	2. Deadlift			2. Deadlift	
Frequency: 2 sessions · wk^{-1}	3. Bench press			3. Bench press	
Design: Total body	4. Lat pull			4. Lat pull	
Workout B	1. Back squat	1. Bench press	Off	1. Back squat	1. Bench press
	2. Deadlift	2. Lat pull		2. Deadlift	2. Lat pull
Frequency: 4 sessions · wk^{-1}	3. DB lunge	3. Arm extension		3. Leg extension	3. Arm extension
Design: Upper–lower split routine	4. Leg curl	4. Arm curl		4. Leg curl	4. Arm curl
Workout C	1. Back squat	1. Bench press	Off	1. Lat pull down	1. Overhead press
	2. Deadlift	2. DB incline press 3. Cable chest press		2. DB bent row	2. Barbell shrug
Frequency: 4 sessions · wk^{-1}	3. DB lunge			3. Cable row	3. Lateral raise
Design: Muscle group split	4. Leg curl	4. Tricep press		4. Bicep curl	4. Rear delt raise
Workout D	1. Back squat	1. Bench press	1. Lat pull down	Off	1. Back squat
	2. Deadlift	2. DB incline press 3. Overhead press	2. DB bent row		2. Deadlift
Frequency: 4 sessions · wk^{-1}	3. DB lunge		3. Cable row		3. Bench press
Design: 3-d Split–combo routine	4. Leg curl	4. Rear delt raise	4. Barbell shrug		4. Lat pull

[a]Workout "C" depicts a muscle group split routine that is commonly used by bodybuilders but not necessarily applicable to athletes. If very high-volume training for specific muscle groups with significant time constraints, Workout "D" is an alternative method more suitable for athletes.

for athlete contact time) could necessitate split routines. Furthermore, the increased volume and subsequent skeletal muscle damage might require greater amounts of rest between sessions. Table 16.1 provides a comparison between various split routines and a combined program. Many other types of split and combination routines have been proposed; the choice of program is dictated primarily by the program goals and time constraints. Muscle group split programs are generally used by body builders and not recommended for athletes. For athletes, combined (total-body) routines are the preferred workout structure, especially as the sport season approaches.

Studies have shown that 2 to 3 sessions · wk^{-1} on alternating days is appropriate for untrained individuals; however, this does not imply that increased frequency is required for intermediate or advanced lifters. The primary advantage of increasing training frequency is that it allows for greater specialization (i.e., greater exercise selection and/or volume per muscle group in accordance with specific goals). For example, compare the four sample workouts in Table 16.1. Workout A uses a total-body exercise design with a frequency of 2 sessions · wk^{-1}. Alternately, workouts B, C, and D employ split routine designs with a frequency of 4 sessions · wk^{-1}. If time restraints allow four exercises to be performed per workout, then using structure B, C, or D permits the athlete to perform more exercises per muscle group per workout compared to structure A. However, the overall weekly time commitment for structure B, C, and D is twice as much for structure A

With this in mind, the following recommendations have been made (12):

- For entire body training, it is recommended that athletes train 2 to 3 d · wk^{-1}.
- For split routine workouts, an overall frequency of 3 to 4 d · wk^{-1} is recommended, while ensuring that each muscle group is trained only 1 to 2 d · wk^{-1} (Box 16.4).

TABLE 16.2 ● RESISTANCE TRAINING FREQUENCY RECOMMENDATIONS BASED ON COMPETITIVE SEASON

PHASE OF COMPETITIVE SEASON	TRAINING FREQUENCY (SESSIONS · WK^{-1})
Off-season	4–6
Preseason	3–4
In season	1–2
Postseason	1–3

Source: Fleck SJ, Kraemer WJ. *Designing Resistance Training Programs*. Champaign, IL: Human Kinetics; 1997; Stone MH, O'Bryant H, Garhammer J, et al. A theoretical model of strength training. *J Strength Cond Res*. 1982;4:36–39; Tan B. Manipulating resistance training program variables to optimize maximum strength in men: a review. *J Strength Cond Res*. 1999;13:289–304.

MUSCLE ACTION

Most resistance exercises include concentric (CON) and ECC muscle actions. CON means that the muscle shortens as it produces force; ECC indicates that the muscle lengthens as it produces force. For example, during the arm curl exercise, the biceps perform a CON action as the weight is lifted and an ECC action as the weight is lowered. Although ECC actions result in more delayed onset muscle soreness than CON actions, improvements in dynamic muscular strength are greatest when ECC actions are included in the repetition movement (as opposed to CON-only movements) (13). Considering that exercises typically used within resistance training programs include CON and ECC muscle actions, that excluding ECC movements reduces gains in strength, and that there is not much potential for variation in this acute program variable, it is recommended that CON and ECC muscle actions are included in all resistance training programs.

Resistance training exercises should include CON and ECC muscle actions.

BOX 16.4

Training Frequency and the Competitive Season

The prescription of resistance training frequency is affected by the phase of the competitive season (e.g., off season, in season). As greater emphasis is placed on sport skills and practice, the strength and conditioning professional must reduce the frequency of resistance training, which reduces the chance of overtraining the athlete and is necessary due to time constraints. See Table 16.2 for frequency recommendations based on competitive season.

REPETITION VELOCITY

Force is equal to mass times acceleration; therefore, performing an exercise slowly reduces the associated muscular forces. Unintentionally and intentionally, slow repetition velocity can occur during resistance exercises. Unintentionally, slow velocities occur when individuals are attempting to exert maximal force but, due to high loading or fatigue, the weight travels at a slow velocity. This phenomenon was demonstrated in a study examining repetition velocity during a 5-RM bench press set. It was shown that the first three repetitions were approximately 1.2 to 1.6 seconds in duration, while the last two repetitions were 2.5 and 3.3 seconds in duration, respectively (14).

Some have proposed the use of intentionally slow velocities with submaximal loads, which allow the individual greater control of the weight. Research has shown that CON force production is significantly lower for an intentionally slow velocity (5-s CON; 5-s ECC) compared to a voluntary velocity (771 vs. 1167 N, respectively) (15). Furthermore, over the course of 10 weeks, use of a very slow velocity (10-s CON; 5-s ECC) compared to a slow velocity (2-s CON; 4-s ECC) program led to significantly less strength gains (16). Compared to slow velocities, moderate and fast velocities have been shown to be more effective for increasing the number of repetitions performed, work and power output, and volume (17) and for increasing the rate of performance gains (17). Therefore, intentionally slow CON velocities are not recommended.

Athletes should intend to perform exercises with a fast lifting velocity, as intentionally slow lifting velocities diminish strength gains.

RESISTANCE TRAINING PRESCRIPTION

After the needs analysis has been performed, the next step in designing a resistance training program is to implement the acute program variables within an individualized regimen. While designing a resistance exercise program, the strength and conditioning practitioner should consider the **SAID principle**: Specific Adaptations to Imposed Demands. Specificity refers to the muscle groups or movements being trained, the velocity of the movement, the kinetics of the exercise, and the metabolic requirements of the exercise. For example, if an athlete requires increased muscular endurance of the lower body extensors to successfully perform his or her sport, then the strength and conditioning coach must implement a program that challenges the metabolic capacity of the lower body extensors to achieve the desired results. Therefore, the following sections discuss the influence of the acute program variables on the trainable characteristics, specifically, strength, power, hypertrophy, and local muscular endurance.

MUSCULAR STRENGTH

Muscular strength is the ability of the neuromuscular system to generate force. The expression of muscular strength is dependent upon the nervous system's ability to recruit motor units and the contractile capabilities of the muscle fibers. Resistance training is commonly prescribed to increase muscular strength because it has been shown to enhance neural function (e.g., increased motor unit recruitment and frequency of stimulation) and increase muscle fiber force-generating capacity via increased cross-sectional area (CSA).

Exercise Selection

Improvements in skeletal muscle strength can be accomplished utilizing single- and multiple-joint exercises. For optimal and efficient strength gains, however, it is recommended that emphasis is placed on multiple-joint exercises (e.g., back squat, bench press, lat pulldown). These exercises are regarded as most effective for increasing overall functional strength because they enable a greater amount of weight to be lifted, stress multiple muscle groups within a single exercise, and are specific to the movement demands of most sports. Alternately, single-joint exercises might be used to target specific muscle groups or to implement specialized injury prevention programs for sports (e.g., lateral neck flexion for football). Single-joint exercises might pose less risk of injury because less skill and technique is involved; however, they do not necessarily stress the neuromuscular system in a sports-specific manner.

> ***For optimal gains in muscular strength, it is recommended that multiple-joint exercises are emphasized.***

Loading

Initial loading prescription depends heavily upon the athlete's training status. This initial phase of strength gain in untrained individuals is characterized by improved motor learning and coordination; therefore, heavy loads might not be required. For novices, loads as low as 45% to 50% of 1-RM have been shown to increase muscular strength. Alternately, for experienced lifters, greater loading is necessary for an overload stimulus and subsequent improvements in muscular strength. Studies indicate that loads greater than approximately 80% to 85% of 1-RM (i.e., 1 to 6-RM) might be more effective for increasing muscular strength (12).

> ***Loading for strength gains is dependent on initial training status; novices might improve with loads as little as 45% to 50% 1-RM, while experienced lifters might require loads of at least 80% to 85% 1-RM.***

Volume

Low-volume (i.e., high loads, low repetitions, and moderate to high number of sets) programs are characteristic of programs designed to improve maximum muscular strength. Research has shown that muscular strength can be improved using one to six or more sets per exercise (18). However, much like training intensity, the optimal training volume is dependent upon training status, age, and other individual factors. A meta-analysis of 140 studies suggested that four sets might be the optimal dose to optimize the work-to-benefit ratio in resistance exercise (18).

Recent studies have compared single-set to multiple-set training programs. In untrained individuals, some studies have reported that single-set training was equally effective as multiple-set programs for increasing muscular strength (19) in the early phases of training. Others, however, have shown that multiple-set programs were more effective for long-term adaptation (20). This is likely due to the fact that early training adaptations are a result of neural adaptations (e.g., improvements in muscle activation and coordination). Trained athletes seem to require higher training volume then untrained athletes. Evidence suggest that multiple-set programs are likely better for improving strength in trained individuals, although some show equivocal findings (21).

Multiple-set programs are recommended for improving muscular strength in all athletes; however, single-set programs might be used during the initial weeks of training in untrained athletes.

Rest Intervals

As previously stated, rest intervals affect physiological and performance responses and adaptations to resistance exercise. Because longitudinal studies have shown greater strength increases with long rest intervals, it is recommended that rest period of at least 2 to 3 minutes is used between sets for **fundamental exercises** (e.g., back squat). For **assistance exercises** (e.g., leg curls), 1 to 2 minutes of rest might suffice.

Improving muscular strength requires long rest periods (i.e., >2 to 3 minutes) between sets and exercises.

Repetition Velocity

Research has shown that muscular strength can be increased using isokinetic repetition training velocities ranging from 30 to 300 degrees · s^{-1}. However, strength increases are specific to the training repetition velocity, with some carryover above and below the training velocity (~30 degrees s^{-1}). Most sports (especially, team sports) and sport-related activities (i.e., running, jumping, throwing) require high-velocity muscle power as opposed to low-velocity strength for success. However, periodized training plans should incorporate both moderate-velocity and high-velocity movements. Regardless of the desired training adaptation (strength or power), the weight should be moved with a high intentional CON velocity.

Regardless of the desired training adaptation, the weight should be moved with a high intentional CON velocity.

MUSCULAR POWER

The expression of muscular power is important from a sport perspective because athletes are typically required to produce a high level of force in a limited amount of time (e.g., swinging a bat or jumping for a rebound). Power is defined as work divided by time or the product of force and velocity. In a practical sense, power is increased by moving more mass in a given amount of time or by moving a given mass at a higher velocity. Neuromuscular contributions to maximal muscle power include maximal rate of force development, muscular strength at slow and fast contraction velocities, stretch-shortening cycle performance, and coordination of movement pattern and skill. Maximal mechanical power output occurs when performing ballistic movements using submaximal loads. For example, during the squat jump exercise, maximal

Q & A from the Field

Q ***The strength coach at a neighboring university trains his athletes using one set to failure for each exercise. I've noticed other strength coaches using a similar philosophy. Is it the best approach for improved athletic performance?***

—undergraduate exercise physiology major

A "One set to failure" programs are used in a few major university strength and conditioning programs; however, this does not mean that it is the best approach to training athletes.

In untrained athletes (e.g., college freshman with little resistance training experience), one set *might* be as good as multiple sets for initial, short-term strength gains (19). However, for athletes with significant resistance training experience, multiple-set routines appear superior for strength gains (22). Therefore, scientific evidence supports the use of multiple-set routines in experienced athletes for long-term gains in strength.

mechanical power occurs using loads ranging from 0% (body weight only) to ~ 45% of 1-RM; however, the optimal load for maximizing mechanical power output depends on the specific exercise used (e.g., power clean, bench throws,etc). Research indicates that training at the load that maximizes mechanical power output in a given exercise might be more beneficial for improving sport-related skills such as sprinting and jumping (23). Power output can be trained at higher or lower percentages of the 1-RM, but translation to maximal mechanical power output should include higher velocity exercise using loads approximately 30% to 45% of 1-RM. Thus, the importance of periodized training with a loading variety is essential for optimal training of power.

Exercise Selection

Multiple-joint, total-body, closed kinetic chain exercises (e.g., power clean, push press) have been used extensively for power training because they require rapid force production in sport-specific movement patterns. The inherent problem with traditional resistance exercises is that the load is decelerated for a significant portion of the movement. Studies examining the bench press indicate that deceleration occurs during 24% to 40% of the CON movement (24); the deceleration phase increases to 52% when performing the lift with a lower percentage (81%) of 1-RM, and the deceleration phase increases when attempting to move the bar rapidly to train at a high movement velocity (24). Ballistic resistance exercises (explosive movements that enable acceleration throughout the full range of motion) limit the deceleration associated with traditional resistance exercises. For instance, loaded jump squats with 30% 1-RM loads have been shown to increase vertical jump performance to a greater extent than traditional back squats (25). Therefore, it is recommended that strength and conditioning coaches choose exercises that allow acceleration throughout the range of motion (e.g., power clean, power snatch, jump squats, plyometrics) to maximize transfer to athletic performance during power training phases.

Multiple-joint ballistic exercises that minimize deceleration are recommended for improving muscular power.

Loading

Research indicates that power can be improved using a traditional resistance training program. However, traditional resistance training might only improve power at slow movement velocities (10). Programs utilizing relatively light loads have been shown to be more effective for improving vertical jump performance than traditional resistance training (26). It appears that the use of light to moderate loads at high velocities increases force output at higher velocities (26).

The optimal load for maximal power output might vary between 30% and 60% of 1-RM depending on the choice of exercise (for review see Kawamori and Haaf (27)). Research using trained athletes has shown that loads of 30% 1-RM maximized performance following ballistic jump squat training (5), whereas loads of 45% to 60% 1-RM maximized power output during single bouts of jump squats and bench press throws (28,29). It is important to note, however, that simultaneously training for strength (i.e., heavy load training) and power (i.e., light load training) provides the basis for optimal power development and continued increases in power output by increasing the force component and the time component of the power equation.

For optimal power development, a periodized program emphasizing strength development (i.e., 85% to 100% 1-RM) with the integration of light load, high-velocity movements (30% to 45% 1-RM) is recommended. Training at a variety of loads and velocities will maximize power output through a continuum of velocities (Fig. 16.2).

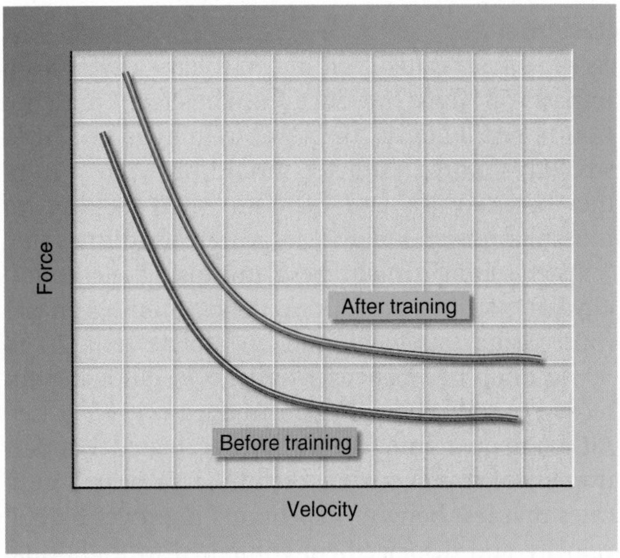

FIGURE 16.2 Impact of power training at fast, moderate, and slow velocities on the force–velocity curve. Training should be at a spectrum of velocities to see increases in power across all movement speeds.

REAL-WORLD APPLICATION

Concentric Force–Velocity Curve

The CON force–velocity curve is an important concept in training for power and maximal athletic performance. All exercises have a power output, some very low and some high. Highest power outputs are seen with moderate (~30% 1RM) weights moved explosively. Power is a critical component of many competitive sports. "A" represents a high-force, low-velocity movement such as a 1-RM max on a squat. "B" represents a low-force, high-velocity movement, such as throwing a baseball at maximal velocity. "C" represents training intentionally slowly, moving away from the force–velocity curve. To shift the force–velocity curve up and to the right (to improve power), training must be as close as possible to the curve. If sport-specific performance is at the high-force, low-velocity end of the curve, as in the case of a powerlifter, for example, training should move to the high-force, low-velocity end of the continuum as the competitive season approaches. If sport-specific performance is at the high-velocity, low-force end of the force–velocity curve, as with a baseball pitcher, for example, training should move to the high-velocity, low-force end of the continuum as the competitive season approaches.

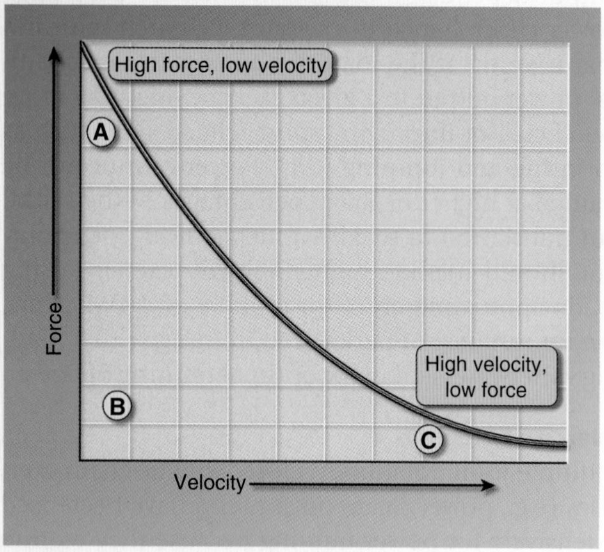

Volume

Recommended volume for power training is similar to strength training. Multiple (three to six) sets of power exercises consisting of one to six repetitions integrated into a strength training program are recommended for maximizing power development (12).

Rest Intervals

As previously stated, rest intervals have a significant impact on force production. Therefore, prescription of rest intervals for power training is similar to strength training. Athletes should rest 2 to 3 minutes between sets and exercises when training for muscular power. Preliminary research indicates that "cluster setting" might be a promising methodology for rest intervals during power training phases (30). Using this technique, an athlete rests 20 to 30 seconds between each repetition, allowing for recovery and optimal performance within a set. Although no training studies have evaluated the effectiveness of cluster setting, preliminary research indicates that rest between repetitions improves barbell velocity and displacement compared to traditional consecutive repetition methods (31). Depending on the time constraints in training, this could be an effective technique, especially for the Olympic lifts.

Repetition Velocity

Though actually performing the repetitions as rapidly as possible is important in power development, the *intent* to perform repetitions quickly is influential regardless of actual movement speed. Studies have shown that performing repetitions with intended maximal concentric acceleration (IMCA) increased power development to a greater extent than lifting the same loads at a volitional (32) or intentionally slow (33) repetition velocity.

Regardless of the load used, when training for muscular power, repetitions should be performed with IMCA.

MUSCULAR HYPERTROPHY

Resistance training increases muscle CSA (Fig. 16.3). Mechanical damage resulting from loaded ECC muscle actions promotes hypertrophy; however, muscle damage is not required for this adaptation. Hypertrophy results from an accumulation of proteins via increased rate of synthesis, decreased degradation, or both (34). Following a bout of resistance exercise, protein synthesis elevates at 2 to 3 hours, peaks at approximately

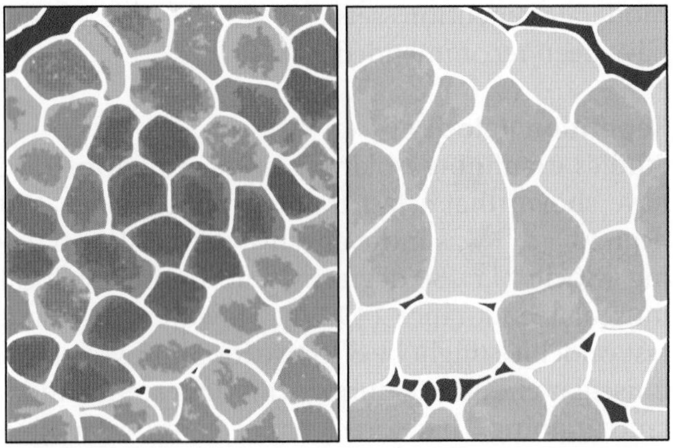

FIGURE 16.3 Micrographs of a muscle biopsy before **(A)** and after 8 weeks **(B)** of resistance training. Muscle fiber is enlarged (hypertrophy) following resistance training.

24 hours, and returns to baseline levels at around 36 to 48 hours after exercise (35). Fast-twitch muscle fibers typically increase CSA to a greater extent than slow-twitch fibers (36).

The time course of muscle hypertrophy has been examined during short-term training periods in previously untrained subjects. During the early weeks of training, it appears that the nervous system plays a primary role in the observed strength increases. Muscle hypertrophy is evident by 6 or 7 weeks of training (37), although changes in the quality of proteins, fiber types, and protein synthetic rates take place much earlier. From this point onward, there appears to be an interaction between neural adaptations and hypertrophy in the expression of strength (38).

Exercise Selection

Single-joint and multiple-joint exercises are effective for muscular hypertrophy. Interestingly, though, the complexity of exercises could affect the time course of muscle hypertrophy. Multiple-joint exercises require a longer neural adaptive phase, which might delay the hypertrophic response (39). However, as previously stated, multiple-joint exercises induce a greater hormonal response, which might be important for maximal gains in muscle size.

Muscular hypertrophy can be induced by single-joint and multiple-joint exercises; however, multiple-joint exercises should be emphasized for maximal long-term gains in muscle size.

Loading and Volume

Various types of resistance training programs have been shown to elicit muscular hypertrophy. However, training programs aimed at maximizing hypertrophy typically emphasize moderate to heavy relative loads (70% to 85% 1-RM) and high volume (8 to 12 repetitions for multiple sets) (1). These programs stimulate greater acute increases in testosterone and growth hormone than high-load, low-volume regimens (i.e., programs that emphasize gains in muscular strength). This has been supported, in part, by greater hypertrophy associated with high-volume, multiple-set programs compared to lower volume, single-set programs in resistance-trained individuals (22,40).

To optimize muscular hypertrophy, resistance training program should emphasize moderate to heavy loads (70% to 85% 1-RM) and high volume (6 to 12 repetitions with multiple sets).

Rest Intervals

Short rest periods (1 to 2 minutes) used in accordance with moderate to high intensity and volume elicit greater acute anabolic hormone responses than programs utilizing very heavy loads and long rest periods (3 minutes) (41,42). However, one study reported no significant difference in muscle girth, skinfolds, or body mass between protocols using 30, 90, and 180 seconds rest between sets in recreationally trained men over 5 weeks (8). Therefore, to date, it is unclear if the use of short rest periods to maximize the anabolic hormonal response to resistance exercise is important for maximizing muscular hypertrophy. Based on this information and the fact that rest periods significantly affect strength gains, we recommend rest periods of 2 to 3 minutes between sets in fundamental exercises and 1 to 2 minutes rest between sets for assistance exercises.

Repetition Velocity

Little is known about the effect of repetition velocity on muscle hypertrophy. It has been suggested that higher velocities of movement pose less of a stimulus for hypertrophy than slow and moderate velocities (43); however, further research is necessary to substantiate this proposition. Therefore, when training for muscular hypertrophy, the prescription of repetition velocity is secondary to the load, repetition number, and goals of the particular exercise.

LOCAL MUSCULAR ENDURANCE

Appropriate prescription of resistance exercise improves local muscular endurance. Resistance training develops absolute muscular endurance, which is the maximal number of repetitions performed with a specific pretraining load (e.g., 150 lb) (44). However, the effects of resistance exercise on relative muscular endurance, which is the maximal number of repetitions performed at a specific relative intensity (e.g., 50% 1-RM), appears limited (45).

Exercise Selection

Exercises stressing multiple or large muscle groups are associated with the greatest acute metabolic responses. This is important because high metabolic demand is a stimulus for adaptations, leading to improved local muscular endurance (e.g., increased mitochondrial density and capillary number, fiber-type transitions, buffering capacity). Therefore, it is recommended that multiple or large muscle group exercises are emphasized in programs aimed at improving local muscular endurance.

Loading and Volume

Light loads used in accordance with high repetitions (20 or more) are most effective for increasing local muscular endurance (44,46). Moderate to heavy loading is also effective for increasing high-intensity and absolute muscular endurance when coupled with short rest periods (44,47). In general, high-volume programs are optimal for endurance performance, especially when multiple sets per exercise are performed.

> ***Light loads, high repetitions, and high overall volume should be emphasized for improving local muscular endurance.***

Rest Intervals

Athletes who typically train using high volume and short rest periods (e.g., body builders) demonstrate significantly lower fatigue rate in comparison with athletes who train with low to moderate volumes and long rest periods (e.g., power lifters) (48). This finding supports the use of short rest periods when training for local muscular endurance. Therefore, rest periods of 1 to 2 minutes for high repetition sets (15 to 20 repetitions) and <1 minute for moderate-repetition sets (10 to 15 repetitions) have been recommended.

Repetition Velocity

Studies examining isokinetic exercise performance have shown that a fast training velocity (i.e., 180 degrees $\cdot$ s^{-1}) was more effective than a slow training velocity (i.e., 30 degrees s^{-1}) for improving local muscular endurance (49,50). However, slow and fast velocities might be effective for improving local muscular endurance during constant external resistance training. Therefore, it has been recommended (4) to employ slow velocities when a moderate number of repetitions (10 to 15 repetitions) are used and moderate to fast velocities when a high number of repetitions (15 or more) are used.

PROGRESSION

Up to this point, we have discussed the implementation of acute program variables to achieve a desired result. It should be noted, however, that these variables require continued and systematic alteration so that long-term progression can occur. **Progression** has been previously defined as "The act of moving forward or advancing toward a specific goal" (4). Although it is impossible to improve at the same rate over the course of a long-term resistance training program, the proper manipulation of acute program variables can limit training plateaus and, consequently, enable achievement of a high level of muscular fitness. The three general principles of progression are progressive overload, variation, and specificity.

PROGRESSIVE OVERLOAD

Progressive overload is the gradual increase of stress placed upon the body during resistance exercise training. As training duration proceeds, there is an increase in exercise tolerance. However, continued gains in performance will only occur if the body's adaptive processes are progressively taxed. Therefore, gradual increases in physiological demands are required for long-term improvements in physical performance.

Progressive overload can be induced by (a) increasing the load, (b) adding repetitions to the current load, (c) altering repetition velocity according to program goals, (d) altering rest period length according to program goals, and/

or (e) increasing volume within reasonable limits (2% to 5% until further adaptation has occurred). In some cases, volume increases may be larger depending upon level of adaptation and starting loads; For example, extremely low starting loads might be rapidly outgrown in early phases of a beginner program where technique was the limiting factor.

VARIATION

Systematic Variation (or periodization) is the purposeful and planned alteration of acute program variables over time. Systematically varying volume and intensity is likely most effective for long-term progression. Therefore, to ensure long-term gains in performance, it is imperative to plan systematic changes in exercise choice, intensity, volume, and repetition velocity. Concepts of **periodization** were discussed in detail in Chapter 14.

SPECIFICITY

Training adaptations are specific to the muscle actions involved, speed of movement, range of motion, muscle groups trained, energy systems involved, and intensity and volume of training (6). These facts provide valuable rationale for performing a needs analysis before prescribing a resistance exercise program. Once the needs of the athlete have been identified, the strength and conditioning practitioner must keep the needs in mind when constructing a resistance exercise regimen to ensure that the desired goals are being met.

In addition, resistance exercise progression should follow a general-to-specific model. For example, if one's goal is to improve vertical jump performance, choice of exercise should progress from general lower body strengthening exercises (e.g., deadlift, back squat) to explosive lower body power exercises (e.g., power clean, jump squat).

PRESCRIBING AND TRACKING DAILY WORKOUTS

Daily exercise prescriptions and athlete progress should be documented to ensure that the athlete is advancing toward his or her training goals. It might be important to develop a "workout log" to give each athlete before a training session. The workout log should include the prescribed exercises, loads, repetition ranges, and exercise order. It could also be important to track daily training volume and volume load. These data might prove useful in the event of abnormal responses to training or injury. For example, if you notice that an athlete is not responding well to training (i.e., there is a noticeable decrease in performance, fatigue, etc.), it could be due to an increase in training volume, volume load, or intensity. If these data are documented in a systematic way, the strength and conditioning coach can quickly evaluate and make alterations to the program to ensure optimal progression and prevent overtraining.

Figure 16.4 provides an example of a theoretical workout log for 1 week of a combined upper and lower body resistance training program with a 3 d wk^{-1} training frequency. In this example, the first 2 days of training within the week are completed. Notice that the training volume and volume load for these sessions is calculated in the right-hand columns. Volume load was higher on training day 1 than on day 2. The prescribed training intensity on day 2 was purposefully lowered to allow recovery from the high training intensity provided on day 1. The final day (day 3) in this example has not been completed by the athlete. Notice that the column for the number of repetitions performed per set is blank, but the training weight has already been prescribed by the strength and conditioning coach and is included on the card. When the athlete performs on the final training day, he or she should record the actual number of repetitions performed with each set. The strength coach can then calculate the daily volume and volume load for the workout and then determine the sum of the 3 days to derive weekly totals.

Summary

The prescription of a resistance exercise program is a sequential process that begins with a needs analysis to identify the specific needs of individual athletes. Identified needs can be met by implementing the acute program variables in a precise manner to produce a desired outcome. Therefore, a sound resistance training program can be developed via a thorough understanding of the acute program variables and their respective impact on trainable characteristics. A detailed summary of the essential components of this chapter can be found in Table 16.3.

Athlete Name												
Day 1												
EXERCISE (120-180s rec)			Set 1		Set 2		Set 3		Set 4		Total	
	Sets	**Reps**	**Reps**	**Load**	**Reps**	**Load**	**Reps**	**Load**	**Reps**	**Load**	**Volume**	**V. Load**
General Warm-up												
Dynamic Flexibility												
Hang Cleans	**4**	**4**	4	205	4	215	4	225	3	235	15	3285
Back Squats	**4**	**4–6**	6	225	6	250	6	275	6	300	24	6300
Lat Pulldown	**4**	**4–6**	6	185	6	195	6	205	5	215	23	4585
Bench Press	**4**	**4–6**	6	185	6	195	6	205	6	215	24	4800
Barbell Lunge	**3**	**4–6**	6	115	6	115	5	115			17	1955
Calf Raises	**2**	**15**	15	300	15	300					30	9000
Ab/Low Back												
Daily Statistics											133	29925
Day 2												
EXERCISE (120-180s rec)			Set 1		Set 2		Set 3		Set 4		Total	
	Sets	**Reps**	**Reps**	**Load**	**Reps**	**Load**	**Reps**	**Load**	**Reps**	**Load**	**Volume**	**V. Load**
General Warm-up												
Dynamic Flexibility												
Hang Cleans	**4**	**4**	4	195	4	195	4	205	4	205	16	3200
Back Squats	**4**	**4–6**	6	225	6	225	6	250	6	250	24	5700
Lat Pulldown	**4**	**4–6**	6	185	6	185	6	195	5	195	23	4365
Bench Press	**4**	**4–6**	6	185	6	185	6	195	6	195	24	4560
Barbell Lunge	**3**	**4–6**	6	95	6	95	6	95			18	1710
Calf Raises	**2**	**15**	15	275	15	275					30	8250
Ab/Low Back												
Daily Statistics											119	24585
Day 3												
EXERCISE (120-180s rec)			Set 1		Set 2		Set 3		Set 4		Total	
	Sets	**Reps**	**Reps**	**Load**	**Reps**	**Load**	**Reps**	**Load**	**Reps**	**Load**	**Volume**	**V. Load**
General Warm-up												
Dynamic Flexibility												
Hang Cleans	**4**	**4**		205		215		225		235	0	0
Back Squats	**4**	**4–6**		225		250		275		300	0	0
Lat Pulldown	**4**	**4–6**		185		195		205		215	0	0
Bench Press	**4**	**4–6**		185		195		205		215	0	0
Barbell Lunge	**3**	**4–6**		115		115		115			0	0
Calf Raises	**2**	**15**		300		300					0	0
Ab/Low Back												
Daily Statistics											0	0

FIGURE 16.4 Sample workout card for 1 week of training. It can be used to prescribe resistance exercise sessions, track athlete progress, and monitor training volume, volume load, and intensity throughout a training cycle.

TABLE 16.3 ● SUMMARY OF RESISTANCE TRAINING EXERCISE PRESCRIPTION

	EXERCISE SELECTION	LOADING	VOLUME	REST INTERVALS	REPETITION VELOCITY
STRENGTH					
Novice	Single-joint and multiple-joint	45%–70% 1-RM	Sets: 1–3 Reps: 8–12	2–3 min for fundamental 1–2 min for assistance	Slow, moderate
Experienced	Emphasize multiple-joint	>80% 1-RM	Sets: multiple Reps : 1–6	2–3 min for fundamental 1–2 min for assistance	Moderate, intentionally fast

TABLE 16.3 ● SUMMARY OF RESISTANCE TRAINING EXERCISE PRESCRIPTION (*Continued*)

	EXERCISE SELECTION	LOADING	VOLUME	REST INTERVALS	REPETITION VELOCITY
POWER					
Novice	Multiple-joint	Strength: >80% 1-RM Velocity: 30%–60% of 1-RM	Sets: 1–3 Reps: 3–6	2–3 min for fundamental 1–2 min for assistance	Intentionally fast
Experienced	Multiple-joint	Strength: >80% 1-RM Velocity: 30%–60% 1-RM	Sets: multiple Reps: 1–6	2–3 min for fundamental 1–2 min for assistance	Intentionally fast
HYPERTROPHY					
Novice	Single-joint and multiple-joint	60%–70% 1-RM	Sets: 1–3 sets Reps: 8–12	1–2 min	Slow, moderate
Experienced	Single-joint and multiple-joint	70%–85% 1-RM	Sets: multiple Reps: 6–12	1–2 min	Slow, moderate
ENDURANCE					
Novice	Single-joint and multiple-joint	50%–70% 1-RM	Sets: 1–3 sets Reps: 10–15	<1 min	Slow, moderate for MR Moderate, fast for HR
Experienced	Emphasize multiple-joint	30%–80% 1-RM	Sets: multiple Reps: 10 or more	1–2 min for high rep ex. <1 min for moderate rep exercise	Slow, moderate for MR Moderate, fast for HR

HR, High Repetitions; MR, Moderate Repetitions.

Maxing Out

1. You are a strength and conditioning coach for a high school football team. During the season, the head football coach instructs you to design an in-season workout that lasts no longer than 45 minutes. You can choose resistance training exercises. List the exercises you would choose and give a brief reason for your choice.
2. You are a strength and conditioning coach in a high school. The school is building a new weight room and the athletic director wants to equip the weight room with various pieces of machine resistance equipment. You have a meeting with the athletic director to discuss your preference of free weights. Outline the major points you will make to the athletic director at this meeting.

CASE EXAMPLE

Designing a Resistance Training Program for a College Football Player

BACKGROUND

You are a strength and conditioning professional at a college and have been asked to design a resistance training program for a football player. The player is a running back entering his junior season and has 5 years of resistance training experience including multiple-joint and Olympic-style lifts. Perform a needs analysis and design an individualized resistance training program.

CONSIDERATIONS

Football is a high-intensity sport with short periods of play (~5 seconds) interspersed with brief rest periods (~30 seconds). Running backs require speed, strength, and power to

(*Continued*)

Designing a Resistance Training Program for a College Football Player

be successful. This specific athlete already possesses adequate muscle mass and minimal body fat; therefore, hypertrophy and/or changes in body mass are not desired. The athlete has no injuries or health concerns.

IMPLEMENTATION

Exercise selection	Multiple-joint, large muscle mass exercises including power exercises should be emphasized
Exercise order	(a) Power exercises; (b) Multiple-joint, large muscle mass exercises; (c) Single-joint, small muscle mass exercises
Loading	Power exercises: 30%–50% 1-RM Strength exercises: >80% 1-RM
Volume	Multiple sets, one to six repetitions per set
Rest intervals	Fundamental exercises: 2 to 3 min Assistance exercises: 1 to 2 min
Frequency	4 sessions · wk^{-1}
Workout structure	Split routine
Muscle actions	CON and ECC
Repetition velocity	Power exercises: intent to perform the repetitions as quickly as possible Strength exercises: volitional speed

RESULTS

Example week of training

Note: This example is for 1 week of training. Follow fundamentals of progression to ensure long-term performance gains.

MONDAY	TUESDAY	WEDNESDAY	THURSDAY	FRIDAY
Bench throws:	Hang cleans:	OFF	Incline press:	Squat jump:
4 sets	3 sets		3 sets	4 sets
3 reps	3 reps		6 reps	3 reps
30% 1-RM	80% 1-RM		6-RM	30% 1-RM
(use medicine ball)				
Bench press:	Deadlift:		Lat pull downs:	Back squat:
3 sets	3 sets		3 sets	3 sets
3 reps	6 reps		6 reps	3 reps
3-RM	6-RM		6-RM	3-RM
Bent-over rows:	Front squat:		Arm extension:	Leg press:
3 sets	3 sets		3 sets	3 sets
6 reps	6 reps		6 reps	6 reps
6-RM	6-RM		6-RM	6-RM
Shoulder press:	Leg extension:		Arm curl:	Calf raises:
3 sets	3 sets		3 sets	3 sets
6 reps	6 reps		6 reps	6 reps
6-RM	6-RM		6-RM	6-RM
Pull-ups:	Leg curls:			
3 sets	3 sets			
6 reps	6 reps			
6-RM	6-RM			

1. The needs analysis determines the goals of the program.
2. The goals of the program determine the implementation of acute program variables.
3. The implementation of acute program variables determines the responses and adaptations to resistance exercise.
4. The adaptations to resistance exercise influence athletic performance.

REFERENCES

1. Kraemer WJ, Ratamess NA. Endocrine responses and adaptations to strength and power training. In: Komi PV, ed. *Strength and Power in Sport*. Malden, MA: Blackwell Science; 2003:361–386.
2. Escamilla RF, Fleisig GS, Zheng N, et al. Biomechanics of the knee during closed kinetic chain and open kinetic chain exercises. *Med Sci Sports Exerc*. 1998;30:556–569.
3. Brennecke A, Guimaraes TM, Leone R, et al. Neuromuscular activity during bench press exercise performed with and without the preexhastion method. *J Strength Cond Res*. 2009;23:1933–1940.
4. Kraemer WJ, Adams K, Cafarelli E, et al.; American College of Sports Medicine position stand. Progression models in resistance training for healthy adults. *Med Sci Sports Exerc*. 2009;41(3):687–708.
5. Willardson JM, Kattenbraker MS, Khairallah M, et al. Research note: effect of load reductions over consecutive sets on repetition performance. *J Strength Cond Res*. 2010;24:879–884.
6. Campos GE, Luecke TJ, Wendeln HK, et al. Muscular adaptations in response to three different resistance-training regimens: specificity of repetition maximum training zones. *Eur J Appl Physiol*. 2002;88:50–60.
7. Pincivero DM, Lephart SM, Karunakara RG. Effects of rest interval on isokinetic strength and functional performance after short-term high intensity training. *Br J Sports Med*. 1997;31:229–234.
8. Robinson JM, Stone MH, Johnson RL, et al. Effects of different weight training exercise/rest intervals on strength, power, and high intensity exercise endurance. *J Strength Cond Res*. 1995;9:216–221.
9. Willardson JM, Burkett LN. The effect of different rest intervals between sets on volume components and strength gains. *J Strength Cond Res*. 2008;22:146–152.
10. Häkkinen K. Neuromuscular fatigue and recovery in women at different ages during heavy resistance loading. *Electromyogr Clin Neurophysiol*. 1995;35:403–413.
11. Häkkinen K, Pakarinen A, Newton RU, et al. Acute hormone responses to heavy resistance lower and upper extremity exercise in young versus old men. *Eur J Appl Physiol*. 1998;77:312–319.
12. Ratamess NA, Alvar BA, Evetoch TK, et al. Progression models in resistance training for healthy adults. *Med Sci Sport Exerc*. 2009;41:687–708
13. Dudley GA, Tesch PA, Miller BJ, et al. Importance of eccentric actions in performance adaptations to resistance training. *Aviat Space Environ Med*. 1991;62:543–550.
14. Mookerjee S, Ratamess NA. Comparison of strength differences and joint action durations between full and partial range-of-motion bench press exercise. *J Strength Cond Res*. 1999;13:76–81.
15. Keogh JWL, Wilson GJ, Weatherby RP. A cross-sectional comparison of different resistance training techniques in the bench press. *J Strength Cond Res*. 1999;13:247–258.
16. Keeler LK, Finkelstein LH, Miller W, et al. Early-phase adaptations of traditional-speed vs. superslow resistance training on strength and aerobic capacity in sedentary individuals. *J Strength Cond Res*. 2001;15:309–314.
17. Morrissey MC, Harman EA, Frykman PN, et al. Early phase differential effects of slow and fast barbell squat training. *Am J Sports Med*. 1998;26:221–230.
18. Rhea MR, Alvar BA, Burkett LN, et al. A meta-analysis to determine the dose response for strength development. *Med Sci Sport Exerc*. 2003;35:456–464.
19. Starkey DB, Pollock ML, Ishida Y, et al. Effect of resistance training volume on strength and muscle thickness. *Med Sci Sports Exerc*. 1996;28:1311–1320.
20. Sanborn K, Boros R, Hruby J, et al. Short-term performance effects of weight training with multiple sets not to failure vs a single set to failure in women. *J Strength Cond Res*. 2000;14:328–331.
21. Hass CJ, Garzarella L, de Hoyos D, et al. Single versus multiple sets in long-term recreational weightlifters. *Med Sci Sports Exerc*. 2000;32:235–242.
22. Kraemer WJ, Ratamess N, Fry AC, et al.; Influence of resistance training volume and periodization on physiological and performance adaptations in collegiate women tennis players. *Am J Sports Med*. 2000;28:626–633.
23. McBride JM, Triplett-McBride T, Davie A, et al. The effect of heavy- vs. light-load jump squats on the development of strength, power, and speed. *J Strength Cond Res*. 2002;16:75–82.
24. Newton RU, Kraemer WJ, Hakkinen K, et al. Kinematics, kinetics, and muscle activation during explosive upper body movements. *J Appl Biomech*. 1996;12:31–43.
25. Wilson GJ, Newton RU, Murphy AJ, et al. The optimal training load for the development of dynamic athletic performance. *Med Sci Sports Exerc*. 1993;25:1279–1286.
26. Häkkinen K, Komi PV. The effect of explosive type strength training on electromyographic and force production characteristics of leg extensor muscles during concentric and various stretch-shortening cycle exercises. *Scand J Sports Sci*. 1985;7:65–76.
27. Kawamori N, Haff GG. The optimal training load for the development of muscular power. *J Strength Cond Res*. 2004;18:675–684.
28. Baker D, Nance S, Moore M. The load that maximizes the average mechanical power output during explosive bench press throws in highly trained athletes. *J Strength Cond Res*. 2001;15:20–24.
29. Baker D, Nance S, Moore M. The load that maximizes the average mechanical power output during jump squats in power-trained athletes. *J Strength Cond Res*. 2001;15:92–97.
30. Haff GG, Hobbs RT, Haff EE, et al. Cluster training: a novel method for introducing training program variation. *Strength Cond J*. 2008;30:67–76.
31. Haff GG, Whitley A, McCoy LB, et al. Effects of different set configurations on barbell velocity and displacement during a clean pull. *J Strength Cond Res*. 2003;17:95–103.

32. Jones K, Hunter G, Fleisig G, et al. The effects of compensatory acceleration on upper-body strength and power in collegiate football players. *J Strength Cond Res.* 1999;13:99–105.
33. Young WB, Bilby GE. The effect of volunatary effort to influence speed of contraction on strength, muscular power, and hypertrophy development. *J Strength Cond Res.* 1993;7:172–178
34. Booth FW, Thomason DB. Molecular and cellular adaptation of muscle in response to exercise: perspectives of various models. *Physiol Rev.* 1991;71:541–585.
35. MacDougall JD, Gibala MJ, Tarnopolsky MA, et al. The time course for elevated muscle protein synthesis following heavy resistance exercise. *Can J Appl Physiol.* 1995;20:480–486.
36. Alway SE, Grumbt WH, Gonyea WJ, et al. Contrasts in muscle and myofibers of elite male and female bodybuilders. *J Appl Physiol.* 1989;67:24–31.
37. Phillips SM. Short-term training: when do repeated bouts of resistance exercise become training? *Can J Appl Physiol.* 2000;25:185–193.
38. Sale DG. Neural adaptations to strength training. In: Komi PV, ed. *Strength and Power in Sport.* Oxford, UK: Blackwell Scientific; 1992:249–265.
39. Chilibeck PD, Calder AW, Sale DG, et al. A comparison of strength and muscle mass increases during resistance training in young women. *Eur J Appl Physiol.* 1998;77:170–175.
40. Kraemer WJ. A series of studies—the physiological basis for strength training in American football: fact over philosophy. *J Strength Cond Res.* 1997;11:131–142.
41. Kraemer WJ, Gordon SE, Fleck SJ, et al. Endogenous anabolic hormonal and growth factor responses to heavy resistance exercise in males and females. *Int J Sports Med.* 1991;12:228–235.
42. Kraemer WJ, Marchitelli L, Gordon SE, et al. Hormonal and growth factor responses to heavy resistance exercise protocols. *J Appl Physiol.* 1990;69:1442–1450.
43. Tesch PA, Komi PV, Hakkinen K. Enzymatic adaptations consequent to long-term strength training. *Int J Sports Med.* 1987;8(suppl 1):66–69.
44. Anderson T, Kearney JT. Effects of three resistance training programs on muscular strength and absolute and relative endurance. *Res Q Exerc Sport.* 1982;53:1–7.
45. Mazzetti SA, Kraemer WJ, Volek JS, et al. The influence of direct supervision of resistance training on strength performance. *Med Sci Sports Exerc.* 2000;32:1175–1184.
46. Stone MH, Coulter SP. Strength/endurance effects from three resistance training protocols with women. *J Strength Cond Res.* 1994;8:231–234.
47. McGee D, Jessee TC, Stone MH, et al. Leg and hip endurance adaptations to three weight-training programs. *J Appl Sport Sci Res.* 1992;6:92–95.
48. Kraemer WJ, Noble BJ, Clark MJ, et al. Physiologic responses to heavy-resistance exercise with very short rest periods. *Int J Sports Med.* 1987;8:247–252.
49. Adeyanju K, Crews TR, Meadors WJ. Effects of two speeds of isokinetic training on muscular strength, power and endurance. *J Sports Med Phys Fitness.* 1983;23:352–356.
50. Moffroid MT, Whipple RH. Specificity of speed of exercise. *Phys Ther.* 1970;50:1692–1700.

CHAPTER 17

Plyometric, Speed, and Agility Exercise Prescription

MARK KOVACS

OBJECTIVES

After reading this chapter, you will be able to:

- Demonstrate an understanding of the role of the stretch-shortening cycle in sprinting, plyometrics, and agility exercises.
- Explain the role of plyometric exercises in injury prevention.
- Discuss the role of plyometric exercises used to increase muscular power.
- Explain the basic concepts involved in improving speed in a linear sprint.
- Discuss the role of reaction time in improving human performance.
- Design a speed, agility, and plyometric training regimen for an athlete.

KEY TERMS

Acceleration Phase
Agility
Attainment Phase
Contractile Elements
Galloping
Hop
Jump
Leap
Maintenance Phase
Mechanical Model
Neural Feed-Forward Mechanism
Neuromuscular Model
Noncontractile Elements
Plyometric Exercises
Reaction Time (RT)
Reciprocal Innervation
Shuffling
Skipping
Stretch-Shortening Cycle (SSC)
Support Phase
Swing Phase
Throwing
Toss

Introduction

In most sports, athletes perform short (5- to 20-yd) or long (20- to 40-yd) sprints, change direction rapidly, or jump for height and/or distance. Therefore, linear acceleration and multidirectional speed; agility; and vertical, horizontal, and lateral jumping movements are essential elements of successful athletic performance. These locomotor skills are learned at young ages as children participate in unstructured playful activities. Maturation and experience will help refine the movement patterns associated with these skills; however, instruction on the mechanical aspects of locomotion is typically required to improve efficiency and performance and to limit the likelihood of injury. Once the global and segmental mechanical aspects of a skill have been mastered, training can focus on improving and ultimately maximizing performance. The types of exercises or drills prescribed to an athlete will be based on identified mechanical flaws or muscular weaknesses. To date, the manipulation of acute training variables for speed, agility, and plyometric training is unclear but will certainly depend on the athletic goals (short and long term), developmental stage, as well as chronological and training age.

To design a training regimen for an athlete, sports performance professionals need to consider aspects from several domains. First, a clear understanding of the sequence of motor development from childhood to adulthood for running, jumping, and changing direction is important. This will help guide the selection of appropriate drills or exercises for inexperienced, mature, and advanced athletes. Second, sports performance professionals should clearly recognize mature movement patterns associated with global and segmental mechanics and understand the specific muscular actions involved. This will help them to identify movement flaws, instruct athletes on appropriate changes, and assist skill improvement during childhood and through adolescence. Finally, understanding how to manipulate acute training program variables (e.g., sets, reps, frequency, volume) will prove to be the most challenging aspect of improving and maximizing performance, since research is scarce regarding sprint, agility, and plyometric training. Nevertheless, appropriate training principles are applied to ensure sufficient stimulation to improve performance while minimizing excessive overload.

This chapter begins with an overview of the stretch-shortening cycle (SSC) and briefly describes factors that impact SSC efficiency. Next, the developmental sequence of sprinting, jumping, and changing direction is illustrated, which includes characteristics for mature motor skill performance. Then a brief list of exercises and drills is provided to help develop and improve sprinting, jumping, and agility skills. Finally, general guidelines for program design are recommended.

THE STRETCH-SHORTENING CYCLE

All explosive movements, whether it is sprinting, jumping, and/or changing direction, have one major component in common: the **stretch-shortening cycle (SSC)**. The SSC can simply be described as the coupling of an eccentric action with a concentric action. In other words, when a muscle or muscle group is eccentrically loaded (i.e., stretched) and is immediately followed by a shortening action, then a SSC has occurred. Although SSCs are common in everyday tasks (e.g., walking), their use in athletics is often intended to enhance performance. By rapidly coupling eccentric–concentric actions, the muscular force and power output during the concentric phase are enhanced (1). This, in turn, allows athletes to run faster, jump higher, and change direction more rapidly.

REAL-WORLD APPLICATION

Muscle Elasticity

Releasing a rubber band from a stretched position will allow it to snap back into its original shape. Similarly, stored elastic energy will provide additional force when muscle shortening is preceded immediately by a stretch. During the stretch, energy is stored in the muscle, just as it is stored in the stretched rubber band. The stored elastic energy of muscle is one reason plyometric exercises increase power output.

Although the SSC has been studied in great detail, the mechanisms responsible for greater power production are still debated (1–5). Two models may contribute to a complex mechanism, which results in enhanced power production during the concentric portion of the SSC. The first is the **mechanical model**, first illustrated by Hill (6), which describes contractile and noncontractile elements (discussed in Chapter 3). The second is the **neuromuscular model**, which outlines the fine interplay of nervous and muscular systems.

Contractile elements are contained within the sarcomere of a muscle and consist of actin and myosin. **Noncontractile elements** consist of the series elastic component (SEC), also known as the muscle–tendon unit (5), and the parallel elastic component (PEC), which consists of the connective tissues surrounding individual fibers, muscle bundles, and the entire muscle (i.e., endomysium, perimysium, and epimysium). The mechanical model states that muscle force is increased due to the reutilization of elastic energy by the SEC (5). In other words, when a muscle is eccentrically loaded (i.e., stretched) and immediately followed by a concentric action, energy will be produced, stored (as potential energy), and ultimately released (kinetic energy) from the muscle–tendon unit and increase force and power output.

On the other hand, the neuromuscular model suggests that preactivation of a muscle or muscle group is partially responsible for the force and power potentiation during the concentric phase of a SSC (1,3). A comparison of jumps initiated from either a static squat position or by beginning with a countermovement shows that there is a greater amount of time to develop force and muscular activation prior to shortening by the contractile element during the countermovement jump (3). In addition, sprinting and agility skills have shown preactivation of a majority of the leg muscles prior to the support phase (7–9), suggesting that movement speed would be dramatically reduced otherwise.

In all likelihood, both models contribute to the enhancement of force and mechanical power output during SSC. In fact, during the early extension phase of a static squat jump, it has been shown that the SEC is stretched only slightly (10). This is most likely due to the large amount of shortening of the contractile element. Just prior to toe-off during a running gait (about 100 milliseconds), there is a reversal in roles where the contractile element does not change in length and the SEC rapidly shortens and releases stored energy (11). Therefore, each model may provide a stimulus during different portions of a given SSC.

The SSC is an important physiological reflex that enhances muscular power output. Both mechanical and neural factors contribute to power potentiation.

Neural control and reflexes of skeletal muscle are governed by two receptors: muscle spindles and Golgi tendon organ (GTO).

Muscle spindles and GTOs are responsible for the enhancement or inhibition of muscular actions by monitoring the rate of stretch and detecting tension in muscle.

IMPACTING FACTORS

In performing exercises that involve SSC, there are several factors that can impact the enhancement of force or power output of the movement.

Another factor affecting SSC, especially during jumping, is the use of the upper extremities. Swinging the arms while performing a countermovement jump creates more downward vertical ground reaction force; consequently, a greater amount of upward vertical force is generated (Newton's law of action–reaction), propelling the body higher or further during flight (12). Arm swing also contributes to takeoff velocity during vertical and horizontal jumping actions (12,13). Swinging the arms during sprinting increases velocity compared to sprinting without arm actions (9). Choosing whether or not to swing the arms can significantly contribute to the execution of SSC drills and consequently affect athletic performance.

Studies have reported gender differences in SSC ability by using indirect measurements such as countermovement jump height or sprinting ability. Typically, boys and men exhibit greater absolute power than girls and women. In addition, larger increases are observed in maximal power for boys compared to girls during adolescence (14). Greater amounts of lean body tissue (i.e., muscle mass) are believed to be responsible for these differences; however, when normalized for body weight, the differences between boys and girls are often minimized (15,16). Reports have shown higher peak velocity during countermovement jumps for men as compared to women (17,18). In fact, one study concluded that the difference in peak power between men and women was solely due to movement velocity (17). Other factors such as fiber-type composition, anaerobic metabolism, and neuromuscular aspects may also contribute to gender differences (14). Although these differences exist, there is no evidence to suggest that men and women respond to SSC training differently; therefore, program design should reflect developmental stage, training experience, and the particular sport rather than gender.

Sprinting, jumping, and changing direction require complex multijoint movements, which must have specific coordination between agonists and antagonists to ensure movement efficiency. There are reflexes that stimulate agonists while simultaneously inhibiting antagonists. This is termed **reciprocal innervation** (19,20). Alterations in this relationship can be impacted by increased strength or fatigue (21–23). For example, strengthening agonists will increase acceleration of the movement, while strengthening antagonists will allow deceleration to occur over a shorter time (24). The overall effect would be a heightened capacity to perform explosive SSC actions.

Fatigue, on the other hand, reduces the effectiveness of the SSC through a host of mechanisms. The mechanisms responsible for altered SSC function may be influenced by whether the fatigue was generated during submaximal or maximal exercise (25,26). Therefore, the duration of recovery from previous training sessions may be heavily dependent on the type and intensity of SSC drills performed.

This brief overview of SSC identifies several aspects that must be considered in designing a training regimen or exercise session. First, the use of arm swing is an integral component of locomotion and should be considered in selecting drills or exercises. For example, proper arm actions should always be implemented for younger, inexperienced athletes who are still learning the fundamental locomotor skills. Second, improving overall strength should be regarded as a priority for improving locomotor skills that require SSC. Children will become stronger through growth and development, but they may still benefit from playful activities or body-weight exercises that can increase strength. Mature athletes can include resistance training to enhance force capacity. Although gender will play a role in the difference of force and power production following puberty, variations between boys and girls at younger ages are minimal. Therefore, children should be taught proper movement mechanics regardless of gender; however, beyond puberty, training regimens should target performance limitations of the individual athlete and may be designed toward particular gender differences. Finally, unless there are specific needs that require an athlete to perform sprints, jumps, or changes in direction in a fatigued state, SSC exercises should be performed early within a training session and appropriate rest given between subsequent training sessions.

Many factors can contribute to SSC function, such as fiber-type distribution, gender, age, muscle activation patterns, fatigue, and arm actions.

PLYOMETRICS

Plyometric exercises are specifically designed to utilize the SSC. Many upper- and lower-body exercises exist; it is beyond the scope of this chapter to include an all-inclusive list, but several examples are provided at the end of the chapter. This section provides a discussion on intended uses, the importance of instructions, complex training outcomes, and proper exercise terminology for plyometric training.

Q & A from the Field

Q ***I work with many youth soccer teams (12- to 14-year-olds) and continually find the need to work on fundamental movement skills, such as sprinting and agility. What are appropriate drills and progressions to use with this age group?***

—high school strength and conditioning coach

A The ability to perform stopping and starting tasks in sports such as soccer is important. Coupling deceleration with reacceleration, however, may be one of the most challenging motor skills to teach younger athletes, since other things like balance, orientation, rhythm, and anticipation will set the foundation for more advanced skills. Nevertheless, an appropriate progression is an important consideration in selecting drills for your athletes.

First, teach your athletes how to accelerate properly. Next, develop their ability to stop or decelerate. Then begin to combine these skills in a linear acceleration, deceleration, and reacceleration sequence. Finally, couple linear stopping with reacceleration in different directions. Each of these steps must start at slow speeds and progress to faster movements, ultimately producing athletes who can start, stop, and restart in a variety of directions at maximal speed. Below are two drills to include in your training plan.

Linear Walk to Stride: Instruct the athletes to transition from walking to a jog and then slow back down again over short distances (5 to 10 yd). Once slower speeds are perfected, have your athletes increase the speed of acceleration. Be sure they use a multiple-step stopping technique when slowing down and avoid using one large step. You can also specify a distance for your athletes to stop within (e.g., 2 to 4 yd) and thereby heighten the intensity.

Jog-Stop-Turn-Jog: Once your athletes can perform linear stopping and starting drills at higher speeds, you can introduce slight changes in direction by having the athletes move between cones. Initially instruct your athletes to completely stop when they reach a cone, plant their outside foot, simultaneously rotate their torso toward the new direction, and finally resume jogging. You should begin with shallow angles (130 to 160 degrees) and progressively make them more challenging (90, 60, and 45 degrees). When your athletes can perform changes in direction at slower speeds with minimal flaws, gradually increase the speed.

Be sure to progress slowly; it may take several months or longer to develop appropriate movement skills. Provide ample practice time when athletes are fresh (at the beginning of practice) and continually give feedback.

TERMINOLOGY

The plyometric literature has yet to clearly define movement skills using the lower extremities to propel the body off the ground. In an effort to clarify the language used by sports performance professionals, terminology from physical education is used in this chapter to describe plyometric motor skills. There are three main movement skills; a few of their derivatives are listed below. First, a **jump** involves a takeoff from one or both feet and a landing on both feet simultaneously. Second, a **leap** (sometimes called a bound) occurs from taking off on one foot and landing on the other. Finally, a **hop** is when the takeoff and landing occur on the same single foot. Other common fundamental skills are the gallop, shuffle, and skip. **Galloping** and **shuffling** are a combination of a step and leap, whereas **skipping** requires combining a step with a hop. It becomes somewhat more difficult to distinguish types of upper-body actions. One distinction that can be used is throwing and tossing. **Throwing** actions will be considered when an overhand movement is used to propel an object, whereas a **toss** occurs when an underhand action is employed. Plyometric exercises also exist for the core. Core exercises can be classified as stability, anterior–posterior flexion and extension, rotation, and lateral flexion and extension.

DEVELOPMENTAL SEQUENCE

Moving from the ground to the air and back down to the ground can be accomplished by three major movement patterns—jumping, leaping, and

REAL-WORLD APPLICATION

Angular Motion and Human Movement

The human body is designed for angular motion around joints, which causes linear motion of the center of gravity of the body. Think about rowing a boat: the blade of an oar enters the water, the oar itself is relatively inflexible, and there is an oarlock providing a pivot point. This lever system works to provide the propulsion that moves the boat forward. Foot contact during the support phase, muscle activation providing stiffness, and motion around the hip joint all ultimately allow horizontal motion.

hopping. All individuals will develop these skills based on experiences throughout childhood, and some will perfect them later in life due to coaching from more knowledgeable instructors. It is important to understand some of the key movement characteristics as well as to be able to identify the developmental difficulties associated with these motor skills. With that said, it is beyond the scope of this chapter to provide all of the criteria to evaluate the different stages of all jumping skills; therefore, a brief overview follows for vertical jumping and horizontal leaping. More detailed information can be found in the references (27,28).

Vertical jumping is common to many sports, and its initiation can begin as early as 2 years of age (28). Many steps are involved in the developmental transition from inefficient jumping actions to proficient movement skills. In younger or inexperienced jumpers, there is only a small preparatory countermovement action. In addition, full extension of the hips, knees, and ankles does not occur. Often the legs are tucked (knee flexion) under during the flight phase, so the center of mass is not elevated. Another characteristic is that there is difficulty jumping and landing on both feet. A small step can usually be observed when a one-footed takeoff and landing occurs. Arm action is also asymmetrical and is not necessarily coordinated with the body or legs. Mature jumping patterns differ dramatically, and changes will occur quickly. For example, there is an appropriate preparatory countermovement action of the legs that is followed by a more forceful extension of the hips, knees, and ankles (28). The movement patterns of the legs are now also coordinated with those of the arms, so that there is an increase in ground reaction forces (preparatory countermovement phase) as well as an improvement in peak vertical velocity (extension phase). During the flight phase, the trunk remains upright; and upon landing, there is appropriate flexion of the hips, knees, and ankles to reduce the forces on impact.

Horizontal leaping (or bounding) is another common jumping skill that is similar to running in that there is an air phase when body weight is transferred from one leg to the other. Unlike running, leaping requires a prolonged air phase with greater vertical height and more horizontal distance covered. Early attempts at leaping typically resemble modestly exaggerated running movements. There is an inability to propel the body upward or for greater horizontal distances (28). There is a high degree of conscious effort to perform this movement; therefore, the entire motion is ineffective and often appears stiff. The arms are not used for generating force but rather for maintaining balance. Mature leaping includes forceful extension of the support leg to maximize horizontal and vertical distances, and the arms are now coordinated and assist in force development.

REAL-WORLD APPLICATION

Absorption of Energy

An egg that has been thrown at you will break when you catch it unless you "give" with it and catch it softly. Similarly, in landing from a jump, or similar movement, the athlete can learn to land softly. Instead of all of the energy dissipating on impact, it is spread out over a larger period. Landing softly decreases the chance of impact-related injuries. The transition from eccentric to concentric muscle action, however, must occur rapidly to utilize the stored elastic energy in the muscle.

Interestingly, chronological age does not guarantee mature jumping or leaping patterns, as adolescents and adults have been found to display immature or ineffective mechanical characteristics. These can range from preparatory, takeoff, and landing inefficiencies. Therefore, sports performance professionals should not assume that movement skills have been mastered simply due to chronological age. A critical examination of these motor skills is important to identify performance deficiencies. Only when proper takeoff and landing characteristics are evident should a training program focus on improving and maximizing performance.

Intended Purpose

Plyometric exercises are used in a variety of settings (e.g., athletic training, strength and conditioning, physical therapy); although no formal classification system has been developed, it is important to understand the purpose and expected outcomes of any plyometric exercises chosen for a training program. For simplicity, the following section describes the instructions used for two very distinct areas of motor development: injury prevention and performance enhancement, both of which are important for any athlete.

Injury Prevention

Some approaches to injury prevention have used plyometric exercises in an attempt to improve neuromuscular control, alter biomechanical risk factors, and provide instructions on general proprioceptive and stability development (29–32). This requires specific instructions that typically focus on reducing landing forces to minimize risk potential. These types of instructions can be effective in a short time (e.g., one to three sessions) (33,34), but they must be used regularly, because adaptations appear temporary.

A common mechanism of injury occurs on landing from a jump. This is often due to improper mechanics, where landing forces are not appropriately dissipated because the hips, knees, or ankles are extended and/or rotated. As an example, these mechanical flaws are associated with noncontact injuries to the anterior cruciate ligament (ACL). By instructing athletes to land with greater hip, knee, and ankle flexion, the landing forces can be significantly reduced (31,35). Although programs using these types of instructions have shown success in reducing landing forces and noncontact ACL injury rates, the effect on performance enhancement is extremely questionable, because no attention is given to maximizing concentric movement velocity. Therefore, these types of instructions for plyometric exercises may be reserved for younger athletes who require proprioceptive and motor development or kept within the context of clinical rehabilitation. Healthy or more advanced athletes might also benefit from this type of work if fundamental motor skills are not fully developed; however, if performance improvement is the intended outcome, other instructions may be necessary.

Improving Power

Plyometric drills are most often incorporated into a strength and conditioning program with the intention of improving SSC capability, power, and ultimately performance (e.g., vertical jump, linear sprint speed). Because power is related to both force and velocity, the question regarding which is more responsible for power improvements is often asked.

It has been reported that the use of plyometric exercises alone can improve jumping ability (36–39). Peak velocity during the concentric phase, however, appears to be the key component for countermovement jump performance (12,13,40). Research has shown that improvements of 12.7% in takeoff velocity accounted for 71% of the observed improvement in jumping performance (13). In addition, the use of light (30% of one-repetition maximum [1-RM]) compared to heavy (80% of 1-RM) squat jump loads has been shown to provide greater velocity specificity and improvements in jumping and acceleration (41). This underscores the importance of instruction for takeoff technique and the ability to take off with maximal velocity. Therefore, landing and jumping mechanics should be viewed as separate motor skills and trained independently.

Plyometric drills used for injury prevention, rehabilitation, or motor skill development should focus on proper jumping and landing mechanics. Training with the intention to improve performance (maximal takeoff velocity) should be the focus.

The performance of SSC drills in isolation during training is not common, and the combination of resistance training and plyometric exercises is often integrated into training regimens. One classic study demonstrated that the combination of resistance and plyometric training caused greater improvements in vertical jump ability than either training modality alone (42). Other research has provided indirect support for this notion by reporting that neither resistance training nor plyometric exercises alone can provide a stimulus any greater than the other when targeting performance enhancement (39). It therefore appears that one cannot increase power simply by becoming stronger and that utilizing any increase in strength at appropriate speeds is the key factor for performance enhancement (43).

The implementation of plyometric exercises at appropriate times to maximize performance for a particular competition requires careful program design. The duration for a given mesocycle may be as short as several weeks and as long as several months. Shorter-duration programs (6 weeks) do not provide adequate stimulation or enough time for major adaptation to occur (44), but interventions implemented over 8 to 12 weeks can improve vertical jump height and power production (37,45). Therefore, a minimum of 8 weeks should be used in designing a training program that includes plyometrics to improve athletic performance.

The combination of resistance and plyometric training provides a significant stimulus for improving performance. The use of high-intensity drills for a minimum of 8 weeks seems necessary.

ACUTE TRAINING VARIABLES

The acute training variables—volume, frequency, and intensity—must be planned on a daily basis and are key components of the exercise, which relate strongly to the potential effectiveness of the training program.

VOLUME

Foot contacts or distance covered are the most common methods for determining plyometric volume. Often volume is prescribed based on classifying the individual as a beginner, intermediate, or advanced athlete (24); however, there is no scientific support for this approach. In fact, studies examining the effects of plyometrics on performance have used between 30 and 200 jumps · d^{-1} (36,39,42,44–48). The volume of work should be based on the intent of the session (i.e., performance vs. learning), the intensity of the drills (i.e., high vs. low), the training age of the athlete (i.e., inexperienced vs. advanced), and other variables, such as the sport itself and the particular goals of the training cycle.

FREQUENCY

The number of plyometric training sessions performed weekly will be governed by many factors. In general, one or two sessions during the season and three to four sessions during the off-season may be sufficient: however, available evidence suggests that 2 to 3 $d \cdot wk^{-1}$ may be optimal for improving performance (36,39,42,44–48). The frequency of plyometric sessions will be dictated by the need for recovery from other training or practice sessions. It may also be affected by the demands of the sport. For example, volleyball and basketball require a large volume of jumps to be performed on a daily basis. Therefore, it may be unreasonable to include in-season plyometric sessions. If plyometric exercises are implemented with the intent to teach proper motor skill development and the demands are small, then more frequent (4 to 5 $d \cdot wk^{-1}$) sessions could be prescribed.

INTENSITY

The intensity of plyometric drills is often qualified with terms such as *high*, *moderate*, or *low intensity*. Unfortunately, no research has quantitatively identified intensity of plyometric exercises by measuring landing forces for a particular exercise. Even if such information existed, there are several factors that will affect the intensity of a plyometric exercise. An athlete with a greater body mass will have greater landing forces. A heavier athlete who lands with greater hip, knee, and ankle flexion, however, might have less landing forces than a lighter athlete who lands with less flexion in those joints. Therefore, landing mechanics will also affect the intensity of plyometric drills. Adding complexity to a drill will alter the intensity. For example, a single-leg hop with rotation will be more intense than a two-leg countermovement jump.

The intensity of the exercises used may impact the outcome in targeting performance enhancement. For example, one study compared depth jump training to countermovement jump training; even though both groups significantly improved jump height, the range of improvement was larger for the individuals performing depth jumps (45).

On the other hand, if injury prevention is the primary focus, it will be helpful to implement a variety of less challenging exercises. Much more research is necessary in this area prior to drawing any definitive conclusions regarding an intensity classification system for plyometrics.

LINEAR SPRINTING

Linear sprint speed is a key component for successful athletic performance in most sports. Linear sprinting can typically be divided into three distinct phases: **acceleration** (0 to 10 yd), **attainment** (10 to 35 yd), and **maintenance** (above 35 yd). These distances will certainly differ between individuals and should be used only as a temporal guide to the various phases. When breaking down the 100-m race, these terms are commonly used for the phases of the race: initial acceleration (0 to 10 yd), acceleration (10 to 40 yd), maximum velocity (40 to 70 yd), and maintenance/deceleration (70 to 100 yd). An understanding of the movements involved and specific muscular actions responsible for creating movement will allow sports performance professionals to design drills and develop training regimens that are appropriate for improving linear sprinting performance. Several key sprint mechanics drills are displayed at the end of this chapter (Table 17.1).

REACTION TIME

Reaction time (RT) is defined as the time from the stimulus (gun signal, ball, opponent movement, etc.) until the production of force by the

TABLE 17.1 ● CHANGES DURING LINEAR SPRINT RUNNING AS ATHLETES INCREASE THEIR VELOCITY (100 METER SPRINT EXAMPLE)

STRIDE LENGTH Short → medium/long and maintain 1.30 m → 1.47 m → 2.35 m (maximum velocity)	Initially, short strides increase to moderate to longer strides throughout the acceleration stage. Once maximum velocity is reached (50–70 m), stride length should be maintained (and not increased).
TOTAL STRIDE TIME Relatively constant throughout the race range from 0.21–0.26 s	Total stride time is the combination of ground contact time and flight time (time in air). Total stride time is relatively constant; however, the percentage of time spent during ground contact and flight time, is vastly different during the different stages of the race.
GROUND CONTACT TIME Long → short → shorter and maintain 0.22 s → 0.11 s → 0.09 s	The amount of time the foot is in contact with ground. Ground contact time moves from long ground contacts at the beginning of acceleration (as a mechanism to generate force into the ground) to very short ground contacts as maximum velocity is reached.
FLIGHT TIME Short → longer → longest 0.03 s → 0.08 s → 0.119 s	The time during each stride spent in the air. Flight time is short during the first few strides of acceleration, but becomes longer as velocity increases.
SHIN ANGLE TO GROUND Small→medium→medium and maintain	The angle between the anterior shaft of the tibia and the ground starts at a very small angle. As stride length increases and body position changes (more upright) as velocity increases, the shin angle to the ground increases to between 70 and 85 degrees.
VELOCITY Slow → fast → fastest → fast ($0\ m \cdot s^{-1} \rightarrow 7\ m \cdot s^{-1} \rightarrow 10\ m \cdot s^{-1} \rightarrow 12\ m \cdot s^{-1}$)	Slow at the onset of the race and increases rapidly over the first 20 m. Velocity increases more gradually for the next 30–40 m until maximum velocity is reached, between 50 and 70 m. Once maximum velocity is reached, it can only be maintained for ~10–20 m.
STRIDE FREQUENCY	Slow stride frequency at the beginning of the race increases rapidly as velocity increases.
HEEL HEIGHT FROM THE GROUND	This is directly related to the height of knee lift throughout each stride. At the beginning of acceleration, the heel height and knee height are rather low. As the athlete increases his or her velocity, the heel and knee heights increase throughout the acceleration period.

Adapted from Kovacs M. *Understanding speed—The Science Behind the 100 meter Sprint*. Birmingham, AL: Metis Publishing; 2005.

athlete. RT has been broken into two separate parts: "premotor" and "motor" time. Premotor time is the time from the stimulus until the first sign of EMG electrical activity in the muscles. Motor time has been defined as the time from the first electrical activity in the muscles until the production of visible force (limb movement) by the muscles (11). To perform the sprint start effectively, the important muscles (gluteals, quadriceps, gastroc–soleus complex) should be activated before any force can be detected against the blocks (49). RT has been recorded to respond quicker in a sprinter's front leg than his or her back leg (49).

After the gun signal, leg extensor muscles, as the producers of the greatest amount of force, must contribute maximally to the production of optimal force. For improving the starting action, it is advisable to recruit all extensor muscles in the lower limbs before any force can be detected against the blocks.

For more than 100 years the accepted figures for simple reaction times for college-age individuals has been about 190 ms (0.19 sec) for light stimuli and about 160 ms (0.16 sec) for sound stimuli (50,51). However, the fastest athletes in the world consistently have RTs <0.15 seconds (49,52). In identical events women have been shown to have longer reaction times than men (53). However, reaction time does not correlate well with sprints lasting longer than a few seconds (49). It is clear that the fastest reaction times do not influence a race over a long distance, and any distance more than 20 m is not typically influenced by an individual's reaction time in elite athletes. However, in sports that cover shorter distances (i.e., racket sports or other short distance sports), an improved reaction time can make a valuable difference.

DEVELOPMENTAL SEQUENCE

The main difference between walking and running is the absence of a double-support phase and the presence of a flight phase, respectively. The earliest attempts to run occur around 2 to 3 years of age or approximately 6 to 7 months after a child learns how to walk (27,28). By observing these movements in young children, one often notes a brief flight phase with a limited range of motion in the legs. This will result in shortened stride length. In addition, the thighs and arms swing away from the body, most likely acting to help stabilize and balance the body during the flight and support phases (27). Also to aid in balance, the stance is often wide. As children mature, they develop movement patterns that are more efficient and powerful. For example, maturity will bring about an increase in muscle mass and strength, which will provide more ground force and increase stride length. Other changes in sprint mechanics include full leg extension, keeping the actions of the extremities in the anterior–posterior plane, and maintaining bent elbows (27). The development of motor skill patterns will impact energy expenditure, fatigue rates, injury risk, and ultimately linear sprint performance.

SPRINTING GAIT

Sprinting is a complex motor skill for which specific kinetic and kinematic patterns emerge. Box 17.1 shows a basic breakdown of leg actions for sprinting. In addition, Figure 17.1 shows the average moments around the hip, knee, and ankle joints during a complete stride. The following discussion briefly outlines the two phases of a sprint: the **swing phase** and **support phase**. This overview describes factors associated with mature movement patterns and should provide a context from which to design drills and develop a training program targeted at improving or maximizing sprinting speed in advanced athletes.

Swing Phase

At toe-off, maximum extension (about 185 degrees) of the hip occurs (55), while knee extension is approximately 145 degrees (56). During early follow-through, both hip flexor and knee

BOX 17.1

Sprinting Gait (54)

1. Swing phase. The time the foot is in midair and not in contact with the ground.
2. Follow-through. From toe-off to maximal hip extension.
3. Forward swing. From the beginning of hip flexion to maximum hip flexion.
4. Foot descent. From maximum hip flexion to foot contact.
5. Support phase. The time the foot is touching the ground.
6. Foot contact. Time of initial foot contact until the acceptance of full body weight.
7. Midsupport. From full weight acceptance until plantar flexion of ankle joint begins.
8. Toe-off. From the onset of plantar flexion to toe-off.

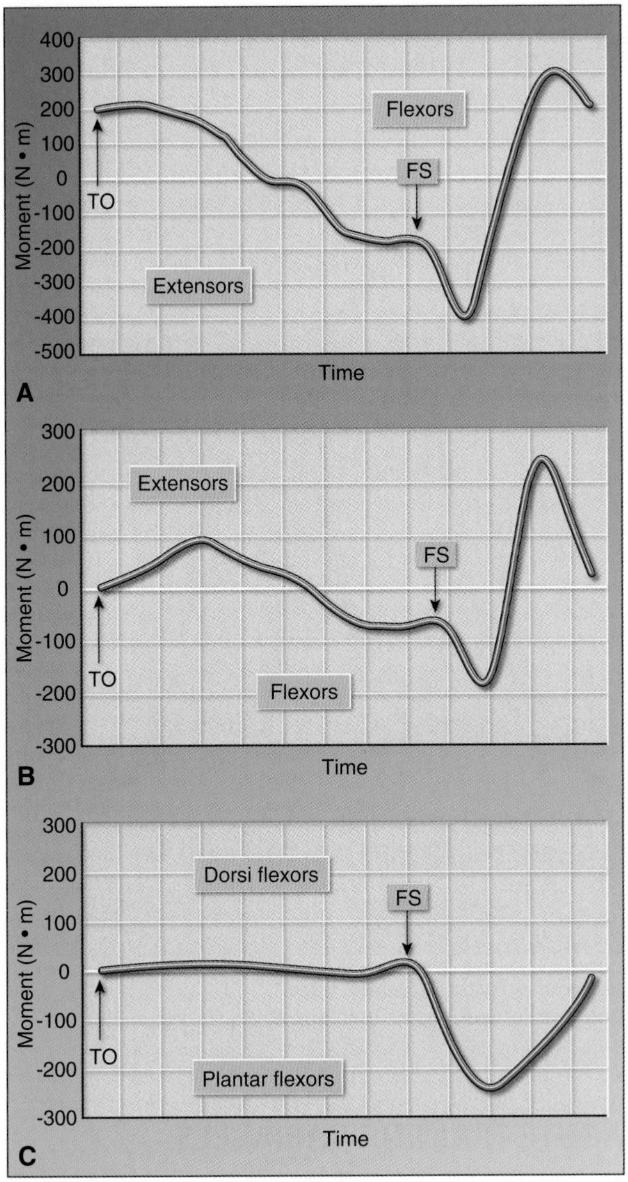

FIGURE 17.1 Muscle dominance during sprinting around the hip **(A)**, knee **(B)**, and ankle **(C)**. TO, toe-off; FS, foot strike. (Modified with permission from Mann RV. A kinetic analysis of sprinting. *Med Sci Sports Exerc*. 1981;13:325–328.)

extensor muscle activity greatly increases, as they are eccentrically loaded. This acts to decelerate leg rotation (57) and helps with quick leg recovery (Fig. 17.2). The transition from follow-through to forward swing is the first SSC observed in the sprint cycle. This is caused by concentric hip flexor action, which rotates the upper leg anteriorly (54). Maximum hip flexion occurs two-thirds of the way through the swing phase and corresponds with contralateral toe-off. About this time, there is a switch from knee flexion to knee extension. Figure 17.2 shows relatively little muscle activation of the quadriceps during this time in the swing cycle (9), indicating that knee extension is mainly brought about by momentum from hip flexion, which provides a whip-like action of the lower leg during the swing phase. The hamstrings now act eccentrically, halting knee extension while simultaneously beginning hip extension during foot descent (58). This is the second SSC observed during the swing phase of the sprinting cycle.

The adductors are active during early follow-through (just after toe-off) and early foot descent, stabilizing the knee by counterbalancing the external rotation and abduction action of the gluteus group (9) (see Fig. 17.2). Tibialis activity begins at toe-off and remains throughout the entire swing phase, whereas gastrocnemius activity is minimal during most of this phase and does not increase until immediately prior to foot contact (59). This preactivity is thought to help prepare the joint to assist in decreasing the vertical forces at foot contact as well as creating a more efficient SSC of the gastrocnemius.

Support Phase

Once the foot has made contact with the ground, hip extensor muscles (e.g., hamstrings and gluteus) act concentrically until midsupport (8). The gluteus maximus is continuously active (60), extending the hip but also stabilizing it (see Fig. 17.2). The hamstrings are responsible for providing the necessary force to propel the body forward and are the key to linear sprint speed (9). Higher-level sprinters have shown the ability to decrease horizontal braking by creating larger forces and generating more power in the hip extensors and knee flexors during early support (57). This extremely brief subphase should be recognized as the most important time of the sprinting cycle, realizing that hip extension is the main action responsible for linear sprinting speed. Therefore, to maximize speed, power must be created as early in the support phase as possible.

A transition of muscle action occurs between midsupport and toe-off when the hip flexors begin to act eccentrically and decelerate leg rotation (57). It appears the main function of the knee joint during the support phase is to transfer power in a proximal-to-distal direction (i.e., hip to ankle). There is a large amount of knee extensor muscle activity up through midsupport to stabilize the knee, transfer forces from the hip to the ankle, and keep the height of the center of mass constant. Lending support to this notion, one study reported negligible power from the knee during midsupport (61). Therefore, during the attainment and maintenance phases of a

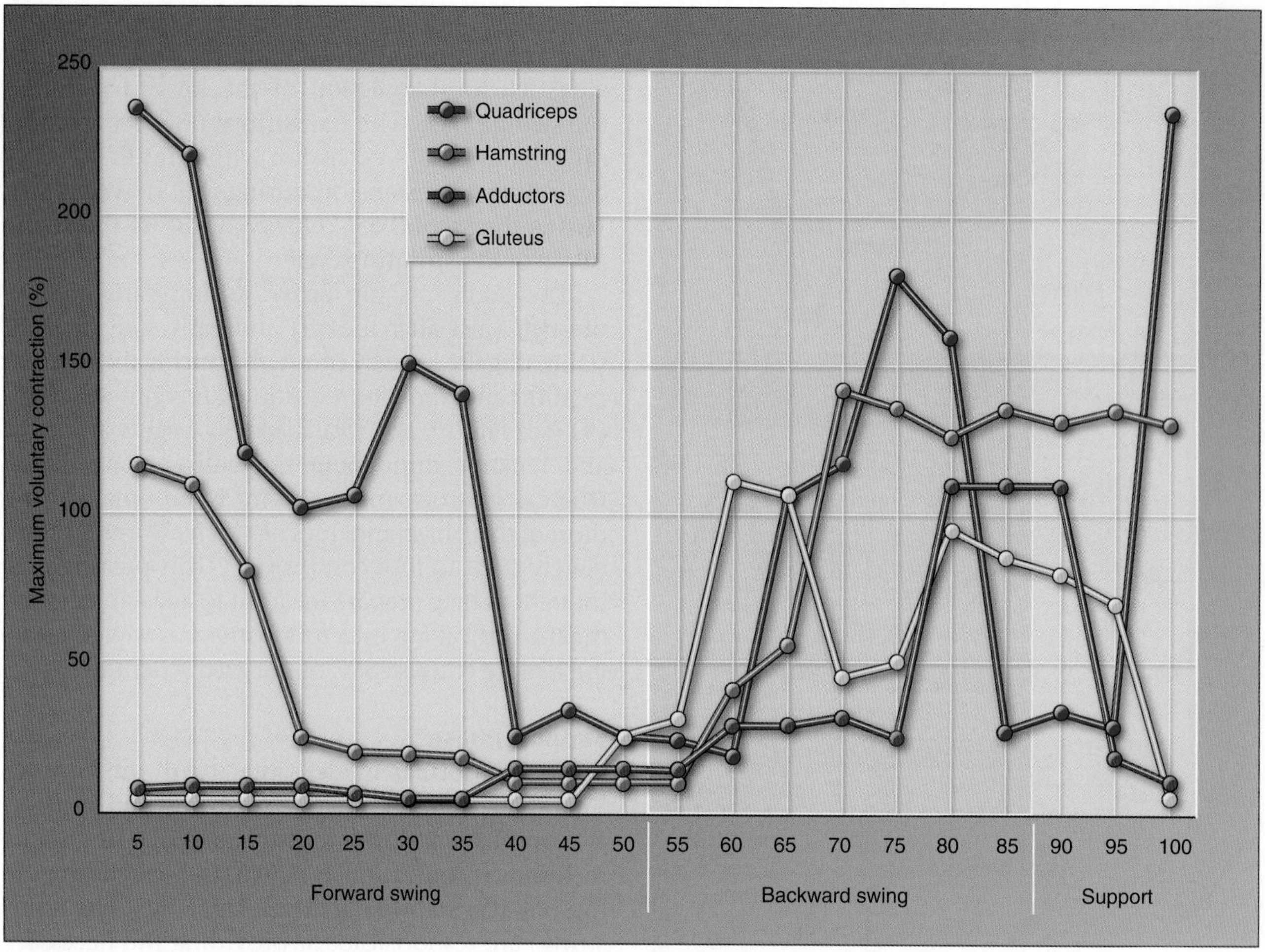

FIGURE 17.2 Relative muscle activation patterns during a sprint stride. (Modified with permission from Wiemann K, Tidow GN. Relative activity of hip and knee extensors in sprinting: implications for training. *New Stud Athlet*. 1995;10(1):29–49.)

sprint, the knee extensors should not be considered a muscle group that produces forward propulsion. In fact, if the knee extensors are activated maximally during support, it would produce a disproportionate upward force rather than forward propulsion. This would lead to a higher and subsequently longer flight phase (9), in turn reducing linear sprinting performance. The primary role of the muscles surrounding the ankle joint is to assist in maintaining the height of the center of mass at foot contact and to provide some thrust, albeit minimal, of the body in the anterior–posterior plane (58,59).

Sprinting requires horizontal power production from the hip extensors and knee flexors to propel the body forward during the early portion of the support phase. Maintaining a stable center of gravity occurs through eccentric actions of the gluteus, quadriceps, and gastrocnemius muscle groups.

ACUTE TRAINING VARIABLES

The acute training variables are the specific variables that are manipulated to produce variation in volume, frequency, and intensity of training. They must be planned on a daily basis and are key components of the exercise, which relate strongly to the potential effectiveness of the training program.

Volume

The volume of linear sprint work will be characterized by the total distance covered during a given training session. It might be beneficial to consider sprint drills (e.g., A-skips, B-skips) and sprint capacity exercises separately. Sprint drills may be included daily during the warm-up routine with a focus on perfecting mechanical technique. On the other hand, the volume of work dedicated to improving sprint capacity will be governed by the characteristics of a given sport and possibly by requirements of a specific position. This includes the metabolic and linear sprint characteristics (i.e., average frequency and distance). There is a great deal of variability in program design, so definitive guidelines on linear sprint volume are limited.

Frequency

Performing high-intensity sprint training is physically demanding; therefore, the number of weekly sessions will depend on recovery from other training and practice sessions. It may be sufficient to schedule 2 to 3 sessions · wk^{-1}, depending on additional demands placed on the athlete.

Intensity

Training to improve sprint capacity will typically involve maximal efforts; however, submaximal bouts of work can be used with inexperienced athletes to develop technique. With that in mind, younger athletes should focus on drills that will enhance mechanics, while more advanced athletes can be prescribed maximal-effort bouts of work, targeting specific linear sprint distances.

Two additional methods often used in sprint training are assisted and resisted sprints. Both of these methods are considered to be of high intensity and should not be prescribed to any athlete who has not mastered linear sprint mechanics. Extreme caution is warranted even for those athletes who have mature movement patterns, since resisted and assisted sprints can have negative consequences that may result in negative movement mechanics and increased injury potential.

Assisted running (e.g., high-speed treadmill exercises, towing, or downhill running) will permit an athlete to run faster than his or her natural pace and is typically prescribed to help increase stride frequency (i.e., improve turnover). In spite of the anecdotal evidence, research clearly shows that running at supramaximal speeds will increase stride length and decrease stride frequency compared with maximal running (62–64). These alterations will consequently cause an increase in the horizontal distance from the foot to the center of mass at ground contact, resulting in greater braking forces during the support phase and increasing the likelihood of injury (63). In addition, high-speed treadmills set below 80% or above 90% of maximal running velocity will cause a breakdown in sprint mechanics (56). Therefore, this type of training should be limited to elite athletes and completely avoided by younger inexperienced athletes.

Resisted running includes dragging a sled or running uphill and is often prescribed to increase force production and consequently stride length during unresisted sprinting. Several mechanical alterations occur with resisted sprints. For example, greater hip, knee, and ankle flexion occurs, which indicates less stiffness in the entire kinetic chain and less potential to maximize sprint velocity. In addition, overall posture is altered when running up slight grades (3 degrees) or pulling minimal weight (12% of body mass) (64,65).

During resisted sprints, a larger amount of the leg cycle is spent in the support phase and there is a decrease in stride length (64–67). These changes in sprint mechanics may be detrimental to linear speed; therefore, extreme caution is warranted in prescribing resisted sprint drills. One error many coaches make is to increase the incline before an athlete is ready (inappropriate training and strength levels) and also increase the angle of incline by an extreme level, which reduces effectiveness and increases chance of injury and/or inappropriate mechanics. Movement mechanics change considerably as the incline is increased. It is advisable to limit inclines to below 6 degrees even with highly developed adult athletes.

Clearly additional research is necessary to determine whether acute changes in sprint mechanics can be permanent if resisted and assisted training methods are chronically integrated into an athlete's regimen. Based on the available information, it would seem prudent to avoid any type of resisted or assisted method with younger and inexperienced athletes.

AGILITY

Changes in direction occur often during many athletic activities and include deceleration followed immediately by reacceleration of the entire body or individual body segment(s). This ability, termed **agility**, has been described as an efficient, coordinated movement in multiple planes performed at multiple velocities (68,69). A fighter dodging a punch or kick, a ballroom dancer performing the mambo or salsa, a wrestler finishing a takedown, tennis player hitting a volley followed by an overhead are all examples of agility. Individuals involved in the development and improvement of sport performance, however, often regard agility as a locomotor skill where an athlete changes direction by decelerating the body and reaccelerating in a new direction (68,69). Although agility has been shown to be an independent athletic attribute (70), additional qualities are considered important, including dynamic balance, spatial awareness, rhythm, and visual processing (71). A high degree of complexity is present within this fundamental athletic motor skill.

DEVELOPMENTAL SEQUENCE

Learning to become agile requires the development of appropriate movement patterns and, more importantly, the ability to integrate locomotor skills efficiently (e.g., running, jumping) with proprioceptive awareness. As children learn to walk fast and run (at 1.5 to 3 years of age), they make attempts to be elusive and change direction when being chased. Their movement efficiency is often poor, however, and associated with awkward arm motion, overall unbalanced posture, and a general lack of timing and coordination. These are all characteristics described earlier in the section on the developmental sequence of sprinting. Because a variety of aspects are included in the ability to change direction, it is difficult to precisely identify a specific developmental sequence, as found in other locomotor skills.

Nevertheless, at particular windows of time, or critical periods, either general or specific drills can be implemented to develop agility appropriately. For instance, children aged 5 to 8 years should perform a large variety of general movement patterns in an effort to develop a foundation of motor skills. This could include arm and leg movements in a stationary position, rhythmic jumps in place, or locomotor drills that incorporate spatial orientation. Learning the temporal characteristics of general movements is extremely beneficial, especially prior to initiating more specific drills or activities. Closed agility drills, where the initiation, execution, and termination of a drill are clearly established, should dominate during this period. Children involved with athletics should be able to perform general drills with minimal flaws prior to advancing to more demanding exercises.

Young athletes will be able to move more quickly as they mature and finish puberty. For reasons of safety and injury prevention, however, they should initially perform drills at submaximal speeds. In addition, drills should not yet include sharp changes in direction but rather involve rounded patterns. Weaving within a set of linear cones, running a figure-eight pattern, or learning how to integrate several locomotor skills into one exercise are all acceptable drills during this stage of development. Drills that include sharp changes in direction performed at high running speeds are unlikely to benefit agility development, especially when mastery has not yet been achieved (72,73). Closed drills should still predominate in this window of time; however, some open drills can be included sparingly to add a reactive component with visual or audio stimuli.

Alterations in body size, structure, and body mass will influence a young athlete's coordination and proprioception. During this stage, take the time to perfect locomotor skills that are already developed, allowing the athlete to become more comfortable with his or her "new" body (68). Greater difficulty and more challenging drills can certainly be added to the training regimen, but throughout this stage, sport specificity should be avoided, as it may hinder overall athletic development.

More complexity and specificity are the focus of agility training during later teenage years (post-puberty) and can now be regularly implemented within the training plan (68). The same drill can be made more difficult simply by using different field conditions, including a partner, or implementing an area or time restriction. These are all acceptable methods to increasingly challenge an athlete's ability to change direction effectively (68). Athletes should perform nearly all of the drills at high speeds, as slower movements have been shown to alter muscle activation patterns (74). However, if muscle mechanics are compromised due to muscle imbalances or technique issues, then these areas should be improved in ancillary movements and exercises, not as part of an agility training session. An example would be an athlete who struggles to change direction effectively and has weak gluteus medius strength should focus on developing gluteus medius strength in the gym, while still working on agility movements close to (or at) game speed.

IMPACTING FACTORS

The ability to coordinate a smooth and rapid transition between stopping and starting is a distinct advantage for athletes performing changes in direction. Inefficient transitions caused by poor deceleration mechanics or an elongated support phase might allow a defender to maintain close proximity, not allowing an offensive player to become open to receive a pass (e.g., football, soccer, lacrosse). Enhanced agility must be developed in concert with many other proprioceptive and kinesthetic skills, such as balance, orientation, reactiveness, rhythm, visual processing, timing, and anticipation (71). With that in mind, several variables will impact how drills and exercises are performed, namely movement velocity, the angle of direction change, and whether a movement is planned (closed skill) or unplanned (open skill).

Effects of Movement Velocity

Agility drills can be performed at slow or fast running speeds. Slower running speeds are associated with greater ground contact time during the deceleration phase compared to faster running speeds (300 vs. 170 milliseconds, respectively) (73–75). As in linear sprinting, preactivation of knee flexors and extensors occurs immediately prior to ground contact, which serves to prepare the joints for eccentric loading during deceleration. An increase in muscle preactivation at higher running speeds has led some to suggest that a neural feed-forward mechanism exists to protect the hip and knee joints from the increased eccentric and rotational loads. A **neural feed-forward mechanism** indicates that the protective musculature would preactivate as a protective mechanism to decrease the chance of injury through neural control. It may also stimulate an increase in SSC ability and enhance the transition from eccentric to concentric muscle actions.

During the support phase, the adductors and gluteus medius are constantly active and are primarily responsible for stabilizing the hip. A highly integrated agonist–antagonist relationship between the quadriceps and hamstrings provides the ability to change direction (74). More specifically, the knee extensors work to decelerate the body upon ground contact, while hip extensor activity predominates during the late support phase. Hip extension provides the necessary horizontal propulsion of the body in the new direction. Recall from the section on linear sprinting that hip extension is important during the early portion of the support phase. This apparent difference from linear sprinting should be considered in developing drills or exercises focused on improving agility performance.

Effects of Angles

Changes in direction can be considered shallow (<45 degrees) or sharp (more than 45 degrees). When athletes are observed in the laboratory and asked to perform sharp changes in direction, there is a large reduction in approaching velocity. Often there is an inability to appropriately execute the drill even with the reduction in approaching velocity (72,73). The fact that these movements are preplanned further highlights the difficulty of performing such maneuvers. It also indicates the need for incorporating drills into training regimens for elite athletes with mature movement skills. Drills that focus on the ability to make drastic changes in movement while maintaining speed will provide the necessary stimulus for adaptation and transfer to competition. On the other hand, inexperienced athletes should focus on more rounded patterns performed at slightly slower speeds and avoid demanding drills.

Changes in direction can be performed with an open or a crossover step. During the early stages of development, it might be beneficial to teach young athletes both movement skills. These steps should be performed at slow speeds, with specific attention given to proper mechanics. An analysis of open-step changes in direction shows internal rotation, whereas crossover steps produce external rotation on the knee. These loads can be up to five times greater than in linear running (72,76). In addition, crossover steps produce varus loads, while open steps show a mixture of varus and valgus loading at the knee (72,76). Changes in direction using an open step increase the activity of the vastus medialis and gluteus medius (73,77). This acts to (a) create stability around the hip joint during stance and (b) to counter the valgus loads associated with this movement. Closely observe your athletes as they perform agility drills to ensure proper mechanics, and include resistance training exercises that target the quadriceps and gluteus muscles, which will help stabilize the knee.

Effects of Anticipation

Whether a skill is preplanned (closed) or unplanned (open) will also impact movement patterns and joint loads. For example, an offensive soccer player may attempt several preplanned cutting maneuvers to elude a defensive player. On the other hand, the defensive player must continually adjust to the visual stimulus and anticipate the movements of the offensive player, making changes of direction reactive, or unplanned. The difference between preplanned and unplanned changes in direction has effects on external varus/valgus and internal/external rotational loading (72,77), muscle activation patterns (77), and body preparation (73).

Compared to an unplanned change in direction, a preplanned open step change in direction shows a slight crossover with the step prior to the pivot foot being planted, an earlier rotation of the pivot foot in the new direction, and a greater body lean (73). Flexion/extension loads are similar in planned and unplanned cutting actions, but there is greater knee flexion when movements are unplanned (76). In addition, a reduction in the whole movement angle occurs during an unplanned change of direction (72). These are all protective mechanisms that provide additional time for appropriate muscle activation, proper joint stabilization, and decreased internal joint forces.

Performing an unplanned cutting maneuver increases the valgus and internal rotation loads by 70% and 90%, respectively. Interestingly, muscle activation only increases by 10% to 20% (72,77). Furthermore, general muscle activation patterns emerge during unplanned changes in direction, indicating nonspecific coordination between anterior/posterior and medial/lateral synergistic muscle pairs (72). On the other hand, preplanned actions produce specific activation patterns of the vastus medialis and biceps femoris to counter the external valgus and internal rotation loads, respectively (72). The inability of the neuromuscular system to initiate the appropriate adjustments during unplanned changes in direction reduces the efficiency and velocity of the movement. Therefore, to enhance the ability to decelerate, include exercises that increase the eccentric ability of muscles (e.g., resistance training) as well as drills that focus on improving reactive ability (e.g., plyometrics).

> *Factors such as velocity of movement, angle of change, or anticipation will impact muscular activation patterns, kinematics, and joint forces. Exercises that develop muscular stability, eccentric muscle strength, and reactive ability should be included for maximal athletic development.*

ACUTE TRAINING VARIABLES

Limited information exists on how to improve agility; however, training for linear speed will not improve the ability to change direction and vice versa (78,79). In fact, linear sprint speed, power, and agility are independent performance characteristics, where ability in one variable is not associated with the others (80). This means that agility training should be an integral component of an athlete's training regimen.

Volume

Specific training sessions dedicated to the development or improvement of agility can utilize guidelines similar to those of linear sprint training, where volume is the total distance covered. Inexperienced athletes may require more time to learn proper mechanics and perform general movement patterns. On the other hand, advanced athletes can perform a greater volume of work. Understanding the relative contribution of changing direction to the sport or position will help to guide the sports performance professional in determining the appropriate volume appropriate for high-level athletes.

There are numerous agility drills; the conditioning specialist is limited only by the imagination when designing these drills. Agility drills should focus on changing direction quickly and using multiple footwork patterns. These drills should also be sport specific in terms of movement patterns, footwork patterns, distances, work intervals, rest intervals, and intensities. Although it would be impossible to make a comprehensive list of agility drills, sample drills are described in Figures 17.19–17.22. These drills can be easily changed from one workout to the next for variety.

Frequency

Inexperienced athletes can include agility daily as a part of a warm-up routine. Regular attention to proper mechanics is vital for the development of appropriate movement skills. Program design for advanced athletes will depend on the time of the year, sport-specific requirements, and other training demands. The intent or focus of exercises can be adjusted to incorporate them more or less frequently.

Intensity

The intensity of agility drills will depend on factors such as running velocity, preplanned (closed) versus unplanned (open) drills, and sharpness of the angles. Young, inexperienced athletes need to perfect general, preplanned motor patterns before performing sport-specific drills. The drills should include rounded patterns performed at slow to moderate speeds. Body-weight resistance exercises and less demanding plyometric drills will also benefit the ability to change direction. As an athlete becomes more advanced, specific movement patterns can be included. The drills can be increasingly reactive and may include a wide variety of angles.

INTEGRATION OF SPEED AND AGILITY DRILLS

Depending on the sport and the time of the training cycle, the focus may be on either speed or agility or possibly both. If the focus is on maximizing forward running speed, 3 to 4 training sessions · wk^{-1} may be devoted to speed. Agility training may be performed occasionally for variety. The opposite will be true if the focus is on agility.

Most sports—soccer, for example—require both speed and agility. If speed and agility are both training goals, 1 to 2 sessions · wk^{-1} can be devoted to speed and 1 to 2 sessions to agility. Well-conditioned athletes may be able to benefit from combined sessions, using both speed and agility exercises. These exercises should be performed early in a training session so that the athlete is fresh. Performing speed and agility exercises while the athlete is fatigued on a regular basis may not be as effective in improving performance.

Speed and Agility Exercises

Plyometric Exercises

Countermovement Jump

Starting Position

The athlete stands with feet shoulder width apart, the body in an upright posture and looking straight ahead (Fig. 17.3A).

Movement Sequence

Begin with a preparatory countermovement by flexing the hips and knees. Maintain an upright body posture (Fig. 17.3B). Once at the bottom position, immediately jump vertically (Fig. 17.3C). Land in same spot from where the jump was

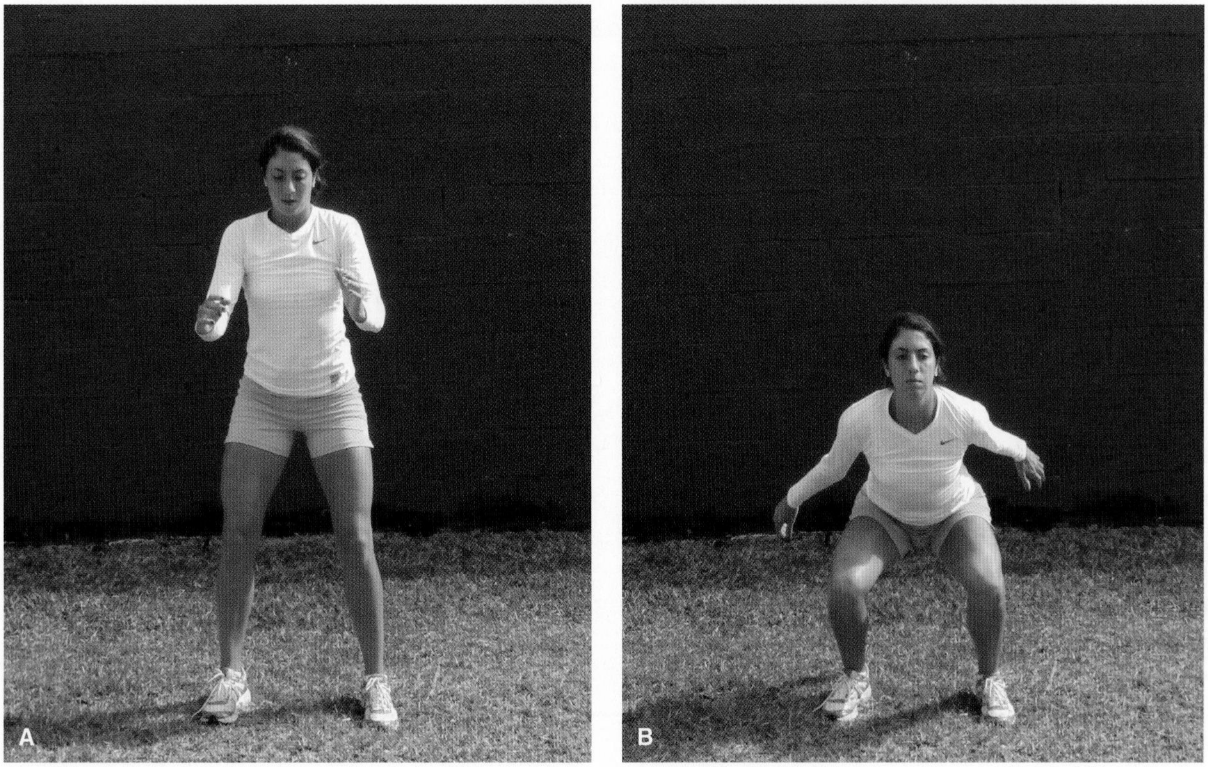

FIGURE 17.3 Countermovement jump. **A.** Starting position. **B.** Countermovement.

(continued)

Plyometric Exercises *(continued)*

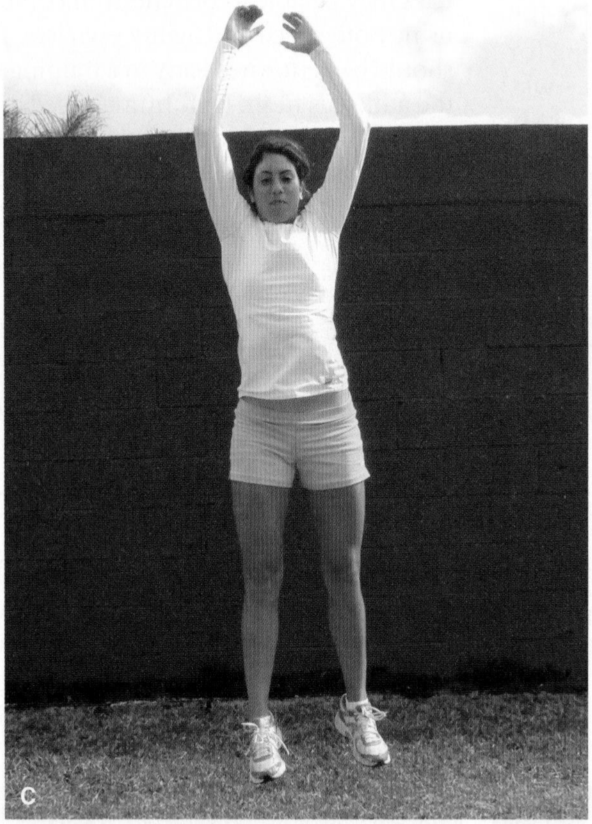

FIGURE 17.3 *(continued)* **C.** Jump.

initiated and flex the hips and knees to reduce landing forces.

Variations

Manipulate the depth of the preparatory countermovement. Keep the hands placed on the hips to eliminate arm swing. Add degrees of rotation so that the athlete will land facing a different direction.

Scissor Jump

Starting Position

The athlete stands with the feet a shoulder width apart, the body in an upright posture, looking straight ahead. Take a half step forward with the right foot and a half step backward with the left.

Movement Sequence

Begin with a preparatory countermovement by flexing the hips and knees. Maintain an upright body posture (Fig. 17.4A). Once at the bottom position, immediately jump vertically (Fig. 17.4B). While in the air, switch the positions of the legs so that the landing will occur with the left leg forward and the right leg behind. Be sure that the knees remain pointed forward and avoid caving inward (Fig. 17.4C).

Variations

Keep the hands placed on the hips to eliminate arm swing. Attempt to perform a double switch of the legs while in the air, so that landing occurs in the same position as the takeoff.

Plyometric Exercises *(continued)*

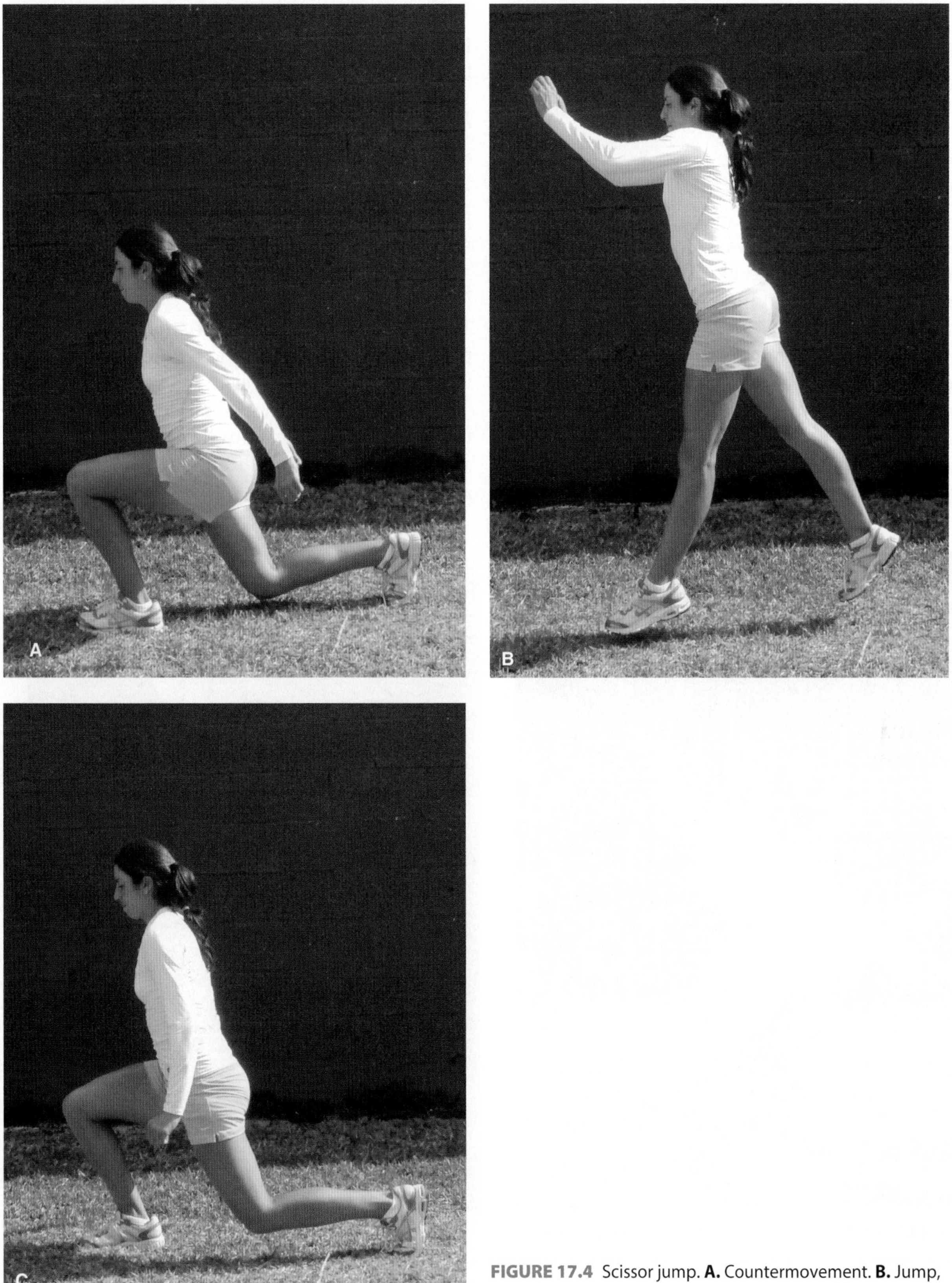

FIGURE 17.4 Scissor jump. **A.** Countermovement. **B.** Jump, with right leg forward. **C.** Landing, with left leg forward.

(continued)

Plyometric Exercises *(continued)*

Broad Jump

Starting Position

The athlete stands with the feet a shoulder width apart, the body in an upright posture, looking straight ahead.

Movement Sequence

Begin with a preparatory countermovement by flexing the hips and knees. During the downward movement, the body will lean slightly forward and the arms should be coordinated with a posterior swing (Fig. 17.5A). At the bottom of the countermovement, jump horizontally in the anterior direction (Fig. 17.5B). Land with an upright body posture and head looking forward. Flex the hips and knees to reduce landing forces and be sure the knees are pointing forward and not caving inward (Fig. 17.5C).

Variations

Eliminate arm swing. Take off from two feet and land on one foot.

Linear Bounds

Starting Position

Although starting from a stationary position is possible, it may be more comfortable by beginning with several lead-in steps.

Movement Sequence

This drill can be compared to an exaggerated run. Forcefully drive off the rear leg (Fig. 17.6A) with the intent to gain as much vertical height and horizontal distance possible (Fig. 17.6B). On landing with the contralateral leg, immediately generate maximal force to propel the body again.

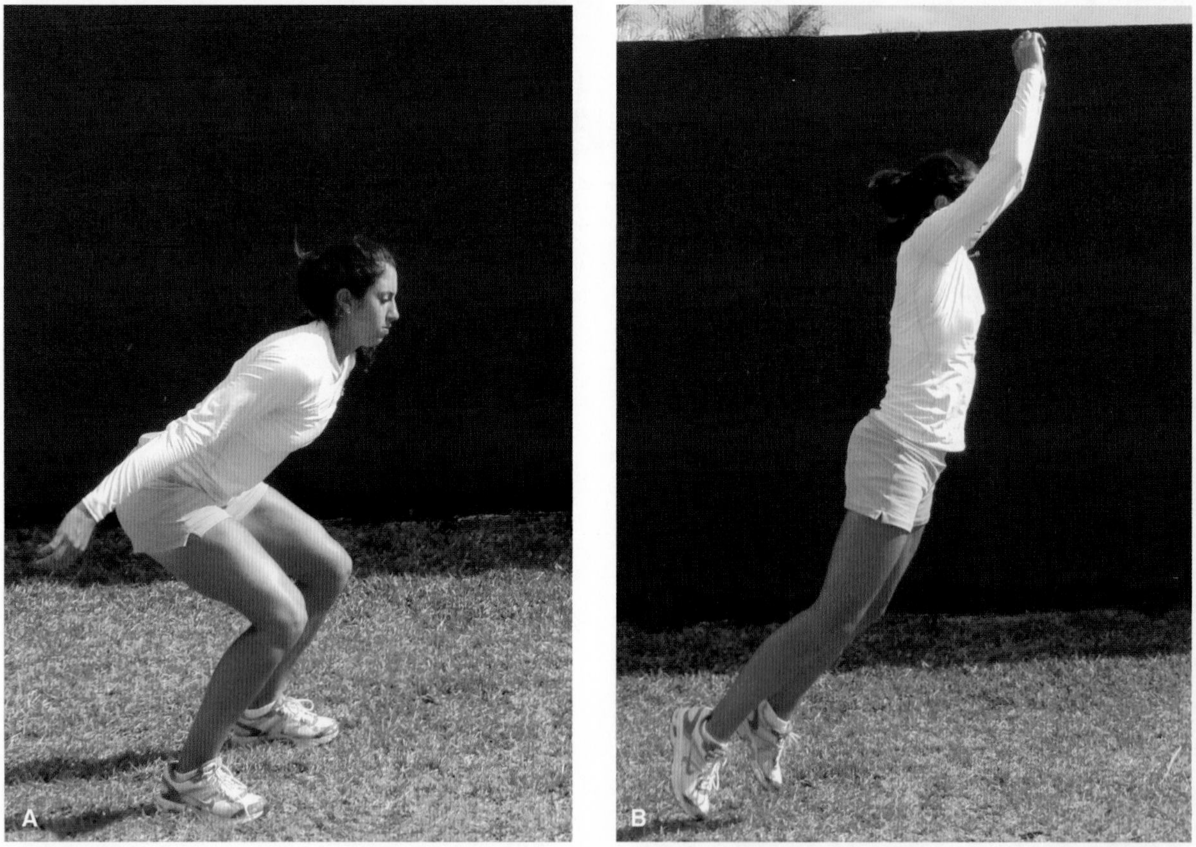

FIGURE 17.5 Broad jump. **A.** Countermovement. **B.** Jump.

Plyometric Exercises *(continued)*

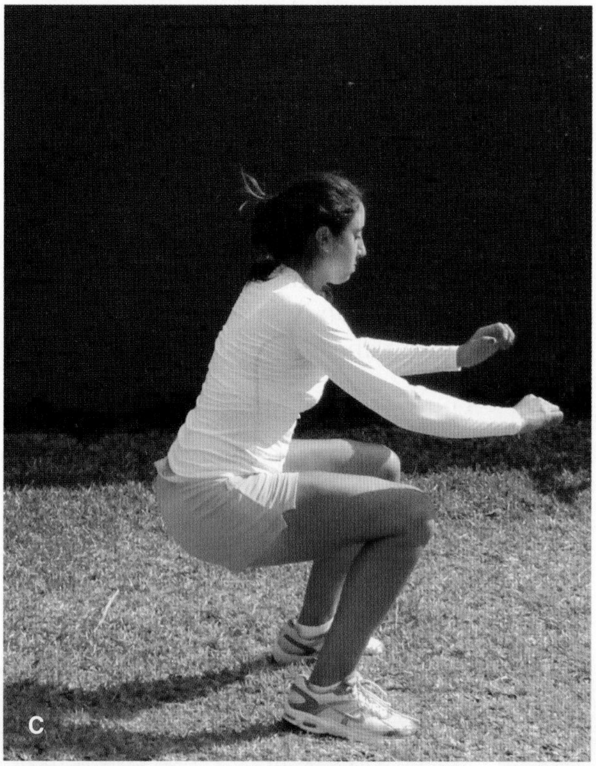

FIGURE 17.5 *(continued)* **C.** Landing.

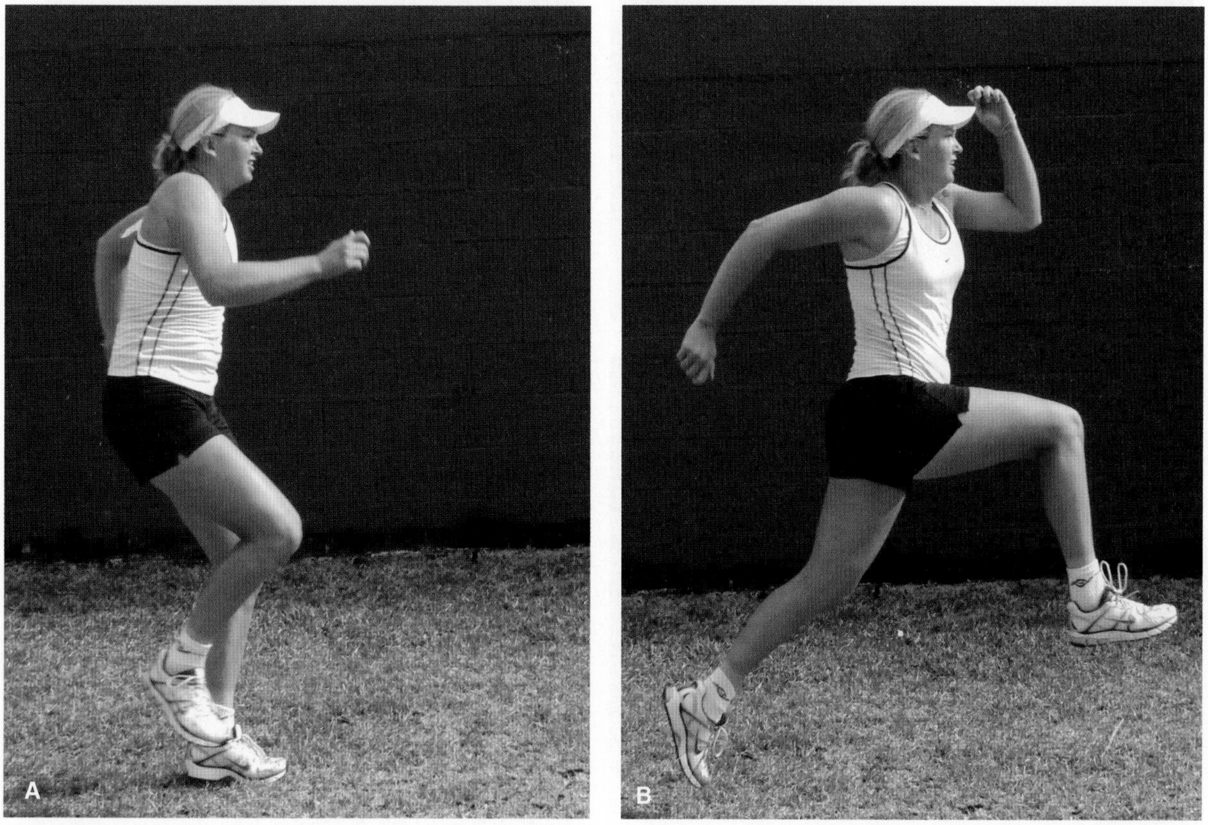

FIGURE 17.6 Linear bound. **A.** Starting position. **B.** Bound.

(continued)

Plyometric Exercises *(continued)*

Lateral Cone Jump

Starting Position

The athlete stands with the feet a shoulder width apart, the body in an upright posture, looking straight ahead, with a cone placed directly to the side.

Movement Sequence

Begin with a preparatory countermovement by flexing the hips and knees (Fig. 17.7A). Maintain an upright body posture. Once at the bottom position, immediately jump, propelling the body vertically as well as laterally (Fig. 17.7B). Land on the opposite side of the cone and flex the hips and knees to reduce landing forces (Fig. 17.7C).

Variations

Keep the hands placed on the hips to eliminate arm swing. Add degrees of rotation so as to land facing in a different direction.

Lateral Bounds

Starting Position

The athlete stands with the feet a shoulder width apart, the body in an upright posture, looking straight ahead.

Movement Sequence

Begin with a preparatory countermovement by flexing the hips and knees. Maintain an upright body posture. During the downward phase, begin to shift the body weight to the left leg (Fig. 17.8A).

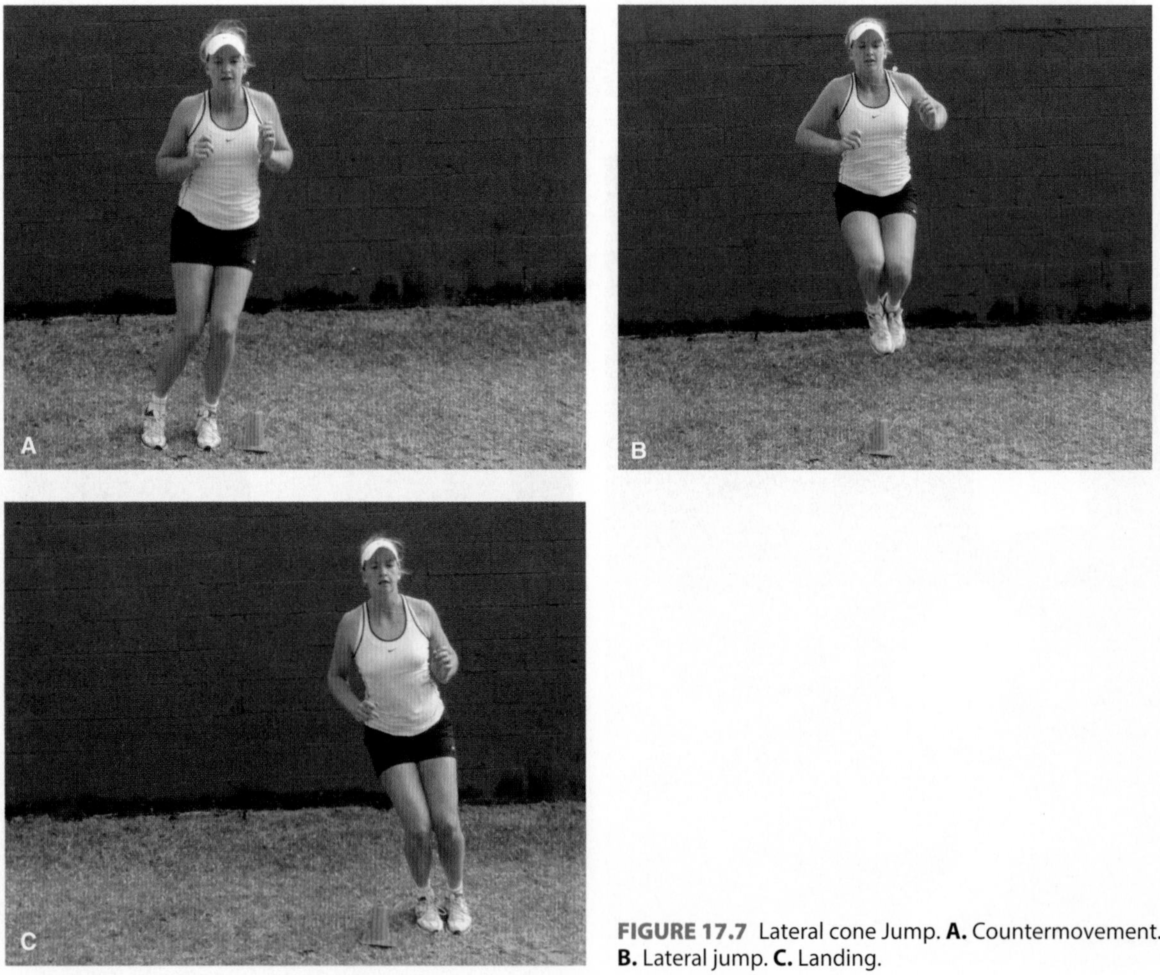

FIGURE 17.7 Lateral cone Jump. **A.** Countermovement. **B.** Lateral jump. **C.** Landing.

Plyometric Exercises *(continued)*

Once at the bottom position, propel the body laterally with the left leg (Fig. 17.8B) and land on the right (Fig. 17.8C). Be sure to flex the hips and knees on landing while also keeping the body inside the vertical plane of the knee (Fig. 17.8D).

Variation

Add anterior movement to this drill where the athlete will follow a zigzag or diagonal pattern with each bound.

Chest Throw

Starting Position

The athlete stands with the feet a shoulder width apart, holding a medicine ball in the center of the chest.

Movement Sequence

Begin with a preparatory countermovement by flexing the hips and knees. Maintain an upright

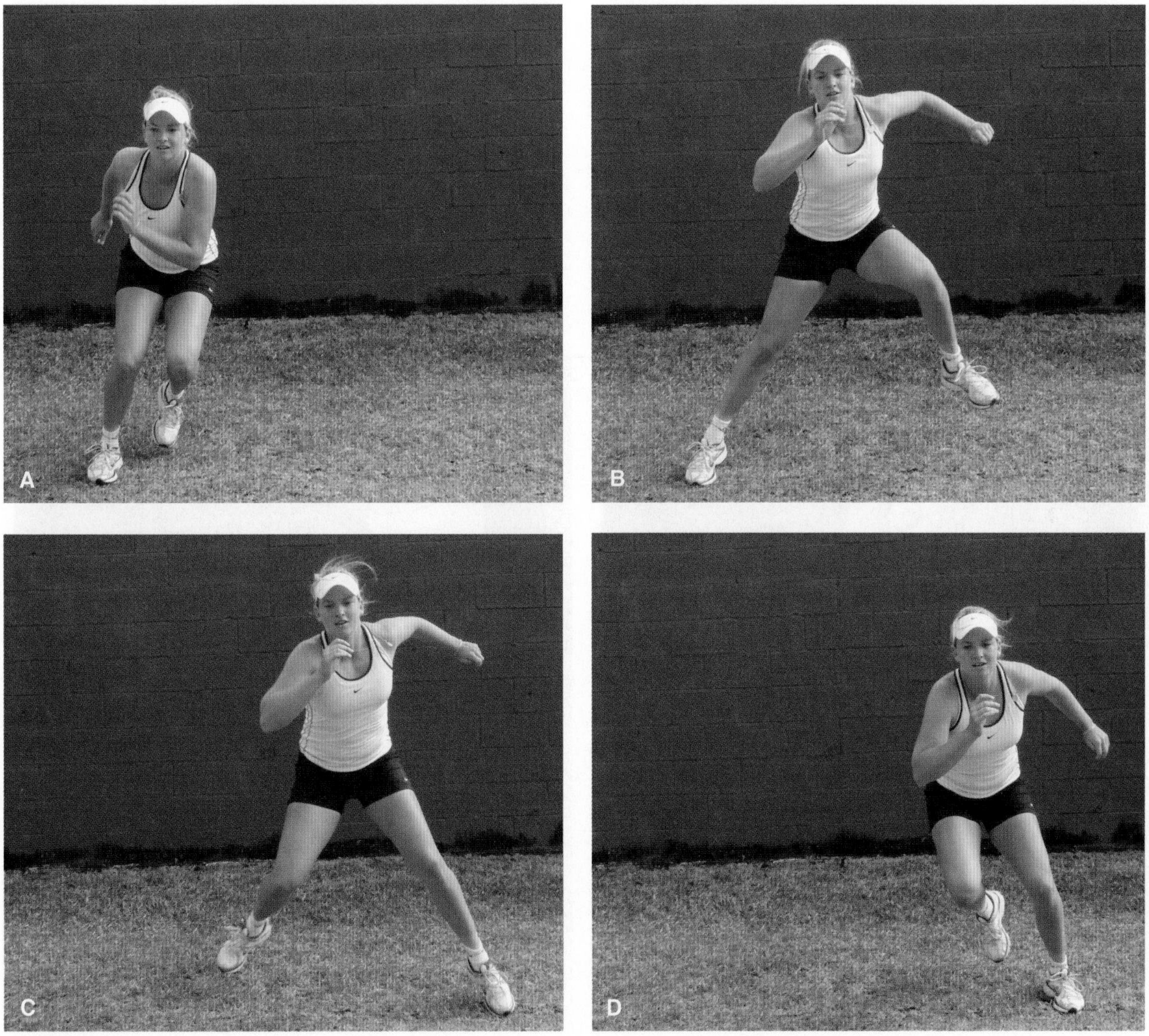

FIGURE 17.8 Lateral bound. **A.** Countermovement. **B.** Lateral movement. **C.** Downward movement. **D.** Landing.

(continued)

Plyometric Exercises *(continued)*

body posture (Fig. 17.9A). During the upward phase, begin to simultaneously extend the arms with the legs. As the legs reach peak extension, the medicine ball is released with the intent of obtaining maximal horizontal distance (Fig. 17.9B).

Variation

Perform this exercise from your knees or with a partner.

Scoop Toss

Starting Position

The athlete stands with the feet a shoulder width apart, holding a medicine ball by the hips with the arms fully extended.

Movement Sequence

Begin with a preparatory countermovement by flexing the hips and knees. Maintain an upright body posture and extended arm position (Fig. 17.10A). During the upward phase, while the legs are extending, begin to flex at the shoulders, keeping the elbows extended (Fig. 17.10B). As full leg extension is reached (Fig. 17.10C), release the medicine ball with the intent of obtaining maximal vertical height (Fig. 17.10D).

Variation

Perform this drill will a partner.

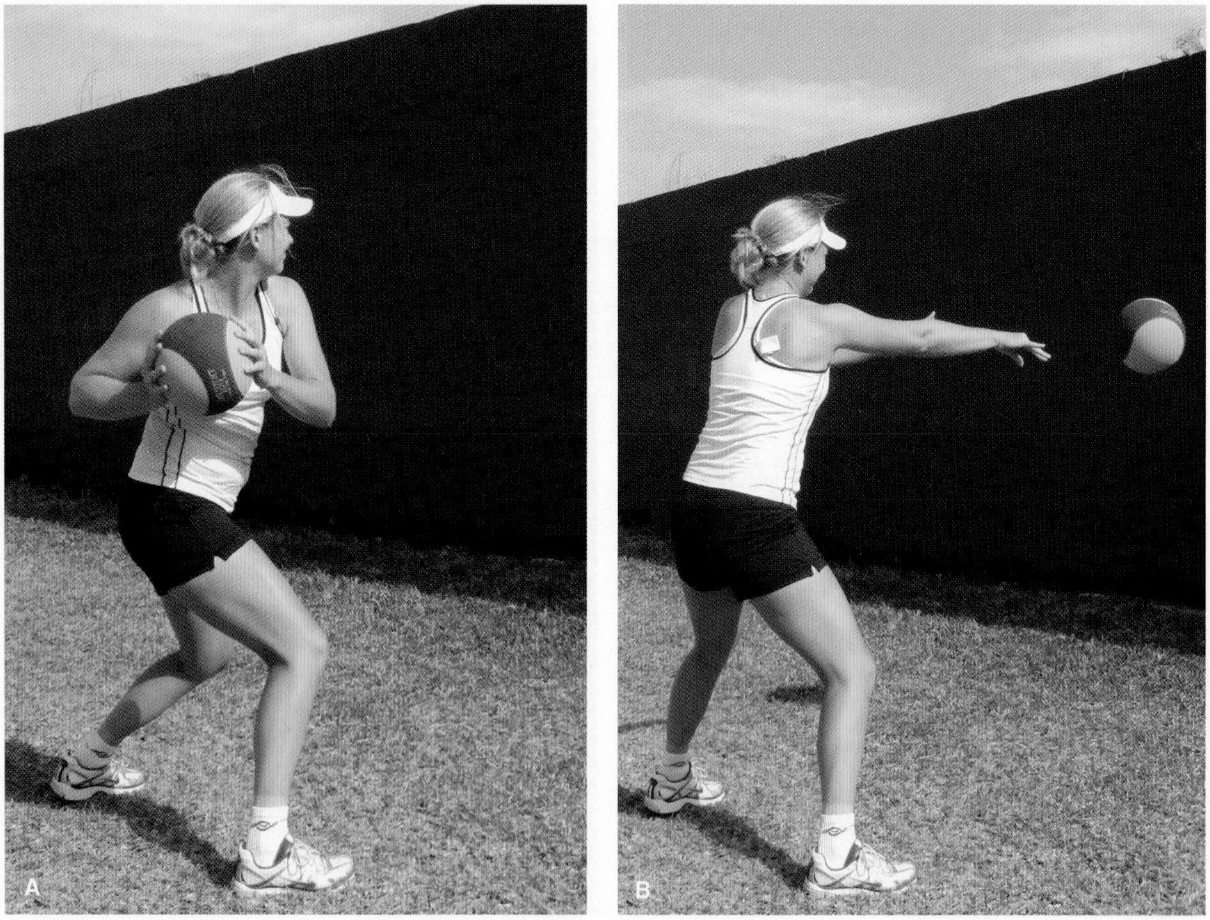

FIGURE 17.9 Chest throw. **A.** Countermovement. **B.** Release.

Plyometric Exercises *(continued)*

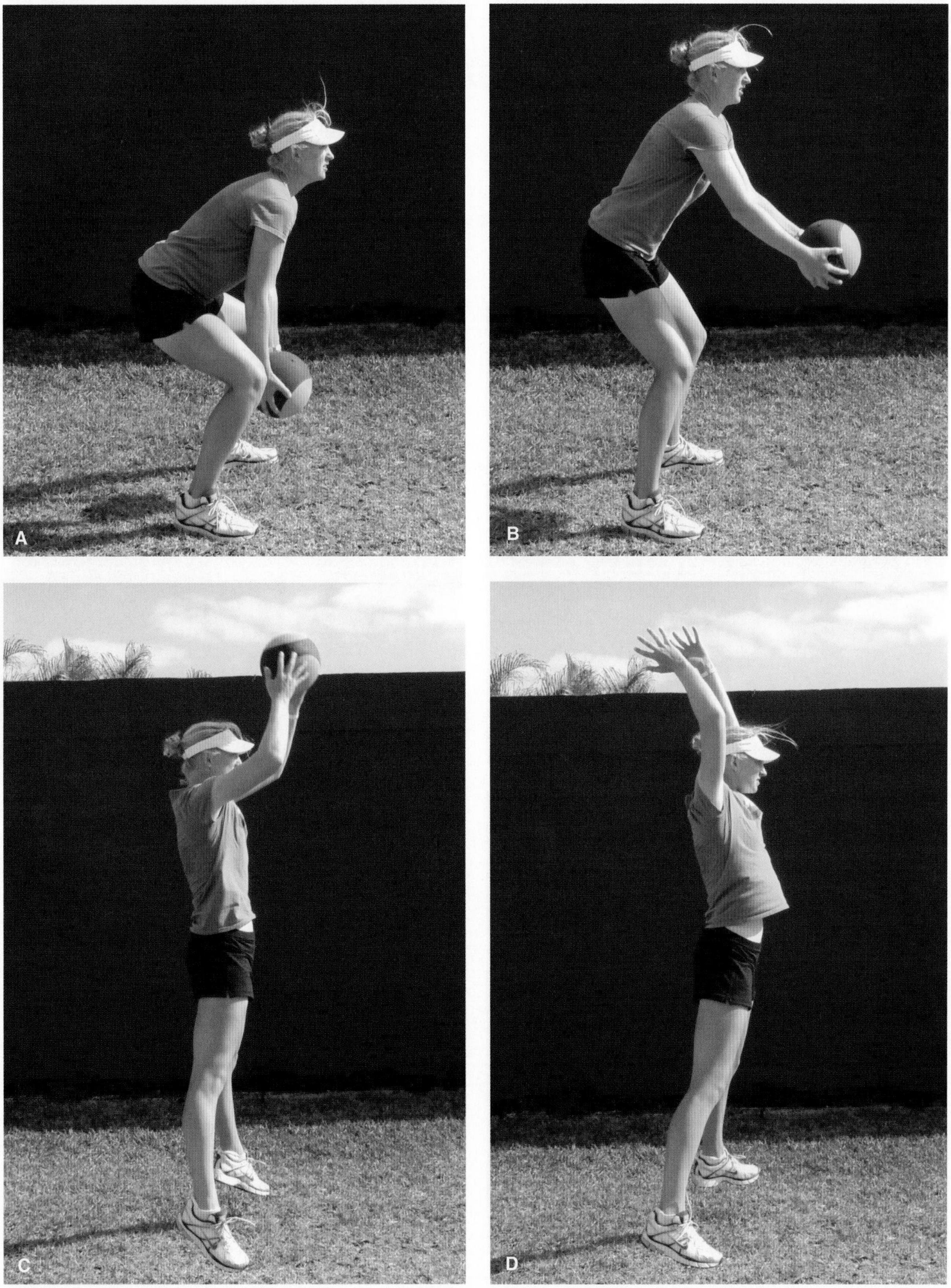

FIGURE 17.10 Scoop toss. **A.** Countermovement. **B.** Upward phase. **C.** Full leg extension. **D.** Release.

(continued)

Plyometric Exercises *(continued)*

Overhead Throw

Starting Position

The athlete stands in a staggered stance, with an upright posture, holding a medicine ball directly overhead with the elbows extended.

Movement Sequence

Begin with a preparatory flexion of the elbows so that the medicine ball is behind the head (Fig. 17.11A). Immediately extend the elbows (Fig. 17.11B) and release the ball toward the wall (Fig. 17.11C). Attempt to hit the wall so that the ball rebounds directly into your hands with your elbows still extended.

Variation

Perform this drill by maintaining extended elbows, moving only from the shoulder.

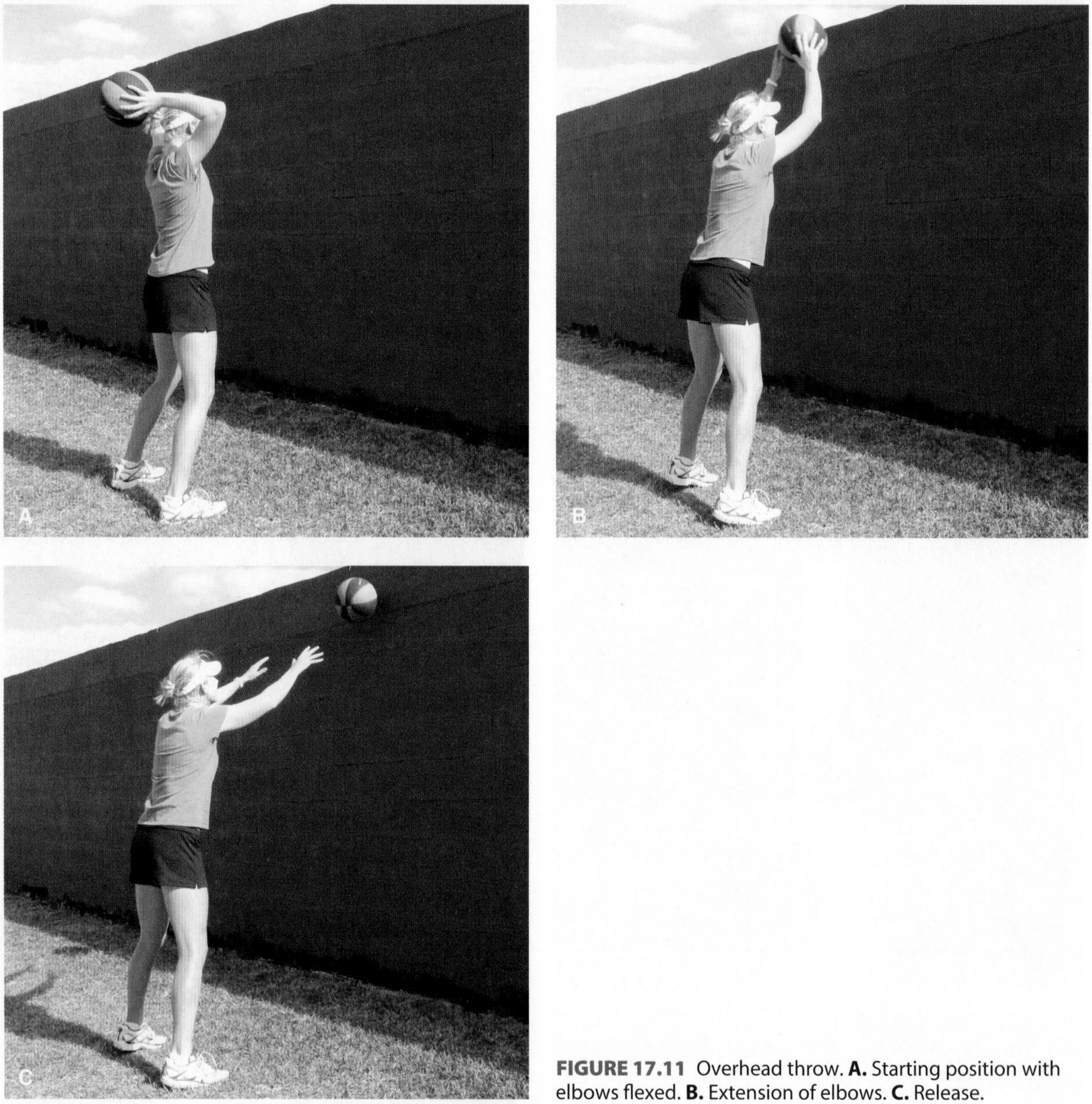

FIGURE 17.11 Overhead throw. **A.** Starting position with elbows flexed. **B.** Extension of elbows. **C.** Release.

Plyometric Exercises *(continued)*

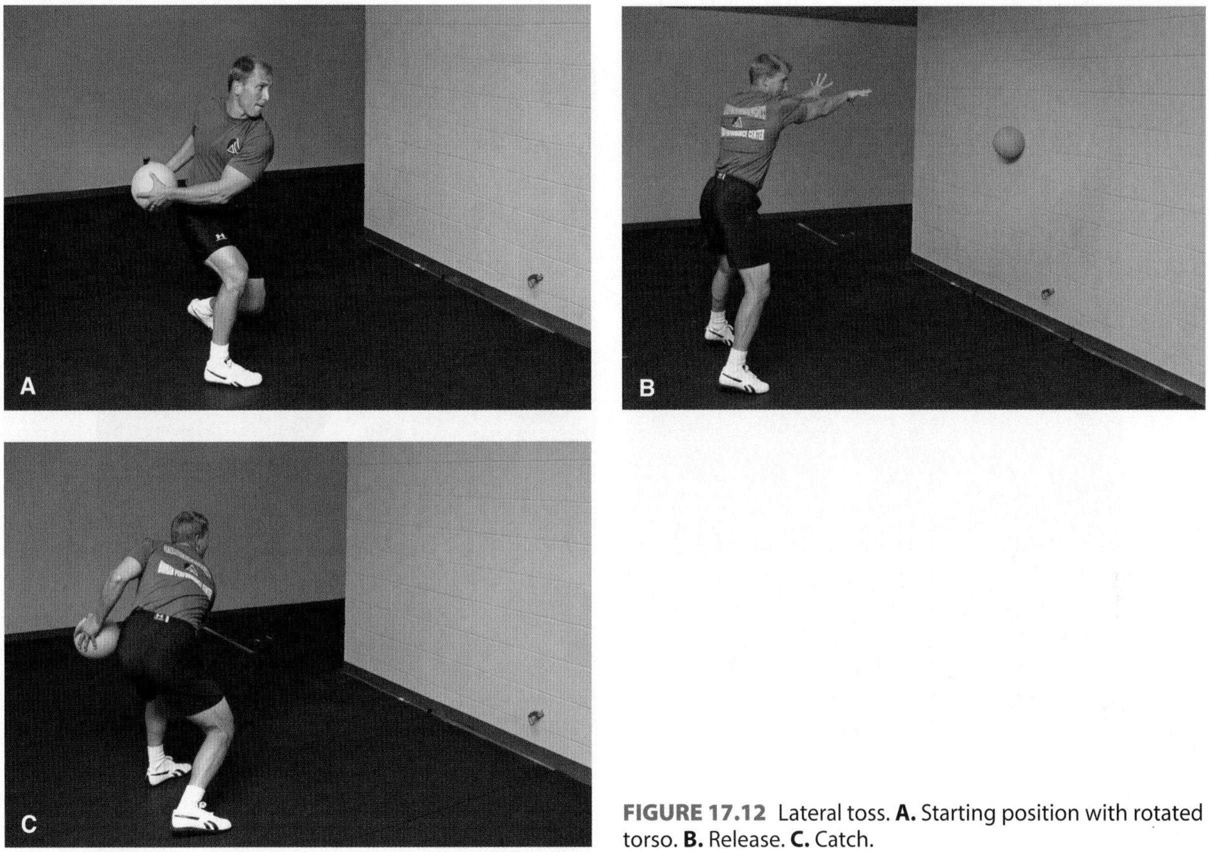

FIGURE 17.12 Lateral toss. **A.** Starting position with rotated torso. **B.** Release. **C.** Catch.

Lateral Toss

Starting Position

The athlete stands with the feet a shoulder width apart and holding a medicine ball by the hips with the arms fully extended.

Movement Sequence

The athlete rotates the torso to the left while simultaneously slightly flexing the hips and knees (Fig. 17.12A). During the return, the hips and knees are extended and the ball is released toward the wall at a slight angle (Fig. 17.12B). As the ball rebounds off the wall, the athlete catches and performs the same action to the opposite side of the body (Fig. 17.12C).

Variations

Perform this drill with a partner. Maintain the rotation to the same side of the body.

Two-Handed Put Throw

Starting Position

The athlete stands with the feet a shoulder width apart, holding a medicine ball in the center of the chest.

Movement Sequence

Begin by rotating the torso to the right (Fig. 17.13A) and flexing the hips and knees into a deep squat position (Fig. 17.13B).

(continued)

Two-Handed Put Throw *(continued)*

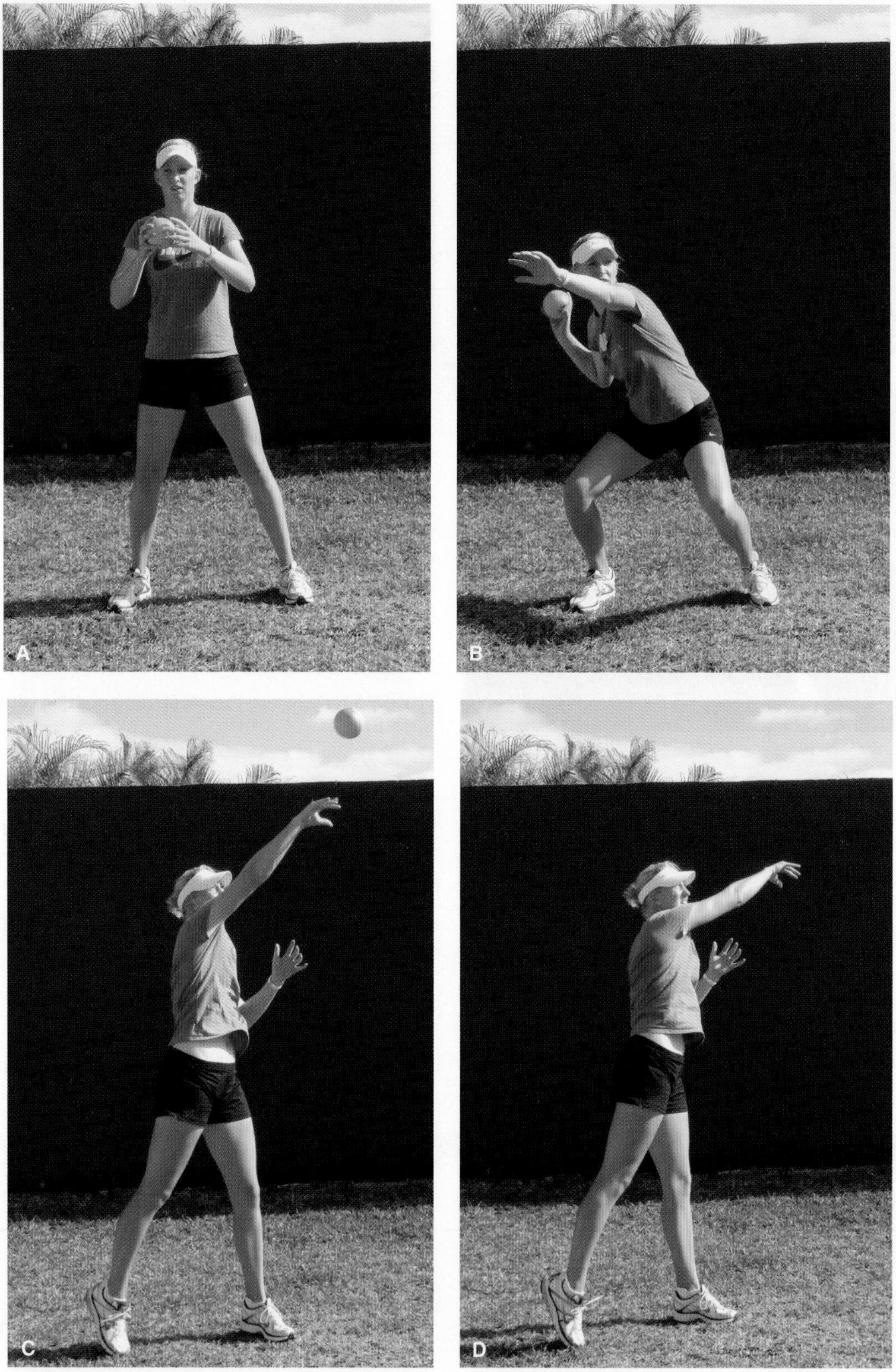

FIGURE 17.13 Two-handed put throw. **A.** Starting position with rotated torso. **B.** Deep squat position. Two-handed put throw. **C.** Full extension and release. **D.** Follow-through.

Two-Handed Put Throw *(continued)*

Once at the bottom, immediately extend the hips and knees while simultaneously rotating toward the starting position. The medicine ball will be thrown with the right hand (guide with the left). Fully extend the hips, knees, and right elbow, attempting to maximize the vertical height of the ball (Fig. 17.13C). Follow through completely by rotating to the left (Fig. 17.13D).

Variation

Perform this drill with a partner.

Wood Chop Throw

Starting Position

The athlete stands with the feet a shoulder width apart, holding a medicine ball at the center of the chest (Fig. 17.14A).

Movement Sequence

Begin by rotating the torso to the right and flexing the hips and knees into a semi-squat position (Fig. 17.14B). Move the ball in an arc from knee height to slightly above the head (Fig. 17.14C). Rotate the torso toward the start position, throwing the ball toward the ground (Fig. 17.14D).

Variation

Attempt to move and position yourself to catch the ball to initiate the next repetition.

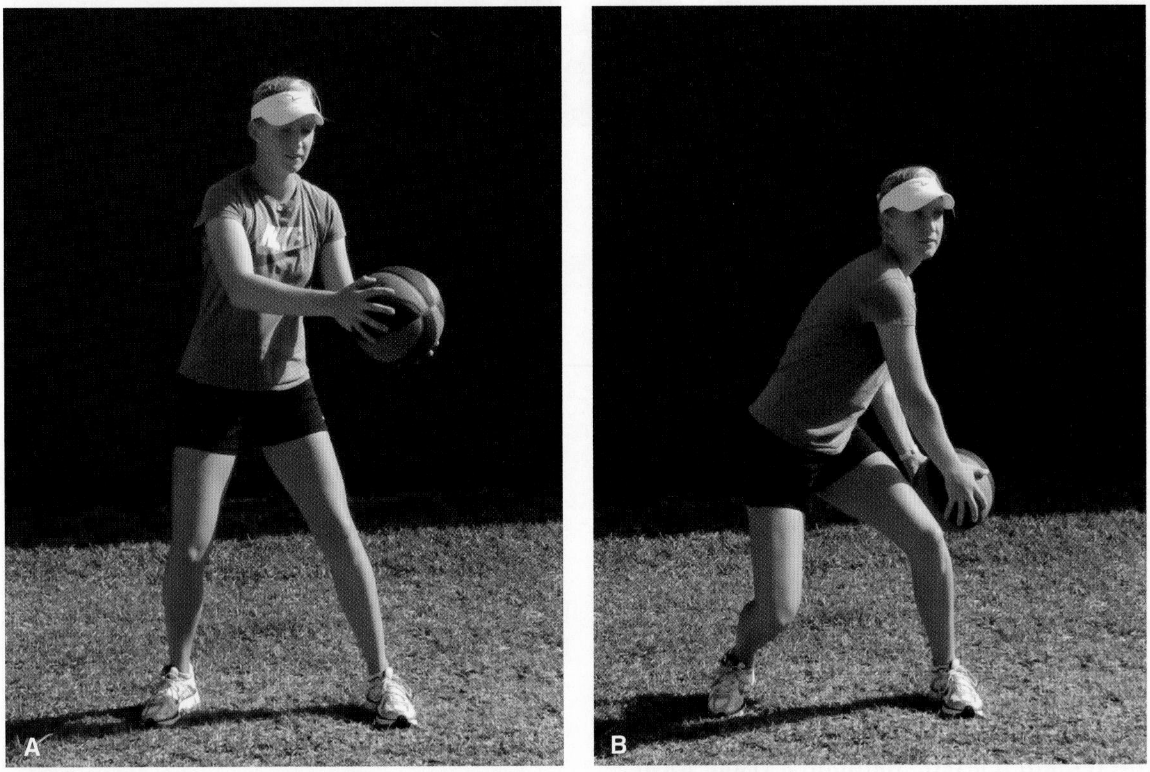

FIGURE 17.14 Wood chop throw. **A.** Starting position. **B.** Semi-squat position.

(continued)

Two-Handed Put Throw *(continued)*

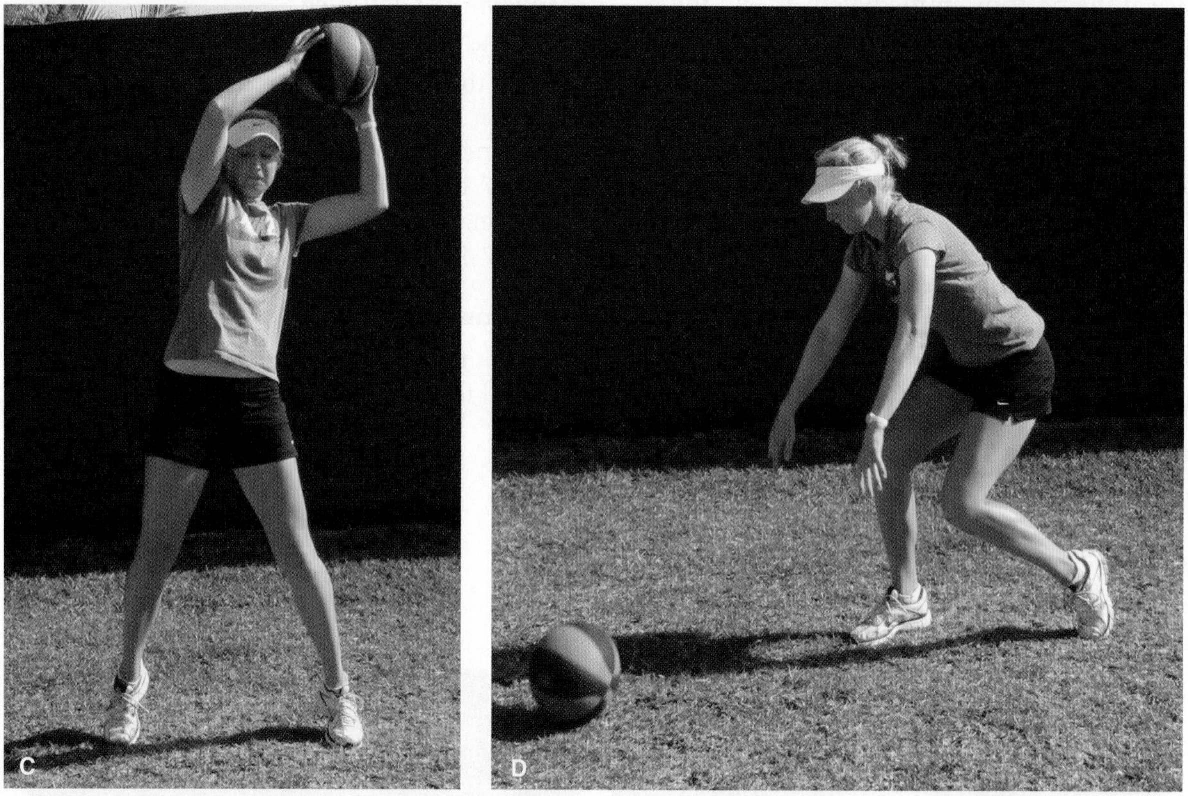

FIGURE 17.14 *(continued)* **C.** Arc movement. **D.** Release.

Sprint Mechanic Drills

Quick Step

Starting Position

This drill begins with the athlete jogging/running in place (Fig. 17.15A).

Movement Sequence

Swing the hands rapidly, being sure to initiate the movement from the shoulder joint. The feet should contact the ground with the ball of the foot during every support phase. Shoulders should remain relaxed. Maintain a visual focal point directed straight ahead (Fig. 17.15B).

The purpose of this drill is to enable the athlete to establish proper movement patterns (e.g., body alignment, support foot position, arm swing) without the mechanical or metabolic loads associated with high-speed horizontal movement.

Variation

Start at slower movement speeds and increase gradually from a jog into a run and finally a sprint.

B-March

Starting Position

The athlete should begin this drill in a "marching" posture facing straight ahead (Fig. 17.16A).

Sprint Mechanic Drills *(continued)*

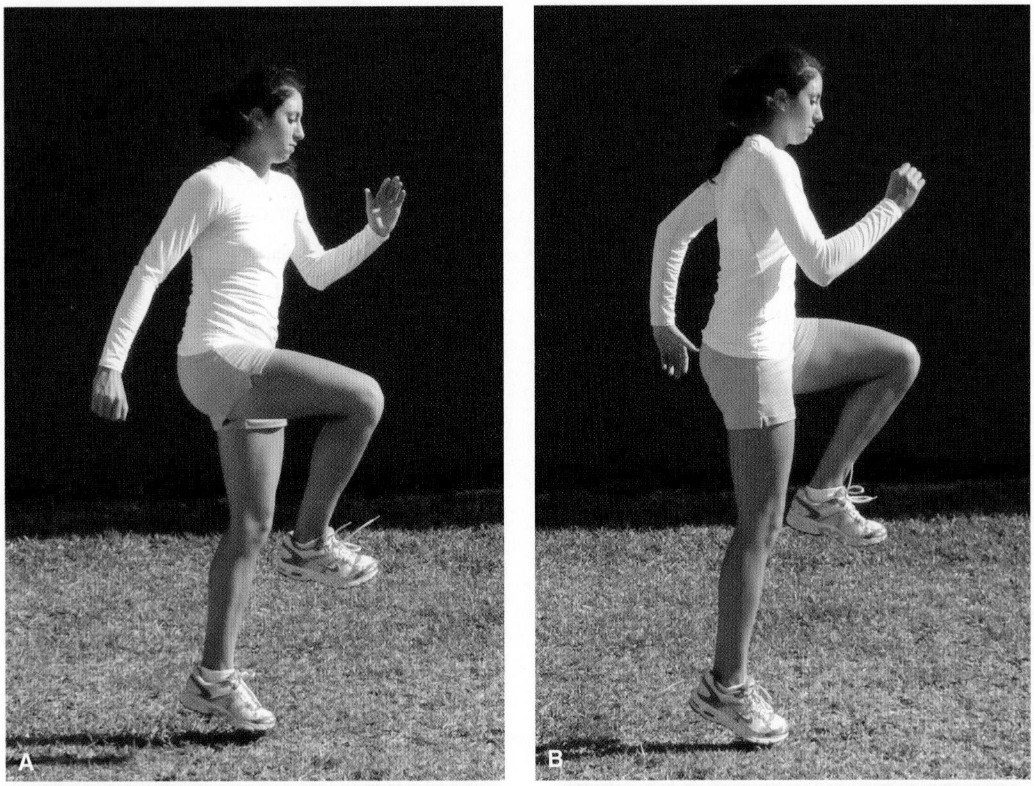

FIGURE 17.15 Quick step. **A.** Starting position. **B.** Step movement.

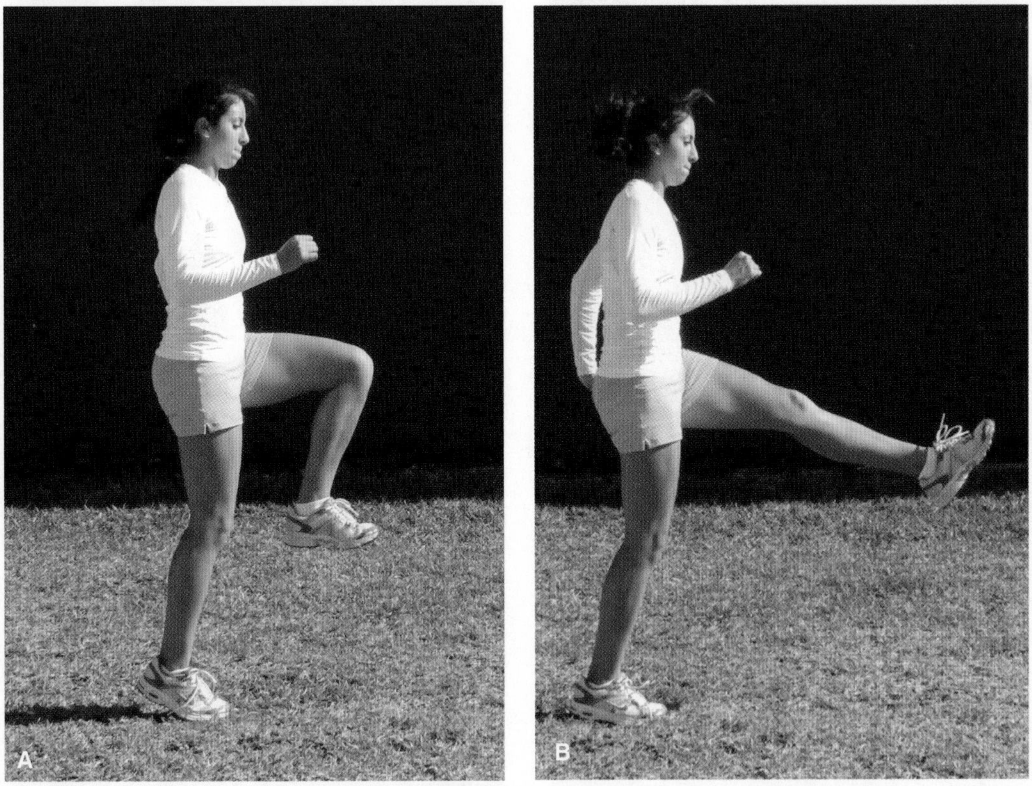

FIGURE 17.16 B-march. **A.** Starting position. **B.** Knee extension.

(continued)

Sprint Mechanic Drills *(continued)*

Movement Sequence

Lift the knee (Fig. 17.16B) and pull the knee back to the ground. Although the knee is lifted and pulled back, it must be understood that the motion originates and is designed to accentuate the action about the hip. Keep the lower leg relaxed (do not kick; the lower leg will naturally have a whip-like motion when relaxed). Contact the ground with the ball of the foot and concentrate on "pulling" the body horizontally. Maintain visual focal point directed straight ahead. Keep shoulders relaxed. Proper arm swing should be maintained throughout.

The purpose of this drill is to create the appropriate muscle activation patterns during late swing through midsupport.

Variation

Start with a marching action and advance into skipping and finally skipping with a transition to a short sprint.

Stride Cycles

Starting Position

The athlete begins this drill by jogging or running forward (Fig. 17.17A).

Movement Sequence

Jog or run on the balls of the feet over a predetermined distance (e.g., 20 to 30 yd) (Fig. 17.17B). At a prescribed number of steps, perform a complete sprint cycle with one leg. Complete this repetition at a higher speed, contacting the ground on the ball of the foot and again "pulling" the body horizontally with hip extension (Fig. 17.17C). Allow the athlete to transition into maximum effort linear sprinting by integrating single-leg full sprint cycles (swing and support phase) at prescribed intervals. All cycles should be performed near or at maximum speed.

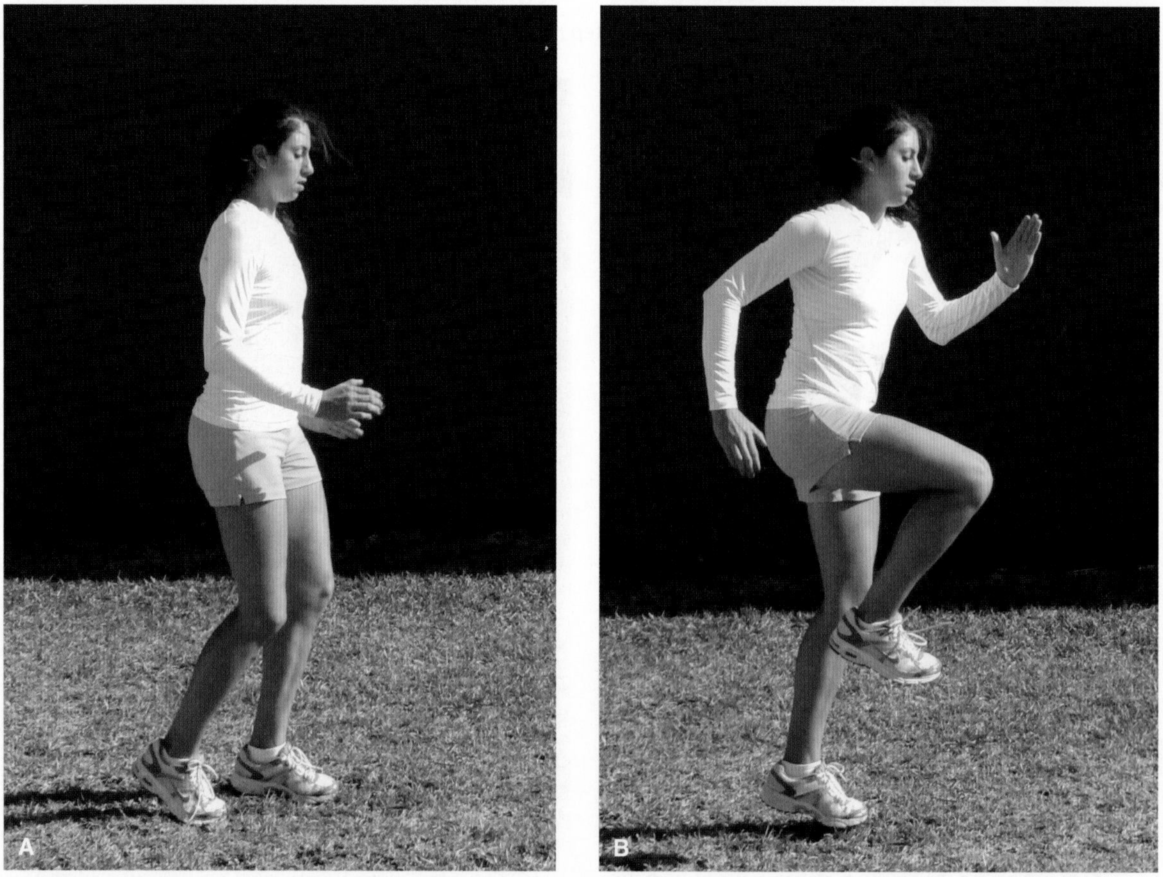

FIGURE 17.17 Stride cycle. **A.** Starting position. **B.** Jogging movement. Stride cycle. **C.** Hip extension.

Speed & Movement Drills

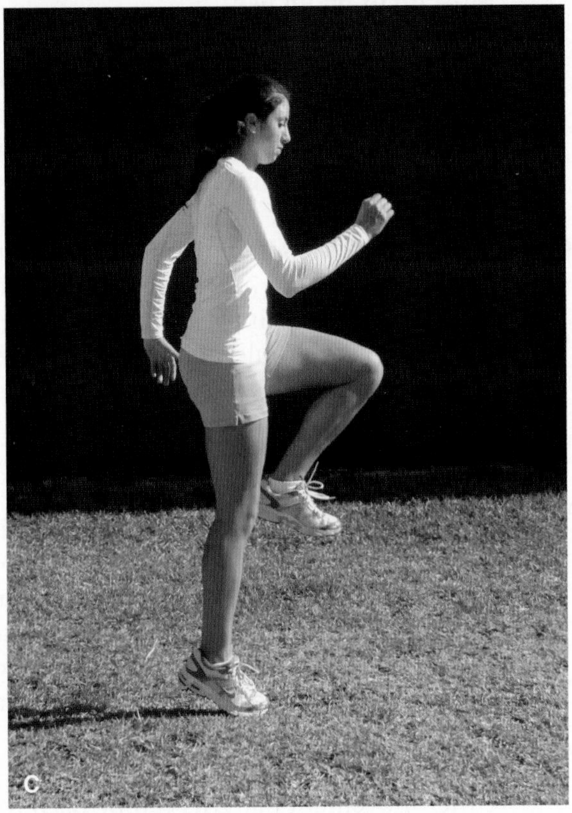

FIGURE 17.17 *(continued)* **C.** Hip extension.

Variation

Start with a high number of jogging/running steps (five to seven) between cycles, gradually reducing this (one to three), and finally coupling into a double cycle (both the left and the right foot complete a cycle without jogging/running steps in between).

Five-Point Agility Run

Starting Position

The athlete should start in an athletic "ready" position facing the direction of the first sprint.

Movement Sequence

Start at position X and run to position 1 as quickly as possible, returning to position X. Continue running to positions two to five, always returning to position X after each one (Fig. 17.18). The purpose of this drill is to improve agility by requiring quick stops, quick starts, rapid accelerations, and changes of direction.

Focus on an explosive start and accelerate to maximum speed as rapidly as possible, keeping the center of gravity low to stop quickly, and keeping the center of gravity on the back edge of the base of support.

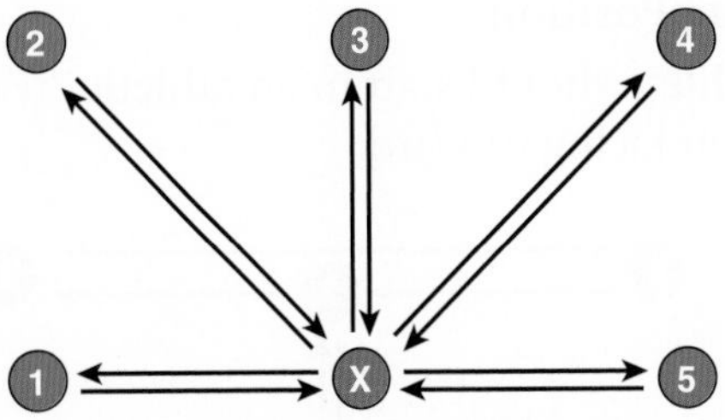

FIGURE 17.18 Five-point agility run.

(continued)

Speed & Movement Drills *(continued)*

Variation

This drill can be performed with various movements including sprinting, shuffling, and backpedaling. It can also be performed both clockwise and counterclockwise, and the distance of each sprint can be varied.

T-Drill for Combining Lateral and Forward/Backward Movement

Starting Position

The athlete should start in an athletic "ready" position facing the direction of the first sprint.

Movement Sequence

Start at cone 1 and sprint to the left side of cone 2. Move around cone 2 and shuffle to the right to and around cone 3. Then shuffle to the left all the way back across to and around cone 4. Then shuffle to the right back to cone 2, then backpedal backward to cone 1 (Fig. 17.19). The purpose of the T-drill is to train the athlete to rapidly and effectively transition from forward/backward, forward/lateral, and backward/lateral movement patterns.

The focus of this drill is not only forward/backward/lateral movements but also the ability to transition from one to the other. The center of gravity should be kept low, and on the back edge of the base of support when changing direction.

Variation

The footwork patterns and the distance between cones can be altered.

Five-Dot Drill

Starting Position

The athlete should start in an athletic "ready" position facing forward.

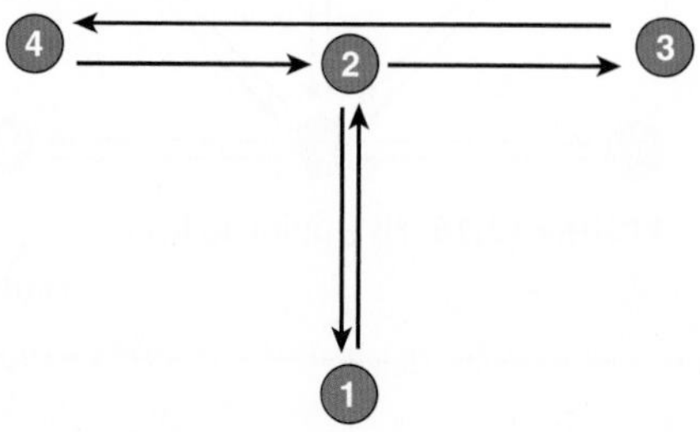

FIGURE 17.19 T-drill for combining lateral and forward/backward movement.

Movement Sequence

There are various movement patterns for this drill. One common pattern is for the athlete to start with one foot on each of the two nearest dots, approximately 2 ft apart. She then jumps in a hopscotch pattern to the two farthest dots, approximately 3 ft away. The athlete then jumps backward in the same manner to the starting position (Fig. 17.20). This movement is repeated as many times as desired.

The athlete should maintain his or her center of gravity as close as possible to the center dot to facilitate rapid movement and maintaining balance. The athlete should maintain an athletic position during the drill with the center of gravity low. Encourage the athlete to move his or her feet as rapidly as possible. The purpose of the five-dot drill is to develop the ability to move the feet quickly while maintaining an athletic balanced position, using both single- and double-leg movements in forward/backward patterns.

Variation

Other movement patterns can be used for this drill, such as jumping with both feet together and jumping to each dot individually. The spacing of the dots can also be increased or decreased. Any variation or combination of movements can be used in one specific drill. The length of time the athlete performs the drill can be modified, or the number of single- or double-leg foot contacts can be used as an estimate of workload.

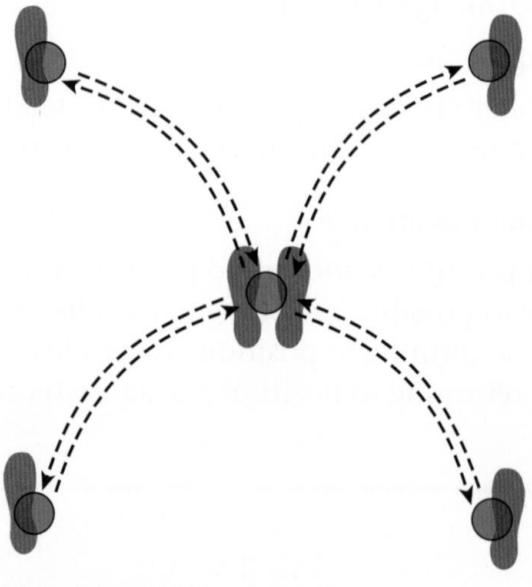

FIGURE 17.20 Five-dot drill.

Speed & Movement Drills *(continued)*

Hexagon Drill

Starting Position

The athlete should start in an athletic "ready" position facing forward in the middle of a hexagon.

Movement Sequence

Jump over one side of the hexagon and return back to the middle. Then jump over each of the six sides of the hexagon in order, always returning to the inside of the hexagon following each jump (Fig. 17.21). The purpose of the hexagon drill is to develop the ability to move the feet quickly while maintaining an athletic balanced position using both single-and double-leg movement patterns.

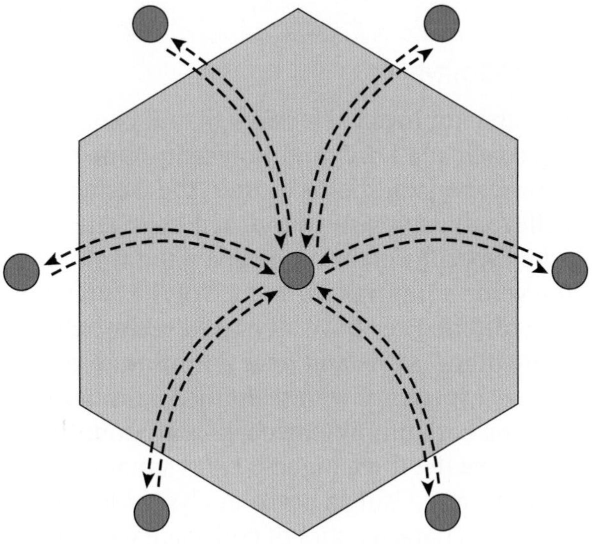

FIGURE 17.21 Hexagon drill.

Variation

The pattern can be performed clockwise or counterclockwise. The size of the hexagon can also be varied.

Summary

Explosive movements such as sprinting, jumping, and changing directions are vital to success in nearly all sports. The effective utilization of the SSC (coupling eccentric and concentric muscle actions) to increase power output and ultimately enhance performance is the major purpose of all explosive training techniques, drills, and exercises. Scientific evidence indicates that both mechanical and neural factors regulate SSC ability. In addition, fiber-type distribution, the use of the upper extremities, gender, age, agonist and antagonist strength, and fatigue can either attenuate or augment the SSC. More importantly, program design and drill selection should weigh heavily on the experience of the athlete(s), with a focus on general motor development (agility, balance, and coordination) for younger athletes and greater sport specificity with relative increases in loads and difficulty for advanced athletes. Training programs utilizing plyometric, sprint, and agility drills should address all these factors in a controlled, technique-focused training program to improve performance and limit the likelihood of injury.

Maxing Out

1. A high school baseball coach asks the new strength and conditioning coach if she will watch his athletes perform their plyometric routine, which includes depth jumps. When they perform the depth jumps, she notices that many of them have poor landing mechanics (e.g., little flexion of the hips and knees, the knees buckling inward). What would be an appropriate suggestion she could make to the coach regarding how the drills should be performed?
2. A varsity track sprinter wants to start lifting weights in an attempt to become faster. He has never been involved in resistance training before. Initially, what muscle groups and what types of exercises would be most beneficial?
3. An elite-level tennis player wants your suggestions for new ways to improve the team's ability to change directions. Which program variables should be the focus of their training and how can they be manipulated to stimulate performance improvements?

CASE EXAMPLE

Designing a Plyometric Training Program for a Women's College Volleyball Player (Outside Hitter)

BACKGROUND

You are employed as a strength and conditioning coach at a Division I university. One of your responsibilities is to train the women's volleyball team year round. The coach has asked specific attention be given to improving the vertical jump performance of the three outside hitters. They have all played volleyball for more than 7 years and have a minimum of 3 years experience with resistance training. Their landing and jumping mechanics are sound and they have the three highest 1-RM squat scores on the team. Using a needs analysis, identify the jumping characteristics of collegiate women's outside hitters and develop an 8-week plyometric cycle leading into the preseason.

RECOMMENDATIONS/CONSIDERATIONS

Begin with a needs analysis of jumping volume for the group of players. Watching several videos from the previous season should provide you with a very reasonable understanding of the types and volumes of jumps performed. You find the maximal number of spikes and blocks performed per game is approximately 34 and 27, respectively. If it is necessary to play four games to determine the outcome of a match, then an outside hitter could expect to perform nearly 250 jumps per match (136 spikes and 108 blocks). A movement analysis indicates that to perform a spike, the athlete must first generate horizontal velocity and transfer it to vertical motion. On the other hand, a block begins from a quasistatic squat position and has only vertical motion.

IMPLEMENTATION

Select exercises that are closely associated with the motor skills. For example, power skips performed for linear distance or maximal height would both provide a suitable stimulus for this group of athletes. Depth jumps could also be used sparingly to develop the ability to decelerate and change directions rapidly, as is found during the spike. Any type of vertical jumping drill would be appropriate to focus on blocking ability. More specifically, the block is started from a quasistatic position; therefore, a drill such as box jumps would fit into the training program. The athletes should be instructed to perform all exercises with maximal takeoff velocity throughout the entire training cycle. An attempt is made to equate the actual volume observed during competition to what is prescribed during training. This should occur over several weeks and only be implemented during select training sessions. Progressive overload and a periodized schedule will allow for proper recovery between training stimuli.

RESULTS

Using appropriate progressions for volume and intensity and providing adequate rest should provide the necessary stimulus for improved performance and greater jumping ability. Regular assessment (~every 2 to 3 weeks) of performance using volleyball-specific vertical jump tests will provide the necessary feedback to monitor your program.

REFERENCES

1. Walshe AD, Wilson GJ, Ettema GJ. Stretch-shorten cycle compared with isometric preload: contributions to enhanced muscular performance. *J Appl Physiol.* 1998;84:97–106.
2. Bobbert MF. Dependence of human squat jump performance on the series elastic compliance of the triceps surae: a simulation study. *J Exp Biol.* 2001;204:533–542.
3. Bobbert MF, Gerristen KG, Litjens MC, et al. Why is countermovement jump height greater than the squat jump height? *Med Sci Sports Exerc.* 1996;28:1402–1412.
4. Ettema GJ. Muscle efficiency: the controversial role of elasticity and mechanical energy conversion in stretch-shortening cycles. *Eur J Appl Physiol.* 2001;85:457–465.
5. Finni T, Ikegawa S, Lepola V, et al. Comparison of force-velocity relationships of vastus lateralis muscle in isokinetic and in stretch-shortening cycle exercises. *Acta Physiol Scand.* 2003;177:483–491.
6. Hill AV. Mechanics of the contractile element of muscle. *Nature.* 1950;166:415–419.
7. Belli A, Kyröläinen H, Komi PV. Moment and power of lower limb joints in running. *Int J Sports Med.* 2002;23:136–141.

8. Kyröläinen H, Komi PV, Belli A. Changes in muscle activity patterns and kinetics with increasing running speed. *J Strength Cond Res.* 1999;13(4):400–406.
9. Wiemann K, Tidow GN. Relative activity of hip and knee extensors in sprinting: implications for training. *New Stud Athlet.* 1995;10(1):29–49.
10. Kurokawa S, Fukunaga T, Fukashiro S. Behavior of fascicles and tendinous structures of human gastrocnemius during vertical jumping. *J Appl Physiol.* 2001;90:1349–1358.
11. Schmidt RA, Lee TD. *Motor Control and Learning.* 3rd ed. Champaign, IL: Human Kinetics; 1999.
12. Harman EA, Rosenstein MT, Frykman PN, et al. The effects of arms and countermovement on vertical jumping. *Med Sci Sports Exerc.* 1990;22:825–833.
13. Ashby BM, Heegaard JH. Role of arm motion in the standing long jump. *J Biomech.* 2002;35:1631–1637.
14. Martin RJ, Dore E, Twisk J, et al. Longitudinal changes of maximal short-term peak power in girls and boys during growth. *Med Sci Sports Exerc.* 2004;36(3):498–503.
15. Kearney JT, Rundell KW, Wilber RL. Measurement of work and power in sport. In: Kirkendall DT, ed. *Exercise and Sport Science.* Philadelphia, PA: Lippincott Williams & Wilkins; 2000.
16. van Praagh E. Development of anaerobic function during childhood and adolescence. *Pediatr Exerc Sci.* 2000; 12:150–173.
17. Caserotti P, Aagaard P, Simonsen EB, et al. Contraction-specific differences in maximal muscle power during stretch-shortening cycle movements in elderly males and females. *Eur J Appl Physiol.* 2001;84:206–212.
18. Harrison AJ, Gaffney S. Motor development and gender effects of stretch-shortening cycle performance. *J Sci Med Sport.* 2001;4:406–415.
19. Fox SI. *Human Phww ysiology.* 8th ed. New York: McGraw-Hill; 2004.
20. Moritani T. Motor unit and motor neuron excitability during explosive movements. In: Komi PV, ed. *Strength and Power in Sport.* Oxford, UK: Blackwell; 2003.
21. Jaric S, Ropret R, Kukolj M, et al. Role of agonist and antagonist muscle strength in performance of rapid movements. *Eur J Appl Physiol Occup Physiol.* 1995;71:464–468.
22. Jaric S. Changes in movement symmetry associated with strengthening and fatigue of agonist and antagonist muscles. *J Motor Behav.* 2000;32:9–15.
23. Avela J, Komi PV. Interaction between muscle stiffness and stretch reflex sensitivity after long-term stretch-shortening cycle exercise. *Muscle Nerve.* 1998;21:1224–1227.
24. Radcliffe JC, Farentinos RC. *High-powered Plyometrics.* Champaign, IL: Human Kinetics; 1999.
25. Strojnik V, Komi PV. Fatigue after submaximal intensive stretch-shortening cycle exercise. *Med Sci Sports Exerc.* 2000;32:1314–1319.
26. Strojnik V, Komi PV. Neuromuscular fatigue after maximal stretch-shortening cycle exercise. *J Appl Physiol.* 1998;84:344–350.
27. Haywood KM, Getchell N. *Life Span Motor Development.* 3rd ed. Champaign, IL: Human Kinetics; 2001.
28. Gallahue DL, John CO. *Understanding Motor Development.* 6th ed. New York: McGraw-Hill; 2006.
29. Caraffa A, Cerulli G, Projetti M, et al. Prevention of anterior cruciate ligament injuries in soccer. A prospective controlled study of proprioceptive training. *Knee Surg Sports Traumatol Arthrosc.* 1996;4:19–21.
30. Griffin LY. The Henning program. In: Griffin LY, ed. *Prevention of Noncontact ACL Injuries.* Rosemont, IL: American Academy of Orthopaedic Surgeons; 2001.
31. Hewett TE, Stroupe AI, Nance TA, et al. Plyometric training in female athletes: decreased impact forces and increased hamstring torques. *Am J Sports Med.* 1996;24:765–773.
32. Silvers HJ, Mandelbaum BR. Preseason conditioning to prevent soccer injuries in young women. *Clin J Sport Med.* 2001;11:206.
33. McNair PJ, Prapavessis H, Callender K. Decreasing landing forces: effect of instruction. *Br J Sports Med.* 2000;34:293–296.
34. Onate JA, Guskiewicz KM, Sullivan RJ. Augmented feedback reduces jump landing forces. *J Orthop Sports Phys Ther.* 2001;31:511–517.
35. Mandelbaum BR, Silvers HJ, Watanabe DS, et al. Effectiveness of a neuromuscular and proprioceptive training program in preventing anterior cruciate ligament injuries in female athletes: 2-year follow-up. *Am J Sports Med.* 2005;33:1003–1010.
36. Brown ME, Mayhew JL, Boleach LW. Effect of plyometric training on vertical jump performance in high school basketball players. *J Sports Med Phys Fitness.* 1986;26:1–4.
37. Fatouros IG, Jamurtas AZ, Leontsini D, et al. Evaluation of plyometric exercise training, weight training, and their combination on vertical jumping performance and leg strength. *J StrengthCond Res.* 2000;14:470–476.
38. Luebbers PE, Potteiger JA, Hulver MW, et al. Effects of plyometric training and recovery on vertical jump performance and anaerobic power. *J Strength Cond Res.* 2003;17:704–709.
39. Wilson GJ, Murphy AJ, Giorgi A. Weight and plyometric training: effects on eccentric and concentric force production. *Can J Appl Physiol.* 1996;21:301–315.
40. Lees A, Rojas J, Ceperos M, et al. How the free limbs are used by elite high jumpers in generating vertical velocity. *Ergonomics.* 2000;43:1622–1636.
41. McBride JM, Triplett McBride T, Davie A, et al. The effect of heavy- vs light-load jump squats on the development of strength, power, and speed. *J Strength Cond Res.* 2002;16:75–82.
42. Adams K, O'Shea J, O'Shea K, et al. The effect of six weeks of squat, plyometric, and squat-plyometric training on power production. *J Appl Sports Sci Res.* 1992; 6:36–41.
43. Bobbert MF, Van Soest AJ. Effects of muscle strengthening on vertical jump height: a simulation study. *Med Sci Sports Exerc.* 1994;26:1012–1020.
44. Young WB, Wilson GJ, Byrne C. A comparison of drop jump training methods: effects on leg extensor strength qualities and jumping performance. *Int J Sports Med.* 1999;20:295–303.
45. Gehri DJ, Ricard MD, Kleiner DM, et al. A comparison of plyometric training techniques for improving vertical jump ability and energy production. *J Strength Cond Res.* 1998;12:85–89.
46. Clutch M, Wilton M. The effect of depth jumps and weight training on leg strength and vertical jump. *Res Q Exerc Sport.* 1983;54:5–10.

47. Diallo O, Dore E, Duche P, et al. Effects of plyometric training followed by a reduced training programme on physical performance in prepubescent soccer players. *J Sports Med Phys Fitness*. 2001;41:342–348.
48. Potteiger J, Lockwood R, Daub M, et al. Muscle power and fiber characteristics following 8 weeks of plyometric training. *J Strength Cond Res*. 1999;13:275–279.
49. Mero A, Komi PV. Reaction time and electromyographic activity during a sprint start. *Eur J Appl Physiol*. 1990;61:73–80.
50. Galton F. On instruments for (1) testing perception of differences of tint and for (2) determining reaction time. *J Anthropol Inst*. 1899;19:27–29.
51. Brebner JT, Welford AT. Introduction and historical background sketch. In: Welford AT, ed. *Reaction Times*. New York: Academic Press; 1980:1–23.
52. Gambetta V, Winckler G. *Sport Specific Speed: The 3S System*. Sarasota, FL: Gambetta Sports Training Systems; 2001.
53. Mero A, Komi PV, Gregor RJ. Biomechanics of sprint running. *Sports Med*. 1992;13(6):376–392.
54. Mann RA, Moran GT, Dougherty SE. Comparative electromyography of the lower extremity in jogging, running, and sprinting. *Am J Sports Med*. 1986;14:501–510.
55. Sinning WE, Forsyth HL. Lower-limb actions while running at different velocities. *Med Sci Sports*. 1970;2:28–34.
56. Kivi DM, Maraj BK, Gervais P. A kinematic analysis of high-speed treadmill sprinting over a range of velocities. *Med Sci Sports Exerc*. 2002;34:662–666.
57. Mann RV. A kinetic analysis of sprinting. *Med Sci Sports Exerc*. 1981;13:325–328.
58. Mann R, Sprague P. A kinetic analysis of the ground leg during sprint running. *Res Q Exerc Sport*. 1980;51:334–348.
59. Dietz V, Schmidtbleicher D, Noth J. Neuronal mechanisms of human locomotion. *J Neurophysiol*. 1979;42:1212–1222.
60. Jacobs R, van Ingen Schenau GJ. Intermuscular coordination in a sprint push-off. *J Biomech*. 1992;25:953–965.
61. Johnson MD, Buckley JG. Muscle power patterns in the mid-acceleration phase of sprinting. *J Sports Sci*. 2001;19:263–272.
62. Bosco C, Vittori C. Biomechanical characteristics of sprint running during maximal and supra-maximal speed. *New Stud Athelet*. 1986;1:39–45.
63. Corn RJ, Knudson D. Effect of elastic-cord towing on the kinematics of the acceleration phase of sprinting. *J Strength Cond Res*. 2003;17:72–75.
64. Paradisis GP, Cooke CB. Kinematic and postural characteristics of sprint running on sloping surfaces. *J Sports Sci*. 2001;19:149–159.
65. Lockie RG, Murphy AJ, Spinks CD. Effects of resisted sled towing on sprint kinematics in field-sport athletes. *J Strength Cond Res*. 2003;17:760–767.
66. Swanson SC, Caldwell GE. An integrated biomechanical analysis of high speed incline and level treadmill running. *Med Sci Sports Exerc*. 2000;32:1146–1155.
67. Zafeiridis A, Saraslanidis P, Manou V, et al. The effects of resisted sled-pulling sprint training on acceleration and maximum speed performance. *J Sports Med Phys Fitness*. 2005;45:284–290.
68. Drabik J. *Children and Sports Training: How Your Future Champions should Exercise to be Healthy, Fit, and Happy*. Island Pond, VT: Stadion; 1996.
69. Verstegen M, Marcello B. Agility and coordination. In: Foran B, ed. *High Performance Sports Conditioning*. Champaign, IL: Human Kinetics; 2001.
70. Little T, Williams AG. Specificity of acceleration, maximal speed and agility in professional soccer players. *J Strength Cond Res*. 2005;19(1):76–78.
71. Ellis L, Gastin P, Lawrence S, et al. Protocols for the physiological assessment of team sports players. In: Gore CJ, ed. *Physiological Tests for Elite Athletes*. Champaign, IL: Human Kinetics; 2000.
72. Besier TF, Lloyd DG, Ackland TR, et al. Anticipatory effects on knee joint loading during running and cutting maneuvers. *Med Sci Sports Exerc*. 2001;33:1176–1181.
73. Rand MK, Ohtsuki T. EMG analysis of lower limb muscles in humans during quick change in running directions. *Gait Posture*. 2000;12:169–183.
74. Neptune RR, Wright IC, van der Bogert AJ. Muscle coordination and function during cutting movements. *Med Sci Sports Exerc*. 1999;31:294–302.
75. Bencke J, Naesborg H, Simonsen EB, et al. Motor pattern of the knee joint muscles during side-step cutting in European team handball. *Scand J Med Sci Sports*. 2000;68–77.
76. Besier TF, Lloyd DG, Cochrane JL, et al. External loading of the knee joint during running and cutting maneuvers. *Med Sci Sports Exerc*. 2001;33:1168–1175.
77. Besier TF, Lloyd DG, Ackland TR. Muscle activation strategies at the knee during running and cutting maneuvers. *Med Sci Sports Exerc*. 2003;35:119–127.
78. Wroble RR, Moxley DP. The effect of winter sports participation on high school football players: strength, power, agility, and body composition. *J Strength Cond Res*. 2001;15:132–135.
79. Young WB, McDowell MH, Scarlett BJ. Specificity of sprint and agility training methods. *J Strength Cond Res*. 2001;15(3):315–319.
80. Mayhew JL, Piper FC, Schwegler TM, et al. Contributions of speed, agility, and body composition to aerobic power measurement in college football players. *J Appl Sports Sci Res*. 1989;3:101–106.

PART

onetwothreefour

Special Topics

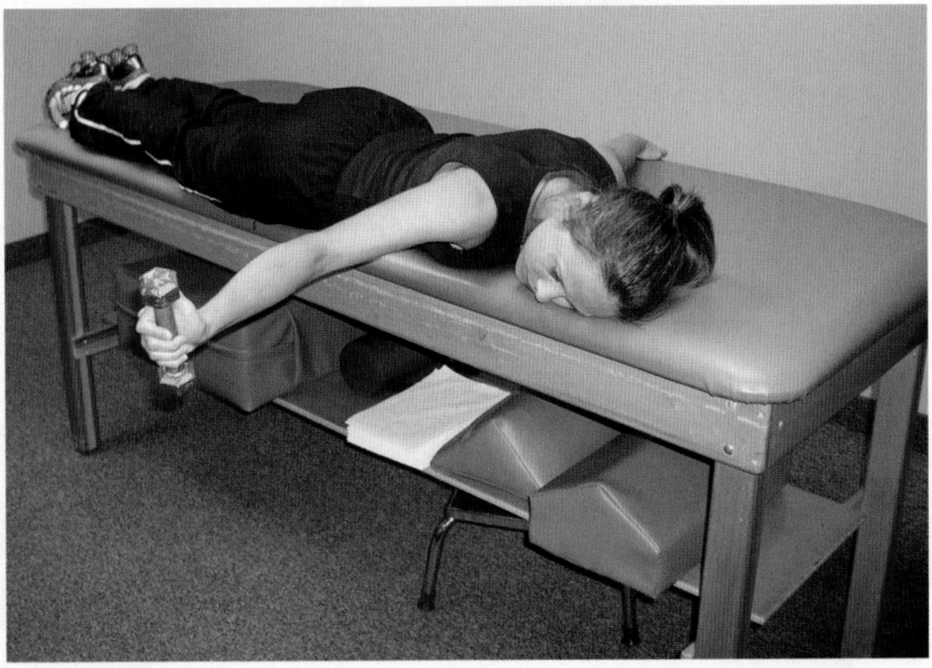

CHAPTER 18

Applied Sport Psychology for the Strength and Conditioning Coach

TRACI A. STATLER

OBJECTIVES

After reading this chapter, you will be able to:

- Understand that the strength and conditioning coach cannot directly motivate athletes.
- Realize that the weight room is an appropriate place for athletes to develop and practice their mental game.
- Set goals.
- Help athletes control their arousal levels.
- Differentiate between a confident athlete and an athlete who is not.
- Notice that most aspects of sports psychology are athlete driven.

KEY TERMS

Achievement Motivation
Broad External Focus
Broad Internal Focus
Concentration
Confidence
Direction of Effort
Emotions
Goal Ladder
Individual Zone of Optimal Functioning (IZOF)
Instructional Self-Talk
Intensity of Effort
Interactional View
Inverted-U Hypothesis
Motivation
Narrow External Focus
Narrow Internal Focus
Negative Self-Talk
Participant-Centered View
Positive Self-Talk
Process-Based Goals
Product-Based Goals
Routine
Self-Talk
Shifting
Situation-Centered View
SMART Goals
Superstition

Introduction

The primary goal of any strength and conditioning coach or personal trainer is to effectively improve athletic performance and fitness using proper strength and conditioning techniques, drawing from the scientific fields of anatomy, exercise physiology, biomechanics, and nutrition. Effective practitioners will be skilled in program design, be adept in the teaching, reinforcement and monitoring of exercise technique, be familiar and comfortable with physical testing and evaluation, and have a variety of organizational and administrative skills (1). The addition of a working understanding of concepts from the field of sport and performance psychology may assist the coach or trainer in the attainment of this primary goal.

It has been argued that the role of sport psychology is to "help athletes achieve more consistent levels of performance at or near their physical potential by carefully managing their physical resources through appropriate psychological strategies and techniques" (2). A basic understanding of these strategies and techniques may help the strength and conditioning coach encourage more consistent effort in the weight room, generate better composure and ability to deal with distractions during workouts, and foster more motivated and confident athletes.

The scientific discipline of sport psychology generally has three major goals: (a) observing and measuring psychological phenomena; (b) investigating the relationship between psychological variables and performance; and (c) applying this theoretical knowledge in performance settings to improve overall athletic performance (2). Therefore, the purpose of this chapter is to focus on the last of these goals, with the aim of helping you—the strength and conditioning coach—effectively integrate some critical sport psychology skills and situational cues into your training programs with the aim of improving your athlete's overall training and performance.

MOTIVATION

As a strength and conditioning coach, you may often find yourself wondering why some athletes you work with seem highly motivated and constantly strive for success in the weight room and on the field of play, whereas others seem to lack this motivation, appearing to simply "Go through the motions" during workouts, practices, and performance situations. Understanding motivation will probably be the most important psychological construct you will need as a strength coach, but it is also one you have little direct control over. You cannot motivate your athletes, but you can help them to better motivate themselves.

Motivation can be defined simply as the intensity and direction of one's effort (3). It is an inner condition that initiates, directs, and sustains a person's behaviors. **Direction of effort** refers to whether an individual will seek out, approach, or be attracted to certain situations (4). For example, an athlete might be attracted to the weight room because he or she understands the relationship between training and sport performance. Along the same lines, an athlete might avoid the weight room because he or she does not enjoy the feeling of fatigue that often results from a hard workout. Both of these examples refer to the direction or one's effort—either toward the weight room or away from it. **Intensity of effort** refers to how much effort a person puts forth in a particular situation (4). For example, an athlete may attend daily workout sessions, but not put forth much effort during that workout. On the other hand, an athlete may only have a short period of access to the training facility yet make the most of every minute. This intensity is an indicator of motivation. Direction and intensity of effort are generally very closely related as those who are drawn to an activity (direction) will often put forth effort in that activity (intensity), and conversely, those who seem lackadaisical about their workouts, often do not have much attraction to the activity in the first place.

Because motivation is "an inner condition," it is not something that you as the coach can give to your athletes. You cannot motivate someone else. However, you may be able to influence them in such a way that they can better motivate themselves.

APPROACHES TO UNDERSTANDING MOTIVATION

Although motivation is something that works differently for everyone, most people can conceptualize how their own motivated behavior comes from a combination of three different orientations. These are the participant-centered view, the situation-centered view, and the interactional view. The **participant-centered view** (sometimes called the trait-centered view) contends that motivated behavior is predominantly a function of individual characteristics, like a person's personality, goals, or needs. Individual characteristics are what determine how motivated a person will be in any given situation. This could, for example, describe those who seem to excel in all areas of their lives. The **situation-centered view** (sometimes called the state-centered view), however, is in direct contrast to this. This view argues that a person's motivation is primarily determined by the situations in which he or she finds himself or herself. You can likely think of situations where you would describe yourself as highly motivated, but others where your motivation is lacking. You are still the same person, but now the situation is different. The reality though is that while there may be some personality characteristics that influence your motivation, and you find yourself motivated in some situations but not others, most of us would generally argue that our motivated behaviors are a function of both our traits (who we are) and our states (how we feel at the moment, in the environment we find ourselves). Therefore, the view of motivation most widely accepted is the interactional view. The **interactional view** of motivation contends that "motivation results neither solely from participant factors nor solely from situational factors" (4). Rather, the best way to understand motivation is to consider both the person and the situation and how these two interact.

The best way to understand motivated behavior is to consider both the person and the situation and examine how these two factors interact with each other.

ACHIEVEMENT MOTIVATION

As a strength coach, understanding that your athletes all participate in their respective sports for different reasons, approach the training expectations for their sports in different ways, and experience motivation for these activities differently, will be critical in enhancing the level of service you can provide. To best tailor your services to the motivations of each athlete, an understanding of what specifically motivates them to act or behave in certain ways is needed. One construct that has emerged from the sport psychology literature to help with this is achievement motivation.

Achievement motivation refers to a person's orientation to strive for task success, persist in the face of failure, and experience pride in accomplishments (5). It is an understanding of this motivation that gives the coach insight into an athlete's desire and willingness to strive for excellence and under what circumstances he or she is willing to do so. As strength coaches, knowing if athletes are motivated to achieve success, even if there is a likelihood of failing, tells us a lot about those athletes. It tells us that these athletes will challenge themselves. They will put in the extra effort to be sure they are getting the most out of every workout, even if they are not seeing immediate results. They will experience a sense of pride when they accomplish goals they have set for themselves, and they will not overly berate themselves when they fail, because they recognize that they have given their all.

Similarly, being able to recognize an athlete who is motivated to avoid failure is also beneficial for the strength coach. While these concepts may sound the same, achieving success and avoiding failure from a motivational perspective are very different. Based on outward behaviors, the athlete motivated to avoid failure may look very similar to the one motivated to achieve success; however, an athlete motivated to avoid failure generally pushes himself or herself for very different reasons. This is a person who strives to avoid situations where failure can be internally attributed. Such athletes will push themselves in the weight room if they perceive that they have the ability to be successful—not because they want to experience the success, but because they do not want to be held accountable for failing. If they perceive a training goal as highly challenging, they will not even make the attempt, because they do not want to take the risk of failing. For these athletes, motivation comes not from a desire to be successful, but more from a desire to protect the ego. They will appear motivated in environments where they can be successful because if they are successful, the ego is safe. However, they may just as likely take on tasks with a very low probability of success, because if they then fail, the ego is still protected—the attitude being that they weren't supposed to be successful in the first place, so why not give it a shot? These athletes will embrace simple tasks and impossible tasks but shy away from anything truly challenging.

Motive to avoid failure is not about avoiding failure—it is about avoiding situations where failure can be attributed internally. It is about protecting one's ego.

Athletes with a motive to succeed will generally focus on the pride and confidence they experience when they are successful. They will often say that things within their control, like high effort and skill, account for their success. When they do fail, they often feel a sense of guilt, because they believe that they have it in their power to do better. On the other hand, athletes with a motive to avoid failure will more often focus on the sense of shame or worry that they experience when they are unsuccessful. They often attribute their failure to things outside of their control, like luck, bad officiating, or the skill of the other team. When they are successful, they will generally feel a sense of relief and feel grateful because they have managed to protect their ego. Paying attention to how your athletes explain or attribute their success and failure and observing their emotional reactions to these situations can tell you a lot about their achievement motivation.

GOAL SETTING

One effective tool for enhancing motivation is by setting and achieving goals we set for ourselves. Additionally, setting goals can provide direction, give feedback, and foster a sense of support as one works toward the attainment of a task. Effective goal setting produces a number of beneficial behavioral changes including more productive training and practice sessions generally resulting in more focused competition behavior.

The weight room is a great place to encourage goal setting. This is one location where the athlete has the most control over his or her own performance and is a place he or she spends concentrated amounts of time. Potential areas in strength and conditioning where goal setting might prove effective include learning appropriate lifting technique and skill refinement, improving overall strength and/or endurance, targeting specific performance markers (i.e., one-repetition maximums [1-RMs], jump heights, sprint times), developing "quality practice" behaviors, and dealing with distractions.

Goal setting can provide direction, enhance motivation, give feedback on progress, and foster a sense of support when used effectively.

PROCESS VERSUS PRODUCT GOALS

There is much discussion within the field of sport psychology about the most effective way to structure or create goal statements. Many have argued that performers should focus more on creating and reinforcing **process-based goals**, or goals that are centered in the present, rather than **product-based goals**, or those that focus more on an outcome. The idea behind this supposition is that if one effectively works toward attaining process-based goals, the probability of achieving the desired outcomes or results correspondingly increases. The outcomes will take care of themselves. Others have stated, however, that in sport settings, the outcome is what really matters, so shouldn't the goal statement then reflect this?

The reality is that every athlete is different. Some are highly motivated by the outcome or product-focused goal, using that to drive their daily behaviors—the proverbial carrot before the horse. Others may be distracted by the product goal, as it is something outside of the present. It is something "out there" and not what I need to be thinking about right now. Some find that outcome-focused goals elevate anxiety, as athletes are fixating on something not entirely within their control. As the coach, understanding how your athletes respond to different types of goal structures and how those varying goal statements help or hinder overall performance can assist you in better structuring your program designs to coincide with that athlete's tendencies.

Both process- and product-based goals can be effective at providing direction and motivating an athlete; however, process-based goals raise the probability that the desired outcomes will occur.

EFFECTIVE STRUCTURE

As the strength coach, you are contributing to, if not fully creating, the daily, weekly, monthly, seasonal, and yearly fitness goals for every athlete on the teams with which you work. As you design the training programs for these athletes, you may choose to discuss with them the rationales behind the plans you generate. Your training plans are in essence a description of the goals you have for these athletes. They fill one main purpose of goal setting: providing direction. Your training programs give athletes the direction they need, every day, week, or month, to attain the long-term strength, fitness, power, or endurance plans you have for them. When athletes take these training programs and begin to implement them, they may wish to create additional goal statements that correspond to the training plan. These goal statements may serve a variety of purposes, including the development of motivation, the enhancement of confidence, and the satisfaction and sense of pride that comes from success.

Goal Ladders

There is a Chinese proverb that states, "A journey of a thousand miles begins with a single step." This idea applies well to the creation of effective goals. Many of us can clearly list a number of long-term goals we have for ourselves—win the championship, get that great job, get an "A" in that class, etc. An understanding of the long-term goal likely also applies to the athletes in your weight room as well (bench x-number of pounds, jump this high, get my $\dot{V}O_{2max}$ to here, etc.). The long-term goal is often easy to conceptualize. It is the understanding of where to go from there—the single steps—that can be challenging. This is where "goal ladders" can be helpful.

Goal ladders are simply conceptual diagrams that outline the steps needed to attain the desired long-term goal. If, for example, the long-term goal for one of your athletes is to improve his or her front squat 1-RM, you will likely have a plan in your head for how you will progressively train that athlete to attain this outcome goal. It is unlikely that you would expect to see improvement in this skill without creating a strategic, periodized training plan that progressively outlines what the athlete will do today, this week, this month, and this season to attain this goal. Goal ladders are specific to the goal for which they are created, but generally follow a structure that includes a series of short-term, medium-range, and long-term goals that all lead to the final outcome goal. Therefore, if the long-term goal is to improve one's 1-RM by 5% by the end of this microcycle, an evaluation of several medium-range and short-term goals must occur. What needs to happen in order for me to improve by 5%? What can I do this week to improve the likelihood of that? What can I do today to take a step toward this? What can I do in this set? The purpose of each goal ladder is to give the performer something he or she can do right now that will take him or her one step closer to that long-term goal.

Goal Ladders are conceptual diagrams that show the progression of goal development along the path toward achieving the long-term goal.

SMART Goals

The acronym **SMART** has often been used to guide people in the effective formation of their goal statements. The letters stand for the following:

- S—Specific—Goals need to be written or conceptualized behaviorally in that they must provide specific guidelines on what to do or think or feel right now. The goal, "I will train with intensity" may sound good, but what does it really mean? What does "with intensity" look like? Rather, "I will focus on proper body alignment in every squat repetition I perform in practice today" is a more effective goal statement.
- M—Measurable—How will you know if you have attained a desired goal if there is no way to determine its attainment? Effective goals should have some way of establishing success or failure built into their wording. At the end of your workout, you should be able to look at your goal statements and definitively determine if you have met them.
- A—Attainable—Goals should be challenging, but attainable. If goals are set "too easy," there is no sense of accomplishment generated when success is attained. If the goal for today's practice is simply, "Complete every repetition indicated in my training plan for

today's workout," and this is an athlete who regularly completes training sessions in full, there is no motivation, reward, or feedback to be garnered from this goal statement.

- R—Realistic—Though goals must be challenging, they cannot be unreachable. If I am an athlete just coming off a lower back injury, and my goal for today's practice is to complete a set of dead lifts at my preinjury weight, I am clearly not going to attain my goal. If goals are set "too hard," the likelihood of failure is high and will thus have a tendency to be demotiviating.
- T—Time Framed—Give yourself a time frame to accomplish your goals. Having a specific window for completion of your goal gives you motivation and structure that may be lacking otherwise. This guideline also corresponds to the "Attainable" and "Realistic" descriptors as well.

ENERGY AND AROUSAL MANAGEMENT

As explained earlier in this book, an understanding of how the human body creates energy to fuel various processes is critical for any effective strength and conditioning coach. As Chandler and Arnold stated in Chapter 1 (Bioenergetics), "human movement requires energy, and energy is vital for athletic performance." Though they were talking specifically about bioenergetics from a physiological perspective, the reality is that in order for athletes to perform effectively, they also need to effectively manage their mental energy.

Mental energy is generated, maintained, depleted, and refreshed via our emotions. **Emotions** are strong feelings, having both physical and psychological manifestations that serve to energize behaviors. These energy-impacting emotions can have both beneficial and detrimental effects on human performance, often depending on how a person interprets them. Emotions are beneficial to performance when they get us excited, cause us to feel motivated, elevate confidence in ourselves, and push us to challenge ourselves in performance. Emotion can be detrimental, however, when there is too much or too little (a performer being too "amped up" or "too flat") or when we lose control of our emotions and cease to function effectively in a performance environment (i.e., an athlete who cannot control his or her anger or frustration).

Emotions are generators of mental energy and can be beneficial or detrimental to performance depending upon how a person interprets them.

FACTORS AFFECTING MENTAL ENERGY

Athletes often pay the most attention to their mental energy levels when it comes time for competition; however, it is also important to recognize how

Q & A from the Field

Q ***I coach a lot of different athletes and don't really have time to sit down with each one more than once a season to discuss their training goals. How can I effectively monitor how they are progressing?***

—DI College Strength and Conditioning Coach

A Providing feedback to your athletes need not be an overly time-consuming process. If you meet with your athletes individually at the start of the season, you can have a discussion about the various fitness and performance goals that athlete will have. If you can periodically review these goals, perhaps just a few each week, you can focus on providing encouragement and support to those athletes at that time. You may also encourage your athletes to share their goals with other members of the team, so they may continually encourage each other and hold each other accountable. Lastly, if you are able to publicly reward or acknowledge athletes who are making respectable progress toward their goals, you will likely find that your athletes' motivation improves, thereby reinforcing the process without you having to do much.

these energy levels affect performance in practice and training conditions as well. Helping your athletes understand what things "drain their battery" prior to beginning their training sessions can help mitigate potential injury. Helping them understand what things "charge their battery" can generate more motivated, focused workouts. This "charging and draining" of one's proverbial battery is simply a way of understanding how arousal levels impact performance. Athletes who are unable to effectively regulate their arousal levels may find themselves experiencing decreases in performance, as well as increased stress and worry. In order to perform at one's best, athletes need to recognize what factors contribute to the most ideal arousal levels for their performances.

A simple tool for evaluating what factors impact your athletes' arousal levels is to have them reflect on what their best performance felt like. Ask them to describe the circumstances of that day, including things like their nutrition, rest, and other physical and mental demands they may have been facing. Then have them compare that to their worst performance (or any day where they felt particularly "off"). What factors were different? What were the same? Ask them which of these factors are things they can control. Once the controllable factors are identified, encourage them to manipulate these factors to help generate an ideal arousal level for performance. If they identify factors outside of their control, remind them that these are things outside of their control, and focusing on those will only "drain their batteries." Instead, ask if there are any tools they can use to compensate for these interfering factors.

"Ain't no use worrying about things beyond your control, because if they're beyond your control, ain't no use worrying....Ain't no use worrying about things within your control, because if they are within your control, ain't no use worrying."—Mickey Rivers

IDENTIFYING EFFECTIVE AROUSAL LEVELS

Before you can help your athletes get to the "right" level of arousal or mental energy for performance, they first need to determine what that right level is for them. Optimum arousal is different for every person, and often differs within that person depending on the situation. For example, think about how much arousal or energy you need to perform a Fartlek workout. Is this the same level you would need for a plyometric test? What about for cardiovascular endurance training? Clearly each of these activities will require a different level of mental energy (as well as physical energy) to perform effectively. It is important for every athlete to know what arousal levels work best for them in different situations. Too much arousal can lead to nervousness, anxiety, muscle tension, and/or overaggressiveness. Too little arousal can lead to distraction, apathy, and concentration problems.

Optimal arousal levels will differ from person to person and from situation to situation. Performers need to identify what arousal levels work best for them in a variety of circumstances.

In an effort to better understand the relationship between energy/arousal levels and performance, many sport psychology professionals turn to the Inverted-U Hypothesis for a basic explanation. The **inverted-U hypothesis** states that performance will improve as arousal levels increase up to some optimal point. Beyond that point, however, further increases in arousal will cause performance to suffer (Fig. 18.1)

When performers are experiencing low arousal or energy levels, they will feel "flat," sluggish, or

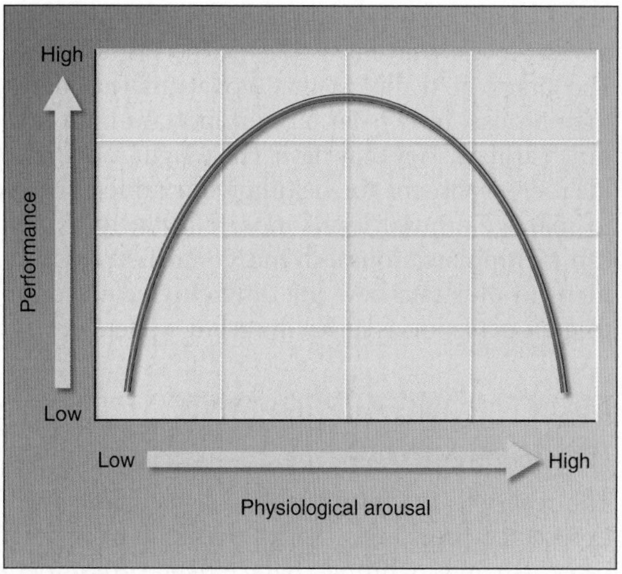

FIGURE 18.1 The inverted-U hypothesis. Performance will improve with increases in arousal levels up to some optimum point, whereupon further increases in arousal will cause a performance decrement.

tired until the energy level rises to a more optimum point. Their attention will wander, they experience a sense of apathy regarding the performance, and their body will feel physically heavy. Then as arousal increases, performers will begin to feel more energetic, motivated, and confident. This ideal performance state will begin to deteriorate, however, if performers cannot keep that mental energy level at the appropriate point. If arousal continues to increase past this ideal state, performance will start to decline, with performers now feeling too "amped up," intense, or frantic. They will feel high levels of muscle tension, have difficulty focusing, may have difficulty breathing, and may feel hyperactive. As the strength coach, you will often be able to see behavioral examples of all of these levels in your athletes. Helping them recognize their arousal levels may help them better manage these variations, thus improving their overall performance during workouts.

It is important to recognize though that not all athletes performing the same tasks will need the same level of mental energy. Every athlete will have his or her own **individual zone of optimal functioning (IZOF)** or state at which his or her best performance occurs. The Inverted-U hypothesis and IZOF constructs can help you better explain this energy–performance relationship to your athletes. Furthermore, having high or low levels of arousal is not always necessarily detrimental. Some athletes report needing to feel really excited in order to perform effectively (i.e., certain extreme sport athletes), and if they are feeling low or even moderate arousal levels, they have difficulty performing well. The practical reality is that how athletes handle their arousal level is far more important than how much arousal they may have. The weight room is an ideal environment for helping your athletes learn to manage arousal levels more effectively, as you can manipulate arousal in this controlled environment to illustrate how the differences correspond to their perceptions of feeling ready to perform.

MAINTAINING APPROPRIATE AROUSAL LEVELS

The reality is that every athlete or performer will experience pressure at some point in his or her career—it is a defining characteristic of competition—but it is the mentally skilled performer who can stay composed enough to perform despite that pressure. When your athletes recognize that they have too much arousal to perform effectively, can they calm themselves down? If they notice that they are too "flat," can they increase their arousal enough to get the job done? These are skills your athletes need on the competitive fields and courts, but having these abilities will also serve them well in the weight room and during training.

When you notice an athlete who seems to be overly pumped, is having difficulty focusing, and seems to be acting in a hyperactive way, you can suggest some very basic relaxation techniques to bring him or her back to that ideal performance zone. These are also effective tools for maximizing training effectiveness. Encouraging athletes to slow down, close their eyes, and take a few deep breaths is a quick method to decrease arousal levels. Another is having them take their pulse and try to actively slow it down. Sometimes the immediate physical feedback from measuring heart rate can help them recognize what overarousal feels like. If athletes can learn to control themselves, "then they have an opportunity to control the situation, instead of letting the situation control them. The athlete must find a relaxation technique that works for them; practice it; master it; and then reap the benefits in...their performance" (6).

Slow, controlled, deep breathing is an effective tool for managing the sensation of too much arousal, and is highly effective at bringing energy levels back to an ideal state.

More than likely, however, you will be confronted with athletes on the opposite side of this spectrum: those who have too little arousal to perform effectively during their workouts. These athletes will look sluggish, will be easily distracted, will be moving slowly, and will lack enthusiasm. When you see this is your weight room, you can suggest some simple activation techniques. First, research shows that mood is often impacted by music (7). If the athlete is too "flat," suggest a more upbeat play list on his or her iPod. Even if you do not allow headphones in your weight room, you likely have some sort of stereo system—crank it up! Respiration rate also impacts arousal level, but rather than using it to calm down, in this instance encourage the athlete to use it to pump up. Increasing one's respiration rate elevates heart rate and increases arousal levels. The use of energizing cue words, self-talk, and creating images of successful attempts can also be useful here. These will be discussed in more depth later in this chapter, but are also fairly typical sport psychology "tools" or skills often described in detail in many sport psychology textbooks.

CONCENTRATION (FOCUS)

"Every athlete quickly recognizes that without appropriate concentration their performances will be inconsistent, error prone, and less than optimal. Concentration therefore is a skill and must be learned" (6). **Concentration** can be defined as the ability to focus on appropriate cues in a given situation and control your responses to these cues for the execution of a particular skill (4). Concentration (or focus), therefore, is a skill athletes will need to perform effectively in competition, but it is also critical for effective performance in practice and conditioning sessions. Unfortunately, it is a skill that often gets overlooked until it is notably absent—that is, it is one of the psychological skill areas that may only become visible when an athlete's behavior reveals a lack of appropriate sport focus (8).

ATTENTION STYLES

One useful framework for understanding how focus or concentration works in performance settings has been Robert Nideffer's model of attention styles. This model suggests that an athlete's focus continually shifts between four quadrants, varying along two intersecting continuums from broad to narrow and from internal to external (9). This then implies that there is not just one type of concentration or attention style; rather, there are several different types that can affect performance. Furthermore, like the previous discussion of arousal levels, there is no one attention style that is best for every person in every situation. Each

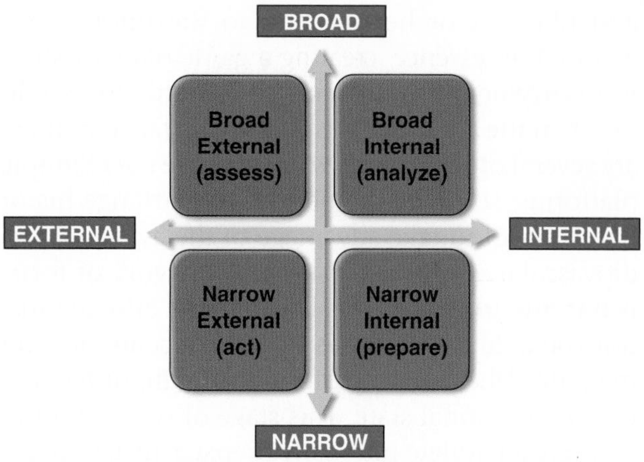

FIGURE 18.2 Nideffer's theory of attentional style. Performers need to master the ability to effectively shift their attention between each of these four quadrants.

type of athletic performance may demand one or several attention styles throughout a performance. Each athletic situation requires a variety of specific attention styles to perform adequately. Even within the same athletic team, the concentration demands on individual athletes may be quite different. It is therefore imperative for an athlete to learn to shift his or her concentration in an appropriate manner as the situation requires. In order to do this effectively, athletes must master the ability to focus in each of the four quadrants as well as be able to shift between each as necessary (9) (Fig. 18.2).

The first attention style is a **broad external focus**, where the performer will rapidly assess a situation, taking in a variety of information from the external environment. In a strength and conditioning context, this would be the necessary focus an athlete would need at the beginning of a workout where he or she would look around the room, identifying things like how many others are present, where the water containers are located, and how loud the music is. The next style is a **broad internal focus**, where the athlete will begin to analyze

REAL-WORLD APPLICATION

A Gymnast is Faced with Maintaining Concentration During Competition

During a gymnastics competition, there are many distractions that occur. There are external variables that may affect an athlete's concentration and may detract from her optimal performance. The gymnast's first event of the meet is the floor exercise. While on the floor, the gymnast has many variables on which to focus. This event involves the playing of music and synchronization of movements to the music. She will have to be able to concentrate on specific cues in the music to stay on point. In addition, competitions tend to have large crowds. Thus, there may be an excess amount of noise. She will have to be able to concentrate on the task at hand and cancel out the noise from the crowd. If she is able to focus, she will most likely perform near or at optimal level.

and plan his or her reaction to the information assessed, in essence, creating a game plan, or strategy. Carrying the same example forward, this would be when the athlete contemplates the fact that there are several other athletes waiting to use the Olympic platforms, so he or she decides to rearrange his or her workout to take advantage of the available cardiovascular equipment. The next category of focus is **narrow internal**. This is where the athlete must now be able to center his or her concentration on mentally rehearsing a performance skill, or regulating an emotional state. This stage of concentration is where an athlete internally prepares to act. In our weight room example, this could be the athlete creating a mental image of himself or herself setting the speed and pitch of the treadmill and creating the necessary energy level for a good cardio session. The fourth category of concentration is **narrow external**, where the athlete will focus entirely on one or two external cues to actually perform the action necessary. This is where the athlete will pay attention to treadmill's display, noting items like miles per hour and METs. The final requirement of attentional style needed for an athlete to perform effectively is referred to as **shifting**. While this is not a separate attentional style in and of itself, it is a critical ability for effective performance. It is absolutely necessary for athletes to have a certain amount of attentional flexibility within any given situation. In essence, they need to be adept at "bouncing" back and forth between the other four categories to assure that they are picking up all relevant cues and filtering out all irrelevant ones. For example, if our athletes on the treadmill were only focused on the display's readout, they might miss the external cue that their coach just came in the weight room looking for them. Clearly, effective concentration requires that you be adept at shifting your focus to the appropriate cues at the appropriate times.

> *Effective concentration requires a performer be adept at shifting between a broad-external, broad-internal, narrow-internal, and narrow-external focus of attention as needed to perform in any given situation.*

DISTRACTIONS

The ability to maintain concentration while immersed in competition or practice drills is critical to effective performance. However, the human brain is not capable of maintaining effective focus for the full duration of an athletic event or workout session. Therefore, we must be able to identify the factors that generate distractions and learn how to effectively deal with them so as not to interfere with performance.

Once you can recognize potential distractions, you can then create a plan for dealing with them. Athletes often report that their distractions come simply from thinking about the wrong things at the wrong times—that they have an inappropriate attentional style. Athletes often come into the weight room still focused on the things that happened earlier in their day, either at practice, or during school, or with relationships they have outside of the sporting arena. Letting go of those thoughts so that you can focus on the appropriate cues will be critical to the attainment of a good workout. Athletes tend to lose their concentration when they choose instead to pay attention to events and experiences that occurred in the past, start thinking about those that will occur in the future, and focus on things outside of their control or on things irrelevant to the task at hand. Furthermore, experiencing excessive anxiety or being overly tired can also cause distraction, as the athlete is then focused on inappropriate cues. As the coach, you can contribute to the creation of an effective performance environment by encouraging your athletes to get enough rest prior to their workouts, create a nonthreatening environment for your athletes, and encourage them to practice their concentration skills while training.

REFOCUSING STRATEGIES

There are several tools or strategies one can use to practice concentration. The weight room is often an ideal environment for this as well because it is usually a location where a multitude of things are going on at the same time, with several people doing different things, and loads of potential distractions present. If athletes can effectively tune their ability to shift between all the needed attentional styles throughout the duration of a workout, chances are pretty high that they will be able to transition those skills out onto the playing fields and courts. The following are some suggestions for practicing concentration skills:

- "Distraction Inoculations"—Create tools that simulate the typical distractions your athletes report. Things like tape recordings of crowd noise, confederate observers watching a practice session as if they were spectators, judges or other coaches on-site, evaluating the athlete as they work out, or negative words or phrases scattered around the facility to invoke negative thoughts will all work. Have the athletes practice maintaining the effective focus despite these distractions, in essence "inoculating" them to their existence.

- Cue words and positive self-talk—Cue words or phrases are things that can be said out loud or in one's head that remind them to focus on specific things. For example, athletes just learning the proper form for a power clean might choose to say the instructional cue words "Scoop!" or "Catch!" to remind themselves to focus on these elements of technique. Others might choose to use more motivational cue words (like "Come on! You've got this!") to get their energy level up and focus themselves on the feeling needed to perform well. The key to cue words is to keep them simple. More on self-talk is provided later in this chapter.
- Routines—Preperformance routines help improve focus by helping athletes transfer their attention from task-irrelevant concepts that might distract them from their preparation to those task-relevant thoughts they need to get ready to perform (4). These can be used before the training session begins (to prepare for your workout), during your workout in preparation for a challenging lift or set, and even after your workout to transition your focus away from the activities in the weight room back to whatever activity is next. Recognize, however, that routines are not the same things as superstitions. A **routine** is a conscious decision to perform an action or series of actions with the express purpose of benefitting performance in some way. A **superstition** is an action taken for fear of what might happen if the action is not taken. Routines direct focus to appropriate cues needed for effective performance. Superstitions draw focus away from these relevant cues, instead focusing on the irrelevant cue of fear of outcomes.
- 2-Minute Drill—The 2-minute drill is one many coaches use in a variety of settings to get their athletes to focus on what they will do in a particular situation. In regard to concentration training, the 2-minute drill is simply telling yourself to focus on whatever action you are performing for the next 2 minutes. At the end of that 2-minute period, you are giving yourself permission to let your attention wander. When the 2 minutes start, you are committing to fully directing your focus to the task-relevant cues needed to perform. You may become aware of internal or external distractions, but as soon as you recognize them, you make a conscious effort to bring your focus back to the task at hand. You are fully committed and fully invested in this thing right here, right now, because you know you only have to focus for 2 little minutes. This is a great exercise for practicing concentration skills because it echoes the realities of many sports. Most sporting events are composed of short bursts of plays, downs, attempts, sets or heats, followed by some sort of brief "rest" period. This occurs in resistance and interval training as well, and presents a great opportunity to challenge athletes to focus for "just this next 10-rep set" or "just this next interval" as this will get them adept at shifting in and out of intense focus.

The skills of concentration are probably the most relevant of all the psychological skills for actual performance, but they can only be mastered if the athlete has learned to control his or her arousal levels first. Concentration, anxiety, arousal, and self-confidence are all intricately interwoven, with each of these factors greatly dependent upon effective concentration skills.

CONFIDENCE AND SELF-TALK

All other things being equal, a confident athlete will perform better than one without confidence (8). **Confidence** is the belief that one's abilities are greater than or equal to the demands placed upon them. It is the belief that you can successfully perform a desired behavior. Confidence is most often situation-specific, though some athletes seem to exhibit confidence across a variety of different domains. More often, however, people are confident in some elements of their lives and less confident in others, or in one skill but not others. Confidence is a critical component for effective sport participation. Confident athletes will

- Set challenging goals for themselves.

- Recover from setbacks, losses, or disappointments fairly quickly.
- Persist when faced with adversity.
- Focus on success and the relevant cues necessary to attain it.
- Stay cool under pressure situations.
- Trust themselves, their perceptions, and their decisions.
- Push themselves past their perceived limits.

An observant strength and conditioning coach will generally be able to spot an athlete lacking in confidence. They will give up easily when situations get challenging, they are generally unwilling to take risks, they will struggle maintaining focus, they will appear tentative, and they protect themselves, both physically and mentally. The good news though is that confidence is a "teachable" skill. Like many of the other sport psychology skills described in this chapter, confidence can be developed through practice, thereby improving overall performance.

All other things being equal, confident athletes will generally outperform one with low confidence because they challenge themselves more, trust in their abilities, and stay focused on the task-relevant cues needed to perform well.

BUILDING, ENHANCING, AND MAINTAINING CONFIDENCE

As a coach, you are in a position to assist athletes in developing, enhancing, and maintaining their confidence levels, both as they relate to their sports as well as in more general aspects of their lives. Although research shows that a large part of a person's confidence is generated from success in past performances, the reality is that several other experiences and sources can contribute to this characteristic as well. Training hard and effectively can contribute to effective performance, which can enhance confidence levels. Breaking down complex skills or tasks into manageable parts and succeeding at these steps can also enhance confidence levels. Recognizing and taking control over the things you can control and letting go of those that you cannot can further enhance confidence. It is important to recognize that it is not just the "big" things that contribute to building confidence—each "little" accomplishment does too. When viewed from this perspective, every successful day in the weight room or hard workout completed can contribute to the development of confidence.

As their strength coach, the ways in which you interact with your athletes can contribute to or deteriorate their confidence in themselves. Be aware of how you communicate with your athletes, both verbally and nonverbally, during your interactions with them. You spend a great deal of time communicating expectations, teaching new skills and behaviors, providing feedback and correcting errors, and encouraging and rewarding achievement. In each of these areas, you have an opportunity to develop and reinforce confidence by acknowledging success (even the small ones) and focusing on the constructive element of criticism, rather than just the critical element. Try to "catch" your athletes being successful, rather than just catching their errors.

TYPES OF SELF-TALK

The internal language athletes use with themselves has the ability to impact everything that has been described thus far in this chapter—the setting of challenging but realistic goals, the initiation and sustaining of motivation, the trust in self to manage arousal levels, and the ability to direct and redirect focus. This internal language—**self-talk**—is essentially the process of thinking and cognition. It is the running dialogue you have going on in your head all the time. Self-talk is closely related to confidence in that a person's self-talk is generally representative of what they believe.

There are basically three types of self-talk—instructional, negative, and positive. Instructional self-talk has already been alluded to earlier in this chapter in the discussion of using cue words to direct focus. **Instructional self-talk** helps the performer focus on technical, tactical, or task-related elements of performance with the goal of improving execution (4). Encouraging your athletes to use instructional self-talk can be beneficial in the development and reinforcement of confidence because each instance can be viewed as a mini attempt at being successful. When athletes give themselves that instructional cue and then are able to follow through on that, they have just experienced success. Knowing their instructional self-talk and reinforcing it is a great way to help your athletes develop their confidence.

The next category, **negative self-talk**, is the most damaging to athletic performance but is difficult to completely avoid or control. It is generally critical and self-demeaning, interfering with a performer's appropriate focus. Anytime negative emotions (distress, anxiety, fear, or frustration) occur, chances are that the vast majority of athletes will respond by talking to themselves negatively. Physical performance can therefore be destroyed by negative self-talk. Negative self-talk and negative thinking are virtually the same thing and are generally caused by fear of failure, fear of success, comparison to others, insecurity, poor confidence, and unrealistic expectations (6). Negative self-talk lessens the control an athlete has over himself or herself, as it inhibits constructive and reinforcing thought patterns, thus eroding confidence and impairing performance.

Positive self-talk, on the other hand, is the type of talk that programs our minds with ideas that enable us to manage situations more effectively. **Positive self-talk** consists of reinforcing statements we say to ourselves generally increasing energy, effort, and positive attitude, but that do not carry any task-specific cues (4). It is solution directed, not problem focused. Positive self-talk focuses on the process, stays in the present moment, and is designed to be uplifting. It is essential for athletes to learn to talk to themselves from a positive perspective, thus enhancing the probability of consistent and optimal performance. Like any skill though, positive self-talk must be practiced to acquire positive, solution-focused inner dialogue. Habits of positive thinking can become integrated and automated by an athlete if they consciously practice developing it.

Summary

It can be argued that the weight room, in and of itself, is a performance environment, with the activities contained therein, the sporting event, and the strength and conditioning coach, the team leader. As such, all of the tools of sport psychology that a sport coach can implement with his or her athletes on the field of play and in performance and practices can be replicated and reinforced in the weight room by the strength and conditioning coach.

The full complement of sport psychology skills and tool that might benefit an athlete during his or her workouts is beyond the scope of this chapter; however, several of the most relevant constructs have been presented here. The concepts of goal setting, motivation, energy and arousal management, concentration, self-talk, and confidence development are all elements of sport psychology training that every athlete can use to better not only their performance, but their experience of that performance as well. Athletes who have practiced with these mental skills are better able to perform more consistently across competitions, recover their composure more quickly after a mistake or distraction, and perform at their best when the pressure is on. As the strength and conditioning coach, you are in a prime position to assist your athletes with these critical constructs.

Maxing Out

1. A head coach indicates that he is concerned about the motivation levels of his athletes for their training sessions. The coach asks the Strength and Conditioning coach to help "pump up" the athletes to get them more motivated for workouts. What does the S & C coach need to understand about motivation? How might they be able to better understand the existing motivation levels of the athletes? What might they be able to do to impact that motivation?
2. A football player tells the Strength and Conditioning coach that his main training goal for the season is simply "to get stronger." How can the coach work with this athlete to improve the structure and phrasing of this goal statement? How might they work together through this process to develop effective short-term and long-term goals to attain this season long mission?
3. Why is it important for an athlete to understand the ideal arousal level needed for them in the weight room? If they find that they are "too low," what might they do to elevate this energy level? If they find they are "too high," how might they get more "pumped up"?
4. Strength and Conditioning training requires different types of attention and focus at different times. When might an athlete need to have a "broad-external" focus? A "broad-internal" one? When would they need a more internal focus?
5. What kinds of self-talk might be beneficial for an athlete during conditioning training? How does an athlete's self-talk relate to their confidence?

CASE EXAMPLE

A Change in Playing Status

BACKGROUND

Mike has been playing soccer for the past 5 years. He is currently a junior and playing for his college team. He had been starting each match; however, he has recently lost his starting position. Mike is not putting as much effort into each practice, being antisocial toward teammates. As well, he has been nonresponsive during practices. What could Mike be suffering from and what might be done to help him?

CONSIDERATIONS/RECOMMENDATIONS

The behaviours exhibited by Mike could illustrate that he is suffering from decreased motivation. The strength and conditioning coach or sport psychology consultant could communicate with Mike to establish his main motivators and possibly reevaluate what he wants from the sport.

IMPLEMENTATIONS

A sport psychology consultant could work in unison with the strength and conditioning coaches and athletes to develop different strategies or techniques to better help athletes find motivation in their sport. Possible ways of accomplishing this would be by setting goals, as well as finding meaning within themselves and their sport. Over time, Mike will hopefully find new motivation within himself to perform at his optimal level, in turn possibly regaining his status within his team.

REFERENCES

1. Triplett NT, Williams C, McHenry P, et al. Strength & Conditioning Professional Standards and Guidelines (on-line). Colorado Springs, CO; NSCA, 2009. Available at: *http://www.nsca-lift.org/publications/SCStandards.pdf.*
2. Hatfield BD, Brody EB. Psychology of athletic preparation and performance. In: Baechle TR, Earle RW, eds. *Essentials of Strength Training and Conditioning*. 3rd ed. Champaign, IL: Human Kinetics; 2008:187–207.
3. Sage G. *Introduction to Motor Behavior: A Neuropsychological Approach*. 2nd ed. Boston, MA: Addison-Wesley; 1977.
4. Weinberg RS, Gould D. *Foundations of Sport and Exercise Psychology*. 4th ed. Champaign, IL: Human Kinetics; 2007.
5. Gill D. *Psychological Dynamics of Sport and Exercise*. Champaign, IL: Human Kinetics; 2000.
6. Henschen KP, Statler TA, Lidor R. Psychological factors of tactical preparation. In: Blumenstein B, Lidor R, Tenenbaum G, eds. *Psychology of Sport Training*. Oxford, UK: Meyer & Meyer; 2007:104–114.
7. Karageorghis C, Terry P. The psychophysical effects of music in sport and exercise: a review. *J Sport Behav*. 1997;20: 54–68.
8. *Sport Psychology Mental Training Manual: Coaches' Guide*. Hoboken, NJ: United States Olympic Committee; 2006.
9. Nideffer RM, Segal M. Concentration and attention control training. In Williams JM, ed. *Applied Sport Psychology: Personal Growth to Peak Performance*. 4th ed. Mountain View, CA: Mayfield; 2001:312–332.

CHAPTER 19

Gender Issues in Strength

TAMMY K. EVETOVICH • KRISTI R. HINNERICHS

OBJECTIVES

After reading this chapter, you will be able to:

- Identify the gender-specific physiological and anatomical considerations that the coach or strength and conditioning professionals may want to consider before designing a training program for their athletes.
- Understand nutritional considerations that are specific to women.
- Be aware of the injury risks and preventative measures that are unique to women.
- Appreciate the effect the menstrual cycle may have on athletic performance.
- Understand all the factors that affect an exercising pregnant woman.
- Recognize the female athlete triad and how it can affect the health of a woman.
- Understand the social and psychological factors that may impact strength training adherence and participation of a female.

KEY TERMS

Aerobic
Amenorrhea
Anaerobic
Anemia
Anterior Cruciate Ligament (ACL)
Ballistic
Basal Metabolic Rate (BMR)
Cardiac Output
Center of Gravity
Corpus Luteum
Decompression Sickness
Disordered Eating
Eating Disorders
Electrolyte
Estrogen
Eumenorrhea
Fast-Twitch Muscle
Follicle-Stimulating Hormone (FSH)
Genu Recurvatum
Gestational Diabetes
Glycogen
Hemoglobin
Hemolysis
Hip Anteversion
Hypertension
Incompetent Cervix
Intercondylar Notch
Isokinetic
Luteinizing Hormone
Macronutrient
Menarche
Menstrual Cycle
Menstruation
Micronutrient
Oral Contraceptive
Osteoporosis
Ovarian Follicle
Patellofemoral Pain Syndrome
Placenta Previa
Posterior Tibial Slope
Postpartum
Preeclampsia
Progesterone
Radiation
Recommended Dietary Allowance (RDA)
Q-Angle
Saturated Fat
Slow-Twitch Muscle
Tibiofemoral Angle
Valsalva Maneuver

Introduction

In 1970, only one out of every 27 high school girls played varsity sports. Today, that figure is one in 2.5. Female high school participation increased from 294,015 in 1971 to 2,472,043 in 1997 to 3,000,000 today. In comparison to men, about one in three high school girls play sports compared with about one in two high school boys. In addition, college participation has more than tripled, from 31,000 to 250,000.

The increase in participation has been largely attributed to Title IX legislation. Title IX is a federal law that states: "No person in the United States shall, on the basis of sex, be excluded from participation in, be denied the benefits of, or be subjected to discrimination under any education program or activity receiving Federal financial assistance…". Although athletic participation was not mentioned, it has become apparent that Title IX prohibits sex discrimination in any educational program or activity at any educational institution that is a recipient of federal funds, including high school, college, and university athletics. In addition, regardless of this important legislation, many organizations have long recognized that women should be afforded the opportunity to compete athletically and participate in all forms of physical and training activities.

National Collegiate Athletic Association (NCAA)

"An athletics program can be considered gender equitable when the participants in both the men's and women's sports programs would accept as fair and equitable the overall program of the other gender. No individual should be discriminated against on the basis of gender, institutionally or nationally, in intercollegiate athletics." (*NCAA Gender-Equity Task Force – www.ncaa.org*).

The Women's Sports Foundation

"…we want equal opportunity for our daughters to play sports so they too can derive the psychological, physiological and sociological benefits of sports participation. Sport has been… important sociocultural learning experiences for boys and men for many years. Those same benefits should be afforded our daughters." (www.womenssportsfoundation.org).

National Association for Sport and Physical Education (NASPE)

"Regard students as having equal rights to education and other professional services, regardless of gender, marital status, race, social class, political convictions, ability level or disability, religion, ethnic background, national origin, sexual orientation, age or other factors irrelevant to human development and well-being" (1).

American Association of University Professors (AAUP)

"Enhancing athletic opportunity for young women and girls is of vital importance because of the significant physical, psychological, and sociological benefits those opportunities provide. A number of studies have recognized the role that athletic opportunities for women provide in promoting greater academic success, responsible social behaviors, and increased personal skills" (2).

Thus, it is evident that women are being encouraged to take part in athletic and recreational activities, and that has led to record participation numbers. This increase in female athletic participation has spurred interest in research examining the effect physical activity has on women. Through this research, it has been shown that the health and social benefits of physical activity to women are similar to those seen in men and may provide some additional benefits specific to the female gender: decreased risk of breast cancer, decreased risk of osteoporosis, decreased likelihood of smoking, decreased teenage pregnancy rates, decreased likelihood to display signs of depression, better performance in the classroom, prevention of heart disease, and healthier body weights.

Not only has a good deal of research been conducted to determine the health benefits of physical activity in women, but there has also been considerable interest in research examining the special case that the female athlete presents to strength and conditioning professionals and coaches. This in turn has led to the question, Should women be trained like men? Do not take this question the wrong way, it is not about equality and whether or not women should be given training and participating in sports. There is no question that women should have equal opportunities to train, participate, and compete. The question is more about whether men and women should be considered separately and uniquely when designing training programs, optimizing nutritional status, and encouraging a healthy psychological profile so that each gender can compete at an optimal level. Thus, the question should more specifically be stated as such: "Should strength and conditioning professionals, athletes, and coaches recognize that men and women have differences anatomically, physiologically, and psychologically that should be given special consideration when training for fitness and competition?" Once the question is stated more specifically, we begin to realize that there are many readily apparent differences between the sexes and that they need to be trained according to their specific needs so that their fitness and athletic potential can be reached. In fact, the National Strength and Conditioning Association (NSCA) released a position statement as follows:

NSCA Position Statement (3)

Strength Training for Female Athletes

The position of NSCA:

> "It appears that proper strength and conditioning exercise programs may increase athletic performance, improve physiological function and reduce risk of injuries. These effects are as beneficial to female athletes as they are to men. The question that has to be addressed is whether female athletes require different training modalities, programs or personnel than those required by male athletes.
> Due to similar physiological responses, it seems that men and women should train for strength in the same basic way, employing similar methodologies, programs and types of exercises. Coaches should assess the needs of each athlete, male or female, individually, and train that athlete accordingly. Coaches should keep in mind that there are many more differences between individuals of the same gender than between men and women. Still, there are many psychological and/or physiological considerations that should be taken into account in training female athletes."

This chapter attempts to address the many physiological, anatomical, sociological, and psychological considerations that come to the forefront when considering women and how they should be trained for fitness and competition.

ANATOMICAL AND PHYSIOLOGICAL DIFFERENCES

There are substantial differences between men and women when considering anatomical and physiological variables that may impact training and performance. Table 19.1 provides a gender comparison for many of these variables. For example, from an anatomical perspective, on an average, women are shorter than men, have higher percent body fat, and have smaller bone mass. Physiologically, compared with men, women have higher resting heart rates, lower lung volumes, unique hormone profiles, and similar muscle fiber type distribution patterns. In addition, women tend to be weaker than men in absolute terms but when strength is expressed per unit of muscle mass the differences begin to disappear.

TABLE 19.1 ● GENDER COMPARISONS OF MEN TO WOMEN

PHYSIOLOGICAL AND ANATOMICAL VARIABLES	GENDER COMPARISON
Height	Women are shorter than men
Weight	Women weigh less than men per kg of body weight Women have more fat weight than men Women have less fat free weight than men
Circumferences	Women generally have smaller circumferences
Diameters	Women generally have smaller diameters with narrower shoulders, smaller chest diameters, but a wider pelvis relative to their body size
% Body fat	Women have higher body fat (average for 20- to 34-year-old men and women is 12% and 28%, respectively)
Bones	Women have smaller bones than men, with peak bone mass occurring around age 25
Ligaments	Women have smaller ligaments and may have differences in ligament laxity due to differences in steroidal hormones
Joints	Women have greater joint laxity
Absolute strength	Women are 35%–80% as strong as men (35%–50% for upper body and 60%–80% for lower body)
Muscle fiber cross-sectional area	Women less than men
Fast-twitch to slow-twitch muscle fiber area	Women less than men
Intramuscular fat and connective tissue	Women greater than men
Strength per unit of muscle cross-sectional area	Women are equal to men for the most part although this is debatable for the upper body whereby women may be less than men.
Resting testosterone levels	Women lower than men
Muscle hypertrophy	The degree to which female muscle hypertrophies is smaller in absolute terms but the relative degree of hypertrophy is equal to that of men.
Resting growth hormone levels	Women greater than men
Rate of muscle force development	Women slower than men in absolute terms but relatively the same (based on a percent of maximal force)
Fiber type	Muscle fiber type (slow vs. fast twitch) distribution patterns are similar for men and women
Posture	Women have greater anterior pelvic tilt, femoral internal rotation, knee hyperextension, and knee valgus.
Q angle	Quadriceps (Q angle) = 8–15 in men and 12–19 in women
Flexibility	Women are more flexible than men at all ages and throughout the lifespan
Lung volume	Women have lower tidal and ventilatory lung volumes
Heart rate	Adult Women have averages 5–10 beats · min^{-1} faster resting heart rates than adult men.
VO_{2max}	Women less than men
Cardiac output	Women less than men
Hemoglobin	Women less than men

TABLE 19.1 ● GENDER COMPARISONS OF MEN TO WOMEN *(continued)*

PHYSIOLOGICAL AND ANATOMICAL VARIABLES	GENDER COMPARISON
Reaction time	Women same as men
Running economy and endurance	At the same submaximal velocity elite male runners are more economical then female runners
Limb length	Women have shorter limb length relative to body length
Pelvis width	Women wider than men
Shoulder width	Women narrower than men
Intercondylar notch	Women narrower notch
Posterior tibial slope	Women greater slope
Surface area to body mass ratio	Larger than men
Sweat rate	Lower rate than men

TRAINING CONSIDERATIONS FOR ANATOMICAL AND PHYSIOLOGICAL GENDER DIFFERENCES

In general, men and women respond similarly when examining strength, hypertrophic, and metabolic responses to training. Both sexes have specific training needs and their programs should be based upon their objectives, activities that they will participate in, and their individual genetic predispositions. However, there are some training considerations that come to light in that many of the anatomical and physiological gender-related differences noted in Table 19.1 could potentially translate into variations in training methods and athletic performance. For example, with regard to resistance training, given that some research has found that women may have lesser upper-body strength, even when taking into consideration strength relative to lean body mass and cross-sectional area, it may behoove the female client/athlete who participates in sports and activities that require strong upper body strength (swimming, power lifting, softball, volleyball) to spend a greater amount of time during training on their upper-body strength (4). In addition, it has been suggested (4) that women should devote more time, particularly during the off-season, to resistance training that causes a high metabolic demand, with high volume and multiple sets with short rest periods (hypertrophic training), given that this may increase the acute hormone response to exercise, stimulate lean body mass, and then further stimulate an acute hormonal response. The increased acute hormonal response during the hypertrophic phase would then result in greater development in the strength and power phases of a training program. Finally, coaches and personal trainers may want to consider altering lifting technique for some women. It is thought that narrow shoulder width observed in women may be cause for concern when performing overhead lifts. Thus, coaches and personal trainers should pay close attention to hand spacing in women. Also, because of differences between the sexes in the Q angle and greater pelvic width, some have suggested that women may want to perform squats with a toe forward stance; however, others have not deemed this change necessary. The strength and conditioning professionals should make their best judgment on what technique and stance is appropriate for each athlete.

Some other sex-related anatomical variations that may lead to altered training and measurement methods include

- Because women have smaller bones and therefore, lower bone mass, strength training and weight-bearing exercises may be particularly important to incorporate into the woman's strength and conditioning routine so that they are not as likely to develop osteoporosis later in life.
- With smaller ligaments there is some thought that this difference may be responsible for the higher incidences of ligament injury found in women, particularly at the knee. In addition, greater joint laxity, possibly due to gender differences in hormone profiles, may increase the risk for injury in women. There are many

conditioning programs aimed at decreasing the risk of joint injury in the female athlete (5–10).
- Body fat and body weight recommendations should be based upon % body fat not body weight. Optimal levels of % body fat are sport specific and coaches/athletes should know that accurate assessment of body fat can be difficult and is dependent upon the type of technique used and the competence of the person doing the measuring. Before any weight loss or gain program is undertaken, coaches and personal trainers need to be aware of the societal signals that may be pressuring women and affecting their assessment of their own body image. **Eating disorders** are observed at a great rate in women and team weigh-ins or other public measurements of weight should be discouraged in order to avoid making the female self-consciousness of her body weight. For athletes, it is recommended that body fat gain and loss programs should be undertaken in the off-season and be under the guidance of a nutritionist or other professional educated on the recommended nutrition levels for **macronutrients** and **micronutrients** so that body fat goals can be met in a healthy manner (11).

There are many anatomical and physiological differences that can impact physical activity and performance when comparing men to women.

ANATOMICAL AND PHYSIOLOGICAL SUMMARY

It is apparent that coaches and trainers should at least consider the dissimilarity in anatomy and physiology when comparing men to women. Although men and women have very similar responses to training there may be some slight modifications in training regimens that can be made to optimize health, fitness, and athletic performance among women.

SOCIAL AND PSYCHOLOGICAL CONSIDERATIONS FOR RESISTANCE TRAINING

It is commendable that so much progress has been made in encouraging women to participate in strength and power training activities and many women have begun to realize the full benefits of participating in these types of activities. However, cultural and sociological pressure is an issue that needs to be considered when expecting the female client to adhere to a strength training program. There are still concerns about feminine appearance, appropriateness of behavior, self-esteem, and self-consciousness both inside and outside the weight room. In addition, there continues to be misinformation about the importance of strength training for maximizing female athletic performance. A recent survey (12) indicated that male student-athletes were more likely to consider weight training an essential part of every training program regardless of sport and were more likely to weight train more days per week with more minutes per training session. Not only are women struggling to decide whether to incorporate resistance training into their days but some coaches of female athletes do not consider it a principal component of an overall conditioning program (12). The same survey mentioned above (12) indicated that weight training was more frequently required by coaches of male student-athletes than by coaches of female student-athletes. The authors of this study went on to say that this difference was an "indication that coaches of women athletes may not consider weight training an important element as part of an athlete's regular training program," and it is clear that we must teach that weight training is important for female and male student-athletes.

There are many points to reflect upon when attempting to understand the social stigmas that women encounter when considering whether to begin and adhere to a strength training program. The following are some general considerations and recommendations when attempting to create an environment that is more socially acceptable and inviting to female resistance trainers:

- Help women realize that it is not physiologically possible (due to their hormonal profile) to amass large amounts of muscle, and large increases in muscle size do not become visually apparent in women. Women who avoid heavy resistance training should know that body circumferences do not increase with the increase in muscle mass that accompanies resistance training. In fact, circumferences may decrease due to a loss of fat with training.
- Having a female role model in the weight room is important for social acceptance,

particularly for young girls. Both male and female strength and conditioning coaches need to be available in all facilities.
- Make sure men and women have equal access to weight room equipment so that they will be more likely to adhere to a program.
- Create a weight room environment and culture that is not intimidating to women.
- Make sure that separate men's and women's weight rooms have equitable types of equipment and machines.
- When setting up fitness room equipment consideration should be given to the outlay of the facility and the ability of a woman to maintain her modesty while lifting. This may mean that certain pieces of equipment should be turned or faced toward a wall or be placed in a more private area so that the woman feels comfortable in the weight room environment.
- Consider not having mirrors on some walls in a fitness facility so that individuals can participate in floor work and face away from the middle of the facility and not be concerned about how their reflection may be viewed by others in the facility.
- Make sure that there is a wide array of weights and machines that can accommodate all levels of weight training and that are the proper dimensions for many different types of body weights, statures, and sizes.
- Remove all magazines and reading materials that may have sexist images or portray women in an unhealthy manner from the weight room and other training facilities.
- Do not allow language in the weight room that someone may find offensive.
- Do not play music or television programs in the weight room that are offensive or sexist.

Although great progress has been made in convincing women that weight training is safe, socially acceptable, and beneficial for maximizing fitness and performance, there is still much work that needs to be done. It can be challenging for educators, personal trainers, and coaches to facilitate adherence to a resistance training program in women. Raising social awareness, erasing myths, confronting negative attitudes, and challenging stereotypes are all important tasks that must be undertaken in order to bolster support so that women can be viewed as athletes and competitors in the weight room without having to sacrifice their femininity.

BOX 19.1

Improving Resistance Training Adherence

A recent article (13) outlined the "Strategies for Improving Resistance Training Adherence in Female Athletes." Although most of the recommendations are true for men and women, the primary objectives outlined in this article are particularly important for women:

- Develop a positive relationship with the athlete.
- Learn about the athlete's history and confidence related to resistance training.
- Learn about the athlete's perceptions, expectations, and goals.
- Educate the athlete.
- Identify constraints and possible reasons for lapses in adherence.
- Develop appropriate goals.
- Start and progress the athlete appropriately.
- Create a program that is conducive to the constraints of the athlete.
- Create alternatives to weight room strength training.
- Create group exercise sessions to provide peer modeling of resistance training.
- Retest strength and functional abilities, reward progress.
- Provide a planned and unplanned feedback system.
- Create an exercise environment conducive to resistance training adherence.

MENSTRUAL CYCLE

Many times coaches, strength and conditioning professionals, athletes, and other active women ask the question, "Does the menstrual cycle affect athletic performance and adherence to physical activity programs in women?" More specifically, these individuals are justifiably asking whether the steroid hormone fluctuations that occur during the menstrual cycle can maximize or hinder performance depending upon the phase of the cycle. Before we can examine this question, however, a basic understanding of the menstrual cycle is necessary.

FOLLICULAR PHASE

The menstrual cycle can be divided up into three phases: the follicular phase, ovulation, and the luteal phase. The follicular phase begins with the onset of **menstruation** (day 1) and lasts through about day 13. During this phase immature eggs called primordial follicles begin to develop into primary follicles, in response to an increase in **follicle-stimulating hormone (FSH)**, which start to produce very low levels of **estrogen**. Although about 20 follicles begin developing during a cycle, only one attains maturity and is released and continues to produce estrogen. The estrogen level continues to increase and peaks about 24 to 48 hours before ovulation. The rising level of estrogen stimulates the hypothalamus to secrete **luteinizing hormone (LH)** so that there is an LH "surge" during the late follicular phase. It is this surge that triggers ovulation. Thus, in summary, FSH is needed to make the follicles mature, the growing follicles release estrogen, which ultimately results in the LH surge. As LH surges, estrogen levels begin to decrease and another hormone, **progesterone**, begins to increase.

OVULATION

The LH surge causes the primary follicle to burst and release its egg (ovulate). This release usually occurs around day 14 of a 28 day cycle.

LUTEAL PHASE

After ovulation the luteal phase begins and continues until the first day of menstruation (beginning of the follicular phase). During this phase the empty follicle is now called the **corpus luteum**, or yellow body, which secretes primarily progesterone. Progesterone levels will reach a peak about 7 days after ovulation. The hormones secreted during this phase prevent new follicles from developing and any further release of eggs so that multiple ovulations do not occur during a cycle. In addition, progesterone is important in supporting a pregnancy should the egg be fertilized and the corpus luteum will continue to support the egg until the placenta can take over. If fertilization does not occur, the corpus luteum will quickly begin to stop functioning as the luteal phase progresses and progesterone levels begin to decrease. It is this decrease in hormone levels that trigger menstruation and allow a new cycle to begin. The menstrual cycle will begin anew and FSH will begin to stimulate the maturation of primordial follicles.

Given our brief discussion on the phases of the menstrual cycle, it is apparent why those working with female athletes wonder whether the menstrual cycle and the evident fluctuations in steroid hormones (estrogen and progesterone in particular) that occur over the cycle, could affect performance. In summary, estrogen starts to increase in the follicular phase, peaking around ovulation, and during the luteal phase both estrogen and progesterone are elevated. It is hypothesized that these fluctuations in hormones could have many physiological ramifications that could affect performance including changes in thermoregulation, respiration, and strength of muscular contraction. Reviews (14–17) have been written over the years examining the effect of menstrual cycle phase on performance. However, although this topic has been examined quite extensively, there is still much research that needs to be conducted to fully understand the effect it has on women and their performance. In fact, given all the confounding factors that could affect the results of this type of research, the issue remains murky. Small sample sizes and case studies, the type of subjects used in the studies (trained vs. untrained; sport specific athletes), different types of exercise testing in the research, study eligibility criteria, method for verification of menstrual cycle phase, examining maximal neural activation versus voluntary muscle actions, **oral contraceptive** usage and dosage, menstrual history, menstrual disturbances, all need to be considered when examining the research. Nevertheless a recent report (17) attempted to provide the most recent findings in the research on this matter for muscle strength and fatigability, maximal oxygen consumption (VO_{2max}), and prolonged aerobic activities.

It is possible that the hormone fluctuations that occur across the menstrual cycle can affect performance.

MUSCLE STRENGTH AND ENDURANCE

It is thought that steroid hormones like estrogen and progesterone may improve strength and deter muscle fatigue at certain phases of the menstrual cycle. Many studies have been conducted on women, yet it is difficult to compare studies when hormone concentrations and menstrual cycle phase were not verified, the maximum force-generating capacity of the muscle was not reached (superimposed electrical stimulation was not applied to the muscle), and/or the subjects were taking some type of oral contraceptive ("the pill"). When limiting this discussion to studies whereby maximal electrical stimulation was applied, hormone level verification was conducted accurately, and subjects were non-pill users, it was concluded (17) that menstrual cycle phase does not affect muscle strength and fatigability. There was a more recent study (18), however, that satisfied all the methodological considerations above and did find a significant increase in strength (isokinetic knee extension and flexion and isometric knee flexion) around ovulation. Thus, although much research has already been conducted in this area of interest, it seems prudent to conclude that the effects of the menstrual cycle on muscular strength remain to be determined.

VO_{2max}

Although there are potentially many factors that could theoretically affect aerobic endurance performance across the menstrual cycle two issues have come to the forefront and have received the most interest: fluid and body temperature changes.

Fluid Fluctuations

There are many potential factors related to body fluids and hormonal fluctuations that could theoretically affect VO_{2max}. For example, changes in body weight due to fluctuations in fluid retention across the cycle could affect VO_{2max}. Fluid fluctuations may also affect plasma volume, which could ultimately affect the ability to transport oxygen (**hemoglobin** concentration) to the working tissues. In addition, blood loss is a factor that many endurance athletes seem to worry about when considering the effect of menstruation on performance.

Unfortunately, not many studies examining this topic have done a good job verifying menstrual cycle phase with hormone measurements and/or did not conduct measurements often enough during the cycle to really give a good indication of whether athletes should be concerned about whether their performance may be affected. However, after examining the literature there may be two potential factors that the coach and athlete may want to consider. First, if daily measurements of body weight are conducted, there may be some indication that a slight increase in body weight may be present during the late luteal and early follicular (during menstruation) phases. In those sports where body weight plays a crucial role, performance may be affected. Secondly, women who lose significant amounts of blood (more than 80 mL) during menstruation have been shown to have a significantly lower hemoglobin concentration (17). For those women, endurance performance may be affected.

Changes in Body Temperature

Body temperature (BT) increases during ovulation and remains elevated during the luteal phase (19). This increase is thought to be caused by the increasing progesterone levels observed during this phase. An increase in BT could affect endurance athletes in many ways such as increasing heart rate and/or creating greater cardiovascular strain (particularly in the heat). An increase in BT causes the brain to send blood to the superficial blood vessels of the skin. As more blood flows through capillaries close to the body surface, more heat can be lost to the environment by **radiation**, which will help to lower body temperature. This means that less blood is available to be sent to working muscles and the heart rate will then increase to maintain **cardiac output**. It has been determined that for every 1-degree increase in BT the resultant increase in HR may be as much as 7 beats $\cdot$ min^{-1}. These changes may seem important when considering whether endurance performance may be affected, however, it should be noted that the increase in BT observed in the luteal phase is only about 0.5 degrees. Thus, as may be expected, most studies report no change in exercising heart rate over the menstrual cycle. But what if you compound the BT increase observed during the luteal phase by exercising in a hot and humid environment? There is some indication that increased body temperature during the luteal phase (due to the increased progesterone levels) may affect prolonged aerobic performance, particularly in the heat, due to the resulting cardiovascular strain (17).

Heat Illness When an individual exercises, heat is produced with muscular activity and if the heat production is compounded with a decreased ability to dissipate the heat (via conduction or radiation) due to a hot or humid environment, there is an increased risk of developing a heat illness. When looking at heat illness from a gender perspective, a woman has some unique characteristics that have led some to theorize that she is at an even greater risk of developing some sort of heat disorder. For example, women have lower sweating rates due to a larger surface-area-to-mass ratio, the threshold for the onset of sweating may be greater during the luteal phase, and as stated earlier, there is a slight increase in core temperature during the luteal phase of a woman's menstrual cycle (16,20,). In addition, women may have fluctuations in body weight with the menstrual cycle and in general have higher body fats and lower $\dot{V}O_{2max}$ values, which may mean that they are working harder than men at a given level of intensity.

After reading above it may seem almost certain that women are suffering from heat illness on a regular basis when compared to men. Interestingly, however, women have been shown to be very tolerant to heat while exercising, even during the luteal phase. In fact, a recent review by Marsh and Jenkins (16) plainly explains the implications for the development of heat illness in women and indicated that the surge in estrogen observed before ovulation may lower the hormonally increased setpoint, which could prove to be a beneficial adaptation for women exercising in the heat at this point in the menstrual cycle. Having said this, however, research into the development of heat illness in women still remains to be conducted and common sense dictates that both men and women should understand the symptoms of heat illness and may want to adjust their training and competition schedule whenever possible so that they are not exercising during the hottest part of the day.

MENSTRUAL CYCLE TRAINING CONSIDERATIONS AND CONCLUSIONS

There are not many indications that there are physiological variables that affect exercise performance across the menstrual cycle for regularly menstruating women who participate in strength-specific or anaerobic/aerobic sports and activities. After much review and reading of the literature, the only potential physiological factor that may be of concern to the coach of a female is that there is possibly a detrimental effect on performance for those women who participate in prolonged exercise in the heat during the luteal phase. In these instances, athletes and coaches may want to adjust their training and competition schedule to the woman's menstrual cycle, so that the time spent in training is used most efficiently.

It should be pointed out that in order to have more control for extraneous variables and to more readily verify menstrual cycle phases, most studies examining the effect of the menstrual cycle on performance only use **eumenorrheic** (regularly menstruating) subjects. With that in mind, most findings suggest that eumenorrheic female athletes should not be affected by menstrual cycle phase, however, we do not know if this statement holds true for those women who have menstrual disturbances. There is much inter- and intraindividual variation with regard to the effect that menstrual cycle can have on each specific woman, and recognition of this individuality should be considered.

Although there are not many physiological indicators that have been shown to affect performance with regard to the menstrual cycle, can we definitively conclude that, for the most part, a woman's menstrual cycle does not affect her performance? Just ask any woman and she will tell you that the effect of the menstrual cycle should not be discounted. Why? Many women report that changes in energy, mood, pain, etc., are apparent during certain phases of their cycle (usually before or during menstruation) and that their performance is affected due to discomfort, lack of motivation, and/or changes in mental status and mood. Thus, coaches and strength and conditioning professionals may want to consider whether there are methods to make the active and competitive woman more comfortable, whether it be the use of ibuprofen to help with pain and discomfort, medications to help regulate the cycle, stress management techniques to help with mood fluctuations, and/or methods to motivate the athlete or recreationally active woman so that she can perform at peak levels. Women usually understand their bodies very well and should experiment with all kinds of methods and techniques and find what works best for them.

USING ORAL CONTRACEPTIVES TO MANIPULATE THE CYCLE

One method that some women utilize if they are concerned about the effect that the menstrual cycle may have on their performance, or if they are looking to control for the symptoms that accompany their menstrual cycle (mood changes, discomfort, etc.), is to use oral (by mouth) contraceptives (OCs). A recent review (21) nicely outlined the prevalence of the use of OCs in female athletes. It was reported through published and anecdotal data collection that the use of OCs has increased from 5% to 12% in the early 1980s to 83% of elite athletes in 2008 (21).

So why do women take OCs and how do they work? OCs are small pills that are taken by mouth daily and are a combination of synthetic estrogen and progesterone. OCs usually come in a package of 28 pills that contain 21 active pills with hormones and 7 placebo pills; however, there are many other formulations. In addition, there are other methods of absorbing these small amounts of hormones into the body (vaginal rings, injection, vaginal inserts) but most research that has been reviewed for this topic involved OC ingestion. Nevertheless, all serve to prevent pregnancy primarily by preventing ovulation. How? Going back to our discussion of the phases of the menstrual cycle, OCs "fool" the body so that it produces less FSH and LH so that the follicle is not developed and released.

So how could OCs potentially help athletic performance? Due to the consistent consumption of these small amounts of hormones on a daily basis it is thought that women are considered to be in a more "stable" hormonal environment (even though there is a placebo week where hormones are withdrawn) and that performance, therefore, will be less affected by hormonal fluctuations. Some have also hypothesized that the small amounts of steroid hormones found in these pills could help build strength. OCs are often prescribed for a variety of reasons including: prevention of pregnancy, to regulate the cycle particularly with **amenorrhea**, to prevent cramping/pain, to regulate heavy flow, to aid in performance, to prevent injury (22), and possibly as a means to prevent menstruation for convenience and psychological reasons. For the most part, however, most users of OCs are taking these synthetic hormones to prevent pregnancy and to alleviate the discomfort associated with menstruation. But what if the pill actually affected performance based upon physiological factors?

A recent review (21) indicated that there is the potential for aerobic capacity, anaerobic capacity, anaerobic power, and reactive strength to vary between users of oral contraceptives when compared to non-OC users. However, it was noted that due to variations in methodological procedures in studies examining this issue (again, small sample sizes in the research studies, the type of subjects used in the studies, and different types formulations of OCs), it is difficult to discern whether OCs affect performance. However, the review did provide some short conclusions:

Anaerobic Activity—it is unclear whether anaerobic performance is affected by OC consumption. There have been some studies that have shown that anaerobic capacity and reactive strength (important in sprinting and jumping performance) (23) could be affected at certain times in the OC cycle.

Muscular Strength—it is generally accepted that the hormones found in OCs do not have enough of an androgenic effect to influence muscular strength over an OC cycle (24).

Aerobic Performance—there is very little evidence to suggest that aerobic performance is affected by OC use, however much research remains to be conducted.

ADVANTAGES AND DISADVANTAGES TO OC USAGE

Confused yet? There are many factors that need to be considered by an athlete and her coach while reviewing the research so that an informed decision can be made as to whether taking an OC would be beneficial. Before deciding, a woman should consider the potential advantages and disadvantages.

Potential Advantages

For those women who do not want to become pregnant the pill may be an acceptable form of contraception.

For those women who are amenorrheic and have the potential for developing **osteoporosis**, OC usage may be beneficial. However, it should be noted that there are conflicting reports as to whether OCs can actually help prevent bone loss in amenorrheic individuals.

For those women who want to manipulate their cycle (delaying or initiating menstruation) for training and competition purposes, the pill may be helpful. It should be noted that this is a controversial use for the pill and some physicians do not condone this method since not menstruating can mask health problems that manifest themselves through changes in the amount of bleeding that is observed.

For those women who would like to experience the convenience of not menstruating there are some OC formulations that limit the number of times per year that menstruation will occur.

For those women who have significant cramping and pain before and during menstruation, OCs may alleviate the discomfort.

For those women who think the menstrual cycle could affect their performance from a physiological standpoint (affecting strength, aerobic capacity, anaerobic performance) and want to have a more stable hormone profile across the cycle, OC use may be for them.

For those endurance athletes who experience severe blood loss during menstruation, OCs may reduce blood loss and decrease the potential for impaired oxygen carrying capacity.

For those women who think that the more stable hormone environment provided by OCs will help prevent injury (22), perhaps they will choose to take the pill, although athletes should not be advised that OCs will definitely reduce the risk of injury.

Potential Disadvantages

Some women who take OCs experience side effects such as fluid retention, breast tenderness, and nausea. In addition, there is the possibility of **hypertension**, cardiovascular disease, and increased risk of breast cancer for some women. Of particular concern for athletes may be the weight gain that for some (not all), can accompany pill usage since that can directly affect performance. In addition, it actually can be a controversial decision, when a woman is deciding whether or not to take the pill. For example, there are some who think that taking a synthetic hormone is considered unethical. These self-named "purists" do not think any exogenous hormones should be put into the body.

Regardless of the reason, an athlete needs to make an informed and individualized decision, in consultation with her strength and conditioning professional and physician as to whether taking the pill is a good decision. Daily consumption of an OC can affect each woman in a different manner. This decision can be affected by an athlete's moral values, type of sport for which she competes, individual physiological response to the pill, level of menstrual discomfort, health profile, etc…and the right of a woman to make this decision on an individualized basis should be respected and not dictated.

FEMALE ATHLETE TRIAD

As mentioned earlier, the menstrual cycle does not, for the most part, affect performance. But does exercising and participating in athletics affect the menstrual cycle? Women involved in intense exercise can experience disturbances in the menstrual cycle including delayed **menarche**, cessation of menstruation, and infertility. In fact, when these disturbances in the menstrual cycle are accompanied by other risk factors (disordered eating, low bone mineral density, inadequate caloric intake) it is referred to as a syndrome known as the female athlete triad. The female athlete triad is a term used to refer to the relationship between low energy intake, menstrual disturbances, and low bone mineral density. The estimated prevalence rate has been reported to be as high as 62% in female athletes (although men can be diagnosed with this syndrome as well) (25). At particular risk are those women who compete in sports and activities where leanness, low body weight, and body image are considered important. It should be noted that it is not just competitive athletes that are at risk but those women and young girls who regularly engage in intense physical activity should also be considered to be at high risk.

The syndrome begins with inadequate dietary intake. This can be a result of severe restriction of calories (due to an intentional reduction in food intake, disordered eating, or intense physical training without a concomitant increase in calories). If low caloric intake continues the athlete can then experience a disrupted menstrual cycle. In addition, the low caloric intake results in the inadequate intake of certain vitamins and minerals (such as vitamin D and calcium) and lower hormone levels (estrogen) that are essential for normal bone growth and building. The inability to reach peak bone mass during the early years of a woman's life may not be reversible and ultimately result in a diagnosis of osteoporosis. The low bone mineral density observed in these women may also put them at greater risk (when compared to eumenorrheic women) for stress fractures (26).

> ***The female athlete triad is a term used to refer to the relationship between low energy intake, menstrual disturbances, and low bone mineral density.***

Coaches and trainers can be instrumental in recognizing the signs and symptoms of this syndrome. Early detection and diagnosis is critical in order to prevent compromised health in the long-term. There are many published guidelines for the recognition, diagnosis, and treatment of the triad (25–28). It is recommended that screening occur during the

BOX 19.2

Signs and Symptoms of an Eating Disorder

Although most coaches and strength and conditioning professionals may not be clinically trained to treat someone with an eating disorder, they should be acquainted with the signs and symptoms of an eating disorder. The following are some signs and symptoms that a strength and conditioning professional or coach may be able to recognize (25):

- Changes in eating habits (unnecessary dieting, not eating, secretive or ritualistic eating habits)
- Changes in exercise behaviors (excessive or unnecessary exercising)
- Exercising while injured despite medically prescribed activity restrictions
- Depression
- Restlessness
- Distorted body image and exhibiting self-criticism
- Intense fear of gaining weight and excessive frequency of weight measurements
- Social withdrawal
- Irritability
- Insomnia
- Concerns about eating in public or frequently eating secretively
- Inflexible thinking and limited spontaneity
- Cold intolerance
- Constipation or other bowel irregularities
- Stress fractures
- Amenorrhea or menstrual dysfunction
- Dry skin
- Brittle hair and nails
- Dizziness
- Low blood pressure
- Irregular heartbeat
- Sores in the mouth or throat
- Damaged teeth or gums
- Use of diet pills, laxatives, or diuretics
- Going to the bathroom immediately after a meal or snack
- Hair loss
- Low heart rate (bradycardia)
- Low blood sugar (hypoglycemia)
- Muscle cramping
- Callus or abrasion on back of hand (from inducing vomiting)
- Fine downy body hair (lanugo)
- Lethargy and fatigue
- Eating until the point of pain or discomfort (binge eating)
- Substance abuse (legal, illegal, prescription, or over-the-counter)

preparticipation exam or annual health screening. Treatment of this disorder requires a multidiscipline approach among the coach, strength and conditioning professional, physician, a dietician, and family. Treatment may involve a combination of nutritional counseling (these women should be carefully monitored for adequate caloric intake and proper nutrition), psychological counseling, family involvement, and pharmacological therapy.

NUTRITION

Caloric intake for an inactive woman should be between 1,600 and 2,000 calories $\cdot$ d^{-1}. However, when a woman exercises, there is a need for increased caloric intake to 2,200 to 2,400 calories $\cdot$ d^{-1} or more and up to 3,000 calories $\cdot$ d^{-1} may be necessary for extremely active competitive athletes. Further, a more specific recommendation of 39 to 44 kcal $\cdot$ kg body weight^{-1} $\cdot$ d^{-1} may be necessary for strength training female athletes (29). It has also been recognized that women may need to consume slightly more kcals during the follicular phase of their menstrual cycle to maintain body weight, given that the resting energy expenditure rate is higher during the luteal phase compared to the follicular phase. For an excellent description of a more detailed method for calculating energy requirements, see the review by Volek et al. (29).

Unfortunately, women are at a great risk for micro- and macronutrient deficiencies. Table 19.2 provides specific recommendations for those nutrients that are commonly important or deficient for women. It is common for women to resist increasing their calorie intake, participate in disordered eating (10 times more prevalent in women than men), eliminate a particular food item from their diet, focus on consuming only certain food items, or participate in severe weight loss practices because of fears of gaining weight and changing their appearance. In addition, there are many sports that are "weight dependent" whereby because athletes' performance is affected by their weight, they try to cut their caloric intake to keep their body weight low. Further, for many athletic competitions there are contour-revealing uniforms or the body appearance is important for scoring. These sports include gymnastics, long distance running, ballet, diving, and skating, to name a few. Women in these sports in particular may be struggling to

TABLE 19.2 ● SOURCES OF KEY NUTRIENTS FOR FEMALE ATHLETES

	GOOD SOURCES	UL OR RDA
Iron	Beans, spinach, dried fruits, meat, liver	15–18 mg · d^{-1}
Calcium	Milk, yogurt, cheese, salmon, sardines, broccoli, spinach, kale	1,000–1,500 mg · d^{-1}
Zinc	Meat, milk, seafood	8 mg · d^{-1}
Magnesium	Nuts, seafood, green leafy vegetables, whole-grains	310–310 mg · d^{-1}
Vitamin D		
B-Vitamins	Lean meats, dairy products, whole grains, eggs	Thiamin 1.1 mg · d^{-1} Riboflavin 1.1 mg · d^{-1} B6 1.3 mg B12 2.4 mg Folate 400 DFE (dietary folate equivalents)
Protein	Lean meats, eggs, milk, yogurt, beans, nuts, soy	1.2–1.7 g · kg body weight · d^{-1}
Carbohydrates	Fruits, vegetables, brown rice, whole grain bread and cereals, potatoes,	6–10 g · kg body weight^{-1} · d^{-1}
Fats	Oils, nuts, seeds, avocados, lean meat, low-fat dairy	20%–35% of daily intake

balance their food intake with concerns about their performance and body image. For these reasons, we may find that the female athlete is deficient in many vitamins and minerals because they just are not eating enough food and/or are not getting enough variety of foods. This ultimately can affect the female athlete's health, performance, and body image. The following is a discussion of only those nutritional considerations that are specific to the female athlete. For a thorough discussion of nutritional consideration for all athletes see the nutrition chapter in this book.

MICRONUTRIENTS (VITAMINS AND MINERALS)

Micronutrients are dietary nutrients like vitamins and minerals needed by the body in small amounts. While most micronutrients can be consumed in adequate amounts from regular food items in the diet, after a dietary analysis a woman may find that a dietary supplement is necessary.

Minerals

Though there are many minerals that are important for athletic performance, the primary minerals that female athletes may need to focus on are iron, calcium, zinc, and magnesium.

Iron Iron is important for helping red blood cells carry oxygen to working muscles and for production of metabolic enzymes. The **recommended daily allowance (RDA)** is 15 mg for teenage women, and 18 mg for adult women. Iron intake in women is often inadequate due to low calorie intake, excessive sweat loss, foot-strike **hemolysis** (particularly for endurance runners), and women may be losing too much iron each month with blood loss due to menstruation. Thus, most women are not aware that they have anemia (low iron levels) and that their performance may be suffering due to lack of iron. Women are at greater risk for anemia then men. It has been reported that 40% to 50% of women have a certain degree of iron depletion even though they may not have overt anemia (30). Runners tend to have a greater risk of having anemia and black adolescent female runners have twice the incidence of anemia when compared to white female runners (30).

Reversing iron deficiency can take several months so prevention is very important. Thus, focusing on iron-rich foods is imperative for women and it may be necessary for the athlete to consume an additional iron supplement to stave off iron depletion and deficiency.

Calcium Calcium is important for building bones and teeth, muscle contraction, nerve impulse conduction, and fluid regulation. Women may find themselves deficient in calcium consumption due to disordered eating, elimination of certain food items from their diet, dieting, low calorie consumption, and menstrual dysfunction. Recommendations for supplementation for these women who may be at risk of calcium deficiency due to the above-mentioned reasons could be as high as 1,500 mg of calcium based upon a dietary analysis (11).

Zinc Zinc is important for growth, bone formation, repair of muscle tissue, energy production, enzyme activity, immunity, wound healing, maintaining thyroid hormone levels, regulating the **basal metabolic rate (BMR)**, cardiorespiratory function, strength, endurance, and protein usage. Thus, it is evident that zinc deficiency could potentially affect athletic performance and it should be noted that women are at particular risk of having low levels (11). The RDA for zinc is 8 mg for women; however, athletes should be careful if considering supplementation as high levels of zinc can have adverse affects in absorption of other nutrients. In addition, recent reviews (31) have indicated that there is no evidence that zinc deficiency impairs performance.

Magnesium Magnesium influences bone formation, is a component of many enzymes, and is important in protein synthesis. The RDA is 310 to 320 mg for women. Magnesium is not normally considered when discussing nutritional considerations for women but a recent position statement by the American College of Sports Medicine (11) has included magnesium as an important mineral when considering the impact it can have upon athletic performance. It notes (11) that in those participating in "body-conscious sports" (such as gymnastics and dance), there has been a report of inadequate consumption of magnesium, which could affect metabolism, hormone function, and cardiovascular indices.

Vitamins

B Vitamins (B_1, or thiamin; B_2, or riboflavin; B_6, or pyridoxine; B_{12}; and folate) are important for protein metabolism, red blood cell and protein synthesis, maintenance of nerve tissue, and tissue repair. Of the B vitamins, thiamin, riboflavin, pyridoxine, folate, and vitamin B_{12} are found to be deficient in female diets (11). There is limited research examining the impact of B-vitamin deficiencies on athletic performance but it may be prudent for endurance athletes in particular to ensure that they get enough B vitamins in their diet. Thiamin (B_1) deficiency has been shown to decrease endurance capacity. Women who start an aerobic training program may need a higher intake of riboflavin (B_2). Those women with anemia (a common problem in endurance runners) may benefit from Vitamin B_{12} supplementation but megadoses are not necessary. Women with low energy intakes may have a B_6 (pyridoxine) deficiency that could impair hemoglobin formation and carbohydrate metabolism. Women using OCs or who are anemic may benefit from folate supplementation (11). For all these reasons, a comprehensive B-vitamin supplement may be warranted if dietary analysis reveals deficiencies.

MACRONUTRIENTS

Macronutrients are dietary nutrients like carbohydrates, protein, fat, and water that are needed by the body in large amounts that can definitely affect

Q & A from the Field

Q ***There are so many forms of calcium supplements on the market. If I determine that my diet is calcium deficient and therefore should take a supplement, which formulation is best?***

A There are many forms such as calcium citrate, calcium carbonate, calcium lactate, calcium gluconate, oyster shells, and bone meal. Calcium citrate is the best absorbed form of calcium although calcium carbonate also absorbs very well in a more acidic environment. Examine labels and look for the elemental calcium content (expressed in mg), not the total content. Some pills may have less elemental calcium, which would require you to take more pills to meet the daily requirement. On the label, you may also see the United States Pharmacopeia (USP) or Consumer Lab (CL) abbreviation, which would indicate that the supplement has voluntarily met the industry standards for quality and purity. Finally, try to take your supplement along with a meal as this increases gastric acidity and slows transit time that promotes calcium absorption.

human performance if not consumed in sufficient amounts.

Protein

The recommended daily requirement for protein intake ranges from 0.9 to 1.0 g · kg body weight^{-1} for healthy adults. However, physically active individuals may require a higher protein intake, particularly for those involved in intense weight training programs (1.2 to 1.4 g · kg^{-1} endurance athletes, 1.6 to 1.8 for anaerobic/resistance-training athletes). Given the lower body weights of women they may need less and can usually meet their requirements through diet alone if their energy intake is sufficient to maintain their body weight.

Carbohydrates

Carbohydrate consumption should be based upon body weight and size and can range from 6 to 10 g · kg^{-1} of body weight (11). Carbohydrate needs are dependent upon the intensity, duration of activity, gender, and type of sport for which the athlete competes. For example, it has been shown that women use significantly less **glycogen** than men during resistance training leading some to argue (29) that high carbohydrate diets may not be desirable for women strength athletes like they are for endurance athletes. In addition, whether this potential difference between men and women should influence the carbohydrate loading strategy of women remains to be determined. It is possible that women strength trainers may want to focus more on protein intake than carbohydrate intake after exercise. Nevertheless, it is clear that all athletes need carbohydrates and should focus on carbohydrates with high fiber and a low glycemic index (fruits, vegetables, brown rice, beans, and oats).

Fat

Many women may believe that they need to cut out fat from their diets because consuming fat will make them deposit fat or gain weight. While consumption of too much fat is not healthy, some fat is essential in a diet in order to provide energy, transport vitamins, and produce hormones. In fact, low dietary fat intake may increase the risk for menstrual disturbances and the incidence of the female athlete triad. Unprocessed sources of fat are the best choice (lean meats, nuts, seeds, fatty fish, avocados, and egg yolks) and avoidance of **saturated fats** is recommended.

As stated earlier there is some indication that women could process fat more efficiently and rely less upon glycogen stores during resistance training. Further, it has been reported that women oxidize more fat than men when active at 65% to 75% of VO_{2max} (19) while other studies report that there is no difference. This potential difference has led some to hypothesize that a higher percentage of fat in the diet may be desirable for women, particularly those involved in low intensity or strength exercises, to enhance energy production from intramuscular fat stores and spare glycogen stores.

Women have specific nutritional requirements that need to be considered for training and competition.

Fluid and Electrolytes

There is some indication that women have lower sweating rates (20) and **electrolyte** losses (due to differences in body size and surface area, fewer number of sweat glands, and lower metabolic rates during a given activity) and may need to partake in varied rehydration practices in order to stay properly hydrated.

Fluid Recommendations It is difficult to recommend fluid consumption rates for all types of activities in that there is no single recommendation that is appropriate for everyone, since body weight, environmental factors, and intensity of exercise make a difference. It is possible to make some general recommendations for staying hydrated:

- Drink at higher rates if heavier and faster and lower rates for slower and lighter persons.
- Adjust fluid intake for environmental temperature and humidity rates.
- Drink when you are thirsty.
- Drink enough so that the urine is slightly yellow.
- Experiment at different fluid consumption levels during training and monitor body weight changes pre- to post-workout to ascertain what rehydration protocol works best for you.
- Consider drinking fluids other than just water, based upon the intensity and duration of exercise. Perhaps a beverage or gel that is a combination of sodium, potassium, and carbohydrates will benefit the athlete and prevent electrolyte imbalance during longer duration activities, particularly in a warmer environment.

Hyponatremia Hyponatremia is a potentially life-threatening condition whereby blood sodium levels are below 130 mmol · L^{-1} (32). It can occur at rest or during exercise (exercise hyponatremia [EH]) when an individual consumes more fluid than is necessary or when large amounts of sodium are lost through sweating. EH can occur with any type of activity but is particularly prevalent when fluids are consumed during an activity of low intensity and lasts for over 4 hours (e.g., a marathon). One study, found that female marathon runners drink more fluids during a race than male runners in proportion to body size, which may simply be due to greater recognition by women of the need to stay hydrated (33). Women may also be at greater risk (some reports indicate as much as three times more likely) due to their small body sizes and lower sweat rates when compared to men (smaller bodies require less fluid to dilute the blood, which makes it easier to over-hydrate).

The International Marathon Medical Directors Association (IMMDA) has provided the following recommendations and warnings with regard to preventing hyponatremia during marathon competitions:

- Runners/walkers planning to spend between 4 to 6 hours or longer on the course are at risk for developing fluid-overload hyponatremia and usually do not need to ingest more than one cup (about 3 to 6 oz: 3 oz if you weigh approximately 100 lb and 6 oz if you weigh approximately 200 lb) of fluid per mile.
- Some participants may find that adjusting their intake to pace or time is easier for them: Adjust the rate of fluid intake to race pace: slower race pace = slower drinking rate; maximum intake of 500 mL · h^{-1} (4 to 6 oz every 20 minute) for runners with >5-hour finishing times (10- to 11-minute · mi^{-1} pace).
- Weight monitoring is also important: if you gain weight during your workout or event, you are drinking too much.
- Remember that thirst is the best method for monitoring hydration status.

NUTRITIONAL SUMMARY

Women have specific nutritional requirements that need to be considered for training and competition. Women have been shown to be at a greater risk for eating disorders and nutritional deficiencies. It is important that a woman complete a nutritional analysis and then, possibly in consultation with a nutritionist or physician, decide to consume additional vitamins and nutrients either through her diet or a supplement so that she can maintain a good health profile and optimize performance. In addition, fluid intake may need to be more closely monitored in women who may be at greater risk for hyponatremia.

PREGNANCY AND THE ATHLETE

It used to be thought that women should not exercise during pregnancy. More recently, numerous studies have shown that the mother and fetus are remarkable at adapting to exercise and the resultant physiological, respiratory, hormonal, and thermoregulatory resultant changes that occur with exercise are conducive to a healthy environment for the fetus to grow and thrive 34–37). Thus, it is generally accepted in today's society and by important organizations (American College of Obstetricians and Gynecologists [ACOG], ACSM, Society of Obstetricians and Gynecologists of Canada [SOGC]) that it is suitable and actually healthy for an expectant mother to exercise. Because of this acceptance and the growing number of women participating in sports, the number of women who may wish to continue to exercise during their pregnancy is increasing. With the approval of their doctor, most women having a normal pregnancy can safely continue to exercise throughout the entire gestational period and, in fact, may be able to initiate an exercise program even though they may have never exercised prior to pregnancy (34). Recommendations for exercise, concerns for pregnant athletes, and contraindications to exercise for a pregnant woman, however, need to be discussed. It is safe to say when making any recommendations for exercise during pregnancy safety is the primary goal and a conservative approach must be followed.

ADVANTAGES TO EXERCISING DURING PREGNANCY

The advantages of incorporating exercise into the life of a pregnant woman are numerous. Not only does it help during the delivery process by strengthening muscle to ease the burden of labor and delivery but it can provide notable reward to a woman during the entire gestational period. For example, the weight gain that accompanies pregnancy can change the center of gravity and put strain on the lower back. It is recommended (34–36) that conditioning and resistance training exercises that target muscles of the back may aid in reducing the low back pain that many women experience, particularly as the pregnancy progresses. Further, although there is a healthy amount of weight that expectant mothers should gain during pregnancy, too much weight gain can be unhealthy. Studies have shown that exercise may serve to limit weight gain so that the expectant mother does not add too many extra pounds (34–36). In addition, exercise during pregnancy can decrease the risk of specific health concerns that can occur with pregnancy such as prevention of **gestational diabetes** and controlling blood pressure (34–36). Finally, there are certain times in a woman's pregnancy where she may feel weary, frustrated, and psychologically stressed and exercise has been shown to significantly improve the mood and outlook of the expectant mother.

There are an ever-increasing number of women who will continue to or begin to exercise during their pregnancy with many benefits to both the mother and developing fetus.

CONTRAINDICATIONS TO EXERCISE

It should be noted that exercising during pregnancy can be healthy in a woman experiencing a normal pregnancy but that there are specific instances whereby it is not recommended that a woman exercise (these are referred to as absolute contraindications). These instances include (34)

- Uncontrolled type I diabetes, cardiovascular disease, respiratory disease, thyroid disease, or systemic disorder
- Incompetent cervix
- Premature labor
- Cervical bleeding
- Intrauterine growth and retardation
- Multiple gestations
- Preeclampsia/eclampsia
- Premature rupture of the membranes
- Placenta previa

This list by no means is comprehensive and each woman's pregnancy has individualized considerations and concerns that must be discussed with her physician. Thus, any pregnant woman who wants to undertake or continue with an exercise program should consult, and keep communicating continually throughout her pregnancy, with her physician providing him/her with updates on changes in intensity and type of activity, symptoms she may be experiencing at rest and during exercise, and other information that may give an indication of her overall health and well-being.

CONSIDERATIONS BEFORE DECIDING TO EXERCISE

The pregnant woman's physician will consider many variables before giving permission to exercise. There are many physiological changes that occur in the mother during pregnancy that could affect exercise capabilities (HR, cardiac output, respirations, etc.). However, a select few have gotten the attention of obstetricians as potential concerns that may need to be considered when determining the safety issues for the exercising mother including increased joint laxity due to hormonal changes, shift in the center of gravity that may increase the risk of falls, redistribution of blood flow away from the fetus to exercising muscles, glucose utilization, increases in maternal core temperature with exercise that could potentially harm the fetus, and soft-tissue swelling (35,36).

For a tool to determine readiness for exercise during pregnancy, the Physical Activity Readiness Medical Examination for Pregnancy (PARmed-X for Pregnancy) can be filled out and then provided to a woman's doctor for review to help make exercise recommendations. It is a tool that was developed by the Canadian Society for Exercise Physiology that can be found at their website.

TRAINING CONSIDERATIONS FOR THE PREGNANT WOMAN

After considering all the typical concerns noted above and after noting the listed advantages to exercising and after receiving permission to exercise from her doctor, many women will choose to exercise during pregnancy. The following are some general recommended training considerations that a woman and her personal trainer should follow when choosing an activity (35,36):

- No quick directional changes—changes in the center of gravity and joint laxity increase the chance for injury and falls.
- No ballistic stretching movements.
- Do not skip having a warm-up and cool-down period.
- Increase caloric intake in the first two trimesters by 150 calories and 300 extra calories during the last trimester and maybe more calories are needed for those who are participating in exercise.
- Monitor hydration status and consume adequate amounts of water.
- If exercising at altitudes >6,000 ft there is greater risk to the mother and fetus. Women should be fully aware of signs of altitude sickness and should stop exercise, descend, and visit their doctor should any of the signs become evident.
- Exercise recommendations are sport-specific and the female athlete should have a detailed conversation with her doctor with regard to the activities she does and the sports for which she is competitive.
- No exercising in extremely hot and humid conditions—maternal core temperature can increase and put the fetus at risk.
- Avoid contact sports (ice hockey, soccer, basketball)—increases risk of trauma to the fetus.
- Avoid sports and activities that increase the risk of falls (gymnastics, horseback riding, downhill skiing, vigorous racquet sports).
- No abdominal crunches—fetus could press on the spine and inferior vena cava restricting blood flow particularly during the latter months of pregnancy.
- No motionless standing—decreases cardiac output.
- No scuba diving—the fetus is not protected from **decompression sickness** and gas embolism.

Aerobic Training Considerations

- Intensity should be in the range of a 12 to 14 rating on the Borg scale.
- Heart rate should not exceed 60% to 80% of max HR.
- No exercising that does not allow a woman to carry on a conversation during exercise (there is a 10- to 15-beat · min^{-1} increase in resting heart rate and a blunted HR response to exercise in pregnant women so intensity must be monitored).

Resistance Training Considerations (38)

- Rep range = 12 to 15 RM. If a woman wants to take an even more conservative route only perform 8 to 10 reps at the 12- to 15-RM load.
- One set of each exercise or more rest in between sets if more sets are performed.
- Machine weights preferred over free weights (if the machine can accommodate the burgeoning belly). There is less risk of injury due to loss of balance, joints are more stabilized so less likely to be injured, and many machines require sitting instead of standing in one spot which can improve cardiac output.
- If machine weights are not an option then light dumbbells, resistance bands, or body weight can be used for resistance.
- Avoid activities that are affected by balance (lunges, stiff-leg dead lifts, and squats) particularly in the last trimester. Changes in the center of gravity and joint laxity increase the chance for injury and falls
- When resistance training, pay particular attention to adductors, abductors, hamstring, gluteals, abdominal, and quadriceps muscles to help with their role in labor and delivery.
- No supine weight lifting, particularly in the second and third trimesters—the weight of the fetus can press on the spine and inferior vena cava.
- During strength training, do not take any position that leaves your abdomen vulnerable to a falling weight. For example, avoid lying flat during the chess press. Incline press or machines are better options.
- No **Valsalva maneuvers** with lifting—blood pressure can dramatically increase with breath holding.

PREVIOUSLY SEDENTARY MOTHERS

The ACOG maintains that previously sedentary pregnant women, in the absence of complications, can adopt the current exercise guidelines put forth by the American College of Sports Medicine (30 minutes or more of moderate exercise a day on most, if not all, days of the week). These women may want to start gradually and work up to 30 minutes. For those women who were sedentary before becoming pregnant, it is recommended that they begin with 15 minutes of continuous exercise 3 times · wk^{-1} and work up to a goal of 30 minutes on most if not all days of the week (34).

PREGNANT ATHLETES

All women who are having a normal, uncomplicated pregnancy can participate in low impact aerobic exercise, resistance training, and moderate intensity activities. For those women who are considered athletes or highly conditioned, in constant consultation with their doctor, they may be able to compete and continue to exercise at higher levels during pregnancy; however, the SOGC do not recommend trying to reach peak fitness during pregnancy. These women should be in consultation with their obstetricians throughout their pregnancy and be sure that they have chosen a doctor who is knowledgeable with regard to the impact of strenuous exercise on the mother and fetus. Again, being conservative in making physical activity recommendations should always be the preferred choice over those decisions that may be more risky.

POSTPARTUM EXERCISE

Most women should be able to continue to exercise in the postpartum period after consulting with their doctors. Most of the physiological and anatomical changes that accompanied the pregnancy disappear within 4 to 6 weeks or earlier for some women. Resumption of activity should be individualized and carries with it many advantages.

Exercise has not been shown to affect the quantity of milk. The quality of milk, however, may be a factor that needs to be considered. There is some indication that lactic acid levels may be greater in breast milk immediately postexercise. Those women who notice that their baby resists breast feeding immediately postexercise may want to consider feeding their babies prior to exercise, waiting an hour after exercise, or pumping milk to be fed after exercise.

MUSCULOSKELETAL INJURIES

NONCONTACT ANTERIOR CRUCIATE LIGAMENT INJURIES

Anterior cruciate ligament (ACL) injuries continue to be the largest single problem in orthopaedic sports medicine. Approximately 70% to 80% of ACL injuries are noncontact in nature (39,40), and these are the ACL injuries that will be referred to throughout this section. Noncontact is defined as forces applied to the knee at the time of injury resulting from the athlete's own movement, not from contact with another athlete or object (40). ACL injuries tend to occur when landing from a jump, cutting or decelerating, where most or all of the force is on a single leg or foot with the foot positioned away from the body's **center of gravity** and involving increased trunk motion (39). Women are more than four times more likely to suffer an ACL injury than men participating in the same sport at the same level of competition. ACL injuries are most prevalent during the high school and college age years (6,39). Isolated ACL injuries occur infrequently as injuries to the articular cartilage, medial collateral ligament, and more often the meniscus are commonly involved (39).

> ***ACL injuries tend to occur when landing from a jump, cutting or decelerating, where most or all of the force is on a single leg or foot with the foot positioned away from the body's center of gravity, and involving increased trunk motion.***

Predisposition to Injury

Predisposition to ACL tears has been organized into three categories: anatomical/structural, hormonal, and neuromuscular/biomechanical (40). Anatomical factors that potentially increase the risk for an ACL injury in women include a narrower intercondylar notch, a smaller ACL, decreased ACL stiffness, less collagen within the ACL, an increased Q-angle, anterior pelvic tilt, **hip anteversion**, **tibiofemoral angle**, **genu recurvatum**, increased posterior tibial slope, anterior knee laxity, general joint laxity, and a different rate of lower extremity alignment development (40). A great number of anatomical factors are not easily corrected. However, it is important to understand their influences on ACL injuries if subjects with an increased risk are to be identified (39).

Even though research has identified sex hormone receptors (estrogen, testosterone, and relaxin) on skeletal muscle and the ACL, little evidence exists to support specific direct or indirect hormonal influences on the ACL. However, mounting evidence supports the idea that women have a significantly greater risk of sustaining an ACL injury during the preovulatory phase of the menstrual cycle than during the postovulatory phase. The mechanical and molecular properties of the ACL are likely influenced not only by estrogen but by the interaction of several sex hormones, secondary messengers, remodeling proteins, and mechanical stresses. Large individual variations in female hormone profiles and a time-dependent effect exist for sex hormones and other remodeling agents to influence a change in ACL tissue characteristics (39).

Knee position and muscle action during dynamic movements are proposed as additional contributors to ACL injures in women (40). Researchers believe that women use different neuromuscular control mechanisms that men and this is the primary reason for the increased incidence of knee injury in female athletes (41). Due to neuromuscular imbalances, women tend to control their knees like ball-and-socket joints, rather than hinge joints. Ligament dominance occurs when there is a decrease in dynamic neuromuscular control of the joint. Joint stability relies more on the ligaments surrounding the joint rather than the muscles during activity. At the knee this can result in increased knee abduction. Quadriceps dominance occurs when there is an increased recruitment of the quadriceps muscles and a decreased recruitment, and quite often strength, of the hamstring muscles. Women with quadriceps dominance tend to perform activities in more of an extended knee position, rather than a deeper knee flexion position. Leg dominance occurs when there are side-to-side differences in strength, flexibility, and coordination, resulting in asymmetrical foot weighting during activity. Core instability can result in increased trunk motion, which is often associated with the foot being placed away from the center of gravity. All four of these altered neuromuscular mechanisms contribute to the increased risk of ACL injuries (41).

> ***Altered neuromuscular control in women can contribute to an increased risk for ACL injuries.***

Identifying women at risk

Identifying athletes at risk for an ACL injury typically involves observing them during normal activities. This allows the coach to identify dangerous positions that put the ACL at greater risk for injury. Some dangerous positions include

- Upright stance during activities, especially landing, cutting, and decelerating movements
- Knee valgus (caving inward), especially during landing, cutting, and decelerating movements
- Stopping with one large step rather than multiple smaller steps
- Landing, cutting, or decelerating with the foot placed away from the line of gravity

Risk Reduction/Prevention Programs

A number of ACL injury prevention programs have been reported in the literature (5–10). Successful programs tend to share a number of common elements. Most include one or more of the following: traditional stretching, strengthening, awareness of high-risk positions, technique modification, aerobic conditioning, sport-specific agilities, proprioceptive and balance training, and plyometrics (39). Programs should include strength and power exercises, neuromuscular training, plyometrics, and agility exercises. Balance training alone has not been shown to decrease the risk of ACL injuries (39).

> ***ACL injury prevention programs should include strength and power exercises, neuromuscular training, plyometrics, and agility exercises.***

Even though ACL injury prevention programs focus on maintaining the knee over the toes, there are a number of additional components that strength and conditioning professionals should also address. Emphasize soft landings, landing softly on the forefoot and rolling back to the rear foot with increased hip and knee flexion (39). At <45 degrees of knee flexion, the quadriceps work as an antagonist to the ACL, increasing the amount of force placed on the ligament during landing. Increasing the depth of the landing beyond 45 degrees of flexion will cause the quadriceps to work as an agonist to the ACL, helping to protect the ACL from increased shear forces. Landing softly with deep knee flexion will also help athletes reprogram peak hamstring/quadriceps firing patterns, increasing co-contractions to help protect the ACL (6).

Emphasize keeping the knees over the toes when cutting and landing (39). The knees should not be allowed to move in multiple directions. Educate athletes on the importance of dynamic control, decreasing knee valgus and only allowing the knees to move in the sagittal plane. During cutting and landing movements, the knees should not move closer together or rotate inward. An increase in hip abductor strength and control can contribute to preventing unwanted side-to-side knee movements. Begin with single plane exercises emphasizing dynamic knee stability and progress to multiplane

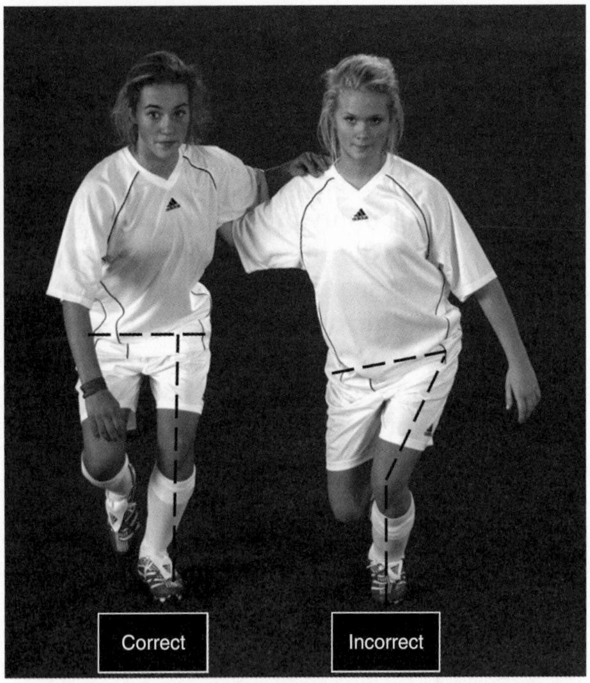

FIGURE 19.1 "Correct" and "incorrect" positions for the single leg squat to demonstrate static knee control in women athletes.

exercises (6). Figure 19.1 demonstrates "correct" and "incorrect" positions for static knee control performing the single leg squat in women athletes.

Improve balance through dynamic balance training (39). Equal leg-to-leg strength, balance, and foot placement should be stressed. Oftentimes women at risk for ACL injuries will exhibit a dominant leg imbalance. Training must progressively emphasize double, then single, leg movements. Core instability can be corrected through progressive neuromuscular training techniques that target the balanced and synchronized turn-on of the dynamic stabilizing musculature of the trunk, pelvis, and hips. Unstable surfaces, single-leg balancing, and unanticipated movement training should be included (6).

Teach proper deceleration technique. Athletes should be instructed to cut, land, and decelerate with increased knee and hip flexion. A rounded cut is recommended over a sharp cutting motion (39). Round off turns when pivoting, keeping the knee inside an imaginary cylinder of the body and not taking any long steps that place the knee outside that cylinder of the upper torso. Decelerate in a more controlled fashion by taking several small steps rather than a sudden single step. Agility exercises can be used to emphasize proper deceleration as well as improve agility and control of dynamic movement (39). Figure 19.2 demonstrates "correct" and "incorrect" form for a cutting maneuver, which is related to dynamic knee stability in women athletes.

Ideally, ACL prevention programs should be implemented as early as possible in the training period. This could be as early as 6 to 10 years of age. Most programs take approximately 4 to 6 weeks for athletes to exhibit changes. However, athletes should participate in maintenance programs before, during, and after sports participation seasons in order to minimize injuries (39).

Prevention program exercises should be conducted at the beginning of training sessions or as separate training session. All drills and exercises should be performed with excellent technique. Neuromuscular fatigue as a result of training may

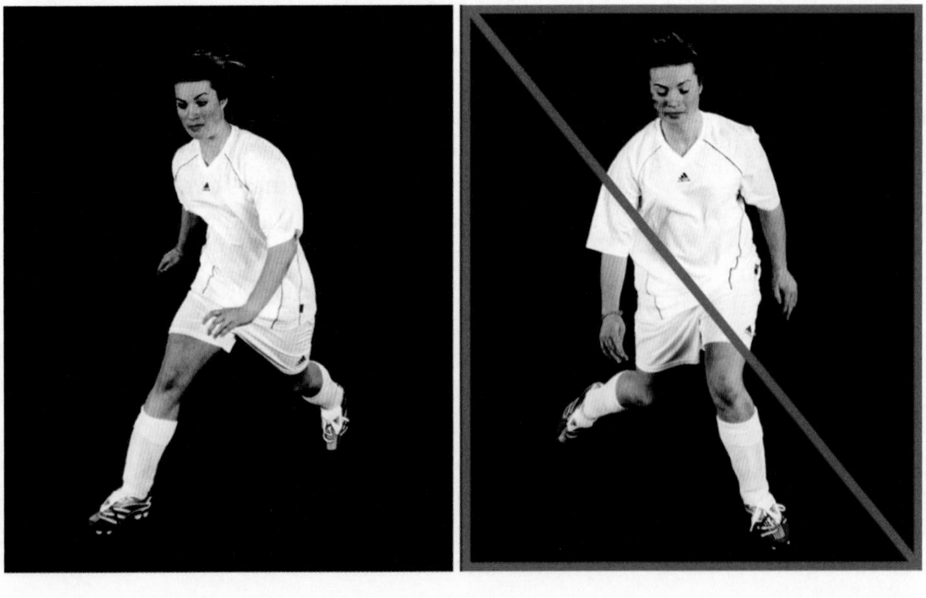

FIGURE 19.2 "Correct" and "incorrect" cutting maneuver demonstrating dynamic knee stability in women athletes.

directly affect the athlete's biomechanical technique and limit any potential prevention benefits (39). Incorporating exercises into the warm-up routine, requiring nothing more than traditional training equipment for the sport, and keeping the time required to perform the exercises to a reasonable length are just a few suggestions for increasing athlete compliance throughout the season. Additional incentive for participating in a prevention program is enhanced performance. Properly executed prevention programs have shown improvements in vertical jump, control of dynamic load of the knee, improved balance, increased hamstring strength, power, and peak torque (39). The drop vertical jump test (Fig. 19.3) can be used to identify athletes at risk of severe knee injuries (47).

Sport-Specific Factors

Little is known about the effect of sport-specific factors (e.g., rules, referees, coaching), meteorological conditions (including shoe-surface interaction), playing surfaces, protective equipment on the risk of suffering an ACL injury. There is also little known about the effect of age, athleticism, skill level, psychological characteristics, and previous knee injury as risk factors for ACL injury (39). More research needs to be conducted in order to better understand all the potential facets to the noncontact ACL injury, especially as it pertains to women.

Although much has been learned about characteristic sex differences relating to ACL injuries, researchers still know very little about the underlying causes of these differences or whether many of the observed differences truly reflect an increased injury risk for the physically active female. It is well accepted that the ACL injury is a multifaceted problem and more integration across risk factors in future research is needed.

PATELLOFEMORAL INJURIES

Patellofemoral pain syndrome (PFPS) is a common orthopedic complaint among active young adults, with a greater occurrence in women (42).

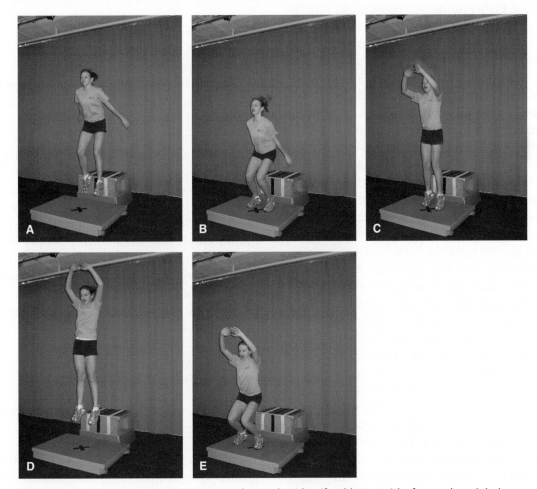

FIGURE 19.3 The drop vertical jump test can be used to identify athletes at risk of severe knee injuries.

A number of factors, categorized into anatomic, hormonal, and neuromuscular groups, have been hypothesized to cause PFPS. These factors include patellar misalignment, increased Q-angle, quadriceps weakness, decreased flexibility in the lower extremity, overuse, and muscle imbalance. Each of these factors has been shown to increase cartilage and subchondral bone stress. However, limited evidence exists to support any of these hypotheses as potential causal factors (42).

Research has shown that women with PFPS tend to exhibit muscular weakness at the hip when compared with healthy controls (42). Strong evidence supports a decrease in hip external rotation, abduction, and extension while moderate evidence supports a decrease in hip flexion and internal rotation. When compared with the unaffected side, rather than a healthy control, these strength deficits decrease, but are still present (42). Due to study designs, it is yet undetermined whether these muscular weaknesses are a cause or result of PFPS. These studies also do not address muscular endurance, which is an important factor to consider since a majority of PFPS complaints come from individuals participating in endurance activities (42).

Weak hip abductors due to decreased abductor strength or activation can result in the opposite hip dropping when standing on one leg. Women with PFPS have been identified as having weak hip abductor muscles. As the opposite hip drops, it has been hypothesized that the weak side iliotibial band will be elongated, thus increasing its tension. Because the iliotibial band in connected to and reinforces the lateral patellar retinaculum, researchers theorize that this increase in length and tension will apply a greater lateral pull to the patella decreasing patellar contact on the femur, resulting in increased stress on the patella and possibly PFPS (43).

Weakness of the hip external rotators and abductors can lead to an increase in hip adduction and internal rotation. An increase in both hip adduction and internal rotation leads to a more lateral tracking of the patella on the femur. As stated earlier, increased lateral tracking can lead to increased patellar stress and possibly PFPS due to decreased patellar contact on the femur (42). When observing women performing weight-bearing activities such as the squat, hip external rotator and abductor weakness can be observed through increased femoral internal rotation and knee valgus (42). However, some women will perform weight-bearing activities with a more externally rotated or toe-out position as a method of compensating for excessive hip internal rotation and adduction (43).

Weak hip external rotators and abductors can lead to an increase in hip adduction and internal rotation, causing a more lateral patellar tracking on the femur.

Researchers suggest patellar maltracking on the femur due to an imbalance of vastus medialis oblique (VMO) and vastus lateralis activity could be a possible cause of PFPS. Delayed and decreased force production by the VMO in relation to the vastus lateralis has been theorized to induce more lateral tracking of the patella on the femur, increasing patellofemoral contact pressure, resulting in articular cartilage pathology and possibly PFPS (44).

Very little research exists to address the treatment and prevention of PFPS. A limited number of case studies do support the use of hip musculature strengthening for the treatment of PFPS. Since women with PFPS exhibit overall hip muscle weakness, it would seem logical to use hip strengthening exercises to address those weaknesses. However, since it is not known whether hip muscle weakness is a cause or effect, hip strengthening has not been a confirmed as a treatment for PFPS (44).

When working with female athletes suffering from PFPS, strength and conditioning professionals should include exercises to address hip strength in all planes. This is not only for potentially decreasing knee pain associated with PFPS, but should be part of a well-rounded strength program. Proper technique during all resistance exercises and conditioning drills should be emphasized. Recommendations addressed in the ACL injury prevention section also apply here. Strength and conditioning professionals should emphasize maintaining proper knee alignment during resistance exercises as well as jump landing, keep knees away from dangerous positions by staying within the body's cylinder, using multiple steps to decelerate, and performing dynamic movements in a deep knee flexion position.

Emphasize correct technique and multi-plane exercises to strengthen the hips.

SHOULDER INJURIES

Anthropometrically, women tend to have narrower shoulders than men. This structural design limits the amount of muscle tissue that can be supported and decreases the mechanical advantage of the upper body muscles when compared with men. Strength and conditioning professionals need to address upper body strength and muscle balance in women. Programs should include a number of back, shoulder, and chest exercises to support correct shoulder posture as well as prepare the shoulder complex for the demands of chosen activities. This is especially true for women who participate in overhead activities. Decreased upper body and core strength can predispose women to a forward or rounded shoulder posture, shoulder instability, and shoulder injury. The rotator cuff should also be addressed in order to reduce the risk of glenohumeral instability and associated overuse injuries (45). For women to partake in more advanced full body exercises, a shoulder strengthening program may be a prerequisite in order to prepare the shoulder complex for the specific demands.

Summary

The number of women participating in exercise programs has grown rapidly over the last few decades. If we look back at where the female athlete was in 1970 versus where they are today, it is evident that great strides have been made in welcoming women into athletic and fitness programs. This creates some important challenges to the coach or trainer working with these individuals. If we return to our original question posed at the beginning of this chapter: "Should trainers, athletes, and coaches recognize that men and women have differences anatomically, physiologically, and psychologically that should be given special consideration when training for fitness and competition?" it is clear that there are many instances when women should be given special consideration when implementing a training and fitness program. Although women respond similarly to most training programs when compared to men, there are specific differences that may need to be addressed when designing and implementing a strength and conditioning regimen.

There are numerous physiological and anatomical differences between men and women that should be considered before exercise. Although many women are participating in strength training programs there still remains a social stigma that must be overcome so that she feels comfortable and accepted in a weight room. Though a woman's menstrual cycle does not, for the most part, affect her performance each woman should be treated as an individual and adjustments to the training and competition schedule may be warranted. When disturbances in the menstrual cycle are observed it may be prudent to screen a woman for the female athlete triad and take appropriate measures to treat or prevent this serious condition. Part of that treatment may involve nutritional and psychological counseling and involvement of many supporting individuals. Women have nutritional needs and requirements that are specific to their gender. They are at risk for disordered eating and nutritional deficiencies for various macro- and micronutrients, particularly if they participate in weight-dependent sports and activities. They may also be at risk for a potentially life-threatening condition called hyponatremia if they consume large amounts of fluids relative to their body weight. Further, women experiencing normal pregnancies should be encouraged to initiate or continue with an exercise program with careful monitoring by their physician. Finally, women have been shown to be at an increased risk for ACL injury, PFPS, and shoulder injuries. There are methods for identifying those women at risk for injury, and there are many programs in the literature that can be incorporated into a strength and conditioning program that can help prevent these injuries and conditions.

Maxing Out

You are working with a group of female long distance runners who want a more specific recommendation with regard to how much fluid they should consume in order to remain hydrated during training and competition. The following protocol may be used to calculate the amount of fluid needed (46):

1. Make sure you are properly hydrated before the workout—your urine should be pale yellow.
2. Do a warm-up run until you begin to sweat, then stop. Urinate if necessary.
3. Weigh yourself naked with a floor scale (accurate to 0.1 kg).
4. Run for 1 hour at an intensity similar to your targeted race or training run.
5. Drink a measured amount of a beverage during the run, if you are thirsty. It is important that you measure exactly how much fluid you consume during the run.
6. Do not urinate until post-body weight is recorded.
7. Weigh yourself naked again on the same scale you used in step 3.
8. You may now urinate and drink fluids as needed.
9. Calculate your fluid need using Table 19.3.

TABLE 19.3 ● CALCULATING FLUID NEEDS FOR PROPER HYDRATION FOR DISTANCE RUNNING

A. Enter your body weight from Step 3 in Kilograms[a] *(To convert from pounds to kilograms, divide pounds by 2.2)*	–	______
B. Enter your body weight from Step 7 in Kilograms[a] *(To convert from pounds to kilograms, divide pounds by 2.2)*		______
C. Subtract B from A	=	______
D. Convert your total in C to grams by multiplying by 1000	x	**1000**
	=	______
E. Enter the amount of fluid you consumed during the run in milliliters *(To convert from ounces to milliliters, multiply ounces by 30)*	+	______
F. Add E to D	=	______
This final figure is the number of milliliters (ml) that you need to consume per hour to remain well-hydrated. If you want to convert milliliters back to ounces, simply divide by 30.		

Adapted from Casa D. Proper hydration for distance running—identifying individual fluid needs. *Track Coach.* 2004;167:5321–5328 with permission.
[a]Weigh

CASE EXAMPLE

Exercise during Pregnancy

BACKGROUND

A personal training client has informed you that she is pregnant. Her exercise routine included biking, lifting weights, body weight exercises, and step aerobics. What are some adaptations that you should incorporate into her routine?

CONSIDERATIONS

Beginning in the second trimester, you should avoid lifting weights while standing still to resist pooling of blood in the legs. Machine leg curls and leg extensions are good substitutes for lunges and squats to avoid falls with the shift in the center of gravity. Some doctors say step aerobics workouts are acceptable if you can lower the height of your step as pregnancy progresses, but caution should be taken as the risk of falls increases. Exercise during cooler parts of the day. Choose stationary biking over land biking. Consider incorporating swimming into her routine. It is a great alternative for staying active.

RESULTS

Some simple adaptations can be made. Beginning in the second trimester, instruct her to sit down when performing lifts whenever possible. Substitute machine leg curls and leg extensions for lunges and squats. She will gradually transition from weight-bearing activities to nonweight-bearing activities (stationary biking, swimming, yoga, weights in an upright or seated position, walking) as the pregnancy progresses. Bike riding and other aerobic activities such as a decreased height step routine will be performed indoors in a controlled temperature environment in the early months of pregnancy. Swimming will be used in increasing amounts as the pregnancy progresses.

REFERENCES

1. National Association for Sport and Physical Education. Position Statement. NASPE Code of Ethics for Professionals in Higher Education; 2009.
2. American Association of University Professors. Position Paper. Title IX: Gender Equity in College Sports, 2003.
3. National Strength and Conditioning Association. Position Paper on Strength Training for Female Athletes. Lincoln, NE NSCA; 1990.
4. Burger ME, Burger TA. Neuromuscular and hormonal adaptations to resistance training: implications for strength development in female athletes. *Strength Cond J.* 2002;24:51–59.
5. Gilchrist J, Mandelbaum BR, Melancon H, et al. A randomized controlled trial to prevent noncontact anterior cruciate ligament injury in female collegiate soccer players. *Am J Sports Med.* 2008;36:1476–1483.
6. Hewett TE, Ford KR, Myer GD. Anterior cruciate ligament injuries in female athletes. *Am J Sports Med.* 2006;34:490–498.
7. Mandelbaum BR, Silvers HJ, Watanabe DS, et al. Effectiveness of a neuromuscular and proprioceptive training program in preventing the incidence of anterior cruciate ligament injuries in female athletes. *Am J Sports Med.* 2005;33:1003–1010.
8. Myer GD, Ford KR, Palumbo JP, et al. Neuromuscular training improves performance and lower-extremity biomechanics in female athletes. *J Strength Cond Res.* 2005; 19:51–60.
9. Myklebust G, Engebretsen L, Braekken IH, et al. Prevention of anterior cruciate ligament injuries in female team handball players: a prospective intervention study over three seasons. *Clin J Sport Med.* 2003;13:71–78.
10. Soligard T, Myklebust G, Steffen K, et al. Comprehensive warm-up programme to prevent injuries in young female footballers: cluster randomized controlled trial. *BMJ.* 2008;337:a2469.
11. American College of Sports Medicine. Position statement. Nutrition and athletic performance; 2009.
12. Poiss CC, Sullivan PA, Paup DC, et al. Perceived importance of weight training to selected NCAA division III men and women student-athletes. *J Strength Cond Res.* 2004;18:108–114.
13. Fischer DV. Strategies for improving resistance training adherence in female athletes. *Strength Cond J.* 2005; 27:62–67.
14. Lebrun C. Effect of the different phases of the menstrual cycle and oral contraceptives on athletic performance. *Sports Med.* 1993;16:400–430.
15. Lebrun C. The effect of the phase of the menstrual cycle and the birth control pill on athletic performance. *Athlet Woman.* 1994;13:419–441.
16. Marsh SA, Jenkins DG. Physiological responses to the menstrual cycle. *Sports Med.* 2002;32:601–614.
17. Xanne AK, de Jonge J. Effects of the menstrual cycle on exercise performance. *Sports Med.* 2003;33:833–851.
18. Bambaeichi E, Reilly T, Cable NT, et al. The isolated and combined effects of menstrual cycle phase and time-of-day on muscle strength of eumenorrheic females. *Chronobiol Int.* 2004;21:645–660.
19. Stephenson LA, Kolka MA. Thermoregulation in women. *Exerc Sport Sci Rev.* 1993;21:231–262.
20. Hazelhurst LT, Claassen N. Gender differences in the sweat response during spinning exercise. *J Strength Cond Res.* 2006;20:723–724.
21. Rechichi C, Dawson B, Goodman C. Athletic performance and the oral contraceptive. *Int J Sports Physiol Perform.* 2009; 4:151–162.
22. Bennell K, White S, Crossley K. The oral contraceptive pill: a revolution for sportswomen? *Br J Sports Med.* 1999;33:231–238.
23. Rechichi C, Dawson B. Effect of oral contraceptive cycle phase on performance in team sports players. *J Sci Med Sport.* 2009;12:190–195.
24. Nichols AW, Hetzler RK, Villanueva RJ, et al. Effects of combination oral contraceptives on strength development in women athletes. *J Strength Cond Res.* 2008;22: 1625–1632.
25. Bonci CM, Bonci LJ, Granger LR, et al. National athletic trainers' association position statement: preventing, detecting, and managing disordered eating in athletes. *J Athlet Train.* 2008;43:80–108.
26. American College of Sports Medicine. Position statement. *The Female Athlete Triad.* Baltimore, MD: Lippincott Williams & Wilkins 2007.
27. Beals KA. *Disordered Eating Among Athletes: A Comprehensive Guide for Health Professionals.* Champaign, IL: Human Kinetics; 2004.
28. Brunet M. *Unique Considerations of the Female Athlete.* Florence, KY: Delmar Cengage Learning; 2010.
29. Volek JS, Forsythe CE, Kraemer WJ. Nutritional aspects of women strength athletes. *Br J Sports Med.* 2006;40:742–748.
30. Ireland ML, Ott SM. Special concerns of the female athlete. *Clin Sports Med.* 2004;23:281–298.
31. Williams M. *Nutrition for Health, Fitness, and Sport.* 8th ed. New York: The McGraw-Hill Companies; 2007:301–302.
32. Ganio MS, Armstrong LE, Casa D, et al. Hyponatremia can happen to anyone. *Strength Cond J.* 2008;30:53–55.
33. Hew TD. Women hydrate more than men during a marathon race: hyponatremia in the Houston marathon: a report on 60 cases. *Sport Med.* 2005;15:148–153.
34. American College of Obstetrics and Gynecology (ACOG). Committee opinion number 267: exercise during pregnancy and the postpartum period. *Obstet Gynecol.* 2002;99: 171–173.
35. DeMaio M, Magann EF. Exercise and pregnancy. *J Am Acad Orthop Surg.* 2009;17:504–514.
36. Olson D, Sikka RS, Hayman J, et al. Exercise in pregnancy. *Am Coll Sports Med.* 2009;8:147–153.
37. Uzendoski AM, Latin RW, Berg KE, et al. Short review: maternal and fetal responses to prenatal exercise. *J Appl Sport Sci Res.* 1989;3:93–100.
38. Pujol TJ, Barnes JT, Elder CL. Resistance training during pregnancy. *Strength Cond J.* 2007;29:44–46.
39. Renstrom P, Ljungqvist A, Arendt E, et al. Non-contact ACL injuries in female athletes: an International Olympic Committee current concepts statement. *Br J Sports Med.* 2008;42:394–412.
40. Shultz SJ, Schmitz RJ, Nguyen AD. Research retreat IV: ACL injuries—the gender bias, April 3–5, 2008, Greensboro, NC. *J Athlet Train.* 2008;43:530–537.

41. Hewett TE, Paterno MV, Myer GD. Strategies for enhancing proprioception and neuromuscular control of the knee. *Clin Orthopaed Relat Res.* 2002;402:76–94.
42. Prins MR, van der Wurff P. Females with patellofemoral pain syndrome have weak hip muscles: a systematic review. *Aus J Physiother.* 2009;55:9–15.
43. Willson JD, Davis IS. Lower extremity mechanics of females with and without patellofemoral pain across activities with progressively greater task demands. *Clin Biomech.* 2008;23:203–211.
44. Fagan V, Delahunt E. Patellofemoral pain syndrome: a review on the associated neuromuscular deficits and current treatment options. *Br J Sports Med.* 2008;42: 789–795.
45. Reeser JC, Verhagen E, Briner WW, et al. Strategies for the prevention of volleyball related injuries. *Br J Sports Med.* 2006;40:594–600.
46. Casa DJ. Proper hydration for distance running – identifying individual fluid needs. *Track Coach.* 2004;167: 5321–5328.
47. Noyes FR, Barber-Westin SD, Fleckenstein C, et al. The drop-jump screening test: Difference in lower limb control by gender and effect on neuromuscular training in female athletes. *Am J Sports Med.* 2005;33:197–207.

CHAPTER 20

Foundations of Strength Training for Special Populations

MOH H. MALEK

OBJECTIVES

After reading this chapter, you shall be able to:

- Identify various populations that will benefit from specific exercise programs.
- Demonstrate an understanding of the roles of cardiovascular training, flexibility training, and resistance training in special populations.
- Discuss the role of resistance training in slowing the natural progression of specific musculoskeletal diseases.
- Discuss the important considerations for youth and seniors when designing an exercise program.
- Work together with other exercise professionals in determining a safe and efficacious training program in special populations.
- Implement an appropriate exercise prescription for various special populations.

KEY TERMS

Acquired Immune Deficiency Syndrome (AIDS)
Adolescents
Cardiovascular Disease
Cancer
Cerebral Palsy (CP)
Children
Chronic Obstructive Pulmonary Disease (COPD)
Down Syndrome
Duchenne Muscular Dystrophy (DMD)
Epiphyseal Plates
Fibromyalgia
Human Immunodeficiency Virus (HIV)
Multiple Sclerosis (MS)
Muscular Dystrophy
Musculoskeletal Diseases
Myopathies
Neuropathies
Osteoarthritis
Osteopenia
Osteoporosis
Pectus Excavatum
Poliomyelitis
Postpolio Syndrome (PPS)
Pregnancy
Progressive Resistance Training (PRT)
Resistance Training
Rheumatoid Arthritis (RA)
Sarcopenia
Spinal Cord Injury (SCI)
Stroke
Type I Diabetes
Type II Diabetes

Introduction

People are living longer, often with one or more chronic diseases. Athletes with disabilities are shattering stereotypes. Physicians are prescribing exercise for their patients to manage medical conditions such as cardiovascular disease and diabetes. Limited insurance coverage may lead a person with hemiplegia out of the physical therapy clinic and into the gym. These are just some of the reasons why exercise management for special populations has become so important.

Venues such as hospital-based wellness centers, fitness centers, and assisted living facilities have a wide mix of clients with special needs. Recently, Malek et al. (1) found that the majority of health fitness instructors surveyed in the Southern California area lacked the level of knowledge needed to safely train special populations. Therefore, the purpose of this chapter is to introduce the reader to a variety of special populations and the current findings related to exercise as a form of intervention. This chapter should be used as a reference by the health fitness instructor rather than a strict guideline (Table 20.1).

As in the case of any training regimen, the health fitness instructor needs to design an individualized program in close consultation with the client. For example, one client with a spinal cord injury (SCI) may desire the strength and endurance to enter athletic competition; another may desire the strength and endurance to be able to get out of bed independently. In any case, it is imperative to work in close communication with the physician, physical therapist, or other primary care personnel to insure the safety of the special population client. The health fitness instructor must understand the client's needs and precautions, where to get more information, and, most importantly, be alert to problems and know when to take action or call for medical help. Though caution is essential, it is equally important not to deny those with special needs the opportunity to reap the benefits of exercise.

This chapter touches upon cardiovascular exercise and flexibility, but the focus is on resistance training. **Resistance training** has become a critical component of exercise programs for athletes, in marked contrast to previous generations who were instructed to avoid resistance training for fear of becoming "muscle bound." More importantly, resistance training has become recognized as an important component for overall health and fitness in the general population (2). There are, however, groups of individuals whose participation in resistance training requires special scrutiny. In this chapter, resistance training for several populations with special needs is discussed, and unique aspects and possible contraindications for resistance training are considered. For those populations where resistance training is appropriate, the general principles of program design are the same as for the general population. That is, factors such as proper warm-up, periodization, and specificity need to be incorporated in all programs. Caution needs to be employed to avoid injury and overwork, but it should be noted that the benefits of resistance training only occur through the application of progressive overload, and high-intensity training (in terms of % one-repetition maximum [1-RM]) is often necessary for optimal benefits even in special populations.

TABLE 20.1 ● DISEASES COMMON AMONG SPECIAL POPULATIONS

DISEASE	WEBSITE
Sacropenia	http://www.nia.nih.gov/
Osteoporosis	http://www.nof.org/
Arthritis	http://www.arthritis.org/
	http://www.niams.nih.gov/
Pectus excavatum	http://my.clevelandclinic.org/disorders/pectus_excavatum/hic_pectus_excavatum.aspx
Cerebral palsy	http://www.ninds.nih.gov/health_and_medical/disorders/cerebral_palsy.htm
Mental retardation/Down syndrome	http://www.ndss.org/
Muscular dystrophy	http://www.mdausa.org/
	http://www.ninds.nih.gov/health_and_medical/disorders/md.htm
Stroke	http://www.ninds.nih.gov/health_and_medical/disorders/stroke.htm
Fibromyalgia	http://fmaware.org/
Post-polio syndrome	http://www.ninds.nih.gov/health_and_medical/disorders/post_polio_short.htm
Multiple sclerosis	http://www.nmss.org/
Spinal cord injury	http://www.asia-spinalinjury.org/
	http://www.spinalcord.uab.edu/
AIDS/HIV	http://www.sis.nlm.nih.gov/HIV/HIVMain.html
Chronic obstructive pulmonary disease	http://www.nhlbi.nih.gov/health/public/lung/other/copd_fact.htm
Obesity	http://www.nhlbi.nih.gov/health/public/heart/obesity/lose_wt/
	http://www.cdc.gov/nccdphp/dnpa/obesity/index.htm
Diabetes mellitus	http://diabetes.niddk.nih.gov/dm/pubs/statistics/index.htm
Cancer	http://www.nci.nih.gov/

GERIATRICS

In 2003, there were almost 36 million people aged 65 and older living in the United States, accounting for just more than 12% of the total population or about one in every eight people. This number will continue to grow over the next two decades as the Baby Boomers age. Persons reaching age 65 have an average life expectancy of an additional 18.2 years, yet many will be dealing with at least one chronic condition that will impact their quality of life. Among those 65 to 74 years old, almost 20% had difficulties with activities of daily living (ADLs), while over half aged 85 years and older had difficulties with ADLs. Unfortunately, only 26% of persons aged 65 to 74 and 16% of persons aged 75 and older report that they engage in regular leisure-time physical activity. (Department of Health and Human Services, Administration on Aging: http://www.aoa.gov/prof/Statistics/statistics.asp). Due to the size of this demographic and their need for physical activity, health fitness professionals will increasingly interact with the geriatric population. The emphasis of many of these clients will be to maintain or improve their abilities to perform daily activities.

NORMAL AGING AND SARCOPENIA

The typical aging process has deleterious effects on human skeletal muscle and is associated with loss of muscle mass, muscle strength and power, and eventually difficulty with ADLs. The progressive loss of muscle mass with advanced age is referred to as **sarcopenia** (3). Age-associated loss of lean body mass and function can not only impact an older person's quality of life but also lead to preventable injuries such as hip fractures. The rate of change in strength can be quite dramatic. Decreases in isokinetic strength occur at a rate of about 1.4% to 2.5% y^{-1} after age 65 depending on muscle group and contraction velocity (4). From ages 20 to 80, there is a loss of muscle fiber number of approximately 40% that is also accompanied by a general reduction in muscle fiber size (5). Some studies have found that between the ages of 20 and 80 years, skeletal muscle mass decreases by 35% to 40% (6,7). The fiber atrophy tends to be greater in type II fibers (5). In addition, sarcopenia is accompanied by loss of motor units. Reinnervation of orphaned muscle fibers by surviving alpha motor neurons leads to whole muscles with fewer total motor units, but with motor units that contain more fibers. Much of the decline in strength results from the loss of muscle mass, but muscle quality (strength per unit of muscle) may also decline (8). The overall effects of sarcopenia likely contribute to the decline in basal metabolic rate with age and progressive increase in percent body fat. It appears that the relative (%) changes in muscle mass and upper body strength may be greater in men than women (9); however, the absolute effects of sarcopenia may be more severe in women. Indeed, approximately 50% of women above age 65 cannot lift 4.5 kg above their head (10).

In order to counteract the effects of sarcopenia, researchers have focused on the effects of resistance training in the elderly (11–13). Fortunately, resistance exercise is a powerful stimulus to ameliorate the effects of sarcopenia in the elderly (3). Moritani and deVries (14) were the first to show that resistance exercise could result in significant increases in muscle strength in the elderly. Since then, numerous studies have shown that resistance training results in significant improvements in muscle strength in older persons. In addition, resistance training can result in significant increases in muscle mass, even in individuals in their 90s (15). For example, Yarasheski et al. (16) examined the effects of a 3-month resistance training program in seventeen 76- to 92-year-old frail adults. The training program was performed on weight machines and consisted of eight different exercises (Fig. 20.1). Subjects lifted weights at 65% to 75% of their 1-RM and gradually progressed to 85% to 100% of their initial 1-RM. Yarasheski et al. (16) found a significant increase in muscle mass in their subjects after 3 months of resistance training. The investigators concluded that, "skeletal muscle proteins maintain the ability to adapt to increased contractile demand even in 76- to 92-year-old physically frail women and men." Trappe et al. (17) examined the effects of maintaining muscle strength and size in the quadriceps muscle following 12 weeks of resistance training in 10 older males (70 ± 4 years). The subjects performed isotonic leg extensions at 80% of their concentric 1-RM leg extension 3 times · wk^{-1}. At the end of 12 weeks, the subjects were divided into two groups, one performing strength training once a week and the other group performing no exercise for 6 months. Trappe et al. (17) found an 11% decrease in 1-RM strength in the no exercise group, but no decrease in the group that exercised once a week. The investigators concluded that training at 80% of 1-RM "is sufficient to preserve both muscle mass and strength characteristics in older adults following 12 weeks of **progressive resistance training (PRT)**."

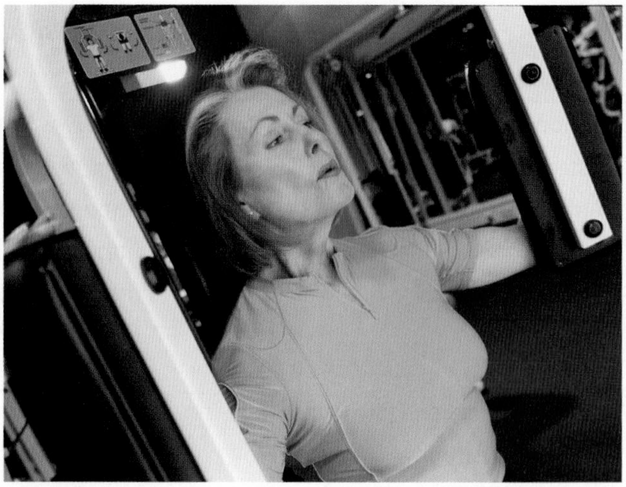

FIGURE 20.1 Weight training among the elderly has been shown to increase muscle mass and preserve strength.

It is clear that resistance training can elicit significant improvements in muscle strength and muscle mass in the elderly. It is less clear whether resistance training improves function in older persons, but measures such as gait speed and the 6-minute walk test tend to show modest improvements with resistance training (18). Given the well-documented benefits of resistance training in older persons, resistance training exercise is now recognized as a critical component of fitness for adults of all ages (2,7). Indeed, it has been noted that "increased muscle strength and mass in the elderly can be the first step toward a lifetime of increased physical activity and a realistic strategy for maintaining functional status and independence" (7). In addition, exercises should specifically target large muscle groups that are used in daily activities (7).

A PRT program for elderly individuals can reduce the effects of sarcopenia by increasing muscle mass and functional capacity and improving quality of life.

OSTEOPOROSIS

Osteoporosis is a systemic process of diminishing bone mass and deterioration of internal bone structure that results in the increased risk of fracture. It is known as a "silent disease" because the first sign of disease may be a fracture, so awareness of risk factors is important (Box 20.1). Diagnosis of osteoporosis is improving, however, with the advent of bone mineral density (BMD) testing. Approximately 44 million Americans, or 55% of people 50 years of age and older, have osteoporosis and almost 34 million more are estimated to be at increased risk. Women are at greater risk due to hormonal changes that lead to rapid depletion of BMD with menopause.

More than 1.5 million fractures annually are attributed to osteoporosis with wrist, hip, and vertebral fractures being the most common. Hip fractures often carry severe consequences; an average of 24% of hip fracture patients aged 50 and older die in the year after their fracture (19). The estimated national direct expenditure (hospitals and nursing homes) for osteoporosis-related fractures was $18 billion in 2002, and the cost is rising, so this is clearly a public health concern (19).

Exercise has become a primary treatment recommendation for osteoporosis. To understand how exercise might affect osteoporosis, consider the process of bone remodeling. Bone is a dynamic tissue in which old, weakened bone tissue is resorbed then replaced by new, stronger material. Peak bone mass is reached during young adult life and then gradually diminishes as more bone is resorbed than created. **Osteopenia** is defined as low bone mass, or BMD between 1.0 and 2.5 standard deviations below the mean of young normal adults. Osteoporosis is defined according to the National Institute of Health as BMD < 2.5 standard deviations below the norm. Since bone responds to physical forces by increasing bone formation, it would be logical to assume that the stresses created during exercise could lead to increased bone density. Research supports this assertion in general, but there is still some variability in findings.

In a meta-analysis that included 18 randomized controlled trials, aerobics, weight bearing, and resistance exercises were all effective on the BMD of the spine. However, studies of resistance training programs varied in intensity, mode, and duration, which led to some variability in findings (20). Nevertheless, the evidence is strong enough to suggest that resistance training and weight-bearing exercise are essential for the client with osteoporosis.

While the ideal training program to improve BMD has yet to be defined, there are practical guidelines that can be incorporated into a structured fitness regime. Avoid spinal flexion during exercise and ADLs by maintaining a straight spine with erect posture. This will minimize increased loads on the vertebral bodies that might cause compression fractures leading to kyphosis. Overhead compressive loads and twisting postures may also jeopardize the spine. Cardiovascular activity should emphasize safety and avoid ballistic movements. Flexibility exercises that improve posture and balance are indicated. Reduce fall hazards through facility safety strategies. Focus on functional exercises that improve leg and core strength and balance to prevent falls. Bone mass attained early in life and maintained with exercise, diet, and lifestyle choices is the best route to prevent osteoporosis, but improvements can be made with a comprehensive program including resistance training (21).

BOX 20.1

Risk factors for Osteoporosis

- Female Sex
- Thin and/or small frame
- Advanced age
- Family history of osteoporosis
- Postmenopausal (including surgically induced)
- Amenorrhea (abnormal absence of menstrual periods)
- Anorexia nervosa
- Low lifetime calcium intake
- Vitamin D deficiency
- Medications (corticosteroids, chemotherapy, and others)
- Inactive lifestyle
- Cigarette smoking
- Excessive use of alcohol
- Low testosterone levels in men

Evidence suggests that resistance training and weight-bearing exercise are essential for the client with osteoporosis.

ARTHRITIS

Musculoskeletal diseases account for approximately $240 billion or 2.9% of the gross national product (22,23). In particular, arthritis is one of the most prevalent chronic conditions worldwide (22) and is projected to affect 60 million individuals by the year 2020 in the United States alone (22). The two most common types are **rheumatoid arthritis (RA)** and **osteoarthritis**.

RA is a chronic, systemic, multijoint disease. It typically affects the joints of the hands, wrists, elbows, shoulders, knees, feet, and cervical spine in a symmetrical pattern. Marked inflammation of the joint synovium can lead to chronic pain, joint damage and deformity, and loss of function. In 20% of the cases, other organ systems such as heart and lung are involved (24). Onset of RA is primarily between ages 30 and 50, but the range extends from children to the elderly. RA affects 1% of the U.S. population or 2.1 million Americans, with 70% being women (25). Though the etiology of RA is unknown, it is classified as an autoimmune disorder (24). As there is no known cure for RA, medical management of the disease focuses on controlling the inflammation with a combination of medications including nonsteroidal anti-inflammatory drugs (NSAIDs), glucocorticoids or prednisone, disease-modifying antirheumatic drugs (DMARDs), biologic response modifiers, and analgesics (25).

Traditionally, the exercise management of RA focused on preserving the joint mobility and minimizing stress placed on the joint. Therefore, range-of-motion exercises and/or non–weight bearing were predominant modes of exercise prescribed by health care professionals. However, the use of dynamic exercise therapy has started to become an alternative approach to treating RA patients (26). While resistance training may seem counterintuitive as a training mode for RA patients, Van den Ende et al. (26) found that dynamic exercise therapy is effective in increasing muscle strength with no negative effects or increase in pain. Evidence regarding the beneficial effects of resistance training is increasing in the literature and may, in the long term, be an alternative to traditional drug therapies that result in substantial cost to the patient (22,23).

More recently, de Jong et al. (27) examined the long-term effects of high-intensity exercise program in a multicenter clinical trial called Rheumatoid Arthritis Patients in Training (RAPIT). Three hundred nine RA patients were recruited for the study and randomly assigned to either a usual care group or the RAPIT group. The RAPIT group consisted of an 80-minute exercise regimen performed biweekly. Each session included an aerobics cycling component (20 minutes), circuit training (20 minutes), and a sport activity/game (20 minutes) such as badminton. The circuit training regimen included exercises to enhance functional living (e.g., turning around in bed) along with resistance training with a light load and high repetitions. De jong et al. (27) found that muscle strength increased significantly in the RAPIT when compared to the usual care group (25% vs. 10%) over the 2-year period. The investigators also found that functional ability, physical capacity increased, and reduced levels of psychological stress as measured by the Hospital Anxiety and Depression Scale (27) significantly improved in the RAPIT group. Munneke et al. (28) evaluated adherence and satisfaction in 146 RA patients who were enrolled in the RAPIT program and found that attendance after 2 years was 74% and by the end of the fifth year, 78% of all patients recommended the program to other RA patients.

Häkkinen et al. (29) examined the effects of a 2-year home-based strength training program in 70 RA patients who were randomly assigned to either a strength training or control group. Patients in the strength training group performed two sets of 8 to 12 repetitions at 50% to 70% intensity for all muscle groups of the arms, legs, and trunk using rubber bands and dumbbells as resistance, whereas the control group performed range-of-motion and stretching exercises. Both groups performed their exercise regimen twice a week. Häkkinen et al. (29) found that strength training significantly increased knee extension strength (59%), grip strength (50%), trunk extension strength (19%), and trunk flexion strength (24%) when compared to the control group. While the control group had an increase in the above-mentioned variables from baseline, the increase was substantially lower than the strength training group. Also, the investigators found that strength levels remained as much as 50% above the baseline levels during a 5-year follow-up period (29). These findings were similar to another study that examined the effects of concurrent strength and endurance training in women with early and longstanding RA (30). As such, researchers have concluded that an individually tailored strength regimen should be part of the standard care when working with clients with RA. Because RA is characterized by periods of exacerbation, joints that are inflamed should be rested other than performing pain-free range of motion. Modifications to build up dumbbells or handles may assist those with a weakened grip.

Another common form of arthritis, especially in the older population, is osteoarthritis, which is also referred to as degenerative joint disease. Osteoarthritis affects more than 20 million individuals in the United States and is predicted to affect 70 million individuals by 2030 (31–33). The disease is characterized by the degeneration of cartilage, which cover the ends of bones in a joint. Although the mechanism causing osteoarthritis is still under investigation, researchers have hypothesized that factors such as being overweight, joint injuries, and the aging process may contribute to the development of osteoarthritis (34). While a number of treatment approaches such as pain-relief techniques, surgery, and/or pharmaceutical interventions exist, recent research has found that exercise is one of the better treatments for osteoarthritis (35), which may also be cost-effective.

Recently, McCarthy et al. (34) examined the effectiveness and cost of providing a home-based exercise program versus home-based exercise that was supplemented with an 8-week class-based exercise program. Over 200 patients, who were diagnosed with knee osteoarthritis as classified by the American College of Rheumatology, were given the home-based exercise program or supplemented with the 8-week class-based exercise program. Both programs involved exercise modalities that included increasing strength of the lower limb as well as improving balance and mobility. All patients were assessed at 6 and 12 months after the exercise intervention. Patients in the supplemented group demonstrated greater improvements in strength, balance, and pain reduction during walking than those patients who received only the home-based exercise program. In addition, McCarthy et al. (34) suggested that the supplement program may be cost-effective for management of patients with knee osteoarthritis. Fransen et al. (36) conducted a meta-analysis of 17 randomized clinical trials that were published in 2002 that examined the effects of various interventions for treating 2,562 osteoarthritis patients. With regard to self-reported physical function and pain rating, the results indicated that class-based programs had a higher effect size for the two indices when compared to individual treatments or home-based programs. Regardless of the exercise training programs, patients with chronic musculoskeletal disease should focus on flexibility development, coordination, muscular strength, balance and mobility, and overall aerobic fitness.

Although strength training for RA patients may seem counterintuitive, studies show increases in functional capacity that can be maintained up to 5 years following training.

PEDIATRICS

Many children are active in competitive sports, but there is a growing number who are sedentary and overweight. The obesity prevalence in adolescents has more than doubled over past 25 years. According to the American Obesity Association (37), approximately 30% of children and adolescents are overweight, and about 15% are obese. With this trend comes an increase in health risk factors such as asthma, diabetes, and hypertension that can follow a child into adulthood, potentially resulting in disease and disability.

Some children are born with a disability, such as cerebral palsy (CP), Down syndrome, or muscular dystrophy. While these conditions are also found in adults, they are included in this section as they first significantly affect physical functioning during childhood. Families and schools may turn to fitness centers as exercise outlets for these children as an adjunct to physical therapy, or when insurance funds are depleted. Health fitness professionals can play a key role in getting the pediatric population started on a lifelong path of physical fitness (Fig. 20.2).

HEALTHY CHILDREN AND ADOLESCENTS

The process of growth and development in **children** (before puberty) and **adolescents** (after puberty) results in increases in muscle size and muscle strength (38–42). Much of the strength increase across age is simply due to increases in muscle size. However, maturation of skeletal muscle and the nervous system lead to increases in muscle strength across age that are larger than can be completely accounted for simply by increased muscle mass (38–42). That is, there is an "age effect" that results

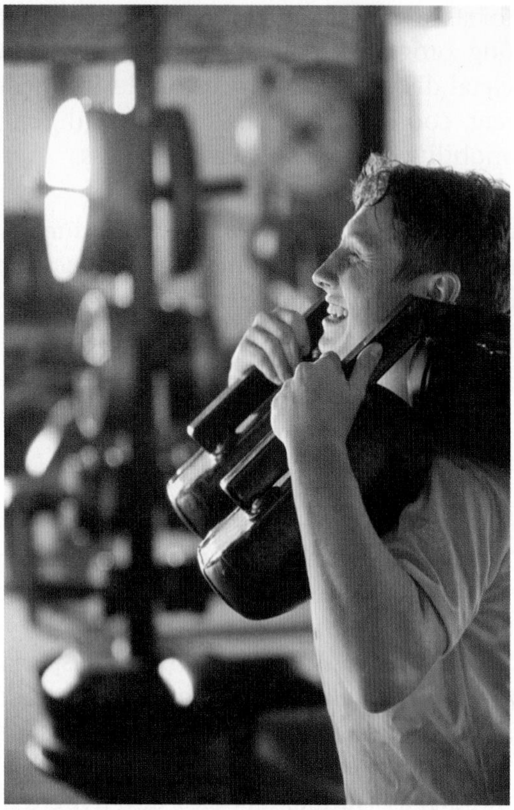

FIGURE 20.2 Encouraging adolescents to weight train will start them on a lifelong path to physical fitness.

in older children and adolescents being stronger, pound for pound, than younger individuals (43).

Of interest have been the effects of resistance training in the context of growth and development. Specifically, can resistance training enhance strength development beyond what would be expected to be seen as a normal consequence of growth and development. Numerous studies have shown that resistance training in children and adolescents is effective in increasing muscle strength (40,42,44). The benefits appear to transfer to performance on other motor skills such as the vertical jump (40). Prior to puberty, anabolic hormone concentrations are quite low, which limits the potential for resistance training to cause significant hypertrophy. Despite this, resistance training does increase muscle strength in this population. This suggests that the dominant effect is via neurological adaptations (40,45). After puberty, both men and women are capable of inducing substantive changes in both muscle size and muscle strength with properly implemented resistance training programs.

A primary concern with youth resistance training is safety; specifically, there is potential for improper resistance training to cause damage to the **epiphyseal plates** (growth plates) at the ends of long bones (39). Fracture of these epiphyseal plates will lead to improper growth of the long bones. In addition, strains and sprains, especially of the low back, are risks associated with resistance training in youths (and adults). However, several studies have been conducted examining resistance training in youths, and found that resistance training is quite safe and has comparable injury risk as resistance training in adults (39,40,45). The position statement of the National Strength and Conditioning Association regarding youth resistance training notes that "There are no justifiable

Q & A from the Field

Q ***A high school athlete wants to improve his strength by beginning a PRT program. However, his parents have read in a popular fitness magazine that resistance training at a young age can be detrimental to the epiphyseal plate. Is it true that resistance training can stunt an adolescent's bone growth?***

A Although popular belief is that resistance training for adolescences can negatively affect bone growth, research does not support this position. Several studies have shown that a properly supervised PRT program does not negatively affect the epiphyseal plate. However, studies have shown that improper techniques and lifting excessive amounts of weight can result in damage to the epiphyseal plate. Therefore, the high school athlete would benefit from a training program that would consist of lifting low to moderate amounts of weight, which can be performed for 8 to 12 repetitions.

safety reasons to preclude prepubescent or adolescents from participating in a properly designed and supervised resistance training program" (40). The key to safe resistance training in youths is to ensure that there is proper supervision for training, and 1-RM or near 1-RM lifts should generally be avoided (45). Instead, lighter weights that allow for relatively high repetitions are preferred for training. However, it has been shown that 1-RM testing is safe (39) and reliable (41). It may also be the case that resistance training can decrease injury risk. In adults, resistance training strengthens structures such as ligaments, tendons, and bones, which lessens the risk of injury. In addition, strength training can be used to correct strength imbalances. Similar outcomes are likely in youths, but limited data are available regarding reduction of injury risk with resistance training in youths.

A properly designed and supervised resistance training program should incorporate periodization principles to vary volume and intensity throughout the year. Each session should include a comprehensive warm-up period. Training programs should target all the major muscle groups and liberally include compound, multijoint exercises. Initial intensity and volume should be relatively light but progress toward 2 to 3 d $\cdot$ wk^{-1} from 1 to 3 sets per exercise at loads that allow 6 to 15 repetitions per set (40). A variety of different training modalities are appropriate, including free weights, body weight resisted calisthenics, and machines. Progression should emphasize increases in repetitions relative to increases in resistance, and very light loads should be employed when learning new movements so that proper technique is learned. Indeed, use of a broomstick in lieu of a weight bar may be appropriate when initially learning proper technique for complex free weight exercises.

A proper supervised resistance training program has been found to be beneficial in the pediatric population with no harm to the epiphyseal plates.

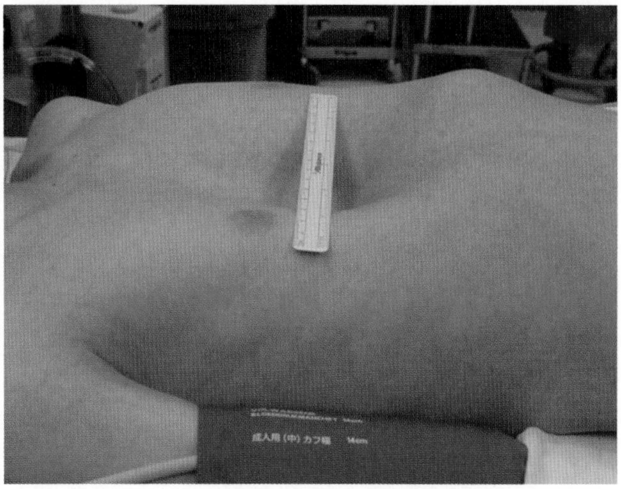

FIGURE 20.3 Patient with pectus excavatum deformity of the chest. (Photo courtesy of Christopher Derby, MD.)

PECTUS EXCAVATUM

Pectus excavatum (or chest wall deformity) is a congenital condition (Fig. 20.3) that occurs in approximately 1 in every 300 births (46) and, therefore, is more common than Down syndrome that occurs approximately 1 in 600 to 1,000 births (47). It has been hypothesized that the pathology of pectus excavatum is the result of unbalanced overgrowth in the costochondral regions of the chest wall, which in turn makes the chest appear to be concave. In addition, the heart is grossly displaced laterally such that it can be palpated underneath the armpit. The severity of pectus excavatum is determined by computed tomography scans that are then used to estimate the inner width of the chest at the widest point and the distance between the posterior surface of the sternum and the anterior surface of the spine. This ratio provides the pectus severity index that ranges from 3.2 (mild) to 12.7 (severe) (46). It should be noted, however, that the normal chest index is approximately 2.5.

Numerous studies by Malek et al. (48–53) have examined the effects of pectus excavatum on cardiorespiratory fitness. For example, in their initial study, Malek et al. (53) examined cardiovascular and respiratory indices during incremental cycle ergometry in aerobically conditioned pectus excavatum patients. The investigators found that although maximal oxygen uptake was in the normal range of predicted normative values, the patient's ability to sustain exercise via aerobic metabolism was compromised as the chest wall deformity became more severe (53). This result indicated that insufficient amount of oxygen was being delivered to the working muscles and, therefore, anaerobic metabolism, during the majority of the exercise test, was being used to sustain the exercise intensity. In a follow-up study, Malek et al. (52) examined cardiovascular and respiratory function during incremental exercise pre- and post-operatively. The concern here was to maintain the same habitual exercise status of the patient before and after the corrective surgery. This would minimize any deconditioning factors that may affect the exercise response. The investigators found that surgery improved the patient's cardiovascular and respiratory functions such that the various physiological indices were in the normative range. These results were supported by a meta-analysis (48) that showed that surgical repair of pectus excavatum significantly improved cardiovascular function.

Pectus excavatum patients are active and try to maintain a level of fitness despite their chest wall deformity. Although surgical repair is the only method of correcting this condition, health fitness instructors need to understand and appreciate the existents of this condition. In addition, it is recommended that prior to and following surgical repair, aerobic and strength exercises be performed to condition the muscles. Training regimens should be individualized and the health fitness instructor needs to work closely with the patient's physician.

CEREBRAL PALSY

Cerebral palsy (CP) is an umbrella term used to describe a group of nonprogressive infant-onset motor disorders typically caused by various sources of cerebral ischemia during the prenatal, perinatal, or postnatal period. Factors such as physical trauma during delivery and metabolic disturbances can lead to CP. Common motor problems include spasticity, hyperreflexia, difficulties with fine motor control, and gait dysfunction (e.g., crouch gait) (54). CP is the most common cause of childhood physical disability and occurs at a rate of between 2.0 and 2.5 cases per 1,000 live births (55).

Muscle weakness is often present in one (hemiplegia) or both limbs (diplegia) in individuals with CP. Quadriceps weakness has been shown to be correlated with poor gait performance in CP (56,57), suggesting that strength training may help improve gait function in CP. A variety of factors appear to contribute to this weakness. Two neural factors appear to be involved. First, individuals with CP have been shown to have higher levels of antagonist co-contraction (58), so that antagonist activation creates an opposing torque across the joint and diminishes the torque expressed at the joint by the agonist. Second, agonist activation appears to be diminished relative to age-matched controls (58), that is, individuals with CP are less able to recruit the motor units that are available in the motor unit pool. In addition, differences in muscle tissue characteristics likely influence strength. First, muscle size tends to be smaller in individuals with CP (58). In addition, higher levels of collagen are present in muscle from individuals with CP (59). Collectively, these observations indicate that less contractile protein can be brought to bear when creating force. Lower levels of specific tension (force per unit of muscle mass) are present in CP, which may reflect changes at both the muscle tissue and in neural activation (recruitment and co-contraction) (58).

Historically, resistance training has been discouraged for individuals with CP, often based on fears that resistance training would exacerbate spasticity (velocity-dependent resistance to stretch). However, there is no evidence in the literature to indicate that resistance training increases spasticity, and several studies have shown that resistance training results in increases in muscle strength in children with CP. Damiano et al. (57,60) showed that a 6-week (3 times · wk^{-1}) strength training program of the quadriceps using ankle weights for resistance (4 sets × 5 repetitions at 65% 1-RM) resulted in significant gains in strength (about 50% over pretraining values) in children (age range, 6 to 14 years) with CP who exhibit spasticity and diplegia. Selected indices of gait function were also improved; however, the effects were much smaller than for the strength gains. Similar results were reported by Damiano and Abel (56) in children with CP exhibiting either hemiplegia or diplegia. Improvements in gait speed with resistance training were primarily influenced by increases in stride frequency with no change in stride length.

While CP occurs in infancy, the effects last throughout life. As noted previously, CP is a disease characterized by symptoms such as spasticity, weakness, elevated antagonist co-contraction, and generally poor motor coordination. Most research regarding resistance training in CP has examined its effects in children and adolescents. Andersson et al. (61) reported that their "experience is that individuals with CP usually stop training after having reached adulthood. They are often tired of physiotherapy after having undergone it all their lives." (p. 220). To date, little data exists regarding the effects of resistance training in adults with CP. Andersson et al. (61) have shown that 10 weeks of 2 times · wk^{-1} training resulted in significant increases in muscle strength. More importantly, there were significant improvements in indices of range of motion, motor function, and ambulation ability. Further, there were no increases in spasticity. While the adult data are limited to one study, it appears that resistance training is effective in improving both muscle strength as well as functional ability in adults with CP.

Resistance training in individuals with CP has been shown to increase muscle strength. These strength increases do not exacerbate symptoms of CP such as spasticity. The strength increases may help improve performance of ADLs.

MENTAL RETARDATION AND DOWN SYNDROME

Several studies have shown that persons with mental retardation have less muscle strength and endurance than age- and sex-matched controls (62,63). One of the major causes of mental retardation is **Down syndrome**. Down syndrome is a genetic disorder that affects approximately 1 in 600 to 1,000 live births (47,64), and is characterized by cognitive delay, distinct facial features such as epicanthal folds of the eyelids and relatively flat occiput and nasal bridge, and short limbs (64). Among its manifestations are low muscle tone (hypotonia) and joint laxity (64,65). These latter factors can lead to increased risk of musculoskeletal and orthopaedic problems (64). In addition, individuals with Down syndrome tend to be less physically active than controls and are at increased risk of obesity, diabetes, and cardiovascular disease (65). Increasing physical activity and fitness in individuals with Down syndrome is an important goal in the management of Down syndrome, especially since the lower fitness associated with Down syndrome, coupled with the typical decline in fitness with aging, will likely leave individuals with Down syndrome at particular risk for prematurely losing the physical ability to perform jobs requiring light work (65).

Individuals with Down syndrome have been shown to be significantly weaker than both age- and sex-matched controls as well as relative to age- and sex-matched individuals with mental retardation other than Down syndrome (62,63). This weakness is correlated with low BMD, and risk for osteoporosis is elevated in those with Down syndrome (62). To date, only a few studies have examined the effects of resistance training in persons with mental retardation generally, or in Down syndrome specifically. Rimmer and Kelly (66) found that a 9-week machine-based resistance training program resulted in large increases in muscle strength (>42%) in adults with mental retardation (IQ range, 40 to 70) other than Down syndrome. Suomi et al. (67) found comparable increases in isokinetic strength following 12 weeks of resistance training (hydraulic machine exercise) in individuals with mild (IQ range, 52 to 67) to moderate (IQ, 36 to 51) mental retardation. Rimmer et al. (68) studied a combined strength and cardiovascular endurance training program in adults (mean age, 39 years) with Down syndrome. Relative to untrained controls, a 12-week program (3 times $\cdot$ wk^{-1}, 10 to 20 repetitions per set) of machine-based exercises including the leg press and bench press resulted in 1-RM strength increases of approximately 40%. Though the data are still limited, these studies suggest that persons with mental retardation are capable of making substantive improvements in muscle strength with resistance training. Given the importance of strength in the vocational skills for persons with mental retardation, the potential for improvement in strength with training is an important observation.

The benefit of resistance training for Down syndrome individuals is an increase in muscle tone and motor activity.

MUSCULAR DYSTROPHY

Muscular dystrophy is an umbrella term that describes a family of genetic muscular diseases that involve dysfunction of the dystrophin glycoprotein complex in skeletal muscle. The muscular dystrophies lead to progressive muscle wasting, weakness, and disability. Of these, by far the most common form is **Duchenne muscular dystrophy (DMD)**. DMD is the most common fatal childhood genetic disease (1 in 3,500 births) and is found only in boys. The gene for the muscle protein dystrophin is found on the X chromosome and is defective in DMD, resulting in a lack of dystrophin. Dystrophin is a filamentous cytoskeletal protein that serves to bind the contractile protein actin to the basement membrane via the dystrophin glycoprotein complex, which is located in the muscle cell membrane (sarcolemma). A lack of dystrophin therefore affects force transmission from the muscle cell to the connective tissue. Dystrophin is present in skeletal muscle, smooth muscle, cardiac muscle, and in brain tissue. Because of the lack of dystrophin, forceful muscle contractions lead to excessive structural damage to the muscle, including the sarcolemma. A hallmark of DMD is high levels of creatine phosphokinase in the blood, which is evidence of sarcolemmal damage since sarolemmal damage allows leaking of muscle proteins to the blood (and is also symptomatic of muscle damage associated with delayed-onset muscle soreness in healthy muscle). In DMD, much of the muscle damage is likely mediated by calcium-activated proteases that are activated by calcium influx following damage to the sarcolemma. Over time, repeated cycles of muscle degeneration and regeneration lead to a net degeneration of the muscle tissue (replaced by fat and connective tissue), weakness, loss of mobility, and eventually death. Death is usually due to secondary complications in the pulmonary and cardiac systems. Relatively few studies have examined the effects of resistance exercise in DMD (69), and the data are not suggestive of a significant benefit. Indeed, individuals with DMD are especially susceptible to damage from eccentric contractions, and resistance training incorporating eccentric contractions may accelerate the progression of DMD and should be avoided.

Alternative forms of a PRT program can build muscle and maintain a healthy body in individuals with DMD.

NEUROMUSCULAR DISEASE

Neuromuscular diseases can be due to damage or dysfunction in the central nervous system (CNS), the peripheral nerves (**neuropathies**), or the muscle tissue itself (**myopathies**). In addition, complex multiple system conditions can occur such as **stroke** and **fibromyalgia**. While specific diseases have primary effects on certain tissues, neurological effects will also lead to changes in the muscle tissue. Common symptoms of neuromuscular diseases include spasticity, which is a velocity-dependent resistance to stretch, rigidity, weakness, and sensory loss. These symptoms can further lead to inactivity and deconditioning, which can then exacerbate motor dysfunction. Historically, activities like resistance exercise have been discouraged for neuromuscular diseases due to concerns about overwork and possible exacerbation of spasticity. However, it is now becoming clear that in many cases the risk of overwork is much less than previously feared, and concerns regarding spasticity exacerbation are unfounded (70,71). Indeed exercise, and in particular resistance exercise, can be a useful tool in the rehabilitation and subsequent management of many neuromuscular conditions, especially for those conditions where weakness is a primary contributor to loss of motor function.

STROKE

It is typically reported that approximately 500,000 people experience a stroke each year in the United States (72,73). However, more recent estimates increase this by 50% to approximately 750,000 (74). Strokes are the third leading cause of death (after heart disease and cancer) in the United States (72,75) and the leading cause of disability in adults (73). Stroke is the second leading cause of death, behind heart disease, worldwide (76). Approximately 31% of first-time strokes result in death within 1 year (77), with the greatest mortality risk occurring within the first 30 days following stroke (78); however, the overall death rate from stroke in the United States has been decreasing (79). The combined direct and indirect costs of stroke are estimated at an annual $30 billion (80).

There are two general categories of stroke. An ischemic stroke is conceptually similar to a myocardial infarction in that occlusion of a cerebral artery occurs as a consequence of plaque formation. In contrast, a hemorrhagic stroke results from the loss of structural integrity of a cerebral blood vessel and subsequent bleeding. Both types of stroke can lead to significant changes in muscle function including weakness and spasticity. The motor symptoms are typically most severe on one side of the body (contralateral to the side of the lesion in the brain), so hemiplegia is common, although even the "good" side frequently shows motor deficits. It was previously thought that motor deficits that were not corrected within the first 6 months of rehabilitation following a stroke were permanent, and there was limited neural plasticity with which improvements in motor function could be effected. It is now clear, however, that the extent of neural plasticity is greater than previously thought, and significant improvements can occur well after the acute stage of stroke recovery.

Historically, resistance training had been discouraged for people following a stroke, often on the argument that resistance training might lead to increased spasticity. However, several studies in individuals following the acute phase of stroke rehabilitation (>6 months after stroke) have shown that spasticity, characterized by a velocity-dependent resistance to passive stretch, is not exacerbated by resistance training (81,82), and individuals who have had a stroke are capable of significant improvements in strength (81–84). Further, several studies have shown that strength training has the potential to improve function. Engardt et al. (83) reported that eccentric-only isokinetic knee extension training of the paretic quadriceps not only increased muscle strength but decreased the asymmetry of body weight distribution across legs during sit-to-stand, while concentric-only isokinetic training improved indices of gait performance. Teixeira-Salmela et al. (84,85) showed that 10 weeks (3 times $\cdot$ wk^{-1}) of combined resistance training and endurance exercise (walking, stepping, cycling) resulted in significant improvements in gait speed, gait kinematics, and questionnaire-based estimates of physical activity and quality of life. In contrast, Moreland et al. (86) found that 6 months of resistance exercise using wrist and leg weights did not result in significant improvements in the 2-minute walk test or a disability index relative to a control group performing the same exercises with only body weight resistance. No information regarding intensity (% 1-RM) or progression of resistance was reported, so it is difficult to judge the efficacy of the intervention.

As with other populations, much of the improvement in strength can be attributed to adaptations in neural control. Engardt et al. (83) showed increases in agonist electromyography following eccentric and concentric-only training from 24% to 33%. The hypertrophic potential of paretic muscle due to stroke has not yet been examined. However, it seems likely that significant adaptations at the muscle level occur, especially given that paretic muscle is significantly deconditioned and would be highly responsive to increased loading. Indeed, Smith et al. (87) have shown significant improvements in isokinetic strength following treadmill gait training in persons with a stroke.

To date, most studies have employed relatively short training periods (≤10 weeks) and longer-term effects are unknown. Further, studies are limited by lack of control group (81–83) or poorly defined resistance training protocol (86). More research needs to be performed to further define the effects of resistance training on motor function poststroke, and to improve understanding of the different resistance training protocols (e.g., optimal intensity range, appropriate frequency and volume of training, unilateral vs. bilateral training) on outcomes. In the meantime, an individualized program focusing on functional activities appears to be a viable option. Particular attention should be afforded to safety and fall prevention; exercise modification may be necessary due to hemiplegia.

> *Structured resistance training programs may improve a poststroke patient's cardiovascular and respiratory efficiency, thus improving their quality of life.*

Fibromyalgia

Fibromyalgia is not a disease per se, but rather is classified as a chronic pain syndrome (fibromyalgia syndrome [FMS]) with a variety of symptoms (88). Chief among these is widespread presence of tender points at sites throughout the body (88,89), typically in muscle tissue. It is estimated that the prevalence of FMS is 2% of the population, and FMS is present predominately in women (89). The prevalence increases with age (89). Individuals with FMS generate over twice the yearly health care costs than health care beneficiaries without FMS (90). Diagnosis of FMS is difficult and requires pain to be present in at least 11 of 18 common sites throughout the body (88,89). In addition, other symptoms such as fatigue (physical and mental), sleep disturbances, and problems with vision are common. A variety of physiological manifestations are also present in FMS. These include endocrine indices such as elevated levels of substance P, diminished levels of serotonin, and suppressed levels of thyroid hormone (89). In addition, autonomic nervous system symptoms include elevated heart rate, low blood pressure, and altered blood flow control during exercise (88). A deconditioning/pain cycle is frequently seen in FMS, as individuals with FMS often avoid physical activity due to FMS-associated pain. This inactivity leads to muscle deconditioning, which makes the muscles more susceptible to damage and further pain (91).

The pathophysiology FMS is still poorly understood, but it appears to be linked with altered processing of afferent information in the CNS, often secondary to previous pain such as from trauma or chronic illness such as cancer. The exposure to the initial pain is believed to cause "central sensitization" of dorsal horn neurons, triggering hyperalgesia (exaggerated response to nociceptive input) and allodynia (interpretation of nonnociceptive input as painful) (92).

Exercise is frequently prescribed as an intervention for FMS (91). Aerobic exercise has been shown to alleviate pain in some individuals with FMS. However, exercise may also exacerbate muscle pain in FMS. Microtrauma to skeletal muscle, such as occurs with eccentric exercise, may lead to increased pain sensory input to the CNS, and "may lead to aggravation of generalized pain through upregulation of nociceptive processing (i.e., central sensitization)" (91).

Recently, studies have been conducted examining the effects of resistance exercise in FMS. Hakkinen et al. (93) found that 21 weeks of traditional weight training (2 times wk^{-1}) in premenopausal women with FMS using exercises such as the squat and bench press resulted in strength increases comparable to age-matched subjects who did not have FMS. These adaptations were accompanied by significant improvements in vertical jump and rate of isometric force development. In addition, the FMS subjects showed significant decreases in neck pain, fatigue, and depression. Similar results from a comparable training program were reported by Valkeinen et al. (94) in older women (60 years old) with FMS. In contrast, Jones et al. (95) did not find significant differences between a strength training group and a strengthening group; however, the strength training intervention was extremely mild (1- to 3-lb hand weights) relative to the protocols of Hakkinen et al. (93) and Valkeinen et al. (94). This suggests that benefits are acquired only when sufficient overload is applied. While more research is needed to further delineate the optimal training protocol and define the long-term benefits and risks of resistance training in FMS, it appears that resistance training is a promising intervention in FMS.

A resistance training program for FMS patients may help reduce pain and maintain muscle tone.

POSTPOLIO SYNDROME

Poliomyelitis is a viral disease in which the polio virus attacks alpha motor neuron cell bodies in the spinal cord and brain stem. Individuals who contracted the virus could be asymptomatic, could develop mild symptoms similar to the flu with possible gastrointestinal distress, or could develop "paralytic" symptoms. Those with the paralytic form developed symptoms that varied depending on the degree of neuronal damage. While death due to respiratory failure was not uncommon, most individuals achieved some level of recovery ranging from various degrees of paralysis to apparent complete recovery. Many of the muscle fibers innervated by degenerated motor neurons were reinnervated by surviving motor neurons, resulting in a smaller total motor unit pool but with larger motor units (more muscle fibers per alpha motor neuron) due to the reinnervation. With advent of the effective vaccines (e.g., Salk vaccine) in the 1950s and 1960s, new cases of poliomyelitis are extremely rare (96).

Individuals with **postpolio syndrome (PPS)** are those who have recovered function after the initial poliomyelitis and subsequently develop symptoms of weakness and fatigue 30 or more years later (69). The development of PPS seems to be a consequence of the prolonged effects of reinnervation. Specifically, because polio survivors have fewer motor units, and each surviving motor unit contains many more muscle fibers than in motor units from control subjects, the consequences of the normal age-related loss of motor neurons are more severe in those with PPS. Further, over time surviving motor units appear to lose the ability to adequately service the large number of muscle fibers that each alpha motor neuron innervates, and neuronal "exhaustion" may contribute to the "new" weakness of PPS. Of primary concern regarding resistance training in PPS has been the possibility of exacerbating symptoms. Specifically, it has been suggested that fatiguing exercise may further contribute to motor neuron loss. In general, however, resistance training has been shown to improve muscle strength in PPS (69,97–99). A significant portion of the strength increase appears to be due to increases in the ability to maximally recruit the available motor units (98). Further, motor unit number estimates have not been shown to be affected by resistance training (98), indicating that resistance training is unlikely to increase the rate of disease progression. Because the literature addressing resistance training in PPS is quite sparse, specific training guidelines are not yet available, and it seems prudent to err on the side of caution, so that the initial training intensity is low and progression occurs slowly.

Studies have found that exercise is safe and effective for individuals with PPS as long as individual tolerance (i.e., one starts to have fatigue or discomfort) is used to monitor the exercise intensity.

MULTIPLE SCLEROSIS

Multiple Sclerosis (MS) is a chronic, inflammatory, autoimmune disease of unknown etiology that affects the CNS. It causes a loss of myelin, the fatty sheath that insulates nerves, resulting in disruption of nerve conduction. Symptoms may include weakness, spasticity, tremor, fatigue, sensory disturbance, heat sensitivity, and impairments of balance, coordination, vision, speech, swallowing, cognition, and bowel and bladder function. Functional losses can range from mild to severe, often exhibit an exacerbation/remission pattern, and are ultimately progressive (100). MS affects approximately 400,000 people in the United States with 200 new cases diagnosed each week, and 2.5 million worldwide. Age of onset is typically 20 to 50 years with the majority being women. There is no known cure, but symptom treatment includes the use of disease-modifying drugs such as interferons, medication for exacerbations such as corticosteroids, rehabilitation, and complementary and alternative medicine such as diet, yoga, and guided imagery (101).

A number of studies have been conducted to support anecdotal reports that exercise is beneficial for people with MS. Individual aerobic exercise programs using stationery cycling were shown to improve the fitness and quality of life of patients with MS (102,103). Group exercise sessions that consisted of a 1-hour class of warm-up, stretch, standing, and mat exercises over 10 weeks were also found to be beneficial (104). Results indicated short-term positive changes on standardized tests for balance, endurance, and fatigue in a group of 10 ambulatory MS patients. Resistance training in combination with aerobic exercise was studied in a randomized controlled trial of 95 individuals with MS (105). The 47 people in the exercise group completed five supervised 30 minutes sessions of aerobic activity in a pool or on a bicycle ergometer at 65% to 70% of age-predicted maximal heart rate. Five supervised resistance training sessions were alternated with the aerobic sessions consisting of circuit training by performing 10 to 15 repetitions at 50% to 60% of 1-RM of circuit training on 10 weight machines that targeted major muscle groups. These sessions were followed by 23 weeks of home exercise program using elastic bands to work the same muscle groups targeted in the resistance training sessions, along with mild aerobic exercise. The 48-member control group continued with their normal ADLs throughout the study. Results indicated that the motor fatigue of knee flexors and extensors of persons in the exercise group was reduced in mildly impaired females with MS when compared to the control group. The clinical message suggested by the authors was that exercise should be as specific as possible, and the outcome will be better in persons with mild to moderate disability.

In summary, studies indicate that people with MS can improve strength, fitness, and quality of life though aerobic and resistance training. Exercise programs should be tailored to the individual taking into account the variability of the disease symptoms, such as balance, sensory loss, spasticity, cognition, and symptom exacerbation. In the case of an symptom exacerbation, focus on stretching and gentle active range of motion; resistance and aerobic exercise should be discontinued until the symptoms have remitted. A potential contraindication for exercise is overheating as persons with MS may have an attenuated or absent sweating response that could result in a temporary exacerbation of symptoms and cause fatigue. Using air conditioning, fans, and proper hydration and clothing will help avoid this problem. For pool therapy, water temperature of 80°F to 84°F is recommended (106). Periods of activity may be alternated with periods of rest to avoid overheating and fatigue. Resistance exercises should target large muscle groups in closed-chain functional exercises.

An aerobic and strength training program may help improve fitness and quality of life in people with MS.

SPINAL CORD INJURY

Spinal Cord Injury (SCI) most often results from motor vehicle accidents (50.4%) and falls (23.8%), followed by violence (11.2%) and sports injuries (9%). According to The Spinal Cord Injury Information Network, there are approximately 247,000 people living with SCI in the United States today with 11,000 new cases $\cdot$ y^{-1} in a 3:1 ratio of men to women. The estimated lifetime cost for a 25-year-old who survives a SCI ranges from $600,000 to more than $2.5 million for complex cases.

Categorization of SCI is complex and depends on not only the level of the injury, but also whether it is complete or incomplete. For a detailed explanation, consult the International *Standards for Classification of Spinal Cord Injury*, updated in 2002. Briefly, C1-T1 injuries result in tetraplegia (formerly quadriplegia) and causes impairments of arms, trunk, legs, and pelvic organs; T2-T12 injuries result in paraplegia and causes impairments of trunk, legs, and pelvic organs. These two groups are considered upper motor neuron injuries and are typified by spastic paralysis and hyperreflexia below the injury. T12 and below injuries result in paraplegia with impairments of the trunk, legs, and pelvic organs and are considered lower neuron injuries typified by flaccid paralysis and areflexia below the level of the injury.

In addition to these primary deficits, those with SCI are at high risk for secondary problems like cardiovascular disease, circulatory insufficiencies, osteoporosis, skin breakdown, musculoskeletal dysfunction, and pain (107). Research has indicated that some of these problems may be mitigated with a structured exercise program incorporating appropriate precautions; however, the effects of exercise conditioning are inversely proportional to the severity of the primary injury (107). For example, those with tetraplegia may require electrical stimulation or passive movements to use an upper-body ergometer resulting in a markedly reduced aerobic training effect (108).

Research on resistance training with SCI has focused on those with paraplegia. Shoulder girdle pain is a common complaint among those with paraplegia, apparently due to the stresses of wheelchair propulsion and transfers, and would indicate the need for strength training (107). Arm ergometry is a common method of endurance training, but used alone it was not sufficient to provide a functional strength gain because it failed to target the scapular muscles necessary for ADLs (109). Improvement in shoulder strength and pain was noted in a study that employed shoulder resistance exercises using elastic bands (110). Circuit resistance training, which incorporates periods of low-intensity, high-repetition movements (such as a free-wheel arm ergometry) interspersed with a series of resistance training exercises (such as free weights, weight machines, or elastic bands), has been shown to be the most effective in improving strength and decreasing pain (107) (Fig. 20.4).

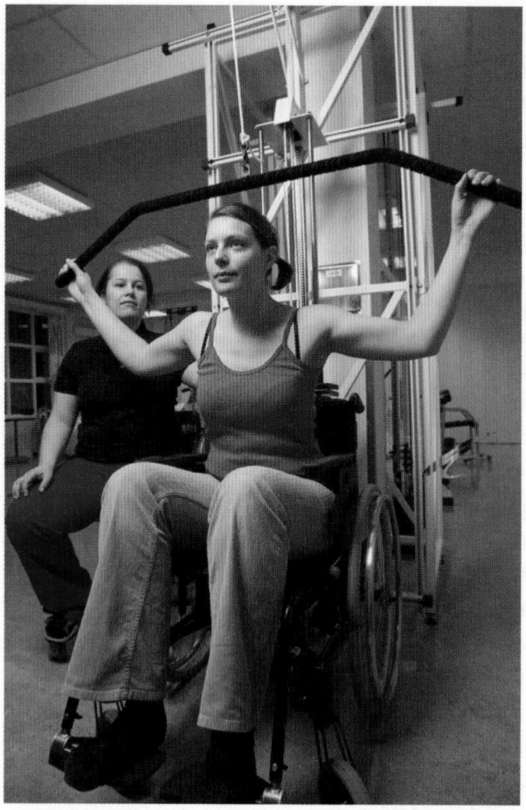

FIGURE 20.4 Resistance training exercise can be an effective way for those with spinal cord injuries to improve their strength and decrease their pain.

In general, the recommendations for resistance and aerobic training for those with SCI are not significantly different than those for the general population and should take into consideration specificity, overload, progression, and regularity (108). However, there are several precautions that must be heeded due to the motor and sensory deficits that result from a SCI. One precaution when working with persons with a T6 or higher SCI is awareness of the potential life-threatening condition known as autonomic dysreflexia (Box 20.2). Symptoms include excessive rise in blood pressure, slowed heart rate, headache, blurred vision, and congestion. It can be set off by a noxious stimulus below the level of the injury, such as pressure to a limb or a full bladder. Immediate intervention consists of identifying and removing the noxious stimuli, monitoring blood pressure, and seeking medical help (108). Other precautions include risk of fracture due to osteoporosis, overuse pain due to muscle imbalance, hypotension, and difficulty maintaining thermal stability (107).

Knowledge of the type of injury and related precautions can minimize the risks and enhance the outcome of exercise programming for persons with SCI.

BOX 20.2

Signs and Symptoms of Autonomic Dysreflexia

- Pounding headache
- Blurred vision
- Nasal congestion
- Piloerection (goose bumps)
- Profuse sweating above level of injury
- Anxiety
- Sudden increase in systolic blood pressure
- Cardiac dysrhythmias

AIDS/HIV

Human immunodeficiency virus (HIV) and **Acquired Immune Deficiency Syndrome (AIDS)** is a pandemic disease that currently has no cure (111). By the end of 2003, approximately 40 million individuals worldwide were diagnosed with HIV/AIDS (112–114). Furthermore, recent reports estimate that 5 million new HIV infections occurred worldwide in 2003 alone (114). In the United States, approximately 40,000 new cases of HIV/AIDS occur each year mostly contracted by males (70%) (112,114). Notwithstanding the effects of HIV/AIDS on the immune system, the disease is also associated with weight loss (i.e., wasting) that is reported to be a strong predictor of mortality (115–117). Wasting is defined as a progressive and unintended loss of more than 10% of the individual's body weight (112). Symptoms of wasting include, but are not limited to, fever, poor appetite, and diarrhea (118–120). Most notably, wasting affects the musculoskeletal system, which results in weakness. As discussed in previous chapters, resistance training increases lean body weight, strengthens connective tissue, and increases skeletal muscle size. Therefore, researchers have examined the effects of resistance training to counteract the effects of wasting along with traditional drug therapies in this population (121–126).

Roubenoff and Wilson (125) examined the effects of a PRT program on functional status in individuals with HIV both with and without muscle wasting. All subjects trained the major muscle groups of the upper and lower body 3 times · wk^{-1} for 8 weeks. The investigators found 5.2% increase in lean body mass following the 8 weeks of training in the group that was experiencing muscle wasting. Additionally, this group increased their strength, as measured by 1-RM, by as much as 57% when compared to baseline. Roubenoff and Wilson (125) concluded that PRT is beneficial in increasing the functional status of individuals with HIV experiencing muscle wasting. Similarly, Bhasin et al. (127) found testosterone treatment and resistance exercise increased gains in lean body weight and muscle mass in HIV-infected men with weight loss and low levels of testosterone. However, the investigators concluded that the combination of testosterone treatment and resistance exercise resulted in no additional gains when compared to either intervention alone (127).

Due to the effects of weight loss during HIV infection and the increases in mortality, the incorporation of resistance training may increase muscle mass and facilitate health benefits.

CHRONIC OBSTRUCTIVE PULMONARY DISEASE

Chronic obstructive pulmonary disease (COPD) is a progressive respiratory illness that is not completely reversible (128). The primary pathology of COPD is expiratory airflow limitation (129). Approximately 12.1 million adults 25 years or older were diagnosed with COPD in 2001 (130). It should be noted that in 2006 the U.S. National Center for Health Statistics reported that death rates due to COPD have continued to increase since 1960, whereas other major diseases such as cardiovascular and cerebrovascular illnesses had decreased during the same time period. Furthermore, a recent economic analysis revealed that the annual societal cost for treating a single COPD patient in the United States and Europe was $5,646 US (131,132). It should be noted that COPD encompasses a number of pulmonary conditions such as asthma, emphysema, and chronic bronchitis. While the condition is mostly associated with chronic cigarette use, other factors such as infection, environmental pollution, and heredity can also bring about COPD (133). Biopsies from the quadriceps muscle of COPD patients has revealed a loss of type I muscle fibers as well as a reduction in oxidative enzymes (134,135). This finding and the increased work of breathing often experienced by COPD patients may explain, in part, the associated fatigue from performing ADLs. The symptoms associated with COPD also include dyspnea with mild exertion and a reduced quality of life. Depending on the severity of the COPD, traditional treatments have included pharmacological intervention, oxygen therapy, lung transplantation, or lung volume reduction surgery (128,129). More recently, pulmonary rehabilitation clinics are incorporating exercise training as a standard part of treating COPD patients.

Interestingly, exercise has been found to a have only a moderate effect on pulmonary functional capacity (136). While most studies have focused on the effects of upper and lower extremity endurance training (137,138), a few studies have examined the effects of resistance training (139,140) as a modality for increasing functional ability and quality of life. Because COPD patients have weakened peripheral and respiratory muscles, resistance training can be used as a countermeasure to stimulate and strengthen the affected musculature (141). While the benefits of this type of exercise have been well documented with other clinical populations (11,142), there is still debate as to the effectiveness of strength training for COPD patients.

Ortega et al. (143) examined the effects of strength and endurance training in 47 patients with moderate to severe COPD ($FEV_1 \leq 41\% \pm 11\%$ of predicted) over a 12-week period. Patients were randomly assigned to an endurance training only, strength training only, or combined endurance and strength training groups. The strength training protocol consisted of five exercises: chest pull, butterfly, neck press, leg flexion, and leg extension. Patients performed four sets of six to eight repetitions for each exercise at an intensity ranging from 70% to 85% of their 1-RM. Adjustments to the workload were made every 2 weeks as the patient's strength increased. Ortega et al. (143) found that patients in the strength training group significantly improved their distance walking (561 m) when compared with the other two training modalities (501 and 493 m, respectively). Additionally, the investigators found that patient's rated their fatigue, dyspnea, and functional impairment scores (as measured by questionnaires) lowest in the strength training group after 12 weeks.

Patton et al. (139) evaluated the effectiveness of a 12-week full-body PRT in nine COPD patients ($FEV_1 \leq 41.9 \pm 16\%$ of predicted) who were undergoing aerobic training as part of their pulmonary rehabilitation. Patients performed three sets of 8 to 12 repetitions at 32% to 64% of their 1-RM on 12 resistance training machines. Exercises included multi-joint (i.e., chest press) as well as single-joint (e.g., biceps curl) movements. Patients had an increase of 5% and 29.2% in lean body mass and total distance completed during the 6-minute walk test, respectively. More importantly, COPD patients who received resistance training improved significantly more than the control group on three of the five physical function assessments (e.g., total arm raises in 1 minute, total standing up and sitting down in 1 minute, and timed climbing stairs). Based on their results, Patton et al. (139) recommended that whole body resistance training should be incorporated with the aerobic training regimen for pulmonary rehabilitation of COPD patients.

A beneficial effect of resistance training for COPD patients is the reduced anxiety and fatigue as well as independence in performing ADLs.

CARDIOVASCULAR DISEASE

Cardiovascular disease, which includes coronary heart disease (CHD) and stroke, remains the leading cause of death among Americans and is estimated to have an economic cost of over $350 billion (144). The major risk factors for cardiovascular disease included hypertension, elevated serum total cholesterol, cigarette smoking, and diabetes mellitus (145). Recent data indicate that approximately 40% of deaths in the United States during 1999 were caused by cardiovascular disease (146,147). In order to reduce the mortality and morbidity associated with cardiovascular disease, researchers have examined the effects of exercise (2,148). Recently, Oguma and Shinoda-Tagawa (149) conducted a meta-analysis examining the dose–response relationship of physical activity on cardiovascular risk factors. The investigators systematically reviewed studies published from 1966 to 2003 in which the effect of exercise was evaluated on cardiovascular risk factors. Oguma and Shinoda-Tagawa (149) found exercise is associated with reducing cardiovascular risk factors in a dose–response manner. That is, higher levels of physical activity were associated with lower risk of developing cardiovascular disease. Furthermore, the investigators found that even 1 h of walking $\cdot$ wk^{-1} resulted in reducing cardiovascular risk factors (149).

The effects of resistance exercise may also reduce cardiovascular risk factors (150). Kelley and Kelley (151) found that resting systolic and diastolic blood pressure decreased by 2% to 4% following dynamic resistance training exercise in adults. Similar results were found for reductions in resting blood pressure for children and adolescents (152). In addition, resistance training improves insulin sensitivity and glucose tolerance and improved muscle strength likely decreases the physiological stress of ADLs (150,153,154).

In addition to reducing cardiovascular disease risk factors, resistance training is increasingly incorporated into comprehensive cardiac rehabilitation programs in those with coronary artery disease. For example, Ades et al. (155) examined the effects of resistance training on functional capacity in older women with CHD. Forty-two CHD subjects were divided into two groups that either performed two sets of eight exercises for the major muscle groups or met three times a week for 40 minutes with a cardiac rehabilitation specialist. The investigators found that those women who in the weight training group improved their function capacity and therefore were able to perform ADLs without adverse effects (155). The principles of resistance training do not differ in those with coronary artery disease than those without, but particular attention must be paid to minimize risk of cardiovascular events during training. Contraindications to resistance training include unstable angina, uncontrolled hypertension (systolic ≥ 160 mm Hg, diastolic ≥ 100 mm Hg), uncontrolled dysrhythmias, severe valvular disease, hypertrophic cardiomyopathy, left ventricular outflow obstruction, and untreated congestive heart failure (150,156). Patients need physician approval prior to training, initial intensity should be low, and progression should be relatively slow. After surgery, up to 3 months may be required before starting resistance training (150).

For those with chronic heart failure (CHF), resistance training may also be a benefit. Individuals with CHF have significant fatigue and shortness of breath with physical activity, and much of the effects seem to be due to changes in skeletal muscle tissue including type I muscle fiber atrophy. Pu et al. (157) found that 10 weeks of resistance training improved muscle strength (43%), muscle endurance (299%), and performance on the 6-minute walk test (13%) in 16 women with CHF. Delgardelle et al. (158) found that combined endurance plus resistance training improved peak Vo_{2max} and left ventricular function more than training with only endurance exercise. Maiorana et al. (159) examined the effects of 8 weeks of aerobic and resistance training on peripheral skeletal muscle vessel function in the forearm in 12 men with CHF. The training sessions consisted of resistance exercise for the upper and lower limbs, whereas cycling on a stationary bicycle comprised the aerobic component of the training intervention. The investigators found that forearm vascular function improved in the trained limb when compared with the untrained limb (159). These findings demonstrated that a combination of aerobic and resistance training exercises are beneficial for improving vascular function in CHF patients. Maiorana et al. (159) stated, "a relatively short program is associated with structural as well as functional changes and that the vascular benefit may be generalized to the circulation rather than limited to the skeletal muscle bed directly involved in the training stimulus."

> *A combination of aerobic exercise and circuit resistance training improves skeletal muscle function, vasculature to skeletal muscle, as well as functional capacity in patients with cardiovascular disease.*

OBESITY

Overweight and obesity are health issues that have reached epidemic proportions within the United States (160). Overweight is defined as having a body mass index (BMI = 25 to 29.9) while obesity is defined as a BMI > 30 (161). A recent study of national costs attributed 5.5% to 9.1% of the total U.S. medical expenditures to overweight and obesity treatments, which is considerably higher than the 2% to 3.5% reported for other countries (162,163). On the state level, obesity-attributed Medicare estimates ranged from $15 million (Wyoming) to $1.7 billion (California) (162). Obesity in the United States is associated with many diseases, such as cancer, type II diabetes, hypertension, hyperinsulinemia, and CHD (160,164,165). Although body size, shape, and composition are influenced by genetics (166–168), studies have found success with caloric restriction regimen (169). The use of resistance training in conjunction with caloric restriction may further aid in the battle against obesity (Fig. 20.5).

Byrne and Wilmore (170) investigated the effects of exercise training on resting metabolic rate in moderately obese women. Subjects were divided into either a resistance training or resistance training plus walking group. The resistance training program was developed to promote increases in strength and fat-free mass. Byrne and Wilmore (170) found that the resistance training only group significantly increased their resting metabolic rate following the training intervention. Thus, they concluded that resistance training has the potential to

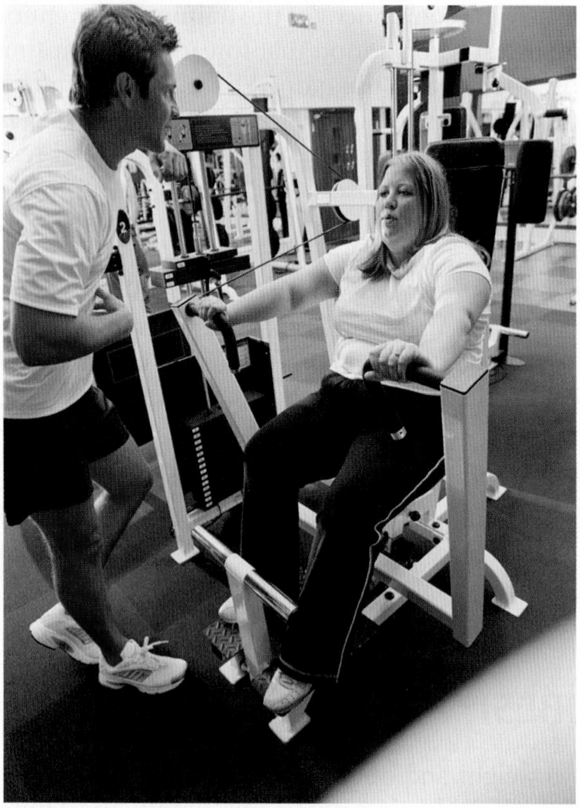

FIGURE 20.5 Resistance training and caloric restriction work together to battle obesity.

increase resting metabolic rate through an increase in fat-free mass. Maziekas et al. (171) systematically analyzed studies that examined the effects of exercise regimens in pediatric obesity and found that exercise, whether aerobic and/or resistance training, accounted for as much as 86% of the variance in changes in body fat percentage at 1 year. The benefits of exercise programs are not limited to body composition. Watts et al. (172) examined the effects of an 8-week circuit training regimen on conduit vessel function in 19 obese adolescents. In addition to the reduction in percent body fat, the investigators found that vascular flow that was impaired prior to the intervention normalized after 8 weeks of circuit training (172). Although we have focused on benefits of resistance training, it should be noted that the combination of aerobic and resistance training exercise (173) as well as caloric restriction are the best approach to reducing body fat in a safe and effective manner (174).

A combination of resistance training, aerobic exercise, and caloric restriction is the optimal method of reducing body fat in a safe and effective manner in obese individuals.

DIABETES MELLITUS

There are two general categories of diabetes mellitus. **Type I diabetes** is a disease characterized by pancreatic damage resulting in diminished insulin secretion from the pancreas. It is typically due to an autoimmune condition in which the immune system attacks the pancreas, but may also stem from pancreatic damage due to other diseases such as pancreatic cancer. Often referred to as juvenile onset diabetes, individuals with type I diabetes require insulin injections to control blood glucose levels. In contrast, **Type II diabetes** is a condition characterized by insulin resistance. That is, a given glucose challenge requires a greater insulin response. Obesity is a prime cause of type II diabetes. The increasing prevalence of obesity is leading to higher incidence of type II diabetes. Notably, increasing rates of childhood obesity are leading to ever more cases of type II diabetes in childhood. In advanced cases, type II diabetes leads to diminished pancreatic function and may lead to the need for exogenous insulin.

It is well established that aerobic exercise can both decrease the risk of developing type II diabetes as well as aid in glycemic control in those with type II diabetes. In addition to the effects of aerobic exercise on body composition and weight control, which decrease insulin resistance, the effects of aerobic exercise on muscle metabolism also contributes to the beneficial effects. Specifically, increases in GLUT4 glucose transporter levels at the muscle cell membrane in response to exercise, and the effects of aerobic exercise on cellular glucose metabolism contribute to the prevention and treatment of type II diabetes.

It is less well appreciated that resistance training can also have significant benefits in the prevention and treatment of type II diabetes (175). Similar to aerobic exercise, studies have shown that resistance exercise improves insulin sensitivity and glucose tolerance (176) and decreases level of glycosylated hemoglobin (177,178), resulting in improved glycemic control in those with type II diabetes. Resistance exercise is recommended for those with type II diabetes by both the American Diabetes Association (179) and the American College of Sports Medicine (180). The specific characteristics of resistance training protocols that optimize the benefits on glucose tolerance, insulin sensitivity, and glycemic control are still unknown; however, it has been suggested that high-intensity resistance training may be more effective than low-intensity, high-volume training (175,177). Nonetheless, significant effects can be had with lower-intensity (40% to 50% 1-RM) training (176), at least in the short term.

The control of overall blood glucose in diabetic patients can be improved by a regular exercise regimen.

CANCER

In 2000, **cancer** was the second leading cause of death in the United States behind heart disease (181). In 2003, it was estimated that 1,334,100 new cases and 556,500 deaths were associated with cancer (182). However, despite these figures, the 5-year relative survival rate for all cancers combined is 62% (182). Generally, the treatment of cancer involved a certain level of radiation, chemotherapy, surgery, or a combination of the above. Because many of these treatments are intensive and affect the individual's physiology function, fatigue, muscle wasting, and energy loss often result (183,184). Studies have found that various forms of physical activity such as aerobic exercise and resistance training are beneficial in minimizing the effects of cancer treatment (183,185).

Durak and Lilliy (186) examined the effects of a 10-week outpatient wellness program on variables of fitness in 20 cancer patients who had a mean age of 50. In addition to performing aerobic exercises, the patients were supervised through a PRT exercise using strength machines. The investigators found that after 10 weeks of training, that muscular strength increased by 45% to 98% depending on the muscle being exercised. Additionally, patients rated their function capacity to perform ADLs (e.g., household tasks, preparing) significantly higher following the 10-week training program. Adamsen et al. (183) found similar results in a study of 23 cancer patients between the ages of 18 and 65 years. Patients engaged in 9 h · wk^{-1} of supervised exercise that included a combination of aerobic and resistance training. The investigators found significant increases in cardiorespiratory endurance and muscular strength (183). For a more extensive review of the effects of physical activity and cancer, we recommend the two recent articles by Thune and Furberg (187) and Oldervoll et al. (188)

Resistance training and aerobic exercise can help counteract the muscle wasting and fatigue associated with cancer treatment.

PREGNANCY

Concerns about exercise during **pregnancy** focus on the potential problems of increased body temperature, impaired uterine blood flow and nutrient supply, and the risk for preterm labor. Studies have shown that for the mother, the benefits outweigh the risks. Moderate, regular exercise during pregnancy has many benefits for the mother, including decreased weight gain, more rapid weight loss after pregnancy, improved sense of well-being, and decreased risk for musculoskeletal pain and gestational diabetes. There are some mild risks to the fetus but, fortunately, the adverse effects of a proper exercise program are minimal if administered prudently (189–191).

The American College of Obstetricians and Gynecologists (ACOG) has established guidelines for exercise during pregnancy. A pregnant woman should always inform and seek guidance from her physician prior to proceeding with an exercise program. If a woman has been exercising prior to pregnancy, she should be able to continue with her program with minor modifications. If a woman has not exercised previously, she may cautiously begin a gentle exercise program during pregnancy, and must be alert to overexertion and complications.

Cardiovascular exercise should consist of 30 minutes or more of moderate exercise most days. Exercise intensity should be judged by ratings of perceived exertion (RPE) in the light to somewhat hard range (RPE 11 to 13), rather than on heart rate, and should allow the participant to pass the "talk test" during exercise. Women may find low-impact activities and water exercise more comfortable due to the increased weight and postural changes that occur with advancing pregnancy. Another musculoskeletal change that occurs during pregnancy is increased ligamentous laxity due increased levels of the hormones estrogen and relaxin. Although research on resistance training is sparse, it appears safe. However, it is prudent to minimize the possibility of strains and sprains by using proper form and a variety of exercises to avoid overuse injuries. Dynamic lifting with lighter weights and multiple repetitions is recommended, while avoiding repetitive isometric or heavy lifting that may result in a Valsava maneuver (192). Supine exercises should be avoided after the first trimester because this position causes mild obstruction of venous return that can affect cardiac output. Motionless standing can lead to venous pooling, so this position should be minimized. Appropriate hydration, avoidance of overheating, and adequate nutrition should be observed.

The ACOG guidelines suggest avoidance of activities that have the potential for impact or falling, such as ice hockey, horseback riding, vigorous racquet sports, kickboxing, and soccer. Exertion at high altitudes or scuba diving is also cautioned against. Exercise of any svort should be terminated immediately if any of the following occurs: vaginal bleeding, dizziness, shortness of breath, headache, chest pain, calf pain or swelling (possible thrombophlebitis), preterm labor, leakage of amniotic fluid, muscle weakness (Box 20.3). A pregnant woman with diabetes, morbid obesity, hypertension, or other high-risk conditions should not exercise until she has been carefully evaluated by her physician and then only with an individualized program.

> *With her physician's approval, a healthy pregnant woman without obstetric or medical risks may safely engage in a moderate, regular exercise program.*

BOX 20.3

Warning Signs to Stop Exercising during Pregnancy

Excessive fatigue
Pain (particularly in the back or pubic area),
Dizziness
Shortness of breath
Heart palpitations
Decreased fetal movement
Persistent contractions
Rupture of membranes
Vaginal bleeding

Summary

Resistance exercise in concert with cardiovascular and flexibility exercises is an important component of exercise programs in the general population. It is increasingly apparent that resistance exercise provides significant benefits to children, adolescents, and the well elderly. Furthermore, resistance exercise appears to provide significant benefits to individuals with a variety of conditions such as COPD, AIDS, diabetes, and neuromuscular diseases. With few exceptions (DMD), the benefits of resistance exercise far outweigh the potential risks, especially when properly designed and supervised. Nonetheless, caution should be applied when introducing progression into a program. Using a team approach with appropriate health care providers can enhance the safety and effectiveness of program. Future research needs to further delineate the program design variables (intensity, frequency, volume, etc.) that maximize benefits (including functional outcomes) while minimizing deleterious effects for different diseases and syndromes. In addition, longer term studies need to be performed to assess the benefits and risks of prolonged resistance exercise for these special populations.

Maxing Out

1. A 30-year-old man wants assistance in designing an exercise program. He is 100 lb overweight, smokes 1 pack of cigarettes · d^{-1}, and complains of knee pain when climbing stairs. What parameters should his program have? Are there any special considerations?
2. An 85-year-old male had a stroke 5 years ago and has some residual right-sided weakness with mild spasticity, although he is able to walk independently and live alone. His daughter has brought him to the gym and wants him to start an exercise program. His goal is to stay as independent as possible. Is it safe to start him on resistance training program? What types of exercise would be most appropriate for him?
3. A 52-year-old female with a history of type II diabetes wants to start exercising. What types of physical problems might this woman have? Are there any precautions that should be considered? Design an appropriate fitness program for this woman.
4. A 44-year-old male volunteer coach for the high school football team wants to start working out with his son who is on the team. He had a heart attack 6 months ago, and has completed cardiac rehabilitation phases 1, 2, and 3. Now he wants to stay fit and asks for some advice. What are some guidelines and precautions for an exercise program?

CASE EXAMPLE

Senior Male Golfer with Knee Pain

BACKGROUND

Mr. Jackson, a 76-year-old avid golfer, complains that he is having increasing difficulty with bending, walking on hills and uneven ground, and getting in and out of the golf cart. He has a history of bilateral knee osteoarthritis controlled with NSAIDs and hypertension controlled with medication. He admits not adhering to exercise programs in the past, but is now motivated because he wants to continue golfing.

INTERVENTION

After having Mr. Jackson complete a health screen questionnaire and getting clearance from his physician, exercise testing is performed as outlined in Chapter 8. The components of the fitness program should focus on strength and flexibility of the lower extremities targeting major muscle groups used in daily activities and golf, aerobic conditioning, and balance and coordination activities. Review sections on sarcopenia, osteoarthritis, and cardiovascular disease for more information.

For resistance training, a 5- to 10-minute warm-up should be followed by strength training for major muscle groups, focusing on lower extremities, but including upper extremities and trunk as all are important for golf and other ADLs. Begin with 65% to 75% of 1-RM, and progress to 85% to 100% of 1-RM as tolerated, 2 to 3 sessions · wk^{-1}, 8 to 12 repetitions. Knee pain should be monitored, and activities modified if increased pain and inflammation is reported. For example, open-chain knee extensions could be replaced with closed-chain leg presses, load could be reduced, or arc of motion modified to a pain-free range. The session would end with stretching to the major muscle groups.

For aerobic conditioning, a combination of activities could be used, including treadmill walking, stationery bicycling, and water activities. Treadmill walking is functional and inclines can be gradually introduced to simulate hill walking. Stationery bicycling has the advantage of providing knee range of motion, which can be increased by lowering the seat height. Water aerobics can provide cardiovascular conditioning while minimizing joint stresses. Mr. Jackson should be taught perceived level of exertion, age-related target heart rate, and advised to monitor his blood pressure. He could be encouraged to join an exercise group to enhance adherence.

Supervised but simple balance and coordination activities such as grapevine walking, single-leg balance, and walking on an exercise mat to simulate uneven ground can become independent once safety is established. Mr. Jackson should be educated on the importance of an ongoing program, warning signs for cardiovascular disease, and osteoarthritis precautions.

REFERENCES

1. Malek MH, Nalbone DP, Berger DE, et al. Importance of health science education for personal fitness trainers. *J Strength Cond Res*. 2002;16(1):19–24.
2. ACSM; American College of Sports Medicine Position Stand. The recommended quantity and quality of exercise for developing and maintaining cardiorespiratory and muscular fitness, and flexibility in healthy adults. *Med Sci Sports Exerc*. 1998;30(6):975–991.
3. Evans WJ. Effects of exercise on senescent muscle. *Clin Orthop Relat Res*. 2002;403S:S211–S220.
4. Frontera WR, Hughes VA, Fielding RA, et al. Aging of skeletal muscle: a 12-yr longitudianl study. *J Appl Physiol*. 2000;88:1321–1326.
5. Lexell J, Taylor CC, Sjostrom M. What is the cause of the ageing atrophy? Total numer, size and proportion of different fiber types studied in whole vastus lateralis muscle from 15- to 83-year-old men. *J Neurol Sci*. 1988;84:275–294.
6. Evans WJ. Effects of exercise on body composition and functional capacity of the elderly. *J Gerontol*. 1995;50A:147–150.
7. Evans WJ. Exercise training guidelines for the elderly. *Med Sci Sports Exerc*. 1999;31:12–17.
8. Frontera WR, Suh D, Krivickas LS, et al. Skeletal muscle fiber quality in older men and women. *Am J Physiol*. 2000;279:C611–C618.
9. Hughes VA, Frontera WR, Wood M, et al. Longitudinal muscle strength changes in older adults: influence of muscle mass, physical activity, and health. *J Gerontol A Biol Sci Med Sci*. 2001;56A:B209–B217.

10. Jette AM, Branch LG. The Framingham Disability Study: II. Physical disability among the aging. *Am J Public Health.* 1981;71:1211–1216.
11. Latham NK, Bennett DA, Stretton CM, et al. Systematic review of progressive resistance strength training in older adults. *J Gerontol A Biol Sci Med Sci.* 2004;59(1):48–61.
12. Villareal DT, Steger-May K, Schechtman KB, et al. Effects of exercise training on bone mineral density in frail older women and men: a randomised controlled trial. *Age Ageing.* 2004;33(3):309–312.
13. Yarasheski KE. Exercise, aging, and muscle protein metabolism. *J Gerontol A Biol Sci Med Sci.* 2003;58(10):M918–M922.
14. Moritani T, deVries HA. Potential for gross muscle hypertrophy in older men. *Am J Phys Med.* 1980;35(5):672–682.
15. Fiatarone MA, Marks EC, Ryan ND, et al. High-intensity strength training in nonagenarians: Effects on skeletal muscle. *J AMA.* 1990;263(22):3029–3034.
16. Yarasheski KE, Pak-Loduca J, Hasten DL, et al. Resistance exercise training increases mixed muscle protein synthesis rate in frail women and men ≥76 yr old. *Am J Physiol.* 1999;277(1 Pt 1):E118–E125.
17. Trappe S, Williamson D, Godard M. Maintenance of whole muscle strength and size following resistance training in older men. *J Gerontol A Biol Sci Med Sci.* 2002;57(4):B138–B143.
18. Latham NK, Bennett DA, Stretton CM, et al. Systematic review of progressive resistance strength training in older adults. *J Gerontol A Biol Sci Med Sci.* 2004;59A(1):48–61.
19. NIH. Osteoporosis prevention, diagnosis, and therapy. *NIH Consens Statement.* 2000;17(1):1–45.
20. Bonaiuti D, Shea B, Iovine R, et al. Exercise for preventing and treating osteoporosis in postmenopausal women. *Cochrane Database Syst Rev.* 2002;(3):CD000333.
21. Helleckson KL. NIH releases statement on osteoporosis prevention, diagnosis, and therapy. *Am Fam Physician.* 2002;66:161–162.
22. Dunlop DD, Manheim LM, Yelin EH, et al. The costs of arthritis. *Arthritis Rheum.* 2003;49(1):101–113.
23. Yelin E. Cost of musculoskeletal diseases: impact of work disability and functional decline. *J Rheumatol Suppl.* 2003;68:8–11.
24. Fassbender HG. *The Pathology and Pathbiology of Rheumatic Disease.* 2nd ed. New York: Springer; 2002.
25. Arthritis-Foundation. http://www.arthritis.org/conditions/diseasecenter/RA/default.asp. Accessed 2004.
26. Van den Ende CH, Vliet Vlieland TP, Munneke M, et al. Dynamic exercise therapy in rheumatoid arthritis: a systematic review. *Br J Rheumatol.* 1998;37(6):677–687.
27. de Jong Z, Munneke M, Zwinderman AH, et al. Is a long-term high-intensity exercise program effective and safe in patients with rheumatoid arthritis? Results of a randomized controlled trial. *Arthritis Rheum.* 2003;48(9):2415–2424.
28. Munneke M, de Jong Z, Zwinderman AH, et al. Adherence and satisfaction of rheumatoid arthritis patients with a long-term intensive dynamic exercise program (RAPIT program). *Arthritis Rheum.* 2003;49(5):665–672.
29. Häkkinen A, Sokka T, Hannonen P. A home-based two-year strength training period in early rheumatoid arthritis led to good long-term compliance: a five-year followup. *Arthritis Rheum.* 2004;51(1):56–62.
30. Hakkinen A, Hannonen P, Nyman K, et al. Effects of concurrent strength and endurance training in women with early or longstanding rheumatoid arthritis: comparison with healthy subjects. *Arthritis Rheum.* 2003;49(6):789–797.
31. Lanes SF, Lanza LL, Radensky PW, et al. Resource utilization and cost of care for rheumatoid arthritis and osteoarthritis in a managed care setting: the importance of drug and surgery costs. *Arthritis Rheum.* 1997;40(8):1475–1481.
32. Liang MH, Cullen KE, Larson MG, et al. Cost-effectiveness of total joint arthroplasty in osteoarthritis. *Arthritis Rheum.* 1986;29(8):937–943.
33. Sevick MA, Bradham DD, Muender M, et al. Cost-effectiveness of aerobic and resistance exercise in seniors with knee osteoarthritis. *Med Sci Sports Exerc.* 2000;32(9):1534–1540.
34. McCarthy CJ, Mills PM, Pullen R, et al. Supplementation of a home-based exercise programme with a class-based programme for people with osteoarthritis of the knees: a randomised controlled trial and health economic analysis. *Health Technol Assess.* 2004;8(46):1–76.
35. Roddy E, Zhang W, Doherty M, et al. Evidence-based recommendations for the role of exercise in the management of osteoarthritis of the hip or knee—the MOVE consensus. *Rheumatology (Oxford).* 2004.
36. Fransen M, McConnell S, Bell M. Exercise for osteoarthritis of the hip or knee. *Cochrane Database Syst Rev.* 2003;(3):CD004286.
37. American-Obesity-Association. http://www.obesity.org/. 2005.
38. Faigenbaum AD, Milliken LA, LaRosa Loud R, et al. Comparison of 1 and 2 days per week of strength training in children. *Res Q Exerc Sport.* 2002;73:416–424.
39. Faigenbaum AD, Milliken LA, Westcott WL. Maximal strength testing in healthy children. *J Strength Cond Res.* 2003;17:162–166.
40. Faigenbaum AD, Kraemer WJ, Cahill B, et al. Youth resistance training: position statement paper and literature review. *Strength Cond J.* 1996;18:62–75.
41. Faigenbaum AD, Westcott WL, Long C, et al. Relationship between repetitions and selected percentages of the one-repetition maximum in healthy children. *Pediatr Phys Ther.* 1998;10:110–113.
42. Falk B, Tenenbaum G. The effectiveness of resistance training in children. *Sports Med.* 1996;22:176–186.
43. Weir JP, Housh TJ, Johnson GO, et al. Allometric scaling of isokinetic peak torque: the Nebraska Wrestling Study. *Eur J Appl Physiol.* 1999;80(3):240–248.
44. Payne VG, Morrow JR Jr, Johnson L, et al. Resistance training in children and youth: a meta-analysis. *Res Q Exerc Sport.* 1997;68:80–88.
45. Bernhardt DT, Gomez J, Johnson MD, et al. Strength training by children and adolescents. *Pediatrics.* 2001;107:1470–1472.
46. Fonkalsrud EW, Dunn JCY, Atkinson JB. Repair of pectus excavatum deformities: 30 years experience with 375 patients. *Ann Surg.* 2000;231:443–448.
47. Hook EB. Epidemiology of Down syndrome. In: SM Pueschel and JE Rynders eds. *Down Syndrome: Advances in Biomedicine and the Behavioral Sciences.* Cambridge,UK: Ware Press; 1982: 11–88.
48. Malek MH, Berger DE, Housh TJ, et al. Cardiovascular function following surgical repair of pectus excavatum: a metaanalysis. *Chest.* 2006;130(2):506–516.

49. Malek MH, Berger DE, Marelich WD, et al. On the application of meta-analysis in pectus excavatum research. *Am J Cardiol.* 2008;101(3):415–417.
50. Malek MH, Berger DE, Marelich WD, et al. Pulmonary function following surgical repair of pectus excavatum: a meta-analysis. *Eur J Cardiothorac Surg.* 2006;30(4):637–643.
51. Malek MH, Coburn JW. Strategies for cardiopulmonary exercise testing of pectus excavatum patients. *Clinics.* 2008;63(2):245–254.
52. Malek MH, Fonkalsrud EW. Cardiorespiratory outcome after corrective surgery for pectus excavatum: a case study. *Med Sci Sports Exerc.* 2004;36(2):183–190.
53. Malek MH, Fonkalsrud EW, Cooper CB. Ventilatory and cardiovascular responses to exercise in patients with pectus excavatum. *Chest.* 2003;124(3):870–882.
54. Padget K. Alterations of neurologic function in children. In: McCance KL, Huether SE, eds. *Pathophysiology. The Biological Basis for Disease in Adults and Children.* St. Louis, MO: Mosby; 1998:566–596.
55. Reddihough DS, Collins KJ. The epidemiology and causes of cerebral palsy. *Aust J Physiother.* 2003;49:7–12.
56. Damiano DL, Abel MF. Functional outcomes of stength training in spastic cerebral palsy. *Arch Phys Med Rehabil.* 1998;79:1998.
57. Damiano DL, Vaughan CL, Abel MF. Muscle response to heavy resistance exercise in children with spastic cerebral palsy. *Dev Med Child Neurol.* 1995;37:731–739.
58. Elder GCB, Kirk J, Stewart G, et al. Contributing factors to muscle weakness in children with cerebral palsy. *Dev Med Child Neurol.* 2003;45:542–550.
59. Booth CM, Cortina-Borja MJ, Theologis TN. Collagen accumulation in muscles of children with cerebral palsy and correlation with severity of spasticity. *Dev Med Child Neurol.* 2001;43(5):314–320.
60. Damiano DL, Kelly LE, Vaughn CL. Effects of quadriceps femoris muscle strengthening on crouch gait in children with spastic diplegia. *Phys Ther.* 1995;75:658–671.
61. Andersson C, Grooten W, Hellsten M, et al. Adults with cerebral palsy: walking ability after progressive strength training. *Dev Med Child Neurol.* 2003;45:220–228.
62. Angelopoulou N, Matziari C, Tsimaris V, et al. Bone mineral density and muscle strength in young men with mental retardation (with and without Down syndrome). *Calcif Tissue Int.* 2000;66:176–180.
63. Carmeli E, Ayalon M, Barchad S, et al. Isokinetic leg strength of institutionalized older adults with mental retardation with and without Down's syndrome. *J Strength Cond Res.* 2002;16:316–320.
64. Goodman CC, Glanzman A. Genetic and developmental disorders. In: Goodman CC Boissonnault WG, Fuller KS, eds. *Pathology. Implications for the Physical Therapist.* 2nd ed. Philadelphia, PA: Saunders; 2003;829–870.
65. Fernhall B. Physical fitness and exercise training of individuals with mental retardation. *Med Sci Sports Exerc.* 1993;25:442–450.
66. Rimmer JH, Kelly LE. Effects of a resistance training program on adults with mental retardation. *Adap Phys Act Q.* 1991;8:146–143.
67. Suomi R, Surburg PR, Lecius P. Effects of hydraulic resistance strength training on isokinetic measures of leg strength in men with mental retardation. *Adap Phys Act Q.* 1995;12:377–387.
68. Rimmer JH, Heller T, Wang E, et al. Improvements in physical fitness in adults with Down syndrome. *Am J Ment Retard.* 2004;109:165–174.
69. Kilmer DD. Response to resistive strengthening exercise training in humans with neuromuscular disease. *Am J Phys Med.* 2002;81(suppl):S121–S126.
70. Curtis CL, Weir JP. Overview of exercise responses in healthy and impaired states. *Neurol Report.* 1996;20:13–19.
71. Forrest G, and X. Qian. Exercise in neuromuscular disease. *NeuroRehabilitation.* 1999;13:135–139.
72. Becker RC. Editorial. Thromboneurology and the search for stroke therapies. *Stroke.* 1997;28:1657–1659.
73. Mayo NE. Wood-Dauphinee S, Ahmed S, et al. Epidemiology and recovery. *Disabil Rehabil.* 1999;21(5–6):258–268. Disablement following stroke.
74. Williams WGR, Jiang JG, Matcher DB, et al. Incidence and occurrence of total (first-ever and recurrent) stroke. *Stroke.* 1999;30:2523–2528.
75. Lackland DT, Bachman DL, Carter TD, et al. The geographic variation in stroke incidence in two areas of the southeastern stroke belt. *Stroke.* 1998;29:2061–2068.
76. Sacco RL, Wolf PA, Gorelick PB. Risk factors and their management for stroke prevention: outlook for 1999 and beyond. *Neurology.* 1999;53(7 suppl 4):S15–S24.
77. Dennis MS, Burn JP, Sandercock PA, et al. Long-term survival after first-ever stroke: the Oxfordshire Community Stroke Project. *Stroke.* 1993;24:796–800.
78. Sacco RL. Risk factors, outcomes, and stroke subtypes for ischemic stroke. *Neurology.* 1997;49(suppl 4):S39–S44.
79. Bonita R. Epidemiology of stroke. *The Lancet.* 1992; 339:342–347.
80. Matchar DB, Duncan PW. The cost of stroke. *Stroke. Clin Updates.* 1994;5:9–12.
81. Badics E, Wittman A, Rupp M, et al. Systematic muscle building exercises in the rehabilitation of stroke patients. *NeuroRehabilitation.* 2002;17:211–214.
82. Sharp SA, Brouwer BJ. Isokinetic strength training of the hemiparetic knee: effects on function and spasticity. *Arch Phys Med Rehabil.* 1997;78:1231–1236.
83. Engardt M, Knutsson E, Jonsson M, et al. Dynamic muscle strength training in stroke patients: effects on knee extension torque, electromyographic activity, and motor function. *Arch Phys Med Rehabil.* 1995;76:419–425.
84. Teixeira-Salmela LF, Olney SJ, Nadeau S, et al. Muscle strengthening and physical conditioning to reduce impairment and disability in chronic stroke survivors. *Arch Phys Med Rehabil.* 1999;80:1211–1218.
85. Teixeira-Salmela LF, Nadeau S, McBride I, et al. Effects of muscle strengthening and physical conditioning training on temporal, kinematic and kinetic variables during gait in chronic stroke survivors. *J Rehabil Med.* 2001;33:53–60.
86. Moreland JD, Goldsmith CH, Huijbregts MP, et al. Progressive resistance strengthening exercises after stroke: a single-blind randomized controlled trial. *Arch Phys Med Rehabil.* 2003;84:1433–1440.
87. Smith GV, Silver KHC, Goldberg AP, et al. "Task-oriented" exercise improves hamstring strength and spastic reflexes in chronic stroke patients. *Stroke.* 1999;30:2112–2118.
88. Goodman CC. The immune system. In: Goodman CC Boissonnault WG, Fuller KS, eds. *Pathology. Implications for the Physical Therapist.* 2nd ed. Philadelphia, PA: Saunders; 2003; 153–193.

89. Wolfe F, Ross K, Anderson J, et al. The prevalence and general characteristics of fibromyalgia in the general population. *Arthritis Rheum*. 1995;38:19–28.
90. Robinson RL, Birnbaum HG, Morley MA, et al. Economic cost and epidemiological characteristics of patients with fibromyalgia claims. *J Rheumatol*. 2003;30:1318–1325.
91. Jones KD, Clark SR. Individualizing the exercise prescription for persons with fibromyalgia. *Rheum Dis Clin N Am*. 2002;28:419–436.
92. Bennett RM. Emerging concepts in the neurobiology of chronic pain: evidence of abnormal processing in fibromyalgia. *Mayo Clin Proc*. 1999;74:385–398.
93. Hakkinen A, Hakkinen K, Hannonen P, et al. Strength training induced adaptations in neuromuscular function in premenopausal women with fibromyalgia: comparison with healthy women. *Ann Rheum Dis*. 2001;60:21–26.
94. Valkeinen H, Alen M, Hannonen P, et al. Changes in knee extension and flexion force, EMG and functional capacity during strength training in older females with fibromyalgia and healthy controls. *Rheumatol*. 2004;43:225–228.
95. Jones KD, Burckhardt CS, Clark SR, et al. A randomized controlled trial of muscle strengthening versus flexibility training in fibromyalgia. *J Rheumatol*. 2002;29:1041–1048.
96. Smith MB. The peripheral nervous system. In: Goodman CC, Boissonnault WG, Fuller KS, eds.. *Pathology. Implications for the Physical Therapist*. Philadelphia, PA: Saunders; 2003: 1161–1162.
97. Agre JC, Rodriquez AA, Franke TM. Strength, endurance, and work capacity after muscle strengthening exercise in postpolio subjects. *Arch Phys Med Rehabil*. 1992;78:681–686.
98. Chan KM, Amirjani N, Sumrain M, et al. Randomized controlled trial of strength training in post-polio. *Muscle Nerve*. 2003;27:332–338.
99. Spector SA, Gordon PL, Feuerstein IM, et al. Strength gains without muscle injury after strength training in patients with postpolio muscular atrophy. *Muscle Nerve*. 1996;19:1282–1290.
100. Klingbeil H, Baer HR, Wilson PE. Aging with a disability. *Arch Phys Med Rehabil*. 2004;85(suppl3):S68–S73.
101. Olek MJ. *Multiple Sclerosis: Etiology, Diagnosis, and New Treatment Strategies*. Totowa, NJ: Humana Press; 2005: XV, 245.
102. Mostert S, Kesselring J. Effects of a short-term exercise training program on aerobic fitness, fatigue, health perception and activity level of subjects with multiple sclerosis. *Mult Scler*. 2002;8(2):161–168.
103. Petajan JH, Gappmaier E, White AT, et al. Impact of aerobic training on fitness and quality of life in multiple sclerosis. *Ann Neurol*. 1996;39(4):432–441.
104. Freeman J, Allison R. Group exercise classes in people with multiple sclerosis: a pilot study. *Physiother Res Intern*. 2004;9(2):104–107.
105. Surakka J, Romberg A, Ruutiainen J, et al. Effects of aerobic and strength exercise on motor fatigue in men and women with multiple sclerosis: a randomized controlled trial. *Clin Rehabil*. 2004;18:737–746.
106. White LJ, Dressendorfer RH. Exercise and multiple sclerosis. *Sports Med*. 2004;34:1077–1100.
107. Jacob PL, Nash MS. Exercise recommendations for individuals with spinal cord injury. *Sports Med*. 2004;34:727–751.
108. Figoni SF. Spinal cord disabilities: paraplegia and tetraplegia. In: Durstine JL, Moore GE, eds. *ACSM's Exercise Management for Persons with Chronic Diseases and Disabilities*. Champaign,IL: Human Kinetics; 2003:247–253.
109. Davis GM, Shepard RJ. Strength training for wheelchair users. *Br J Sports Med*. 1990;24:25–30.
110. Curtis KA, Tyner TM, Zachery L. Effect of a standard exercise protocol on shoulder pain in long-term wheelchair users. *Spinal Cord*. 1999;37:421–429.
111. Wheeler DA. The human immunodeficiency virus. *Cutis*. 1995;55(2):81–83.
112. CDC. HIV and AIDS-United States 1981–2001. *MMWR Morb Mortal Wkly Rep*. 2001;50:430–434.
113. Fleming PL. HIV prevalence in the United States, 2000. In *Proceedings of the 9th Conference on Retroviruses and Opportunistic Infections*. 2002; Seattle, WA.
114. UNAIDS; *AIDS Epidemic Update*. Geneva, Switzerland: UNAIDS Information Centre; 2003:1–39.
115. Sherlekar S, Udipi SA. Role of nutrition in the management of HIV infection/AIDS. *J Indian Med Assoc*. 2002;100(6):385–390.
116. Wheeler DA. Weight loss and disease progression in HIV infection. *AIDS Read*. 1999;9(5):347–353.
117. Wheeler DA, Gibert CL, Launer CA, et al. Weight loss as a predictor of survival and disease progression in HIV infection. Terry Beirn Community Programs for Clinical Research on AIDS. *J Acquir Immune Defic Syndr*. 1998;18(1):80–85.
118. MaCallan DC. Metabolic abnormalities and the "wasting syndrome" in HIV infection. *Nutrition*. 1996;12(9):641–642.
119. Macallan DC. Wasting in HIV infection and AIDS. *J Nutr*. 1999;129(1S suppl):238S–242S.
120. Macallan DC, Griffin GE. Metabolic disturbances in AIDS. *N Engl J Med*. 1992;327(21):1530–1531.
121. Bhasin S, Storer TW. Exercise regimens for men with HIV. *JAMA*. 2000;284(2):175–176.
122. Dudgeon WD, Phillips KD, Bopp CM, et al. Physiological and psychological effects of exercise interventions in HIV disease. *AIDS Patient Care STDS*. 2004;18(2):81–98.
123. McDermott AY, Shevitz A, Knox T, et al. Effect of highly active antiretroviral therapy on fat, lean, and bone mass in HIV-seropositive men and women. *Am J Clin Nutr*. 2001;74(5):679–686.
124. Roubenoff R, Abad LW, Lundgren N. Effect of acquired immune deficiency syndrome wasting on the protein metabolic response to acute exercise. *Metabolism*. 2001;50(3):288–292.
125. Roubenoff R, Wilson IB. Effect of resistance training on self-reported physical functioning in HIV infection. *Med Sci Sports Exerc*. 2001;33(11):1811–1817.
126. Sattler FR, Jaque SV, Schroeder ET, et al. Effects of pharmacological doses of nandrolone decanoate and progressive resistance training in immunodeficient patients infected with human immunodeficiency virus. *J Clin Endocrinol Metab*. 1999;84(4):1268–1276.

127. Bhasin S, Storer TW, Javanbakht M, et al. Testosterone replacement and resistance exercise in HIV-infected men with weight loss and low testosterone levels. *JAMA.* 2000;283(6):763–770.
128. ATS. Pulmonary rehabilitation—1999. American Thoracic Society. *Am J Respir Crit Care Med.* 1999;159(5 pt 1):1666–1682.
129. ATS/ERS. Skeletal muscle dysfunction in chronic obstructive pulmonary disease. A statement of the American Thoracic Society and European Respiratory Society. *Am J Respir Crit Care Med.* 1999;159(4 pt 2):S1–S40.
130. NIH National Heart, Lung, and Blood Institute (NHLBI). *Chronic Obstructive Pulmonary Disease (COPD) Data Fact Sheet.* Bethesda, MD; 2003:1–6.
131. Halpern MT, Stanford RH, Borker R. The burden of COPD in the U.S.A.: results from the Confronting COPD survey. *Respir Med.* 2003;97(suppl C):S81–S89.
132. Ramsey SD, Sullivan SD. The burden of illness and economic evaluation for COPD. *Eur Respir J.* 2003;41(suppl):29s–35s.
133. Trupin L, Earnest G, San Pedro M, et al. The occupational burden of chronic obstructive pulmonary disease. *Eur Respir J.* 2003;22(3):462–469.
134. Jakobsson P, Jorfeldt L, Brundin A. Skeletal muscle metabolites and fibre types in patients with advanced chronic obstructive pulmonary disease (COPD), with and without chronic respiratory failure. *Eur Respir J.* 1990;3(2):192–196.
135. Maltais F, Simard AA, Simard C, et al. Oxidative capacity of the skeletal muscle and lactic acid kinetics during exercise in normal subjects and in patients with COPD. *Am J Respir Crit Care Med.* 1996;153(1):288–293.
136. Lacasse Y, Wong E, Guyatt GH, et al. Meta-analysis of respiratory rehabilitation in chronic obstructive pulmonary disease. *Lancet.* 1996;348(9035):1115–1119.
137. Mador MJ, Kufel TJ, Pineda LA, et al. Effect of pulmonary rehabilitation on quadriceps fatiguability during exercise. *Am J Respir Crit Care Med.* 2001;163(4):930–935.
138. Maltais F, LeBlanc P, Simard C, et al. Skeletal muscle adaptation to endurance training in patients with chronic obstructive pulmonary disease. *Am J Respir Crit Care Med.* 1996;154(2 pt 1):442–447.
139. Panton LB, Golden J, Broeder CE, et al. The effects of resistance training on functional outcomes in patients with chronic obstructive pulmonary disease. *Eur J Appl Physiol.* 2004;91(4):443–449.
140. Storer TW. Exercise in chronic pulmonary disease: resistance exercise prescription. *Med Sci Sports Exerc.* 2001;33(7 suppl):S680–S692.
141. Mador MJ. Muscle mass, not body weight, predicts outcome in patients with chronic obstructive pulmonary disease. *Am J Respir Crit Care Med.* 2002;166(6):787–789.
142. Fenicchia LM L, Kanaley JA J, Azevedo JL J Jr, et al. Influence of resistance exercise training on glucose control in women with type 2 diabetes. *Metabolism.* 2004;53(3):284–289.
143. Ortega F, Toral J, Cejudo P, et al. Comparison of effects of strength and endurance training in patients with chronic obstructive pulmonary disease. *Am J Respir Crit Care Med.* 2002;166(5):669–674.
144. Chobanian AV, Bakris GL, Black HR, et al. Seventh report of the Joint National Committee on prevention, detection, evaluation, and treatment of high blood pressure. *Hypertension.* 2003;42(6):1206–1252.
145. American College of Sports Medicine; Franklin BA, Whaley MH, Howley ET,et al. *ACSM's Guidelines for Exercise Testing and Prescription.* Philadelphia, PA: Lippincott Williams & Wilkins; 2000;33–130.
146. Anderson RN. Deaths: leading causes for 1999. *Natl Vital Stat Rep.* 2001;49(11):1–87.
147. NIH. NIH develops consensus statement on the role of physical activity for cardiovascular health. *Am Fam Physician.* 1996;54(2):763–764, 767.
148. Kelley GA, Kelley KS, Tran ZV. Walking and resting blood pressure in adults: a meta-analysis. *Prev Med.* 2001;33(2 pt 1):120–127.
149. Oguma Y, Shinoda-Tagawa T. Physical activity decreases cardiovascular disease risk in women: review and meta-analysis. *Am J Prev Med.* 2004;26(5):407–418.
150. Pollock ML, Franklin BA, Balady GJ, et al. AHA Science Advisory. Resistance exercise in individuals with and without cardiovascular disease: benefits, rationale, safety, and prescription: an advisory from the Committee on Exercise, Rehabilitation, and Prevention, Council on Clinical Cardiology, American Heart Association; Position paper endorsed by the American College of Sports Medicine. *Circulation.* 2000;101(7):828–833.
151. Kelley GA, Kelley KS. Progressive resistance exercise and resting blood pressure: a meta-analysis of randomized controlled trials. *Hypertension.* 2000;35(3):838–843.
152. Kelley GA, Kelley KS, Tran ZV. The effects of exercise on resting blood pressure in children and adolescents: a meta-analysis of randomized controlled trials. *Prev Cardiol.* 2003;6(1):8–16.
153. Goldberg L, Elliot DL, Keuhl KS. Cardiovascular changes at rest and during mixed static and dynamic exercises after weight training. *J Appl Sport Sci Res.* 1988;2:42–45.
154. McCartney N, McKelvie RS, Martin J, et al. Weight training induced attenuation of the circulatory response of older males to weight lifting. *J Appl Physiol.* 1993;74:1056–1060.
155. Ades PA, Savage PD, Cress ME, et al. Resistance training on physical performance in disabled older female cardiac patients. *Med Sci Sports Exerc.* 2003;35(8):1265–1270.
156. American College of Sports Medicine; Whaley MH, Brubaker PH, Otto RM, et al. *ACSM's Guidelines for Exercise Testing and Prescription.* 7th, 30th Anniversary ed. Philadelphia, PA: Lippincott Williams & Wilkins; 2006: 366.
157. Pu CT, Johnson MT, Forman DE, et al. Randomized trial of progressive resistance training to counteract the myopathy of chronic heart failure. *J Appl Physiol.* 2001;90:2341–2350.
158. Delagardelle C, Feiereisen P, Autier P, et al. Strength/endurance training versus endurance training in congestive heart failure. *Med Sci Sports Exerc.* 2002;34:1868–1872.
159. Maiorana A, O'Driscoll G, Dembo L, et al. Effect of aerobic and resistance exercise training on vascular function in heart failure. *Am J Physiol Heart Circ Physiol.* 2000;279(4):H1999–H2005.
160. Calle EE, Rodriguez C, Walker-Thurmond K, et al. Overweight, obesity, and mortality from cancer in a prospectively studied cohort of U.S. adults. *N Engl J Med.* 2003;348(17):1625–1638.

161. NIH. *Clinical Guidelines on the Identification, Evaluation, and Treatment of Overweight and Obesity in Adults*. Bethesda, MD: National Institutes of Health, National Heart, Lung, and Blood Institute; 1998.
162. Finklestein EA, Fiebelkorn IC, Wang G. National medical spending attributable to overweight and obesity: How much, and who's paying? *Health Affairs*. 2003;W3:219–226.
163. Thompson D, Wolf AM. The medical-care cost burden of obesity. *Obes Rev*. 2001;2(3):189–197.
164. NIH. *The Surgeon General's Call to Action to Prevent and Decrease Overweight and Obesity 2001*. Rockville, MD: U.S. Department of Health and Human Services; 2001:1–39.
165. Stunkard AJ, Wadden TA. *Obesity: Theory and Therapy*. New York: Raven Press; 1993.
166. Schousboe K, Visscher PM, Erbas B, et al. Twin study of genetic and environmental influences on adult body size, shape, and composition. *Int J Obes Relat Metab Disord*. 2004;28(1):39–48.
167. Schousboe K, Willemsen G, Kyvik KO, et al. Sex differences in heritability of BMI: a comparative study of results from twin studies in eight countries. *Twin Res*. 2003;6(5):409–421.
168. Whitaker RC, Wright JA, Pepe MS, et al. Predicting obesity in young adulthood from childhood and parental obesity. *N Engl J Med*. 1997;337(13):869–873.
169. Taylor E, Missik E, Hurley R, et al. Obesity treatment: broadening our perspective. *Am J Health Behav*. 2004;28(3):242–249.
170. Byrne HK, Wilmore JH. The effects of a 20-week exercise training program on resting metabolic rate in previously sedentary, moderately obese women. *Int J Sport Nutr Exerc Metab*. 2001;11(1):15–31.
171. Maziekas MT, LeMura LM, Stoddard NM, et al. Follow up exercise studies in paediatric obesity: implications for long term effectiveness. *Br J Sports Med*. 2003;37(5):425–429.
172. Watts K, Beye P, Siafarikas A, et al. Exercise training normalizes vascular dysfunction and improves central adiposity in obese adolescents. *J Am Coll Cardiol*. 2004;43(10):1823–1827.
173. Park SK, Park JH, Kwon YC, et al. The effect of combined aerobic and resistance exercise training on abdominal fat in obese middle-aged women. *J Physiol Anthropol Appl Human Sci*. 2003;22(3):129–135.
174. Wing RR. Physical activity in the treatment of the adulthood overweight and obesity: current evidence and research issues. *Med Sci Sports Exerc*. 1999;31(11 suppl):S547–S552.
175. Willey KA, Fiatarone Singh MA. Battling insulin resistance in elderly obese people with type 2 diabetes. Bring on the heavy weights. *Diabetes Care*. 2003;26(5):1580–1588.
176. Ishii T, Yamakita T, Sato T, et al. Resistance training improves insulin sensitivity in NIDDM subjects without altering maximal oxygen uptake. *Diabetes Care*. 1998;21:1353–1355.
177. Castaneda C, Layne JE, Munoz-Orians L, et al. An randomized controlled trial of resistance exercise training to improve glycemic control in older adults with type 2 diabetes. *Diabetes Care*. 2002;25:2335–2341.
178. Dunstan DW, Daly RM, Owen N, et al. High-intensity resistance training improves glycemic control in older patients with Type 2 diabetes. *Diabetes Care*. 2002;25:1729–1736.
179. Association AD. Diabetes mellitus and exercise. *Diabetes Care*. 2002;25(suppl 1):S64–S68.
180. Albright A, Franz M, Hornsby G, et al. American College of Sports Medicine position stand: exercise and type 2 diabetes. *Med Sci Sports Exerc*. 2000;32:1345–1360.
181. Mokdad AH, Marks JS, Stroup DF, et al. Actual causes of death in the United States, 2000. *JAMA*. 2004;291(10):1238–1245.
182. American Cancer Society; *Cancer Facts and Figures 2003*. Atlanta, GA: American Cancer Society; 2003:1–48.
183. Adamsen L, Midtgaard J, Rorth M, et al. Feasibility, physical capacity, and health benefits of a multidimensional exercise program for cancer patients undergoing chemotherapy. *Support Care Cancer*. 2003;11(11):707–716.
184. Oldervoll LM, Kaasa S, Knobel H, et al. Exercise reduces fatigue in chronic fatigued Hodgkins disease survivors—results from a pilot study. *Eur J Cancer*. 2003;39(1):57–63.
185. Friendenreich CM, Courneya KS. Exercise as rehabilitation for cancer patients. *Clin J Sport Med*. 1996;6(4):237–244.
186. Durak EP, Lilliy PC. The application of an exercise and wellness program for cancer patients: a preliminary outcomes report. *J Strength Cond Res*. 1998;12:3–6.
187. Thune I, Furberg AS. Physical activity and cancer risk: dose-response and cancer, all sites and site-specific. *Med Sci Sports Exerc*. 2001;33(6 suppl):S530–S550, discussion S609–S610.
188. Oldervoll LM, Kaasa S, Hjermstad MJ, et al. Physical exercise results in the improved subjective well-being of a few or is effective rehabilitation for all cancer patients? *Eur J Cancer*. 2004;40(7):951–962.
189. ACOG. ACOG Committee opinion. Number 267, January 2002: exercise during pregnancy and the postpartum period. *Obstet Gynecol*. 2002;99(1):171–173.
190. Kramer MS. Aerobic exercise for women during pregnancy. *Cochrane Database Syst Rev*. 2002;(2):CD000180.
191. SMA. SMA statement the benefits and risks of exercise during pregnancy. Sport Medicine Australia. *J Sci Med Sport*. 2002;5(1):11–19.
192. Artal R, O'Toole M. Guidelines of the American College of Obstetricians and Gynecologists for exercise during pregnancy and the postpartum period. *Br J Sports Med*. 2003;37(1):6–12, discussion

CHAPTER 21

Principles of Injury Prevention and Rehabilitation

TODD S. ELLENBECKER • SUSAN MERRIMAN • JAKE BLEACHER

OBJECTIVES

After reading this chapter, you shall be able to:

- Identify key structural deficits and strength and flexibility deficiencies, which can decrease the risk of injury or reinjury. Understand the role of the strength and conditioning professional as a part of the sports medicine team.
- Understand and articulate the phases of injury and the role of the PRICE method in treating injury.
- Demonstrate an understanding of the role of the strength and conditioning professional in the "return to activity" phase of rehabilitation from injury.
- Apply the concept of core stabilization for enhancing performance and preventing injury in designing appropriate strength and conditioning programs for athletes using various methods. Design appropriate sport-specific conditioning programs based on an understanding of the biomechanical concepts of the knee, shoulder, and spine and be able to provide specific exercise applications based on the inherent joint biomechanical characteristics.`
- Demonstrate awareness of the stress placed on body tissues during strengthening exercises to minimize injury risk.

KEY TERMS

Articular Cartilage
Closed Kinetic Chain
Contusion
Core Stabilization Training
Coupling Patterns
Force Couple
Functional Tests
Inflammation
Inflammatory Phase
Interval Sport Return Program
Lumbar–Pelvic Rhythm
Macrotrauma
Microtrauma
Neutral Spine
Open Kinetic Chain
Patellofemoral Pain Syndrome
Preparticipation Physical
PRICE Method
Proprioception
Remodeling Phase
Repair Phase
Scapular Plane Position
Scapulohumeral Rhythm
SHARP
Shoulder Impingement
Spinal Segment
Sprain
Strain
Tendonitis
Tendonosis
Vastus Medialis Oblique

Introduction

The purpose of this chapter is to overview the role of strength and conditioning in the prevention of injuries. Included in this chapter is an overview of the sports medicine professionals responsible for providing care for the athlete, as well as the stages of recovery and healing from a musculoskeletal injury. Basic definitions of musculoskeletal injuries are also be included along with more detailed descriptions of shoulder, knee, and spinal anatomy, and biomechanics, along with common injury patterns, and exercise implications applicable for strength and conditioning professionals working with athletes with a history of musculoskeletal injury, and especially with those athletes hoping to prevent them.

Some of the most basic principles of injury prevention have the most profound influence for strength and conditioning professionals as well as other clinicians in sports medicine. These include adequate preactivity development of muscular strength, endurance and balance, proper flexibility, and often most importantly, proper sport biomechanics or technique (1). As is covered later in this chapter, many injuries in athletes occur from overtraining and overuse (2). Improper levels of muscular strength and endurance are often cited as critical factors in the development of injuries such as rotator cuff tendonitis (3), humeral epicondylitis (4), as well as patellofemoral pain and shin splints (5).

Additionally, sports medicine research profiling various populations of athletes has also identified characteristic patterns of muscular development that create muscular imbalances and can lead to injury (6). One example of a muscular imbalance identified with isokinetic testing of the glenohumeral joint of overhead athletes was reported by Ellenbecker (7) whereby significant increases in the strength of the internal rotators was measured on the dominant arm of professional baseball pitchers without concomitant increases in strength of the external rotator musculature creating a muscular imbalance. Similar studies in elite level tennis players (8,9) have identified similar muscle imbalances between the internal and external rotators.

Careful evaluation and application of stretching programs are other important factors in injury prevention. While studies directly linking flexibility training and injury prevention are not clear-cut, the general consensus among sports medicine professionals is that muscular inflexibility can inhibit optimal performance and can lead to joint and muscle tendon injury in the repetitive environment athletic individuals train and compete in (1). Despite recent changes in the application of static and dynamic stretching programs, sport scientists still believe specific types of flexibility training to be important in both performance enhancement and injury prevention.

Finally, the use of proper sport technique and biomechanics is a critical factor in the prevention of injury. The link between improper use of the kinetic chain in throwing and racquet sports and arm injury has been outlined by Kibler (10). The use of sport technique that optimizes power generation from the lower extremity and trunk and allows for the transfer of force from the ground reaction forces up through the lower extremities and trunk to the upper extremity is recommended. While in many cases the strength and conditioning professional cannot directly evaluate this facet of the injury prevention program, referral of athletes to qualified individuals such as high-level sport-specific coaches and sport biomechanists is highly recommended.

PREPARTICIPATION PHYSICALS

Though it is beyond the scope of this chapter to completely outline all facets of the **preparticipation physical**, the basic premise of the physical as well as key components should be discussed. Several complete references on preparticipation physicals can serve as excellent resources when designing or developing a preparticipation physical (10,11). In general, the preparticipation physical is an integral part of the injury prevention process. The actual physical is designed to evaluate the athlete's body using a specific series of evaluation methods or tests that screen or identify key factors that could lead to an injury if the athlete were to participate in that sport without rehabilitation or other preparative measures.

Preparticipation physicals are an important part of the comprehensive care of the athlete. Using a structured evaluation process, key structural deficits and strength and flexibility deficiencies can be identified that can decrease the risk of injury or reinjury.

Though some of the basic tests are provided in nearly all physicals (measurement of height, weight, heart rate, blood pressure, etc.), most physicals are made specific to the sport or activity that athlete or group of athletes is participating in. One example would be the careful evaluation of rotator cuff strength and shoulder flexibility in baseball and tennis players as well as swimmers. This area would not be emphasized as heavily for soccer players or other primarily lower body athletes. Careful development of the actual components of the preparticipation physical with the entire sports medicine team is necessary since many specialists and types of clinicians are needed to ensure that the most thorough evaluation is made. Additionally, the important role follow-up, tracking, and, ultimately, retesting play cannot be overlooked.

ROLES OF HEALTH CARE PROFESSIONALS INVOLVED IN INJURY PREVENTION AND REHABILITATION

Numerous health care professions are involved in sports injury management. Depending on the sports program (e.g., high school, college, professional team, community recreation), professionals in medicine, chiropractic, psychology, biomechanics, exercise physiology, nutrition, physical therapy, athletic training, and strength and conditioning may be involved in injury management. The diversity of health professionals involved in injury management allows the athlete to recover not only physically but also emotionally and socially.

The areas of injury prevention, recognition, and rehabilitation are common interests to professionals including physicians, physical therapists, athletic trainers, and strength and conditioning professionals. These four professions commonly have extensive involvement throughout the rehabilitation process and are further discussed below.

- *Physicians:* The physician is responsible for the health care of an injured athlete, including diagnosing and treating injuries. When an injury occurs, the physician makes the ultimate decision on when it is safe to return to sport activities. The physician guides other members of the team throughout the rehabilitation process.
- *Physical Therapists:* According to the American Physical Therapy Association, the scope of practice for a physical therapist includes providing services to patients who have impairments, functional limitations, disabilities, or changes in physical function and health status resulting from injury, disease, or other causes; interaction and practicing in collaboration with a variety of professionals; addressing risk factors and behavior that may impede optimal functioning; providing prevention and promoting health, wellness, and fitness; consulting, educating, engaging in critical inquiry, and administration; and directing and supervising support personnel (12). Physical therapists practice in a wide variety of settings including hospitals, outpatient clinics, research centers, fitness centers, and sports training facilities. Physical therapists can receive specialist certifications in seven different areas including both orthopedics and sports through the American Board of Physical Therapy Specialties.
- *Athletic Trainers*: Performance domains of the certified athletic trainer as defined by the National Athletic Trainers' Association Board of Certification include prevention of athletic injuries; recognition, evaluation, and

immediate care of injuries; rehabilitation and reconditioning of athletic injuries; health care administration; and professional development and responsibility (2). School districts, colleges and universities, sports medicine clinics, professional teams, and industrial settings may employ athletic trainers. The athletic trainer is often present at sport practices and games and is therefore likely to be the first person to evaluate an injury and provide acute treatment. Their daily presence at sport practices also allows athletic trainers extensive involvement throughout the entire rehabilitation process.

- *Strength and Conditioning Professionals*: Strength and conditioning professionals have the knowledge of appropriate exercise techniques to work in conjunction with other members of the health care team to develop and supervise reconditioning programs. It is important that strength and conditioning professionals be informed of injuries and any precautions to exercise as they may be the only ones involved with the athlete once return to sport has occurred. Strength and conditioning professionals play an important role in the transition from a controlled, supervised rehabilitation program to a lifelong, independent exercise program.

The strength and conditioning professional plays a key role in injury prevention by developing a sport-specific exercise plan that may decrease the risk of injuries common in a specific sport. The strength and conditioning professional, by working closely with the sports medicine team, also plays an important role in the transition from a rehabilitation program to full participation in the sport.

Because sports injury management involves a multidisciplinary team, it is essential to have good communication to allow a safe return to athletic activity as soon as possible. Within each individual sports medicine team, there should be agreement on the specific role for each member. The roles of sports medicine professionals are increasingly overlapping as practitioners extend from the "traditional" work settings, complete continuing education, and attain specialist certifications. However, each professional brings his or her unique expertise to the sports medicine team that will enhance injury prevention, recognition, and rehabilitation. Despite research evidence, sports medicine (including injury management and return to play criteria) is not an exact science. The sports medicine team must discuss varying philosophies and theories to provide consistent, up-to-date care. Communication must also occur with the athlete, coach, team, and family members when appropriate. To allow optimal injury recovery, responsibilities of all professionals involved in injury management include communication, continuing education, promoting athlete safety, and understanding the mental and physical demands of sport.

To work in the field of sports medicine requires teamwork, and optimal knowledge and understanding of the roles of all of the members of the sports medicine team is required to best serve the athlete.

INJURY CLASSIFICATION

Injuries occur on a regular basis in sporting activities. In successfully treating athletic injuries in a rehabilitation setting, the health professional needs to understand the mechanism and type of injury that has occurred. When classifying an injury, we use various definitions to outline the extent and severity of the injury in order to adopt the appropriate methods of treatment at the appropriate stages of healing.

Overuse injuries are often a result of **microtrauma**, where the involved tissue becomes inflamed and painful over an indeterminate amount of time, secondary to forces that exceed the strength and healing rate of the tendon or involved structure. **Tendonitis** refers to inflammation of the tendon and associated sheath, whereas **tendonosis** involves degeneration of the tendon (13).

Injuries that occur at a single point in time, with an identifiable source, are termed **macrotrauma**. There are varying degrees of macrotraumatic events, and they can be categorized as intrinsic or extrinsic. Intrinsic injuries are the result of forces (mechanical, environmental, or situational) that supersede the ability of the athlete to respond and avoid injury (1,2,14). A shot-putter who ruptures his pectoralis tendon while attempting to best his opponent's distance is an example of an intrinsic injury. Extrinsic injuries occur when an identifiable source outside of the athlete's control is the primary cause of trauma. A running back tackled directly at his knee by an opponent's helmet causing rupture of the knee ligaments is an example of an extrinsic injury.

There exists a continuum when classifying injury severity. A **strain** occurs when the involved tissue(s) is subject to forces invoking a graded local inflammatory response, without disrupting the structural integrity of the tissue. A baseball pitcher who throws 100 pitches in a game at high velocities experiences local soreness in the shoulder girdle secondary to placing a strain on the contractile tissue around the shoulder. The healing rate with a strain is usually several days to a week, if further immediate stressors are avoided.

A **sprain** occurs when contractile or noncontractile tissue is subject to forces exceeding the inherent strength of the tissue, causing pain, local or diffuse inflammation, and varying degrees of functional and structural tissue loss. Different classification systems for sprains exist. Typically classified with a numerical scale (1,13,15), the lower numbers indicate the least amount of tissue damage, and the higher numbers usually indicate a complete rupture or functional loss of the structure. For example, a grade 1 ankle sprain according to Hershman and Nicholas involves microscopic tearing of the ligament without loss of function, and may take weeks to heal, and a grade III ankle sprain involves a complete tearing of the ligament with complete loss of function and will likely require surgical intervention (15). Treatment of the athlete then varies based on the degree of severity of the injury.

Contusions can occur to muscle, bone, and cartilage, and are typically the result of a collision with an outside force such as an opponent, the ground, or a foreign object. Contusions to muscle tissue can also be classified by severity based on the amount of hemorrhage, pain, ROM limitations, and the extent of tissue involvement. The grading system is similar to ligamentous injuries with grade I injuries involving mild pain and limitations, and grade III injuries being the most severe, with herniation of the muscle through the fascial envelope along with possible bruising of the underlying bone. Severe contusions may require surgery or evacuation of the hematoma. Care must be taken with moderate to severe muscle contusions to avoid further complications, such as functional loss of the muscle or myositis ossificans, which is a condition involving calcification within the muscle tissue as a result of additional inflammation or trauma (2). **Articular cartilage** is a thin layer of specialized tissue covering joint surfaces in synovial joints such as the knee or hip. The cartilage promotes normal movement between joint surfaces, and reduces potentially harmful forces such as shear or compression between the joint surfaces. Articular cartilage receives nutrition through components within the synovial fluid that bathe the joint during normal movement. Injuries to articular cartilage pose a challenge, due to the lack of a direct blood supply and limited ability to self-repair. When injuries to articular cartilage or synovial joints do occur, the goals should be to promote healing by decreasing joint effusion and maintaining ROM and movement between joint surfaces, while preventing overloading to the joint surfaces (14).

PHASES OF TISSUE HEALING: CLINICAL TREATMENT AND EXERCISE CONSIDERATIONS

After an acute musculoskeletal injury, there are three phases of tissue healing: inflammation, proliferation/repair, and maturation/remodeling. Health professionals need to identify the healing phase in order to determine appropriate treatment and exercise. Although each phase is defined by certain characteristics, healing occurs along a continuum and phases overlap. Phase durations are given only as guidelines and vary based on factors including type of tissue and injury severity. Clinical judgment must be used to determine appropriate treatment as healing progresses. Signs and symptoms should be continually monitored throughout the healing phases and treatment adjusted as necessary. The physiology, signs and symptoms, treatment, and exercise considerations are described for each phase.

INFLAMMATION PHASE

Inflammation is the body's first response to injury and is necessary to begin the healing process. The **inflammation phase** begins immediately after injury and can last up to approximately 6 days (16). The purposes of inflammation are to protect the body against foreign material, destroy and remove foreign materials (e.g., bacteria, damaged cells, dead tissue), localize the injury, and ultimately promote tissue healing and regeneration (16,17). Although inflammation is necessary to recognize an injury has occurred and to begin the healing process, it can become undesirable as it is a nonspecific response that can occur in an excessive amount. For example, the same inflammatory response occurs whether there is foreign material present (e.g., infection) or no foreign material is present (e.g., ankle sprain). Another example involves the inflammatory response of scar tissue formation. This response is useful when damage such as a muscle tear occurs, but can be detrimental to the tissue and decrease function in chronic inflammatory conditions. Prompt recognition and treatment of an injury will help control the inflammatory response, optimize the healing environment, and allow earlier return to activity.

Physiology

After tissue damage and cell death from an injury, chemicals are released that cause several vascular and cellular changes. Immediately following trauma, the first cells to arrive at the injured site are platelets (2). Platelets release serotonin, responsible for immediate vasoconstriction at the injured site. Following the brief period of vasoconstriction, histamine is released from mast cells (connective tissue cells). Histamine increases vascular permeability and causes vasodilatation, resulting in increased swelling. Bradykinin is another chemical released by injured tissue that increases permeability. Increased vascular permeability increases swelling by allowing fluids and proteins out of the capillaries and into the tissues. An osmotic pressure imbalance is created as blood and plasma proteins enter the interstitial space. Swelling results as more fluid moves into the area to return pressure to normal. Prostaglandins and leukotrienes are two other chemicals causing increased permeability and vasodilatation, resulting in swelling and pain. Prostaglandins are produced in nearly all tissues and released in response to damaged cells. Many pain and anti-inflammatory medications work by affecting prostaglandin synthesis.

The cellular response consists of increased leukocytes (white blood cells) in the injured area due to increased permeability. Neutrophils and macrophages are two kinds of leukocytes found at the injury site. They are responsible for phagocytosis and removal of debris. Neutrophils destroy bacteria when present (17).

To control the amount of fluid in the tissue area and localize injury, blood coagulation must occur. This process begins with damaged cells releasing thromboplastin, which causes prothrombin to be converted into thrombin. Next, fibrinogen is converted into a fibrin clot that shuts off blood supply to the injured area. This prevents the spread of infection by blocking off the area, keeps foreign agents at the site with greatest white blood cell activity, forms a clot to stop bleeding, and gives a framework for tissue repair (18).

Signs and Symptoms

Signs and symptoms used to identify the physiologic changes of inflammation phase are remembered by using the acronym **SHARP**: Swelling, Heat, Altered function, Redness, and Pain. Swelling is assessed visually, through palpation, and with anthropometric measurements (measurements taken circumferentially around an extremity). Intensity of the inflammatory response and swelling is usually proportional to amount of tissue damage; however, amount of swelling is not always an accurate predictor of injury severity. Skin that is warm to the touch is another sign of the inflammation process. Altered function is a consequence of damaged tissue, swelling, heat, and pain. Redness is assessed visually with bilateral comparison. Pain is a subjective measure. Quantitative pain rating scales (e.g., visual analog scale—rating pain on a scale from 0 to 10) can be used to monitor pain levels throughout the rehabilitation process.

Treatment

Goals of clinical treatment and exercise during the inflammation phase include

- Preventing further injury
- Decreasing swelling and pain
- Establishing baseline measurements of signs and symptoms (pain level, swelling, ROM, strength, functional ability)
- Maintaining overall fitness level

Many of these goals are accomplished by following the **PRICE method** of protection, rest, ice, compression, and elevation.

- *Protection:* Based on injury location and severity, protection of the injured area can be accomplished through the use of a splint, sling, brace, or assistive device such as crutches. Splinting assists in decreasing muscle guarding and breaking the pain-spasm-pain cycle.

- *Rest*: Rest is often applied as "relative rest" or "restricted function". Based on injury severity, clinical judgment is used to determine the balance between protection and safe, early mobilization. Although injured tissue needs to be protected and immobilized, prolonged rest can lead to tissue contractures and loss of range of motion. Even if the injured area needs to be immobilized, appropriate exercise can be performed with uninjured areas to minimize losses in overall fitness level (see Exercise Considerations below).
- *Ice/Cryotherapy*: The primary goal of cryotherapy is to decrease tissue temperature (17). The decreased temperature subsequently results in other physiological changes to promote healing. Decreased metabolism is one of the main benefits of cryotherapy used for acute injuries. Decreased metabolism minimizes secondary hypoxic injury by decreasing the oxygen need of the cell. Secondary hypoxic injury is tissue death that occurs after the initial injury due to lack of oxygen supply. Tissues near the injured site die because the inflammatory process decreases blood flow. With decreased blood flow, cells that survived the initial injury die because they cannot get enough oxygen or get rid of waste products. Other benefits of cryotherapy are decreased vascular permeability and vasoconstriction. Cryotherapy should be applied as soon as possible after evaluation of an acute injury. However, it is important to do an adequate evaluation before muscle spasm, pain, and stiffness increase. Prompt application of cryotherapy cannot reverse the initial trauma, but decreasing secondary hypoxic injury will decrease the overall amount of injured tissue. Cryotherapy should be applied with a cooling to rewarming ratio of 1:2; initially ice may be applied approximately 30 minutes every 1½ to 2 hours (17).
- *Compression*: Compression can be applied via an intermittent compression pump or elastic bandage. Compression controls edema formation and decreases swelling by promoting reabsorption of fluid.
- *Elevation*: Elevation decreases capillary hydrostatic pressure, which forces fluid out of the capillary in an uninjured state.

The strength and conditioning professional should be aware of the PRICE method of treating injuries. Some of these treatment methods may also be utilized during the postinjury transition from rehabilitation to full participation in the sport.

In addition to the treatments already discussed, health care professionals may use a variety of other modalities to promote healing and control the inflammatory process. A common form of electrical stimulation used for control of acute pain is sensory level stimulation. TENS (transcutaneous electrical nerve stimulation) units are devices that provide sensory level stimulation. One disadvantage of this modality is that symptom relief occurs only while the TENS device is being used (19) (Fig. 21.1).

Ultrasound is another modality that may be used to promote healing. During the inflammatory phase, pulsed ultrasound should be used for its nonthermal effects including altered membrane permeability to promote tissue healing (16). The use of continuous ultrasound produces heat in the tissues and is contraindicated during

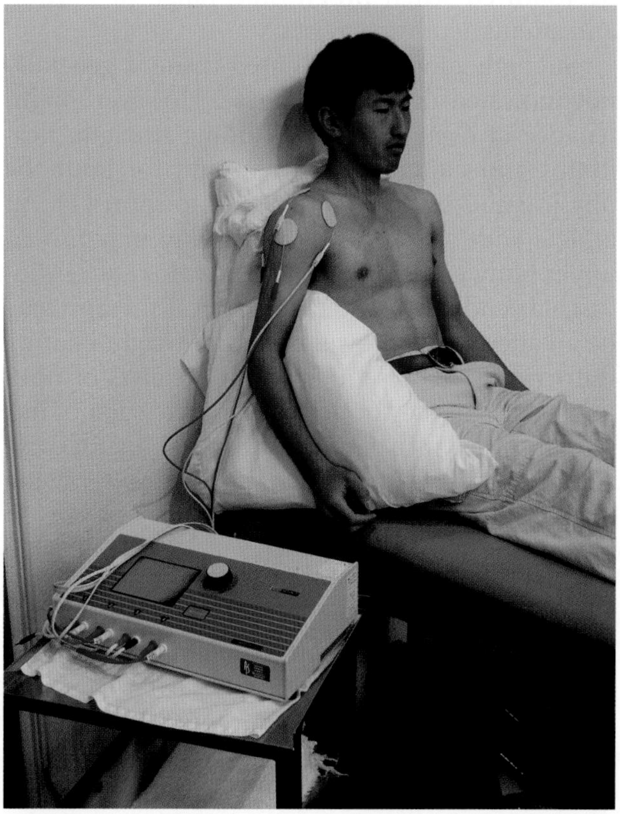

FIGURE 21.1 Modality setup used to treat a patient with rotator cuff tendonitis.

the inflammatory phase. Various applications of electrical stimulation and ultrasound may be used to facilitate delivery of a topical drugin to the tissues, known as iontophoresis and phonophoresis, respectively. Use of any of the above modalities is decided upon by an appropriately trained health care professional.

Exercise Considerations

Based on injury severity, gentle range of motion of exercises may be indicated near the end of the inflammatory phase. Performing early range of motion will decrease the negative effects of immobilization. Each type of tissue responds differently to immobilization and remobilization. Negative effects of immobilization on muscle include decreased muscle fiber size, decrease in size and number of mitochondria, decrease in muscle tension produced, increase in lactate concentration with exercise, and a decrease in total muscle weight (14). Early controlled passive or active motion may be used postoperatively to retard muscle atrophy and tissue contracture. It also allows for diffusion of synovial fluid to nourish articular cartilage, meniscus, and ligaments. In postoperative cases, the physician protocol must be followed when progressing range of motion and strengthening exercises.

Strengthening of the injured tissue is generally not indicated during this phase. However, maintenance of overall fitness including strength, flexibility, and endurance is important for both the physical and psychological return to sport (1). An athlete with a lower extremity injury may use an upper body ergometer to minimize loss of cardiovascular endurance. Aquatic physical therapy may be an alternative if lower extremity weight-bearing restrictions are present. Strength exercises of noninvolved areas may be performed if they do not risk reinjury. A balance between strengthening for overall fitness and rest must be maintained to allow the body to heal and prevent fatigue.

REPAIR PHASE

The **repair phase** begins once inflammatory debris has been removed, approximately 3 to 20 days after injury (16). According to some sources, the repair phase may last up to 6 weeks (2). Events during the repair phase include scar formation, tissue regeneration, and tissue repair, which increase strength at the injured site.

Physiology

A lack of oxygen at the injured site stimulates neovascularization, the formation of new capillaries. The formation of new capillaries increases blood flow, oxygen, and nutrients at the injured site. Collagen synthesis occurs as fibroblastic cells begin producing collagen fibers. During this phase, the collagen is laid down randomly and is weak in structure.

The formation of scar tissue after injury is a normal response; however excessive collagen deposition and scar formation can hinder the healing process. As scar tissue matures, it becomes inelastic and firm, and lacks blood flow. This type of tissue forms adhesions, which decrease range of motion and function. Therefore, it is important to promote proper healing and decrease the amount of scar tissue formation.

Signs and Symptoms

During the repair phase, the signs and symptoms of the inflammation response subside. The amount of swelling remains constant or begins to subside. Skin temperature and color approaches that of the contralateral side. Although pain decreases overall, palpable tenderness or pain with specific movements may still be present. Skin color is similar to the contralateral extremity; however, ecchymosis may be present. Function slowly improves throughout the repair phase.

Treatment

Goals of treatment during the repair phase include

- Continuing to decrease inflammation
- Maintaining ROM by minimizing contracture and adhesion formation
- Regaining strength and function

Modalities should be used as needed to increase exercise tolerance and continue to promote healing. In addition to controlling pain, modalities are used to increase circulation prior to exercise and decrease circulation (and swelling) afterward. Thermotherapy, which was contraindicated in the inflammation phase, is safe to use once there is no active swelling. Monitoring the signs and symptoms of the inflammatory response will help determine when swelling is no longer active and begins to decrease. Thermotherapy promotes healing by increasing circulation, decreasing pain, and increasing collagen extensibility. Common forms of thermotherapy include moist hot packs, warm whirlpools, and continuous ultrasound. After exercise, many of the same treatment interventions used during the inflammation phase should be continued. Cryotherapy, electrical stimulation, compression, and elevation will control pain and swelling that may result from exercise.

In addition to modalities, manual therapy techniques including passive range of motion and joint mobilizations may be used to further decrease pain and increase range of motion. Joint mobilizations will help restore normal joint motion when range of motion is limited due to joint capsule tightness (14).

Exercise Considerations

Active-assisted and active range of motion exercises should be initiated if not already included in treatment at the end of the inflammation phase. Range of motion is performed under controlled, supervised conditions, as the collagen is still weak during this phase. As soon as pain and swelling are controlled, strengthening exercises for the injured area can be initiated. Proper exercise progression will aid healing by increasing circulation, increasing oxygen, and optimizing collagen realignment. Range of motion and strengthening exercises promote optimal healing of soft tissue and collagen by causing realignment along lines of stress in a similar manner as bone responds to stress according to Wolff's law.

Exercise should place progressively increasing amounts of stress on the healing tissues. Davies (20) described an exercise progression continuum to be used during rehabilitation. Although all stages are listed here, the later stages are not appropriate until the repair phase due to increased stress placed on the tissue. The exercise progression is as follows: submaximal multiple angle isometrics, maximal multiple angle isometrics, submaximal short arc exercises, maximal short arc exercises, submaximal full ROM exercises, maximal full ROM exercises.

Multiple angle and short arc exercises are performed to allow exercise throughout pain-free range of motion. In addition to strengthening muscles at the range of motion where the exercise is performed, strengthening also occurs up to 10 degrees (isometric) or 15 degrees (isokinetic) on either side of the range of motion at which the exercise is performed (20). Therefore, performing exercises in a safe, pain-free range of motion will increase strength into the affected areas (Fig. 21.2).

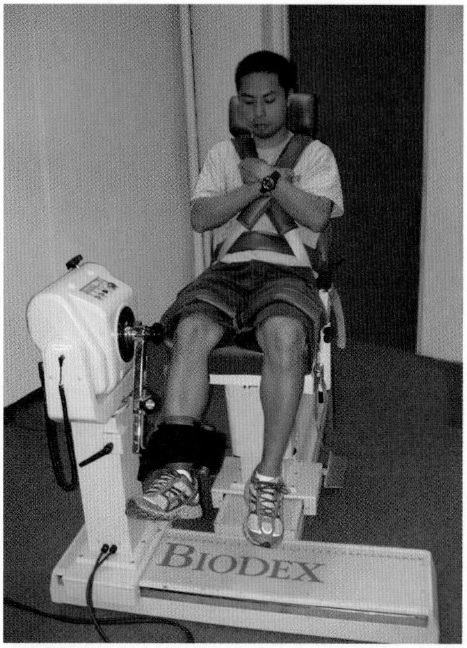

FIGURE 21.2 Biodex isokinetic knee extension exercise using a short arc of range of motion between 90 and 60 degrees.

In addition to strengthening, proprioceptive exercises should be included. The term **proprioception** describes the sensation of joint movement (kinesthesia) and joint position (joint position sense) (21). Proprioception is decreased after trauma to tissues containing mechanoreceptors, such as muscles, ligaments, and joints. A joint with decreased proprioceptive feedback and joint position sense is at greater risk for reinjury. By incorporating proprioceptive exercises into a rehabilitation program, the neuromuscular control and dynamic joint stabilization needed for athletic activities are improved (21). Examples of basic proprioceptive exercises include single leg balance and balance board activities (Fig. 21.3).

Tissue response to exercise should be constantly monitored. Increased pain and swelling imply that too much stress has been placed on the tissue. When signs and symptoms of inflammation reoccur or increase, exercise should be decreased and treatment discussed during the inflammation phase as indicated.

REMODELING PHASE

The last stage in the healing process is the **remodeling phase**. Even though a person may have returned to prior level of function, the remodeling phase can continue more than a year after the initial injury (18).

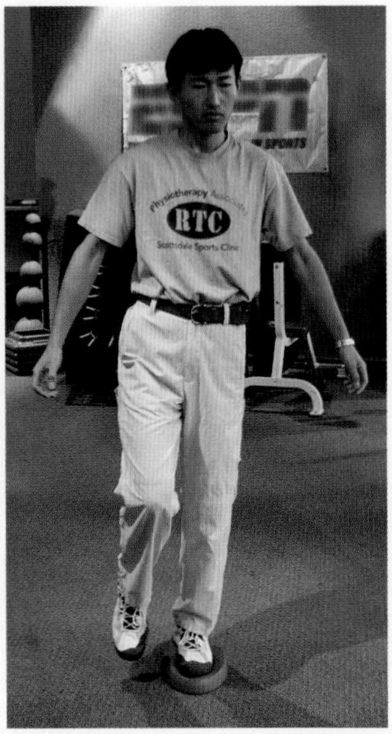

FIGURE 21.3 Unilateral lower extremity proprioception exercise using a Theraband stability trainer.

Physiology

Near the end of the repair phase, the tensile strength of the collagen increases and the number of fibroblasts diminishes, signaling the start of the maturation phase. According to Davis' law, realignment and remodeling of the collagen fibers results from tensile forces. As stress to the collagen is increased, the fibers realign in a position of maximum efficiency, parallel to the lines of tension. Collagen becomes more organized and its strength increases.

Signs and Symptoms

Signs and symptoms present since the inflammation phase will continue to decrease and eventually disappear by the end of the remodeling phase. There will be minimal to no swelling, pain with motion, and pain with palpation. Function continues to approach preinjury levels. Initial measurements, including swelling, ROM, and strength, should be reevaluated.

Treatment

The primary goal of treatment during the remodeling phase is to regain the prior level of function of the injured tissue. Modalities will be continued as in the repair phase as needed to maintain optimal healing environments and assist in regaining full range of motion. However, modality use is decreased as exercise tolerance increases. Manual therapy and joint mobilizations should be continued until full range of motion is achieved. Collagen will continue to realign along the lines of stress applied by range of motion and strengthening activities.

Exercise Considerations

Regaining full strength is an emphasis during the remodeling phase. Exercises are progressed as discussed in the repair phase. Signs and symptoms are monitored to prevent placing too much stress on the tissue and risking reinjury. Proprioceptive exercise should also be progressed. As strength and proprioception are increased, functional activities simulating work or sport requirements should be included. Speed of movement, type of muscle contraction, and length of activity are important factors to consider when developing functional activities. Functional and sport-specific exercises are incorporated into the Return to Activity Phase discussed in the next section.

Phases of healing must be kept in mind as health professionals continue to push earlier return to sport. Clinical judgment will determine appropriate exercise and treatment progression through the healing phases to allow optimal return to sport. Since return to competitive sport activities often occurs before the healing phases are complete, continued strengthening and bracing should be incorporated as necessary to prevent further injury. A strength and conditioning professional is able to assist the transition from the controlled, supervised environment of a rehabilitation clinic to a lifelong independent exercise program for injury prevention.

RETURN-TO-ACTIVITY PHASE: THE ROLE OF THE INTERVAL PROGRAM

Of all the stages in the rehabilitation process, the return to sport or full activity is easily the most anticipated for all persons in the sports medicine team and clearly the most anticipated both physically and mentally by the patient. Despite the popularity of this stage of the recovery process, this phase is probably the least well defined, and filled with guidelines and ambiguous rules that often are not predicated on research, functional outcomes, or evidence-based practice themes. Many methods can be used to define or determine whether the athlete is ready for a return to full activity. Most clinicians and sports scientists recommend the inclusion of as much objectively based testing that is possible. Use of clinical testing comes in two primary categories. These categories are subjective and objective. Subjective tests are designed to be completed by patients themselves and typically involve questions geared at obtaining patients' perceived level of function.

The return-to-activity phase is an extremely critical part of the rehabilitation process that should be based on function rather than time or symptoms. The strength and conditioning professional should have a defined role in this phase of the recovery process.

Objective testing is performed in several areas to determine the appropriateness of a return to sport. Determination of a return of range of motion of the injured joint or joints is carefully performed with a goniometer, or additional flexibility testing can be done using standardized tests like the sit and reach maneuver, which measures low back and hamstring flexibility. Typically, a return of range of motion equal to the contralateral or uninjured extremity is striven for. Exceptions to matching range of motion or strength to the opposite side must include injury to the opposite side, or presence or either exceptional range of motion or strength on one side from playing a unilateral sport such as tennis or baseball. In most patients, however, using a goal of achieving at least the range of motion or strength levels of the uninjured side is an appropriate goal.

A determination of strength must also be made before the patient can be returned to sport or aggressive activities without injury. Typical strength comparisons again use the opposite side as a baseline, and employ either manual muscle testing techniques or more sophisticated equipment like isokinetic or handheld dynamometers that further objectify strength levels and are capable of reliably testing strength at multiple velocities that more appropriately match the speeds at which the muscles and joints function during ADLs or some sport activities. Initiation of return-to-sport programs such as running and throwing is not recommended when deficits in muscular strength are 20% or more (20). Therefore, while these isolated types of muscle performance tests cannot simulate all functional demands, they provide the clinician with a valid and reliable measure or indicator of muscular performance around an injured joint.

In addition to the objective tests for strength and range of motion, testing specifically designed to assess the function of the limb or individual as a whole are recommended. These are typically called **functional tests**. Examples of functional tests are hop and jump tests like the one-leg hop test and vertical jump test. One particularly popular test is the one leg hop test. In patients with an injured knee, this test can be performed simply in a clinic using a tape measure and piece of tape to delineate starting position. The patient takes off and lands on the same limb with comparison of one limb to the other performed. Failure to reach the distance generated on the contralateral side indicates often an inability to generate gross lower extremity power in the lower extremity, as well as very often a hesitancy in landing and having the eccentric control necessary to absorb the load following the jump. In addition to the actual distance, quantitative assessment of these patients often provides valuable insight as to the patient's readiness to absorb the impact load on landing, and ability to land on one leg. Often patients will land on both legs in an effort to shield the injured extremity from the stress and eccentric overload inherent in landing. Information gleaned during functional testing is imperative for the clinical decision-making process that must be undertaken when considering a patient for a full return to activity.

THE INTERVAL SPORT PROGRAM

Several key components are inherent in an **interval sport return program**. These are warm-up, alternate-day performance scheduling, integration with conditioning, progressive stages of intensity, proper biomechanics and evaluation of mechanics, and cool-down or aftercare. Each of these important components forms the currently used interval sport return programs and can easily be adapted into nearly any sport or activity.

WARM-UP

Despite the understandable anticipation that a patient has upon returning to a sport following the hiatus required following injury or during rehabilitation, a proper warm-up must precede actual performance in the interval program. Despite recent evidence that the acute effects of stretching may diminish jump and power performance for a period of up to 20 minutes (22,23), the potential injury prevention or reinjury benefits of stretching and warm-up make this an important initial stage in the interval program. Typically, the warm-up consists of a light cardiovascular workout to elevate local tissue temperature, and increase blood flow to the peripheral aspects of the limbs (24). This warm-up is then followed by static stretches with isolated positioning of the muscles' origin and insertion such that controlled and static elongation occurs. Hold times of 15 to 30 seconds have been reported to produce plastic deformation of the tissue and enhance the flexibility and range of motion of the hamstrings and other muscles (24).

ALTERNATE-DAY PERFORMANCE SCHEDULE

Interval sport performance programs typically have an alternate-day performance schedule. This is designed to allow the musculature and static restraint mechanisms surrounding the injured joint or joints a period of recovery before sport activity is again administered. Additionally, the day off following performance allows the patient and clinician time to determine the tolerance of the body to the previous day's level of performance. Close monitoring of all subjective symptoms and objective signs is an important part of determining when the next stage or intensity or activity is initiated. Therefore, alternate-day performance of the interval program is recommended.

INTEGRATION WITH OTHER CONDITIONING

This is perhaps one of the most difficult aspects of returning a patient to his or her sport. The importance of continuing with strength and range of motion exercises during the interval program is widely recognized. Restoration of final muscular balance and obtaining the last few degrees of flexibility and motion around a formally restricted joint are all aspects that require continued rehabilitative exercise and conditioning during this phase. Though there is limited work published in this area, several clinical suggestions or guidelines are typically followed. Performance of sport-specific activity is recommended before or prior to any strength or power training. This is to ensure that the body's musculature, which provides the dynamic stability for the joints, is properly functioning and not fatigued during the functional performance. Additionally, exercises to segments even far away from the injured segment may complicate functional performance.

PROGRESSIVE STAGES OF INTENSITY

For a program to truly be interval in nature, it must contain progressive stages of gradually increasing intensity. These progressive stages allow patients and clinicians to responsibly progress the stresses applied to the postoperative or postinjury tissue. One example is an interval throwing program. The interval throwing program contains gradually progressive stages or steps of both increasing distance, and volume (number of throws). Careful monitoring of patients through this program finds them increasing distance from as little as 30 to 45 ft initially, to as much 120 to 150 ft based on the type of position they play in baseball. Within each distance is a progression in the number of throws as well. This allows for independent increases in the intensity of the throwing (longer distance) as well as an increase in the number of repetitions, which challenges the patients' ability to withstand repeated stresses and builds endurance. For a complete description of an interval throwing program used in shoulder rehabilitation, see Andrews and Wilk (7). Interval tennis programs follow similar guidelines and can be found in Ellenbecker (3).

PROPER BIOMECHANICS AND EVALUATION OF MECHANICS

Another critical part of the interval return process is the emphasis on proper biomechanics. Many times, returning from an injury or surgery leaves the athlete with deficits in muscle balance, range of motion, and proprioception or kinesthetic awareness in the limb or affected joint and hence sets the athlete up for compensatory movement patterns. Often these movement patterns can lead to injury in the segment being rehabilitated or in adjoining segments. A perfect example of this is when someone is returning to tennis play after a knee arthroscopy and they develop tennis elbow because of problems with lower body movement and an increase in the contribution and loading on the arm. Another example would be illustrated in the athlete returning to throw after a shoulder injury and due to a loss in external rotation range of motion "short-arms" the ball resulting in greater loading on the inside (medial aspect) of the elbow joint (25).

Therefore, careful monitoring of the athlete's mechanics is indicated during the return-to-activity phase. This can be accomplished by having the health care clinician observe the interval process, as well as having the interval process performed in the presence of a coach or even sports biomechanist.

AFTERCARE

Equally important as the warm-up, the cool-down or aftercare after the interval return program is an essential part of this process. In the earlier phases of the interval program, where oftentimes a physical therapist or athletic trainer is supervising the program being executed in the clinical setting, the remainder of a rehabilitation program is typically completed on the same day as the interval sport return program. So, following the throwing or running or whatever the sport activity is, rehabilitation exercises geared at restoring optimal muscle balance and fatigue resistance, joint range of motion, as well as proprioception and balance are commenced. This allows the athlete to continue perfecting the injured areas during the interval return process and ensures that a day of nearly complete recovery can be followed on the day following the interval program and rehabilitative exercise session. Aftercare in this situation is guided by the rehabilitation professional.

During the later stages of the interval program, athletes are typically performing these activities independently off-site. Therefore, strict instruction regarding the amount, intensity, and duration of maintenance exercise must be shared with the athlete as well as the specific instructions for post-session stretching and icing. The use of ice to create vasoconstriction in the affected area is widely accepted in clinical medicine and sports medicine arenas. The amount of time that ice is used after an injury or following a return to full activity varies and has not been formally studied. Current recommendations are typically for application of ice following postworkout stretching. Following an organized and consistent program of aftercare will ensure that off-site interval program execution mirrors the program initially designed in the clinical setting and is thought to minimize the risk of reinjury and facilitate the return to activity.

OVERVIEW OF KNEE MECHANICS AND EXERCISE APPLICATIONS

KNEE ANATOMY AND BIOMECHANICS

The knee joint is commonly injured during athletic activities. Knowledge of knee anatomy and biomechanics should be considered when designing exercise programs to prevent and rehabilitate lower extremity injuries. The knee joint is classified as a synovial joint and consists of the tibiofemoral and patellofemoral articulations. Motion at the tibiofemoral joint occurs in flexion, extension, and internal and external rotation. The screw home mechanism occurs at terminal knee extension and involves the tibia externally rotating on a fixed femur in open kinetic chain activity.

There are four main ligaments providing stability to the knee joint: anterior cruciate ligament, posterior cruciate ligament, medial collateral ligament, and the lateral collateral ligament. Another commonly injured structure in the knee is the meniscus. The knee has a lateral and medial meniscus, with the medial meniscus having a higher incidence of injury. The meniscus functions to absorb shock by dissipating forces over a larger surface area, aid in joint lubrication, and increase joint congruency and stability (26).

COMMON KNEE INJURIES AND EXERCISE CONSIDERATIONS

In general, rehabilitation for knee injuries will include strengthening exercises for the quadriceps and hamstring muscles, total leg strengthening, and proprioceptive exercises. Restoring the balance between knee flexion and extension strength is an important rehabilitation goal. A 2:3 ratio of knee flexion to extension strength is desirable (27). As is further discussed below, total leg strengthening is indicated as proximal muscle weakness is often found with distal lower extremity injuries. Proprioceptive exercises are often indicated after a lower extremity injury because trauma to tissues containing mechanoreceptors will decrease proprioception. These rehabilitation principles are further discussed below in relation to two common knee injuries, patellofemoral pain syndrome and anterior cruciate ligament (ACL) injury.

Patellofemoral Pain Syndrome

Related Knee Anatomy and Biomechanics The patella is a sesamoid bone that functions to optimize the extensor mechanism by increasing the force capability of quadriceps muscles (26). Different areas of the patella contact the femur as the knee joint moves through full range of motion. The injured area of the patellar surface will determine the symptomatic ranges of motion. Symptoms occur because of a compressive force on the patellofemoral joint as the quadriceps muscle contracts to extend the knee. The quadriceps muscle pulls the patella superiorly, and the resistance from the patellar tendon pulls the patella inferiorly. The resultant force is compression of the patella against the femur. Dynamic and static restraints, such as the quadriceps muscles and retinaculum, will affect medial and lateral tracking of the patella.

Etiology of Injury Patellofemoral pain syndrome is the name often given to the symptom of anterior knee pain. There are several possible causes of anterior knee pain. Specific diagnoses that may be included under this general term include chondromalacia patella, patellar tendonitis, patellofemoral malalignment, plica syndrome, and Osgood–Schlatter disease (28).

Success in treating this syndrome is dependent on determining the cause of the pain, which can often be multifactorial. Only after identifying the cause(s) of patellofemoral pain can appropriate treatment be determined. A classification system of patellofemoral disorders has been developed by Wilk et al. (29) to serve as a foundation for clinical interventions. Categories within this classification system include: patellar compression syndromes, patellar instability, biomechanical dysfunction, direct patellar trauma, soft tissue lesions, overuse syndromes, osteochondritis diseases, and neurologic disorders. Pathological findings that may need to be addressed when treating patellofemoral pain syndrome include patellar alignment, patellar hypomobility or hypermobility, **vastus medialis oblique** (VMO) weakness, and muscle strength/flexibility imbalances. Rehabilitation for patellofemoral pain syndrome commonly includes the following: VMO strengthening, addressing muscle strength and flexibility imbalances throughout the entire lower extremity, orthotic devices, stretching the lateral retinaculum, aerobic conditioning, taping, and bracing (5). Patellofemoral pain often occurs as a secondary injury. Therefore, it is necessary to consider the patellofemoral joint during all knee joint rehabilitation programs to prevent causing additional injuries.

Exercise Considerations Exercises for patellofemoral pain syndrome should be related to the specific pathological findings of the evaluation. The following are general exercise suggestions that apply to developing strength programs to treat and prevent patellofemoral pain syndrome.

- *Perform exercises only through pain-free ranges of motion.* Relatively safe ranges of motion in which to perform patellofemoral rehabilitation have been recommended. Due to the different effects of gravity in the open and closed kinetic chain positions, it has been recommended to perform open kinetic chain forces between the angles of 90 and 50 degrees and 10 to 0 degrees of knee flexion. Activities in the closed kinetic chain should be performed between 50 and 0 degrees (14). Wallace et al. (30) found an increase in patellofemoral joint reaction forces as flexion angle increased during a squat exercise. These researchers also recommend avoiding knee flexion angles greater than approximately 60 degrees in an attempt to reduce patellofemoral compression during closed kinetic chain activities such as the squat exercise. Multiple angle isometrics and short arc exercises can be used for strengthening in pain-free ranges of motion.
- *Emphasize VMO strengthening.* After an injury, pain and swelling lead to selective reflex inhibition of the VMO muscle. With decreased medial force on the patella from the VMO, the lateral quadriceps muscles cause excessive lateral tracking of the patella during extension. This maltracking will alter patellofemoral joint mechanics and increase symptoms. Despite numerous research studies, there is little consensus on the most effective exercises to maximize VMO muscle recruitment. Although selective activation of the VMO muscle is controversial, exercises can be performed

in an attempt to maximize VMO activation. Suggested exercises for VMO strengthening include biofeedback to monitor VMO contraction used in conjunction with open and closed kinetic chain exercises, short arc quadriceps exercises, and hip adduction performed in conjunction with a squat exercise (28).

- *Incorporate exercises for total leg strengthening.* Exercises for proximal lower extremity muscles should be included as indicated by the evaluation. Strengthening of the hip flexor muscles and hamstring muscles is often indicated (28). It has also been shown that the hip external rotators (5,31) and hip abductors (31) may require strengthening, especially in females. Examples of exercises for total leg strengthening that often do not increase symptoms include stationary bicycling with a high seat, supine straight leg raises, lateral step-ups, and retro step-ups.

Anterior Cruciate Ligament Injury

Related Knee Anatomy/Biomechanics One of the most common injuries to the knee during athletic injuries is a torn ACL. The ACL is the primary restraint to anterior translation of the tibia on the femur in the open kinetic chain. In the closed kinetic chain, the ACL functions to prevent posterior displacement of the femur on the tibia. Depending on the direction and amount of force, injury to the medial collateral, lateral collateral, and posterior cruciate ligaments or menisci may also occur with a torn ACL. Depending on the severity of injury and activity level of an individual, operative or nonoperative treatment may be chosen. For active individuals with a torn ACL, surgical reconstruction is usually the treatment of choice.

After reconstructive surgery, the emphasis of rehabilitation progresses from range of motion to strength and proprioception. Regaining full knee extension is important for normal knee biomechanics during gait and to prevent secondary complications. Once strengthening exercises are initiated, it is important to consider strain on the ACL during lower extremity strength exercises. The greatest amount of strain is placed on the ACL between 0 and 30 degrees of knee flexion. Guidelines for strengthening exercises are discussed below.

Rehabilitation after ACL injury Goals of ACL reconstruction and rehabilitation include restoration of knee stability, preservation of knee cartilage, expedient return to daily activities including sport participation, and early recognition of complications (32). Exercise progression will be based on the orthopedic surgeon's protocol. Factors that may influence healing rate and exercise progression are preoperative condition of the knee, type of graft used, and concomitant injuries. General exercise guidelines after ACL reconstruction are as follows:

- **Regain knee flexion and extension strength.** The hamstring muscles are the dynamic restraint to anterior translation of the tibia on femur. Increasing the strength and control of the hamstring muscles will increase dynamic stability of the knee joint and decrease ACL strain. The quadriceps must also be strengthened as atrophy occurs due to pain and swelling. Regaining strength of the quadriceps muscles is needed for control of the knee joint. As mentioned above, the ratio of knee flexion to extension strengthening should be at least 2:3 (27).
- **Incorporate proprioceptive exercises.** Lower extremity proprioceptive exercises are indicated since decreased proprioception occurs after ACL injury. Mechanoreceptors, which provide input from the knee to the central nervous system, are injured after a torn ACL. This causes decreased input from the knee joint to the central nervous system (33). The resulting decreased neuromuscular control and proprioception increase reinjury risk. There are numerous exercises to improve proprioception including single-leg balance activities on surfaces such as foam and balance boards.
- **Include unilateral exercises.** A study by Neitzel et al. (34) found subjects that had undergone ACL reconstruction significantly unloaded the involved extremity when performing a parallel squat exercise 6 to 7 months postoperatively. Not until 12 to 15 months postoperatively did bilateral weight bearing normalize. Therefore, unilateral strength exercises should be performed to achieve maximal strength gains in the involved extremity.
- **Strengthen muscles in both the closed and open kinetic chain.** Strengthening exercises should simulate functional activities. Both regular daily activities such as gait and sport activities require muscles to function in the **open kinetic chain** (OKC) and **closed kinetic chain** (CKC). CKC exercises involve cocontraction of the muscles surrounding a joint and are

characterized by a linear stress pattern and fixture of the distal segment of the extremity to the ground of supportive surface (35). CKC exercises utilize multiple joints and joint axes. One prime example of a CKC exercise is the squat or lunge. CKC exercise in lower extremity involves cocontraction of the quadriceps and hamstring muscles. Anterior translation of the tibia on the femur is minimized by hamstring contraction, decreasing strain on the ACL. OKC exercise is characterized by a rotator stress pattern, and isolated joint and muscle function. The distal aspect is technically allowed to swing freely in space. One example of an OKC exercise is the knee extension exercise. Open kinetic chain exercises are needed to provide isolated quadriceps strengthening. Due to increased strain on the ACL from approximately 0 to 30 degrees of knee extension in the open kinetic chain, exercises must be performed with appropriate modifications (limit last 30 degrees of knee extension) (Fig. 21.4).

Nonoperative Treatment Nonoperative treatment is usually chosen only by less active individuals. The laxity from a torn ACL increases the risk of future meniscal and articular cartilage damage. Cartilage damage will continue to increase knee pain and limit function over time. Similar to the postoperative rehabilitation goals, nonoperative goals include regaining hamstring and quadriceps muscle strength and lower extremity proprioception. The same exercise principles discussed above for postoperative strengthening can be applied.

ANATOMY AND BIOMECHANICS OF THE SHOULDER

The shoulder or glenohumeral joint is the most mobile joint in the human body. The shoulder complex is comprised of several joints; however, the discussion here will be primarily focused on the glenohumeral and scapulothoracic joints. Codman (36) identified the delicate balance

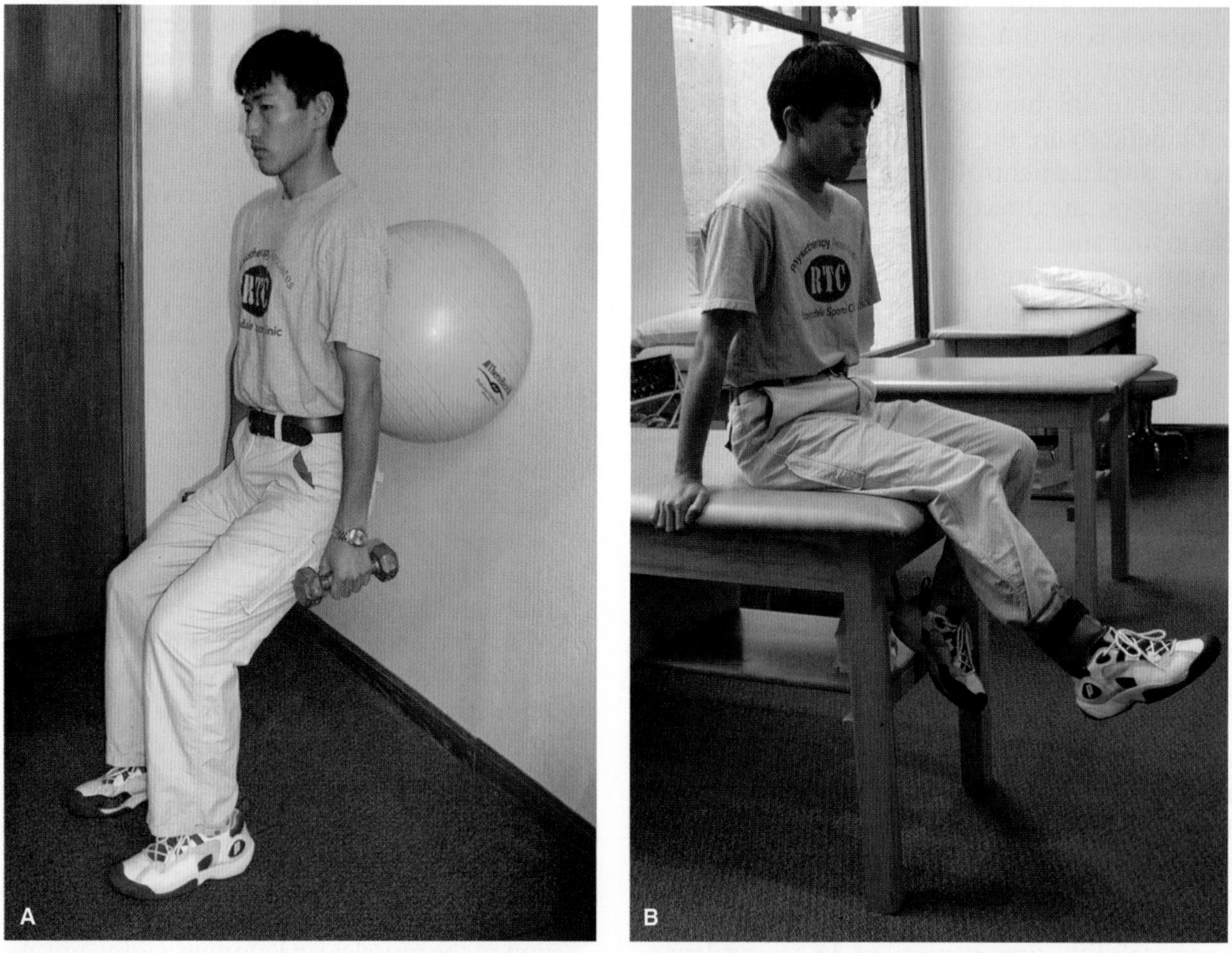

FIGURE 21.4 **A.** Closed kinetic chain exercise using a stability ball. **B.** Open-chain knee extension exercise.

during upper extremity elevation between the glenohumeral and scapulothoracic joints. He termed this the **scapulohumeral rhythm**. According to Codman (36), for every 2 degrees of glenohumeral joint motion, 1 degree of scapulothoracic motion occurs. This relationship points out the important role the scapulothoracic joint plays in shoulder function and how important proper strength and endurance of the muscles that stabilize the scapula are for normal function. The muscles that stabilize the scapula include the serratus anterior, trapezius, rhomboids, and levator scapulae. The important upward rotation of the scapula that the serratus anterior and trapezius perform is required to optimize the length–tension relationship of the rotator cuff muscle tendon units as well as move the acromion from the path of the elevating humerus (10).

The stability of the glenohumeral joint's "ball and socket" articulation is provided by both static and dynamic elements. The static elements include the glenoid labrum, articular capsule as well as negative intra-articular pressure (7). The dynamic stabilizers of the glenohumeral joint include the four rotator cuff muscle tendon units and the biceps long head (37).

One of the most important biomechanical principles in shoulder function is the deltoid rotator cuff force couple. This phenomenon known as a **force couple** explains how the rotator cuff and deltoid muscles work together to provide arm movements (38). The deltoid provides force primarily in a superior direction when contracting unopposed during arm elevation. The rotator cuff must provide both compressive force as well as an inferiorly directed force to prevent impingement of the rotator cuff tendons against the overlying acromion. Failure of the rotator cuff to maintain humeral congruency leads to glenohumeral joint instability, rotator cuff tendon pathology, and labral injury (7). Imbalances in the deltoid–rotator cuff force couple that primarily occur during inappropriate training and development of the deltoid without strengthening of the rotator cuff and exacerbate the superior migration of the humeral head provided by the deltoid and lead to impingement. The exercises shown in Figure 21.5 can be applied to ensure that a balanced training program for the shoulder and upper extremity is followed, which is particularly important for overhead athletes such as baseball players, tennis players and swimmers.

Common Injuries of the Shoulder

In the early 1970s, Neer (39) introduced the concept of **shoulder impingement**. Impingement refers to the mechanical impingement or compression of the rotator cuff tendons between the humeral head and the acromion. The subacromial space is only reported at 6 to 14 mm in normal subjects (40), and with muscular imbalance and/or fatigue, capsular range of motion restriction, and repeated overuse in overhead positions, rotator cuff impingement occurs producing a progression of disability. This progression, according to Neer (39), starts with edema and hemorrhage initially and, with continued overuse, could result in partial- and full-thickness tears from the mechanical stresses of compression and impingement. Impingement typically responds to nonoperative rehabilitation, which consists of modalities to decrease inflammation and pain, as well as proper exercises that activate and strengthen the rotator cuff muscles using positions that do not place the rotator cuff in a compressed or impinged position to allow for healing.

Most recently, medical professionals and scientists have understood the important role glenohumeral joint instability plays in rotator cuff disease. Impingement of the rotator cuff against the acromion may occur secondary to glenohumeral joint instability from attenuation of the static stabilizers such as capsular laxity, labral pathology, and abnormal work or sport biomechanics (41–43). Excessive translation or subluxation of the humeral head relative to the glenoid can occur in athletes and individuals with capsular laxity, often developed from repetitive overuse in the overhead movement patterns used in throwing or serving (41). Additionally, shoulder instability can occur from a traumatic event such as a fall on an outstretched arm or the combined movement of abduction and external rotation in contact sports. This can result in a full dislocation of the humeral head from the glenoid. Careful application of rotator cuff and scapular exercises are again indicated in these patients to improve dynamic stabilization.

Application of Resistive Exercise for the Glenohumeral Joint

The anatomical and biomechanical concepts outlined earlier in this chapter provide framework for the clinician to choose exercise positions and movement patterns to increase both strength and muscular endurance in patients and individuals with shoulder injury or weakness. In addition to the concepts such as the **scapular plane position**, avoidance of impingement positions, and the important role force couples play in producing controlled glenohumeral joint motion, electromyographic (EMG) studies should be considered that specifically measure individual muscular activity patterns with traditionally utilized exercise patterns.

Blackburn et al. (44) used electromyography to measure muscular activity in the posterior rotator cuff during traditional shoulder exercise using isotonic weights. The authors identified a position that has been referred to as the "Blackburn Position," which consists of prone horizontal abduction with 100 degrees of abduction and an externally rotated humeral position. This position was reported to involve high levels of muscular activity in the supraspinatus muscle, infraspinatus, teres minor, and scapular stabilizers (44–46). This prone position has become a classic exercise in many rehabilitation programs for both glenohumeral joint impingement and instability (44). Modification of this exercise using only 90 degrees of abduction to decrease potential subacromial contact and compression has been recommended (3,47).

In addition to the Blackburn et al. study (44), Townsend et al. (45) has provided the most comprehensive analysis of shoulder muscle activity during traditional exercises used during rehabilitation programs. Examples of exercises used during rotator cuff rehabilitation are pictured in Figure 21.5. These exercises utilize positions outlined in this chapter and have confirmed high levels of muscle activation of the rotator cuff while placing the shoulder in a comfortable "nonimpingement position." Exercises to improve strength and muscular endurance are also recommended for the scapular stabilizers. Moseley et al. (48) has outlined the muscular activation patterns of the scapular muscles during rehabilitation exercises. Application of seated rows and push-up with a "plus" that involves accentuating scapular protractions are considered "core scapular" exercises based on this research.

The use of exercises with 90 degrees of abduction are indicated to provide sport-specific conditioning of the rotator cuff (3). Figure 21.6 shows how external rotation can be performed with the shoulder elevated 90 degrees in the scapular plane. The scapular plane position is the plane 30 degrees anterior to the coronal or frontal plane of the body and is a position that is characterized by high levels of bony congruity between the humeral head and glenoid as well as neutral tension in the glenohumeral capsule (49). The use of the scapular plane position is highly recommended during rehabilitation.

Finally, modification of traditional exercises performed by many athletes and active individuals in the gym is followed and recommended. Limiting shoulder forward and lateral raises to only 90 degrees is highly recommended along with performing lat pull-downs in front of the head rather than behind (50). Limiting the range of motion during bench presses and "pec deck" exercise to positions in front of the scapular plane to decrease stress on the front of the shoulder is also widely recommended (50).

THE SPINE

Anatomy

The spine consists of 33 segments divided into five regions (cervical, thoracic, lumbar, sacral, and coccygeal), with the first 24 or presacral vertebrae having the most clinical relevance. The S-shaped curve of the spine allows increased shock absorption and overall flexibility and is due to the cervical and lumbar lordosis combined with the thoracic and sacral kyphosis. The spine has several key functions from an anatomical and biomechanical standpoint. It serves to house and protect the spinal cord and vital organs. It functions to dissipate weight-bearing forces of the head and trunk to the pelvis and allows controlled movement of the spine against gravity. The spine can be divided into individual blocks or units called spinal segments. The **spinal segment** is considered the functional (Fig. 21.7) unit within the spinal column and consists of the disc–vertebral body interface, the facets or zygapophyseal joints, and the ligaments, muscles, and vessels that innervate the segment. Together the individual functional units or spinal segments function as a whole to allow for coordinated movement (51).

The size and mass of the spinal segment increases from the cervical to the lumbar spine to allow for increased weight bearing on the lower segments. In addition, regional differences in the structure of the spine exist to accommodate for the functional demands and movement patterns that are unique to a particular area of the spine. In the cervical spine, for example, the orientation and shape of the joint surfaces allows for greater

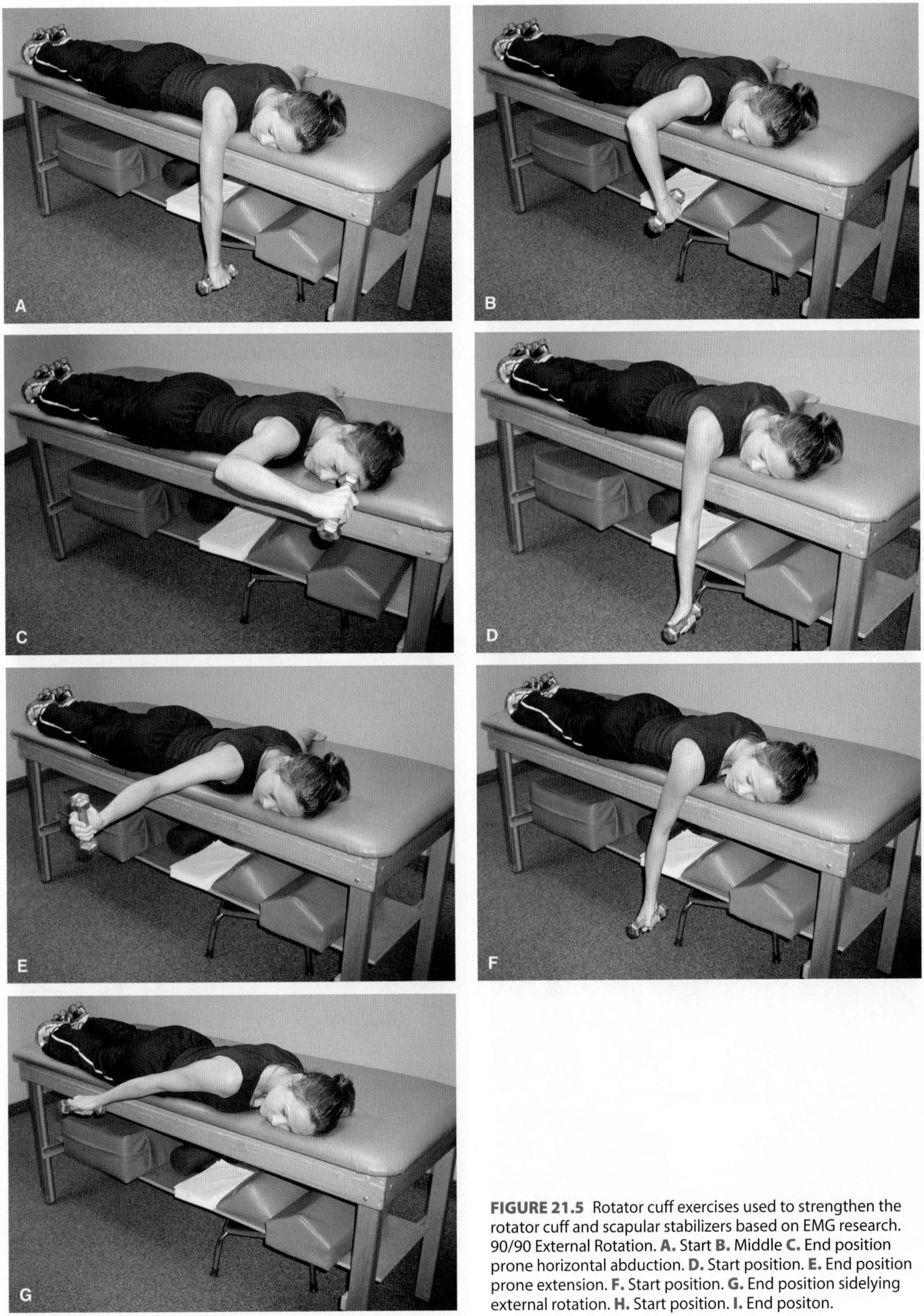

FIGURE 21.5 Rotator cuff exercises used to strengthen the rotator cuff and scapular stabilizers based on EMG research. 90/90 External Rotation. **A.** Start **B.** Middle **C.** End position prone horizontal abduction. **D.** Start position. **E.** End position prone extension. **F.** Start position. **G.** End position sidelying external rotation. **H.** Start position. **I.** End positon.

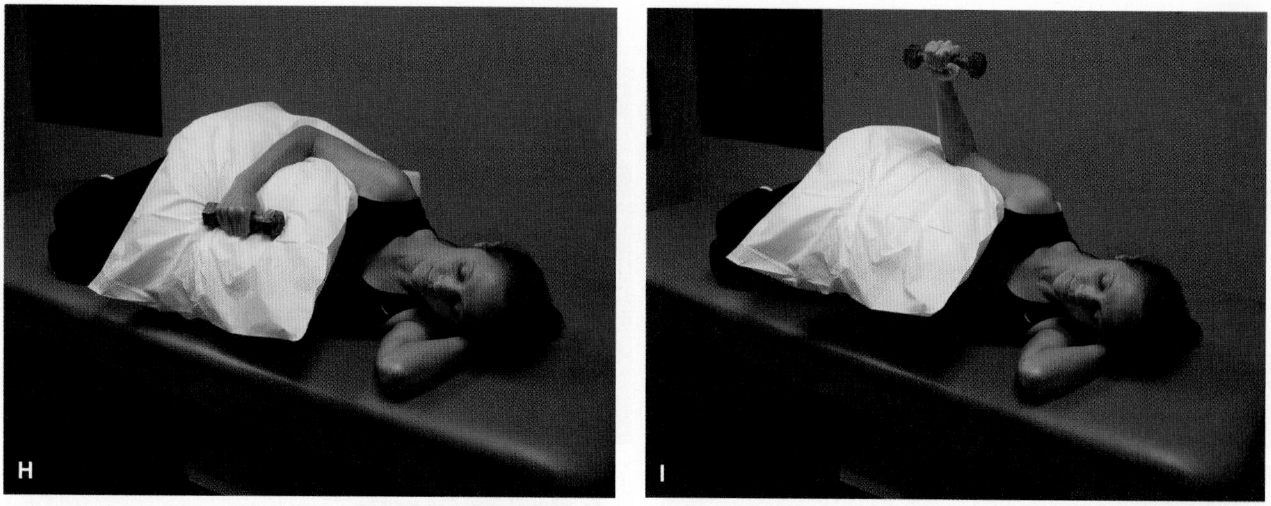

FIGURE 21.5 *(Continued)*

freedom of movement allowing for positioning of the head in space. In contrast, the thoracic spine has significantly less total ROM, due to the articulation of the ribs and the shape of the spinal motion segment, and this is due to the primary role being protection of vital organs and increasing respiratory efficiency. In the lumbar spine, the size and shape of the discs are larger to allow for increased weight bearing, and the orientation of the facet joints are primarily in the sagittal plane, allowing for greater flexion and extension movements with minimal rotation (51).

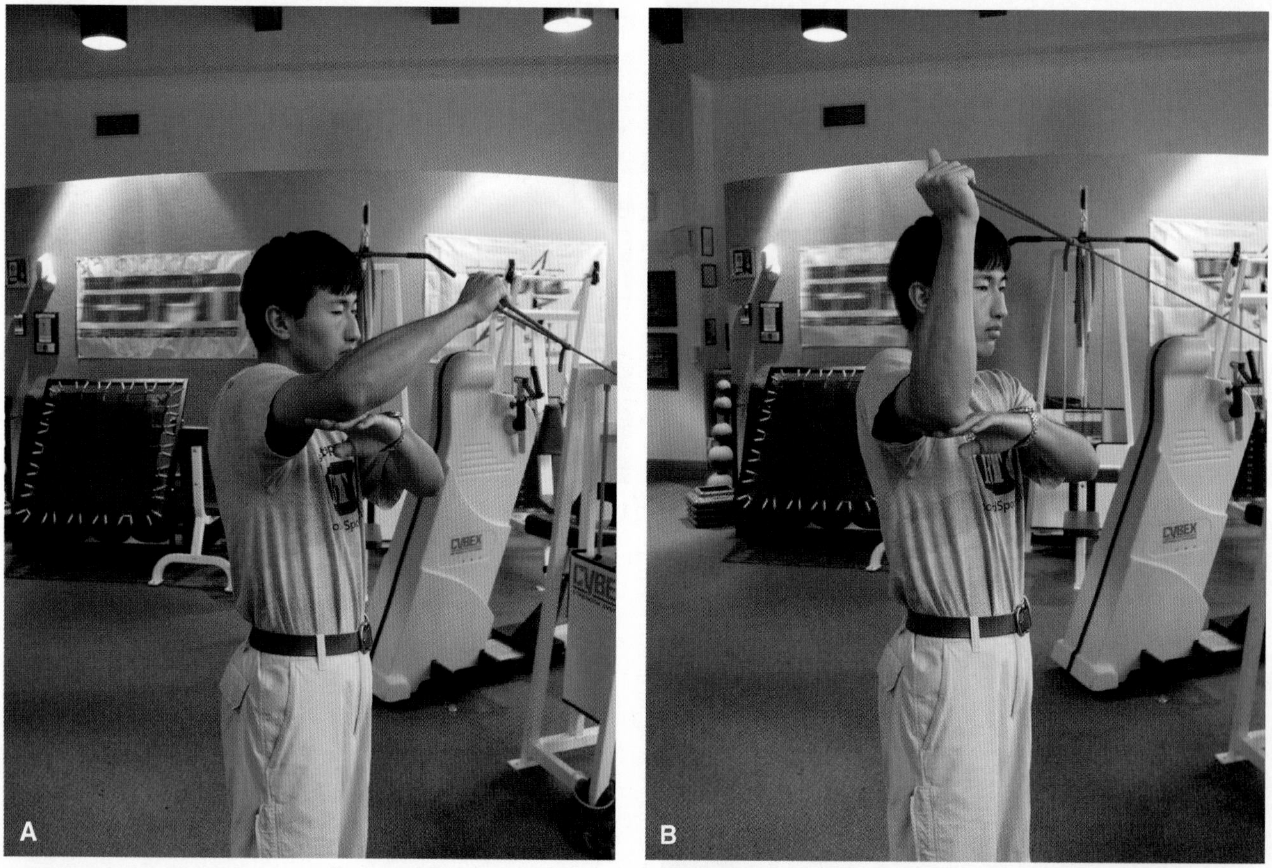

FIGURE 21.6 External rotation exercise with Theraband using 90 degrees of elevation in the scapular plane. **A.** Starting position. **B.** Ending position.

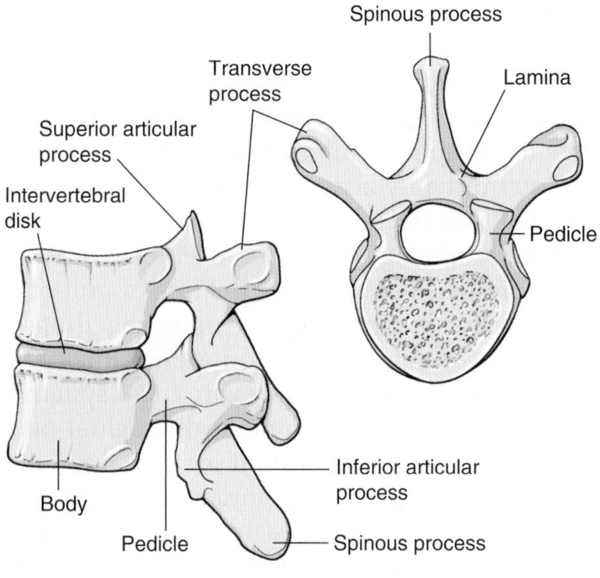

FIGURE 21.7 Anatomy of the vertebrae.

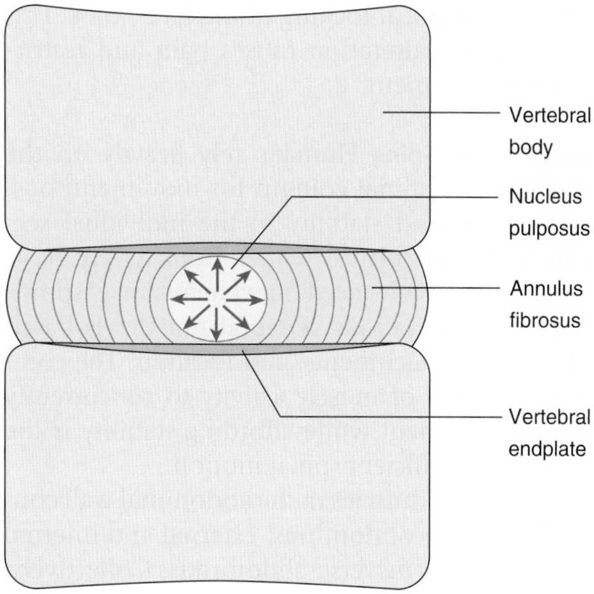

FIGURE 21.8 Structure of the intervertebral disc.

In a normal upright standing posture, 84% of the weight-bearing forces are transmitted through the vertebral body, and disc–vertebral body interface, with the remaining 16% being borne by the articular facet joints. The intervertebral disc interface consists of the cartilaginous vertebral endplates on the superior and inferior surfaces of the vertebral body, and the interposed disc. The disc consists of the nucleus pulposus at the center, composed of a mucoid material with a water-binding capacity giving it a gelatinous composition. The nucleus is surrounded by the annulus fibrosis composed of concentric layers of collagen and fibrocartilage designed to resist tensile, torsion, and compressive loads imparted to the disc (52) (Fig. 21.8). The oblique orientation of the annular fibers reinforces the strength of the disc, allowing resistance to the directional forces and movements exerted by the nucleus. Based on the design of the disc, it is thought to have characteristics of a hydraulic system, where the self-contained nucleus cannot be compressed, and therefore exerts pressure outwards toward the vertebral endplates and annular rings (53). Due to the relative avascularity of the disc, most disc nutrition occurs through diffusion via the vertebral endplate during cycles of loading and unloading, allowing for adequate exchange of nutrients and waste products. With age, the composition of the nucleus becomes less distinct from the annular fibers due to changes in the chemical composition in the nucleus.

Biomechanics

Movement in the spine occurs in a three-dimensional model where the individual segments have six degrees of freedom or motion components. On a basic level, movement at the spinal segments has varying degrees of translation and rotation that occur when cardinal movements are produced such as flexion, extension, side bending, and rotation. The term used to describe the accompanying movements between the vertebrae as primary movements are produced is termed coupling patterns. The **coupling patterns** are the result of the geometry of the individual vertebrae, connecting ligaments, and discs. For example, when the spine is flexed, there is accompanying superior and inferior translation or gliding of the individual segments accounting for the coupling movements. Another example of coupling occurs when the cervical spine is side bent or laterally flexed; the vertebral segments will rotate in the same direction as the side-bending motion (54). Coupling patterns need to occur for normal spinal movement, and the degree and types of patterns vary based on the region of the spine, and spinal posture when the movement is produced (54).

Clinical manifestation of coupling patterns becomes relevant when dysfunction occurs due to either degeneration or mechanical locking of the joint. This frequently happens when one attempts to perform a combined movement such as retrieving an object by bending forward and rotating causing mechanical locking of the facet joint. This biomechanical alteration causes pain and restriction with movement.

Muscles of the Spine Humans rely heavily on the muscles of the spinal column for movement, postural control, and stability of the individual segments as we perform activities from a very basic level to highly advanced movements like sports. The role of the various vertebral muscles is based on their size, attachments, and location. The complex interaction of muscle activity to concurrently produce movement while affording stability is the foundation of efficient spinal motion.

The anterior muscles in the abdominal wall consist of the rectus abdominus, external and internal obliques, and transverse abdominus. Collectively, the primary movements produced by these muscles are flexion and rotation of the trunk, with minimal muscle activity during normal erect standing (55). These muscles also act to regulate pelvic position by counterbalancing the pull of the back extensors. The transverse abdominus plays a key role in achieving spinal stabilization by forming a rigid cylinder, increasing intra-abdominal pressure when contracted. The horizontal orientation of the fibers and the attachment into the thoracolumbar fascia provide this stabilizing role (Fig. 21.9).

The erector spinae muscles are posteriorly situated to the spine, run the entire length of the spine, and consist of the superficial and deep divisions. Together, the erector spinae muscles act to extend the spine while lifting, and consequently are intermittently active to counteract the gravitational flexion line of pull on the body (55).

The stabilizing role of the deep erector spinae is evident when considering the line of pull of the deep erector spinae and the opposing iliopsoas (52). The contralateral anteroposterior line of pull in these muscles acts as a guy wire check system for stability of the lumbar spine in the sagittal plane. The multifidus is an important segmental stabilizer in the lumbar spine. It is present throughout the entire spine, but is thickest in the lumbar region. With the segmental attachment, along with their orientation of pull, the multifidus muscles are thought to act as important stabilizers in the lumbar spine during lifting and rotational movements of the trunk (15).

Back Injuries from and Functional Implications of Lifting Injuries in the spine occur frequently, with an estimated 80% of the general population experiencing low back pain at some point in their life (15). The etiology of back pain is not clearly understood, and oftentimes, identifying the source or

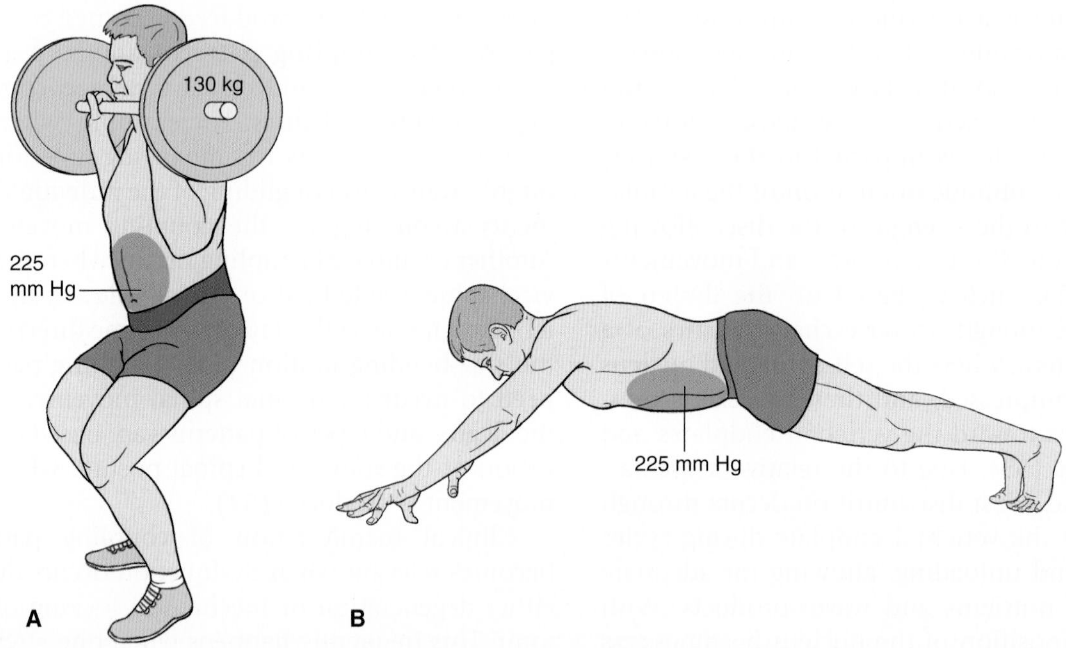

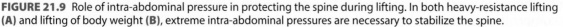

FIGURE 21.9 Role of intra-abdominal pressure in protecting the spine during lifting. In both heavy-resistance lifting **(A)** and lifting of body weight **(B)**, extreme intra-abdominal pressures are necessary to stabilize the spine.

cause of back pain is difficult. However, in many cases, mechanical back pain is a result of faulty body mechanics, postural habits, and repetitive stresses that may be avoided.

The **neutral spine** is a posture, which reduces the stress to the static structures of the spine, and minimizes muscular effort by optimally aligning the segments in their most natural resting position. The neutral spine is achieved through finding the neutral position of the pelvis. This is done by flexing and extending the pelvis to end ranges, appreciating the sense of the extremes, and finding the middle range, where there is the least amount of strain to the spine. Maintaining this neutral spine position provides optimal position of the spinal curves for muscle length and joint position sense, and equally distributes the forces along the spinal segment(s).

When lifting weights or performing functional lifting, several concepts should be followed to avoid risk of injury. Minimizing the distance of the object to be lifted by keeping it close to the body reduces the joint reaction forces, and intradiscal pressure within the spine. By holding a weighted object away from the body, the lever arm is dramatically increased, requiring higher muscle forces to maintain equilibrium, while significantly increasing intradiscal pressure (14) (Fig. 21.10). For example, while performing front raises with dumbbells with the elbows extended, the intradiscal pressure is exceedingly high. By simply flexing the elbows and keeping the dumbbells closer to the body, the lever arm is reduced, thereby lessening the forces acting on the spine. The role of obesity and the development of lower back problems are also related to having a larger lever arm acting on the low back when the abdomen protrudes anteriorly.

Studies have demonstrated the importance of generating large intra-abdominal pressures within the spine through the contraction of the stabilizing muscles of the paraspinals and abdominals when lifting heavy weights, and when performing pushing movements against heavy resistance (5). The amount of weight, as well as the speed at which the lift is performed correlates with the increase in intra-abdominal pressures to support the spine, reinforcing the importance of the role of the stabilizing muscles of the trunk when lifting or pushing (see Fig. 21.9). Some of the more common lifts requiring adequate stabilization to reduce the risk of injury are the weighted squat and dead lift.

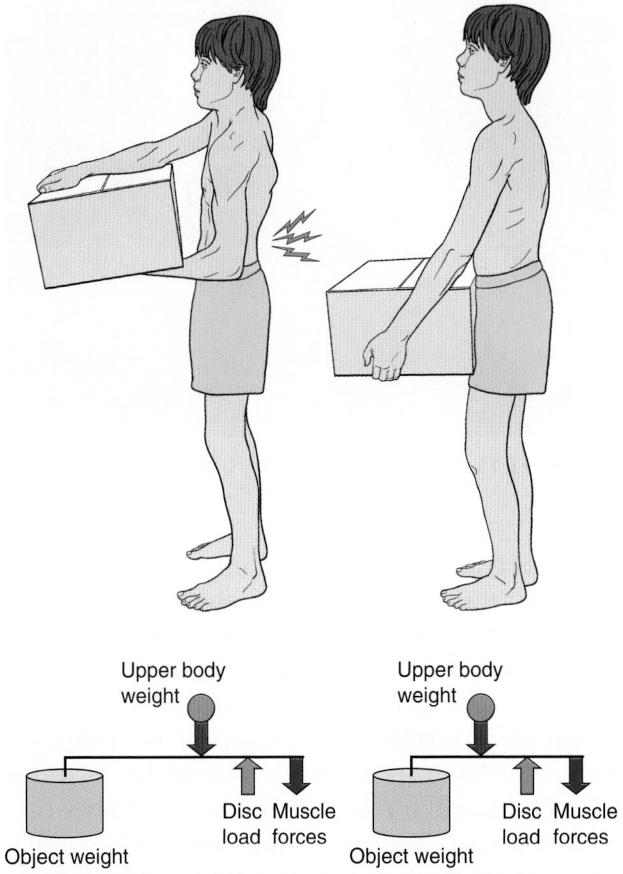

FIGURE 21.10 Proper lifting mechanics. Minimizing the distance of the object being lifted to the body reduces joint reaction forces and intradiscal pressure within the spine.

While performing a weighted squat or dead lift, it is important to maintain the spine in a neutral position, avoiding excess lumbar flexion or extension throughout the movement, by increasing intra-abdominal pressure through contraction of the abdominal and paraspinal stabilization muscles. This concept of back stabilization through muscular contraction should be utilized with any type of resistance training where the spine lacks adequate stabilization, and is the forefront of core stabilization training.

Core stabilization is an important concept for the strength and conditioning professional in terms of both performance and injury prevention. A number of appropriate methods can be utilized to train the core.

Core stabilization training has reached new levels of popularity within athletic and exercise training circles due to the fact that it has been shown

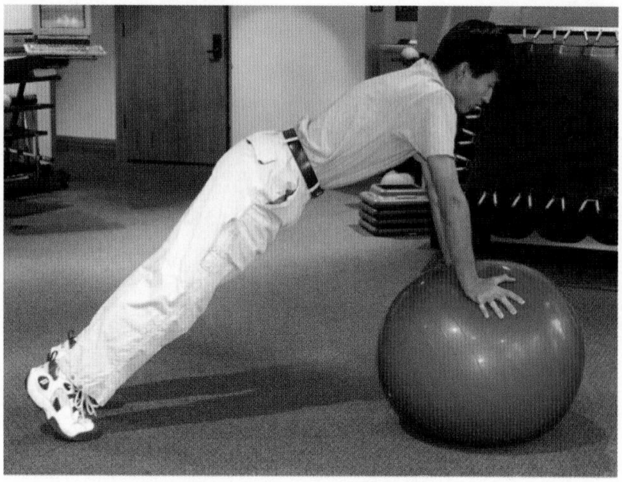

FIGURE 21.11 Push-up over a stability ball.

that this type of training not only reduces the risk of injury through focusing on the important role of the stabilization muscles but also enhances muscular control and efficiency. Traditional lifting methods have been supplemented with exercises utilizing core training to improve performance. Supplemental core exercises should be included with traditional lifting exercises during daily workouts to engage these very important trunk muscles. Some of the more common exercises include

- Push-ups with feet or hands on a ball (Fig. 21.11)
- Bench press with back on ball, unsupported at the hips (Fig. 21.12)
- Reverse sit-up with feet on ball

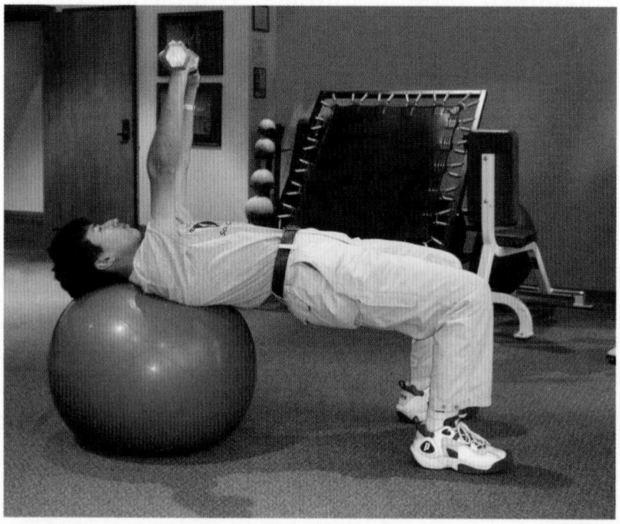

FIGURE 21.12 Bench press exercise performed using a stability ball to increase the muscle activity of the core.

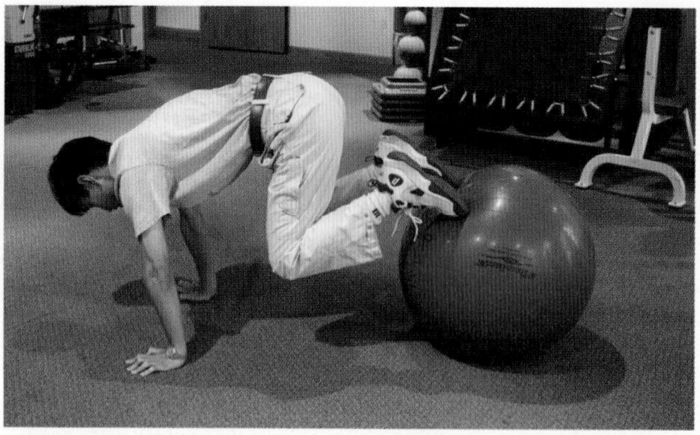

FIGURE 21.13 Knee to chest exercise using a stability ball.

- Trunk rotation in standing or sitting on a ball
- Opposite arm and leg in quadruped
- Prone isometric abdominals
- Bridging with feet on a ball (Fig. 21.13)
- Lunges with trunk rotation
- Theraband sidestepping
- Side-lying plange with unilateral row (Fig. 21.14)

Maintaining adequate flexibility in the muscles of the low back and lower extremities is also very important due to the influence they have with pelvic alignment and control. Tight hamstrings, paraspinals, or hip flexors can adversely position

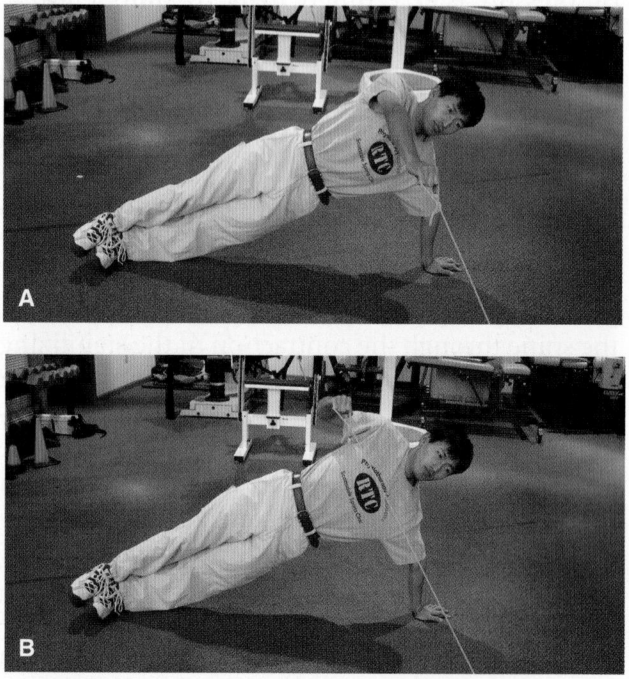

FIGURE 21.14 Plange with unilateral row using elastic resistance. A. Starting position. B. Ending position.

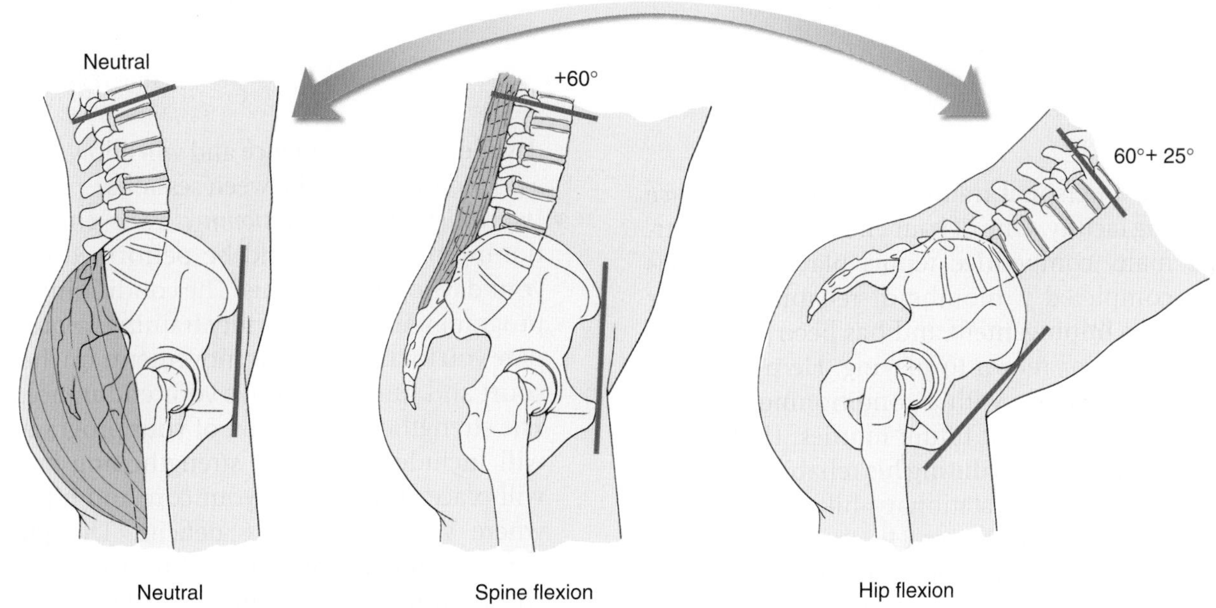

FIGURE 21.15 Muscle activity in forward bending. Bending forward is a two-part movement involving both the spine and the pelvis. Part one involves the first 60 degrees of movement, and part two involves an additional 25 degrees of forward trunk flexion.

the pelvis in too much flexion or extension predisposing one to injury or degenerative changes over longer periods. An example of this need for adequate flexibility can be demonstrated in what is termed **lumbar–pelvic rhythm**, which is a sequential sharing of motion between the paraspinals and hip extensors in the act of bending forward to touch your toes. During the initial bending movement, the pelvis is locked by the hip extensors for approximately the first 60 degrees of motion with movement primarily coming from the lumbar segments. This is followed by approximately 25 degrees of hip motion when the paraspinal muscles become more active, to allow for the additional motion to achieve full forward bending. The reverse sequence occurs with return from full flexion, with lumbar extension, followed by pelvic extension. The implications are that with inadequate range of motion or muscle activation in either area, injury may result from motion compensations due to an abnormal lumbar–pelvic rhythm (Fig. 21.15).

Summary

Injury prevention and rehabilitation involve a coordinated effort from various health care professionals. Strength and conditioning professionals must be aware of the stress placed on body tissues during strengthening exercises to minimize injury risk. When pain or injury does occur, activity needs to be modified, and referral to an appropriate health care professional should be made as needed. Communication between sports medicine professionals is vital in transitioning an athlete from a supervised rehabilitation program to a return-to-sport interval program, and ultimately an independent conditioning program. Conducting preparticipation physicals, identifying muscular strength and endurance deficits, awareness of joint and body mechanics during strengthening exercises, and appropriate activity progression after injury are all ways to minimize injury risk and maximize sport performance.

Maxing Out

1. A basketball player at a rural high school sustains an ankle sprain. There is no health care professional present at the time of the injury. What actions should be taken?
2. What muscles should be addressed by exercises in a core stabilization program?

CASE EXAMPLE

Designing a Return to Sport Conditioning Program for a Personal Training Client

BACKGROUND

You are a personal trainer at sport performance training facility. One of your clients is an 18-year-old male, competitive tennis player, who has just completed 2 months of rehabilitation for shoulder impingement and has been cleared by his doctor for return to playing. He presents to you for assistance with a conditioning program to help him prevent future injuries. He has not been playing tennis during his rehabilitation but has been riding a stationary bike to maintain cardiovascular endurance. His shoulder pain has dissipated, and he is eager to return to the court. You perform an assessment of his musculoskeletal durability to assist with the development of a conditioning program for the client and offer advice on a return-to-sport program.

CONSIDERATIONS

Your musculoskeletal durability assessment includes testing for the core, lower extremities, and upper extremities. You make note of the client's core and hip strength deficits as well as his lower extremity flexibility limitations and include exercises appropriate to address these areas. You also take into consideration the client's history of shoulder impingement and ensure that modifications are made to traditional upper extremity exercises to avoid reaggravation of his shoulder. While the client reports maintaining cardiovascular endurance by cycling for the past 2 months, you feel that a more sport-specific agility program would be ideal for preparing him for a return to the dynamic movement patterns performed on the court.

IMPLEMENTATION

You take into consideration the key components of an interval return to sport program and prescribe the following for this client:

- *Warm-Up:* Prior to stepping onto the court, perform 5 minutes of jumping rope, followed by a stretching program I have designed to target your lower extremities.
- *Alternate Day Performance Scheduling:* Schedule your return to tennis sessions for every other day. Your days off from tennis will allow you to determine your tolerance to the previous day's level of performance and will allow you a period of recovery between sessions.
- *Integration with Conditioning:* Your conditioning program should be performed on your days off from tennis. The conditioning program will include agility training to prepare you for the dynamic movements on the court and further improve your endurance. The strengthening portion of your program will include total body strengthening but will place emphasis on your core and hips, where you demonstrate deficits. Though your shoulder pain has diminished, it will be important to continue rotator cuff strengthening during your return to tennis to ensure that the strength you developed while in rehabilitation is not lost.
- *Progressive Stages of Intensity:* Your return to tennis should follow a schedule of gradually progressed intensity. You should follow the progression as listed in the return to tennis protocol given to you by your physician or therapist and closely monitor your tolerance to each stage of progression.
- *Proper Biomechanics:* Performing your return to tennis program with your coach is essential to ensure that proper mechanics are maintained.
- *Cool Down:* Following your interval tennis program performance, you should again perform the stretching program targeting your lower extremities and commence with ice to your shoulder as you have been doing in rehabilitation.

RESULTS

Because of your advice, your client was compliant with the interval return to tennis program supervised by his coach and maintained an alternate-day schedule that allowed him to closely monitor his response to each stage of progression. He was able to demonstrate steady improvements in core strength, LE flexibility, and agility. Two months following his return to tennis, he was able to admit that he was not only able to return to competitive tennis without pain, but was performing at a higher level than prior to his shoulder injury secondary to his improved agility and increased power with his serves.

REFERENCES

1. Taylor J, Stone R, Mullin MJ, et al. *Comprehensive Sports Injury Management: From Examination of Injury to Return to Sport*. 2nd ed. Austin, TX: PRO-ED Inc.; 2003.
2. Arnheim DA, Prentice WE. *Principles of Athletic Training*. 9th ed. St. Louis, MO: McGraw-Hill Companies; 1997.
3. Ellenbecker TS. Rehabilitation of shoulder and elbow injuries in tennis players. *Clin Sports Med*. 1995;14(1):87–109.
4. Nirschl RP, Sobel J. Conservative treatment of tennis elbow. *Phys Sports Med*. 1981;9:43–54.
5. Fulkerson JP. Diagnosis and treatment of patients with patellofemoral pain. *Am J Sports Med*. 2002;30(3):447–456.
6. Chandler TJ, Kibler WB, Stracener EC, et al. Shoulder strength, power, and endurance in college tennis players. *Am J Sports Med*. 1992;20:455–458.
7. Wilk KE, Arrigo CA. Interval sport programs for the shoulder. In Andrews JR, Wilk KE. *The Athletes Shoulder*. New York, NY: Churchill Livingstone; 1994.
8. Ellenbecker TS. Shoulder internal and external rotation strength and range of motion in highly skilled tennis players. *Isok Exer Sci*. 1992;2:1–8.
9. Ellenbecker TS, Roetert EP. Age specific isokinetic glenohumeral internal and external rotation strength in elite junior tennis players. *J Sci Med Sport*. 2003;6(1):63–70.
10. Kibler WB. The role of the scapula in athletic shoulder function. *Am J Sports Med*. 1998;26(2):325–337.
11. American College of Sports Medicine. Position statement on pre-participation physicals. Indianapolis, IN: ACSM.
12. *Guide to Physical Therapist Practice*. 2nd ed. Alexandria, VA: American Physical Therapy Association; 2001.
13. Kraushaar BS, Nirschl RP. Tendonosis of the elbow (tennis elbow): Clinical features and findings of histological, immunohistochemical, and electron microscopy studies. *J Bone Joint Surg*. 1999;81-A(2):259–278.
14. Andrews JR, Harrelson GL, Wilk KE, eds. *Physical Rehabilitation of the Injured Athlete*. 3rd ed. Philadelphia, PA: W.B. Saunders Co; 2004.
15. Richardson JK, Iglarsh A. *Clinical Orthopaedic Physical Therapy*. Philadelphia, PA: W.B. Saunders Co; 1994.
16. Cameron MH (ed). *Physical Agents in Rehabilitation: From Research to Practice*. Philadelphia, PA: W.B. Saunders Company; 1999.
17. Knight KL. *Cryotherapy in Sports Injury Management*. Champaign, IL: Human Kinetics; 1995.
18. Prentice WE. The healing process and the pathophysiology of musculoskeletal injuries. In: Prentice WE, ed. *Rehabilitation Techniques in Sports Medicine*. 2nd ed. St. Louis, MO: Mosby-Yearbook; 1994.
19. Robinson AJ, Snyder-Mackler L. *Clinical Electrophysiology: Electrotherapy and Electrophysiologic Testing*. 2nd ed. Philadelphia, PA: Lippincott Williams & Wilkins; 1995.
20. Davies GJ. *A Compendium of Isokinetics in Clinical Usage and Rehabilitation Techniques*. 4th ed. Onalaska, WI: S & S Publishers; 1992.
21. Lephart SM, Pincivero DM, Giraldo JL, et al. The role of proprioception in the management and rehabilitation of athletic injuries. *Am J Sports Med*. 1997;25:130–137.
22. Avela J, Kyrolainen J, Komi P. Altered reflex sensitivity after repeated and prolonged passive muscle stretching. *Am J Phys Med*. 1999;86:1283–1291.
23. Kokkonen J, Nelson A, Cornwell A. Acute muscle stretching inhibits maximal strength performance. *Res Q Exer Sport*. 1998;69(4):411–415.
24. Zachazewski JE, Reischl S. Flexibility for the runner: specific program considerations. *Top Acute Care Trauma Rehabil*. 1986;1:9–27.
25. Marshall RN, Elliott BC. Long-axis rotation: the missing link in proximal to distal sequencing. *J Sports Sci*. 2000;18:247–254.
26. Magee DJ. *Orthopedic Physical Assessment*. 3rd ed. Philadelphia, PA: W.B. Saunders Co; 1997.
27. Davies GJ, Heidersceit BC, Clark M. Open kinetic chain assessment and rehabilitation. *Athl Train Sports Health Care Perspect*. 1995;1(4):347–370.
28. Davies GJ, Manske RC, Slamma K, et al. Selective activation of the vastus medialis oblique: what does the literature really tell us? *Physiother Can*. 2001;100–115.
29. Wilk KE, Davies GJ, Mangine RE, et al. Patellofemoral disorders: a classification system and clinical guidelines for nonoperative rehabilitation. *J Orthop Sports Phys Ther*. 1998;28(5):307–322.
30. Wallace DA, Salem GJ, Salinas R, et al. Patellofemoral joint kinetics while squatting with and without an external load. *J Orthop Sports Phys Ther*. 2002;32(4):141–148.
31. Ireland ML, Willson JD, Ballantyne BT, Davis IM. Hip strength in females with and without patellofemoral pain. *J Orthop Sports Phys Ther*. 2002;33(11):671–676.
32. DeCarlo M, Klootwyk T, Oneacre K. Anterior cruciate ligament. In Ellenbecker TS, ed. *Knee Ligament Rehabilitation*. Philadelphia, PA: Churchill Livingstone; 2000.
33. Beynnon BD, Ryder SH, Konradsen L, et al. Effect of anterior cruciate ligament trauma and bracing on knee proprioception. *Am J Sports Med*. 1999;27(2):150–155.
34. Neitzel JA, Kernozek TW, Davies GJ. Loading response following anterior cruciate ligament reconstruction during the parallel squat exercise. *Clin Biomech*. 2002;7(7):551–554.
35. Ellenbecker TS, Davies GJ. The application of isokinetics in testing and rehabilitation of the shoulder complex. *J Athl Train*. 2000;35(3):338–350.
36. Codman EA. *The Shoulder: Privately Printed*. Boston; 1934.
37. Rodosky MW, Harner CD, Fu F. The role of the long head of the biceps muscle and superior glenoid labrum in anterior stability of the shoulder. *Am J Sports Med*. 1994;22:121–130.
38. Inman VT, Saunders JB, Abbott LC. Observations on the function of the shoulder joint. *J Bone Joint Surg*. 1944; 26(1):1–30.
39. Neer CS. Anterior acromioplasty for the chronic impingement syndrome in the shoulder. *J Bone Joint Surg Am*. 1972;54A:41–50.
40. Cotton RE, Rideout DF. Tears of the humeral rotator cuff: a radiological and pathological necropsy survey. *J Bone Joint Surg*. 1964;46B:314.
41. Jobe FW, Kivitne RS. Shoulder pain in the overhand or throwing athlete. *Orthop Rev*. 1989;18:963–975.
42. Walch G, Boileau P, Noel E, Donell ST. Impingement of the deep surface of the supraspinatus tendon on the posterosuperior glenoid rim: an arthroscopic study. *J Shoulder Elbow Surg*. 1992;1:238-X.
43. Burkhart SS, Morgan CD, Kibler WB. The disabled throwing shoulder: spectrum of pathology. Part I: pathoanatomy and biomechanics. *Arthroscopy*. 2003;19(4):404–420.

44. Blackburn TA, McLeod WD, White B, et al. EMG analysis of posterior rotator cuff exercises. *Athl Train.* 1990;25:40.
45. Townsend H, Jobe FW, Pink M, et al. Electomyographic analysis of the glenohumeral muscles during a baseball rehabilitation program. *Am J Sports Med.* 1991;19:264–272.
46. Ballantyne BT, O'Hare SJ, Paschall JL, et al. Electromyographic activity of selected shoulder muscles in commonly used therapeutic exercises. *Phys Ther.* 1993;73:668.
47. Ellenbecker TS. *Clinical Examination of the Shoulder.* Philadelphia, PA: Elsevier Saunders; 2004.
48. Moseley JB, Jobe FW, Pink M. EMG analysis of the scapular muscles during a shoulder rehabilitation program. *Am J Sports Med.* 1992;20:128–134.
49. Saha AK. Mechanism of shoulder movements and a plea for the recognition of "zero position" of glenohumeral joint. *Clin Orthop* 1983;173:3–10.
50. Gross ML, Brenner Sl, Esformes I, et al. Anterior shoulder instability in weight lifters. *Am J Sports Med.* 1993;21(4):599–603.
51. Hertling D, Kessler RM. (Chapter 18) Spine: general structure and biomechanical considerations. In: *Management of Common Musculoskeletal Disorders: Physical Therapy Principles and Methods.* 4th ed. Baltimore, MD: Lippincott Williams & Wilkins; 2006.
52. Porterfield JA, DeRosa C. *Mechanical Low Back Pain: Perspectives in Functional Anatomy.* Philadelphia, PA: W.B. Saunders Co; 1991.
53. Cailliet R. *Low Back Pain Syndrome.* 2nd ed. Philadelphia, PA: F.A. Davis; 1981.
54. White AA, Panjabi MM. *Clinical Biomechanics of the Spine.* 2nd ed. Philadelphia, PA: J.B. Lippincott; 1990.
55. Norkin CC, Levangie PK. *Joint Structure and Function.* 2nd ed. Philadelphia, PA: F.A. Davis; 1992.

CHAPTER 22

Ergogenic Aids

LEM TAYLOR • COLIN WILBORN • ABBIE SMITH • JOSÉ ANTONIO

OBJECTIVES

After reading this chapter, you will be able to:

- Define and explain the role of ergogenic aids in sports.
- Discuss and advise athletes on the role of creatine and exercise.
- Discuss and advise athletes on the role of caffeine and exercise.
- Demonstrate an understanding of the role of anabolic–androgenic steroids (AASs) in sports.
- Discuss and advise athletes on the role of fluid replacement beverages before, during, and after exercise.
- Discuss and advise athletes on the role of other potential ergogenic aids for specific events.

KEY TERMS

Adenosine Triphosphate (ATP)
Anabolic
Anticatabolic Agent
Beta-Hydroxy-Beta-Methylbutyrate (HMB)
Branched-Chain Amino Acids (BCAAs)
Caffeine
Creatine
Creatinine
Dehydration
Epigallocatechin Gallate (EGCG)
Ergogenic Aids
Essential Amino Acids (EAAs)
Glucosamine
Glutamine
Glycogenolysis
Glucose–Alanine Cycle
Hypohydration
Isocaloric
Loading Cycle
Lipolysis
Osteoarthritis (OA)
Sports Drinks
Thermogenic
Muscle Dysmorphia
Anticatabolic Properties

Introduction

Ergogenic aids are substances (including nutrients, nutritional supplements, and drugs) that improve athletic performance. *Nutritional ergogenic aids* include substances that contain fats, carbohydrates, proteins, vitamins, and/or minerals. Fats, carbohydrates, and proteins provide energy (calories) to produce **adenosine triphosphate (ATP)**. Vitamins and minerals regulate energy-producing metabolic pathways. *Nutritional supplements* are nutrients in a concentrated form. Drugs can have an effect on cellular function that can directly or indirectly improve performance.

Numerous substances have been studied in the quest for improved athletic performance in multiple sports and athletic events. The conditions under which a substance might have a positive effect vary depending on metabolic requirements of the exercise, as well as the environmental conditions. The list of nutritional supplements that do not work would be endless. This chapter, however, focuses on several supplements that have been shown to have a positive effect and have been supported by research in a variety of settings to be ergogenic.

β-ALANINE

β-Alanine is a naturally occurring non-EAA that is found in many common food sources, such as chicken and turkey. β-alanine is thought to be a rate-limiting precursor to intramuscular carnosine synthesis. Carnosine, a natural buffer, is synthesized within the muscle but is dependent upon the levels of histidine and, more specifically, β-alanine. Because of this fact, the utilization of β-alanine supplementation has become prevalent. β-alanine supplementation does in fact result in an increase in muscle carnosine levels and has been shown to potentially decrease fatigue and improve performance in high-intensity exercise settings by buffering hydrogen ions (H^+). Thus supplementation of β-alanine leads to increased levels of intracellular muscular carnosine, which can have a buffering effect and potentially delay the onset of muscular fatigue and enhance performance (1).

The research around supplementation of β-alanine has been developed quite extensively over the past 5 years. A more detailed review of this research can be seen in a review article by Sales and associates (1). Overall, β-alanine supplementation has been reported to increase muscular strength and power, increase training volume, and delay fatigue, and thus improving performance in both aerobic and anaerobic settings. Specifically, a recent study by Smith et al. (2) found that β-alanine supplementation ($6 \text{ g} \cdot \text{d}^{-1}$ for days 1 to 21; $3 \text{ g} \cdot \text{d}^{-1}$ for days 22 to 42) for 6 weeks resulted in increases in $\dot{V}O_{2peak}$, time to exhaustion, training volume, and lean body mass (LBM) when combined with high-intensity interval training. It should be noted that the increases in performance that occurred with the β-alanine supplementation occurred in the last 3 weeks of the training period, in which no further increases were observed in the placebo group on the same performance markers. Despite the fact that more research is needed on different aspects and issues of β-alanine supplementation, it is safe to say that there is sound evidence to support the use of β-alanine as an ergogenic aid.

β-alanine may provide an indirect ergogenic effect by increasing carnosine levels in skeletal muscle; thus increasing the buffering capacity which can enhance performance and training volume.

BRANCHED-CHAIN AMINO ACIDS

Amino acids are the building blocks of proteins. The amino acids leucine, isoleucine, and valine are collectively known as the **branched-chain amino acids (BCAAs)**. Supplementation with BCAAs does not seem to improve short-term exercise performance, but may reduce muscle breakdown during clinical conditions of wasting (e.g., starvation, post-surgery, burns) and periods of prolonged exercise.

According to the "central fatigue hypothesis," during prolonged exercise, the plasma levels of BCAAs decrease and levels of fatty acids increase. The increase in fatty acids causes an increase in the levels of free tryptophan, which is a precursor to serotonin, a neurotransmitter that causes feelings of sleepiness and depression. In other words, decreases in BCAAs during prolonged exercise can, in theory, increase the mental effort necessary to perform. Use of BCAAs as an ergogenic aid may attenuate the increase in serotonin, thus reducing perceived exertion and mental fatigue during prolonged exercise. Although there is some support for these effects during prolonged cycling, marathon running, and time trials, an equal number of studies have shown no beneficial effect from BCAA supplementation. Since the side effects from BCAAs appear to be minimal, individuals competing in events lasting 2 or more hours, especially events in the heat, may wish to experiment with repeated liquid doses of BCAAs. One approach that has yielded positive effects is to ingest a total of 5 to 10 g of BCAAs dissolved in 1 L of fluid (i.e., drinking 150 mL of the solution every 10 to 20 minutes) (3).

Another interesting aspect of BCAAs, that has only recently been explored, is their potential effect on weight loss. During a moderate-protein (1.5 g · kg body weight^{-1} · d^{-1}), lower carbohydrate (100 to 200 g · d^{-1}) diet, the increased intake of BCAAs (especially leucine) is thought to have positive effects on muscle protein synthesis, insulin signaling, and sparing of glucose use by stimulation of the **glucose–alanine cycle**. This leads to more fat loss and a greater sparing of lean tissue compared to an isoenergetic, higher carbohydrate diet (4). Additional research regarding the effects of BCAAs on changes in body composition is warranted, but this notion is supported by the fact that **isocaloric** replacement of carbohydrates with lean protein sources does elicit benefits on improving body composition.

BCAAs may have positive ergogenic effects related to their anticatabolic effect; however, fairly large doses must be consumed to achieve this.

CAFFEINE

Caffeine is a bitter white alkaloid ($C_8H_{10}N_4O_2$) often derived from tea or coffee. Perhaps the most commonly consumed drug in the United States, caffeine is an effective ergogenic aid. Research on caffeine is easily accessible and is typically focused on caffeine's role in promoting lipolysis and energy expenditure (1), stimulating the central nervous system, and acting as a performance-enhancing aid for many types of athletic activity (5,6). Both older (65 to 80 years of age) and younger (19 to 26 years of age) men show a similar **thermogenic** response to caffeine ingestion, but the increase does seem to be blunted as age increases. Caffeine ingestion has been shown to stimulate both **lipolysis** and energy expenditure (1). It is not clear whether the lipolytic effect of caffeine is associated with increased lipid oxidation or futile cycling between triglycerides and free fatty acids (FFAs). Also, it is not known whether the effects of caffeine are mediated via the sympathetic nervous system.

Caffeine can also act as a potent ergogenic aid in multiple settings. Caffeine has been removed from the World Anti-Doping Agency's (WADA) banned list update. Ingesting caffeine (5 mg · kg body weight^{-1}) can significantly increase exercise time to exhaustion and moderate intensities (6). Caffeine ingestion can also improve maximal anaerobic power and sprint-swimming performance in trained swimmers among various other things. For a complete review of the effects that caffeine has on performance see the position stand from the International Society of Sports Nutrition (7). Table 22.1 lists the caffeine content of various beverages.

TABLE 22.1 ● CAFFEINE CONTENT OF VARIOUS PRODUCTS (8)

PRODUCT	SERVING (OZ)	CAFFEINE (MG)
Starbucks (tall) Coffee	12	375
Red Bull	12	120
Mountain Dew	12	55
Diet Coke	12	45
Dr. Pepper	12	41
Sunkist Orange	12	41
Starbucks Espresso	1	35
Coca-Cola Classic	12	34
Nestea Sweetened Iced Tea	12	26
Barqs Root Beer	12	22
Hot Chocolate	12	8

A large volume of data supports the ergogenic effects of caffeine as well as its thermogenic properties.

COLOSTRUM

Colostrum is a component of human breast milk or cow's milk, found at its highest concentration 2 to 3 days after a female gives birth. It is a rich source of protein, antibodies, and growth factors. Several compelling studies demonstrate an ergogenic effect of colostrum supplementation (9,10). Such supplementation (20 g · d^{-1} for 8 weeks) combined with aerobic and heavy resistance training significantly increased bone-free LBM (mean increase of 1.49 kg) compared to whey protein (9).

Another investigation demonstrated the potential ergogenic effects of colostrum supplementation by comparing the effects of bovine colostrums to whey protein powder. Using a randomized, double-blind, placebo-controlled parallel design, 51 men completed 8 weeks of resistance and plyometric training while consuming 60 g · d^{-1} of bovine colostrum or concentrated whey protein powder. By week 8, peak vertical jump power and peak cycle power were significantly greater in the colostrum group as opposed to the whey protein group. Interestingly, there were no differences between groups with regard to anaerobic work capacity, 1 RM or plasma insulin-like growth factor I (IGF-I) (10).

Data for colostrum supplementation support daily doses ranging from 20 to 60 g to enhance performance as well as to promote gains in LBM.

CREATINE

Creatine is a naturally occurring nitrogenous compound made in the liver, kidneys, and pancreas from the amino acids arginine, glycine, and methionine. Creatine is found in relatively high amounts in meat, fish, and poultry. In fact, adults and teenagers who regularly consume these foods typically eat 1 to 2 g creatine · d^{-1}, an amount equal to its natural rate of excretion by the kidneys, where creatine is converted to **creatinine**. Vegetarians who do not consume meat or fish have reduced body stores of creatine. Interestingly, when these individuals are fed creatine, they retain more of it in their bodies (in comparison to nonvegetarians), suggesting that creatine might actually be "essential" to a normal diet. In a 154-lb adult man, about 120 g of creatine is found in the body, 95% of which is in the skeletal muscle (11).

A large body of literature demonstrates the ergogenic properties of creatine (12–14). This literature is summarized in a recent position stand on creatine (15). The following discussion is by no means a comprehensive discussion of creatine; however, it does give the reader insight into this effective ergogenic aid.

On ingestion, creatine is absorbed into the bloodstream through the small intestine and reaches peak levels 60 to 90 minutes later (11). Creatine is thought to serve at least four vital functions:

1. It stores energy that can be used to regenerate ATP.
2. It enhances energy transfer between the mitochondria and muscle fibers.
3. It serves as a buffer against intracellular acidosis during exercise.
4. It stimulates **glycogenolysis** (glycogen breakdown) during exercise.

Collectively, these effects underscore creatine's central role in energy metabolism and explain why this substance has been the subject of intensive study (12,14).

A common analogy used by exercise scientists is that creatine is to the weight lifter/sprinter what carbohydrate is to the distance runner. Of the well-controlled human trials on creatine, about two-thirds have shown benefits from its use. Depending on the initial fitness level of the subjects, these have included the following:

- Increased dynamic strength and power (~5% to 15%)
- Increased body weight and LBM (~2% to 5%)
- Increased sprint performance (~1% to 5%)

As little as 3 days of creatine supplementation (0.35 g · kg fat-free $mass^{-1}$) can increase thigh muscle volume and may enhance cycle sprint performance in elite power athletes, with the effects being greater in females as sprints are repeated (16). Creatine supplementation in conjunction with heavy resistance training increased total body mass, fat-free mass, thigh volume, muscle strength, and myofibrillar protein (17).

Creatine is considered beneficial to weight lifters and athletes involved in sports requiring short, repeated bursts of high power (e.g., wrestling, rowing, sprint running/swimming/cycling, football, rugby, volleyball, soccer, hockey, lacrosse). Additionally, a growing body of evidence points to the health/medical benefits of oral administration of creatine monohydrate. For instance, creatine supplementation may protect against neuronal degeneration in amyotrophic lateral sclerosis and Huntington's disease and in chemically mediated neurotoxicity (18). Creatine may protect the immature brain from hypoxic–ischemic injury. Also, creatine supplementation has a "significant positive effect on working memory (backward digit span) and intelligence (Raven's Advanced Progressive Matrices), both tasks that require speed of processing" (19). Creatine supplementation has applications that extend beyond the athletic realm. The health benefits of creatine may indeed be a positive area of research in the future.

What are the potential risks (side effects) of using creatine? The only consistently reported "side effect" in humans has been weight gain. Despite inflammatory reports in the media of a link between creatine use and muscle cramps/pulls, dehydration/heat exhaustion, and kidney/liver disorders, these effects have not been documented by independent research. To the contrary, studies have either reported no effect (on kidney/liver function or musculotendinous stiffness) or an improved response from creatine use (a lower incidence of muscle cramps/pulls) (20). In one study of 98 athletes, long-term supplementation with creatine (up to 21 months) did not adversely affect a 69-item panel of serum, whole blood, or urinary markers of clinical health status (13). A long-standing myth holds that creatine supplementation is harmful to the kidneys. This is clearly not the case. Short-, medium-, or long-term oral creatine supplementation causes detrimental effects on the kidneys of healthy individuals (21).

In a lay article published on the Internet, a comparison of 28 creatine distributors revealed that over half were selling products containing contaminants. The overall purity of each product averaged about 90%, but there were dramatic differences in the amount of several potentially toxic impurities. Athletes considering creatine use should exercise the following precautions:

1. A "**loading cycle**" is not needed. Rather than ingesting 20 to 30 g for the first 5 to 7 days and then 5 g · d^{-1} thereafter, take only about 3 to 5 g daily.
2. Cycle periods of use (4 to 8 weeks) with periods of nonuse (4 weeks).
3. Purchase the product from a reputable manufacturer who is able to provide a "certificate of analysis," including all of the following information:
   - Appearance (should be white to pale cream)
   - Assay (should be at least 95% creatine)
   - Moisture content (should be ≤12.5%)
   - Residue on ignition (should be ≤1%)
   - Microbial/pathogenic contamination (should be negative for *Escherichia coli*, *Staphylococcus aureus*, and *Salmonella*)
   - Yeasts and molds (should be <50 g^{-1})
   - Poisons/heavy metals (should be <10 ppm for lead and mercury)
   - Other contaminants (should be <3 ppm for arsenic, 30 ppm for dicyandiamide, and nondetectable for dihydrotriazine)

Creatine is the most widely studied ergogenic aid over the past 20 years. Creatine used for regular supplementation, has been shown to increase skeletal muscle mass and muscle fiber size and improve anaerobic exercise performance. No evidence is available that regular creatine supplementation is harmful to otherwise healthy individuals.

ESSENTIAL AMINO ACIDS

Of the 20 amino acids used to form proteins, nine are considered **essential amino acids (EAAs)** because your body does not produce them and you need to consume them in your daily diet. A growing body of literature demonstrates the efficacy of EAA supplementation in enhancing physical performance (22–24). The **anabolic** response to the consumption of an oral cocktail containing EAAs plus carbohydrate (EAC) before versus after heavy resistance exercise was studied (24). Six healthy subjects (three men and three women; average age 30.2 years, height 1.71 m, weight 66 kg) consumed the EAC (6 g of EAAs plus 35 g of sucrose in 500-mL water) either immediately before or after exercise (in a randomized order). The exercise bout consisted of 10 sets of eight reps of the leg press (80% of 1 RM), and 8 sets of eight reps of the leg extension

(80% of 1 RM). The rest interval was about 2 minutes, with the total exercise time roughly 45 minutes. The investigators then examined phenylalanine uptake across the leg as a measure of muscle protein accretion. Over a 3-hour period, taking the EAC before exercise resulted in a net phenylalanine uptake that was about 160% greater than that noted when the EAC was taken after exercise. Furthermore, work from the same laboratory found that the non-EAAs are not required to stimulate protein synthesis. Finally, there is a dose-dependent effect of EAA ingestion on muscle protein synthesis (22). Thus, a relatively small dose (6 g) of EAA may confer a significant anabolic response.

The EAAs play a critical role in promoting skeletal muscle anabolism and should be a component of most meals and snacks throughout the day.

GLUCOSAMINE

Glucosamine is a combination of glutamine and glucose (amino polysaccharide). Following ingestion and absorption of glucosamine, it is incorporated into molecules called proteoglycans, which are part of the joint cartilage. This process is thought to help maintain the integrity of the joint as well as to repair damaged cartilage. Glucosamine may also stimulate chondrocytes, or cartilage-producing cells, to make new cartilage. The regular consumption of glucosamine may alleviate the signs and symptoms of **osteoarthritis (OA)**. Glucosamine supplementation may provide some degree of pain relief and improved function in persons experiencing regular knee pain, which may be caused by prior cartilage injury and/or OA. At a dosage of 2,000 mg $\cdot$ d^{-1}, most of the noted improvement occurs within 8 weeks (25). A meta-analysis examined clinical trials of glucosamine from January 1980 to March 2002. This study demonstrated that glucosamine (alone or in combination with chondroitin sulfate [CS]) reduced pain and damage to the knee joint. No differences were found in adverse events between placebo and glucosamine, indicating that the supplement appears to be safe (26).

Regular supplementation of glucosamine may decrease the symptoms associated with OA.

GLUTAMINE

Glutamine is the most plentiful non-EAA in the human body, particularly in the plasma and skeletal muscle, and has numerous physiological functions. Although the body can synthesize glutamine, it does become a "conditionally" EAA in cases of major trauma such as surgery, illness, and overtraining. Even an intense workout or multiple intense workouts that lead to overtraining are a cause for decreased glutamine levels. Among other things, glutamine acts as a cell-volume regulator (27) and has **anticatabolic properties**. It may stimulate muscle protein synthesis (28) and support immune function. Although more research is necessary, there are limited data to support its ability to increase cellular hydration and stimulate protein synthesis, and most show that glutamine supplementation does not lead to increases in muscle mass, improvements in body composition, strength, and/or improvements in exercise performance (29).

Clinical evidence for the exogenous use of glutamine supplementation in critically ill patients for the maintenance of muscle mass and immune function is well supported. Glutamine's role as an ergogenic aid as it relates to immune function may be of greater significance to athletes than its ability to increase muscle mass. Glutamine use may modify the apparent immunosuppression that is observed after prolonged, exhausting exercise. After such strenuous exercise, the concentration of glutamine in the blood is severely decreased. Supplementation of glutamine in this situation may decrease the incidence of illness in these athletes. The influence of glutamine on time to exhaustion and power before and after a prolonged bout of exercise has been examined (30). One group ingested a carbohydrate-plus-glutamine (Glu) beverage and a placebo group ingested a carbohydrate-only beverage (Pl). The Glu group significantly increased time to exhaustion compared to Pl. Peak power in the Glu group was similar in both trials, whereas the Pl group was still significantly lower after the second trial 6 days later. Therefore, glutamine supplementation seemed to help the Glu group exercise longer and recover quicker than the Pl group.

There is a sound physiological rationale and some evidence that glutamine supplementation can have a positive impact on muscle mass and strength gains in athletes. More convincing,

Q & A from the Field

Q ***I am concerned about my boyfriend. He wants to lift weights every day. He is always looking in the mirror and flexing his muscles. He spends a lot of time lifting weights and his muscles are extremely well developed. He is taking lots of different supplements. What is muscle dysmorphia, and what can we do for him if he has it?***

A Let me offer an example. Joe, a man 5 ft 10 in tall with extremely hypertrophied muscles, walks over to the squat rack, his eyes focused and his concentration fierce. He is a regular at the gym and is admired for his well-developed pecs, lats so large that his arms appear uncomfortably pushed inches away from his body, and powerful quads. Yet at 230 lb, Joe feels scrawny. He is embarrassed by what he perceives to be an underdeveloped body and tormented by the fear of losing the muscle he has if he doesn't work out for hours daily and follow a strict muscle-building diet. His kitchen is filled with large canisters of protein powder, a cupboard full of supplements touted to build muscles, and a scale to measure everything, but Joe is still displeased with his body.

Joe suffers from **muscle dysmorphia**, a preoccupation with his body image and the feeling that his body is not muscular enough. Like many other men who suffer from this disorder, Joe actually has a well-defined, muscular physique. Because of its striking similarity to other body-image distortions, muscle dysmorphia has been referred to as *reverse anorexia* or *bigorexia* and is considered to be a type of body dysmorphic disorder seen primarily in men. It is not surprising that an individual with body dysmorphia would take a lot of supplements to help him reach his goal.

Men suffering from muscle dysmorphia often lift weights for hours, pay meticulous attention to their diet, use various ergogenic aids, frequently check their bodies out in mirrors, and may spend more than 5 hours daily obsessing about their musculature. Like those who suffer from anorexia or other body-image disorders, these individuals are often depressed and may also experience anxiety, especially at the thought of anything disrupting their workout or diet regimen.

It isn't known how many men suffer from muscle dysmorphia, since large-scale studies have not been conducted. In addition, the etiology of muscle dysmorphia is unclear, though many theories have been presented; researchers believe that it may follow a psychosocial model with an underlying biological or genetic predisposition combined with social influences. The sociocultural theory is also believed to be a significant contributing factor. This view describes the societal pressures placed on men to fit media images of masculinity that include a fit, muscular physique. For years, women have been subjected to images of how a desirable female "should" look. Similarly unrealistic expectations for men, however, have become popular only in recent years.

Those who suffer from muscle dysmorphia rarely seek help for many reasons, including embarrassment over their preoccupation, the anxiety they feel at the thought of having to reduce their gym time during treatment, and the fear of a potential decrease in muscle mass once they start treatment. Proposed treatment options include cognitive behavioral therapy and the use of antidepressant medication.

—Marie Spano, MS, RD

though, is evidence that supports exogenous glutamine supplementation for immune system function, especially with prolonged, exhausting exercise.

Glutamine is an amino acid that may be needed in greater quantities during times of severe stress. Despite the various important roles of glutamine, current evidence does not support that glutamine supplementation can increase muscle mass or body composition.

GREEN TEA EXTRACT

Green tea extract has a high content of caffeine and catechin polyphenols, which could increase 24-hour energy expenditure and fat oxidation in humans. **Epigallocatechin gallate (EGCG)** is a purified catechin derived from green tea and is the main active component of the biological activity of tea polyphenols. For instance, one study compared three treatments: green tea extract (50-mg caffeine and 90-mg EGCG), caffeine (50 mg), and placebo, which were ingested at breakfast, lunch, and dinner.

Green tea extract resulted in a significant increase in 24-hour energy expenditure as well as a decrease in respiratory quotient, indicating a greater reliance on fatty acid oxidation. Green tea has thermogenic properties and promotes fat oxidation beyond that explained by its caffeine content. Green tea extract may play a role in the control of body composition by thermogenesis, fat oxidation, or both, but the results to this date are mixed at best.

EGCG is one of the primary active components of green tea. To this date, it seems that EGCG supplementation does not have a clear-cut ergogenic effect directly related to performance. However, research supports its use as an agent to increase energy expenditure and fat oxidation.

BETA-HYDROXY-BETA-METHYLBUTYRATE

Beta-hydroxy-beta-methylbutyrate (HMB) is a natural component of fish and milk. As a breakdown product of the EAA leucine, HMB is thought to increase strength and LBM by acting as an **anticatabolic agent** in muscle (i.e., decreasing muscle protein breakdown) (31). Studies have verified these beneficial effects, particularly in untrained men and women who consume 1.5 to 3.0 g HMB $\cdot$ d^{-1}, divided into two doses, for at least 4 weeks. One study suggested that its effects on strength and LBM can be further enhanced by coingesting creatine (Cr dose: 20 g $\cdot$ d^{-1} for 7 days followed by 10 g $\cdot$ d^{-1} thereafter) (32). Although the exact mechanism(s) behind its effects are unclear, the research suggests that the effects on body composition are not significant and there tends to be a more substantial effect on lower body strength than upper body strength, and these responses do not seem to occur in previously resistance-trained men (33). Ingestion of HMB appears to be safe and may even have beneficial effects on cardiovascular health (e.g., decreasing total cholesterol, low-density lipoprotein [LDL] cholesterol, and blood pressure) when doses of at least 3 g $\cdot$ d^{-1} are ingested for up to 8 weeks (31).

HMB supplementation may have an anticatabolic effect and increase strength, but the effects seem to be limited to untrained individuals.

HYDRATION

Dehydration has negative effects on performance (34). Inadequate hydration can refer to either **hypohydration** (being dehydrated prior to exercise) or exercise-induced dehydration, which occurs during exercise. Either state of dehydration can negatively impact muscle metabolism, body temperature regulation, and cardiovascular function, with performance decrements occurring with as little as a 1% to 2% reduction in body weight.

Water and commercial **sports drinks** can be very effective in maintaining performance or delaying the inevitable decrease in performance, especially in endurance or team sports that last longer than 1 hour. It is recommended that individuals consume a nutritionally balanced diet and drink adequate fluids in the 24-hour period prior to training or competition. The American College of Sports Medicine (ACSM) Position Statement on Exercise and Fluid Replacement (1996) also recommends the consumption of about 500 mL of fluid 2 hours prior to training or competition to promote adequate hydration and allow for excretion of excess fluid. Maintaining proper hydration prior to exercise is simple and generally should not be an issue if prudent measures are followed.

Fluid replacement during exercise is extremely critical not only to exercise performance but also to health. Without proper fluid replacement during prolonged exercise or exercise in a hot and humid environment, heat-related illness and cardiovascular issues can become life threatening. To minimize these conditions, it is recommended that water losses via sweating be replaced at a rate equal to the sweat rate. Athletes should replace the weight lost during exercise by drinking fluid. Unfortunately, individuals generally do not sufficiently replace lost fluid at a rate equal to water loss. This is referred to as *voluntary dehydration*. Water alone is not always sufficient to replace the fluid deficit incurred due to exercise, especially long-duration exercise with high sweat rates. Complete restoration of fluid lost during exercise cannot occur without replacement of electrolytes, primarily sodium.

Along with sodium, the addition of carbohydrates to fluid replacement solutions can enhance the intestinal absorption of water (35). More importantly, though, ingestion of a carbohydrate-containing beverage during exercise will help maintain blood glucose concentration and thus delay reliance on muscle glycogen stores as well as ultimately delaying fatigue (36). This is especially true in sessions lasting longer than 1 hour. An optimal carbohydrate solution of

4% to 8% helps maintain blood glucose concentrations and replace fluid lost via sweating. The inclusion of carbohydrates in rehydration solutions is necessary to maintain blood glucose concentrations for optimal performance in exercise lasting longer than 1 hour. It is also important to note that fructose should not be the predominant carbohydrate in a fluid replacement solution due to its low glycemic index and the associated relatively slow increase in blood glucose. Frequent ingestion of water and commercial sports drinks (containing electrolytes and carbohydrates) during exercise is certainly one of the simplest and most beneficial ergogenic aids available.

Hydration is a critical factor governing exercise performance in the heat. Both water and sports drinks are effective tools to help prevent, maintain, and replenish hydration status in athletic populations.

NUTRITION BEFORE AND AFTER WORKOUTS

Strenuous exercise, whether aerobic or anaerobic, can reduce various energy substrates (glycogen, protein, stored phosphagens [ATP, phosphocreatine], intracellular triglycerides), increase muscle protein breakdown, damage cell membranes, cause fluid loss, and temporarily impair immune function. The manner in which these physiological changes occur and how they respond to different interventions has provided clues to researchers as to what and when to eat with regard to optimizing performance.

Assuming that body hydration and muscle glycogen levels are adequate, a successful preexercise strategy is to provide a small amount of carbohydrate (25 to 50 g) along with 6 g of EAAs (or 40 g of complete protein) approximately 15 minutes prior to resistance training (23,24). This specific combination of carbohydrates and EAAs has been shown to increase muscle protein synthesis 160% more than ingesting the same cocktail postexercise (14). In this case, the exercise bout was for the lower body only (i.e., 10 sets of eight reps of leg press at 80% of 1 RM and 8 sets of eight reps of leg extension at 80% of 1 RM). Interestingly, research from the same lab found that adding non-EAAs to the mix does not increase protein synthesis. In other words, only the EAAs are needed to promote anabolic processes in muscle (22).

Nutrition during the postexercise period accomplishes three goals: (a) it puts the brakes on protein degradation, (b) it increases muscle protein synthesis, and (c) it rapidly initiates the process of muscle glycogen regeneration. An "optimal" food/beverage has yet to be identified. Based on research conducted over the past few years (3), however, a carbohydrate-to-protein ratio that ranges from 4:1 to approximately 1:1 may expedite recovery as well as enhance muscle glycogen synthesis *and* net protein status (23,24,37). Athletes should use a lower ratio of carbohydrate to protein when the volume of work (sets times reps) being performed is low and a higher ratio when the volume of work being performed is high. Practically, this means that athletes interested in increasing LBM as well as muscular strength and power should consume a postworkout beverage containing at least 100 cal and as much as 500 cal (and a combination of protein and carbohydrate) within

REAL-WORLD APPLICATION

Supplements Versus Foods

1. Eat about six meals each day. Healthy foods are the basis of sound nutrition. Frequent small meals increase metabolism.
2. Supplements should be treated only as an additional "tool" for achieving your goals. They are not magic potions that will cure the adverse effects of poor training and diet. When combined with sound nutrition, supplements could help athletes make substantial improvements in performance, recovery, and immunity.
3. Creatine is clearly a safe and effective supplement that can enhance LBM, muscle strength, and power with little to no side effects.
4. Always consume a postworkout carbohydrate–protein shake within 30 minutes of completing exercise (strength and endurance) to expedite recovery and promote gains in LBM.
5. Supplements should *never* take the place of real food.

Q & A from the Field

Q ***I've been hearing a lot of talk about using myostatin blockers. I am not familiar with these. What are they, and how effective are they? Do they pose any dangers?***

A I have seen these supplements in health food stores; they have been marketed with claims that they bind to serum myostatin and inhibit it. Myostatin causes muscle atrophy and wasting. Therefore, myostatin blockers could basically remove the inhibition of muscle growth and allow unlimited potential in muscle mass. One study has recently shown that *Cystoseira canariensis*, a brown sea algae that is the active ingredient in myostatin blockers, does exhibit binding specificity for serum myostatin (38). We have recently shown that *C. canariensis* binds myostatin; however, when combined with heavy weight training, 1,200 mg · d^{-1} of *C. canariensis* had no effect in reducing the level of serum myostatin or in preferentially increasing muscle strength and mass and decreasing fat mass (39). Therefore, the results from this study suggest that there is no apparent anabolic benefit from ingesting myostatin-blocking supplements.

Myostatin appears to negatively regulate skeletal muscle growth. In the blood, myostatin appears to work in part by slowing down and inhibiting the growth of muscle.

Recent studies with adult rodents showed that antibodies were created against myostatin, increasing total body mass, muscle mass, muscle size, and absolute muscle strength. The implication is that a myostatin blocker could conceivably provide benefits as an ergogenic aid or in the treatment of patients with muscle-wasting diseases.

—Darryn Willoughby, PhD, CSCS, FISSN, Baylor University

30 minutes of exercise. It is critical to consume this immediately after training or competition.

Anecdotally, many athletes find that adding 3 to 5 g of creatine and 5 to 10 g of BCAAs to their pre- and/or postworkout beverages provides an enormous benefit.

Consuming a combination of carbohydrate and protein immediately after exercise will expedite recovery and perhaps improve subsequent performance.

OTHER POTENTIAL ERGOGENIC AIDS

Ergogenic aids will always be a part of sports and athletic performance. A number of additional ergogenic aids have become popular from time to time. Myostatin blockers (Table 22.2), for example, have been purported to enhance muscle hypertrophy, but research currently does not support that claim.

TABLE 22.1 ● SUMMARY OF ERGOGENIC AIDS

NUTRIENT/ SUPPLEMENT	ACTIONS	DOSAGE	COMMENTS	REFERENCES
Aromatase inhibitors	Block the aromatase activity thus increasing endogenous levels of serum testosterone.	~75 mg · d^{-1} (hydroxyandrost-4-ene-6,17-dioxo-3-THP ether and 3,17-diketo-androst-1,4,6-triene)	Research has confirmed that aromatase inhibitors can increase serum testosterone levels with supplementation. One trial also found a significant decrease in fat mass during supplementation.	(40)
BCAA	May increase fat-free mass; anticatabolic effect; may ameliorate performance decrement.	BCAA (12–14 g · d^{-1}; 50% L-leucine, 25% L-isoleucine, 25% L-valine)	High-dose BCAA supplementation may be ergogenic.	

TABLE 22.1 ● SUMMARY OF ERGOGENIC AIDS (*Continued*)

NUTRIENT/ SUPPLEMENT	ACTIONS	DOSAGE	COMMENTS	REFERENCES
Caffeine	Lipolytic agent; increases mental alertness; increases thermogenesis; may enhance performance.	200–400 mg (acute dose)	No longer a banned substance; most commonly consumed drug.	(1,7)
Colostrum	May increase LBM; may enhance performance.	20–60 g · d^{-1} for several weeks	Compared to whey protein, may be more anabolic.	(9,10)
Creatine	May increase LBM; may enhance performance (i.e., sprints, 1 RM, repeated anaerobic exercise bouts, etc.).	3–5 g · d^{-1}; for loading phase (if chosen), 20–25 g · d^{-1} for about a week	Enormous scientific support for ergogenic effect.	(14–16,41)
EAA	May increase muscle protein accretion.	6 g (acute dose increases net muscle protein balance)	Has greater anabolic effects when taken preworkout vs. postworkout.	(22,23)
EGCG	A component of green tea; may increase thermogenesis beyond the normal effects of caffeine.	270 mg · d^{-1}	May have antioxidant and anticarcinogenic effects; data show enhanced thermogenesis.	(42)
Glucosamine	May treat symptoms of OA.	1,500 mg of glucosamine hydrochloride (GH) and 1,200 mg of CS daily	May ameliorate symptoms of OA.	(43)
Glutamine	Increases immune function.	6–10 g	May be more effective as immune function supporter in times of severe stress (exercise).	(29)
HMB	May alleviate the exercise-induced proteolysis and/or muscle damage; may increase muscle mass/function.	3 g · d^{-1}	May work best in untrained individuals.	(31)
Myostatin blockers	Purported to block the action of myostatin, which is a negative regulator of skeletal muscle mass.	1,200 mg · d^{-1} of *C. canariensis*	Research does NOT support the supplementation of purposed myostatin inhibitors.	(39)
Pre- and postworkout supplements	Increase muscle mass; increase muscle glycogen repletion; increase recovery.	Supplement containing 80-g CHO, 28-g Pro, 6-g fat immediately after exercise (10 min) and 2 h postexercise as little as 100 cal may help (17); 6 g of EAAs consumed preworkout is effective	Timing of ingestion is critical. Need to consume a carbohydrate–protein beverage immediately postexercise.	(24,37)
Prohormones	Proposed to increase testosterone levels and have effects on anabolism.	Dosage varies based on individual prohormone	May increase testosterone, but NO evidence to support that prohormones have an effect on muscle mass. No ergogenic effect; may also increase estrogen levels.	(44)

(*Continued*)

TABLE 22.1 ● SUMMARY OF ERGOGENIC AIDS (*Continued*)

NUTRIENT/ SUPPLEMENT	ACTIONS	DOSAGE	COMMENTS	REFERENCES
Sodium bicarbonate	Buffers the increase in H^+ ions that increase acidity (lowers pH) and impact fatigue.	0.3 g · kg body weight^{-1}	Potentially effective in maximal exercise lasting 2–5 min; may improve sprint performance.	(45,46)
Sports drinks	Carbohydrates necessary to maintain blood glucose to delay fatigue; electrolytes (sodium) help with absorption and complete fluid restoration.	4%–8% carbohydrate solution	Dehydration causes decrease in performance; may be only effective when exercise duration exceeds 1 h; fluid and electrolyte loss due to sweat is variable and dependent upon individual sweat rates; sports drinks without added protein are inadequate for promoting skeletal muscle recovery.	(36,47)

Q & A from the Field

Q ***A friend in my class says he is taking a supplement containing nitric oxide (NO). He says he has gained 10 lb of muscle in a month. What does research say about NO stimulators (arginine and arginine alpha-ketoglutarate)? Is there any evidence that they might help athletes gain muscle mass?***

A The problem here is that you have some fairly complex physiology being thrown around about NO without any substantive human data showing an effect on exercise performance or body composition. For instance, we know that arginine is an amino acid that participates in the maintenance of muscle and lean tissue throughout the body. It can be converted into ornithine, another amino acid. Its presence can stimulate the release of certain endogenous anabolic hormones, such as growth hormone and IGF. There is supposedly a better-absorbed form of arginine on the market called arginine alpha-ketoglutarate. This supplement is marketed under various names with claims that it accelerates the body's natural production of NO, vastly augmenting blood flow to muscles. It is also claimed that this product adds new muscle fibers, not muscle water, and that this addition of lean muscle combined with ingestion of the supplement will decrease body fat and enhance recovery. Unfortunately, there appear to be no scientific studies to validate any of these claims. Future research will reveal the effectiveness of this supplement.

Based on the current research, pure arginine may be better and more effective than arginine alpha-ketoglutarate. Arginine has been well researched and has many beneficial effects, especially in terms of cardiovascular health. Its main mechanism of action lies in boosting NO. NO is a signaling molecule within muscle cells that may have many anabolic effects, including increased nutrient transport and vasodilatation. Arginine boosts NO by stimulating NO synthase, the enzyme that makes NO. Research suggests it may help improve exercise performance, support protein synthesis, boost growth hormone levels at higher doses, and even help replenish postworkout glycogen stores.

OKG (ornithine ketoglutarate) (a salt formed from one molecule of alpha-ketoglutarate and two molecules of ornithine) is a metabolic regulator and precursor for glutamine and arginine. Glutamine promotes protein synthesis in skeletal muscle. OKG is also a precursor for other amino acids and ketoacids, which are important for protein synthesis. OKG stimulates the secretion of hormones such as insulin and human growth hormone and has an anabolic effect on muscles. It can also help with ammonia detoxification. This could be of significance, since high levels of ammonia are prevalent among body builders and other athletes. Therefore, OKG has been marketed as a sports supplement for helping to build muscle.

—Darryn Willoughby, PhD, CSCS, FISSN, Baylor University

BOX 22.1

Anabolic–Androgenic Steroids in Sports

AASs are synthetic forms of testosterone, the primary male hormone. Testosterone is responsible for both anabolic (muscle growth) and androgenic (secondary sex characteristics) effects that begin at puberty in males. The anabolic and androgenic characteristics of the drug go hand in hand, thus the name anabolic–androgenic steroids. The androgenic properties of the drug are responsible for many of the negative side effects reported.

AASs are generally effective in promoting muscle growth. Although some forms of AASs can be obtained as a legal prescription drug for certain medical conditions, they are illegal for possession without a prescription. AASs can be prescribed for males with delayed puberty and inadequate endogenous testosterone production and for individuals with muscle-wasting diseases. AASs are against the rules of most sport-governing bodies. Because of their pronounced effect on muscle size and strength, these drugs are widely used and abused by athletes, particularly in strength and power sports.

Abuse of AASs, however, can lead to potentially serious health problems, some irreversible. In addition to using AASs to improve athletic performance, many individuals are using AASs simply to improve physical appearance. Anabolic steroids come in both oral and injectable forms. Athletes, in an attempt to maximize the benefits of AAS use, will cycle the drugs rather than use them continuously. Cycling means taking multiple doses of steroids over a period of time and then going off them for a period of time before starting again. One concern is that athletes often combine several different types of steroids in an effort to maximize their effectiveness and minimize negative effects (referred to as *stacking*). Many of the studies looking at the negative effects of AAS use are looking at the effects of a prescription dose, not a dose that is stacked and/or cycled. It is quite possible that the larger doses used by athletes would cause the side effects to be even more pronounced.

The side effects from abusing AASs may include liver tumors (usually benign), negative blood lipid changes (increases in LDL [bad] cholesterol, and decreases in high-density lipoprotein [HDL] [good] cholesterol), fluid retention, high blood pressure, and severe acne. Since AASs are male hormones, they produce different side effects in males, females, and adolescents. In males, common side effects are shrinking testicles, reduced sperm count, infertility, baldness, gynecomastia (breast development), and an increased risk of prostate cancer. In females, anabolic steroids can cause male hair growth patterns on the face and body, male-pattern baldness, enlargement of the clitoris, and a deepened voice. Adolescents may experience premature closure of epiphyseal discs, causing stunted growth. Negative side effects are likely a result of the type of AAS used, the dose, frequency, and duration of use. Notice that males tend to develop feminine side effects and females tend to develop masculine side effects. In males, excess androgens (excess testosterone) are converted to estrogen, a primary female hormone. It is the estrogen production in males that is related to the feminine side effects. Many, but not all, of the side effects are irreversible when the athlete stops taking AAS.

What does all this mean to the strength and conditioning professional? First of all, we should be aware that the athletes we work with may be using AASs to enhance performance or appearance. Second, we must be able to provide sound advice to athletes and parents based on the legality of using AASs. Third, competition and sports should be based on the concept of fair play. The use of AASs by athletes to enhance performance crosses this line and jeopardizes the athlete's safety.

NO stimulators (arginine and arginine alpha-ketoglutarate) are currently popular to build muscle mass. Up to now, controlled research studies have not demonstrated a benefit from this supplement.

The focus of this chapter has been on legal ergogenic aids that have been shown to be potentially effective and apparently safe, although illegal substances such as anabolic–androgenic steroids (AASs) are commonly used (Box 22.1).

Summary

Table 22.2 summarizes the main ergogenic aids discussed in this chapter and a few more that are not as promising in regards to their beneficial effects. Strength and conditioning professionals should be aware of the various ergogenic aids potentially available to athletes. The research on a specific substance will likely always be equivocal, as the efficacy of ergogenic aids will be specific to their mechanism of action. Future research should continue to focus on both the safety and efficacy of these substances.

Maxing Out

1. A football running back for a division I college football team asks for your advice regarding his nutrition and supplementation program. He currently eats two to three very large meals each day (lunch and dinner). He often skips breakfast because he is not hungry, and he drinks coffee. His meals are mainly fast food (e.g., burgers, fries, and regular cola) as well as pizza and beer on late-night binges. At 5 ft 10 in tall, weighing 200 lb, and 18 years of age, he consumes approximately 3,000 cal · d^{-1}. His workouts for football are quite rigorous, and the day after a game he feels extremely lethargic. He wants to know how he can improve his diet as well as whether supplements might improve his performance and help him gain LBM.
2. There are literally thousands of purported ergogenic aids, all of which cannot be covered in a single chapter. Using the Internet or a library resource, investigate a familiar substance that is a purported ergogenic aid. Answer the following questions relative to that substance:
   a. Is there a logical "mechanism of action" by which this substance may have a positive effect on human performance?
   b. If this substance were to improve performance, what sports or events would be most likely to be improved?
   c. What information can you find regarding the effectiveness of this ergogenic aid? Positive/negative results? Dosing requirements?
   d. What information can you find regarding the safety of this ergogenic aid? Adverse events? Specific side effects? Any long-term health consequences?
3. It is difficult to address the ethical considerations of using ergogenic aids. Most will agree that there is a line we should not cross in recommending ergogenic aids. Write your own definition of an ergogenic aid. Then make a determination of whether or not these substances should be allowed to be used by athletes under your definition:
   a. Amino acids
   b. Creatine monohydrate
   c. Concentrated glucose replacement beverage
   d. Testosterone and related compounds
   e. Insulin
   f. Insulin-like growth factor
   g. Growth hormone
   h. Vitamin concentrates
   i. Mineral concentrates
   j. Coffee and concentrated caffeine beverages or tablets
   k. Vitamin B_{12} injections
   l. Protein bars

CASE EXAMPLE

Professional Boxer

BACKGROUND

You are a sports nutritionist who has been asked by a professional boxer how to best enhance his performance. He fights in the heavyweight division at 200 lb (he is 6 ft tall and 26 years old). He is preparing for an upcoming fight in 3 months and needs advice on how to improve his punching power/speed with new nutrition strategies. He is currently working with a top strength and conditioning specialist to improve his conditioning. This upcoming fight is 10 rounds (3-minute rounds), with 1 minute of rest between rounds.

RECOMMENDATIONS/CONSIDERATIONS

Because he is a heavyweight, he can add extra LBM and not worry about exceeding a weight limit. Also, he is "light" for a heavyweight boxer and likely needs to maintain his body weight while gaining more LBM.

IMPLEMENTATION

Descriptive information. Gathering basic information such as height, weight, body fat percentage (using skinfolds), age, and training history is essential. Examine past fights to see how he fared at different body weights and to determine at what rounds his strength/power subside. Determine, if possible, whether he has an "ideal" boxing weight.

Diet analysis. Have the subject keep a record of his food intake over the next 7 days to assess whether he is currently meeting his energy needs as well as macronutrient requirements. It is important to ensure an adequate intake of protein and essential fatty acids.

CASE EXAMPLE (*Continued*)

Professional Boxer

Supplements. Is this athlete taking any supplements? Again, you can determine this from the interview and his food diary. Perhaps creatine monohydrate supplementation is needed.

Rest. How much rest is the athlete getting?

Conditioning Program. Is he training properly for the fight? Is his training program periodized, matching up with his competition schedule? Does his regime include core training, and are his workouts sports specific? Work with his strength and conditioning coach to answer these questions.

Results. Based on the information obtained from this process, you make the following recommendations:

1. Increase daily caloric intake to 4,000 kcal $\cdot$ d^{-1}, utilizing a weight gain supplement if needed to obtain the desired intake.
2. Maintain a protein intake of 1 g $\cdot$ lb body $weight^{-1}$ d^{-1}.
3. Consume a preworkout beverage containing EAAs plus carbohydrate.
4. Consume a postworkout carbohydrate–protein shake to expedite recovery and promote gains in LBM.
5. Consume 3 to 5 g of creatine monohydrate as a daily supplement.
6. Get 7 to 8 hours of sleep every night.

SUGGESTED READINGS

Buford TW, Kreider RB, Stout JR, et al. International Society of Sports Nutrition position stand: creatine supplementation and exercise. *J Int Soc Sports Nutr*. 2007;4:6.

Campbell B, Kreider RB, Ziegenfuss T, et al. International Society of Sports Nutrition position stand: protein and exercise. *J Int Soc Sports Nutr*. 2007;4:8.

Goldstein ER, Ziegenfuss T, Kalman D, et al. International society of sports nutrition position stand: caffeine and performance. *J Int Soc Sports Nutr*. 2010;7:5.

Kerksick C, Harvey T, Stout J, et al. International Society of Sports Nutrition position stand: Nutrient timing. *J Int Soc Sports Nutr*. 2008;5:17.

Kreider RB, Wilborn CD, Taylor L, et al. ISSN exercise & sports nutrition review: research & recommendations. *J Int Soc Sports Nutr*. 2010;7:7.

REFERENCES

1. Acheson KJ, Gremaud G, Meirim I, et al. Metabolic effects of caffeine in humans: lipid oxidation or futile cycling? *Am J Clin Nutr*. 2004;79:40–46.
2. Smith, AE, Walter, AA, Graef JL, et al. Effects of beta-alanine supplementation and high-intensity interval training on endurance performance and body composition in men; a double-blind trial. *J Int Soc Sports Nutr*. 2009;6(5).
3. Blomstrand E, Saltin B. BCAA intake affects protein metabolism in muscle after but not during exercise in humans. *Am J Physiol Endocrinol Metab*. 2001;281:E365–E374.
4. Layman DK, Baum JI. Dietary protein impact on glycemic control during weight loss. *J Nutr*. 2004;134:968S–973S.
5. Armstrong LE. Caffeine, body fluid-electrolyte balance, and exercise performance. *Int J Sport Nutr Exerc Metab*. 2002;12:189–206.
6. Bell DG, McLellan TM. Effect of repeated caffeine ingestion on repeated exhaustive exercise endurance. *Med Sci Sports Exerc*. 2003;35:1348–1354.
7. Goldstein ER, Ziegenfuss T, Kalman D, et al. International society of sports nutrition position stand: caffeine and performance. *J Inter Soc of Sports Nutr*. 2010;7:5.
8. Mayo Clinic. Caffeine content of common beverages. http://www.mayoclinic.com/health/drug-information/DR202105. Accessed June 26, 2006.
9. Antonio J, Sanders MS, Van Gammeren D. The effects of bovine colostrum supplementation on body composition and exercise performance in active men and women. *Nutrition*. 2001;17:243–247.
10. Buckley JD, Brinkworth GD, Abbott MJ. Effect of bovine colostrum on anaerobic exercise performance and plasma insulin-like growth factor I. *J Sports Sci*. 2003;21:577–588.
11. Terjung RL, Clarkson P, Eichner ER, et al. American College of Sports Medicine roundtable. The physiological and health effects of oral creatine supplementation. *Med Sci Sports Exerc*. 2000;32:706–717.
12. Kraemer WJ, Volek JS. Creatine supplementation. Its role in human performance. *Clin Sports Med*. 1999;18:651–666, ix.
13. Kreider RB, Melton C, Rasmussen CJ, et al. Long-term creatine supplementation does not significantly affect clinical markers of health in athletes. *Mol Cell Biochem*. 2003;244:95–104.
14. Volek JS, Rawson ES. Scientific basis and practical aspects of creatine supplementation for athletes. *Nutrition*. 2004;20:609–614.

15. Buford TW, Kreider RB, Stout JR, et al. International Society of Sports Nutrition position stand: creatine supplementation and exercise. *J Int Soc of Sports Nutr*. 2007;4:6.
16. Ziegenfuss TN, Rogers M, Lowery L, et al. Effect of creatine loading on anaerobic performance and skeletal muscle volume in NCAA Division I athletes. *Nutrition*. 2002;18:397–402.
17. Willoughby DS, Rosene J. Effects of oral creatine and resistance training on myosin heavy chain expression. *Med Sci Sports Exerc*. 2001;33:1674–1681.
18. Tarnopolsky MA, Beal MF. Potential for creatine and other therapies targeting cellular energy dysfunction in neurological disorders. *Ann Neurol*. 2001;49:561–574.
19. Rae C, Digney AL, McEwan SR, et al. Oral creatine monohydrate supplementation improves brain performance: a double-blind, placebo-controlled, cross-over trial. *Proc R Soc Lond B Biol Sci*. 2003;270:2147–2150.
20. Watsford ML, Murphy AJ, Spinks WL, et al. Creatine supplementation and its effect on musculotendinous stiffness and performance. *J Strength Cond Res*. 2003;17:26–33.
21. Poortmans JR, Francaux M. Long-term oral creatine supplementation does not impair renal function in healthy athletes. *Med Sci Sports Exerc*. 1999;31:1108–1110.
22. Borsheim E, Tipton KD, Wolf SE, et al. Essential amino acids and muscle protein recovery from resistance exercise. *Am J Physiol Endocrinol Metab*. 2002;283:E648–E657.
23. Tipton KD, Borsheim E, Wolf SE, et al. Acute response of net muscle protein balance reflects 24-h balance after exercise and amino acid ingestion. *Am J Physiol Endocrinol Metab*. 2003;284:E76–E89.
24. Tipton KD, Rasmussen BB, Miller SL, et al. Timing of amino acid-carbohydrate ingestion alters anabolic response of muscle to resistance exercise. *Am J Physiol Endocrinol Metab*. 2001;281:E197–E206.
25. Braham R, Dawson B, Goodman C. The effect of glucosamine supplementation on people experiencing regular knee pain. *Br J Sports Med*. 2003;37:45–49; discussion 49.
26. Richy F, Bruyere O, Ethgen O, et al. Structural and symptomatic efficacy of glucosamine and chondroitin in knee osteoarthritis: a comprehensive meta-analysis. *Arch Intern Med*. 2003;163:1514–1522.
27. Rennie MJ, Low SY, Taylor PM, et al. Amino acid transport during muscle contraction and its relevance to exercise. *Adv Exp Med Biol*. 1998;441:299–305.
28. Rennie MJ. Glutamine metabolism and transport in skeletal muscle and heart and their clinical relevance. *J Nutr*. 1996;126:1142S–1149S.
29. Candow DG, Chilibeck PD, Burke DG, et al. Effect of glutamine supplementation combined with resistance training in young adults. *Eur J Appl Physiol*. 2001;86(2):142–149.
30. Piattoly T, Welsch MA. L-Glutamine supplementation: effects on recovery from exercise. *Med Sci Sports Exerc*. 2004;36:S127.
31. Nissen S, Sharp RL, Panton L, et al. Beta-hydroxy-beta-methylbutyrate (HMB) supplementation in humans is safe and may decrease cardiovascular risk factors. *J Nutr*. 2000;130:1937–1945.
32. Jowko E, Ostaszewski P, Jank M, et al. Creatine and beta-hydroxy-beta-methylbutyrate (HMB) additively increase lean body mass and muscle strength during a weight-training program. *Nutrition*. 2001;17:558–566.
33. Rowlands DS, Thomson JS. Effects of beta-hydroxy-beta-methylbutyrate supplementation during resistance training on strength, body composition, and muscle damage in trained and untrained young men: a meta-analysis. *J Strength Cond Res*. 2009;23(3):836–846.
34. Schoffstall JE et al. Effects of dehydration a nd rehydration on the one-repetition maximum bench press of weight-trained males. *J Strength Cond Res*. 2001;15:102–108.
35. Schedl HP, Maughan RJ, Gisolfi CV. Intestinal absorption during rest and exercise: implications for formulating an oral rehydration solution (ORS). *Med Sci Sports Exerc*. 1994;26:267–280.
36. Coggan AR, Coyle EF. Carbohydrate ingestion during prolonged exercise: effects on metabolism and performance. *Exerc Sport Sci Rev*. 1991;19:1–40.
37. Ivy JL, Res PT, Sprague RC, et al. Effect of a carbohydrate-protein supplement on endurance performance during exercise of varying intensity. *Int J Sport Nutr Exerc Metab*. 2003;13:382–395.
38. Ramazov, Z, Jimenez del Rio M, Ziegenfuss T. Sulfated polysaccharides of brown seaweed *Cystoseira canariensis* bind to serum myostatin protein. *Acta Physiol Pharmacol*. 2003;27:1–6.
39. Willoughby DS. Effects of an alleged myostatin binding supplement and heavy resistance training on serum myostatin, muscle strength and mass, and body composition. *Int J Sports Nutr Exerc Metab*. 2004;14(4):461–472.
40. Willoughby DS, Wilborn C, Taylor L, et al. Eight weeks of aromatase inhibition using the nutritional supplement Novedex XT: effects in young, eugonadal men. *Int J Sport Nutr Exerc Metab*. 2007;17(1):92–108.
41. Bermon S, Venembre P, Sachet C, et al. Effects of creatine monohydrate ingestion in sedentary and weight-trained older adults. *Acta Physiol Scand*. 1998;164:147–155.
42. Rietveld A, Wiseman S. Antioxidant effects of tea: evidence from human clinical trials. *J Nutr*. 2003;133:3285S–3292S.
43. Segal L, Day SE, Chapman AB, et al. Can we reduce disease burden from osteoarthritis? *Med J Aust*. 2004;180:S11–S17.
44. King DS, Sharp RL, Vukovich MD, et al. Effect of oral androstenedione on serum testosterone and adaptations to resistance training in young men: a randomized controlled trial. *JAMA*. 1999;281(21):2020–2028.
45. Lindh AM, Peyrebrune MC, Ingham SA, et al. Sodium bicarbonate improves swimming performance. *Int J Sports Med*. 2008;29(6):519–523.
46. McNaughton L, Thompson D. Acute versus chronic sodium bicarbonate ingestion and anaerobic work and power output. *J Sports Med Phys Fitness*. 2001;41:456–462.
47. Maughan RJ, Leiper JB. Limitations to fluid replacement during exercise. *Can J Appl Physiol*. 1999;24:173–187.

CHAPTER 23

Implement Training

ALLEN HEDRICK

OBJECTIVES

After reading this chapter, you will be able to:

- Understand the concepts of fluid resistance, tires, chains, and other lifting implements.
- Discuss the integration of implement training with more traditional resistance training exercises.
- Understand the concept of transferability as it relates to implement training and sports performance.
- Design sport-specific conditioning programs for athletes incorporating various implements appropriately.

KEY TERMS

Active fluid resistance
Chains
Implements
Kegs
Logs
Tires
Water-Filled Implements
Water-Filled Dumbbells

Introduction

In competitive athletics, today, more than ever, a tremendous emphasis is placed on strength and conditioning as a method to improve athletic performance. More and more frequently, financial resources are directed toward building bigger and better strength and conditioning facilities. In addition, through educational and professional organizations, the knowledge base of strength and conditioning coaches continues to improve.

Resistance training is recognized as a necessary component of any training program designed to improve athletic performance.

SIMILARITY IN TRAINING PROGRAMS

Though there are exceptions, the majority of strength and conditioning programs meant to improve athletic performance emphasize free weights as the preferred method of training (1–4). Further, many of those programs emphasizing free weight training place a priority on performing the Olympic-style exercises (5–8). In addition, most strength and conditioning coaches design their training programs based on the concept of periodization, organizing their training programs into cycles. Each of these cycles has a specific physiological goal, with the ultimate goal to bring athletes to a peak at the appropriate point in the competitive season (9–12). There are variations in the periodization model used from program to program. However, if you reviewed the training programs used in strength and conditioning facilities across the country, you would likely find many similarities in the programs designed from facility to facility.

As a result, there are a significant number of athletes training in high-quality facilities being directed by well-educated strength and conditioning professionals employing programs that have similarities in design. Thus it becomes difficult to provide your athletes a significant competitive edge through their strength and conditioning programs. The challenge for the strength and conditioning coach is to find ways to manipulate the strength and conditioning programs they design to provide their athletes a competitive advantage.

The majority of strength and conditioning coaches accentuate free weight training and performance of the Olympic-style exercises following a periodized training program. As a result, it is difficult to design training programs that provide your athletes with a competitive advantage.

RELYING ON SCIENCE

The amount of research in the field of sports science has dramatically increased, evaluating a broad spectrum of topics. Because of this, it is important that the strength and conditioning coach take advantage of the available information and apply it appropriately. The majority of any training program should be based on what sports science has determined to be the best approach to achieving the desired goal (27).

Because of the wide spectrum of research occurring in the area of sports science, the majority of any training program should be based on science.

LACK OF IMPLEMENT TRAINING RESEARCH

However, there are still methods of training used to improve athletic performance that has little or no scientific evidence to support or refute. One such area that is lacking scientific research is the value of training with **implements** (nonstandard resistance training modes, such as kegs, tires, or sandbags) as compared to the more traditional barbell, dumbbell, or strength-training machine. Based on a review of literature, little research has been conducted evaluating the effectiveness of training with nonstandard equipment, such as tires, logs, kegs, stones, and similar, for lack of a better term, strongman-type implements (13). Despite this lack of research, the use of strongman-type training is becoming more common in strength and conditioning programs (13–15). This is not surprising given that most strength and conditioning professionals are diligent in exploring alternative training strategies as a means to gaining an advantage (13).

One area that is lacking research is the value of performing strength training activities with nontraditional resistance training implements.

TRAINING PRINCIPLES

Despite this lack of research, the same principles that apply to traditional training methods can be used to guide the use of implement training. Perhaps most important is the concept of training movements, not muscle groups (12,16–18). That is, increases in strength and or power will occur primarily in the movement used during training. The more similar the movement pattern is to the target sport or activity, the more valuable such training becomes. As a result, it becomes obvious that activities such as a fireman's carry, where the athlete carries a heavy implement in each hand over a prescribed distance or time, does not transfer well to the movement patterns found in most athletic activities. Similarly, lifting heavy stones and placing them on an elevated stand, because of the opportunity for injury and the need for strict technique, may be time better spent performing more traditional-type training.

Although there is a lack of research evaluating implement training, the same principles that are applicable to conventional training modes can be applied to implement training.

TRANSFERABILITY OF IMPLEMENT TRAINING TO SPORTS PERFORMANCE

On the other hand, some nontraditional training methods transfer very effectively to athletic performance, and its inclusion in an athletic strength and conditioning program can be of value for two primary reasons. First, the movement pattern can be similar to the movement pattern seen during competition (e.g., the movement of flipping a tire transfers well to blocking, tackling, wrestling and so on). Secondly, implement training increases variation in the training program, reducing the physiological and psychological staleness that can occur when performing the same strength training movements repetitively over weeks and months.

Some nontraditional training methods can be used to effectively train sport-specific movements and provide variation in the training program.

WATER-FILLED IMPLEMENTS

One implement training method that theoretically seems as if it could be of value in the training programs of certain types of athletes (i.e., football, hockey, wrestling) is the use of **water-filled implements** (water-filled implements are objects such as kegs or specially designed training logs or dumbbells in which the majority of the resistance is provided by water contained within the implement). Water as a form of resistance provides a unique

Q & A from the Field

Q ***Differences of opinion exist in the field about training modalities and the use of various implements. Many of the implements lack a solid foundation in the research literature in terms of effectiveness. Should we, as professionals, be concerned about that fact? How should we deal with questions about the lack of research when speaking with administrators, coaches, and parents?***

A Admittedly, there is a lack of research on many of the implements discussed in this chapter. Does that mean that we must wait for that research to be done before using these implements? Not really. As long as we apply safe and effective principles of training, implement training can be safely added to any training program. To justify the exercise as related to a specific sport, the concepts of specificity and transferability can be used.

Future research will provide additional evidence related to the effectiveness of the various implements discussed in this chapter. As professionals, even though we do not need to wait on that research to utilize these innovative methods of training, we must keep up with new research and be willing to adjust our training programs accordingly. We must also consider the entire body of research on a specific topic. A single study is unlikely to "prove" or "disprove" the effectiveness of a single training implement.

training stimulus because water provides an **active fluid resistance** (the water contained within the object is constantly moving during performance of the exercise, providing an active resistance) rather than a static resistance (14,19). Contrast that to a typical exercise where the resistance (in the form of a weight stack, barbell, or dumbbell) is relatively static, that is, there's very little if any extraneous movement occurring.

Unfortunately there is little if any research evaluating the value of training with an active fluid resistance. But, applying the concept of specificity, it makes logical sense that training with an active fluid resistance provides a highly sport-specific method of training (for certain types of athletes) as compared to lifting exclusively with a static resistance. This is because in many situations, athletes encounter dynamic resistance (in the form of an opponent) as compared to a static resistance. Further, because the active fluid resistance enhances the need for stability and control, this type of training may reduce the opportunity for injury because of improved joint stability.

Water-filled implements provide the athlete the opportunity to train against an active fluid resistance rather than the static resistance that most traditional training methods provide.

IMPLEMENT TRAINING SHOULD SUPPLEMENT TRADITIONAL METHODS

It is not being suggested that implement training become the primary form of resistance training for athletes. Barbells and dumbbells are proven tools that have been shown to be very effective at developing increases in strength and power. However, if the goal of training is to gain a competitive edge, then supplementing traditional training with implement training may be a viable option.

Implement training should be used to supplement traditional exercises (i.e., exercise machine, barbell, and dumbbell exercises) that make up the typical athletic resistance training program.

PROGRAM DESIGN

Examples of supplementing traditional training methods with implement training are provided in Tables 23.1 through 23.3. The following list provides explanation of the abbreviations used in the workouts presented in the tables below.

- TB: Total body exercise; this is one of the Olympic-style lifts or related training exercise

REAL-WORLD APPLICATION

Unstable Resistance or Unstable Surface?

This chapter discusses several forms of implements used in training programs that provide an unstable resistance: kegs, sandbags, etc. Implements are available that provide an unstable surface or an unstable base from which the athlete is required to produce force. One question then becomes which modality is more appropriate: an unstable resistance or an unstable surface?

The answer to this question is most certainly sport specific. One point of consideration will be the degree to which a supporting surface is "unstable" while performing sport-specific activities.

A stability ball is a common piece of equipment used in training athletes today. A "balance disk" or "wobble board" is used in some cases to provide an unstable surface underneath a planted foot. As a strength and conditioning professional, you must be able to evaluate these exercise modalities and determine whether they are specific to the sport for which the athlete is training.

In many sports, the ground is the primary surface the athlete uses to generate ground reaction force. In some cases, the ground is slippery (wet grass) or allows sliding (a clay tennis court). Is a slippery surface the same as an unstable surface? Probably not.

Although this does not mean that an unstable surface should never be used, you as a strength and conditioning professional should have a reason for using any piece of equipment. These modalities may be very useful in the rehabilitation of specific injuries. Since conditioning programs should progress from general to specific, it may be that unstable surfaces are useful in the general conditioning phase but not applicable to the sport-specific phase.

Before using an unstable surface in a sport-specific conditioning phase, evaluate the sport and have a specific rationale for using the modality.

TABLE 23.1 ● HOCKEY: STRENGTH CYCLE I

DATES: April 28–May 25
CYCLE: Strength 1
GOAL: To increase muscle strength, because of the positive relationship between strength and power
LENGTH: 4 wk
INTENSITY: Complete the full number of required repetitions on the first set only prior to increasing resistance
PACE: *Total* body lifts performed as explosively as possible. All other exercises lift explosively, lower in 2 s
REST: 2:30 between total body lifts, 2:00 between all other exercises
SETS/REPS:
April 28–May 4: TB = 4 × 5, CL = 4 × 7, AL = 3 × 8
May 5–May 11: TB = 4 × 2, CL = 4 × 4, AL = 3 × 8
May 12–May 18: TB = 4 × 5, CL = 4 × 7, AL = 3 × 8
May 19–May 25: TB = 4 × 2, CL = 4 × 4, AL = 3 × 8

MONDAY	WEDNESDAY	FRIDAY
TOTAL BODY	**TOTAL BODY**	**TOTAL BODY**
Squat Clean **(Floor)** TB	DB Hang Clean/Tire Flip TB	Hang Alt Foot Snatch TB
LOWER BODY	**LOWER BODY**	**CHEST**
Squat CL	DB/Keg/Log 1-Leg Squat CL	Bench Press **(1-Set Standing)** CL
Keg/Log Lateral Squat CL	DB/Keg/Log Hockey Lunge CL	
60-s Stabilization		
TRUNK	**TRUNK**	**TRUNK**
WT Decline Twist Pushdown 3 × 15	MB Trunk Twist 3 × 15	WT Russian Twist 3 × 15
WT Reverse Back Ext 3 × 12	DB/Keg/Log Straight Leg Dead Lift 3 × 12	WT Toe Touchers 3 × 15
UPPER BACK	**CHEST**	**SHOULDERS**
MR Row 2 × 8	DB/Keg/Log Bench Press CL	Keg/Log Shoulder Press CL
		MR Front Raise 2 × 8
NECK	**UPPER BACK**	**NECK**
MR Lat Flexion 2 × 8	DB/Keg/Log Row CL	MR Flex/Ext 2 × 8

- CL: Core lift; this is a multijoint exercise such as a squat
- AL: Auxiliary lift; this is a single-joint exercise such as a biceps curl
- DB: Dumbbell; the exercise is performed with a dumbbell
- WT: Weighted; the exercise is performed with an external resistance to provide added intensity
- MR: Manual resistance; the exercise uses a partner as the form of resistance
- MB: Medicine ball; the exercise is performed with a medicine ball
- Alt: Alternating; the exercise is performed alternating legs or alternating arms (depending on the exercise being performed).
- DB/Tire Squat Clean: On the days our athletes perform dumbbell hang squat cleans, we provide them the opportunity to perform a tire flip. This tire flip is performed with a movement similar to the pull sequence seen when performing a clean.

DESCRIPTION OF SUGGESTED TRAINING IMPLEMENTS

KEGS

The number of **kegs** needed in the training program, and the range of weights from the lightest to heaviest keg, will depend on the number of athletes training with kegs at one time and the types of keg exercises placed into the training program. You can think of each keg as a training station; ideally you will want no more than three athletes per keg. Certain exercises, such as a keg front raise, requires a fairly light

TABLE 23.2 ● RUNNING BACKS/WIDE RECEIVERS: STRENGTH CYCLE 2

DATES: March 29–May 2
CYCLE: Strength 2
GOAL: Increase muscle strength, because of the positive relationship between strength and power
LENGTH: 5 wk
INTENSITY: Select a resistance that allows completion of the full number of required repetitions on the ***first*** set only prior to increasing resistance
PACE: Total body lifts performed explosively. All other exercises lift explosively, lower in 2 s
REST: 2:30 between total body exercises, 2:00 between all other sets and exercises
SETS/REPS:
March 29–April 4: TB = 4 × 5, CL = 4 × 6, AL = 3 × 6
April 5–April 11: TB = 4 × 3, CL = 4 × 4, AL = 3 × 6
April 12–April 18: TB = 4 × 5, CL = 4 × 6, AL = 3 × 6
April 19–April 25: TB = 4 × 3, CL = 4 × 4, AL = 3 × 6
April 26–May 2: TB = 4 × 5, CL = 4 × 6, AL = 3 × 6

MONDAY	WEDNESDAY	FRIDAY
TOTAL BODY	**TOTAL BODY**	**TOTAL BODY**
Squat Clean **(Floor)** TB	DB Hang Clean/Tire Flip TB	Split Alt Ft Snatch Balance TB
Split Alter Foot Jerks TB		
CHEST	**LOWER BODY**	**LOWER BODY**
Bench Press CL	DB/Keg/Log 1-Leg Squat CL	Squats CL
	DB/Keg/Log Lateral Squat CL	Keg/Log Walking Lunges CL
	Leg Curl AL	1 × 60-s stabilization
TRUNK	**TRUNK**	**TRUNK**
MB Decline 1-Arm Throws 3 × 15	MB Pushdowns 3 × 15	WT Alter V-Ups/with MB 3 × 15
MR Reverse Back Ext 3 × 12	MB Twist Pushdowns 3 × 15	MR Reverse Back Ext 3 × 12
SHOULDERS	**CHEST**	**UPPER BACK**
MR Front Raise	DB/Keg/Log Incline Press CL	Pulldowns CL
UPPER BACK	**ARMS**	**NECK**
Bent Row CL	MR Stand Triceps 2 × 8	MR Flex/Ext 2 × 8
MR Up-Right Row		
NECK		
MR Lateral Flex 2 × 8		

weight (e.g., 20 lb) while some athletes may be able to go as heavy as 280 to 300 lb on a keg squat.

Be aware that because of the additional balance and stability requirements, athletes will not be able to use the same amount of weight in a keg exercise that they will performing the same exercise with a barbell. Though initially this may seem to compromise potential increases in strength, consider that the athletes may be building a higher level of transferable strength, that is, strength that can be used effectively during competition.

The kegs can be filled to the desired weight by removing the cap, placing the keg on a scale, and using a hose to fill the keg with water until the desired weight is reached. Another technique that can be used to fill the keg is to cut off the spout of the keg, pour the desired amount of water and sand into the keg, and weld the spout back on; a full-size keg, filled with water, will weigh about 160 lb. To further increase the weight of the keg, sand can be mixed in with water. Sand is advantageous because it is inexpensive and, because it stays wet inside the keg, it maintains its dynamic characteristics, moving inside the keg as the exercise is performed.

Keg stands can be built to make it easier to perform exercises such as squats, lunges, or shoulder

TABLE 23.3 ● VOLLEYBALL: POWER CYCLE 2

DATES: May 31–June 27
CYCLE: Power 2
GOAL: Increases in muscle power, because of the positive relationship between muscle power and performance
LENGTH: 4 wk
INTENSITY: Complete the full number of repetitions in good form on the first set only prior to increasing resistance
PACE: Total body lifts performed as explosively as possible. Timed lifts performed at a pace that allows completion of the required number of repetitions in the specified time period
REST: 3:00 between total body sets and exercises, 2:30 between all other sets and exercises
SETS/REPS:
May 31–June 6: TB = 5 × 2, TL = 4 × 4 @ 5 s (1.3)
June 7–June 13: TB = 5 × 3, TL = 4 × 6 @ 9 s (1.5)
June 14–June 20: TB = 5 × 2, TL = 4 × 4 @ 5 s (1.3)
June 21–June 27: TB = 5 × 3, TL = 4 × 6 @ 9 s (1.5)

MONDAY	WEDNESDAY	FRIDAY
TOTAL BODY	**TOTAL BODY**	**TOTAL BODY**
Hang Squat Clean TB	DB Split Alt Ft Alt Snatch Balance TB	Scoop Split Alt Ft Snatch TB
	DB Hang Split Alt Ft Alt Snatch TB	Split Alt Ft Jerks TB
LOWER BODY	**LOWER BODY**	**CHEST**
Squats (2 sets) TL	DB/Log 1-Leg Front Squats TL	Bench Press (2 sets) TL
Keg/Log Squats (2 sets) CL	DB/Keg/Log Arch Lunge TL	Bench Press (2 sets) CL
Keg/Log Side Lunge TL	60-s Stabilization	DB Pullovers TL
TRUNK	**TRUNK**	**TRUNK**
Stand 2-Hand Bar Twist 3 × 10	MB Ankle Chop/Twist 3 × 10	MB Decline 2-Hand Arm Throw 3 × 10
WT Back Ext 3 × 8	WT Twist Back Ext 3 × 8	
UPPER BACK	**CHEST/SHOULDER**	**SHOULDERS**
Bar/Keg/Log Bent Row TL	DB Alt Bench Press TL	Keg/Log Shoulder Press TL
ROTATOR CUFF	**ROTATOR CUFF**	**ROTATOR CUFF**
Internal Rotation 2 × 12	Empty Cans 2 × 12	Functional Rotation 2 × 12 MB Overhead Throw 2 × 12

press. The purpose of these stands is to securely hold the keg in place at shoulder height to make it easier to place the keg in the correct position to perform the selected exercise. You can think of the keg stands as being similar to a squat rack where the bar is held in place at about shoulder height so that the athlete can place it on the back to perform a squat.

Most kegs are built with a handle on the top end. The bottom end is typically built with a lip that allows the user to more effectively grip that end of the keg. By gripping the handle at the top end and using the lip at the bottom end, a secure grip can be achieved when handling the keg. However, caution must still be taken when using the kegs to perform resistance training exercises. The ability to grip the keg is not as secure as when using a barbell or dumbbell. Further, the water movement within the keg creates a difficult resistance to control. The spotter must take great care when a keg exercise is being performed, and the lifter must remember to use a lighter resistance than would be used when performing the same exercise with a barbell or dumbbell.

The number of kegs needed to supplement the strength training program, and the range of poundage needed in the kegs, will depend on the number of athletes training and the types of keg exercises being performed. It is important to remember that exercises performed with the kegs are more difficult than the same exercise performed with a barbell or dumbbell. Because of this, the athlete will have to reduce the training weight when performing a keg exercise as compared to the same exercise performed with a barbell or dumbbell.

LOGS

The **logs** (6-ft-long "tubes" with a 12-in circumference) are filled with water. Extending out from each tube is piping the size of a standard barbell so that additional weight plates can be attached to the log. The ability to rapidly change the weight of the log limits the need to have a large number of logs available at various weights.

The logs are designed with handles to make it easier to hold on to the implement. Because of the length of the logs, the water has the opportunity to travel a significant distance as compared to the kegs increasing the dynamic nature of the movement.

Similar to the kegs, because of the instability of the implement, athletes will not be able to perform exercises performed with the log with the same weight that they would perform the identical exercise with a barbell. Err on the side of caution, and slowly increase the weight lifted with this type of training as the athlete demonstrates the ability to control the implement during exercise.

Because the logs are 6 ft long, the water contained within the log can move a significant distance, increasing the dynamic characteristics of the exercise and thus the degree of difficulty of the movement.

WATER-FILLED DUMBBELLS

These **water-filled dumbbells** (smaller versions of the water-filled logs) are used as a typical dumbbell. Water displacement is less than what occurs when using the logs because the length of the dumbbells is much shorter than that of the logs. However, the movement of the water still provides an additional challenge to the athlete as compared to a typical dumbbell. Water-filled dumbbells provide a unique training stimulus and thus have the potential to provide the athlete with a competitive advantage.

Although less dynamic resistance occurs using water-filled dumbbells as compared to the kegs or logs (because the dumbbells are shorter than the kegs or logs and thus provides less opportunity for dynamic movement of the water), water-filled dumbbells still provide a unique training stimulus for the athlete.

TIRES

The **tires** (used truck and heavy equipment tires) can be modified so that athletes can attach additional weight in the center of the tire to adjust the resistance to their specific strength levels. Unlike the kegs, logs, and water-filled dumbbell with which a variety of exercises can be performed, the tires are only flipped. The tire flip requires a heavy tire be flipped end over end as quickly as possible (20). To perform the movement, the athlete crouches down in front of the tire, grabs the underside of the tire with a supinated grip approximately shoulder-width apart, and forcefully extends the ankle, knee, hip to flip the tire over.

One common technique used to flip the tire that could increase the likelihood of injury is the use of a single leg support position when repositioning the hands to push the tire over. This technique places a high degree of stress on the supporting leg and should be avoided.

However, if done correctly, using the tires does provide some advantages. First, flipping the tire provides athletes greater variety in their training program, which is a positive. Secondly, strongman exercises such as the tire flip, along with more common lifts such as the power clean, snatch, and squat may improve trunk stability (15).

An additional advantage of including tire flips in the workout is that athletes who have an injury (typically wrist, elbow, shoulder, or back) that prevents them from performing the Olympic-style exercises safely and pain free may still be able to perform a tire flip without aggravating the injury. Finally, because there is no catch phase in flipping a tire, the athlete sometimes feels better able to concentrate on the explosion phase of the movement.

The tires provide a unique and challenging variation for athletes who regularly perform cleans or high pulls as a part of their workout.

CHAINS

One mode of training that has become increasingly popular is adding lengths of chain to the end of the barbell (21–26,28). The rationale for the use of chains is that the chain provides a variable resistance. When performing a typical barbell exercise, the weight remains constant throughout the performance of the exercise (7). Theoretically, chain training provides a variable resistance throughout the range of motion of the exercise (22–26), For example, when performing a squat or clean, the chains collect on the floor at the bottom of the movement, adding the least amount of additional resistance at this point of the exercises (which is the point where the muscle is able to generate the least amount of force; Fig. 23.1). As the bar is lifted out of this low position, the bar gets progressively heavier as more and more links of chain are lifted off the floor until the bar gets to its heaviest point, which is where the muscles generate the greatest amount of force (24).

However, despite the increasing popularity of using chains, and the widespread belief that the use of chains provides an advantage, these claims remain mostly anecdotal (22–25). While it has been suggested that the use of chains promote power, acceleration, motor control, stabilization, and enhanced neurological adaptation (25), these claims are primarily anecdotal because only a limited number of studies have been conducted evaluating what effect, if any, chains provide during training and these studies have provided mixed results in terms of the effectiveness of using chains (22,25).

Despite these mixed study results and primarily anecdotal claims, athletes who make use of chains during training believe that chains positively affect their training, increase performance, and require greater effort (22). If an athlete believes chain training is more difficult and requires greater effort during training, this may lead to increased performance over time.

DESCRIPTION OF IMPLEMENT EXERCISES PROVIDED IN EXAMPLE WORKOUTS

The list of exercise descriptions provided below is not an all-inclusive list of the exercises that can be performed with the implements discussed in this chapter. Rather, this list is a description of the implement exercises included in the example workouts provided above. Most of the implement exercises are performed very similarly to the same exercises performed with traditional strength training equipment.

It is important to note that the Olympic-style exercises are not performed with either kegs or logs. Because of the technical difficulty of performing these types of exercises, and the awkwardness of using these implements, the chance of injury performing these types of exercises with these implements is too great. However, all of the Olympic-style exercises can be safely performed with the water-filled dumbbells by those athletes who have good technique when performing these exercises with standard dumbbells.

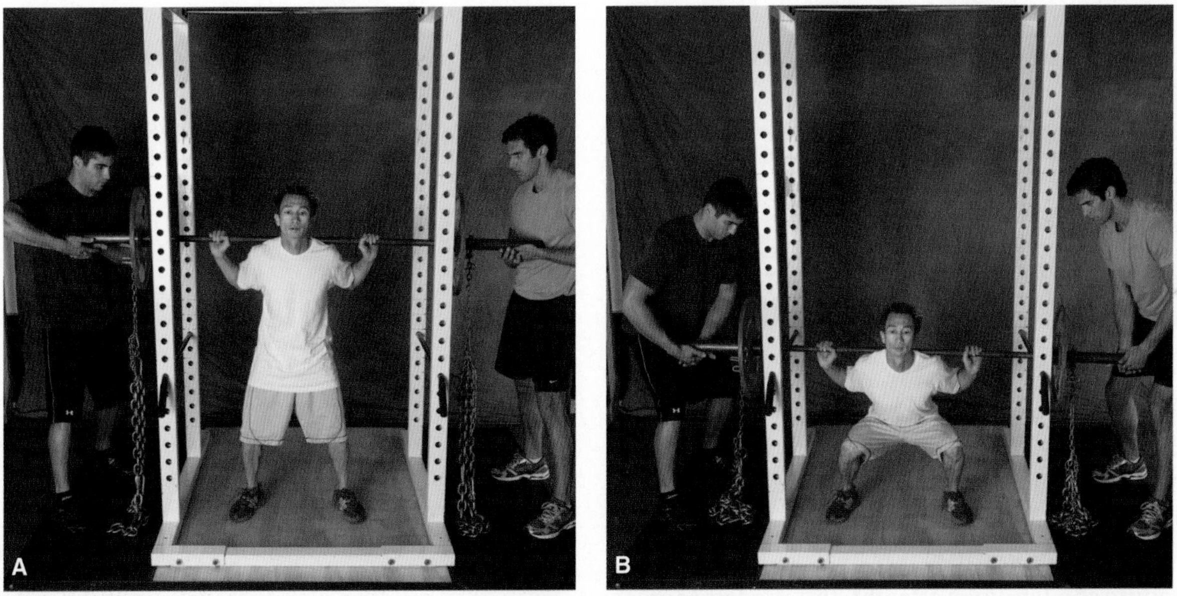

FIGURE 23.1 A. Starting Position. Hang the chains on the bar so that the ends of the chains just barely touch the floor when the bar is placed on the back. Place the bar on the back in a normal barbell squat position. **B. Movement Sequence.** Keeping the back arched, initiate the movement by sitting back at the hips, not allowing the knees to drift excessively forward of the feet. Continue to sit back until the mid thigh has achieved a parallel position. Maintaining an arched back position, return to the starting position.

Remember that in all of the exercises performed with implements, the training weight must be reduced in comparison to what athletes would use with a traditional barbell or dumbbell.

Exercise descriptions for the water-filled dumbbells are not included in this list. Movements using the water-filled dumbbells are identical to movements using standard dumbbells and so are not described.

Implement Exercises

Keg/Log Lateral Squat (Fig. 23.2)

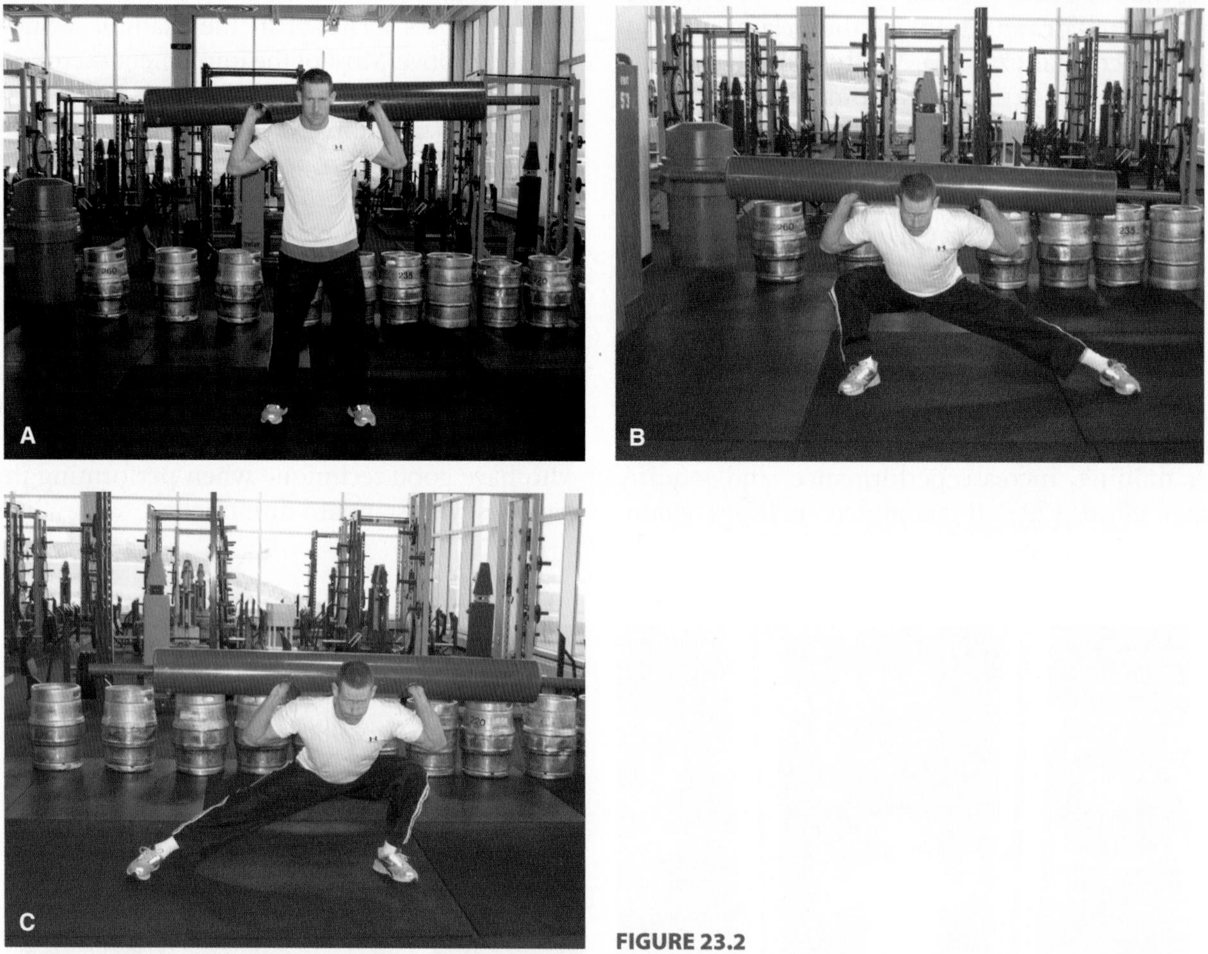

FIGURE 23.2

Starting Position

Place the keg or log on the back, as when performing barbell squats. Place the feet 10 to 12 in wider than shoulder width.

Movement Sequence

Keeping the left knee straight and the left foot planted, flex the right knee while sitting back at the hips and moving the hips laterally to the right. Return to the starting position, and alternate the movement to the opposite side until the required number of repetitions has been performed

Tire Flip (Fig. 23.3)

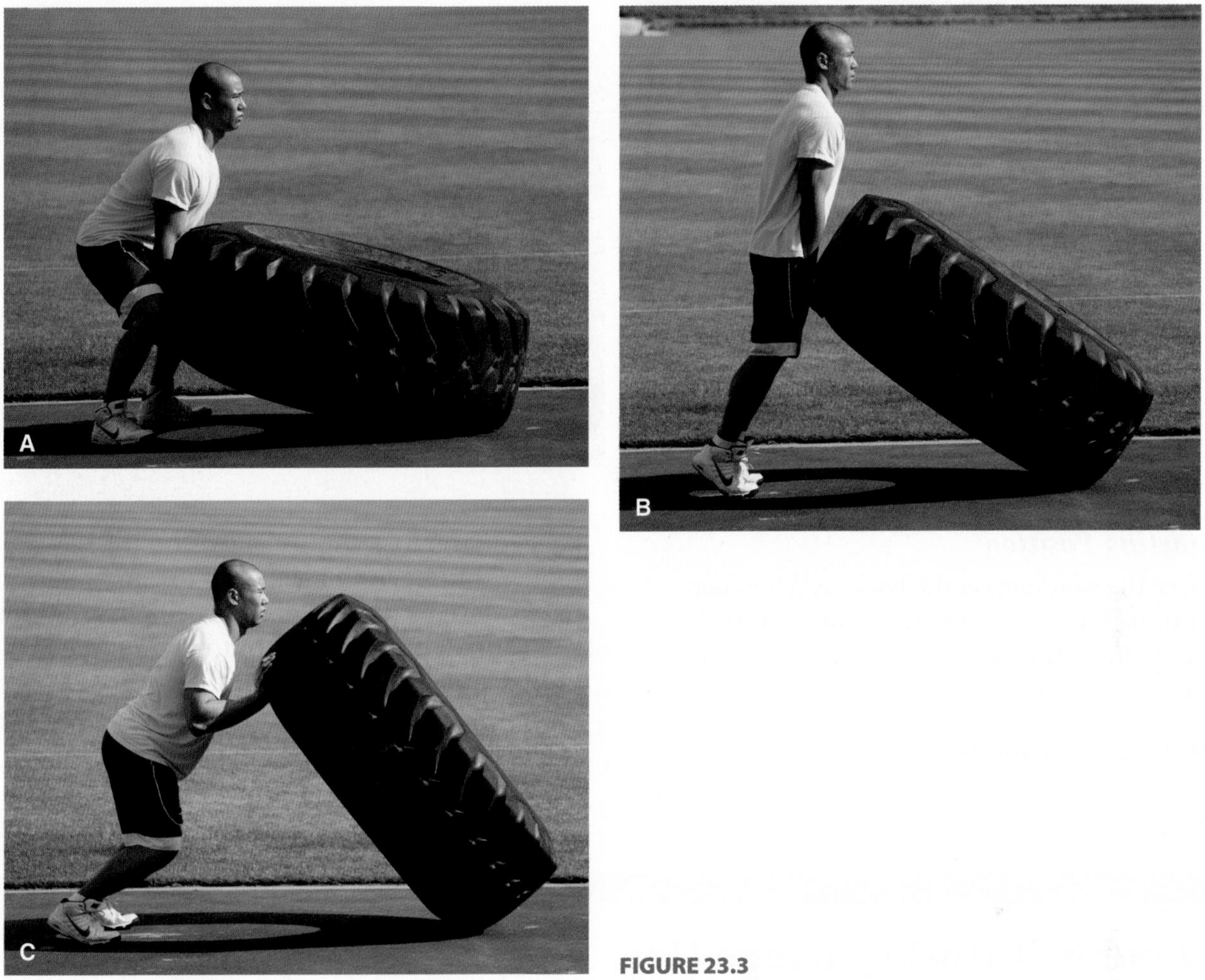

FIGURE 23.3

Starting Position

Place the feet about shoulder-width apart. Keeping the back arched, sit back at the hips (not allowing the knees to drift forward of the toes), and assume an underhand grip on the tire. The hands should be slightly wider than shoulder-width apart.

Movement Sequence

Use the legs to lift the tire so that the hands are raised to a mid-thigh position. The arms should be fully extended, the back arched, and the feet flat on the floor. Using a jumping action, explode up through the legs and flip the tire onto its side, remembering to keep the back arched through the entire movement. Once the tire has been flipped onto its side, step forward and aggressively push the tire onto its opposite side

Sandbag One-Leg Squat (Fig. 23.4) *(continued)*

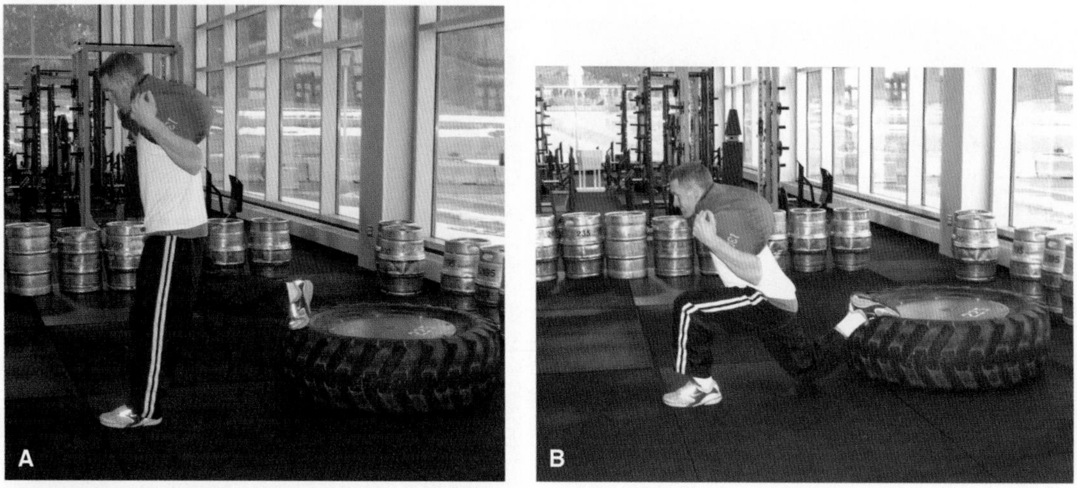

FIGURE 23.4

Starting Position

Place the sandbag on the back, as when performing barbell squats. Stand about a stride's length away from a utility bench. Reach back with one leg, and place the foot on the bench.

Movement Sequence

Keeping the back arched, initiate the movement by sitting back at the hips, not allowing the knee to drop forward of the toes on the forward foot. Continue to sit back until the mid thigh has achieved a parallel position. Maintaining an arched back position, return to the starting position. Repeat with the opposite leg.

Dumbbell Hockey Lunge (Fig. 23.5)

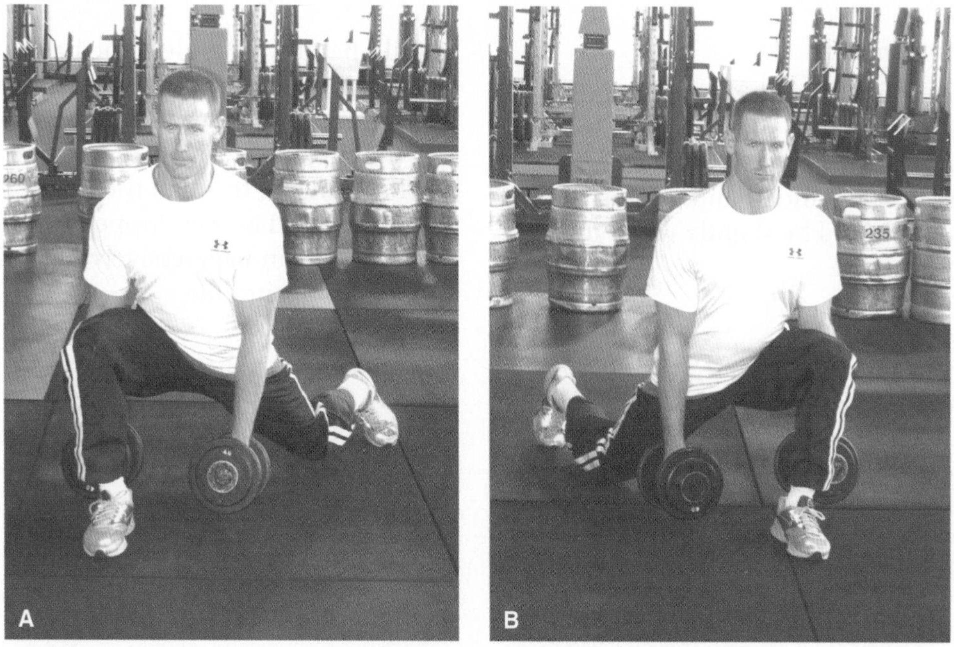

FIGURE 23.5

Dumbbell Hockey Lunge (Fig. 23.5) *(continued)*

Starting Position

Place the dumbbell on the back, as when performing barbell squats.

Movement Sequence

Take an exaggerated stride with the right leg, stepping forward so that the right foot is 14″ to 16″ wider than the right shoulder, and then lower the body so that the right knee is behind the toes on the right foot and the left leg is bent with the left knee just off the floor. From that bottom position, stride forward in one continuous movement with the left leg and take an exaggerated stride with the left leg as described above; the right leg is bent, and the right knee is just off the floor. It is important to keep the back arched during the entire performance of this exercise.

Keg/Log Straight Leg Dead Lift (Fig. 23.6)

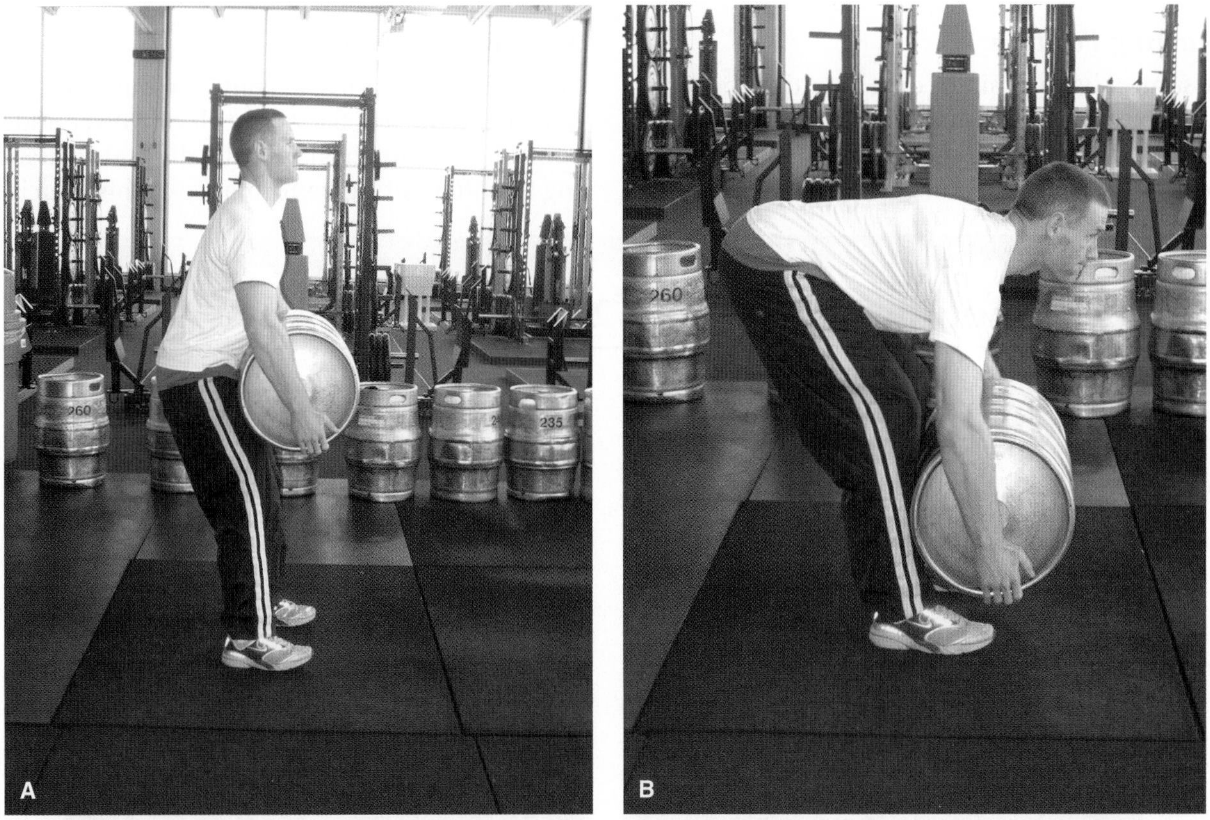

FIGURE 23.6

Starting Position

Stand on a pair of plyometric boxes, 18″ to 20″ high. The keg should be sitting on end between the two boxes.

Movement Sequence

Squat down and, keeping the back arched, pick up the keg. Holding the keg at arm's length in front of the body, bend the knees slightly. Maintaining that slight knee bend and the arch in the back, rotate forward at the hips, lower the keg to a point just short of touching the floor directly underneath the feet, and then return to the starting position.

Keg/Log Bench Press (Fig. 23.7)

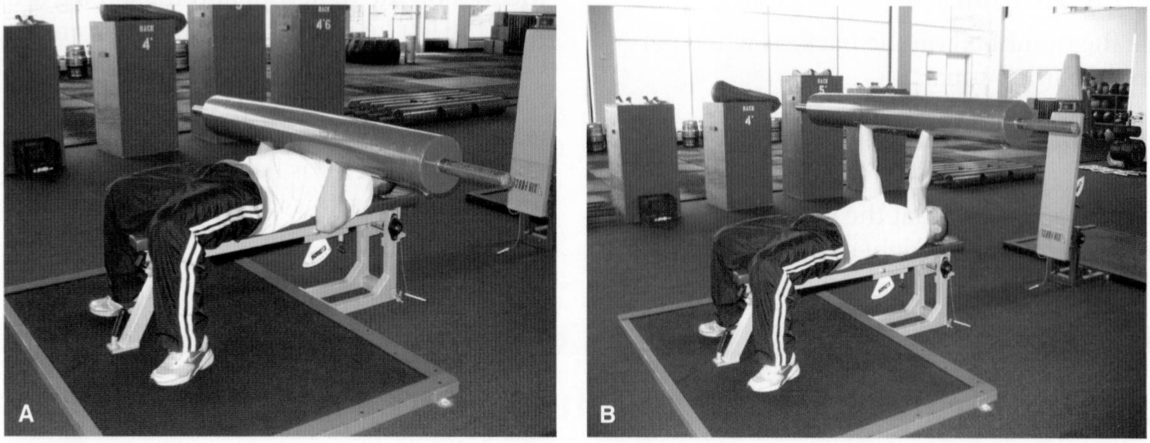

FIGURE 23.7

Starting Position

Assume a lying position on a flat utility bench, feet on the floor and butt on the bench. Place the keg or log on the chest as when performing a barbell bench press, and grip the implement.

Movement Sequence

Fully extend the arms, keeping the butt on the bench and the feet flat on the floor. Lower under control. The spotter(s) must be diligent in assisting the lifter during performance of this exercise.

Keg/Log Shoulder Press (Fig. 23.8)

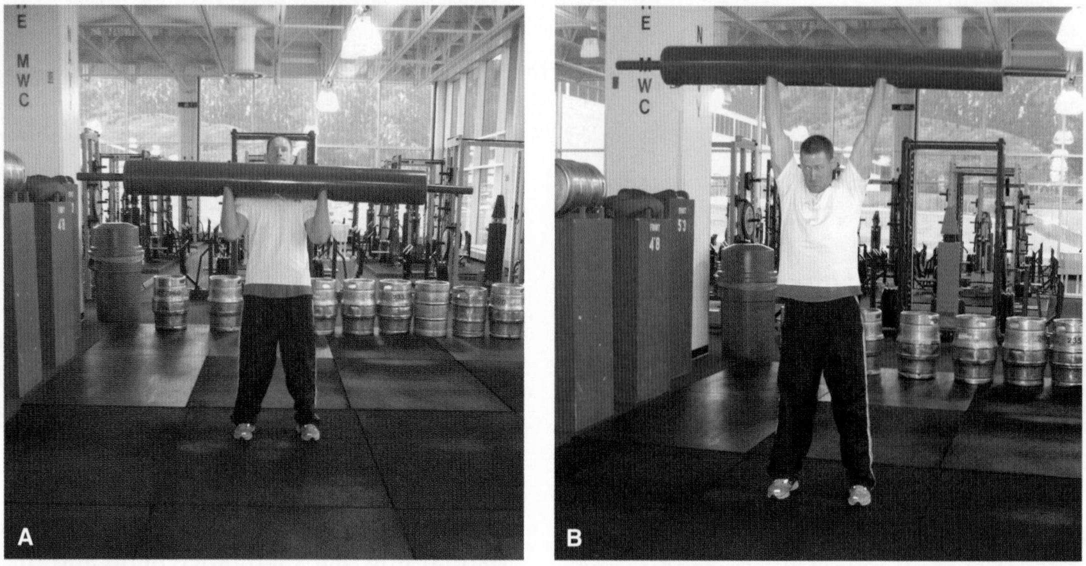

FIGURE 23.8

Starting Position

Grip the keg or log high on the chest.

Movement Sequence

Using a shoulder-width split stance with the feet, press the keg or log directly overhead until the arms are fully extended, and then lower under control. It is important to not lean back while performing the exercise; the back should remain straight. Lower through the full comfortable range of motion.

Sandbag Incline Press (Fig. 23.9)

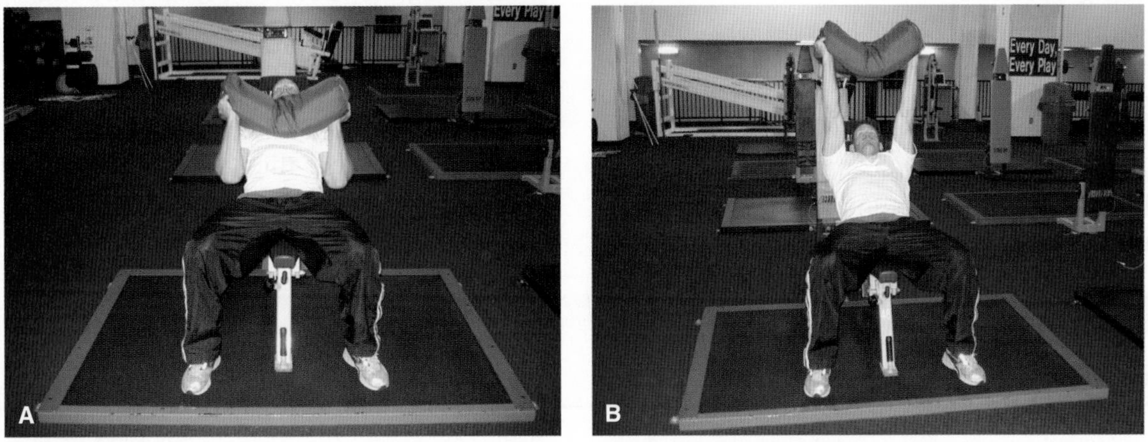

FIGURE 23.9

Starting Position

Assume a lying position on an incline bench, with the feet on the floor and the buttocks on the bench. Place the sandbag on the chest as when performing a barbell incline press, and grip the implement.

Movement Sequence

Fully extend the arms, keeping the butt on the bench and the feet flat on the floor. Lower under control. The spotter(s) must be diligent in assisting the lifter during performance of this exercise.

Keg/Log Walking Lunges (Fig. 23.10)

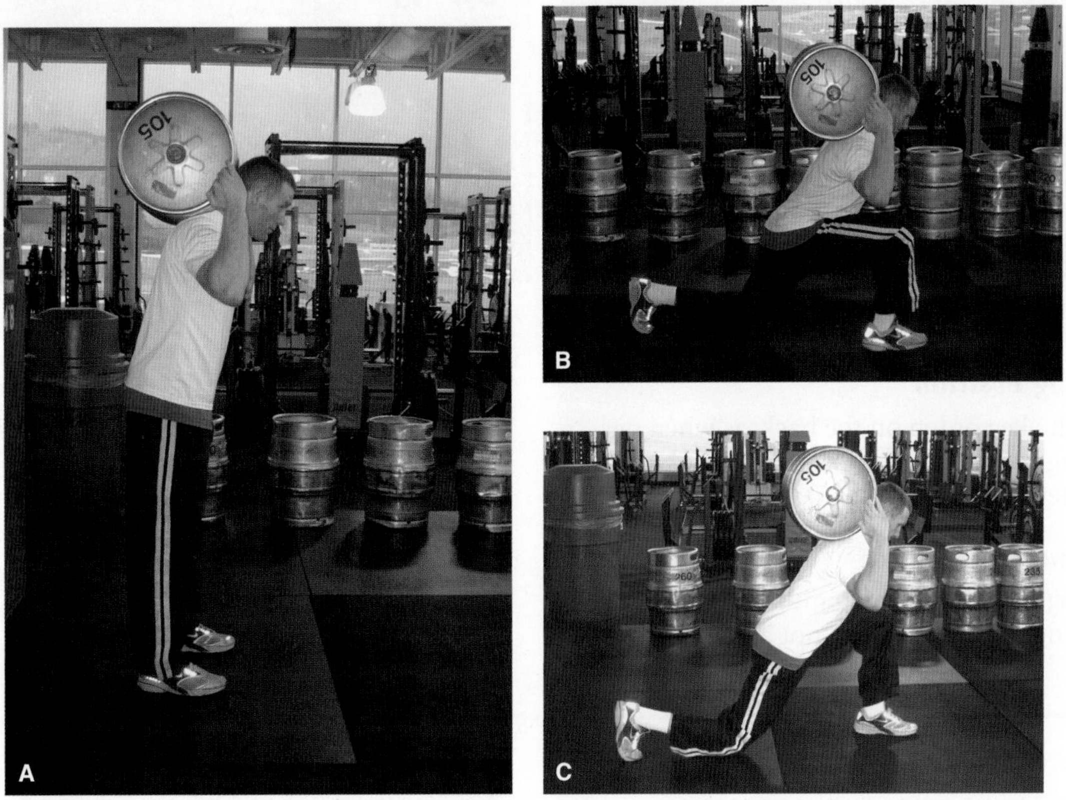

FIGURE 23.10

(continued)

Keg/Log Walking Lunges (Fig. 23.10) *(continued)*

Starting Position

Place the keg or log on the back, as when performing barbell squats.

Movement Sequence

Take an exaggerated stride with the right leg, and then lower the body so that the right knee is behind the toes on the right foot and the left leg is bent with the left knee just off the floor. From that bottom position, stride forward in one continuous movement with the left leg, and take an exaggerated stride with the left leg; the right leg is bent and the right knee is just off the floor. It is important to keep the back arched during the entire performance of this exercise.

Keg/Log Squats (Fig. 23.11)

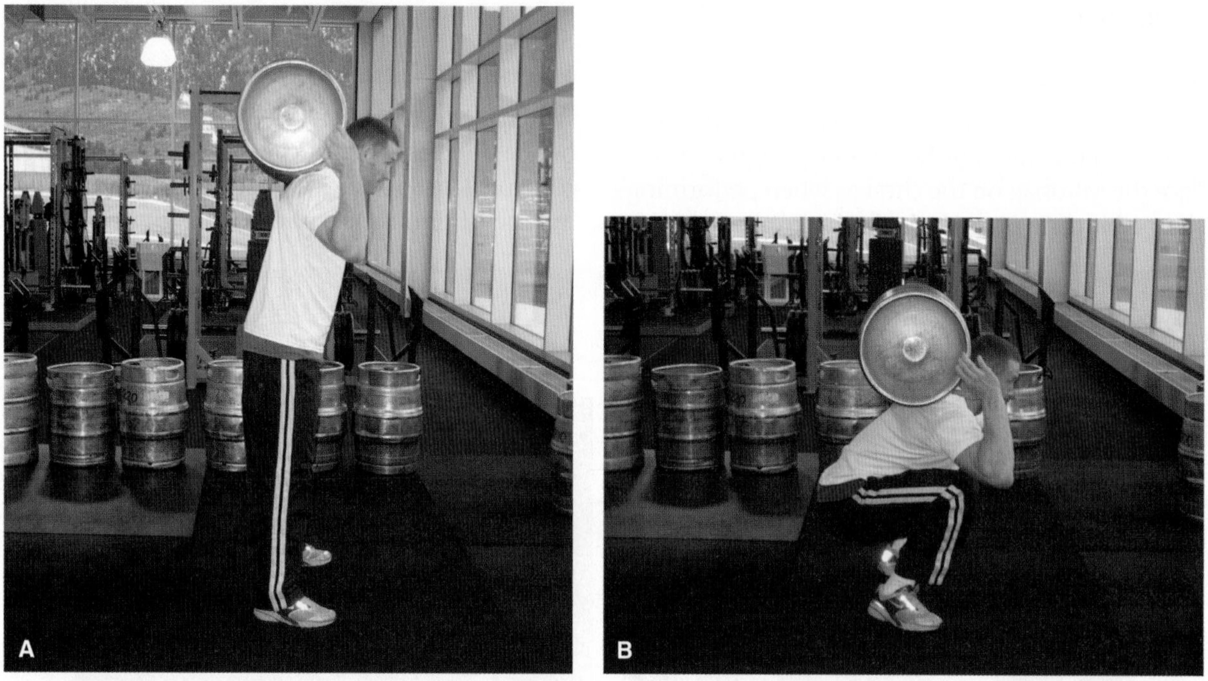

FIGURE 23.11

Starting Position

Place the keg or log on the back, as when performing barbell squats. Place the feet about shoulder-width apart.

Movement Sequence

Keeping the back arched, initiate the movement by sitting back at the hips, not allowing the knees to drop forward of the toes. Continue to sit back until the mid thigh has achieved a parallel position. Maintaining an arched back position, return to the starting position.

Variation: Log Front Squats

Starting Position

Place the log high on the chest, with the log supported on the deltoids and the elbows high, identical to a typical front squat or clean catch position. Place the feet about shoulder-width apart.

Movement Sequence

Keeping the back arched, initiate the movement by sitting back at the hips, not allowing the knees to drop forward of the toes. Continue to sit back until the mid thigh has achieved a parallel position. Maintaining an arched back and high elbow position, return to the starting position.

Keg/Log Side Lunge (Fig. 23.12)

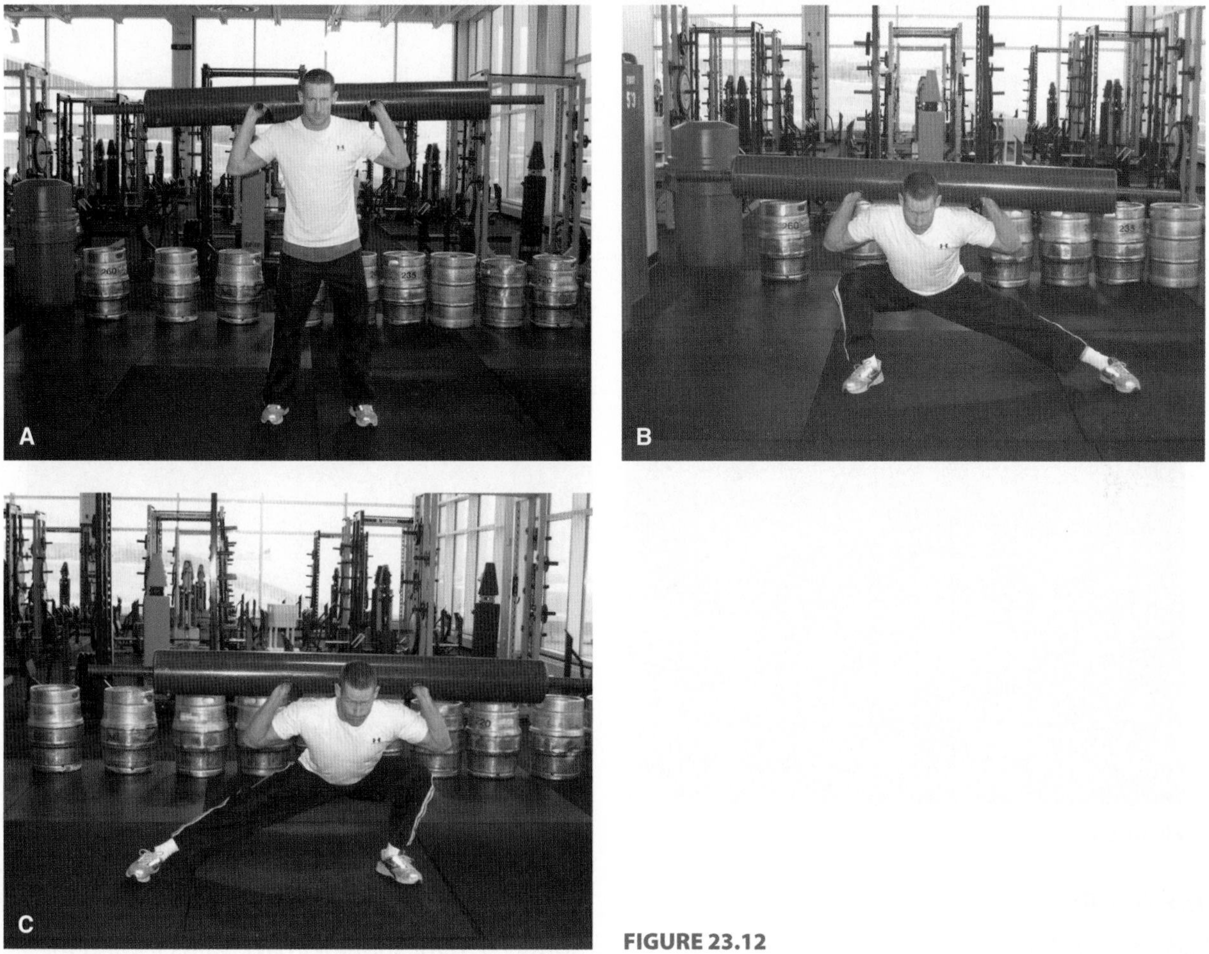

FIGURE 23.12

(continued)

Keg/Log Side Lunge (Fig. 23.12) *(continued)*

Starting Position

Place the keg or log on the back, as when performing barbell squats. Place the feet about shoulder-width apart.

Movement Sequence

Step directly laterally with the right foot through a comfortable range of motion, Keeping the left knee straight and the left foot planted, flex the right knee while sitting back at the hips and moving the hips laterally to the right. Return to the starting position, and alternate the movement to the opposite side until the required number of repetitions has been completed.

Kettle Bell Bent Row (Fig. 23.13)

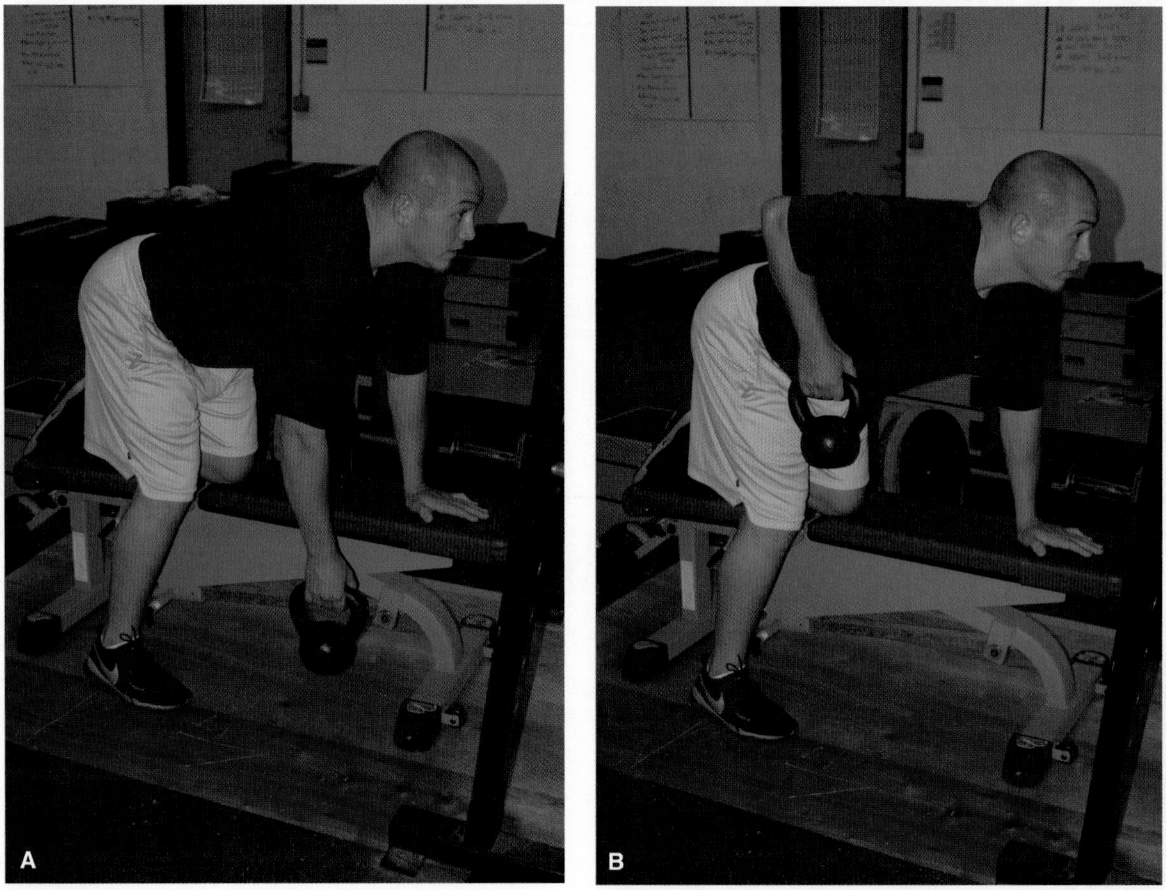

FIGURE 23.13

Starting Position

Place the left knee on an exercise bench, with the palm of the left hand flat on the bench. The left hip joint should be straight above the left knee. The back should be flat and the head up. Grasp the handle of the kettlebell in the right hand (Fig 23.13A)

Movement Sequence

Shrug the right shoulder backwards toward the ceiling, seeing how high you can lift the kettlebell without bending the right elbow. At the top of the shrug, finish by pulling the kettlebell with the right arm from the outside of the rib cage (Fig 23.13B). Reverse the position and repeat with the left arm.

Variation: Keg/Log Bent Row

Starting Position

Place a keg on its side in front of the body or stand behind a log, depending upon which implement is to be used. Bend the knees slightly and rotate at the hips to lower the upper body so the shoulders are parallel with the hips. The shoulders should be directly over the implement.

Movement Sequence

Keeping the back arched, reach down and grasp the implement. Pull the arms back so that each elbow slides along the rib cage, and lift the implement to the chest; then return to the starting position.

Sandbag Arch Lunge (Fig. 23.14)

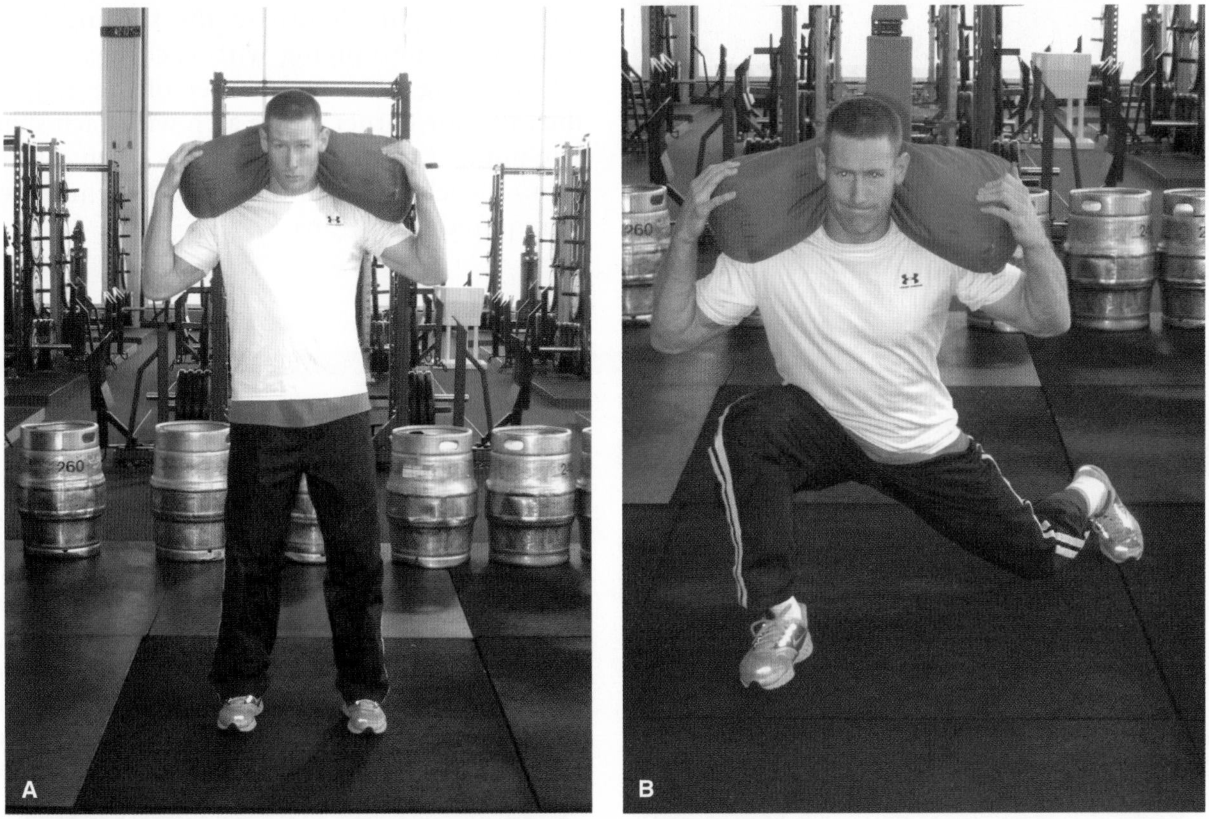

FIGURE 23.14

(continued)

Keg/Log Arch Lunge (Fig. 23.14) *(continued)*

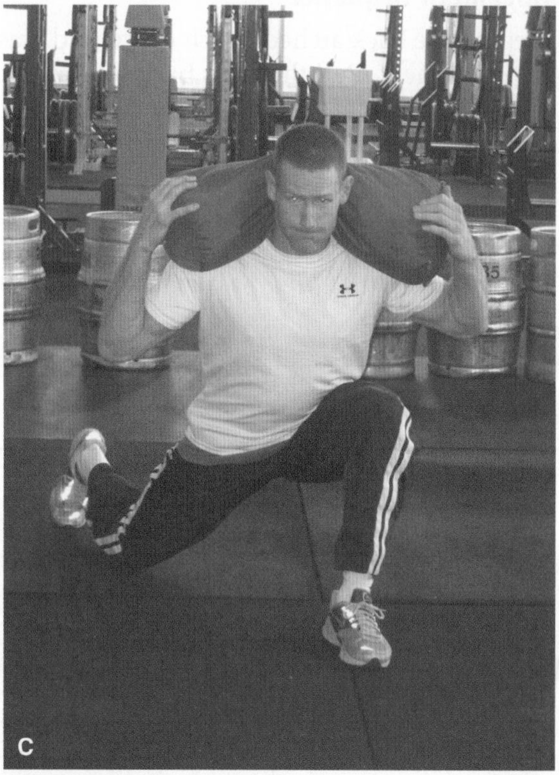

FIGURE 23.14 (Continued)

Starting Position

Place the keg or log on the back, as when performing barbell squats. Place the feet about shoulder-width apart.

Movement Sequence

Imagine an arch on the floor in front of where you are standing, starting a stride length away directly lateral of the right foot and ending a stride length away directly lateral of the left foot. Initiate the movement by lunging directly laterally with the right foot to the right edge of the arch while keeping the right knee behind the toes on the right foot and the left leg straight. Return to the starting position. Alternate lunging with each leg, gradually working from one corner of the arch to the opposite corner of the arch with each step. The number of steps and the placement of the foot on each step will depend on the number of required repetitions.

Maxing Out

1. You are introducing a new implement in your conditioning program for baseball players. Name the implement, briefly discuss how you will introduce it into the conditioning program over the next 4 weeks, briefly describe the exercises you will use with the implement, and explain how you expect this form of training to benefit your athletes.
2. In evaluating the athletic ability of a high school basketball player, his coach tells you he needs better balance and stability. He is already performing resistance training using a standard free-weight resistance. Would you consider using a training modality that incorporates an active fluid resistance? Why or why not?
3. Some of the athletes in your program are complaining of low back pain. The only significant change in the program is an increase in the volume and intensity of power cleans over the past 2 weeks. Would you consider tire flipping as an alternative to power cleans? Why or why not?

CASE EXAMPLE

Using implement training in an athletic strength and conditioning program

BRYAN

Background Bryan is a 6 ft, 215-lb sophomore division I running back. His test results are as follows:

a. Bench press: 370 lb
b. Squat: 500 lb
c. Clean: 330 lb
d. Forty-yard dash: 4.5
e. Vertical jump: 38 in

He is very committed to his strength and conditioning program and rarely misses a training session. Despite his impressive testing results, he is looking for ways to improve his athletic performance, and his position coach feels he needs to develop more functional strength to reach his potential as a football player. What are some training techniques that could be used to help this athlete achieve his goals?

Recommendations/Considerations. With his superior strength levels, it is doubtful that further enhancing his strength levels will have a positive effect on performance. For example, he could focus on increasing his squat from 500 to 525 lb, but it is questionable if this would have the effect of improving on-the-field performance.

What might be more effective at improving performance is to integrate water-filled implement exercises into his training program, giving him the opportunity to train using an active fluid resistance. For example, exercises such as keg bench press (to help pass blocking and straight arm capabilities) and log lunges (to help him maintain balance during contact) could be worked into his training program to help improve his athletic performance, converting his "weight room strength" to "functional strength".

TYRONE

Tyrone is a 6′11″, 230-lb sophomore who is the starting center for his division I college basketball team. During the last game, Tyrone landed awkwardly after coming down with a rebound and strained his lower back. Tyrone is able to complete the majority of his resistance training program without aggravating his back condition. However, he has found that the catch phase when performing a clean does cause him some pain. He is concerned because he has found that performing cleans does help his vertical jump ability and makes him feel more explosive on the court. What is a possible alternative exercise that he could perform that would mimic the triple extension jumping action that occurs when performing a clean without aggravating his strained low back?

Recommendations/Considerations. To mimic the jumping action that occurs when performing a clean and to eliminate the pain that occurs during the catch phase, Tyrone could be instructed on how to properly flip a tire. Once he has learned the correct movement pattern, he could attempt the movement on a lightweight unloaded tire to make sure the exercise did not cause any pain in his strained low back. From there, a gradual increase in training intensity could occur, making sure that he maintained good technique and that he continued to be able to perform the movement pain free.

REFERENCES

1. Coker CA, Berning JM, Briggs DL. A preliminary investigation of the biomechanical and perceptual influence of chain resistance on the performance of the snatch. *J Strength Cond Res*. 2006;20(4):887–891.
2. Neelly KR, Terry JG, Morris MJ. A mechanical comparison of linear and double-looped hung supplemental heavy chain resistance to the back squat: a case study. *J Strength Cond Res*. 2010;24(1):278–281.
3. Siff MC. Functional training revisited. *Strength Cond J*. 2002;24(5):42–46.
4. Waller W, Piper T, Townsend R. Strongman events and strength and conditioning programs. *Strength Cond J*. 2003;25(5):44–52.
5. Allerheiligen B. In-season strength training for power athletes. *Strength Cond J*. 2003;25(3):23–28.
6. Gadeken SB. Off-season strength, power, and plyometric training for Kansas State volleyball. *Strength Cond J*. 1999;21(5):49–55
7. Hedrick A. Using uncommon implements in the training programs of athletes. *Strength Cond*. 2003;25(4):18–22.
8. Pollitt D. Sled dzragging for hockey training. *Strength Cond J*. 2003;25(5):7–16.
9. Baker D. Applying the in-season periodization of strength and power training for football. *Strength Cond*. 1998;20(2):18–24.
10. Kraemer WJ, Vescovi JD, Dixon P. The physiological basis of wrestling: implications for conditioning programs. *Strength Cond J*. 2004;26(2):10–15.

11. Krough JWL, Payne AL, Anderson BB, Atkins PJ. A brief description of the biomechanics of a strongman event: the tire flip. *J Strength Cond Res*. 2010;24(5):1223–1228.
12. Young W, Pryor J. Resistance training for short sprints and maximum-speed sprints. *Strength Cond J*. 2001;23(2):7–13.
13. Berning JM, Adams KJ, Climstein M, et al. Metabolic demands of "junkyard" training: pushing and pulling a motor vehicle. *J Strength Cond Res*. 2007;21(3):853–856.
14. Hedrick A. Athlete strongman. *Pure Power* 2003;3(5):66–74.
15. Kirksey B, Stone MH. Periodizing a college sprint program: theory and practice. *Strength Cond*. 1998;20(3):42–47.
16. Keough JWL, Payne AL, Anderson BB, Atkins P. A brief description of the biomechanics and physiology of a strongman event: the tire flip. *J Strength Cond Res*. 2010;24(5):1223–1228.
17. Rosene JM. In-season, off-ice conditioning for minor league professional ice hockey players. *Strength Cond J*. 2002;24(1):22–28.
18. Szymanski DJ, Fredrick GA. College baseball/softball periodized torso program. *Strength Cond J*. 1999;21(4):42–47.
19. Keogh J. Lower body resistance training: increasing functional performance with lunges. *Strength Cond J*. 1999; 21(1):67–72.
20. McGill SM, McDermott A, Fenwick CMJ. Comparison of different strongman events: trunk muscle activation and lumbar spine motion, load, and stiffness. *J Strength Cond Res*. 2009;23(4):1148–1161.
21. Baker DG, Newton RU. Effect of kinetically altering a repetition via the use of chain resistance on velocity during the bench press. *J Strength Cond Res*. 2009;23(7):1941–1946.
22. Berning JM, Coker CA, Briggs D. The biomechanical and perceptual influence of chain resistance on the performance of the Olympic clean. *J Strength Cond Res*. 2008;22(2):390–395.
23. Berning JM, Adams KJ. Using chain for strength and conditioning. *Strength Cond J*. 2004;26(5):80–84.
24. DeGarmo R. University of Nebraska in-season resistance training for horizontal jumper. *Strength Cond J*. 2000;22(3):23–26.
25. Murlasits Z, Langley J. In-season resistance training for high school football. *Strength Cond J*. 2002;24(4):65–68.
26. Parakh AA, Domowitz FR. Strength training for men's and women's ice hockey. *Strength Cond J*. 2000;22(6):42–45.
27. Brooks TJ. Women's collegiate gymnastics: a multifactorial approach to training and conditioning. *Strength Cond J*. 2003;25(2):23–37.
28. McMaster DT, Cronin J, McGuigan M. Forms of variable resistance training. *Strength Cond J*. 2008;31(1):50–54.

INDEX

Note: Page numbers followed by f denote figures; those followed by t denote tables.